Surgical Management of Cerebrovascular Disease

Second Edition

Surgical Management of Cerebrovascular Disease

Second Edition

Robert G. Ojemann, M.D.
Professor of Surgery, Harvard Medical School
Visiting Neurosurgeon, Massachusetts General Hospital
Boston, Massachusetts

Roberto C. Heros, M.D.
Associate Professor of Surgery, Harvard Medical School
Director of Cerebrovascular Surgery, Massachusetts General Hospital
Boston, Massachusetts

Robert M. Crowell, M.D.
Professor and Head, Department of Neurosurgery
University of Illinois at Chicago
Chicago, Illinois

Illustrations by
EDITH TAGRIN
Chief, Medical Art Unit
Massachusetts General Hospital
Boston, Massachusetts

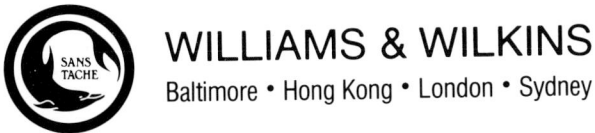

WILLIAMS & WILKINS
Baltimore • Hong Kong • London • Sydney

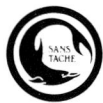

Editor: Carol-Lynn Brown
Associate Editor: Victoria M. Vaughn
Design: Norman W. Och
Production: Theda Harris

Copyright © 1988
Williams & Wilkins
428 East Preston Street
Baltimore, MD 21202, U.S.A.

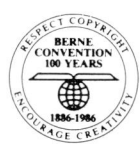

All rights reserved. This book is protected by copyright. No part of this book may be reproduced in any form or by any means, including photocopying, or utilized by any information storage and retrieval system without written permission from the copyright owner.

Accurate indications, adverse reactions, and dosage schedules for drugs are provided in this book, but it is possible that they may change. The reader is urged to review the package information data of the manufacturers of the medications mentioned.

Printed in the United States of America
First Edition, 1983

Library of Congress Cataloging-in-Publication Data

Surgical management of cerebrovascular disease.

   Rev. ed. of: Surgical management of cerebrovascular disease / Robert G. Ojemann, Robert M. Crowell. © 1983.
   Includes index.
   1. Cerebrovascular disease—Surgery. I. Ojemann, Robert G. (Robert Gerdes), 1931–   . II. Heros, Roberto C. III. Crowell, Robert M. IV. Ojemann, Robert G. (Robert Gerdes), 1931–   . Surgical management of cerebrovascular disease.
[DNLM: 1. Cerebrovascular Disorders—surgery. WL 355 S961]
RD594.2.S87   1987   617'.481   87-10694
ISBN 0-683-06640-4

                            88 89 90 91 92
                      10 9 8 7 6 5 4 3 2 1

DEDICATION

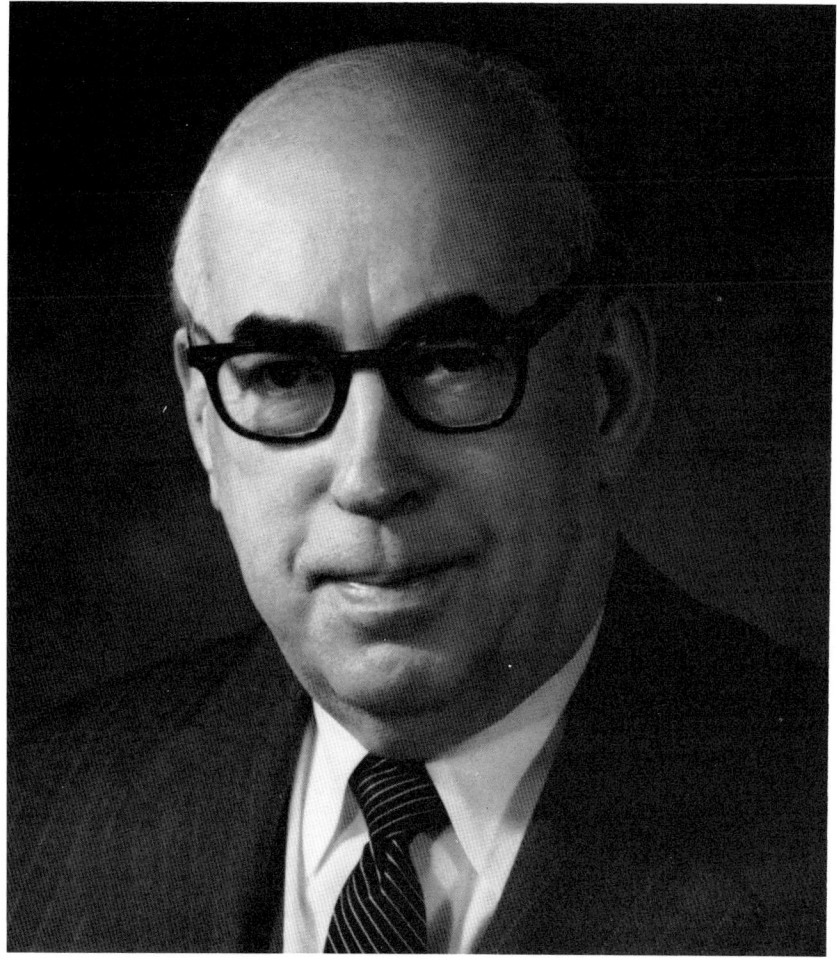

C. Miller Fisher, M.D.

For his remarkable accomplishments in the field of cerebrovascular disease, we dedicate this book to Dr. C. Miller Fisher. His ability to observe and describe clinical phenomenon, his insistence on establishing, whenever possible, a definite diagnosis in the stroke patient and to then plan a rational program of treatment, his publications, and his teaching have all done as much to advance the field of cerebrovascular disease as any other single factor.

We are fortunate to be able to continue a most pleasant association which began many years ago with this outstanding dedicated physician. Every discussion of a patient's problem is a learning experience, for each case will be reviewed in relationship to his vast background. His unique ability to organize clinical observations into well-ordered patterns has led to a method and style which have been a constant inspiration.

As one listens to his teachings, a series of basic principles emerge which he has followed in the practice of medicine. Caplan has nicely summarized these into "Fisher's Rules" (1):

1. The bedside can be your laboratory. Study the patient seriously.
2. Settle an issue as it arises at the bedside.

3. Make a hypothesis and then try as hard as you can to disprove it or find the exception before accepting it as valid.
4. Always be working on one or more projects; it will make the daily routine more meaningful.
5. In arriving at a clinical diagnosis, think of the five most common findings (historical, physical, or laboratory) found in a given disorder.
6. Describe quantitatively and precisely.
7. The details of the case are important; their analysis distinguishes the expert from the journeyman.
8. Collect and categorize phenomena; their mechanism and meaning may become clearer later if enough cases are gathered.
9. Fully accept what you have heard or read only when you have verified it yourself.
10. Learn from your own past experience and that of others (literature and experienced colleagues).
11. Didactic talks benefit most the lecturer. We teach others best by listening, questioning, and demonstrating.
12. Write often and carefully. Let others gain from your work and ideas.
13. Pay particular attention to the specifics of the patient with a known diagnosis; it will be helpful later when similar phenomena occur in an unknown case.
14. Be a good listener; even from the mouths of beginners may come wisdom.
15. Resist the temptation to prematurely place a case or disorder into a diagnostic cubbyhole that fits poorly.
16. The patient is always doing the best he can.
17. Maintain a lively interest in patients as people.

A review of C. Miller Fisher's publications from the past three decades reveals the range of his accomplishments in cerebrovascular disease. His clinical and pathological studies beginning in 1951 established the clinical syndrome related to carotid artery atherosclerosis which was the foundation for development of the surgical treatment of carotid artery occlusive disease. He called attention to the frequency and pathology of cerebral embolism, described syndromes associated with lacunar disease and vertebrovascular disease, studied the clinical manifestations of vasospasm and carotid dissection, described the syndromes and pathology of brain hemorrhage, and reported numerous other observations pertaining to cerebrovascular disease. He has also made many other important contributions to the field of neurology, and these have been summarized by Adams and Richardson in a "Salute to C. Miller Fisher" (2).

1. Caplan LR: Fisher's rules. *Arch Neurol* 39:389–390, 1982.
2. Adams RD, Richardson EP: Salute to C. Miller Fisher. *Arch Neurol* 38:137–139, 1981.

C. Miller Fisher's Publications on Cerebrovascular Disease (1951–1986)

1. Fisher CM: Occlusion of the internal carotid artery. *Arch Neurol Psychiatry* 65:346–377, 1951.
2. Fisher CM, Adams RD: Observation on brain embolism. *J Neuropathol Exp Neurol* 10:92, 1951.
3. Fisher CM, Vander Eecken HM, Adams RD: The arterial anastomoses of the human brain and their importance in the delimitation of human brain infarction. *J Neuropathol Exp Neurol* 11:91, 1952.
4. Fisher CM: Transient monocular blindness associated with hemiplegia. *Arch Ophthalmol* 47:167–203, 1952.
5. Fisher CM: Concerning strokes. *Can Med Assoc J* 69:257–268, 1953.
6. Fisher CM, Cameron DG: Concerning cerebral vasospasm. *Neurology* 3:468–473, 1953.
7. Fisher CM: Concerning cerebral arteriosclerosis. *J Am Geriatr Soc* 2:1–18, 1954.
8. Fisher CM: Occlusion of the carotid arteries. *Arch Neurol Psychiatry* 72:187–204, 1954.
9. Fisher CM: Clinical picture of cerebral arteriosclerosis. *Minn Med* 38:839–851, 1955.
10. Fisher CM: Left hemiplegia and motor impersistence. *J Nerv Ment Dis* 123:201–218, 1956.
11. Fisher CM: Cranial bruit associated with occlusion of the internal carotid artery. *Neurology* 7:299–306, 1957.
12. Hakim S, Fisher CM: A new technique for the microscopic examination of cerebral vessels in vivo. *J Neurosurg* 14:405–412, 1957.
13. Fisher CM: Cerebral thromboangitis obliterans. *Medicine* 36:169–209, 1957.
14. Fisher CM, Adams RD: Transient global amnesia. *Trans Am Neurol Assoc* 83:143–146, 1958.
15. Fisher CM: The use of anticoagulants in cerebral thrombosis. *Neurology* 8:311–332, 1958.
16. Fisher CM: Cerebrovascular diseases: Pathophysiology, diagnosis, and treatment. *J Chronic Dis* 8:419–447, 1958.
17. Fisher CM: Intermittent cerebral ischemia. In Wright and Millikan (eds): *Cerebral Vascular Disease (Second Conference)*. New York, Grune & Stratton, 1958, pp 81–97.
18. Fisher CM, Karp HR, Adams RD: Cerebrovascular diseases. In Harrison TR, et al (eds): *Principles of Internal Medicine*, ed 3. New York, McGraw-Hill, 1958, pp 1560–1606.
19. Fisher CM: Cerebral embolism. In Conn HF (ed): *Current Therapy*. Philadelphia, WB Saunders, 1958, pp 548–550.
20. Fisher CM: Early-life carotid-artery occlusion associated with late intracranial hemorrhage. Observations on the ischemic pathogenesis of mantle sclerosis. *Lab Invest* 8:680–700, 1959.
21. Fisher CM: Observations of the fundus oculi in transient monocular blindness. *Neurology* 9:337–347, 1959.
22. Fisher CM: The pathologic and clinical aspects of thalamic hemorrhage. *Trans Am Neurol Assoc* 84:56–59, 1959.
23. Fisher CM: Ocular palsy in temporal arteritis. *Minn Med* 42:1258–1268, 1430–1437, 1617–1630, 1959.
24. Fisher CM: Present trends in the treatment of the cerebral vascular diseases. *R I Med J* 43:27–34, 44, 1960.
25. Fisher CM, Adams RD: Subarachnoid hemorrhage due to ruptured aneurysm. In HF Conn (ed): *Current Therapy*. Philadelphia, WB Saunders, 1960, pp 523–524.
26. Fisher CM: Clinical syndromes in cerebral arterial occlusion.

In WS Fields (ed): *Pathogenesis and Treatment of Cerebrovascular Disease.* Springfield, IL, Charles C Thomas, 1961, pp 151–177.
27. Adams RD, Fisher CM: Pathology of cerebral arterial occlusion. In Fields WS (ed): *Pathogenesis and Treatment of Cerebrovascular Disease.* Springfield, IL, Charles C Thomas, 1961, pp 126–142.
28. Fisher CM: Clinical syndromes in cerebral hemorrhage. In Fields WS (ed): *Pathogenesis and Treatment of Cerebrovascular Disease.* Springfield, IL, Charles C Thomas, 1961, pp 318–338.
29. Fisher CM: The pathology and pathogenesis of intracerebral hemorrhage. In Fields WS (ed): *Pathogenesis and Treatment of Cerebrovascular Disease.* Springfield, IL, Charles C Thomas, 1961, pp 295–311.
30. Fisher CM: Palpation of arteries in temporal arteritis. *JAMA* 175:325, 1961.
31. Fisher CM: Anticoagulant therapy in cerebral thrombosis and cerebral embolism. *Neurology* 11:119–131, 1961.
32. Fisher CM, Karnes WE, Kubik CS: Lateral medullary infarction—the pattern of vascular occlusion. *J Neuropathol Exp Neurol* 20:323–379, 1961.
33. Fisher CM, Dalal PM, Adams RD: Cerebrovascular disease and the stroke syndrome. In Harrison TR, et al (eds): *Principles of Internal Medicine*, ed 4. New York, McGraw-Hill, 1962, pp 1746–1795.
34. Fisher CM: Concerning recurrent transient cerebral ischemic attacks. *Can Med Assoc* 86:1091–1099, 1962.
35. Fisher CM: Cerebral arterial occlusion—remarks on pathology, pathophysiology, and diagnosis. *Clin Neurosurg* 9:88–105, 1963.
36. Fisher CM, Curry HB: Pure motor hemiplegia. *Trans Am Neurol Assoc* 89:94–97, 1964.
37. Fisher CM: Pure sensory stroke involving face, arm, and leg. *Neurology* 15:76–80, 1965.
38. Fisher CM: The circle of Willis: Anatomical variations. *Vasc Dis* 2:99–105, 1965.
39. Fisher CM, Picard EH, Polak A, Dalal P, Ojemann RG: Acute hypertensive cerebellar hemorrhage: Diagnosis and surgical treatment. *J Nerv Ment Dis* 140:38–57, 1965.
40. Fisher CM, Cole M: Homolateral ataxia and crural paresis: A vascular syndrome. *J Neurol Neurosurg Psychiatry* 28:48–55, 1965.
41. Fisher CM, Curry HB: Pure motor hemiplegia of vascular origin. *Arch Neurol* 13:130–140, 1965.
42. Fisher CM, Gore I, Okabe N, White PD: Atherosclerosis of the carotid and vertebral arteries—extracranial and intracranial. *J Neuropathol Exp Neurol* 24:455–476, 1965.
43. Fisher CM: Lacunes: Small, deep cerebral infarcts. *Neurology* 15:774–784, 1965.
44. Fisher CM, Gore I, White PD, Okabe N: Calcification of the carotid siphon. *Circulation* 32:538–548, 1965.
45. Fisher CM: Diagnosis and management of cerebrovascular disease. *Postgrad Med* 38:130–140, 1965.
46. Fisher CM: The vascular lesion in lacunae. *Trans Am Neurol Assoc* 90:243–245, 1965.
47. Fisher CM: Augmentation bruit of the vertebral artery. *J Neurol Neurosurg Psychiatry* 29:343–345, 1966.
48. Fisher CM: Capsular infarcts—the underlying vascular lesions. *Trans Am Neurol Assoc* 91:227–229, 1966.
49. Fisher CM: Dilated pupil in carotid occlusion. *Trans Am Neurol Assoc* 91:230–231, 1966.
50. Fisher CM: Vertigo in cerebrovascular disease. *Arch Otolaryngol* 85:529–534, 1967.
51. Fisher CM: A lacunar stroke. The dysarthria-clumsy hand syndrome. *Neurology* 17:614–617, 1967.
52. Fisher CM, Pearlman A: The nonsudden onset of cerebral embolism. *Neurology* 17:1025–1032, 1967.
53. Fisher CM: Some neuro-ophtalmological observations. *J Neurol Neurosurg Psychiatry* 30:383–392, 1967.
54. Fisher CM: Headache in cerebrovascular disease. In Vinken PJ, Bruyn GW (eds): *Handbook of Clinical Neurology.* Amsterdam, North-Holland, 1967, pp 124–156
55. Fisher CM: Dementia in cerebral vascular disease. In: *Cerebral Vascular Disease (Sixth Princeton Conference).* New York, Grune & Stratton, 1968, pp 232–236.
56. Fisher CM: Migraine accompaniments versus arteriosclerotic ischemia. *Trans Am Neurol Assoc* 93:211–213, 1968.
57. Fisher CM: The arterial lesions underlying lacunae. *Acta Neuropathol* 12:1–15, 1969.
58. Fisher CM: Occlusion of the vertebral arteries. *Arch Neurol* 22:13–19, 1970.
59. Fisher CM: Facial pulses in internal carotid artery occlusion. *Neurology* 20:476–478, 1970.
60. Fisher CM, Mohr JP, Adams RD: Cerebrovascular diseases. In Harrison TR, et al (eds): *Principles of Internal Medicine*, ed 6. New York, McGraw-Hill, 1970, pp 1727–1764.
61. Fisher CM, Kaplan LR: Basilar artery branch occlusion—a cause of pontine infarction. *Neurology* 21:900–905, 1971.
62. Fisher CM: Cerebral ischemia—less familiar types. *Clin Neurosurg* 18:267–336, 1971.
63. Fisher CM: Pathological observations in hypertensive cerebral hemorrhage. *J Neuropathol Exp Neurol* 30:536–550, 1971.
64. Fisher CM: Cerebral miliary aneurysms in hypertension. *Am J Pathol* 66:313–324, 1972.
65. Ojemann RG, Fisher CM, Rich JC: Spontaneous dissecting aneurysm of the internal carotid artery. *Stroke* 3:434–440, 1972.
66. Fisher CM: Acute headache and tender scalp arteries in the elderly. *Trans Am Neurol Assoc* 97:280–281, 1972.
67. Hochberg FH, Fisher CM, Roberson GH: Subarachnoid hemorrhage from a small non-aneurysmal artery. *Neurology* 24:319–321, 1974.
68. Duncan GW, Parker SW, Fisher CM: Acute cerebellar infarction in the PICA territory. *Arch Neurol* 32:364–368, 1975.
69. Hochberg FH, Bean CS, Fisher CM, Roberson GH: Stroke in a 15 year old girl secondary to terminal carotid dissection. *Neurology* 25:725–729, 1975.
70. Fisher CM: Clinical syndromes in cerebral thrombosis, hypertensive hemorrhage and ruptured saccular aneurysm. *Clin Neurosurg* 22:117–147, 1975.
71. Fisher CM: Anatomy and pathology of cerebral vasculature. In Meyer JJ (ed): *Modern Concepts of Cerebrovascular Disease.* New York, Spectrum, 1975.
72. Ojemann RG, Crowell RM, Roberson GH, Fisher CM: Surgical treatment of extracranial carotid occlusive disease. *Clin Neurosurg* 22:214–263, 1975.
73. Altemus LR, Roberson GH, Fisher CM, Pessin M: Embolic occlusion of the superior and inferior divisions of the middle cerebral artery with angiographic-clinical correlation. *Am J Roentgenol Radium Ther Nucl Med* 126:576–581, 1976.
74. Fisher CM: The microembolic theory of transient ischemic attacks. In: *Cerebrovascular Disease, Princeton Conference.* New York, Grune & Stratton, 1976, pp 50–53.
75. Fisher CM, Roberson GH, Ojemann RG: Cerebral vasospasm with ruptured saccular aneurysm—the clinical manifestations. *Neurosurgery* 1:245–248, 1977.
76. Walshe TM, Davis KR, Fisher CM: Thalamic hemorrhage: A computed tomographic-clinical correlation. *Neurology* 27:217–222, 1977.
77. Groothuis DR, Duncan GW, Fisher CM: The human thalamocortical sensory path in the internal capsule: Evidence from a small capsular hemorrhage causing a pure sensory stroke. *Ann Neurol* 2:328–331, 1977.
78. Fisher CM: Bilateral occlusion of basilar artery branches. *Neurol Neurosurg Psychiatry* 40:1182–1189, 1977.
79. Hinton R, Kistler JP, Fallon JT, Friedlich A, Fisher CM: Influence of etiology of atrial fibrillation on incidence of systemic embolism. *Am J Cardiol* 40:509–513, 1977.
80. Fisher CM, Ojemann RG, Roberson GH: Spontaneous dissection of cervico-cerebral arteries. *Can J Neurol Sci* 5:9–19, 1978.

81. Fisher CM, Ojemann RG: Basal rupture of saccular aneurysm. *J Neurosurg* 48:642–644, 1978.
82. Mohr JP, Kase CS, Meckler MD, Fisher CM: Sensorimotor stroke due to thalamocapsular ischemia. *Arch Neurol* 34:739–741, 1977.
83. Fisher CM: Thalamic pure sensory stroke: A pathologic study. *Neurology* 28:1141–1144, 1978.
84. Fisher CM: Bilateral capsular infarcts—the mechanism of recovery from hemiplegia. *J Neuropathol Exp Neurol* 37:613, 1978.
85. Ropper AH, Fisher CM, Kleinman GM: Pyramidal infarction in the medulla: A cause of pure motor hemiplegia sparing the face. *Neurology* 29:91–95, 1979.
86. Fisher CM: Reducing risks of cerebral embolism. *Geriatrics* 34:59–66, 1979.
87. Fisher CM: Capsular infarcts—the underlying vascular lesions. *Arch Neurol* 36:65–73, 1979.
88. Hinton RC, Mohr JP, Ackerman RH, Adair LB, Fisher CM: Symptomatic middle cerebral artery stenosis. *Ann Neurol* 5:152–157, 1979.
89. Fisher CM: Late-life migraine accompaniments as a cause of unexplained transient ischemic attacks. *Can J Neurol Sci* 7:9–17, 1980.
90. Fisher CM, Kistler JP, Davis JM: Relation of cerebral vasospasm to subarachnoid hemorrhage visualized by computerized tomographic scanning. *Neurosurgery* 6:1–9, 1980.
91. Beal MF, Park TS, Fisher CM: Cerebral atheromatous embolism following carotid sinus pressure. *Arch Neurol* 38:310–312, 1981.
92. Fisher CM: Visual disturbances associated with quinidine and quinine. *Neurology* 31:1569–1571, 1981.
93. Fisher CM: The headache and pain of spontaneous carotid dissection. *Headache* 22:60–65, 1982.
94. Fisher CM: Embolism in atrial fibrillation. In Kulbertus HE, Olsson SB, Schlepper M (eds): *Atrial Fibrillation*. Sweden, AB Hässle, 1982, pp 192–210.
95. Fisher CM: Lacunar strokes and infarcts: A review. *Neurology* 32:871–876, 1982.
96. Fisher CM: Atherosclerosis: The correlation of antemortem angiography and pathology. In Bond GM, Insull W Jr, Glagov S, Chandler AB, Cornhill JF (eds): *Clinical Diagnosis of Atherosclerosis*. New York, Springer-Verlag, 1982.
97. Fisher CM: Pure sensory stroke and allied conditions. *Stroke* 13:434–447, 1982.
98. Fisher CM: The management of occlusive cerebrovascular disease. In Ropper AH, Kennedy SK, Zervas NT (eds): *Neurological and Neurosurgical Intensive Care*. Baltimore, University Park Press, 1983.
99. Beal MF, Fisher CM: Neoplastic angioendotheliosis. *J Neurol* 53:359–375, 1982.
100. Fisher CM: Transient global amnesia. Precipitating activities and other observations. *Arch Neurol* 39:605–608, 1982.
101. Fisher CM, Ojemann RG: The reduplication of transient symptoms with recurrences of carotid stenosis. *Ann Neurol* 12:85, 1982.
102. Fisher CM: Abulia minor versus agitated behavior. *Clin Neurosurg* 31:9–31, 1984.
103. Fisher CM: Painful states. A neurological commentary. *Clin Neurosurg* 31:32–53, 1984.
104. Fisher CM: Remarks to neurosurgical residents. *Clin Neurosurg* 31:54–57, 1984.
105. Kistler JP, Buonanno FS, DeWitt LD, Davis KR, Brady TJ, Fisher CM: Vertebral-basilar posterior cerebral territory stroke delineation by proton nuclear magnetic resonance imaging. *Stroke* 15:417–426, 1984.
106. Fisher CM: Vascular disease, senility and dementia. Letter to editor. *Lancet* 1:173, 1985.
107. Fisher CM: The ascendancy of diastolic blood pressure over systolic. *Lancet* 2:1349–1350, 1985.
108. Fisher CM: Unusual vascular events in the territory of the posterior cerebral artery. *Can J Neurol Sci* 13:1–7, 1986.
109. Fisher CM, Ojemann RG: A clinico-pathologic study of carotid endarterectomy plaques. *Rev Neurol (Paris)* 142:573–589, 1986.
110. Fisher CM: The posterior cerebral artery syndrome. *Can J Neurol Sci* 13:232–239, 1986.
111. Fisher CM: An unusual case of migraine accompaniments with permanent sequela—a case report. *Headache J* 26:266–270, 1986.
112. Fisher CM: Late-life migraine accompaniments—Further experience. *Stroke* 17:1033–1042, 1986.

PREFACE

The purpose of the first edition of this book was to give the reader a concise summary of those cerebrovascular disorders that might require consideration for surgical treatment. Included were the clinical presentation, diagnostic studies, indications for surgical treatment, illustrated details of operative management, handling of complications, results, and appropriate pertinent references.

During the 5 years since that edition was published, understanding of these disease processes has increased, and new diagnostic procedures and improved surgical techniques have been developed. In this second edition, the same general format used previously is continued. The guidelines and the results of surgical management of the diseases presented continue to be based on the clinical experience of the authors at the Massachusetts General Hospital, Boston. To this end, Roberto C. Heros, M.D., Director of Cerebrovascular Surgery at the Massachusetts General Hospital since 1980, has joined us as co-author. Dr. Robert Crowell, who preceded Dr. Heros, continues to provide valuable information.

This edition has been considerably expanded, and many new illustrations have been added. Every chapter has been thoroughly revised. The chapters on giant aneurysms and arteriovenous malformations have been enlarged and completely rewritten. A new chapter on spinal arteriovenous malformations has been added. We have illustrated many of the operative procedures step by step, going into considerable detail for the more common operations and supplementing the illustrations with a full description in the text. The references have been updated to include the pertinent literature through 1986.

ACKNOWLEDGMENTS

It is not possible to acknowledge the contributions from all who helped with this book or to list all those from the clinical services at the Massachusetts General Hospital who participated in the care of the patients with cerebrovascular disease. We would like to thank Dr. Nicholas T. Zervas, Chief of Neurological Surgery at the Massachusetts General Hospital, Dr. Kenneth Davis, Chief of the Neuroradiology Service, and Dr. Gerard Debrun for their invaluable help.

For the beautifully detailed drawings, we are indebted to Edith Tagrin, Chief of the Medical Art Unit at the Massachusetts General Hospital, who spent countless hours attending to every aspect of the illustrations. Thanks also go to Stanley Bennett, Chief of the Photography Unit at the Massachusetts General Hospital, who did the reproductions of the radiographic studies.

The staff at Williams & Wilkins was a great help to us. We want to mention especially Carol-Lynn Brown (Editor), Vicki Vaughn (Associate Editor), and Theda Harris (Production Coordinator).

Finally, we thank Barbara Marino, Jean Ojemann, and Suzanne Sampson for their assistance in preparation of the manuscript.

CONTENTS

Dedication .... *v*
Preface .... *ix*
Acknowledgments .... *xi*

SECTION 1: Occlusive Cerebrovascular Disease

1. Atherosclerosis of the Carotid Circulation: Evaluation and Management 1
2. Carotid Endarterectomy 35
3. Asymptomatic Carotid Bruit and Stenosis 77
4. Extracranial to Middle Cerebral Artery Bypass Graft 83
5. Atherosclerosis of the Vertebrobasilar Circulation: Evaluation, Management, and Operative Procedures 103
6. Fibromuscular Dysplasia of the Internal Carotid Artery 121
7. Dissection of Internal Carotid, Vertebral, and Intracranial Arteries 125
8. Embolism 137
9. Cerebral and Cerebellar Infarction 143

SECTION 2: Intracranial Aneurysms, Arteriovenous Malformations, and Brain Hemorrhage

10. Intracranial Aneurysms and Subarachnoid Hemorrhage: Incidence, Pathology, Clinical Features, and Perioperative Management 147
11. Intracranial Aneurysms: General Aspects of Surgical Treatment 163
12. Internal Carotid Artery Aneurysms 179
13. Paraclinoid Aneurysms 199
14. Anterior Communicating Artery Aneurysms 217
15. Distal Anterior Cerebral Artery Aneurysms 235
16. Middle Cerebral Artery Aneurysms 241
17. Basilar Bifurcation, Posterior Cerebral, and Superior Cerebellar Artery Aneurysms 253
18. Basilar Trunk and Vertebral Artery Aneurysms 271
19. Multiple, Unruptured, and Asymptomatic Aneurysms 287
20. Giant Aneurysms 297
21. Infectious Aneurysms 337
22. Arteriovenous Malformations of the Brain 347
23. Dural Arteriovenous Malformations 415
24. Carotid-Cavernous Fistula 427
25. Brain Hemorrhage 435

SECTION 3: Spinal Arteriovenous Malformations

26. Arteriovenous Malformations of the Spinal Cord 451

Index *467*

Section 1 OCCLUSIVE CEREBROVASCULAR DISEASE

1

Atherosclerosis of the Carotid Circulation: Evaluation and Management

DIAGNOSIS

Clinical Presentation

Clinical syndromes associated with atherosclerosis of the carotid circulation include transient ischemic attacks (TIAs) and neurologic deficits due to cerebral infarction. In the latter category there may be prolonged reversible ischemic neurologic deficits and acute or completed strokes. TIAs include transient monocular blindness, transient hemispheral attacks, or both. When they are caused by carotid atherosclerosis, the most frequent site of pathology is the region of the common carotid bifurcation and proximal internal carotid artery in the neck, but stenosis, ulceration, and/or occlusion also occur in the carotid siphon, distal internal carotid artery, and proximal middle cerebral artery.

TIAs usually last from a few seconds to several minutes and rarely last longer than 30 minutes (47). Occasionally, the duration may be up to 8 hours, which has been suggested as the upper limit for a TIA. The history may be of only one attack or several hundred, but most patients have had fewer than five attacks when first seen. Recurrent attacks are usually of the same general type (92). On rare occasion, a patient will present with syncope, dizziness, or seizures, but when this is the case a cerebrovascular etiology is not the primary concern.

Transient monocular blindness may be total or partial. The characteristic description is the sudden onset of a gray-black shade or curtain, gradually and painlessly descending or ascending to obscure all or part of monocular vision and then gradually recovering with the sensation that the shade is receding. Some patients complain of a fog, blurriness, or blindness of one eye. Others will note one or a shower of specks of bright light or sparks that dart across the field of vision.

The most frequent transient hemispheral attacks consist of numbness of the fingers followed in decreasing order of prevalence by speech disturbance, numbness and weakness of the hand and arm, weakness of the arm and leg, weakness of the hand, numbness and weakness of the arm and leg, and numbness of the face (44). When the history indicates that both transient monocular blindness and transient hemispheral attacks have been present in the same patient, the transient monocular blindness usually occurs first, and the transient hemispheral attacks and transient monocular blindness do not occur simultaneously (92).

The pathophysiology of the transient cerebral and ocular symptoms associated with carotid atherosclerosis is unsettled. Fisher brought attention to the relationship between carotid occlusive disease and stroke, and it was thought that the major mechanism of stroke related to inadequate distal cerebral perfusion (43–45). Fisher has emphasized that low flow is particularly likely when the spell comes on with standing up or when the limbs (especially the leg) shake on one side. Subsequently, more attention has been focused on the possible role of embolization from the carotid bifurcation to the intracranial arteries as a mechanism of stroke (8, 76, 93).

However, in a study of 95 consecutive patients with unilateral carotid TIAs who had been examined angiographically no correlation was found with ulcerations of the carotid artery (92). In a detailed study of a patient with severe carotid stenosis, a minor stroke, and TIAs, cerebral blood flow measurements demonstrated a hemodynamic cause (119). Fisher has listed several reasons why the multiple, stereotyped, short-lasting focal TIAs are probably due to a hemodynamic cause and not emboli (46). The authors believe that either hemodynamic flow or embolism can be the underlying cause of TIAs and stroke.

The neurologic examination in a patient with TIAs is usually normal. A bruit is sometimes heard over the neck. Careful auscultation over the entire course of the carotid artery from the clavicle to the angle of the jaw can often determine the point of maximum intensity. Bruits associated with internal carotid artery stenosis are usually localized in the midcervical region and are not heard in the low neck and chest. In general, the higher the pitch of the bruit, the tighter the stenosis, and a severe stenosis is suggested if the bruit extends into diastole. However, with a very tight stenosis, the bruit may become less intense and even disappear as the rate of blood flow is reduced. On occasion, platelet or cholesterol emboli may be seen in the retina.

A significant number of patients who have had a stroke will also have atheromatous occlusive disease. In the patient with a prolonged reversible ischemic neurologic deficit, the symptoms usually resolve within a few days, although computed tomography (CT) may show a small area of infarction. The distressing fact is that in a group of patients who developed a permanent moderate to severe neurologic deficit due to carotid occlusion, 60% had a prior history of TIAs that might have led to preventive treatment; 20% were associated with a fluctuating or stepwise progression that might have allowed time for treatment, and 20% came on suddenly without warning (44). In the authors' pathologic evaluation, 23 of 51 patients had TIAs before a persistent deficit (see Chapter 2). Clearly, careful attention must be paid to any patient who has a history of TIAs.

On examination, the patient who has had a stroke may also have a bruit. The neurologic deficit will depend on the area of brain infarction. Occasionally, the only permanent deficit in a patient with carotid occlusive disease is impaired vision due to a retinal artery embolus. A small but separate group of patients are those who have venous stasis retinopathy or ischemic oculopathy due to ischemia from carotid occlusive disease (23). Usually there is occlusion or severe stenosis of one and often both internal carotid arteries. Very frequently these patients have ipsilateral or bilateral external carotid or common carotid artery disease. The ocular ischemia may progress to intractable neurovascular glaucoma and blindness.

Diagnostic Studies

Guidelines for Planning Studies

The patient with a TIA and a carotid bruit on the side appropriate to explain the symptoms should have selective angiography. It has been suggested that patients with TIAs also have a computerized tomographic (CT) scan as part of the initial evaluation because of the evidence of silent cerebral infarction in 20–30% in these patients, which is reported to be associated with an increased risk of operation (118). When there is a typical transient monocular blindness and no bruit, noninvasive carotid studies are done; if a significant lesion is found, angiography is indicated.

The patient with transient hemispheral attacks and no bruit should have a CT scan done first because an occasional patient with a tumor, especially a metastatic lesion, subdural hematoma, or aneurysm, may present with transient ischemic attacks. If the CT is not diagnostic, angiography is indicated. Angiography is also indicated when the clinical examination and noninvasive studies suggest significant carotid disease in patients who have presented with dizziness, syncope, or seizure.

For patients who have had a completed stroke, a CT scan is usually done first to define the extent of the infarction, if any, and to exclude hemorrhage as a cause of the problem. When the history and examination suggest carotid occlusive disease, angiography is indicated.

If the problem is an acute stroke with mild to moderate deficit or a fluctuating or progressive stroke, CT scan and immediate angiography are done. The patient with a massive stroke with altered level of consciousness will have a CT scan, but angiography is usually not done unless significant improvement occurs because these patients do not benefit from surgery. If the CT scan on a patient with stroke does not show pathology and angiography is normal, diagnostic possibilities include embolus from a cardiac source and lacunar disease. Pure motor or sensory transient ischemic hemispheral symptoms are characteristic of the lacunar stroke syndrome. A history of hypertension suggests this as a cause. The CT scan may or may not show the small deep area of infarction. Magnetic reasonance imaging (MRI) will better define this pathology. Angiography is usually negative.

With improved noninvasive diagnostic tests, carotid endarterectomy has been done based on the results of these tests without angiography (28, 113). Situations where this has been done include stenosis documented by previous angiography that has progressed, acute stroke problems with severe stenosis, the presence of severe peripheral vasuclar disease, a history of dye allergy, and severe medical problems, such as impaired renal function and unstable angina. The authors have performed surgery without angiography on rare occasions for these indications or when the patient has refused the angiogram because of the risk involved. Some have concluded that angiography adds little in evaluating those patients with classical TIAs and demonstration of an unequivocal lesion on noninvasive testing (97, 113). However, it is emphasized that angiography is indicated if the noninvasive study suggests a long lesion extending up the internal carotid artery, a nonstenotic ulcerative plaque, or an unidentifiable lesion (113). At the present time the authors still recommend angiography for the majority of these patients in order to define the extent of the stenosis, to determine if there is intraluminal thrombus, to detect areas of ulceration, and to demonstrate any area of intracranial stenosis.

Noninvasive ultrasound tests have been useful in assessment of hemodynamic change and follow-up in patients with asymptomatic bruits (see Chapter 3), the study of patients with central retinal occlusion, evaluation of patients with atypical or vague symptoms and possible carotid disease, and some patients with completed strokes.

Angiography

Angiography must include visualization of both carotid bifurcations, the intracranial carotid circulation, and, in some patients, the vertebrobasilar system. The study is best done by retrograde femoral catheterization with selective carotid injection and serial films. In some cases, subtraction studies give additional information. Aortic arch injections usually do not clearly define the pathology and do not help in patient management (50). If there is significant disease in the distal aorta or its branches, a right brachial or axillary artery injection may be used.

What constitutes a significant degree of narrowing of the internal carotid artery on the angiogram? Most publications refer to a percentage narrowing of the internal carotid artery lumen. In many angiograms this percentage is hard to determine because the internal carotid artery diameter is not uniform (Fig. 1.1) and the distal artery may narrow when pressure is reduced (slim sign) (70) (Fig. 1.2). Therefore, the authors prefer to measure the lumen diameter in millimeters at the point of maximum narrowing with correction for magnification. In general, a residual internal carotid artery diameter of 2 mm represents at least a 70% narrowing of the lumen diameter. As the lumen narrows below this diameter, a hemodynamic change usually begins to occur in the artery distal to the stenosis (30). Another point to remember is that in some patients the severity of the stenosis (Fig. 1.3) or degree of ulceration (Fig. 1.4) may not be seen unless the area is visualized in two planes.

The vast majority of patients with TIAs and a carotid bruit will have a severe stenosis (<1.5 mm lumen diameter) on the angiogram. The stenosis may occur anywhere from the common carotid bifurcation to a point in the internal carotid artery 3–4 cm distal to the bifurcation, and narrowing may be short or long (Fig. 1.5A–D). In a small number of patients with TIAs, an ulcer may be the principal pathology (Figs. 1.4 and 1.13). Some patients have both stenosis and ulceration (Fig. 1.6). A few have complete internal carotid artery occlusion.

It is important that serial films be done for up to 10–15 seconds. These films may demonstrate collateral flow in cases of severe internal carotid artery stenosis (Fig. 1.7) or occlusion. One must be careful in evaluating intracranial occlusion or stenosis on a single injection when there is significant collateral circulation into the hemisphere because an intraluminal defect may be due to washout (83) (Fig. 1.8). Late films may also show dye in an ulcer crater, indicating an area of stagnation and potential thrombus formation (Fig. 1.9). One may see varying degrees of retrograde flow down the internal carotid artery in patients with complete occlusion (Figs. 1.8 and 1.20).

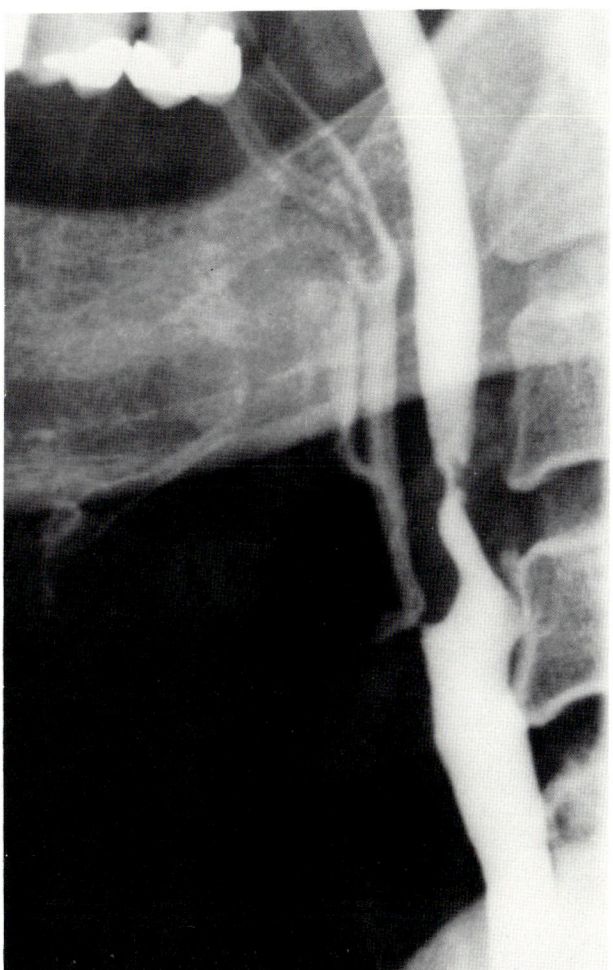

Figure 1.1. Measuring degree of stenosis. Lateral angiogram showing the carotid bifurcation with severe stenosis in the proximal internal carotid artery and markedly severe stenosis at the origin of the external carotid artery with reduced flow. Comment: The authors prefer to describe the degree of stenosis by measuring the lumen diameter at the narrowest point corrected for magnification, here 1.0 mm in the internal carotid artery. Using a percentage narrowing for description has been avoided because it is often difficult to decide what value to use for the denominator. Here the widest diameter distal to the stenosis is 9 mm and the narrowest is 7 mm.

There may be delayed flow through an area of severe stenosis ("pseudo-occlusion") (Fig. 1.10) or evidence of embolic occlusion of an anterior or middle cerebral artery branch (101).

In patients with internal carotid artery occlusion, the appearance of the proximal end does not accurately predict the age of the occlusion. In a report of patients with acute stroke and angiography done within 6 days of the onset, three configurations were found, in descending order of frequency: a sharp pointed stump, virtual absence of the artery, and a rounded blunt stump (91).

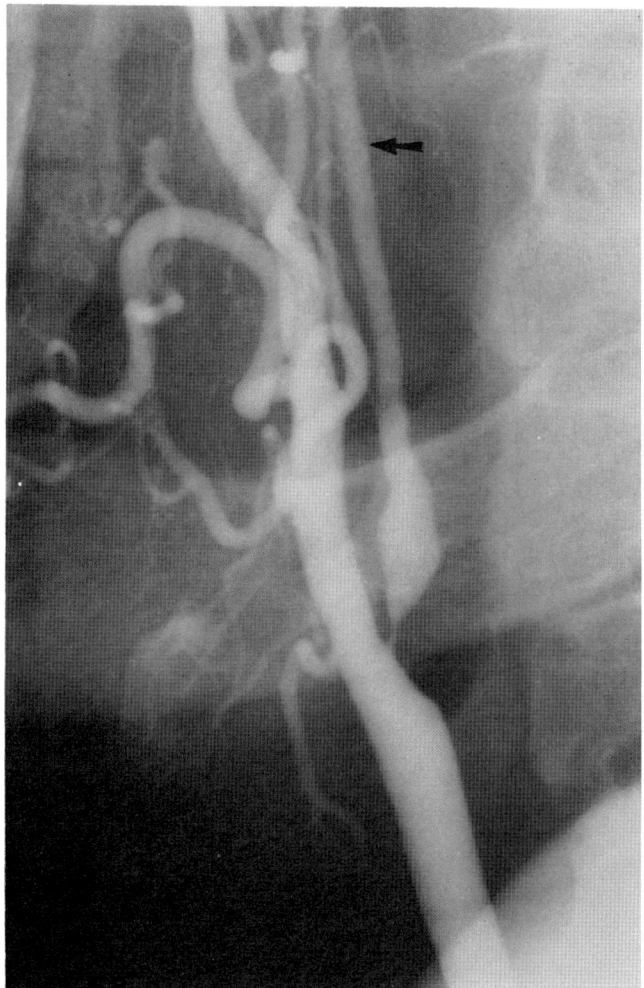

Figure 1.2. Carotid "slim" sign. Left carotid angiogram showing stenosis at the origin of the internal carotid artery. The stenosis is severe with a residual lumen diameter of less than 1 mm and a poststenotic dilatation. The distal internal carotid artery is small (*arrow*) with a diameter less than the external carotid artery diameter, a finding noted when the pressure is reduced distal to the stenosis (slim sign). This sign does not indicate distal atherosclerosis or hypoplasia of the artery.

In a consecutive series of patients who had angiography for TIAs, 37% had a severe stenosis (lumen <2 mm diameter) of the carotid bifurcation or proximal internal carotid artery; 12% had a complete internal carotid artery occlusion; 3% had severe stenosis distal to the bifurcation; 6% had moderate stenosis at the bifurcation (3–5 mm diameter lumen); 23% showed minimal stenosis at the carotid bifurcation (6–8 mm diameter lumen), and 19% had a normal carotid bifurcation and proximal internal carotid artery (92). A few patients with severe stenosis also had ulceration at the carotid bifurcation, and a few had intracranial branch occlusion. In the patients with a normal carotid bifurcation region, 22% had nonobstructive irregularity of the common carotid artery and 17% had intracranial branch occlusion. In the patients with minimal stenosis, 27% had ulcerative lesions and 20% had intracranial branch occlusion. No correlation between most of the clinical features of the ischemic attack and a specific angiographic finding was noted. If a transient hemispheral attack was longer than 60 minutes, there was more chance of finding a nonsignificant carotid stenosis and an intracranial branch occlusion, suggesting an embolic cause for the problem. When the patient had both transient monocular blindness and transient hemispheral attack, a severe carotid stenosis was more likely.

The major deterrent to cerebral angiography is the risk of a lasting neurologic complication. In the best hands, 0.5% serious complications can be anticipated, including iliofemoral occlusion and cerebral infarction.

Digital Subtraction Angiography

The initial enthusiasm for intravenous digital subtraction angiography has been tempered by clinical experience (90). The proposed advantages of intravenous digital subtraction angiography were possible lower risk in most patients, the ability to perform the study on an outpatient basis, and the decreased cost. In some patients the degree of stenosis and the presence of ulceration can be seen (Fig. 1.11A and B). However, the disadvantages include decreased resolution, the failure to visualize the arteries of interest adequately in a significant percentage of patients, the inability to evaluate intracranial and collateral circulation, and the risks involved with the high volume of contrast material used (6). The authors rarely recommend intravenous digital subtraction angiography for evaluation of cerebrovascular occlusive disease.

Digital subtraction angiography by arterial injection, on the other hand, has been used with increasing frequency (90). The advantages over conventional angiography include the fact that because of the contrast resolution provided by computer enhancement, smaller volumes of dilute contrast material can be given through smaller, softer catheters and injections can often be made near origins of arteries without selective catheterization. This makes the examination shorter and safer with a reduction in cost.

Computerized Tomography

The CT scan is done to determine the presence and extent of infarction and to exclude other pathology. The characteristic appearance of an infarct is an area of low density with sharp margins extending to the surface of the brain and involving both gray and white matter. There is no characteristic on the CT scan that will definitely establish the diagnosis of an infarct or its age (33, 100, 115) (Fig. 1.12). An infarct is

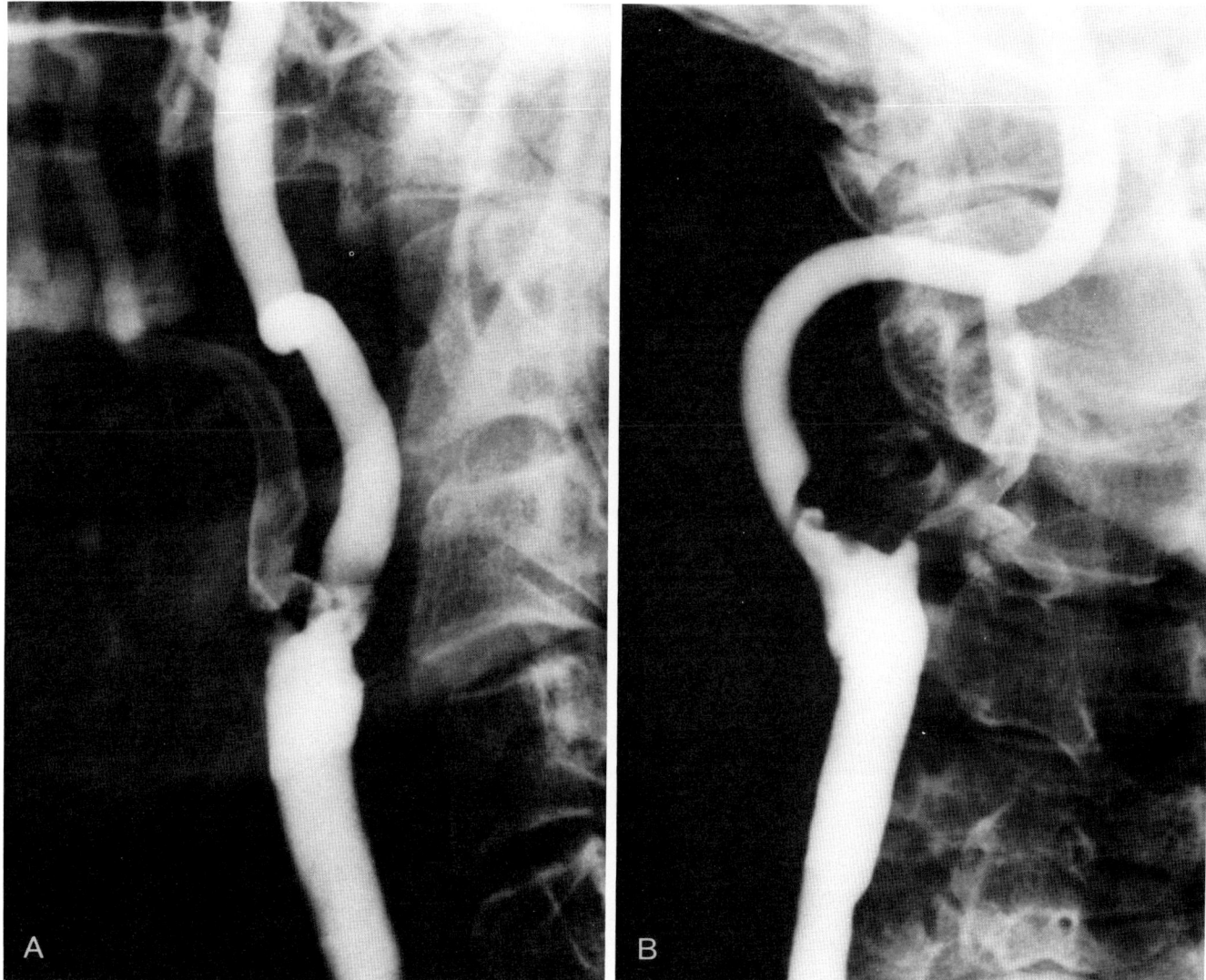

Figure 1.3. Two planes of view are necessary in some cases of stenosis. **A**, Lateral angiogram of the carotid bifurcation showing severe stenosis and reduced flow at the origin of the external carotid artery and marked irregularity at the internal carotid origin. **B**, Anteroposterior angiogram reveals the true degree of stenosis at the internal carotid artery origin.

usually not seen on the CT scan for at least 24 hours, but with improved spatial and contrast resolution of the new scanners, evidence of infarction may be seen within 24 hours (117).

The hypodensity usually becomes better defined on the third or fourth day after stroke (Fig. 1.13). In some patients this change may lessen in the second or third week and the infarcted area becomes indistinguishable from normal brain tissue (100). This does not indicate that recovery of tissue has occurred; this is the period when macrophages invade the area and proliferation of capillaries occurs. As the healing process continues, the infarcted area gradually becomes replaced by cystic spaces, and the CT scan again shows a low-density area that is sharply demarcated. The CT scan may not differentiate hemorrhagic infarction from hematoma (75). CT scanning of the cervical internal carotid artery has been able to detect stenosis, thrombosis, intramural hemorrhage, ulceration, and dissection (60). Further experience is needed to define their indications.

Contrast enhancement of the area of the infarction occurs in some patients, usually within 1–4 weeks after the onset of clinical symptoms. However, enhancement may be seen as early as the first day or it may not appear until several months after the event. When there is enhancement, the area of infarction may revert to a nonenhanced appearance over several months, but on occasion it may persist indefinitely. In an occasional patient, contrast enhancement is the only manifestation of infarction. An enhanced infarct can be confused with glioma, metastatic tumor, or

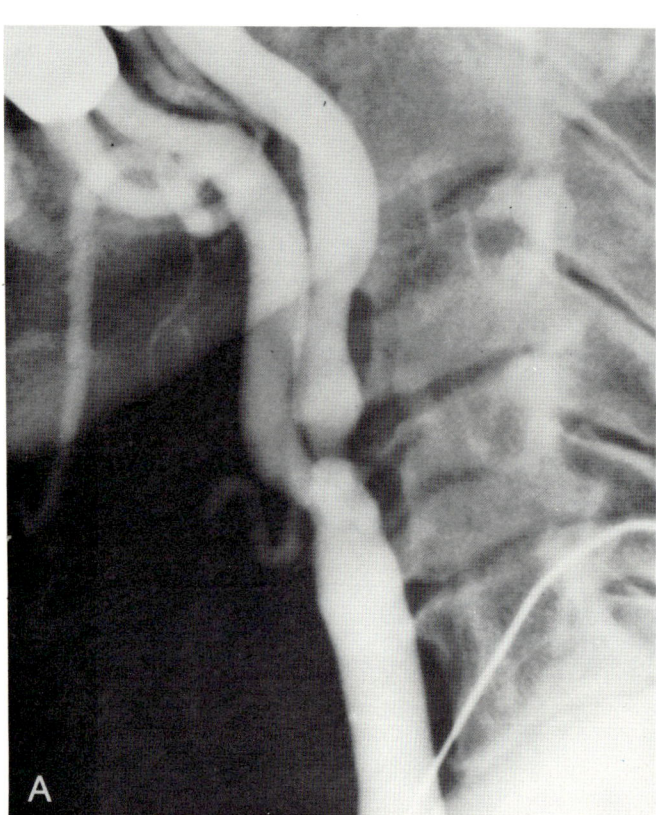 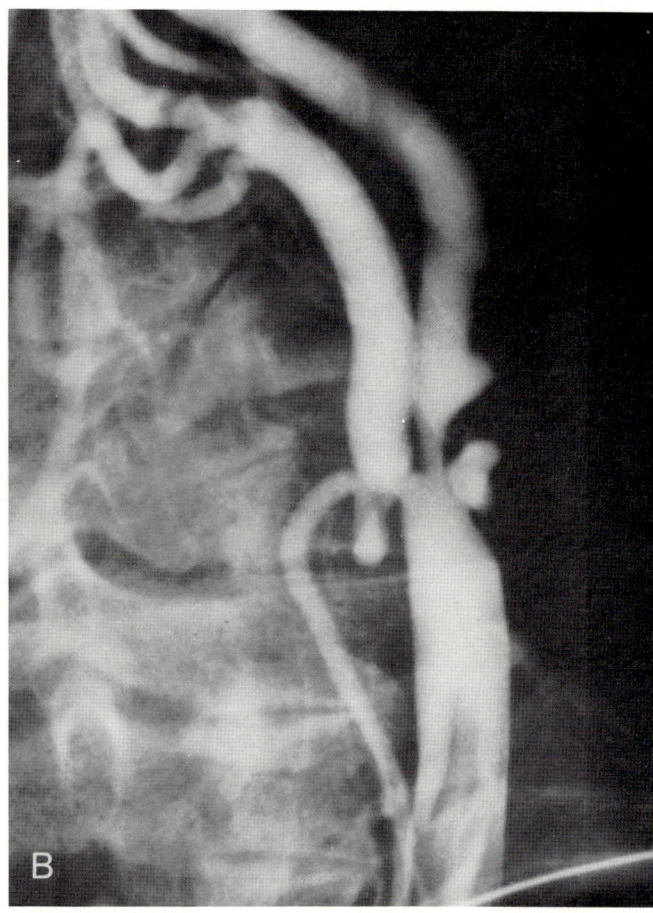

Figure 1.4. There is a need for two planes of view in some cases of ulceration and stenosis. **A**, Lateral angiogram of carotid bifurcation does not show significant stenosis (diameter 5.0 mm) in the proximal internal carotid artery. Careful inspection reveals a double density at the bifurcation suggesting an ulcer. **B**, Anteroposterior (AP) angiogram reveals that stenosis is 2 mm at narrowest point and a large ulcer crater is seen. Comment: The patient presented with episodes of weakness in the upper extremity. The true pathology is apparent only on the AP view.

arteriovenous malformation. Concern has been expressed by some about the possible hazard of using contrast media in patients with infarction (100).

Magnetic Resonance Imaging (MRI)

The place of this form of imaging in the evaluation of stroke patients being considered for surgical treatment remains to be determined (18). MRI may be more sensitive than CT in detecting ischemic pathologic conditions because of the precise demonstration of anatomic detail, lack of bone artifact, and ability to visualize infarctions within the first few days of the event. In one report MRI was more accurate than CT in detecting cerebellar infarction, particularly during the first 24 hours when the CT scan is likely to be negative (104). MRI has also demonstrated internal carotid artery occlusion (4).

Noninvasive Ultrasound Studies of Carotid Circulation

The use and limitation of noninvasive ultrasound studies of the carotid circulation have been reviewed in detail (1, 2, 29, 48, 64, 69, 75). Two types of ultrasound instruments demonstrate the anatomy of the carotid bifurcation. The B mode scan uses data on tissue composition to construct an anatomic field that includes the carotid artery (2). B mode scanning will show stenosis severe enough to create a bruit and will demonstrate which artery is responsible for the bruit (75). The duplex Doppler scanner uses physiologic data to construct profiles of a moving blood column to outline the vessel wall and combines this information with an analysis of the presence, direction, and nature of the flow at any point within the image (69). Difficulties in interpretation may be caused by calcification in the wall of the artery, a deep vessel, a high or low bifurcation, a thrombus being isodense with blood, and a severe stenosis mistaken for occlusion.

Phonoangiography is another test that gives useful information in evaluation of a carotid bruit (38, 65, 66, 69). Quantitative phonoangiography records the bruit, does a computer analysis, and plots the bruit

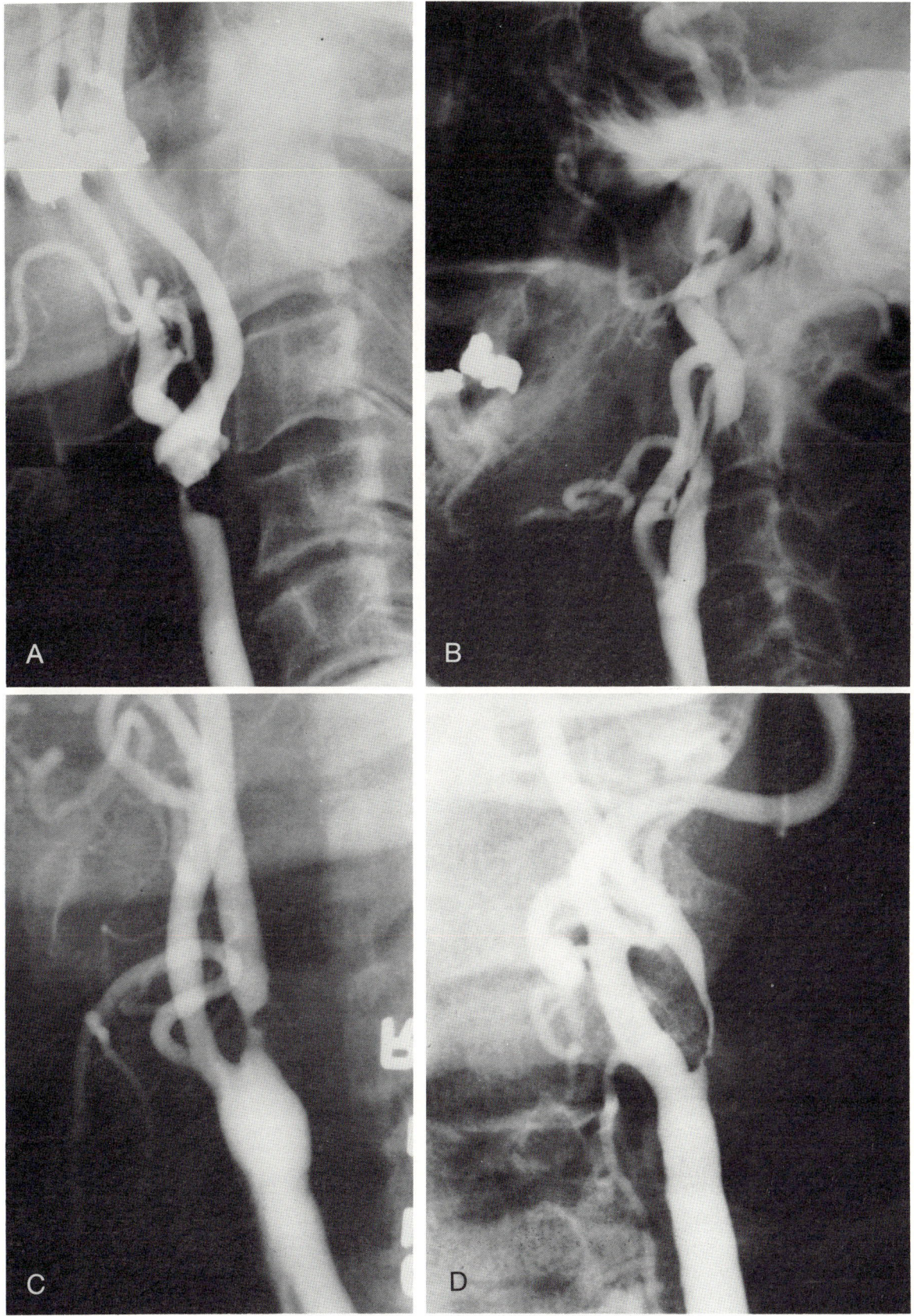

Figure 1.5. Varieties of internal carotid artery stenosis. Angiograms of carotid bifurcation. The stenosis may be located from the common carotid bifurcation (**A**) to a point 3–4 cm distal in the internal carotid artery (**B**). The length of the lesion may be short (**C**) or long (**D**). Comment: All of these patients presented with TIAs.

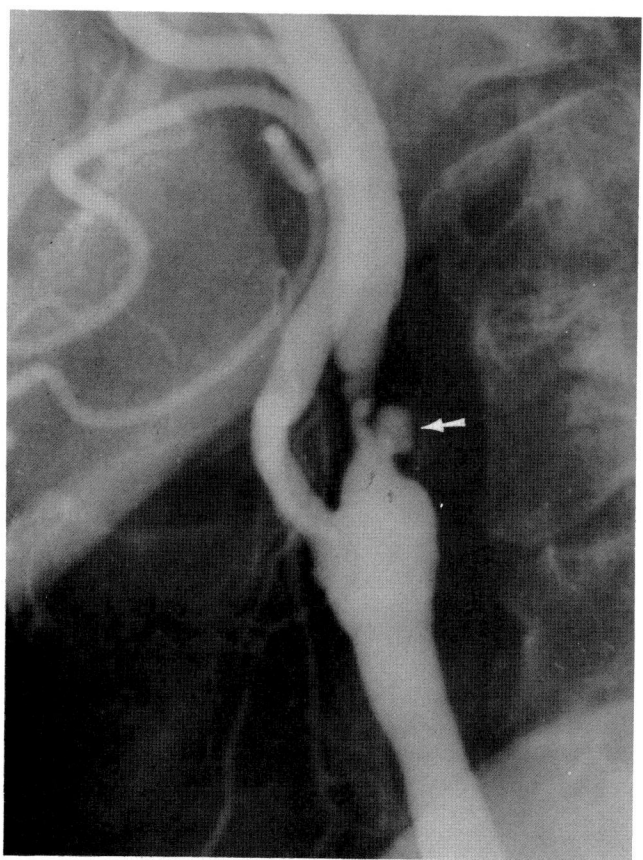

Figure 1.6. Internal carotid artery stenosis and ulceration. Left carotid angiogram showing severe stenosis in the proximal internal carotid artery with associated large ulcer (*arrow*). Both the degree of the stenosis and the size of the ulcer are of concern. Comment: Patient presented with TIAs. At operation a thrombus was noted in the ulcer. The symptoms were relieved.

intensity against frequency. The frequency with maximum intensity (break frequency) is proportional to the residual lumen diameter. The residual lumen diameter at the point of stenosis can be accurately estimated in about 90% of these patients (38, 66). Serial studies over time can identify progressive stenosis (see Chapter 3). In addition, this test can be used to differentiate between bruits originating at the carotid bifurcation and those emanating from the thorax.

Other tests help to determine if there is a hemodynamically significant lesion (1, 2). Periorbital Doppler ultrasonography reveals the direction of flow in external carotid branches on the brow. Reversal of flow indicates reduced pressure in the internal carotid artery system. The test requires careful positioning of probes and can be influenced by external carotid stenosis. It is the best test for studying the superficial orbital circulation. Oculoplethysmography measures the relative arrival time of the ocular pulse in each eye (64). A delay of greater than 20 milliseconds is significant. This is the most useful test to study the deep orbital circulation. Results are difficult to interpret in 10–20% of patients because of technical artifacts. For internal carotid artery occlusion, oculoplethysmography is 95% accurate (2).

MANAGEMENT AND INDICATIONS FOR SURGICAL TREATMENT

Transient Ischemic Attacks

Transient Ischemic Attacks with Unilateral Carotid Stenosis and/or Ulceration

Carotid endarterectomy is usually indicated for the patient with TIAs and severe stenosis (lumen less that 1.5 mm diameter) and/or severe ulceration in the common carotid bifurcation or proximal internal carotid artery (Figs. 1.1 and 1.6). These attacks are warnings of possible impending disaster. In 29 patients with persistent moderate to severe neurologic deficits due to carotid occlusion, 60% had prior TIAs (44).

If the angiogram shows severe stenosis with reduced flow in the internal carotid artery (Figs. 1.7 and 1.14) or a thrombus in the lumen (Fig. 1.15A) or if the clinical picture includes increasingly severe attacks in the preceding days, attention should be directed to performing the surgery as soon as possible. If there will be a delay of more than 12–24 hours, the patient should be heparinized. This drug seems to be effective in preventing stroke from intraluminal thrombus (21, 89).

If ulceration is found with a nonobstructive plaque, decision regarding endarterectomy or medical therapy will be made based on the severity of the lesion. In the past, carotid endarterectomy has been recommended for patients with TIAs who were found to have an area of ulceration even though the lumen diameter was greater than 1.5 mm (Fig. 1.16). However, the authors' clinicopathologic studies (see Chapter 2) suggest that ulceration is only rarely associated with major clinical events (57). There is also evidence that many ulcerating lesions associated with nonobstructive atherosclerosis may have a very low risk of future stroke (56, 67). Such patients may be treated with antiplatelet therapy and be followed by noninvasive tests. The area of ulceration may heal (105). Should there be evidence of development of stenosis or should TIAs continue, then surgery is indicated. If the ulceration is deep (Fig. 1.6) or if dye remains in the ulcer crater on delayed films (Fig. 1.9), carotid endarterectomy may be indicated. Evidence has been presented to suggest that deep and irregular ulceration may be associated with a higher incidence of stroke (78), but this was not found in another series (56).

In the authors' series of elective carotid endarterectomies the mortality rate was 1%, the incidence of

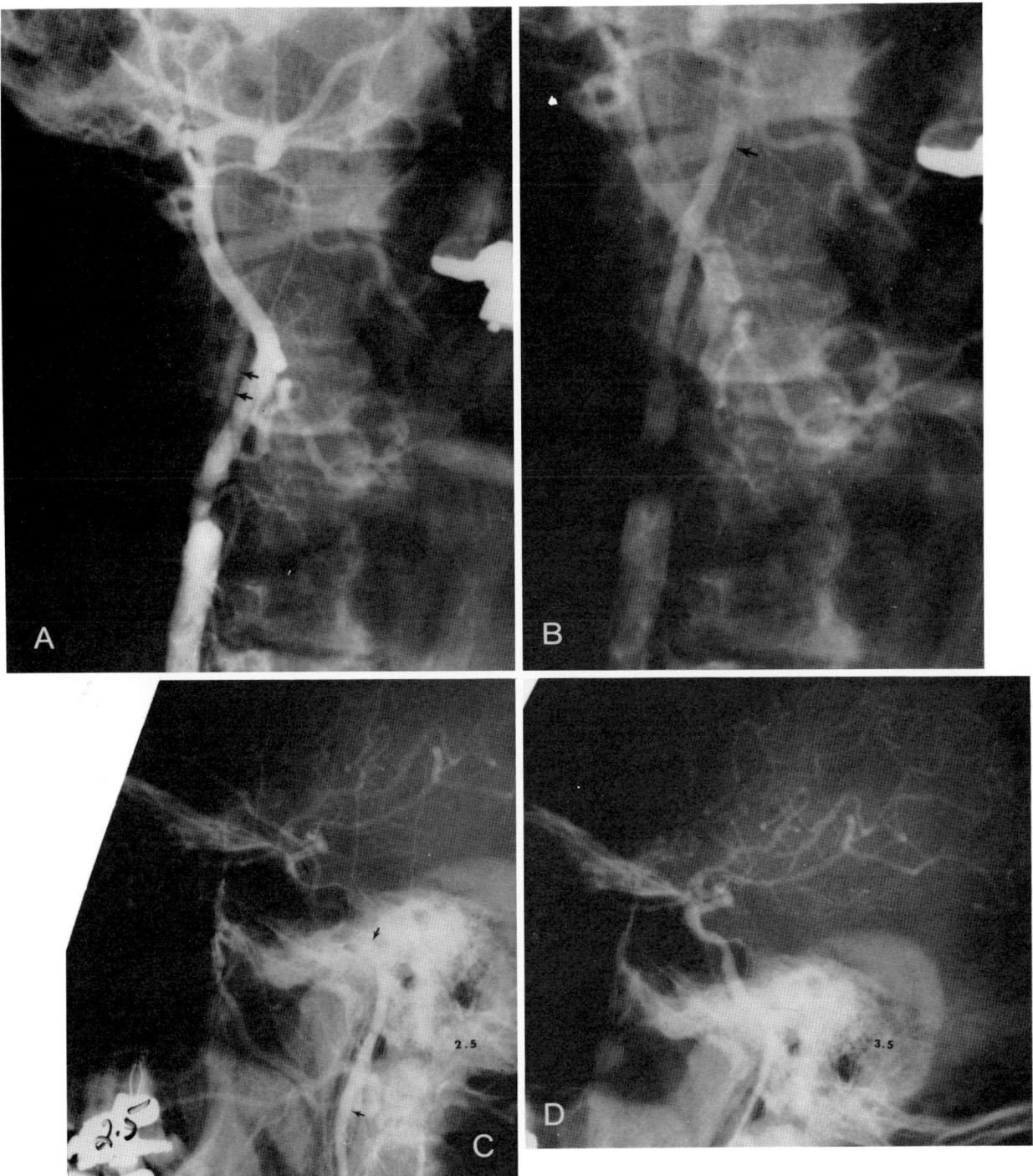

Figure 1.7. Importance of delayed films: slow internal carotid artery flow and ophthalmic collateral. **A**, The right internal carotid artery (*arrows*) fills slowly and faintly due to severe stenosis at its origin. Rapid, normal flow is seen in the external carotid artery. **B**, 2 seconds later, contrast in the internal carotid artery (*arrow*) is shown flowing upward as the external carotid artery opacification is clearing. **C**, An early film of the lateral cranial series shows opacification of the supraclinoid internal carotid artery and distal carotid siphon by ophthalmic artery collateral flow (*upper arrow*), prior to the arrival of contrast from delayed antegrade flow in the internal carotid artery (*lower arrow*). **D**, 1 second later, the internal carotid artery is completely opacified as the two streams of flow combine. Comment: This patient reported that 3 days before admission he had an episode of weakness in the left upper extremity and numbness in the left thigh. On the morning of admission he had severe weakness in the left foot for 30 minutes and in the left arm for several hours. Admission examination was normal and there was no right carotid bruit. Operation was done on an urgent basis a few hours after the angiogram. There was full recovery. (From Ojemann RG, Crowell RM, Roberson GH, Fisher CM: Surgical treatment of extracranial carotid occlusive disease. In: *Clinical Neurosurgery*. Baltimore, Williams & Wilkins, 1974, vol 22, chap 14.)

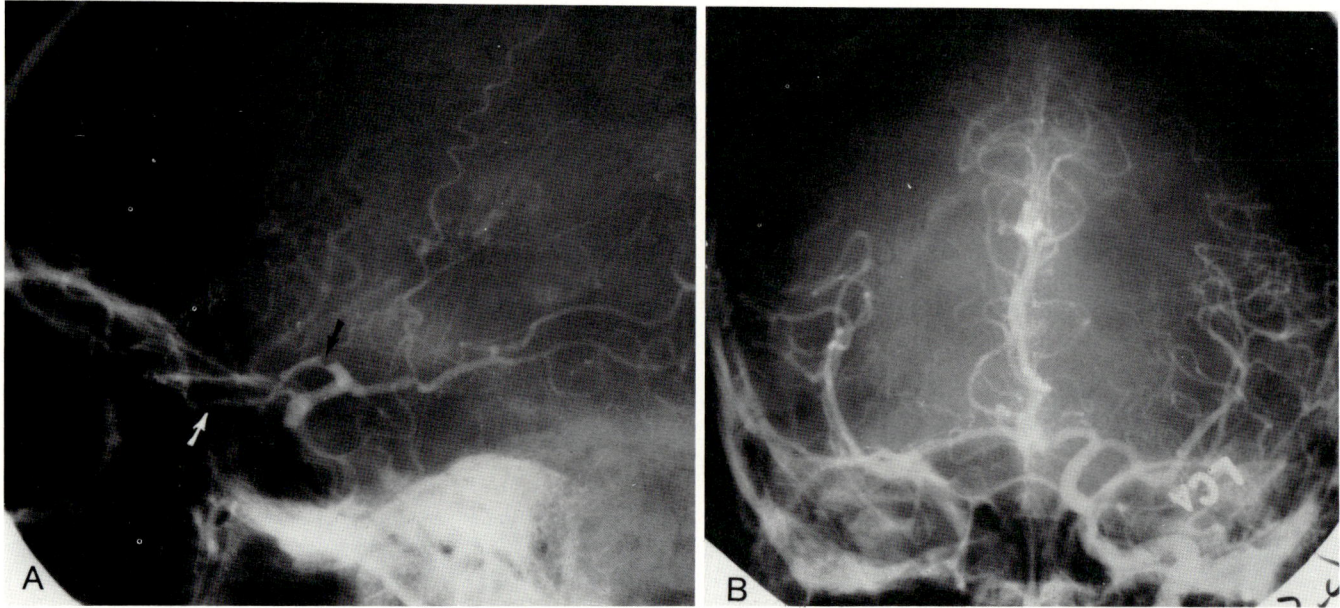

Figure 1.8. Internal carotid occlusion, collateral circulation, and intracranial "pseudostenosis." **A**, Right carotid angiogram showed complete occlusion of the internal carotid artery at its origin. The distal internal carotid artery is supplied by collateral through the ophthalmic artery (*white arrow*). There is retrograde flow for a few millimeters to the distal end of the occlusion and filling of the posterior cerebral artery and faint filling of middle cerebral artery branches. The *black arrow* points to a pseudostenosis due to washout from cross-circulation from the opposite side. **B**, Left carotid injection shows cross-filling into both right anterior and middle cerebral arteries. Comment: Patient had history of transient monocular blindness in the right eye followed by a mild stroke. The artery cannot be reopened. Bypass graft is not indicated. The patient should be treated with anticoagulation to prevent emboli. Care must be taken in interpretation of a single angiogram film. Patients with the finding seen in *A* have been referred for bypass graft because of the presumed intracranial stenosis.

major stroke was 1%, and the incidence of minor strokes was 1% (31). Virtually all other patients returned to their previous level of activity free of attacks. In the report of 1935 cases of carotid endarterectomy from the Mayo Clinic, the results were the same: minor morbidity 1%, major morbidity 1%, and mortality 1% (111). Several other reports of patients who have had elective carotid endarterectomy for TIAs have documented a similar low morbidity and mortality rate in experienced hands (5, 11, 13, 20, 30, 39–41, 49, 54, 59, 85, 86, 113, 121). The presence of a significant medical risk factor slightly increases the morbidity and mortality (109). This is discussed in Chapter 2. Age by itself has not usually been a determining factor, the decision for surgery being made on the basis of physiologic rather than chronologic age (87, 99).

The question is frequently asked as to whether carotid endarterectomy for TIAs prevents stroke. The incidence of stroke following the onset of a TIA is reported to be about 10% in the first 6 months and then averages 6%/year without surgery (119). A long-term study of stroke mortality after carotid endarterectomy from the Mayo Clinic reported 151 consecutive patients with TIAs and unilateral stenosis (120). There was an operative mortality of less than 1% and a stroke operative morbidity of 3%. During a 5-year follow-up the ischemic stroke rate was 1.4%/year ipsilateral to the endarterectomy and 0.6% on the unoperated side. The importance of collateral circulation was also emphasized in this study, where it was found that no patient who had a cerebral blood flow of 40 ml or greater per 100 g of brain per minute during occlusion for the endarterectomy had a stroke during operation or during 4.5 years of follow-up. In other reports 64 patients followed for a mean of 6 years (1–13 years) had an annual stroke rate of 1.6% on the operated side and 0.8% in the territory of the unoperated internal carotid artery (81). For 329 patients followed a minimum of 10 years the incidence of late stroke involving the operated side was 1.1% (58). These studies suggest that carotid endarterectomy done by experienced surgeons decreases but does not abolish the frequency of ipsilateral stroke.

Transient Ischemic Attacks with Bilateral Carotid Stenosis

Occasionally, a patient may present with a history of TIAs related to both carotid arteries. More often, the patient is studied because of symptoms due to stenosis in one artery, and significant narrowing of the internal carotid artery is found on the opposite

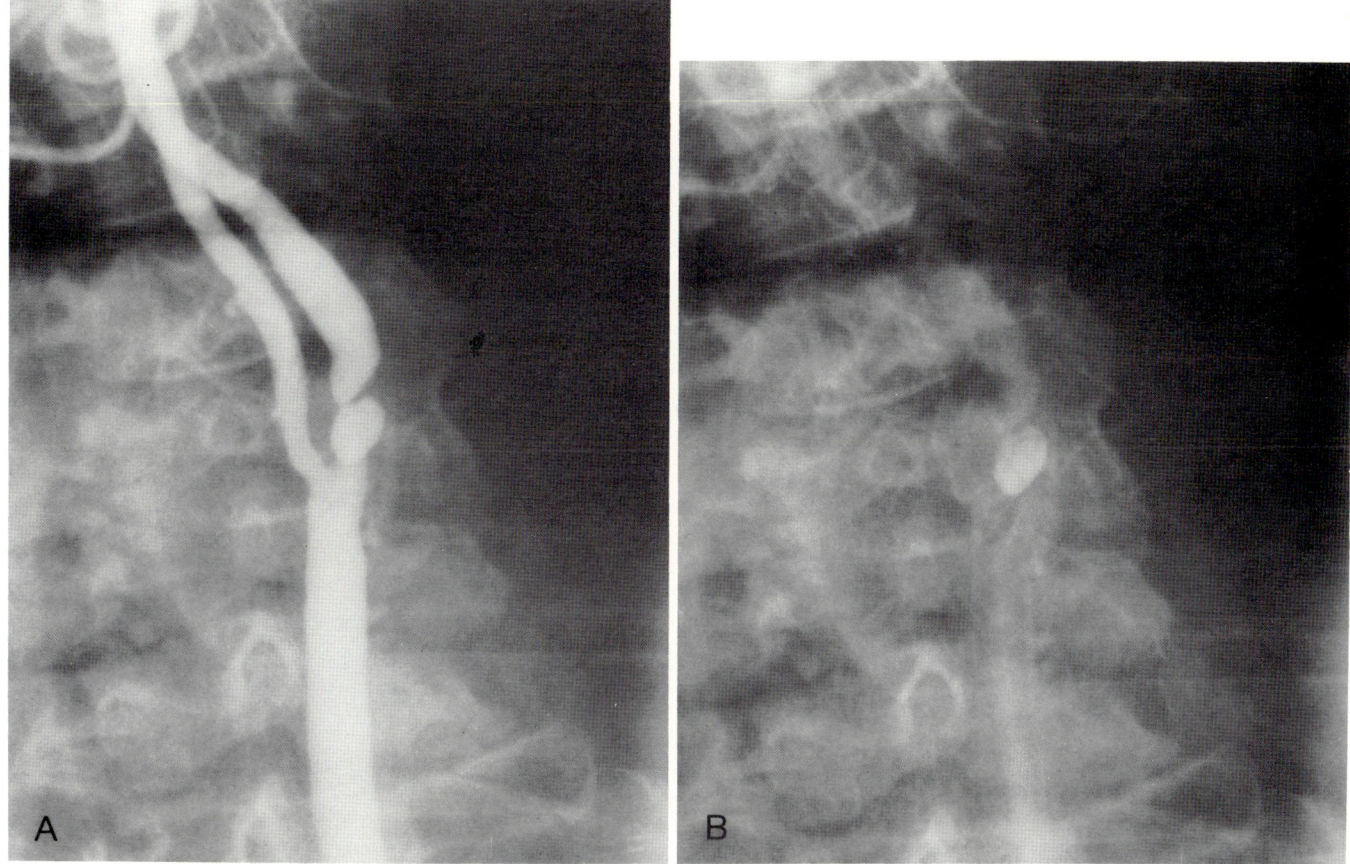

Figure 1.9. Delayed films highlight carotid ulceration. Angiogram of the carotid bifurcation. **A**, At the origin of the internal carotid artery, there is a pocket of dye suggesting an ulcer crater. Just distal to this is a severe stenosis. **B**, At 2.5 seconds after injection, the artery is faintly outlined but dye remains in the large ulcer crater. Comment: The patient presented with an episode of difficulty with speech, dizziness, and light-headedness. The endarterectomy specimen confirmed the angiogram findings. No further attacks occurred following the operation.

side. There may be bilateral carotid bruits. Angiography documents the pathology. Noninvasive studies may be necessary to help determine the hemodynamic significance of the lesions.

Carotid endarterectomy is indicated for the hemodynamically significant lesions. When only one side is symptomatic, it is generally treated first unless the asymptomatic side has a tighter stenosis with a more severe hemodynamic lesion, as demonstrated by angiography and noninvasive tests (Fig. 1.17). If both sides are symptomatic, the side with the most severe hemodynamic lesion is operated first. The second side is usually done within 7–14 days unless there is a neurologic complication or vocal cord paresis. When the second stenosis is very severe, heparin therapy may be indicated until the second operation is done. The case illustrated in Figure 1.18 indicates why these guidelines should be followed and emphasizes that TIAs and severe stenosis may be warnings of impending disaster.

Transient Ischemic Attacks with Ipsilateral Carotid Stenosis and Contralateral Carotid Occlusion

Most patients with this combination of lesions present with TIAs related to the internal carotid artery stenosis. Occasionally, patients will have had neurologic symptoms related to the contralateral internal carotid artery occlusion. There may be a bruit localized over the carotid bifurcation region. The neurologic examination is usually normal, but there may be a residual deficit if there was a stroke related to the carotid occlusion.

The indications for surgery are the same as for TIAs associated with unilateral internal carotid artery stenosis. The patient with a contralateral internal carotid artery occlusion is more likely to have an EEG change and need a shunt at the time of the carotid clamping for the endarterectomy than is the patient with a normal contralateral internal carotid artery (85, 88). However, in the authors' experience, as well

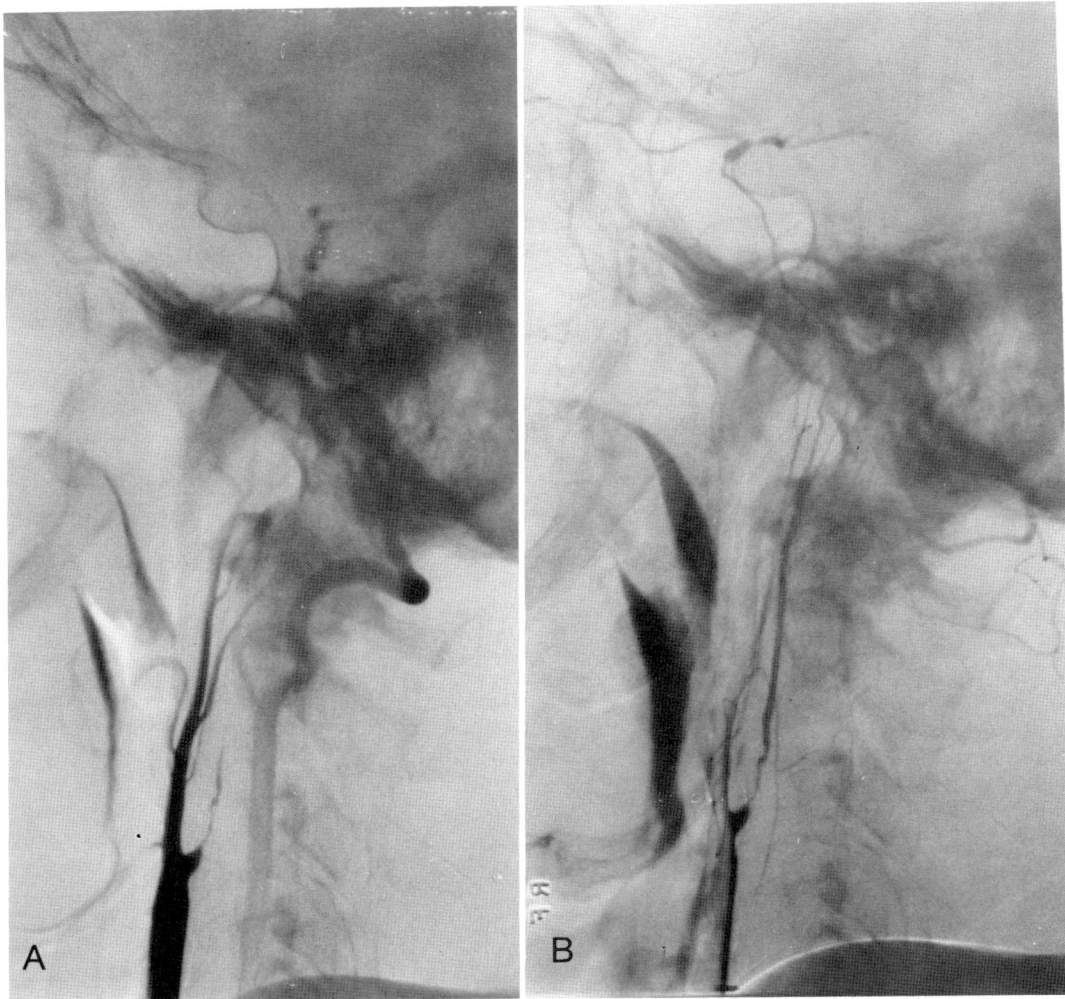

Figure 1.10. Pseudo-occlusion of the internal carotid artery. **A**, At 1 second the internal carotid artery appears to be occluded with a thin column of dye entering the proximal artery. **B**, At 10 seconds the long thin column of dye is filling the intracranial internal carotid and ophthalmic arteries.

as in that of others, there is no increase in neurologic complications in patients with contralateral internal carotid artery occlusion or stenosis 77, 88, 94).

Transient Ischemic Attacks with Internal Carotid Stenosis in the Neck and in the Siphon (Tandem Lesions)

No unusual clinical features are present in a patient with more than one lesion in the internal carotid artery. Angiography will show one area of stenosis in the carotid bifurcation or proximal internal carotid artery and another stenosis in the intracavernous or intracranial portion of the internal carotid artery (Fig. 1.19). The occurrence of this problem emphasizes the importance of complete angiography. Usually the stenosis in the neck is more severe than the distal lesion (98). If the residual lumen in the neck is less than 1.5 mm, carotid endarterectomy is indicated for TIAs even if the distal lesion is also significantly stenotic. Postoperatively, a decision is made between anticoagulation or antiplatelet therapy. In one report there was no relationship found between the presence or the severity of the siphon disease and the risks of recurrent symptoms associated with carotid endarterectomy (98), but another study indicated a high risk of cerebral infarction and myocardial infarction in patients with significant siphon stenosis (27).

Transient Ischemic Attacks with Ipsilateral Carotid Occlusion

TIAs can occur in the territory normally supplied by a completely occluded internal carotid artery (9, 15, 19, 55, 61, 85, 103). The cause of symptoms may be an embolus from the distal end of a thrombus in the occluded internal carotid artery, an embolus passing through the external carotid artery circulation from atheromatous stenosis of the external or

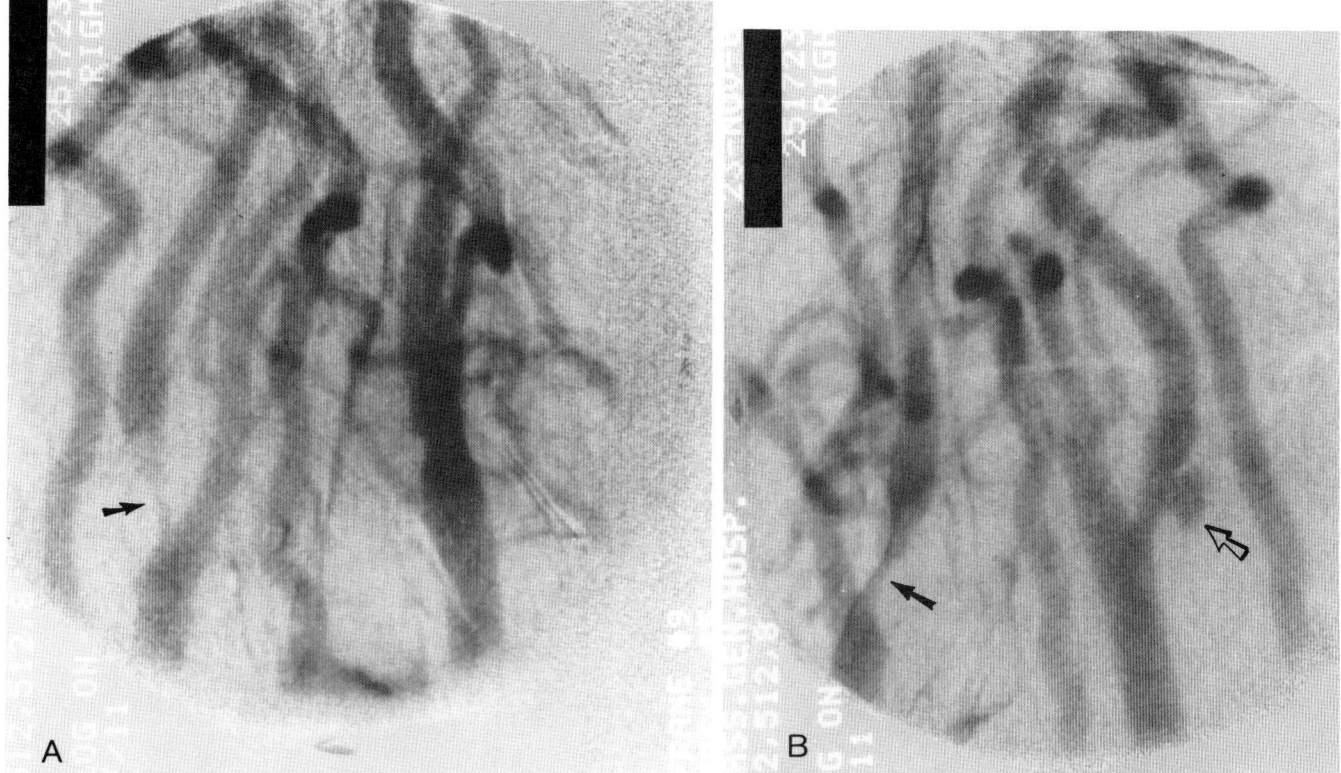

Figure 1.11. Stenosis and ulceration demonstrated by digtal subtraction angiography. **A** and **B**, Right and left oblique views. There is severe stenosis at the origin of the right internal carotid artery (*closed arrow*) and slight stenosis, but a large ulcer at the origin of the left internal carotid artery (*open arrow*).

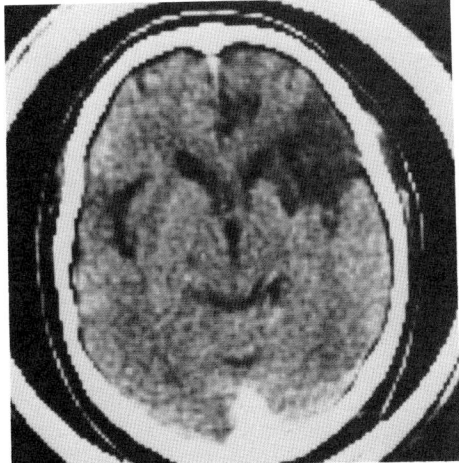

Figure 1.12. Cerebral infarction. This patient had a stroke several months prior to this scan. There is no enhancement. Note the characteristic appearance of an infarct with low density, sharp margins, triangular or quadrilateral shape, extending to the surface of the brain, and a tendency to narrow medially.

distal common carotid artery or from the stump proximal to the occlusion in the internal carotid artery, or a reduction of flow to the eye and/or cerebral hemisphere.

Angiography should include evaluation of the collateral circulation from the opposite carotid artery and, in many patients, the vertebrobasilar circulation. Lateral serial films of the head and neck for several seconds and subtraction studies help to determine the collateral flow and show how far down the internal carotid artery dye flows (3, 84, 101). This is important in deciding about the etiology of the symptoms and the probability of reopening the complete occlusion.

In a report of 35 patients (61), the angiographic visualization of the internal carotid artery distal to the occlusion was categorized as follows:

1. No visualization of the internal carotid artery;
2. Visualization of the internal carotid artery from the posterior communicating artery distally;
3. Visualization from the ophthalmic artery distally;

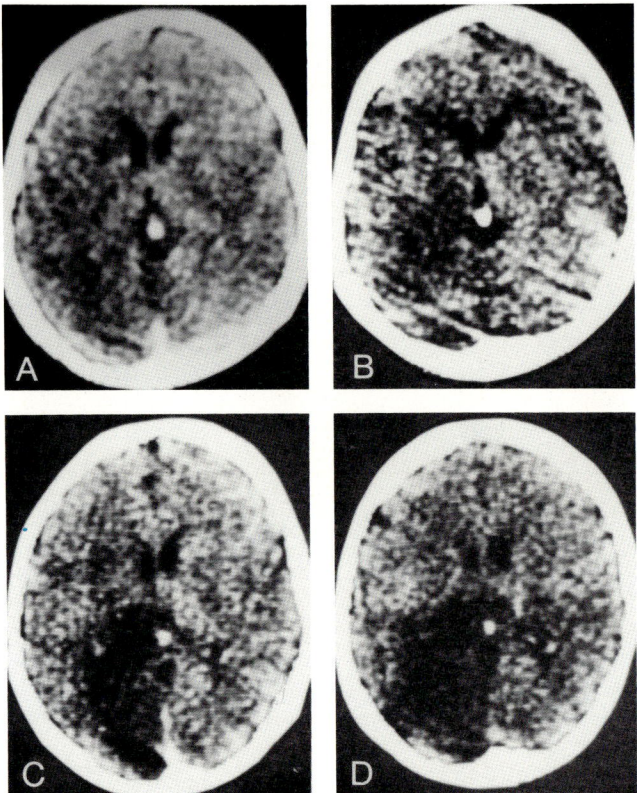

Figure 1.13. Serial CT scans following infarction in left posterior cerebral artery territory. **A**, Day 1, slight low density noted. **B**, Day 2, more pronounced low-density area seen. **C**, Day 4, sharply demarcated low-density region is more prominent. **D**, Day 7, area of low density somewhat larger than seen on previous scan.

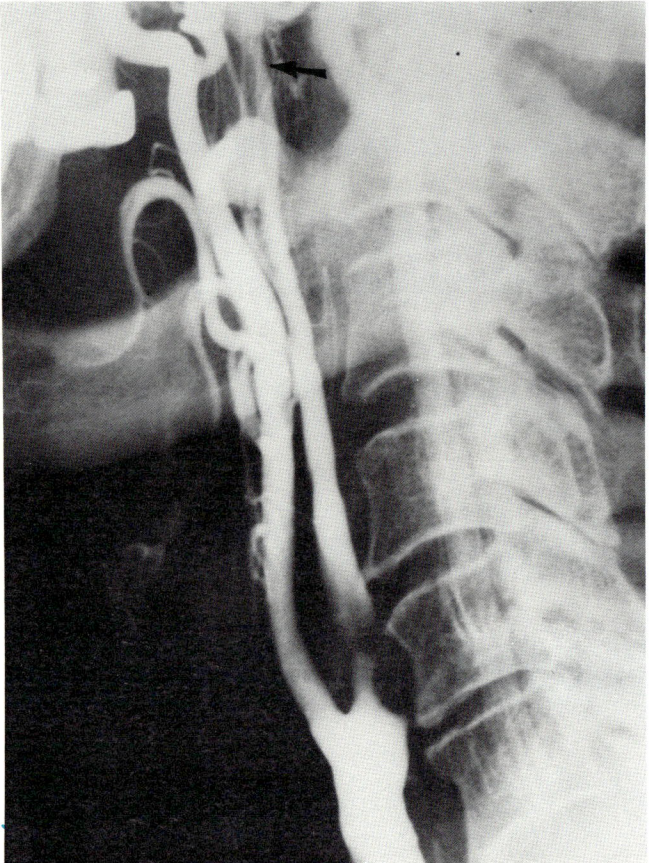

Figure 1.14. Severe internal carotid artery stenosis with delayed flow. Angiogram of carotid bifurcation region shows severe stenosis at the origin of the internal carotid artery with delayed flow beyond this area (*arrow*). The dye is less dense and the diameter smaller than that seen in the external carotid artery. Comment: The patient presented with TIAs. This is a worrisome situation because of ischemia, as well as possible occlusion or thrombus formation and embolus.

4. Retrograde flow to a point even with the floor of the sella turcica;
5. Retrograde flow into the carotid canal to near the base of the skull.

None of the category 1 patterns could be reopened even with immediate surgery. In categories 2 and 3, only six of 18 arteries could be reopened, and five of the six were operated within 7 days of the occlusion. In category 4, four of six arteries were reopened, and the two failures had been occluded 7 months and 3 years. All of the category 5 patients were reopened regardless of the time of occlusion (Fig. 1.20).

In two of the authors' patients, angiography revealed an occluded internal carotid artery several weeks before they saw the patient (85). Reevaluation of the x-rays with subtraction and repeat angiography were done because of continuing transient spells, and these revealed retrograde flow almost to the base of the skull. The arteries were reopened and the symptoms relieved. Others have reported similar cases (103). Even after a month of occlusion, there may be a reasonable chance of reopening the internal carotid artery if the occlusion does not extend too far distally (55, 61). When it has been decided that a complete occlusion cannot be reopened, anticoagulation is indicated. Even if there is good collateral circulation, the authors have favored this treatment because of the risks of embolization (16, 42).

If the angiogram shows a significant proximal stump in the occluded internal carotid artery in the neck and external carotid artery to ophthalmic artery collateral, this may be the source of embolus and the cause of TIAs, transient monocular blindness, or infarction (stump syndrome) (5, 9, 10). The evidence that emboli can pass through the external carotid artery circulation has been summarized (19). The presence of a stump is commonplace, but the incidence of the stump syndrome is uncommon. A stump that is causing symptoms is difficult to recognize angiographically, but suspicion should be directed

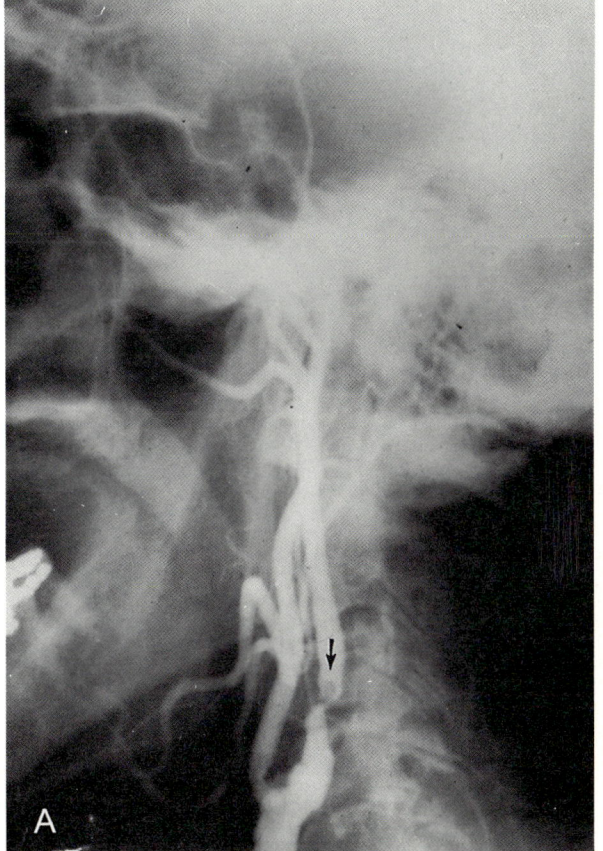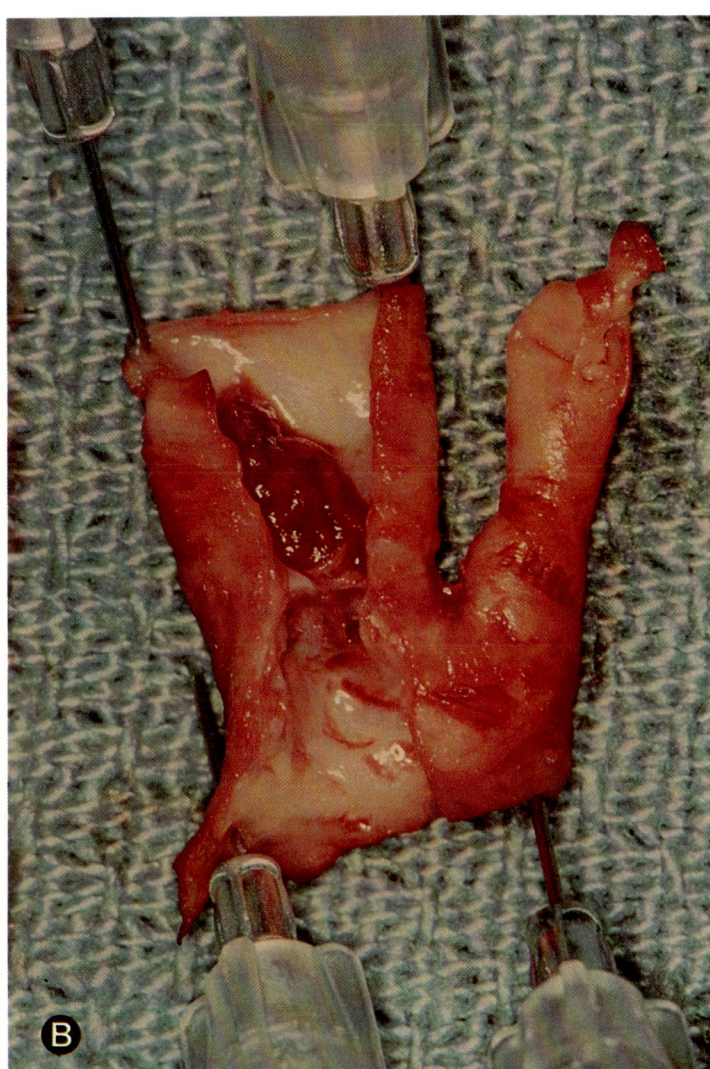

Figure 1.15. Stenosis with thrombus formation. **A**, Angiogram of carotid bifurcation showing severe stenosis with thrombus projecting distally into the internal carotid artery lumen from the stenosis (*arrow*). Note that there is also slight delay in internal carotid artery flow with the superficial temporal artery filling ahead of the intracranial circulation. **B**, Specimen removed at surgery. The thrombus is adherent to the distal end of the stenosis as it almost always is when present.

to those that are long and irregular in shape (Fig. 1.21). The natural history of this problem is unknown. Treatment has usually been surgical, but some patients have been followed on antiplatelet therapy (10).

Transient Ischemic Attacks with External Carotid Stenosis or Occlusion

Collateral circulation to the brain from the external carotid artery system can occur by flow through the ophthalmic system or the caroticotympanic branches or meningeal branches of the internal carotid artery (44). when the internal carotid artery is occluded, stenosis at the origin of the external carotid artery may be associated with TIAs (15, 35, 44, 82, 102). In a report of 22 patients with internal carotid artery occlusion and external carotid artery collateral flow, 10 patients with no significant atherosclerotic narrowing or ulceration of the external carotid artery remained free of symptoms over 6–40 months (24). In the other 12 patients, delayed recurrent cerebral or retinal symptoms developed ipsilateral to the internal carotid artery occlusion, and all were found to have stenosis or ulceration involving the common and/or external carotid artery. Subsequently, 17 patients with amaurosis fugax were reported to have the same findings (25). Endarterectomy completely stopped the symptoms. Occasionally, opening of a severely stenotic external carotid artery may be helpful in halting the progression of ischemic retinopa-

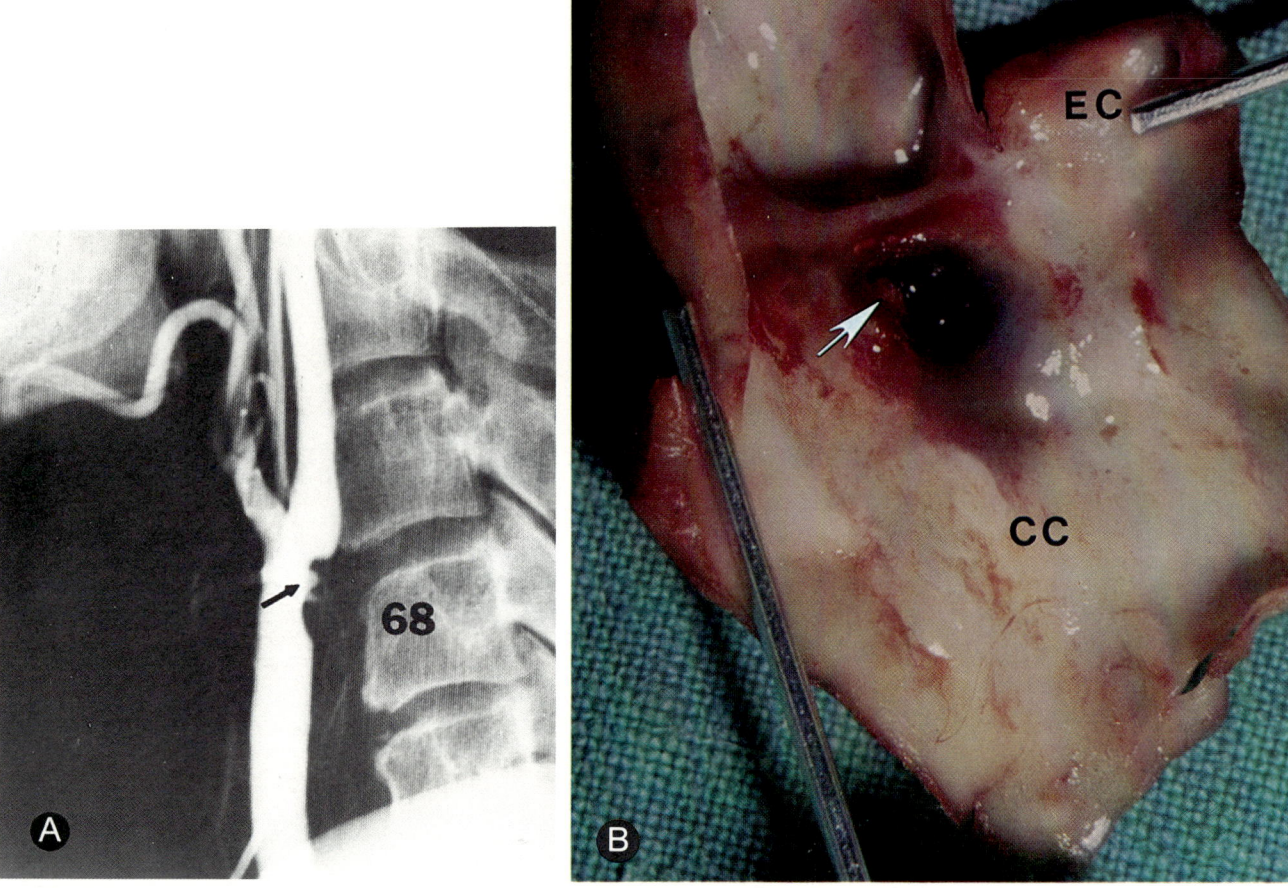

Figure 1.16. TIAs from ulcerated plaque with thrombus. **A,** Angiogram of carotid bifurcation shows no significant stenosis, but there is a discrete ulceration (*arrow*) within a plaque along the posterior wall of the distal common and proximal internal carotid artery. **B,** Atheromatous plaque removed intact at operation and then opened longitudinally on the anterior wall. *CC*, common carotid artery; *EC*, external carotid artery; *IC*, internal carotid artery. The *arrow* points to a thrombus in the well-circumscribed ulceration. Comment: The patient presented with TIAs. There was no bruit. Neurologic examination and noninvasive studies were normal. No further attacks were noted after surgery, and follow-up angiogram 4 years later, when he had attacks referable to the opposite side, showed a normal artery. (From Ojemann RG, Crowell RM, Roberson GH, Fisher CM: Surgical treatment of extracranial carotid occlusive disease. In: *Clinical Neurosurgery*. Baltimore, Williams & Wilkins, 1974, vol 22, chap 14.)

thy. When the internal carotid artery is open, external carotid artery stenosis or occlusion usually does not cause significant clinical symptoms. However, an occluded external carotid artery can be the source of a stump embolus into the internal carotid artery (26). The authors had a case in which they believe that an embolus into the internal carotid artery formed in the proximal pouch of a very tight, almost completely occluded external carotid artery (Fig. 1.22).

Posterior Circulation Transient Ischemic Attacks with Carotid Stenosis

Occasionally, patients will present with posterior circulation TIAs secondary to carotid stenosis. Diagnosis is more difficult because of the diverse clinical presentations. The most characteristic symptoms of TIA in the vertebrobasilar circulation are diplopia, dysarthria, dizziness, and weakness or numbness of part or all of one or both sides of the body (47). Other manifestations include headache, staggering, veering to one side, blurred vision, blindness, ptosis, dysphagia, confusion, and memory lapse. Occasionally, patients will have both cerebral and vertebrobasilar TIAs.

When there is evidence of carotid artery disease from either physical examination or noninvasive studies in a patient with posterior circulation TIAs, angiography is indicated. This should include both

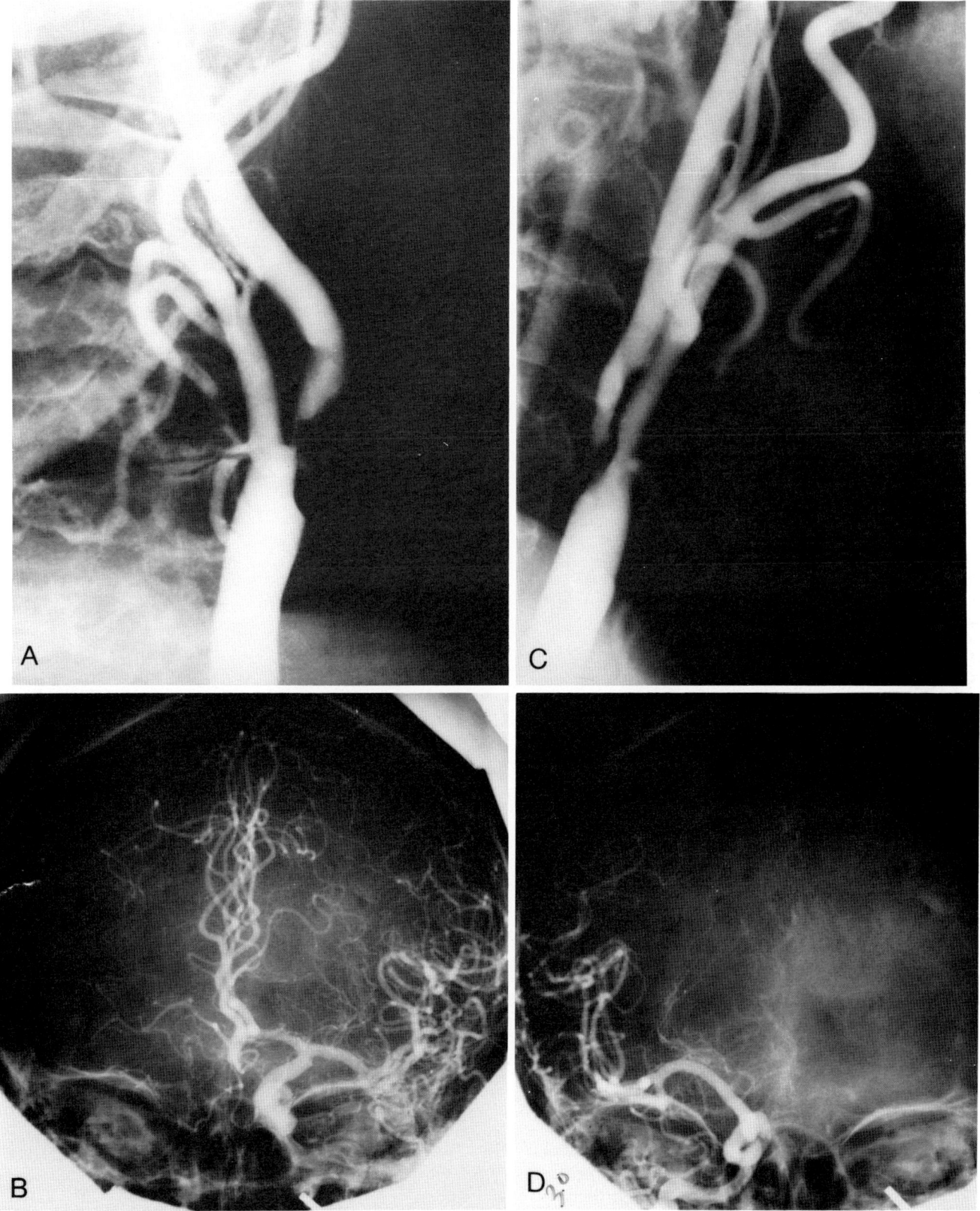

Figure 1.17. Bilateral carotid artery stenosis with unilateral TIAs. **A**, Left carotid angiogram showing severe stenosis at the origin of the internal carotid artery. **B**, Anteroposterior (AP) view reveals that this left internal carotid artery supplies both anterior cerebral arteries with flow into the watershed area on the right. **C**, Right carotid angiogram showing stenosis so severe that one can hardly see the dye going through. **D**, AP view shows only slight filling of anterior cerebral complex. Comment: The patient presented with left brain TIAs. The angiogram indicates that the most severely involved artery is the asymptomatic right side. The recommendation would be to do right carotid endarterectomy followed within a week by an operation on the left side.

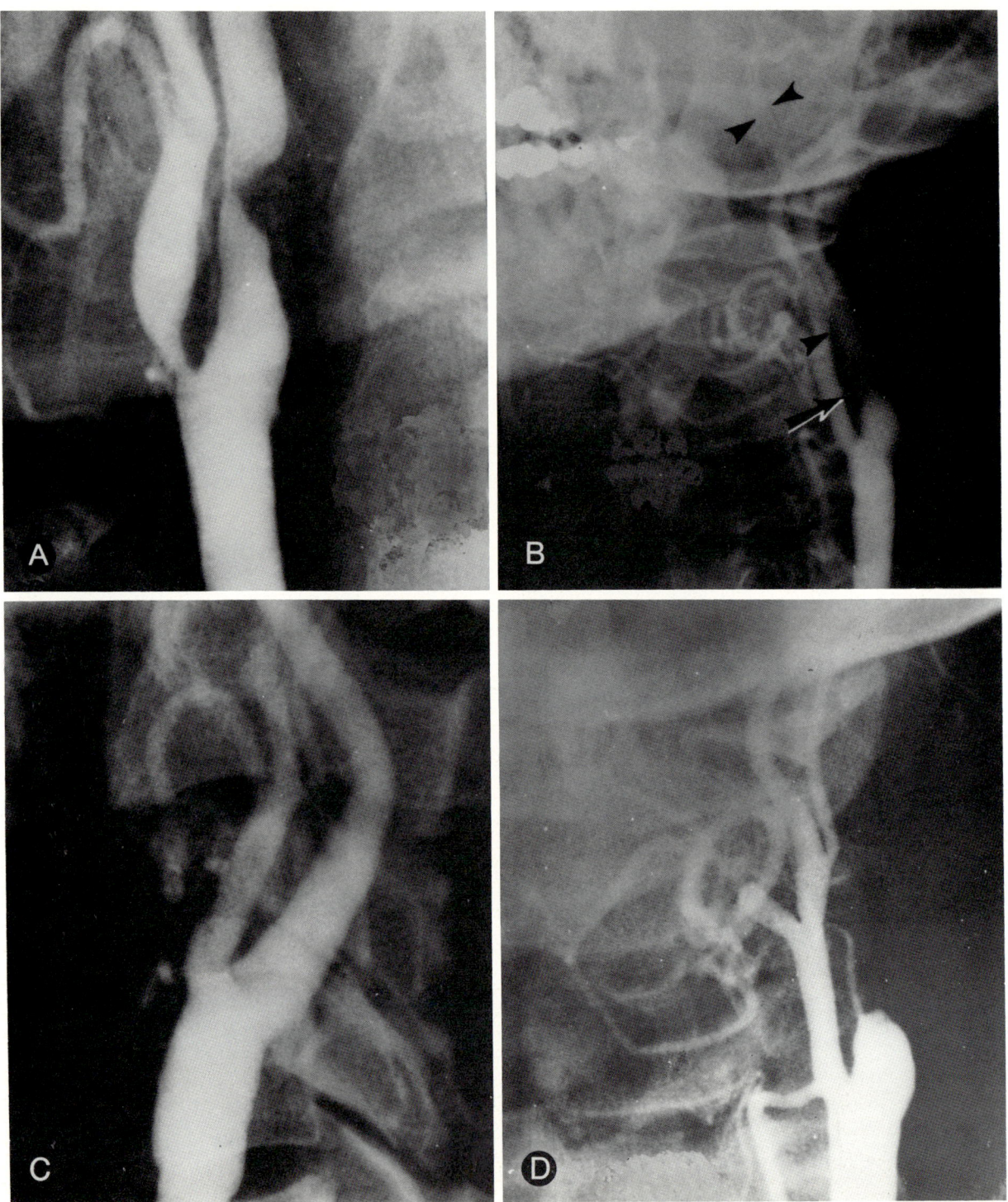

Figure 1.18. Bilateral carotid artery stenosis with bilateral TIAs: operate the tighter stenosis first. **A**, Right carotid angiogram showing localized plaque on the posterior wall 2 cm above the bifurcation. Stenosis is also present in the external carotid artery. **B**, Left carotid angiogram shows a more severe stenosis with reduced flow in the internal carotid artery. **B**, Right carotid angiogram 1 month after operation, showing normal restoration of both external and internal carotid lumens. The slight widening at the ends of the entarterectomy is normal. **D**, Left carotid angiogram with complete occlusion of the internal carotid artery. Comment: The patient presented with a history of TIAs relative to the left carotid artery beginning 1 year before admission, but none had occurred for 9 months. In the weeks before admission, TIAs relative to the right carotid circulation were noted. Bilateral carotid bruits were present, and the examination was normal. This patient was seen early in the authors' series, and the most recent symptomatic side was operated. He then declined the second operation planned a week later. One month after operation, he developed a stroke related to the left hemisphere. (From Ojemann RG, Crowell RM, Roberson GH, Fisher CM: Surgical treatment of extracranial carotid occlusive disease. In: *Clinical Neurosurgery*. Baltimore, Williams & Wilkins, 1974, vol 22, chap 14.)

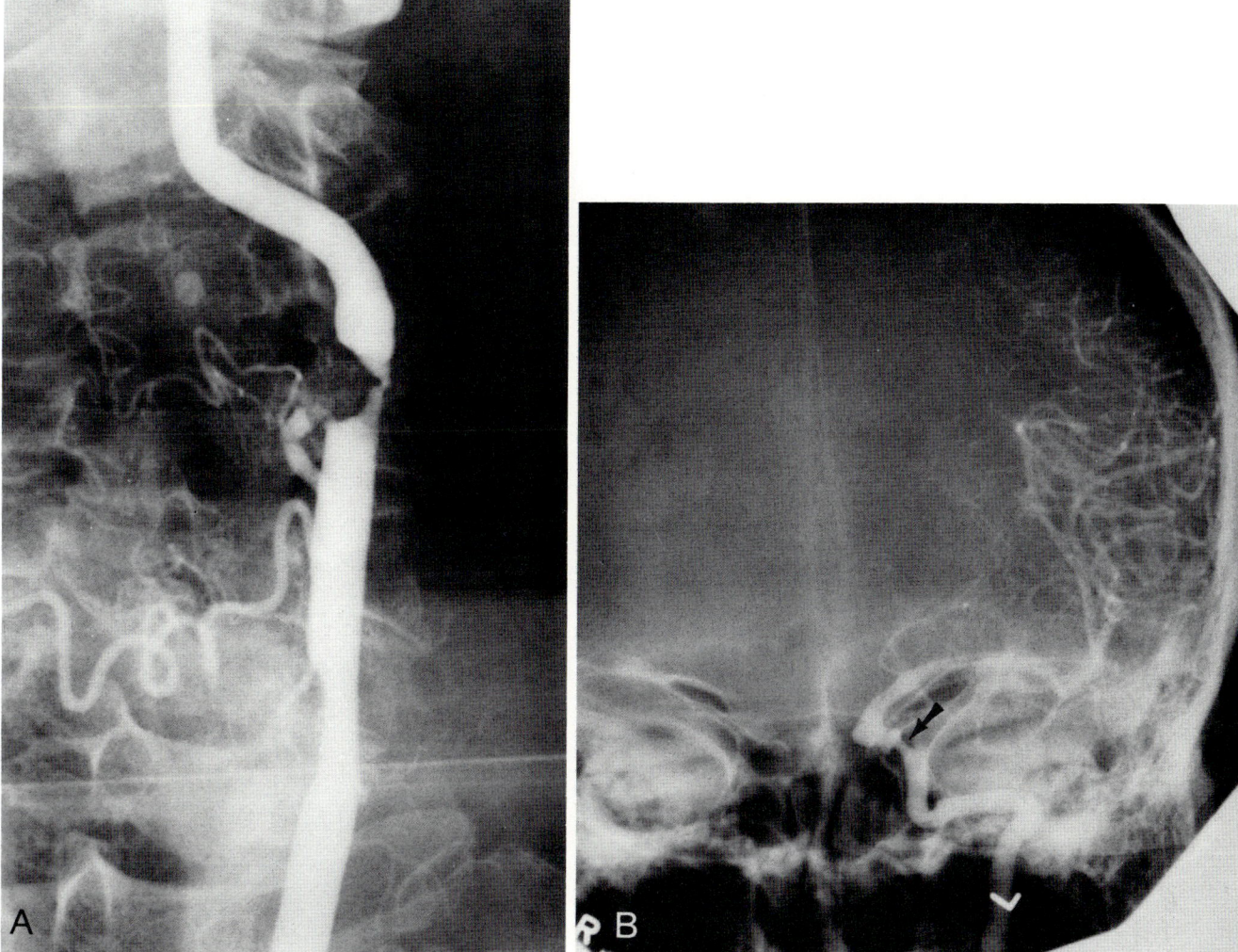

Figure 1.19. Tandem internal carotid artery stenosis. **A**, Severe stenosis at the origin of the internal carotid artery (residual lumen 1 mm) with occlusion of much of external carotid artery. Slight narrowing in the common carotid artery is also noted. **B**, Severe stenosis in the carotid siphon (*arrow*) with residual lumen of a little over 1 mm. Comment: Carotid endarterectomy may be indicated to remove the severe stenosis at the origin of the internal carotid artery and to reopen the external carotid artery. After surgery, a program of medical therapy is started.

the carotid and posterior circulation. Carotid endarterectomy is usually indicated if the angiogram shows filling of the posterior cerebral artery via the stenotic internal carotid artery, or filling of the posterior circulation from the internal carotid artery because of vertebral artery occlusive disease (Fig. 1.23), or a persistent hypoglossal or trigeminal artery (106), or there is evidence of a steal of blood with posterior to anterior circulation by flow through the posterior communicating artery (14). The authors have not been convinced that carotid endarterectomy will alter vertebrobasilar symptoms unless one of the conditions noted above is found on the angiogram, and this has also been the experience of others (72). When severe carotid stenosis is present with no filling of the posterior circulation from that artery, one considers the problem as an asymptomatic carotid stenosis. The optimal treatment for this lesion is correlated with management of the vertebrobasilar occlusive disease.

Intracranial Aneurysm with Carotid Stenosis

Severe internal carotid artery stenosis may be found in association with an intracranial aneurysm on the ipsilateral intracranial circulation (85). In patients with TIAs it is presumed that the stenosis is the cause of the symptoms, and relief of symptoms has usually followed endarterectomy. It is recognized, however, that an aneurysm can be the source of an embolus that causes the transient attack. Occasionally, asymptomatic carotid stenosis is found in a patient being studied for subarachnoid hemorrhage.

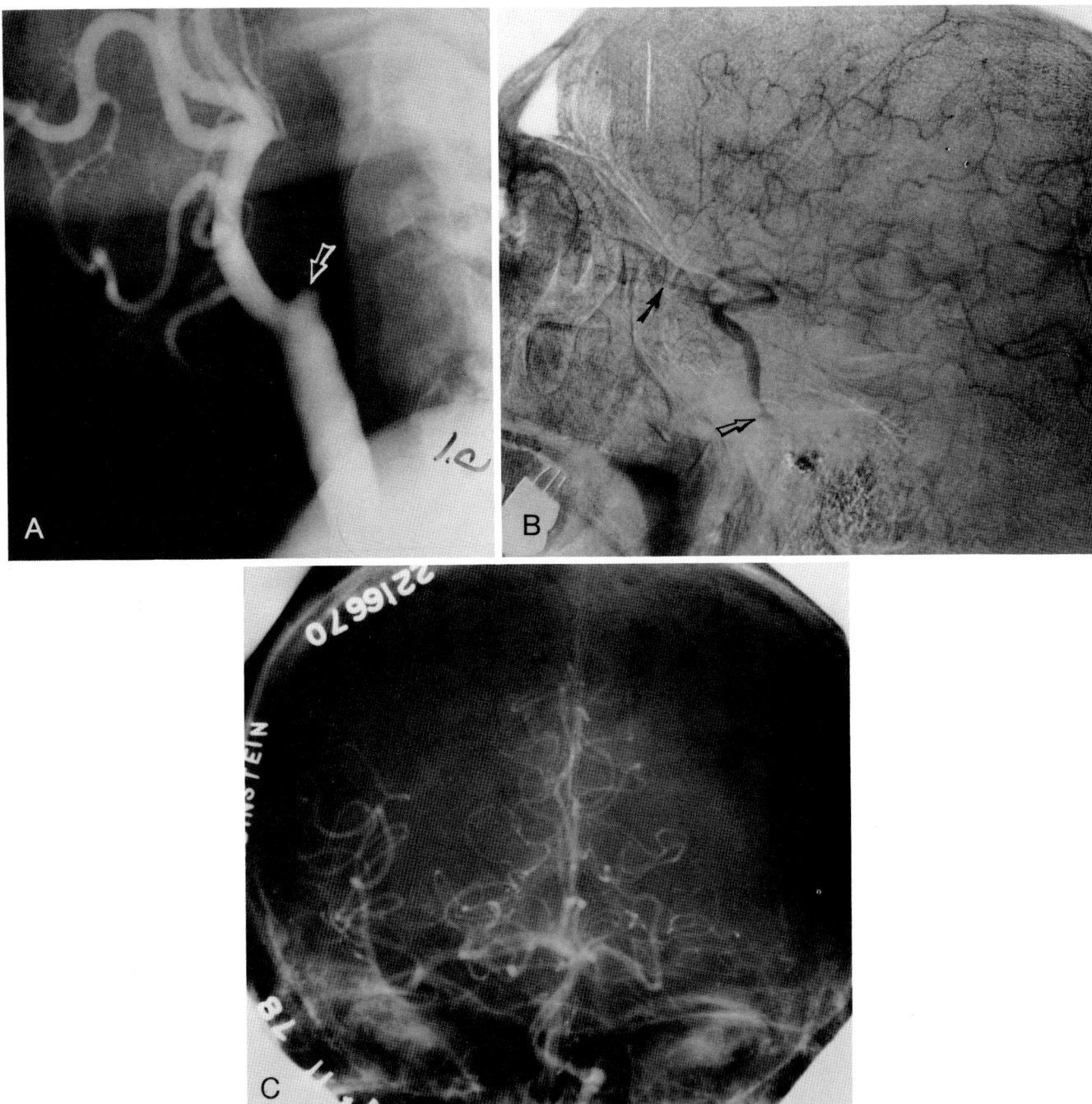

Figure 1.20. Reopening an internal carotid artery occlusion. **A**, Complete occlusion of right internal carotid artery (*arrow*). **B**, Subtraction lateral view several seconds after injection showing collateral flow through the ophthalmic artery (*solid arrow*) into the internal carotid artery with retrograde flow toward the base of the skull (*open arrow*). This finding means that there is a good chance of reopening the artery. **C**, Good collateral flow into the right middle and anterior cerebral arteries from the vertebral injection. This collateral circulation does not protect the patient from possible serious neurologic deficits due to emboli. Comment: Patient presented with right cerebral TIA. Carotid endarterectomy restored right internal carotid artery flow; no TIAs occurred after operation.

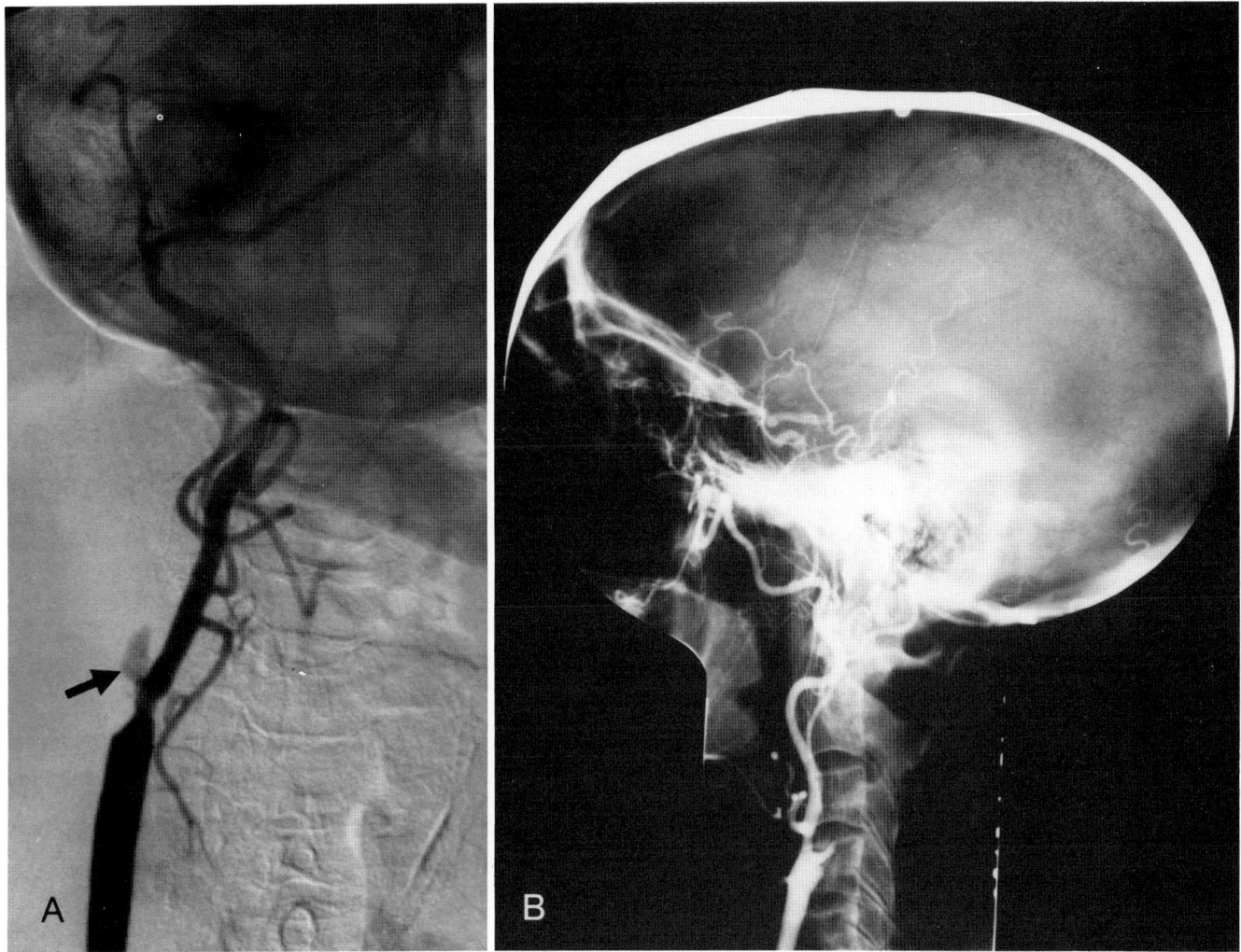

Figure 1.21. Proximal internal carotid artery stump as a source of embolism. **A**, There is no characteristic angiographic appearance of such a stump, but a long irregular pouch is suspicious (*arrow*). **B**, A long stump is present and there is collateral flow through the ophthalmic artery into the intracranial internal carotid artery. In both patients a thrombus was found in the stump and TIAs ceased after operation.

A review of 20 patients (from one institution) with extracranial stenosis and intracranial aneurysm revealed that 15 had TIAs and an incidental aneurysm and five presented with symptoms referable to the aneurysm and were found to have asymptomatic carotid stenosis (107). It was concluded that there was no additional risk in performing carotid endarterectomy in patients with asymptomatic aneurysm. However, there was considerable risk when endarterectomy was performed after subarachnoid hemorrhage, and it was recommended that the aneurysm be treated before the endarterectomy is performed in these patients. In another report there were no complications in treating 19 patients with carotid stenosis and asymptomatic aneurysm (68).

The authors' experience in a smaller series substantiates the conclusion that carotid endarterectomy can be performed safely in a patient with an asymptomatic aneurysm. Intraoperative hypertension is avoided and a shunt used if necessary, with temporary heparinization during cross-clamping. A decision regarding treatment of the asymptomatic stenosis is based on guidelines discussed in Chapter 19. When there is subarachnoid hemorrhage, priority must be given to treating the aneurysm. A decision regarding treatment of the asymptomatic stenosis is based on guidelines discussed in Chapter 3. On rare occasion both lesions are treated under the same anesthesia (Fig. 1.24).

Transient Ischemic Attacks with Common Carotid Stenosis or Occlusion

Stenosis at the origin of the common carotid artery is rare and is not often a cause of transient ischemic

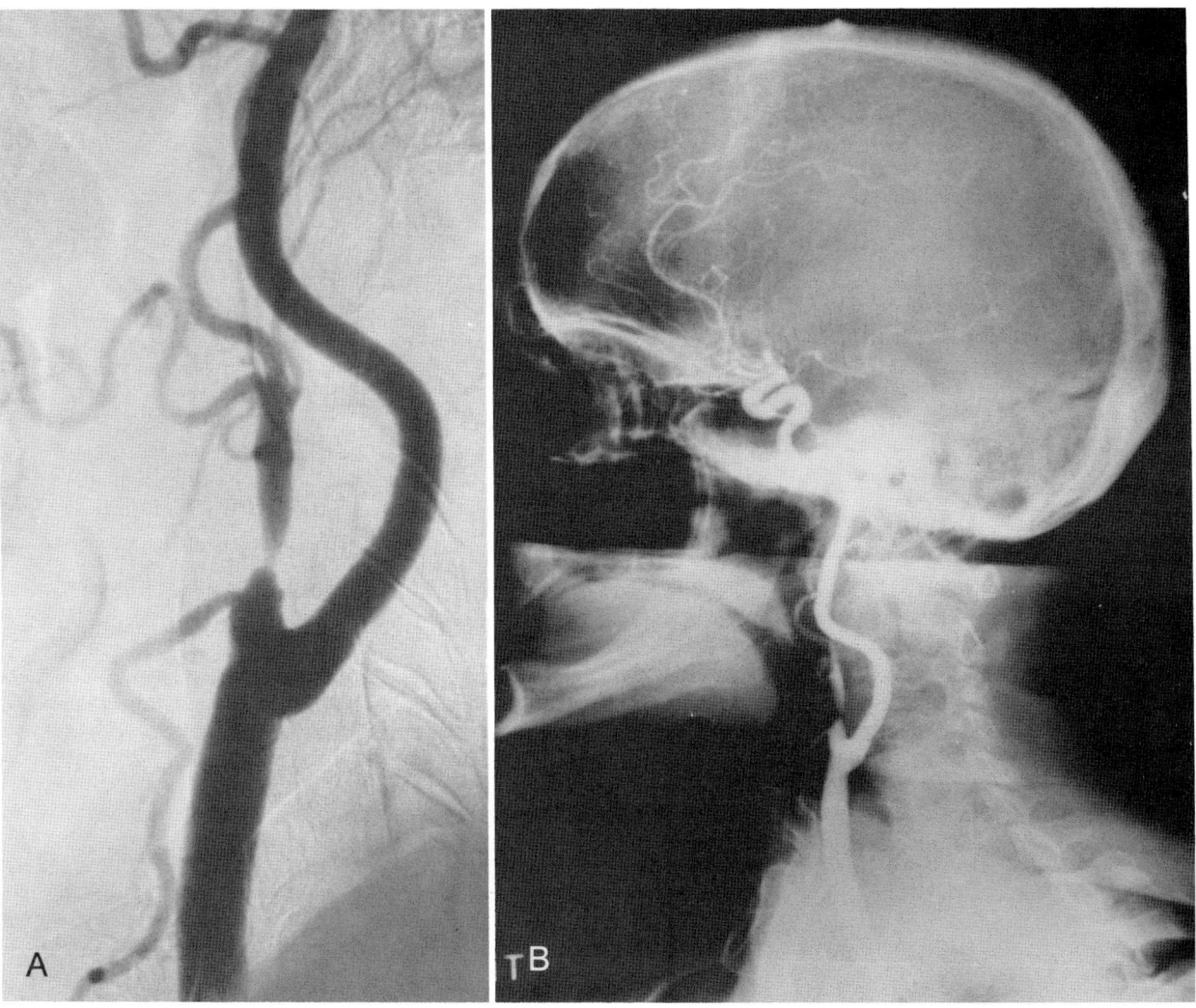

Figure 1.22. TIAs with external carotid stenosis. **A**, Angiogram shows severe stenosis in the proxial external carotid artery. **B**, Marked delayed flow in the external carotid artery and left middle cerebral artery occlusion, thought to be due to embolus, are seen. No other source for embolus was found. At operation an irregular plaque with mural thrombus was removed.

attacks. More frequently the distal common carotid artery is involved at the bifurcation (Fig. 1.5A). Occasionally, significant stenosis may involve the midportion of the common carotid artery (Fig. 1.25). Occlusion of the common carotid artery may be due to retrograde thrombosis superimposed on the atherosclerosis at the carotid bifurcation or antegrade thrombosis from atherosclerosis at the origin of the artery from the aortic arch. Radiographic evaluation requires the assessment of the patency of the internal carotid artery. This is best seen by delayed films following vertebral or contralateral carotid injection, which may fill the internal carotid artery by retrograde collateral flow into the external carotid system (Fig. 1.26). This determination of patency of the distal internal carotid artery in the neck is essential in planning an operative approach. A reconstructive procedure to restore antegrade flow to the internal carotid artery is almost always possible when the internal carotid artery is patent.

In a review of 12 patients with angiographic demonstration of common carotid occlusion, it was found that only three had hemispheric TIAs, one had a hemispheric stroke, five had vertebrobasilar TIAs, and three were completely asymptomatic (96). There were often multiple vessels involved. In six of nine patients explored, both the external and internal carotid arteries were found to be open.

The indication for surgery is continuation of symptoms in spite of medical therapy. The operative technique is discussed in Chapter 2.

Completed Stroke

Evaluation of patients who have had a stroke and have a neurologic deficit will lead to the finding of

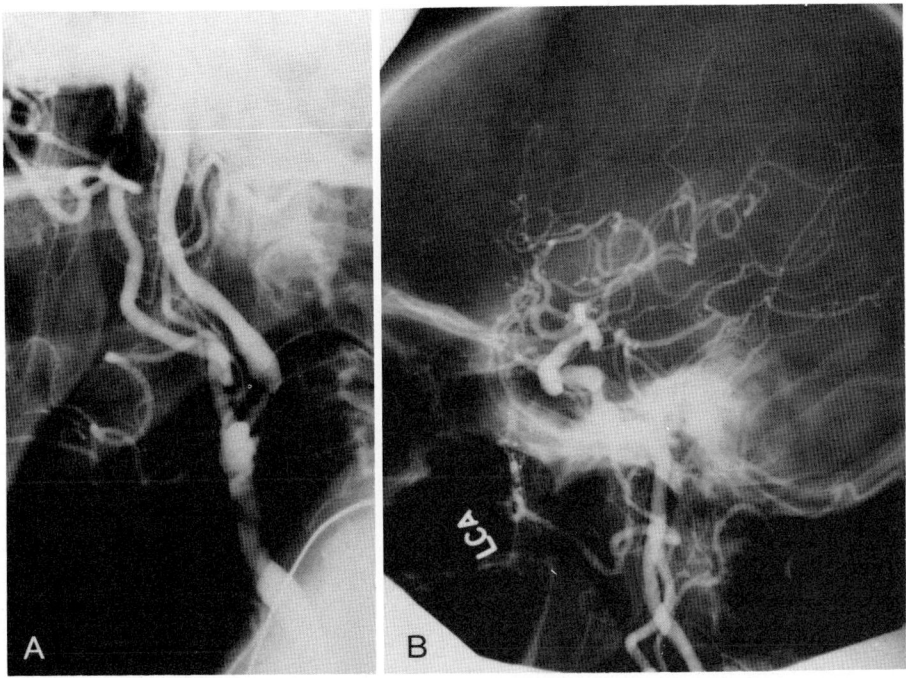

Figure 1.23. Carotid stenosis and vertebrobasilar TIAs. **A,** Lateral angiogram of neck showing severe stenosis at the origin of the left internal carotid artery, as well as some disease in the common carotid artery. **B,** Lateral angiogram of head showing filling of posterior cerebral and basilar arteries from the carotid circulation. Other films showed occlusion of both vertebral arteries. Comment: Patient presented with TIAs related to both the left middle cerebral and vertebrobasilar circulation. Carotid endarterectomy was done with a shunt. There were no further attacks.

carotid artery disease in a significant number. Often, carotid occlusive disease is suggested by the history. In a group of patients whom the authors treated who had suffered a stroke and were found to have carotid disease, more than half had a prior history of TIAs due to carotid stenosis that had not brought the patient to medical attention (30). In a group of 29 patients with a persistent neurologic deficit following carotid occlusion, 60% had a prior history of TIAs, 20% were associated with a fluctuating or stepwise deficit, and 20% developed deficits suddenly without warning (44).

In the past a patient with a stroke and mild or moderate neurologic deficit lasting longer than 24 hours was usually thought to have had an infarction and was often followed for several weeks before considering angiography and surgery. However, these patients are at risk for a second stroke. In one study, four of 19 patients (21%) suffered a second stroke during the 4–6-week waiting period (37). Because of this risk and to help establish a definitive diagnosis, all of these patients should have a high resolution CT scan. In the same study referred to above, 171 of 245 patients (70%) with mild or moderate neurologic deficit lasting longer than 24 hours were found to have a negative CT scan, and 64% had carotid lesions on angiography (37). When the CT scan does not show infarction, the neurologic deficit is not severe, and the patient's level of consciousness is normal, angiography and surgery should be considered without delay. When there is an area of infarction on the CT scan, angiography and surgery may be delayed unless noninvasive carotid studies suggest a critical stenosis.

How long one should delay has not been established. Some have advocated waiting several weeks to reduce the possible chance of postoperative brain hemorrhage (22). If the neurologic deficit is mild, the authors would operate within a few days. If the deficit is moderate to severe, the patient will usually have CT evidence of an infarct. In this circumstance, the authors would wait 2–4 weeks to allow maximum recovery. Surgery can then be done safely as long as there is careful control of postoperative blood pressure.

The long-term natural history of patients with a permanent neurologic deficit has not been well defined. However, one study found a significant incidence of recurrent deficits over a 6-year period (71). It is likely that some of these deficits could have been prevented by carotid endarterectomy. The angiographic indications for surgery are the same as outlined for TIAs: a severe stenosis with residual lumen of 1.5 or less, deep ulceration, and in some patients, complete occlusion. The risk of carotid endarterectomy when the CT scan does not show infarction is

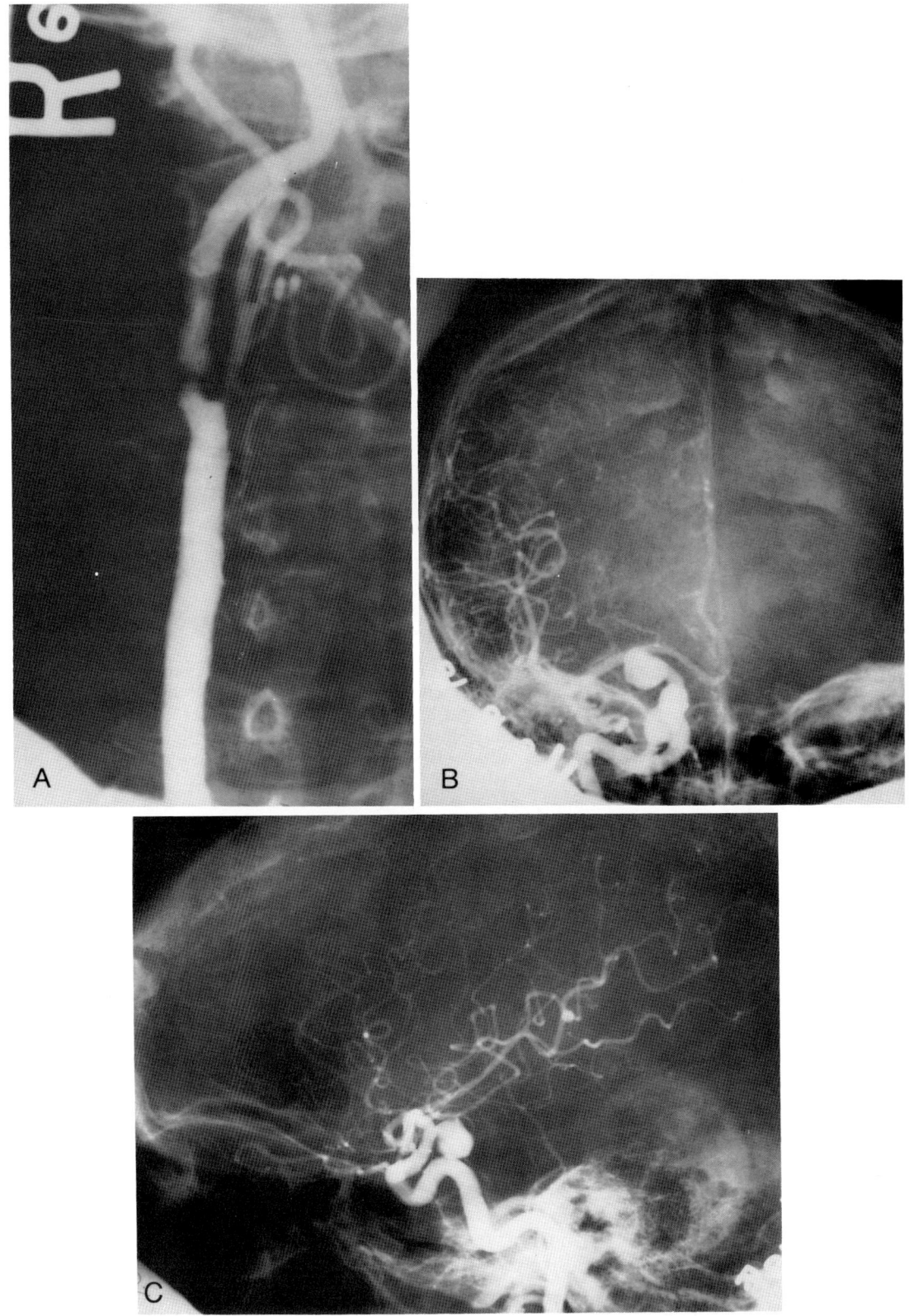

Figure 1.24. Intracranial aneurysm with carotid stenosis. **A**, Right carotid angiogram showing severe stenosis at the origin of the internal carotid artery. **B** and **C**, Anteroposterior and lateral angiograms of the head revealing a large internal carotid-posterior communicating artery aneurysm. Comment: This patient presented with TIAs. Her neurologic examination was normal. There had been no symptoms referable to the aneurysm. She was treated with carotid endarterectomy and intracranial microsurgical occlusion of the aneurysm under the same anesthesia.

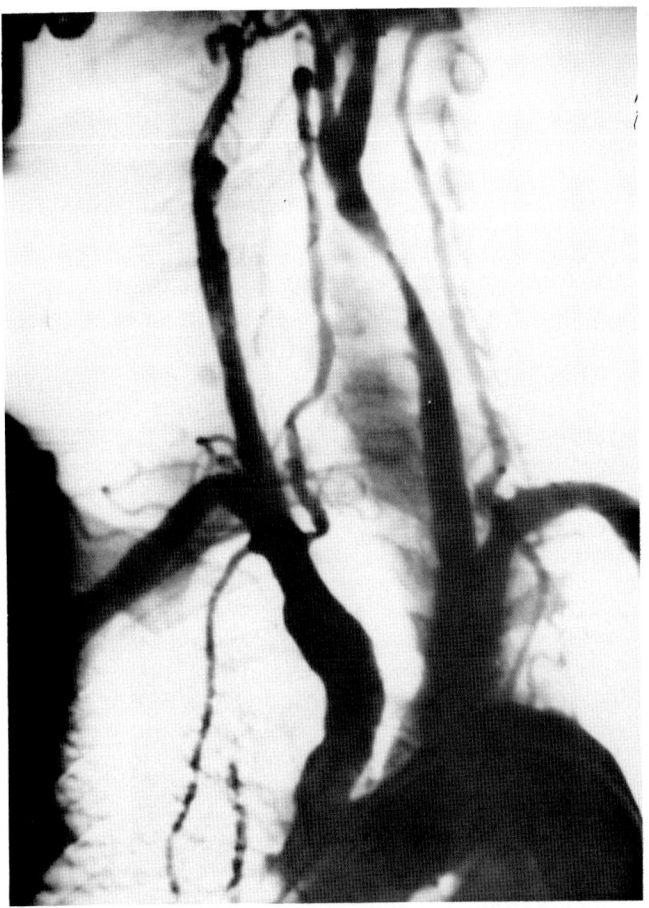

Figure 1.25. Stenosis of common carotid artery. Arch angiogram. Subtraction study showing stenosis in the common carotid artery. The patient had TIAs, which ceased after operation.

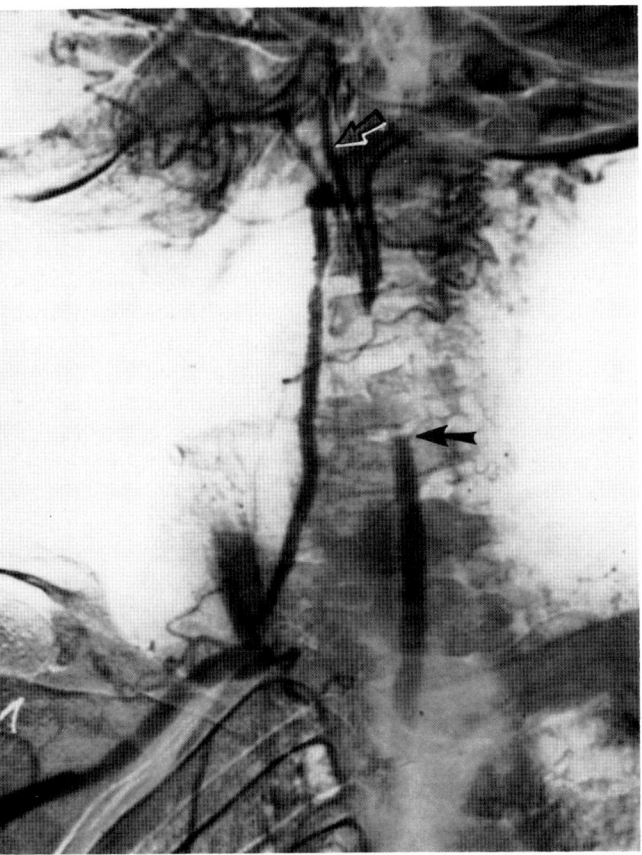

Figure 1.26. Common carotid artery occlusion. Right innominate artery injection. The subtraction study shows complete occlusion of the distal common carotid artery (*solid arrow*) with reconstitution of the internal carotid artery (*open arrow*) from the external carotid artery branches via thyrocervical and vertebral artery collateral flow. Comment: Operation revealed atherosclerosis at the carotid bifurcation with thrombosis. Flow was restored following surgery.

no higher than that for patients with TIAs (37). However, when there has been an infarction the operative risk is somewhat higher (7, 31, 53, 54, 59).

If the patient has had a massive stroke with a severe fixed deficit, evaluation may be limited to a CT scan. These patients cannot be helped by carotid endarterectomy. Angiography is done if significant improvement occurs.

Two types of patients with multiple neck vessel occlusions are rarely encountered. In one there will be a reduction in memory and mental capabilities that improves after carotid endarterectomy (62), and in the other there is a slowly progressive neurologic deficit with no evidence of a mass lesion on CT scan (98, 112). Both are thought to be due to chronic cerebral ischemia due to low cerebral blood flow. Hypoperfusion can be documented with cerebral blood flow measurements with xenon washout.

Acute Stroke and Indications for Emergency Carotid Endarterectomy

Laboratory investigations using different animal models of temporary middle cerebral artery occlusion have provided a rationale for considering emergency revascularization (32, 63, 74, 79, 110). These studies have shown that several hours of reduced cerebral blood flow can be tolerated without permanent infarction and that variations in the time of tolerated ischemia depend to a great extent on collateral circulation.

The natural history of patients with acute stroke and/or angiographic findings who might be considered for emergency carotid endarterectomy is hard to define. In addition to collateral circulation the prognosis is influenced by systemic factors that influence the cerebral circulation.

Many clinicians have concluded that a patient with an acute ischemic stroke should be treated symptomatically and no attempt made to establish a diagnosis in the acute phases of the illness because of the concern of increased morbidity with angiography and surgery. However, some patients will have unstable neurologic syndromes of mild to moderate degree that may progress to a severe disability without treatment. For such problems, the authors believe a diagnosis should be established at the time of admission, using whatever tests are indicated, and then a rational program of treatment instituted (85). In addition, some stable patients have a worrisome angiographic finding and should be considered for emergency surgery. Other centers have reported encouraging results in the surgical treatment of selected acute stroke patients (34, 36, 51, 52, 73, 74, 80, 95, 109).

A careful history and examination will lead to the correct diagnosis in a high percentage of patients. Almost every patient admitted with an acute stroke problem should have an electrocardiogram and immediate CT scan to differentiate between infarction and hemorrhage (17). Laboratory tests should include blood count, blood chemistries, and coagulation studies.

If the history and/or findings suggest carotid disease, then immediate angiography should be done. This is especially important if the patient has had increasing TIAs in preceding days (crescendo TIAs), or the sudden onset of a mild to moderate neurologic deficit with or without prior TIAs, or has a progressive or fluctuating deficit. TIAs which last more than 1 hour or TIAs involving face, arm, and leg are particularly worrisome and should be promptly investigated.

During the period of initial evaluation the patient may be helped by medical therapy. Clinical studies have shown that in patients with acute ischemia of less than 48 hours' duration hemodilution has been of value (108). Infusion of serum albumin is adjusted to keep the hematocrit between 30–35% and maintain the central venous pressure between 8–12 cm H_2O (122).

Emergency carotid endarterectomy is considered for two general categories of patients: (a) those patients with an acute neurologic deficit and angiographic findings of severe stenosis with delay in flow, stenosis with presumed thrombus in the lumen, or internal carotid artery occlusion, especially if there is reflux to the intrapetrous segment of the internal carotid artery; (b) those patients undergoing scheduled angiography for evaluation of a cerebrovascular problem who are found to have one of the above angiographic findings.

The authors' experience with emergency carotid endarterectomy has been summarized (84, 85, 118). The most recent summary included 64 patients not previously reported (118). They attempted to classify the patients into categories of TIAs, stroke in evolution, and acute stroke. However, in many patients with acute neurologic deficits it was difficult to determine from the history whether the deficit was stable, progressive, or fluctuating because the time interval between onset and treatment did not allow this assessment. Therefore, they classified the preoperative neurologic status in terms of the deficits alone as intact, mild, moderate, or severe. Intact patients had a history of TIAs. Mild deficits were those that caused only slight impairment of normal activity. Moderate deficits significantly impaired the patients' function but would allow them to perform activities of daily living. Severe deficits were associated with a major loss of neurologic function that would significantly impair daily activities.

The overall results at the time of discharge are recorded in Table 1.1. Patients were the same or improved following surgery in 92% who were intact or had a mild preoperative deficit, 80% who had a moderate deficit, and 77% who had a severe deficit. In the four deaths, two could be attributed to cardiac causes and two to complications of an unrelated disease process. Six patients developed their acute deficit in relationship to angiography: all four with a severe deficit improved to moderate disability, one of the others had a moderate deficit with improvement, and the other died.

Twelve patients were intact prior to operation and all had TIAs. The reason for the operation was a severe stenosis and marked delay in flow in 10 (Fig. 1.27), one of whom was having TIAs on heparin; stenosis with a filling deficit in the lumen in one who had crescendo TIAs on heparin; and a 1.5-mm stenosis with the opposite internal carotid artery occluded in another. Eleven patients were intact at discharge. The one patient with crescendo TIAs had a moderate deficit, and the postoperative angiogram did not disclose a cause.

Twenty-four patients had a mild acute persistent deficit, often with a history of TIAs. In 19 the primary indication for surgery was the angiographic finding: severe stenosis and marked delay in flow in 10, se-

Table 1.1.
Results of Emergency Carotid Endarterectomy

Preoperative Deficit[a]	Status at Discharge				Total
	Improved	Same	Worse	Dead	
Intact	0	11	1	0	12
Mild	15	7	2	0	24
Moderate	11	1	2	1	15
Severe (alert)	6	1	0	3	10
Severe (not alert)	3	0	0	0	3
Total	35 (55%)	20 (31%)	5 (8%)	4 (6%)	64

[a]See text for definitions of deficits.

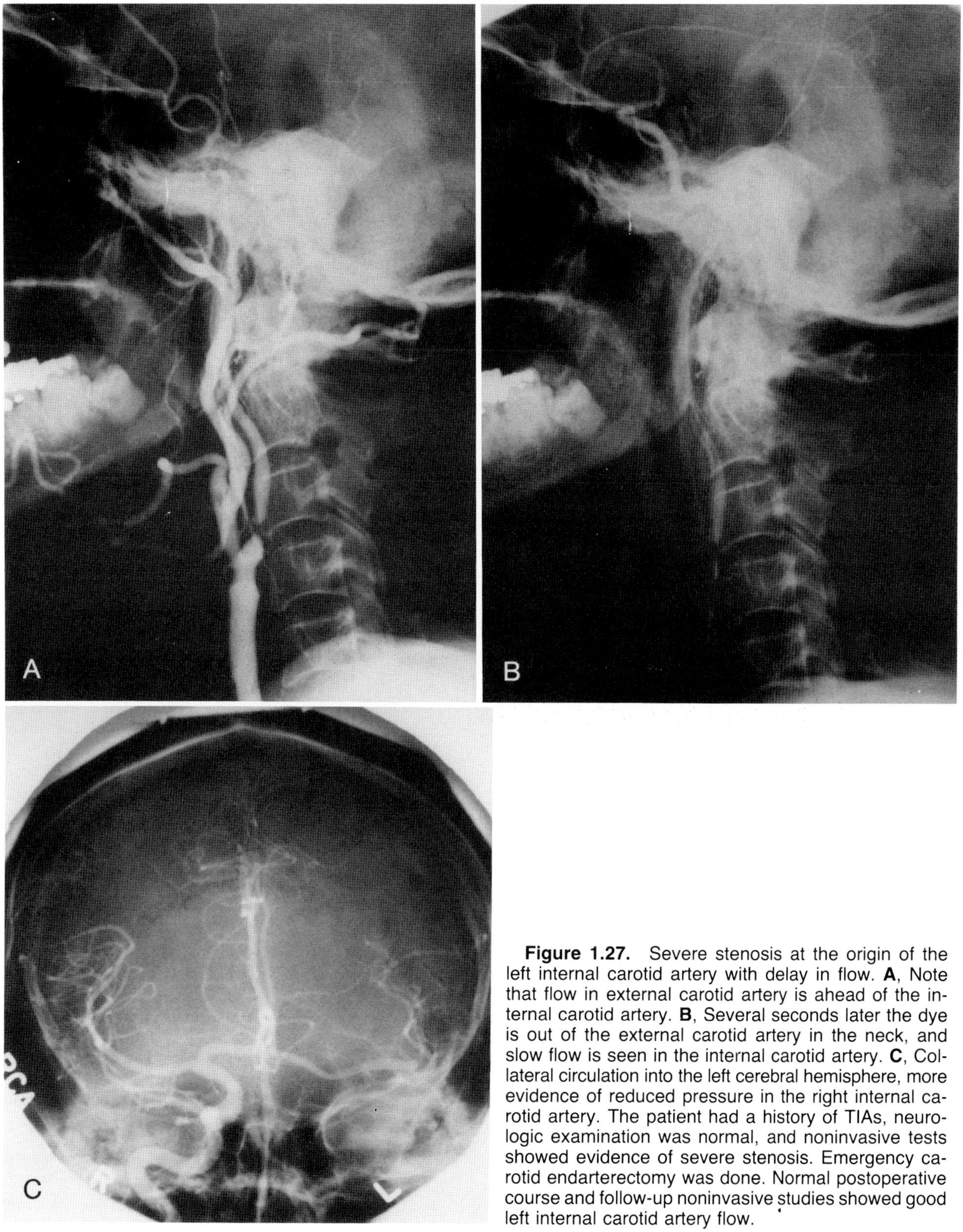

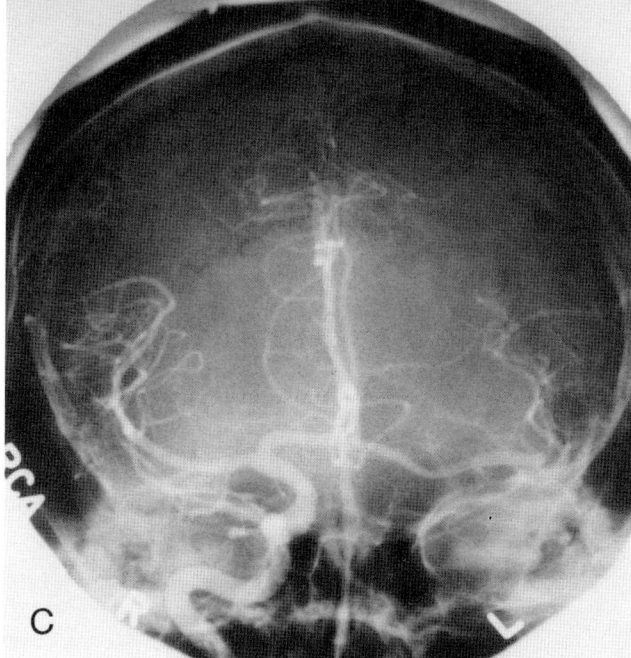

Figure 1.27. Severe stenosis at the origin of the left internal carotid artery with delay in flow. **A**, Note that flow in external carotid artery is ahead of the internal carotid artery. **B**, Several seconds later the dye is out of the external carotid artery in the neck, and slow flow is seen in the internal carotid artery. **C**, Collateral circulation into the left cerebral hemisphere, more evidence of reduced pressure in the right internal carotid artery. The patient had a history of TIAs, neurologic examination was normal, and noninvasive tests showed evidence of severe stenosis. Emergency carotid endarterectomy was done. Normal postoperative course and follow-up noninvasive studies showed good left internal carotid artery flow.

vere stenosis and intraluminal filling defect in five, and complete internal carotid artery occlusion in four. In the other five the indications for surgery were fluctuating deficit on heparin in two (Fig. 1.28), an acute deficit associated with moderate stenosis in two, and a severely ulcerated plaque in one. At discharge 15 were improved, five of whom were intact, seven were the same, and two were worse (one had a slight increase in a mild deficit and one a moderate deficit associated with postoperative hypotension).

Fifteen patients had a moderate deficit preoperatively. Thirteen had the onset outside the hospital, and two became worse during or shortly after the angiogram. The indication for surgery was the neurologic deficit and angiographic finding. At discharge 11 were improved, two of whom were intact, one was the same, two were worse, and one died of myocardial infarction.

Thirteen patients had a severe deficit. Only three were not alert, and all of these developed the deficit in relationship to angiography. The absence of other patients in the series who were drowsy reflects the authors' previously published policy regarding such patients (84). In the group of 10 patients who were alert, two had the sudden onset of a severe neurologic deficit with loss of carotid bruit while in the hospital and both made a full recovery. Five patients had the sudden onset of the deficit outside the hospital. Three remained with severe but improved deficits, and two died—one from complications of ulcerative colitis and the other from myocardial infarction. Three other patients had the onset in the hospital—one after angiography, one (who subsequently died from an acute abdomen) after urologic surgery, and one while awaiting evaluation.

The results of emergency endarterectomy can also be analyzed in relationship to the angiographic findings (Tables 1.2–1.5). Table 1.2 shows that 25 of 27 patients with severe stenosis, often with delay in flow, were intact or had a mild to moderate deficit. In these patients the primary indication for surgery was usually concern that the patient would develop a more severe deficit from progression of the stenosis to occlusion. No patient in this group died, and 25 of the 27 were the same or improved after surgery. Table 1.3 shows the results in patients in whom the indication for emergency endarterectomy was the finding of an intraluminal filling defect at angiog-

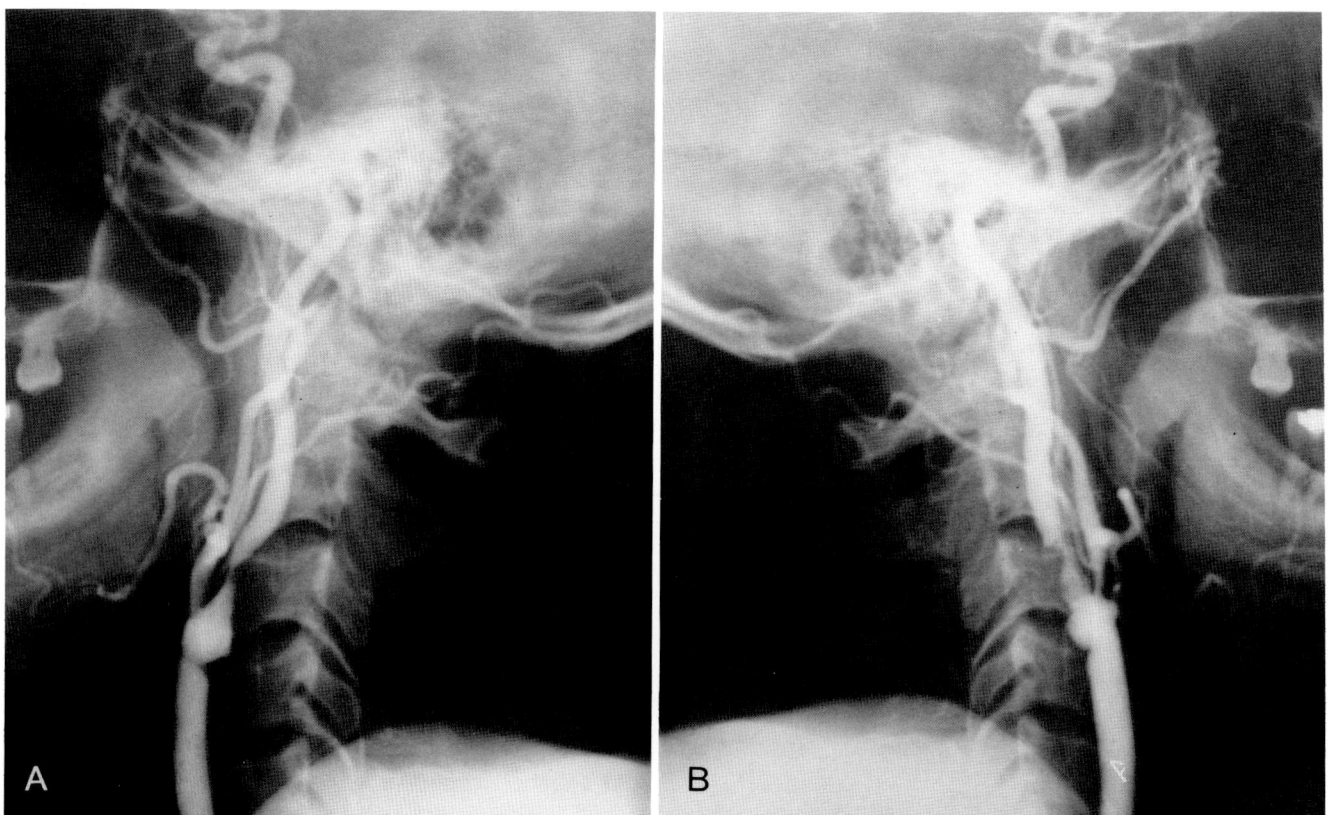

Figure 1.28. TIAs and fluctuating deficit on heparin. **A**, Right carotid angiogram showing severe stenosis in the proximal internal carotid artery. **B**, Left carotid angiogram showing a stenosis that is not quite as severe as on the right. Patient presented with TIAs and fluctuating deficit in the left hand. Emergency right carotid endarterectomy was followed by full recovery. The left side was operated electively a few weeks later.

Table 1.2.
Severe Stenosis with Delay in Flow

Preoperative Deficit	Status at Discharge				Total
	Improved	Same	Worse	Dead	
Intact	0	9	0	0	9
Mild	6	3	1	0	10
Moderate	5	0	1	0	6
Severe (alert)	1	0	0	0	1
Severe (not alert)	1	0	0	0	1
Total	13 (49%)	12 (44%)	2 (7%)	0	27

Table 1.3.
Stenosis with Intraluminal Filling Defect

Preoperative Deficit	Status at Discharge				Total
	Improved	Same	Worse	Dead	
Intact	0	0	1	0	1
Mild	4	1	0	0	5
Moderate	3	0	0	1	4
Severe	0	0	0	1	1
Total	7 (64%)	1 (9%)	1 (9%)	2 (18%)	11

Table 1.4.
Complete Occlusion

Preoperative Deficit	Status at Discharge				Total
	Improved	Same	Worse	Dead	
Mild	1	3	0	0	4
Moderate	2	1	1	0	4
Severe (alert)	4	1	0	1	6
Severe (not alert)	2	0	0	0	2
Total	9 (57%)	5 (31%)	1 (6%)	1 (6%)	16

Table 1.5.
Moderate to Severe Stenosis and/or Severe Ulceration

Preoperative Deficit	Status at Discharge				Total
	Improved	Same	Worse	Dead	
Intact	0	2	0	0	2
Mild	4	0	1	0	5
Moderate	1	0	0	0	1
Severe (alert)	1	0	0	1	2
Total	6 (60%)	2 (20%)	1 (10%)	1 (10%)	10

raphy. Only six of these patients were found at surgery to have an intraluminal clot (Fig. 1.29); in the rest the defect was due to atheromatous material (Fig. 1.30). In this group, nine improved or were unchanged and two died—one due to complications following intraoperative myocardial infarction and one following emergency colectomy. Table 1.4 gives the results in all patients operated with an acute complete occlusion. In a few cases the finding proved to be a pseudo-occlusion (94). Flow through the internal carotid artery was established by endarterectomy in all cases. In this group 14 of 16 were unchanged or improved by surgery, one was worse, and one died from a cardiopulmonary arrest on postoperative day 24.

There were nine patients with moderate to severe stenosis without delay in flow and one patient with a severely ulcerated plaque who underwent emergency endarterectomy because of the onset of an acute fixed or fluctuating neurologic deficit or because of persistence of TIAs in spite of adequate heparinization (Table 1.5). There was one death from non-neurologic complications, and eight patients were unchanged or improved.

The proposed indications for emergency carotid endarterectomy are based on the authors' experience and review of the literature. The indications are as follows:

1. Sudden onset of neurologic deficit with loss of carotid bruit—Most of these patients will already be hospitalized. Angiography is not needed. The patient should be taken immediately to the operating room where a complete or nearly complete occlusion is usually found. It is the authors' experience as well as that of others that these patients generally have a good prognosis (36, 74, 80, 118).
2. Sudden onset of a neurologic deficit with occlusion during angiography—Several reports document benefit from emergency operations in these patients when the operation is done within 1–2 hours of the occlusion unless there has been an associated middle cerebral artery embolus (31, 80, 84, 110).
3. The presence of TIAs or an acute spontaneous, neurologic deficit that is apparently stable, progressing, or fluctuating with one of the following angiographic findings:
   a. Severe stenosis in the proximal internal carotid artery with marked delay in flow;
   b. Stenosis in the proximal internal carotid artery with an intraluminal thrombus;
   c. Complete occlusion of the internal carotid artery.

Patients with TIAs may need emergency surgery based on the severity of the angiographic finding or on the clinical situation of recurrence of TIAs while on heparin, or crescendo TIAs, and the finding of a significant stenosis (41, 51, 52, 73, 84, 95).

Patients with an acute mild or moderate stable deficit are usually considered for emergency carotid endarterectomy because of the angiographic indication since their overall prognosis is good. When there is severe stenosis at the internal carotid artery origin and marked delay in flow, the patients are at signif-

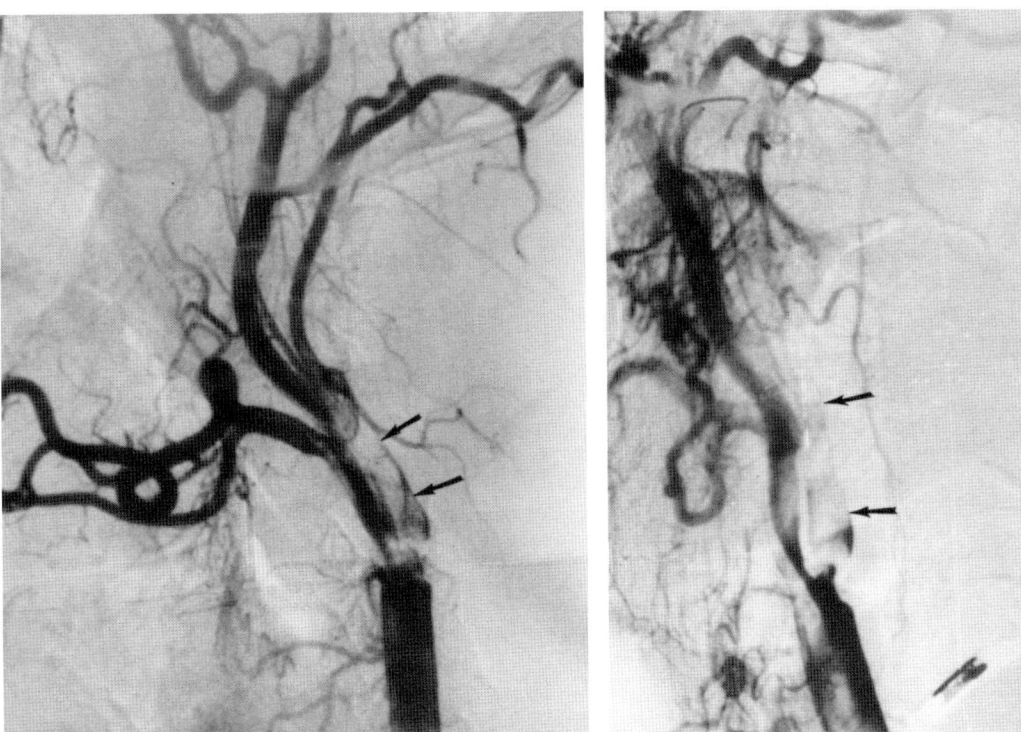

Figure 1.29. Typical angiographic appearance of large intraluminal thrombus in the internal carotid artery with dye streaking around the sides of the clot (*arrows*). At operation a severe stenosis was present at the origin of the internal carotid artery and a large thrombus was removed with excellent backflow from the distal internal carotid artery.

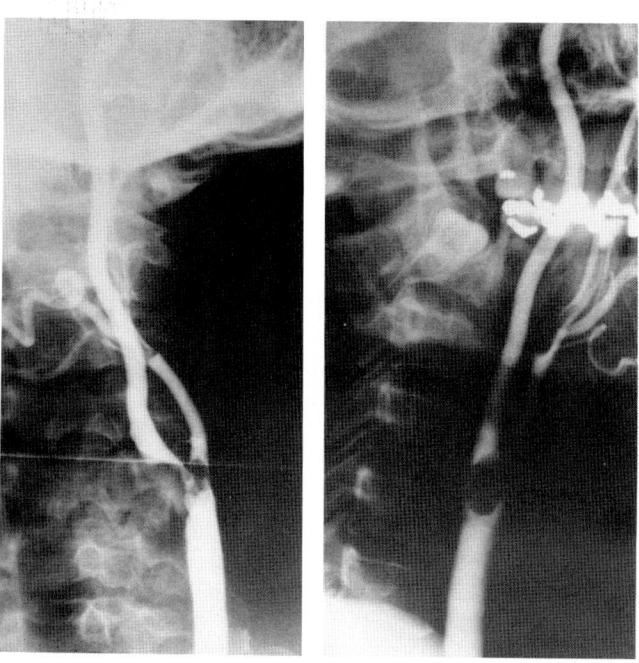

Figure 1.30. Angiographic picture of an intraluminal filling defect that proved to be atheromatous debris rather than a thrombus. Emergency carotid endarterectomy was followed by an uncomplicated course.

icant risk for further ischemia. Some have recommended that surgery be delayed for up to 4–6 weeks in patients with mild to moderate fixed deficits. However, in one study it was found that during this waiting period there was a 21% incidence of recurrent stroke (37). It was recommended that these patients have a CT scan and if it was normal, which it was in 70% of the patients, that angiography and surgery be done without delay. The results are good in these patients.

The authors' data suggest that those with a mild or moderate deficit and an intraluminal thrombus should also be considered for surgery to prevent neurologic worsening. In a summary of 20 reported patients who had carotid endarterectomy when there was an intraluminal thrombus, there was no postoperative worsening (21). However, this recommendation may need to be modified in light of other reports (12, 89). In a series of eight patients with angiographically demonstrated intraluminal thrombus associated with significant atherosclerosis of the carotid bifurcation, the thrombus resolved with heparin therapy in seven and with aspirin therapy in one (89). There were no new permanent neurologic events while they were undergoing medical therapy, and six patients subsequently had a delayed endarterectomy.

The patient with a severe deficit presents a more difficult challenge. Clearly some patients benefit with dramatic improvement in their deficit, but selection is a problem. The incidence of postoperative intracerebral hemorrhage has been markedly reduced with the careful control of blood pressure. If there is a significantly depressed level of consciousness an infarct has probably already occurred and revascularization will usually not be of benefit and is associated with high morbidity and mortality (34, 55, 85, 95). If the patient with a severe deficit is alert and particularly if there has been a fluctuating or progressive history, emergency operation may be of benefit (34, 51, 52, 73, 84, 95).

The angiographic criteria for suggesting which patients with complete internal carotid artery occlusion have a good chance of reestablishing flow are discussed earlier in this chapter. The authors' previous reports show a good correlation between the ability to reestablish flow and outcome (84). In one report emergency carotid endarterectomy was done in 34 patients already in the hospital who had the onset of acute occlusion and a profound neurologic deficit (74). In this group 13 (38.3%) had a dramatic improvement with nine making an essentially full recovery. The mortality was 20%, which is lower than would have been expected. Where documentation was available, the prognosis was worse when collateral flow was poor or there was a middle cerebral embolus.

REFERENCES

1. Ackerman RH: Non-invasive carotid evaluation. Stroke 11:675–678, 1980.
2. Ackerman RH: Clinical evaluation of cerebrovascular physiology. In Fein JM, Flamm ES (eds): *Cerebrovascular Surgery.* New York, Springer-Verlag, 1985, vol 1, pp 181–211.
3. Ahn HS, Rosenbaum AE, Allen GS, Prezios TJ, Shilliton JS, Heros RC, Baker RA: Occluded but non-thrombosed internal carotid artery: An indication for endarterectomy. AJNR 4:286–288, 1983.
4. Alvarez O, Edwards JH, Hyman RA: MR recognition of internal carotid artery occlusion. AJNR 7:356–361, 1986.
5. Baker WH, Littooy FN, Hayes AC, Dorner DB, Stubbs D: Carotid endarterectomy without a shunt. The control series. J Vasc Surg 1:50–56, 1984.
6. Ball JB Jr, Lukin RR, Tomsick TA, Chambers AA: Complications of intravenous digital subtraction angiography. Arch Neurol 42: 969–972, 1985.
7. Bardin JA, Bernstein EF, Humber PB, Collins GM, Dilley RB, Devin JB, Stuart SH: Is carotid endarterectomy beneficial in prevention of recurrent stroke? Arch Surg 117:1401–1407, 1982.
8. Barnett HJM: The pathophysiology of transient cerebral ischemic attacks. Med Clin North Am 63:649–680, 1979.
9. Barnett HJM, Peerless SJ, Kaufmann JCE: "Stump" of internal carotid artery: A source for further cerebral embolic ischemia. Stroke 9:448–456, 1978.
10. Barnett HJM, Peerless SJ, Sutherland GR: The stump syndrome. In Smith RR (ed): *Stroke and the Extracranial Vessels.* New York, Raven Press, 1984, pp 219–225.
11. Bernstein EF, Humber PB, Collins GM, Dilley RB, Devin JB, Stuart SH: Life expectancy and late stroke following carotid endarterectomy. Ann Surg 198:80–86, 1983.
12. Biller J, Adams HP, Boarini D, Godersky JC, Smokey WRK, Kongable G: Intraluminal clot of the carotid artery. Surg Neurol 25:467–477, 1986.
13. Bland JE, Lazar ML: Carotid endarterectomy without shunt. Neurosurgery 8:153–157, 1981.
14. Bogousslavsky J, Regli F: Vertebrobasilar transient ischemic attacks in internal carotid artery occlusion or tight stenosis. Arch Neurol 42:64–68, 1985.
15. Bogousslavsky J, Regli F, Hungerbuhler JP, Chrzanowski R: Transient ischemic attacks and external carotid artery. Stroke 12:627–630, 1981.
16. Britton M: Progression of stroke after arrival at hospital. Stroke 16:629–632, 1985.
17. Buonanno F, Toole JF: Management of patients with established ("completed") cerebral infarction. Stroke 12:7–16, 1981.
18. Buonanno FS, Fossel ET, Kistler JP: Nuclear magnetic resonance in stroke. In Barnett HJM, Mohr JP, Stein BM, Yatsu FM (eds): *Stroke.* New York, Churchill Livingstone, 1986, pp 165–180.
19. Burnbaum MD, Selhorst JB, Harbison JW, Brush JJ: Amaurosis fugax from disease of the external carotid artery. Arch Neurol 34:532–535, 1977.
20. Callow AD: An overview of the stroke problem in the carotid territory. Am J Surg 140:181–191, 1980.
21. Caplan L, Stein R, Patel D, Anmico L, Cashman N, Gewertz B: Intraluminal clot of the carotid artery detached radiographically. Neurology 34:1175–1181, 1984.
22. Caplan LR, Skillman J, Ojemann R, Fields WS: Intracerebral hemorrhage following carotid endarterectomy: A hypertensive complication? Stroke 9:457–460, 1978.
23. Carter JE: Chronic ocular ischemia and carotid vascular disease. Stroke 16:721–728, 1985.
24. Countee RW, Vijayanathan T: External carotid artery in internal carotid artery occlusion. Angiographic, therapeutic and prognostic considerations. Stroke 10:450–460, 1979.
25. Countee RW, Vijayanathan T, Chavis P: Recurrent retinal ischemia beyond cervical carotid occlusions. J Neurosurg 55:532–542, 1981.
26. Countee RW, Vijayanathan T, Wa SZ: External carotid occlusion as a cause of recurrent ischemia after carotid endarterectomy. Neurosurgery 11:518–521, 1982.
27. Craig DR, Maguro K, Watridge C, Roberston JT, Barnett HJM, Fox AJ: Intracranial internal carotid artery stenosis. Stroke 13:823–828, 1982.
28. Crew JR, Dean M, Johnson JM, Knighton D, Bashour TT, Ellertson D, Hassa ES: Carotid surgery without angiography. Am J Surg 148:217–220, 1984.
29. Crowell RM, Kistler JP, Ojemann RG, Thompson RA: Non-invasive techniques in cerebrovascular disease. Clin Neurosurg 29:489–510, 1982.
30. Crowell RM, Ojemann RG: Extracranial cerebrovascular disease. In Hoff JT (ed): *Practice of Surgery.* Philadelphia, Harper and Row, 1981, chap 28.
31. Crowell RM, Ojemann RG: Results and complications of carotid endarterectomy. In Smith RR (ed): *Stroke and the Extracranial Vessels.* New York, Raven Press, 1984, pp 203–211.
32. Crowell RM, Olsson Y, Klatzo I, Ommaya A: Temporary occlusion of the middle cerebral artery in the monkey: Clinical and pathological observations. Stroke 1:439–448, 1970.
33. Davis KR, Ackerman RH, Kistler JP, Mohr JP: Computed tomography of cerebral infarction: Hemorrhage, contrast enhancement and time of appearance. Comput Tomogr 1:71–86, 1977.
34. DeWeese JA: Management of acute stroke. Surg Clin North Am 62:467–472, 1982.
35. Ditmore QM, Watts C: External carotid endarterectomy. In

Smith RR (ed): *Stroke and the Extracranial Vessels.* New York, Raven Press, 1984, pp 219–225.

36. Donaldson MC, Drezner AD: Surgery for acute carotid occlusion. *Arch Surg* 118:1266–1268, 1983.
37. Dosick JM, Whaler RC, Gale SS, Brown DW: Carotid endarterectomy in the stroke patient—computerized axial tomography to determine timing. *J Vasc Surg* 2:214–219, 1985.
38. Duncan GW, Gruber JO, Dewey CF, Meyers GS, Lees RS: Evaluation of carotid stenosis by phonoangiography. *N Engl J Med* 293:1124–1128, 1975.
39. Easton JD, Sherman DG: Stroke and mortality rate in carotid endarterectomy: 228 consecutive operations. *Stroke* 8:565–568, 1977.
40. Ennix CL Jr, Lawrie GM, Morris GC Jr, Crawford ES, Howell JF, Reardon MJ, Weatherford SC: Improved results of carotid endarterectomy in patients with symptomatic coronary disease: An analysis of 1546 consecutive carotid operations. *Stroke* 10:122–125, 1979.
41. Ferguson GG: Extracranial carotid artery surgery. *Clin Neurosurg* 29:543–574, 1982.
42. Finklestein S, Kleinman GM, Cuneo R, Baringer JR: Delayed stroke following carotid occlusion. *Neurology* 30:84–88, 1980.
43. Fisher CM: Occlusion of the internal carotid artery. *Arch Neurol Psychiatry* 69:346–377, 1951.
44. Fisher CM: Clinical syndromes in cerebral thrombosis, hypertensive hemorrhage, and ruptured saccular aneurysm. *Clin Neurosurg* 22:117–147, 1975.
45. Fisher CM: The natural history of carotid occlusion. In Austin GM (ed): *Microneurosurgical Anastomoses for Cerebral Ischemia.* Springfield, IL, Charles C Thomas, 1976, pp 194–201.
46. Fisher CM: Discussion at Princeton Conference, 1976. In Schemberg P (ed): *Cerebrovascular Disease. X Research (Princeton) Conference.* New York, Raven Press, 1976, pp 50–52.
47. Fisher CM, Dalal PM, Adams RD: Cerebrovascular disease and stroke syndrome. In Harrison TR, Bennett IL Jr, Resnik WH, Thorn GW, Wintrobe MM (eds): *Principles of Internal Medicine.* New York, McGraw-Hill, 1962.
48. Gee W, Oller DW, Wylie EJ: Non-invasive diagnosis of carotid occlusion by ocular pneumoplethysmography. *Stroke* 7:18–21, 1976.
49. Giannotta SL, Dicks RE III, Kindt GW: Carotid endarterectomy: Technical improvements. *Neurosurgery* 7:309–312, 1980.
50. Goldstein SJ, Fried AM, Young B, Tibbs PA. Limited usefulness of aortic arch angiography in the evaluation of carotid occlusive disease. *Neurosci Res* 2:559–564, 1981.
51. Goldstone J, Effeney DJ: The role of carotid endarterectomy in the treatment of acute neurologic deficit. *Prog Cardiovasc Dis* 22:415–422, 1980.
52. Goldstone J, Moore WS: A new look at emergency carotid artery operations for the treatment of cerebrovascular insufficiency: Current concepts of cerebrovascular disease. *Stroke* 9:599–602, 1978.
53. Graber JN, Vollman RW, Johnson WC, Levine H, Butler R, Scott RM, Nabseth DC: Stroke after carotid endarterectomy: Risk as predicted by preoperative computerized tomography. *Am J Surg* 147:492–497, 1984.
54. Green RM, Messick WJ, Ricotta JJ, Charlton MH, Satran R, McBride MM, DeWeese JA: Benefits, shortcomings and costs of EEG monitoring. *Ann Surg* 201:785–792, 1985.
55. Hafner CD, Tew JM: Surgical management of totally occluded internal carotid artery: A ten-year study. *Surgery* 89:710–717, 1981.
56. Harward TR, Kroener JM, Wickbom IG, Bernstein EF: Natural history of asymptomatic ulcerating plagues of the carotid bifurcation. *A J Surg* 146:208–210, 1983.
57. Heros R, Grundy BL: Ischemic cerebrovascular disease. In Katz J, Matjasko J (eds): *Controversy in Neurosurgical Anesthesia.* New York, Academic Press, in press.
58. Hertzer NR, Arison R: Cumulative stroke and survival ten years after carotid endarterectomy. *J Vasc Surg* 2:661–668, 1985.
59. Hertzer NR, Beven EG, Modic MT, O'Hara PJ, Vogt DP, Weinstein MA: Early patency of the carotid artery after endarterectomy: Digital subtraction angiography after two hundred sixty-two operations. *Surgery* 92:1049–1057, 1982.
60. Hodge CJ, Cacayorin AD, Leeson M, Iliya A: CT evaluation of extracranial carotid artery disease. In press.
61. Hugenholtz H, Elgie RG: Carotid thromboendarterectomy: A reappraisal. Criteria for patient selection. *J Neurosurg* 53:776–783, 1980.
62. Jacobs LA, Ganji S, Shirley JG, Morrell RM, Brinkman SD: Cognitive improvement after extracranial reconstruction for the low-flow-endangered brain. *Surgery* 93:683–687, 1983.
63. Jones TH, Morawetz RB, Crowell RM, Marcoux FW, Fitzgibbon SJ, DeGirolami U, Ojemann RG: Threshold of focal cerebral ischemia in awake monkey. *J Neurosurg* 54:773–782, 1981.
64. Kartchner MM, McRae LP: Noninvasive evaluation and management of the "asymptomatic" carotid bruit. *Surgery* 82:840–847, 1977.
65. Kistler JP, Lees RS, Friedman J, Pessin M, Mohr JP, Roberson GS, Ojemann RG: The bruit of carotid stenosis versus radiated basal heart murmurs: Differentiation by phonoangiography. *Circulation* 57:975:981, 1978.
66. Kistler JP, Lees RS, Miller A, Crowell RM, Roberson G: Correlation of spectral phonoangiography and carotid angiography with gross pathology in carotid stenosis. *N Engl J Med* 305:417–419, 1981.
67. Kroener JM, Dorn PL, Shoor PM, Wickbom IG, Bernstein EF: Prognosis of asymptomatic ulcerating carotid lesions. *Arch Surg* 115:1387–1392, 1980.
68. Ladowski JS, Webster MW, Youas HO, Steed DL: Carotid endarterectomy in patients with asymptomatic intracranial aneurysm. *Ann Surg* 200:70–73, 1984.
69. Lees RS, Kistler JP: Non-invasive diagnosis of extracranial cerebrovascular disease. In Barnett HJM, Mohr JP, Stein BM, Yatsu FM (eds): *Stroke.* New York, Churchill Livingstone, 1986, pp 257–268.
70. Lippman HH, Sundt TM Jr, Holman CB: The post stenotic carotid slim sign; spurious internal carotid hypoplasia. *Mayo Clin Proc* 45:762–767, 1970.
71. McCullough JL, Mentzer RM Jr, Harman PK, Kaiser DL, Kron IL, Crosby IK: Carotid endarterectomy after a completed stroke: Reduction in long-term neurologic deterioration. *J Vasc Surg* 2:7–14, 1985.
72. McNamara JO, Heyman A, Silver D, Mandel ME: The value of carotid endarterectomy in treating transient cerebral ischemia of the posterior circulation. *Neurology* 27:682–684, 1977.
73. Mentzer RM Jr, Finkelmeier BA, Crosby IK, Welions HA Jr: Emergency carotid endarterectomy for fluctuating neurologic deficits. *Surgery* 89:60–66, 1981.
74. Meyer FB, Sundt TM Jr, Piepgras DG, Sandok BA, Forbes G: Emergency carotid endarterectomy for patients with acute carotid occlusion and profound neurological deficits. *Ann Surg* 203:82–89, 1986.
75. Mohr JP: Overview of laboratory studies. In Barnett HJM, Mohr JP, Stein BM, Yatsu EM (eds): *Stroke.* New York, Churchill Livingstone, 1986, pp 183–188.
76. Mohr JP, Caplan LR, Milski JM, Goldstein RJ, Duncan GW, Kistler JP, Pessin MS, Bleich HL: The Harvard cooperative stroke registry: A prospective registry. *Neurology* 28:754–762, 1978.
77. Moore DJ, Modi JR, Finch WT, Sumner DS: Influence of the contralateral carotid artery on neurologic complications following carotid endarterectomy. *J Vasc Surg* 1:409–414, 1984.
78. Moore WS: Surgical significance and management of the ulcerated carotid plaque. In Bergan JJ, Yao JT (eds): *Cere-*

brovascular Insufficiency. New York, Grune & Stratton, 1983, pp 199–211.
79. Morawetz RB, DeGirolami U, Ojemann RG, Marcon FEW, Crowell RM: Cerebral blood flow determined by hydrogen clearance during middle cerebral artery occlusion in unanesthetized monkeys. Stroke 9:143–149, 1978.
80. Najafi H, Javid H, Dye WS, Hunter JA, Wideman FE, Julian OC: Emergency carotid thromboendarterectomy. Arch Surg 103:610–613, 1971.
81. Norrving B, Nilsson E, Olsson JE: Progression of carotid disease after endarterectomy: A Doppler ultrasound study. Ann Neurol 12:548–552, 1982.
82. O'Hara PJ, Hertzer NR, Beven EG: External carotid revascularization: Review of a ten-year experience. J Vasc Surg 2:709–714, 1985.
83. Ojemann RG: Comment on paper. Little JR, Sawhyn B, Weinstein M: Pseudo-tandem stenosis of the internal carotid artery. Neurosurgery 7:577, 1980.
84. Ojemann RG, Crowell RM: *Surgical Management of Cerebrovascular Disease*. Baltimore, Williams & Wilkins, 1983, pp 25–26.
85. Ojemann RG, Crowell RM, Roberson GH, Fisher CM: Surgical treatment of extracranial carotid occlusive disease. Clin Neurosurg 22:214–263, 1975.
86. Ott DA, Cooley DA, Chapa L, Coelho A: Carotid endarterectomy without temporary intraluminal shunt. Arch Surg 191:708–714, 1980.
87. Ouriel K, Penn TE, Ricotta JJ, May AG, Green RM, DeWeese JA: Carotid endarterectomy in the elderly patient. Surg Gynecol Obstet 102:334–336, 1986.
88. Patterson RH Jr: Risk of carotid surgery with occlusion of the contralateral carotid artery. Arch Neurol 30:188–189, 1974.
89. Pelz DM, Buchan A, Fox AJ, Barnett HJM, Vinuela F: Intraluminal thrombus of the internal carotid artery: Angiographic demonstration of resolution with anticoagulant therapy alone. Radiology, in press.
90. Pelz DM, Fox AJ, Vinuela F: Digital subtraction angiography: Current clinical applications. Stroke 16:528–539, 1985.
91. Pessin MS, Duncan GW, Davis KR, Hinton RC, Roberson GH, Mohr JP: Angiographic appearance of carotid occlusion in acute stroke. Stroke 11:485–487, 1980.
92. Pessin MS, Duncan GW, Mohr JP, Poskanzer DC: Clinical and angiographic features of carotid transient ischemic attacks. N Engl J Med 296:358–362, 1977.
93. Pessin MS, Hinton RC, Davis KR, Duncan GW, Roberson GH, Ackerman RH, Mohr JP: Mechanism of acute carotid stroke. Ann Neurol 6:245–252, 1979.
94. Phillips MR, Johnson WC, Scott RM, Vollman RW, Levine H, Nabseth DC: Carotid endarterectomy in the presence of contralateral carotid occlusion. The role of EEG and intraluminal shunting. Arch Surg 114:1232–1239, 1979.
95. Pistolese GR, Ventura M, Speziale F, Fiorani P: Emergency carotid endarterectomy. Int Surg 69:231–234, 1984.
96. Podore PC, Rob CG, DeWeese JA, Green RM: Chronic common carotid occlusion. Stroke 12:98–100, 1981.
97. Ricotta JJ, Holen J, Schenk E, Plasssche W, Green RM, Gramiak R, DeWeese JA: Is routine angiography necessary prior to carotid endarterectomy? J Vasc Surg 1:96–102, 1984.
98. Roederer GO, Langlois YE, Chan AR, Chikos PM, Thiele BL: Is siphon disease important in predicting outcome of carotid endarterectomy? Arch Surg 118:1177–1181, 1983.
99. Rosenthal D, Rudderman RH, Jones DH, Clark MD, Stanton PE Jr, Lamis PA, Daniels WW: Carotid endarterectomy in the octogenarian: Is it appropriate? J Vasc Surg 3:782–787, 1986.
100. Savojardo M: CT scanning. In Barnett HJM, Mohr JP, Stein BM, Yatsu FM (eds): *Stroke*. New York, Churchill Livingstone, 1986, pp 189–219.
101. Sekhar LN, Heros RC, Lotz PR, Rosenbaum AE: Atheromatous pseudo-occlusion of the internal carotid artery. J Neurosurg 52:782–794, 1980.
102. Sekhar LN, Heros RC, Wolfson SK, Segal RC, Dujovny M: External carotid endarterectomy for cerebral and ocular ischemia. Vasc Surg 16:185–203, 1982.
103. Shucart WA, Garrido E: Reopening some occluded carotid arteries. J Neurosurg 45:442–446, 1976.
104. Simmons Z, Biller J, Adams HP Jr, Dunn V, Jacoby CG: Cerebellar infarction: Comparison of computed tomography and magnetic resonance imaging. Ann Neurol 19:291–293, 1986.
105. Smith RR, Janford RA: Spontaneous healing of carotid artery ulcerations. Neurosurgery 4:549, 1979.
106. Stern J, Correll JW, Bryan N: Persistent hypoglossal artery and persistent trigeminal artery presenting with posterior fossa transient ischemic attacks. Report of two cases. J Neurosurg 51:614–619, 1979.
107. Stern J, Whelan M, Brisman R, Correll JW: Management of extracranial carotid stenosis and intracranial aneurysm. J Neurosurg 51:147–150, 1979.
108. Strand T, Splund K, Eriksson J, Hugg E, Lithner F, Webster PO: A randomized controlled trial of hemodilution therapy in acute ischemic stroke. Stroke 15:980–989, 1984.
109. Sundt TM Jr, Sandok BA, Whisnant JP: Carotid endarterectomy. Complications and preoperative assessment of risk. Mayo Clin Proc 50:301–306, 1975.
110. Sundt TM Jr, Sharbrough FW, Anderson RE, Michenfelder JD: Cerebral blood flow measurements and electroencephalograms during carotid endarterectomy. J Neurosurg 41:310–320, 1974.
111. Sundt TMJ, Sharbrough FW, Marsh WR, Ebersold MJ, Piepgras DG, Messick JM Jr: The risk-benefit ratio of intraoperative shunting during carotid endarterectomy. Ann Surg 203:196–204, 1986.
112. Sundt TM Jr, Sharbrough FW, Piepgras DG, Kearns TP, Messick JM Jr, O'Fallen WM: Correlation of cerebral blood flow and electroencephalographic changes during carotid endarterectomy. With results of surgery and hemodynamics of cerebral ischemia. Mayo Clin Proc 56:533–543, 1981.
113. Thomas GI, Jones TW, Stavney LJ, Manhas DR, Spencer MP: Carotid endarterectomy after Doppler ultrasonographic examination without angiography. Am J Surg 151:616–619, 1986.
114. Thompson JE: Protection of the brain during carotid endarterectomy. I. Routine shunting. Anesthesiol Clin 22:129–135, 1984.
115. Vollman RW, Eldrup-Jorgensen J, Hoffman MA: The role of cranial computed tomography in carotid surgery. Vasc Surg 2:255–268, 1986.
116. Vorstrup S, Engell HC, Linderwald H, Lassen NA: Hemodynamically significant stenosis of the internal carotid artery treated with endarterectomy. Case report. J Neurosurg 60:1070–1075, 1984.
117. Wall SD, Brant-Zawadzki M, Jeffrey RB, Barnes B: High frequency CT findings within 24 hours after cerebral infarction. AJNR 2:553–557, 1981.
118. Walters BB, Ojemann RG, Heros RC: Emergency carotid endarterectomy. J Neurosurg, in press.
119. Whisnant JP: The role of the neurologist in the decline of stroke. Ann Neurol 14:1–7, 1983.
120. Whisnant JP, Sandok BA, Sundt TM Jr: Carotid endarterectomy for unilateral carotid system transient cerebral ischemia. Mayo Clin Proc 58:171–175, 1983.
121. Whittemore AD, Kauffman JL, Kohler TR, Mannick JA: Routine electroencephalographic (EEG) monitoring during carotid endarterectomy. Ann Surg 197:707–713, 1983.
122. Wood JN, Kee DB Jr: Hemorheology of the cerebral circulation in stroke. Stroke 16:765–772, 1985.

2

Carotid Endarterectomy

PREOPERATIVE EVALUATION

Many patients with carotid atherosclerosis have significant medical risk factors. These include the presence of symptomatic coronary artery disease, myocardial infarction, severe peripheral arterial disease, rheumatic heart disease, congestive heart failure, severe hypertension (blood pressure more than 180/110 mm Hg), chronic obstructive pulmonary disease, diabetes, hyperlipidemia, renal insufficiency, and obesity. Previous publications have documented that the operative risks are higher in these patients (20, 81). In one report involving patients who were neurologically stable but had significant medical risk factors, the morbidity and mortality rate was 7%, primarily related to cardiac disease (81).

All patients being considered for operation for carotid occlusive disease are evaluated with a complete blood count, blood sugar, blood urea nitrogen, serum electrolytes, clotting studies [prothrombin time (PT), partial thromboplastin time (PTT), and platelet count], electrocardiogram (ECG), and chest x-ray. Blood cholesterol and triglycerides are also checked. Preoperative pulmonary function tests are obtained in patients with pulmonary dysfunction.

When there is a question about cardiac reserve a stress test is done. If this shows significant abnormality coronary angiography may be indicated. A history of myocardial infarction within 6 months or evidence of overt left ventricular failure are strong but not absolute contraindications to surgery.

Severe hypertension should be treated preoperatively but care must be taken not to lower the blood pressure too much (90). It is probably satisfactory to aim to keep the blood pressure below 170/90 (35). Patients receiving diuretic medication should have serum potassium checked and any deficiency should be treated.

Many patients will have mild renal insufficiency which may be worsened if large amounts of dye have been used at angiography and fluids restricted (35). It is essential to maintain adequate hydration.

Indications for intraoperative monitoring with a pulmonary artery catheter include impaired cardiac reserve, left ventricular failure, a recent myocardial infarction, severe mitral valvular disease, and persistent angina after a coronary artery bypass. Patients with symptomatic heart block undergo placement of a temporary intravenous pacer.

In a group of over 400 carotid endarterectomies, we found 86 patients who were judged to have evidence of increased cardiopulmonary risk (15). They underwent 95 endarterectomies. Coronary artery disease was the most common risk factor, being present in 72 patients, with previous coronary bypass surgery in five, serious arrhythmias in two, and previous cardiac arrest during anesthetic induction in one. The other risk factors were chronic obstructive pulmonary disease in nine and rheumatic valvular disease in five. Recognition of these factors, careful preoperative evaluation and preparation, an experienced anesthesia team, and well-staffed intensive care unit (ICU) have made it possible to keep the morbidity and mortality low in this group (about 4%).

Several reports indicate that patients who have symptomatic carotid artery stenosis, as well as severe coronary artery disease, and who are candidates for myocardial revascularization, should have both operations done under the same anesthesia to reduce the risk of coronary occlusion (19, 20, 47, 69). In one report, it was found that the perioperative mortality up to 30 days after operation was 1.5% in 1306 consecutive endarterectomies done in 1026 patients without symptomatic coronary artery disease (20). Those patients with significant cardiac symptoms were divided into two groups. In one, 85 carotid endarterectomies performed in 77 patients without prior coronary bypass operation had a perioperative mortality of 18.2%. In the other group, 155 operations in 135 patients who were treated with either prior coronary artery bypass (84 patients) or simultaneous carotid endarterectomy and coronary artery bypass (51 patients) had an operative mortality of only 3%.

If the carotid stenosis or occlusion is asymptomatic in a patient who is to have coronary or peripheral arterial reconstruction, there is reported to be no increased risk of stroke, and prophylactic or simultaneous carotid endarterectomy is usually not recommended (3, 45, 47, 91). However, in one study where the degree of internal carotid artery stenosis was considered, those patients with a severe internal carotid artery stenosis, as indicated by noninvasive tests, had a higher rate of perioperative cerebral ischemic events after major surgery (49). Therefore, patients with a residual lumen of less than 1 mm and distal hemodynamic change may need to be considered in the same category as those with symptomatic stenosis when planning a major surgical procedure.

PREOPERATIVE MEDICATION

Many patients will be on drugs for treatment of cardiovascular disease. Usually these are continued. If the patient is on heparin, this is continued until the patient leaves the floor for the operating room.

Because of the fragile cardiovascular status of many of these patients, preoperative medication is kept to a minimum. A sedative like diazepam (10–15 mg for a 70kg adult) is recommended. In rare cases a narcotic may be used. Use of atropine and scopolamine is optional.

It has been shown in the laboratory that preoperative use of aspirin reduces the incidence of postoperative thrombus formation following carotid endarterectomy (21). In a prospective, randomized, double-blind study of 22 patients undergoing carotid endarterectomy and randomly assigned to perioperative administration of an aspirin/dipyridamole combination or placebo, it was found that platelet deposition at the endarterectomy site, as measured by autologous indium-lll-labeled platelets, was significantly reduced in the treated group (26). In recent years the authors have used 300 mg of aspirin daily preoperatively and no increased problems with wound hematoma have been evident.

ANESTHETIC MANAGEMENT

Of major importance for successful results is a team approach to the surgical and anesthetic management of these cases. The authors prefer general endotracheal anesthesia. This technique provides good airway control, maintenance of normal arterial blood gases, maximum patient comfort, optimal surgical exposure, and some protection against cerebral ischemia.

As soon as the patient arrives in the operating room, blood pressure is recorded, a peripheral intravenous (IV) infusion is started, and an intraarterial cannula is inserted percutaneously into the radial artery for direct blood pressure recording and for blood gas measurement. If there is any indication of low blood volume or hypotension, central venous pressure (CVP) is recorded and the patient is given fluid or colloid to raise the CVP to 8–10 cm of H_2O. A vasopressor IV infusion is prepared, usually with 10 mg of phenylephrine hydrochloride in 250 ml of saline, and administered as needed through a pediatric microdrop set to maintain an adequate blood pressure. All patients receive prophylactic antibiotics. Electroencephalogram (EEG) electrodes are attached to the scalp and ECG leads are placed. Other monitoring includes a pulse oximeter, temperature probe, twitch (blockade) monitor, and end-tidal CO_2 monitor.

After preoxygenation, a sleep dose of Pentothal (100–300 mg) is given slowly. At times this is preceded by a narcotic —often fentanyl (100–400 mg). Once the patient is asleep and the airway can be adequately maintained, a long-acting muscle relaxant (pancuronium 0.1 mg/kg) is given IV and the patient is ventilated until total paralysis is established. To prevent an acute cardiovascular response, IV Xylocaine (1.5 mg/kg) is given before intubation. In some patients a slow infusion of nitroglycerin may be needed.

Anesthesia is maintained with O_2/N_2O at a ratio of 30/70%. Ventilation is controlled to keep the pCO_2 near normal. Intravenous narcotics (fentanyl) may be given at appropriate times. In some patients, to smooth the anesthetic course and to prevent acute fluctuations in blood pressure, a background inhalation agent (isoflurane) is commonly used.

During carotid clamping a sudden decrease in pressure within the carotid bifurcation may produce an ischemia response from the sinus resulting in hypertension and tachycardia. Control of this response is especially important in patients with coronary artery disease. Deepening the anesthesia with IV narcotics or inhalation agents or use of nitroglycerin infusion may be needed.

Release of the clamps after the endarterectomy is completed often causes a transient fall in blood pressure due to sudden rise in pressure on the sinus. Use of a pressor or infusion of crystalloid may be needed.

Reversal of the muscle relaxant is monitored carefully. Atropine is avoided because of its effect on the heart in patients with coronary artery disease. Glycopyrolate is used instead.

During the procedure, arterial blood gas measurements are done to assure adequate ventilation and to maintain the arterial pCO_2 in the range of 36–40 mm Hg. Blood replacement is usually not necessary.

BRAIN PROTECTION AND MONITORING

The best method of maintaining adequate cerebral circulation during the operation is to combine the benefits of general anesthesia with the maintenance of adequate blood volume and a normal or slightly elevated arterial pressure. At the time of carotid clamping for the endarterectomy, the arterial pressure is elevated to an average systolic level of 170 mm Hg if there is no cardiac contraindication. In the normal brain, constant cerebral blood flow (CBF) is maintained by autoregulation over a wide range of arterial pressures. However, in areas of focal cerebral ischemia, autoregulation of CBF may be lost and flow becomes passively dependent on the perfusion pressure and blood volume.

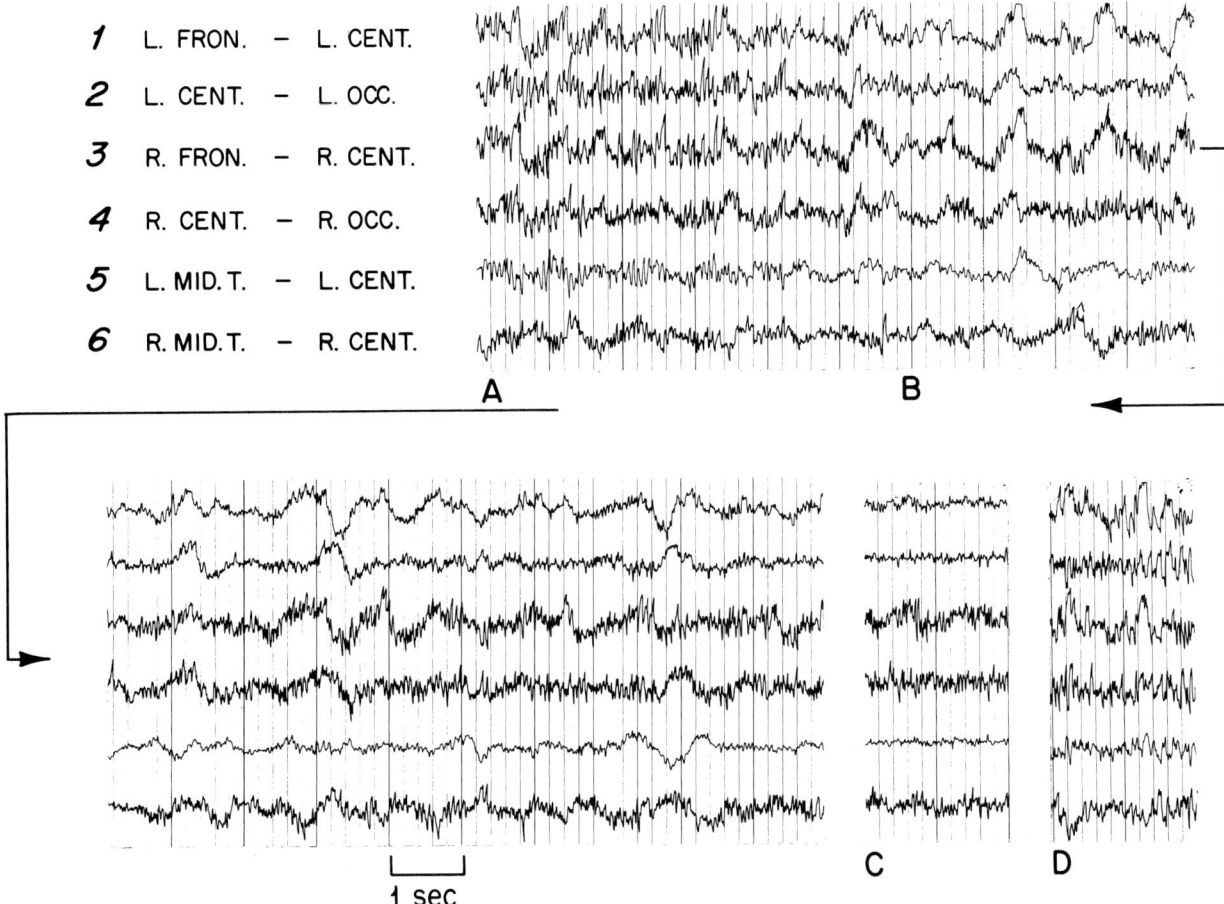

Figure 2.1. EEG recording during carotid endarterectomy. At **A**, the carotid circulation is occluded. Blood pressure is 170-180 mm Hg systolic. By 6 seconds (**B**), definite slowing and reduced voltage are noted in the left side recordings (*lines 1, 2, and 5*). The changes are more pronounced over the next several seconds. At 1 minute (**C**), the left midtemporal to central tracing is almost flat (*line 5*). One minute after insertion of the shunt, a normal record is restored (**D**).

The most effective method of monitoring the intracranial circulation during the time of clamping for the carotid endarterectomy is continuous EEG recording with a full set of leads from both sides of the head (8, 11, 14, 57, 63, 76). If the EEG shows minor slowing and/or a slight decrease in voltage, usually nothing needs to be done. The surgeon must check and be sure the blood pressure is being maintained over 170 mm Hg if there is no cardiac contraindication. In most patients with significant EEG abnormality, the change occurs soon after the arteries are occluded and comes on over a period of a few seconds to less than a minute (Fig. 2.1). When this occurs, a shunt should be placed promptly.

A high degree of correlation has been found between CBF measurements during carotid occlusion and changes in the EEG (76, 82). In these studies, the critical CBF (flow required to maintain a normal EEG) was approximately 30% (15 ml/100 gm/min) of normal flow (50 ml/100 gm/min). The degree of EEG change reflected the severity of flow reduction. This change was reversed with placement of a shunt which was done if the CBF was less than 18 to 20 ml/100 gm/min. In an evaluation of 1935 cases undergoing carotid endarterectomy, the need for shunting was based on a correlation between EEG changes and a fall in CBF below the critical level required for adequate perfusion during the period of carotid occlusion (80). Based on the severity of reductions in CBF during the period of carotid occlusion, it was concluded that 12% of all patients would have sustained a major deficit and 15% would have had a minor or transient deficit without shunting. The risk of shunting was 0.5%. In another study where regional anesthesia was used, 7.6% of the patients could not tolerate occlusion without the appearance of a neurologic deficit in 10–30 seconds and in most, insertion of a shunt was needed to prevent the deficit (42).

In our consecutive series of 173 elective operations for carotid stenosis, 10 patients showed a significant change in EEG tracing at some point after carotid occlusion (63). In four, further elevations of blood pressure resulted in improvement in the EEG, but six patients required a shunt. All 10 patients recovered with no neurologic deficit. The EEG will not tell if an embolus has occluded a perforating artery, but it will tell if the hemisphere needs more blood. Other methods have been advocated for monitoring, including measurement of stump pressure and sampling of jugular venous pCO_2 but these tests have not been as reliable (42, 50, 59, 70).

The question of whether a temporary shunt is indicated during carotid endarterectomy has been the subject of several articles. Some surgeons routinely use a shunt for cerebral protection (31, 87, 88, 90, 93). Others believe a shunt is not needed, and some use a shunt only when monitoring indicates a need for it (23–25, 33, 63–65, 78, 83, 94). The use of a shunt carries with it a small risk of embolization and injury to the distal intima, and it does make the technical removal of the distal end of the plaque in the internal carotid artery a little more difficult. Everything should be done to reduce the morbidity of the operation to as low a level as possible. Every patient should be monitored. In only a small percentage of patients will a shunt be needed, but when it is indicated, it should be used.

In some patients, the surgeon will know preoperatively that there is a high probability a shunt will be needed. These include patients where the vertebrobasilar circulation depends on the carotid artery (Fig. 1.23) or where there are multiple occlusions of major extracranial vessels. In two series of patients with contralateral internal carotid artery occlusion, EEG changes were found in 18% and 37% (63, 78).

OPERATIVE TECHNIQUE

Since the original description of the author's operative approach, the technique gradually has been revised and refined (62, 63). The patient is placed in the supine position with a thyroid bag inflated under the shoulders. The head is slightly extended and turned away from the side of the operation. The entire operation is done using a headlight and magnifying loupes.

Figure 2.2 outlines the setup in the operating room for a left carotid endarterectomy. The important points to note are: (a) the nurse stands directly opposite the surgeon, (b) the EEG is where the surgeon can see the tracing if necessary, and (c) the anesthesiologist has full access to the head and right arm.

It is important to mark the incision beginning along the anterior border of the sternocleidomastoid muscle. Between 1 and 2 cm below the level of the angle of the jaw the incision should be curved over the muscle posteriorly and superiorly toward the mastoid process (Fig. 2.3A). This will allow maximum exposure to the base of the skull beneath the parotid gland and helps avoid injury to the mandibular branch of the facial nerve near the angle of the jaw.

After the skin incision is made, the platysma is incised. The external jugular vein is ligated, small transverse cervical nerves divided, and the great auricular nerve identified at the upper end of the exposure (Fig. 2.3B). This nerve, which usually crosses the upper portion of the incision just beneath the platysma muscle, is preserved, if possible, thus avoiding unpleasant numbness of the ear.

Dissection is continued along the anterior border of the sternocleidomastoid muscle (Fig. 2.4). Self-retaining retractors are used to aid the exposure. The medial blades must be kept on the subcutaneous tissue and platysma. If they are placed too deeply against the paratracheal muscles, the recurrent laryngeal nerve may be injured.

The internal jugular vein is identified just medial and deep to the sternocleidomastoid muscle (Fig. 2.5). The dissection then extends along the medial border of the internal jugular vein; medial draining branches are ligated as necessary. The most prominent of these is usually the common facial vein. The descendens hypoglossi nerve is often seen in the tissue just medial to the internal jugular vein and overlying the common carotid artery. This nerve is reflected medially.

The common carotid artery is exposed medial to the internal jugular vein in the lower part of the incision (Fig. 2.6). Often the vein may overlie the artery. A tape is placed around the artery which maintains its exposure and facilitates the further dissection. On rare occasions, the vagus nerve lies anteriorly on the common carotid artery and one must be alert for this possibility.

The dissection is then extended superiorly along the medial border of the internal jugular vein (Fig. 2.7). The descendens hypoglossi nerve is kept medially and leads one to the hypoglossal nerve, which may swing low into the neck across the carotid bifurcation or lie high beneath the edge of the posterior belly of the digastric muscle. Often it lies just beneath the common facial vein and may be adherent to this vessel. In some patients, nerve branches will come around the lateral side of the common carotid artery to enter the descendens hypoglossi nerve. Usually these branches are from the cervical plexus, but on rare occasions they come from the vagus nerve. In most cases, they can be divided to allow the descendens hypoglossi nerve to be reflected medially. However, if the branch is large or is coming from the vagus nerve, the descendens hypoglossi nerve is divided close to the hypoglossal nerve and the branch from the vagus nerve is reflected laterally.

To give adequate exposure, it may be necessary to remove a group of lymph nodes which are commonly present over the region of the carotid bifurcation.

Carotid Endarterectomy

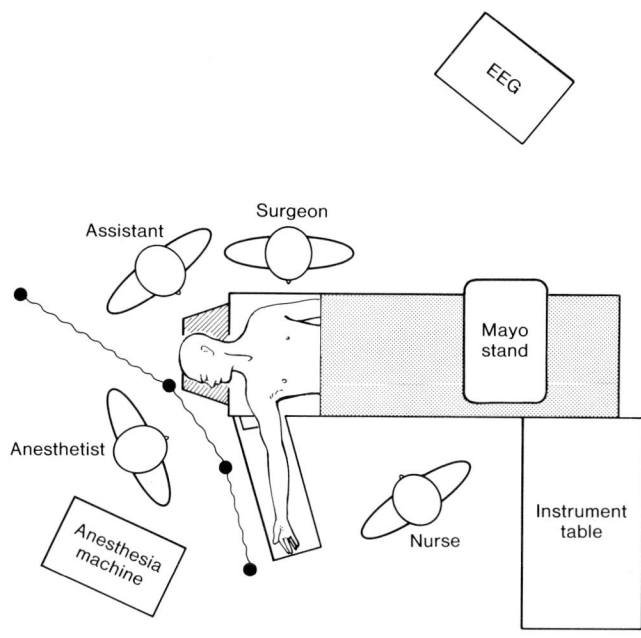

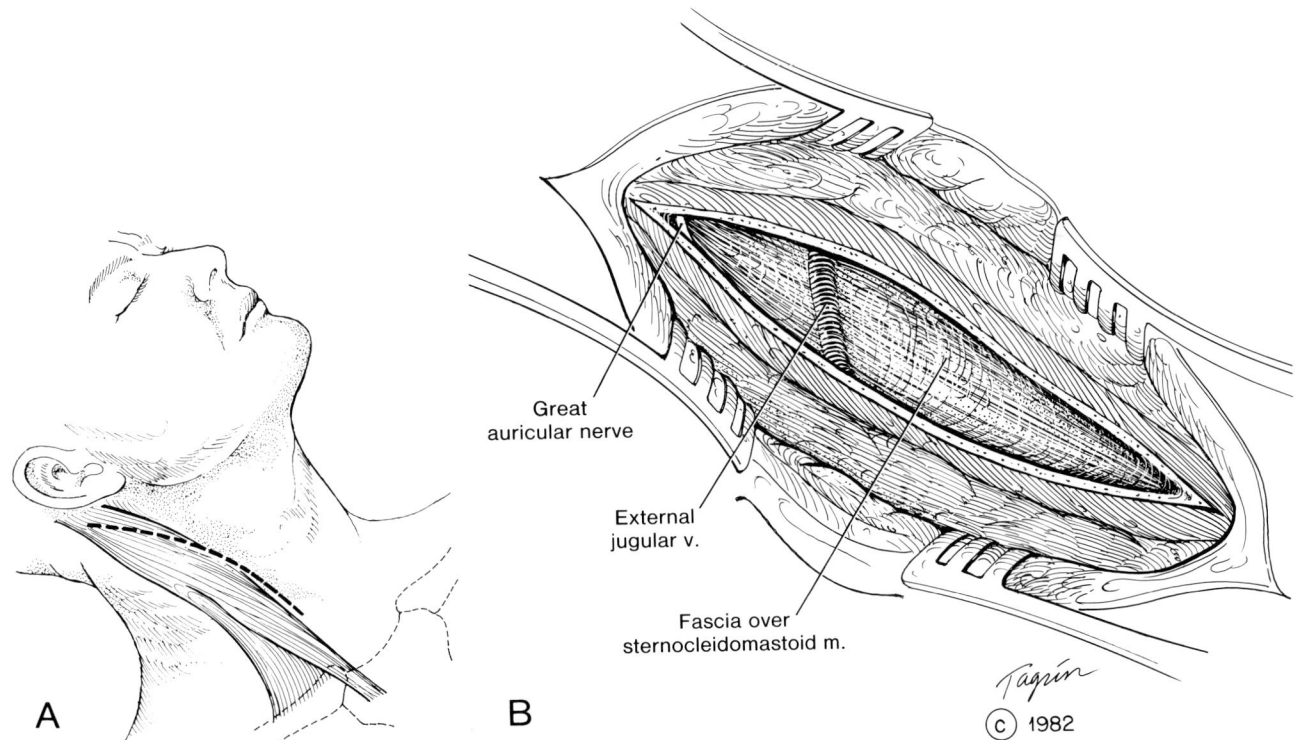

Figure 2.2. Operating room setup for left carotid endarterectomy. Note (a) the position of the nurse so she can see and act as a second assistant, (b) the location of the EEG so the surgeon can view the tracing if necessary, (c) the position of the first assistant (we find this is much better than having him on the opposite side of the table), and (d) the anesthesiologist has full access to the head and right arm.

Figure 2.3. Carotid endarterectomy. Skin incision and initial exposure. **A**, Note that the upper end of the incision curves over the sternocleidomastoid muscle toward the mastoid process. **B**, The skin incision has been made and the platysma incised in line with the anterior border of the sternocleidomastoid muscle.

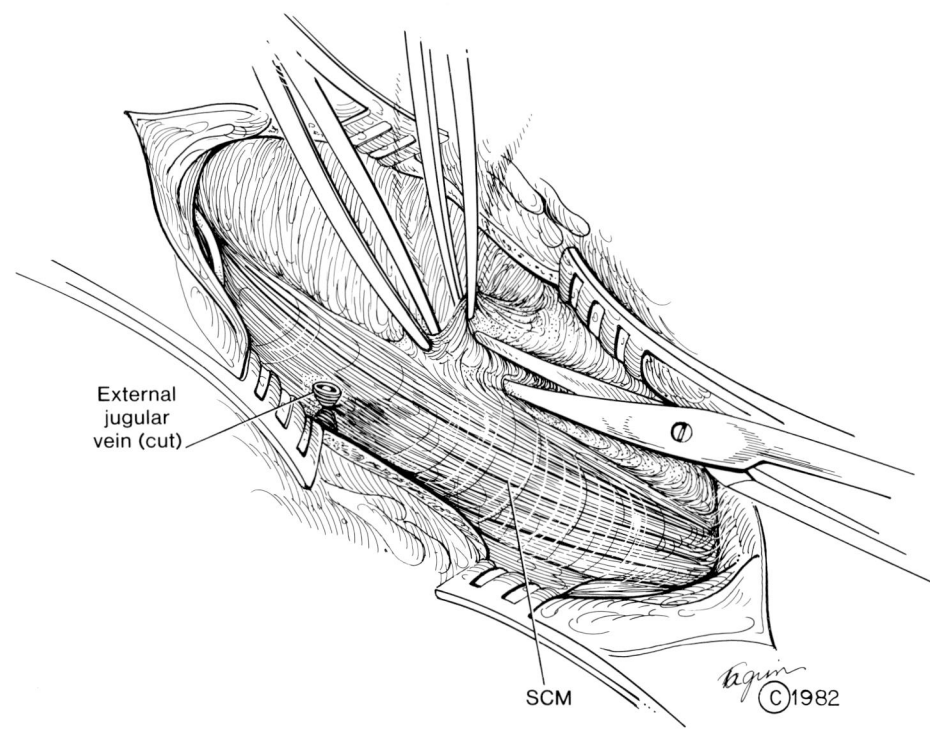

Figure 2.4. Carotid endarterectomy. Opening of fascia along anterior border of sternocleidomastoid muscle.

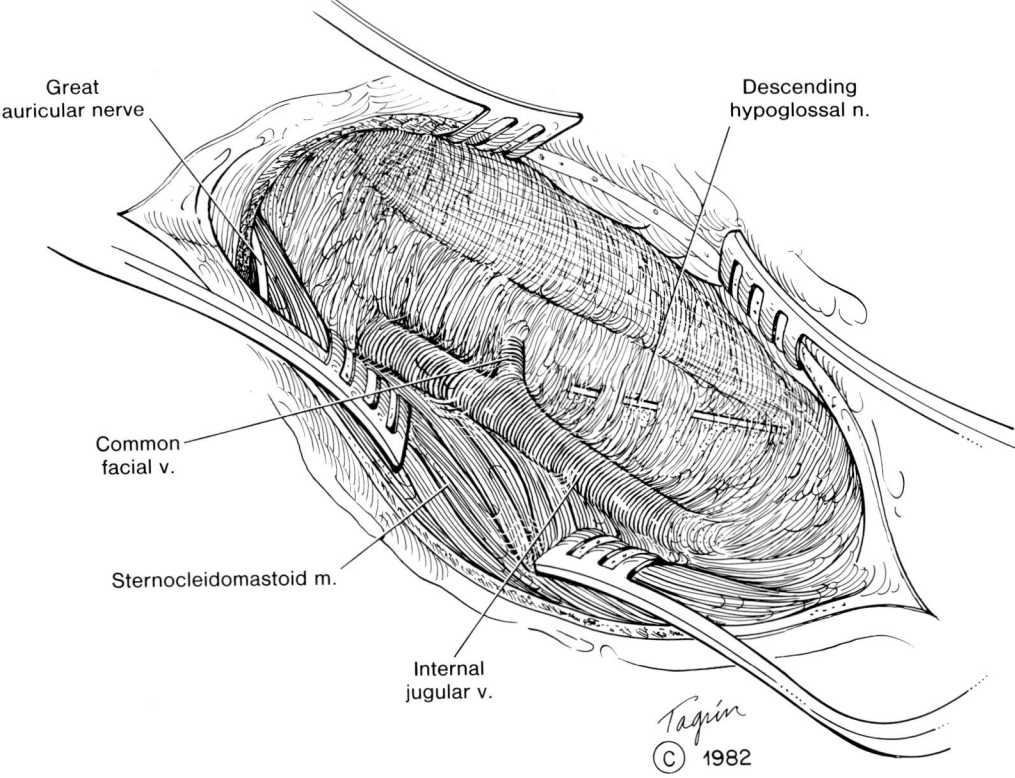

Figure 2.5. Carotid endarterectomy. The anterior border of the sternocleidomastoid muscle has been retracted laterally and the anterior and medial aspect of the internal jugular vein brought into view.

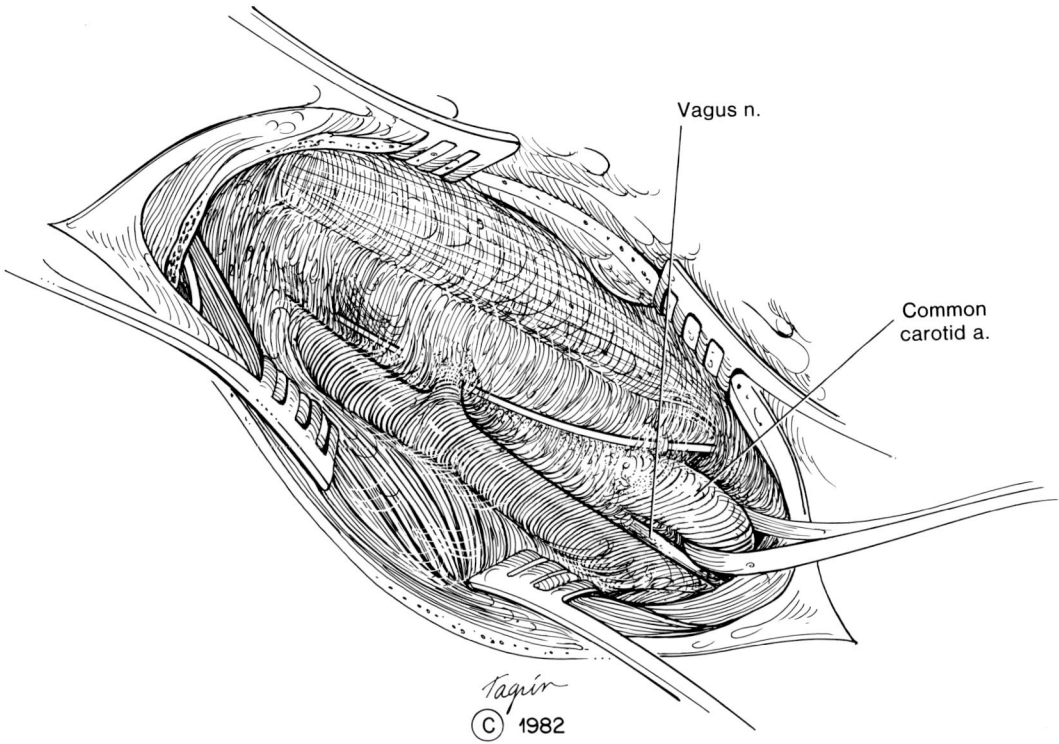

Figure 2.6. Carotid endarterectomy. The proximal common carotid artery is exposed and a tape passed around it.

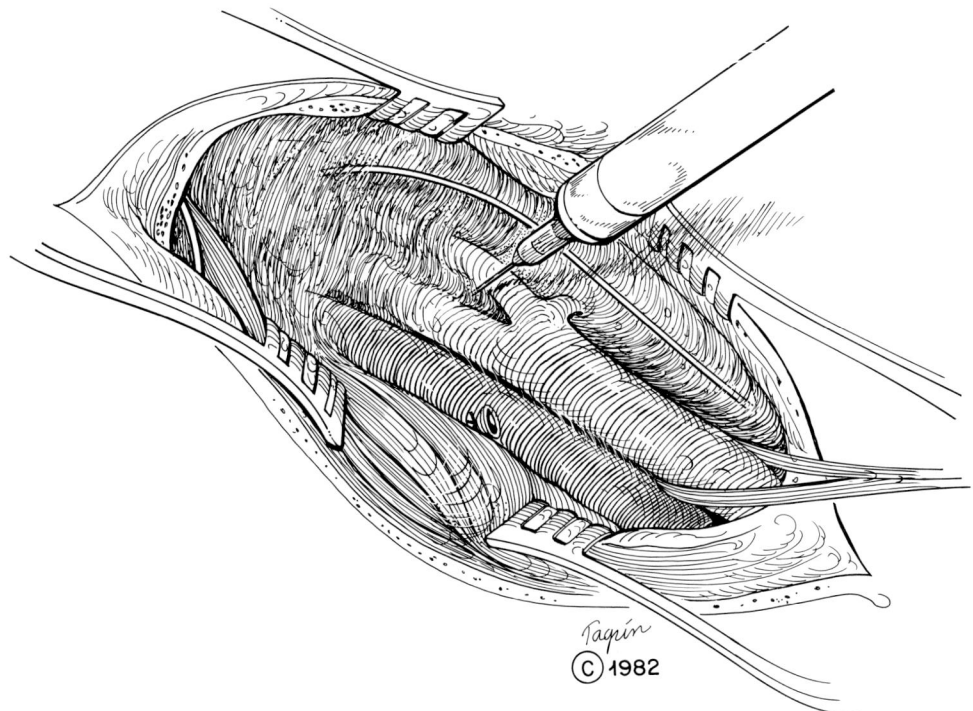

Figure 2.7. Carotid endarterectomy. The bifurcation of the common carotid artery has been exposed by staying along the medial border of the internal jugular vein and reflecting the descending hypoglossal nerve medially. The region of the carotid sinus is blocked with lidocaine hydrochloride.

When the carotid bifurcation is exposed, the region of the carotid sinus is blocked with lidocaine hydrochloride to avoid hypotension and carotid sinus reflex bradycardia (Fig. 2.7). Care is taken to leave the region of the distal common carotid artery, carotid bifurcation, and proximal internal carotid artery adherent to the posterior tissue. This avoids undue manipulation of the area reducing the possibility of dislodging an embolus, lessening the chance of carotid sinus stimulation, and avoiding possible injury to the superior laryngeal nerve.

The distal internal carotid artery is carefully exposed, staying in the tissue plane between the hypoglossal nerve or descendens hypoglossi nerve medially and the internal jugular vein laterally (Fig. 2.8). If one follows these guidelines, the distal internal carotid artery can be nicely exposed. As the hypoglossal nerve swings medially, an arterial branch often comes across the inner side of the curve of the nerve and passes posteriorly. This fairly constant sternocleidomastoid artery, often accompanied by a vein, is occluded and divided. In patients with a high bifurcation the hypoglossal nerve and, if necessary, the descendens hypoglossi nerve may be gently reflected medially with a soft rubber band tape to facilitate the exposure. If the carotid bifurcation is located high in the neck, dissection is carried along the medial border of the internal jugular vein and beneath the parotid gland. It may be necessary to retract the posterior belly of the digastric muscle.

Rarely will it need to be divided. On occasion, the occipital artery must be divided to free the hypoglossal nerve in order to expose the distal internal carotid artery.

The superior thyroid artery is identified on the medial wall of the distal common or proximal external carotid artery and a tape placed around it (Fig. 2.9). The external carotid artery is exposed to the level of the first major branching of this vessel and a tape placed at this point. If the angiogram shows an ascending pharyngeal artery coming off the region of the bifurcation, this will have to be separately exposed and controlled. The exposure of the distal internal carotid artery is carried to a point at least 1 cm above the distal end of the plaque. In many patients the atheromatous plaque extends several millimeters further up the posterior wall of the internal carotid artery than it does the anterior wall. Great care is taken in exposing this vessel to avoid any undue pressure or manipulation of the artery. The vagus nerve may be closely adherent to the posterior wall of the internal carotid artery; occasionally it will be lateral or anterior to the artery. It must be carefully dissected free before placing the tape around the vessel. A second tape is placed around the common carotid artery several millimeters distal to the original tape. Tourniquets are placed on this tape, as well as on the internal carotid artery tape in case a shunt is needed.

When hemostasis has been obtained, the patient is

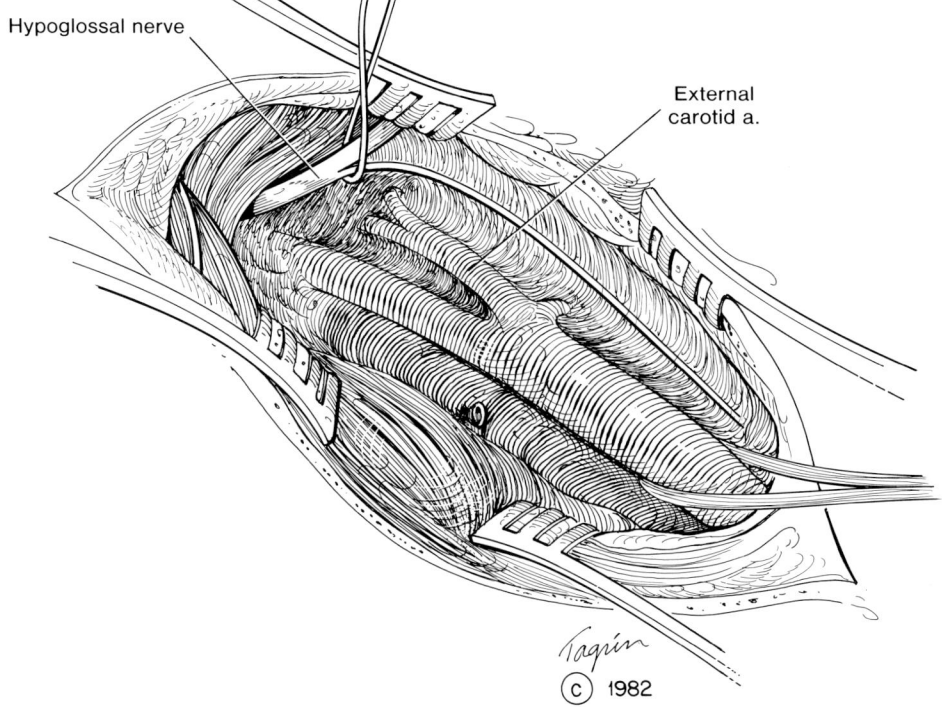

Figure 2.8. Carotid endarterectomy. The internal carotid, external carotid, and superior thyroid arteries have been isolated.

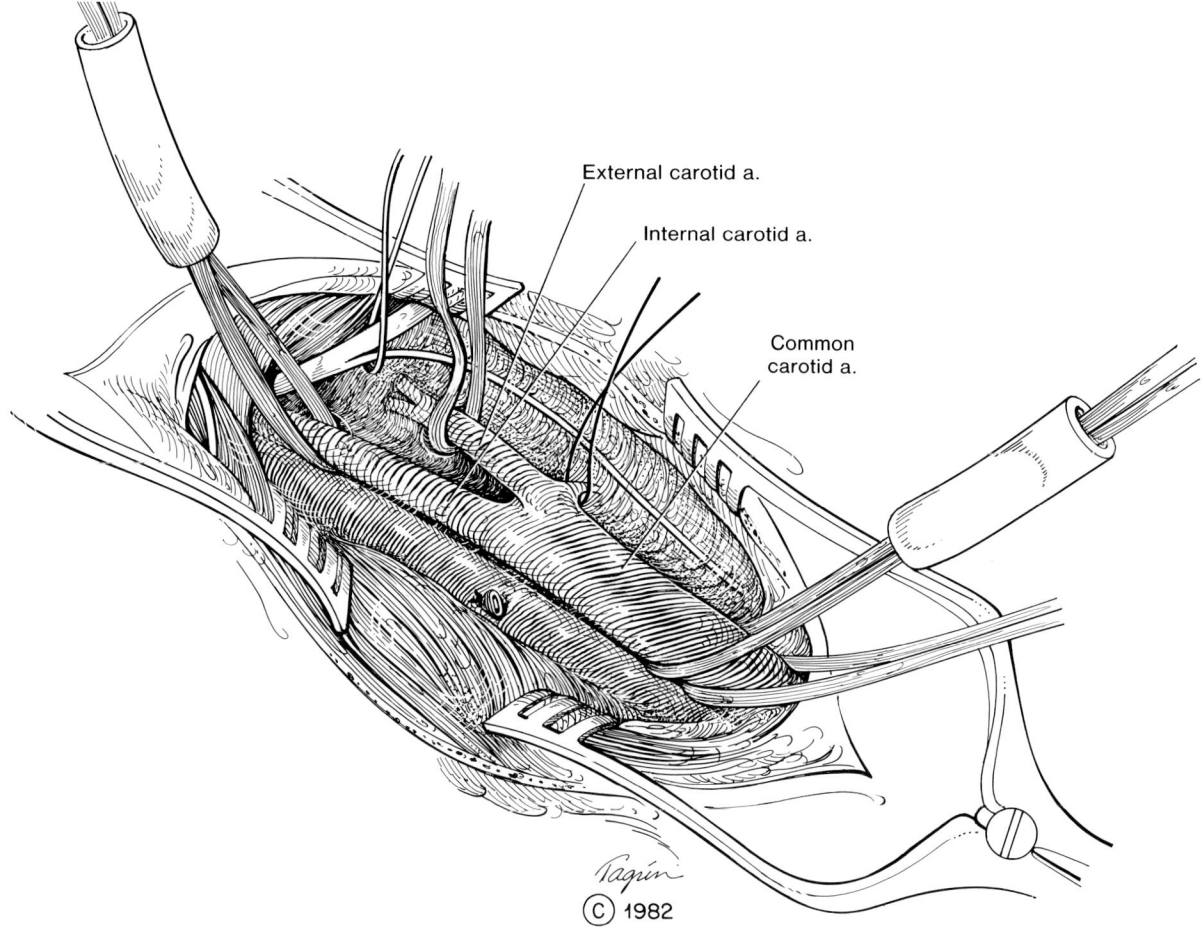

Figure 2.9. Carotid endarterectomy. Appropriate tapes and tourniquets have been placed.

given an IV bolus of 5000 units of heparin. If the blood pressure is not already elevated with the anesthetic technique being used, a phenylephrine hydrochloride drip may be necessary to raise the blood pressure to approximately 170 mm Hg systolic if the patient has no cardiac contraindication. The EEG is monitored continuously. The surgeon should check to be sure that the shunt tubing is available.

The common carotid artery is then occluded with an appropriate vascular clamp being careful to avoid injury to the underlying vagus nerve (Fig. 2.10). A Fogerty clamp is usually used. The authors prefer to use medium and long straight Heifetz aneurysm clips to occlude the other arteries, but on occasion a large internal or external carotid artery will require the use of a small bulldog clamp. Because of its small size, it is advantageous to use the Heifetz clip on the internal carotid artery for it can be placed several millimeters more distally on the artery. Care must also be taken to avoid injury to the vagus nerve at this point because it lies in the tissue just behind the internal carotid artery. The clip on the external carotid artery is placed as far distally as possible, usually at or just below the first major bifurcation.

A longitudinal incision is made in the distal common carotid artery with a no. 15 knife blade (Fig. 2.11). The incision is carried through the wall of the artery until the shiny yellow surface of the atheromatous plaque is seen. A Penfield no. 4 dissector is then used to separate the plane between the atheroma and outer arterial wall (Fig. 2.12). Often the atheroma is adherent to a relatively thin outer wall at the bifurcation. Great care must be taken to avoid an unduly superficial plane of dissection. It is best to separate the plaque for a few millimeters and then extend the incision superiorly with Potts scissors before attempting further dissection (Fig. 2.13). The distal end of the incision extends up the internal carotid artery to approximately the distal end of the plaque. The proximal extent of the incision can be estimated from the angiogram. The incision usually does not need to be more than 1–2 cm below the bifurcation. A thin layer of atheromatous plaque will usually extend proximally in the common carotid artery and

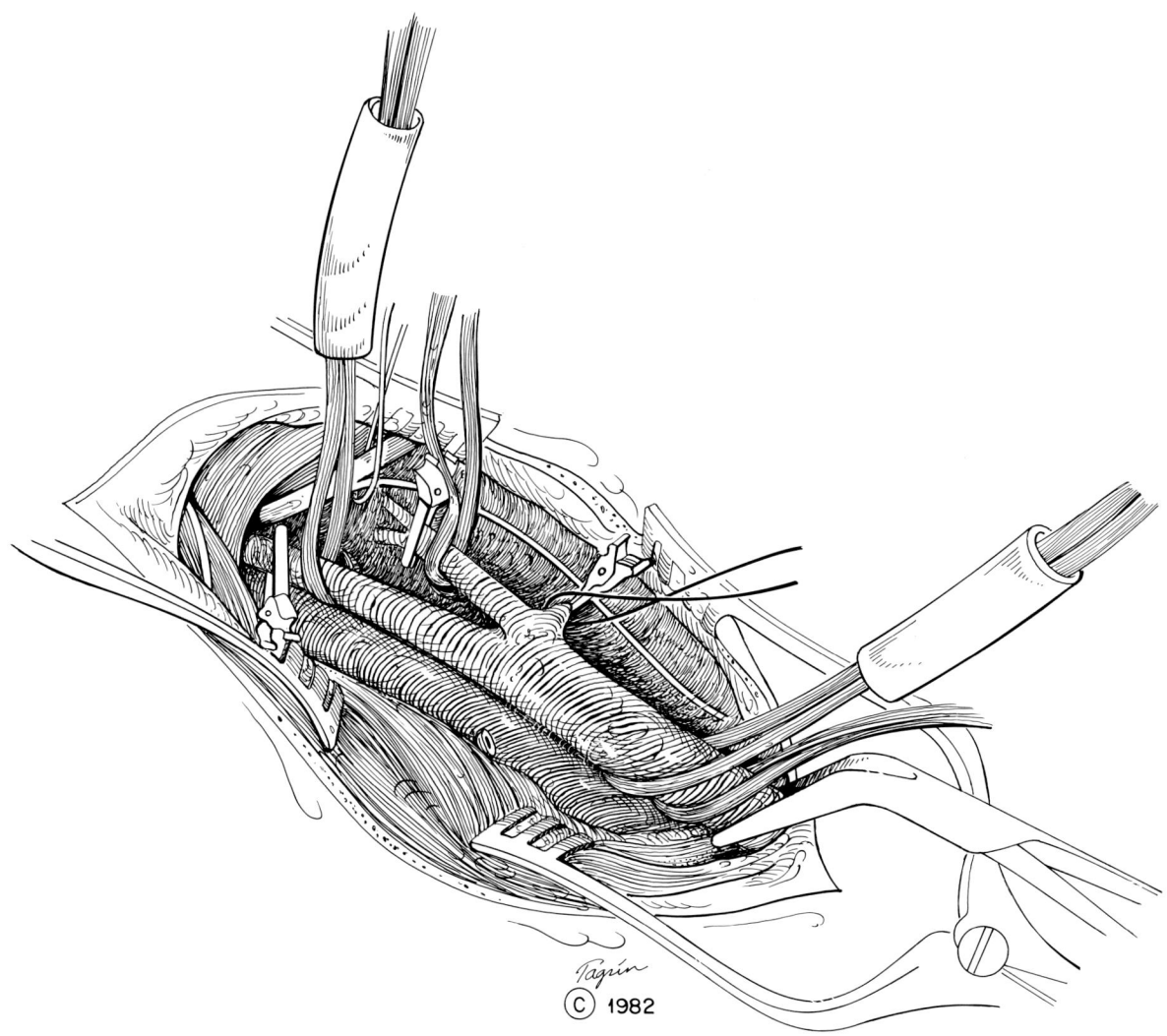

Figure 2.10. Carotid endarterectomy. The circulation has been occluded. Heifetz clips are used on the distal vessels when possible.

does not need to be of concern as long as one is proximal to the stenosis.

The atheromatous plaque is then carefully separated from the outer arterial wall in the common carotid artery with a Penfield dissector. A right-angled clamp is placed around the plaque and the plaque is cut off sharply at the proximal end of the arteriotomy in the common carotid artery with a no. 15 knife blade (Fig. 2.14). If the cut across the plaque reveals a residual area of stenosis, the incision is extended as far proximal as is necessary. In some cases the edge of the intima in the common carotid artery may require trimming with a microscissors. The plaque is kept intact and is removed first from the origin of the superior thyroid artery and the proximal external carotid artery (Fig. 2.15). In some patients it is necessary to open the clamp temporarily on the external carotid artery to remove the plaque which may extend quite far distally. Once this removal has been accomplished, the atheroma is carefully dissected from the outer wall of the internal carotid artery which, on occasion, may be exceedingly thin. Usually there is a very clean dissection plane. Great care is taken as the distal end of the plaque is reached. With gentle traction on the intact plaque, the wall of the internal carotid artery can be slightly everted and the dissection carried distally pushing the media away from the plaque until normal intima is reached (Fig. 2.16). Usually the plaque will extend distally several millimeters further along the posterior wall of the artery. Care must be taken to remove this portion of the atheroma. Once the plaque has been separated, it usually comes away cleanly at the junction with normal intima and does not leave an intimal flap. Only on rare occasions is it necessary to place one or two sutures to tuck a distal intima flap (Fig. 2.17). The intima adjacent to and beyond the distal end of the plaque is usually

Carotid Endarterectomy

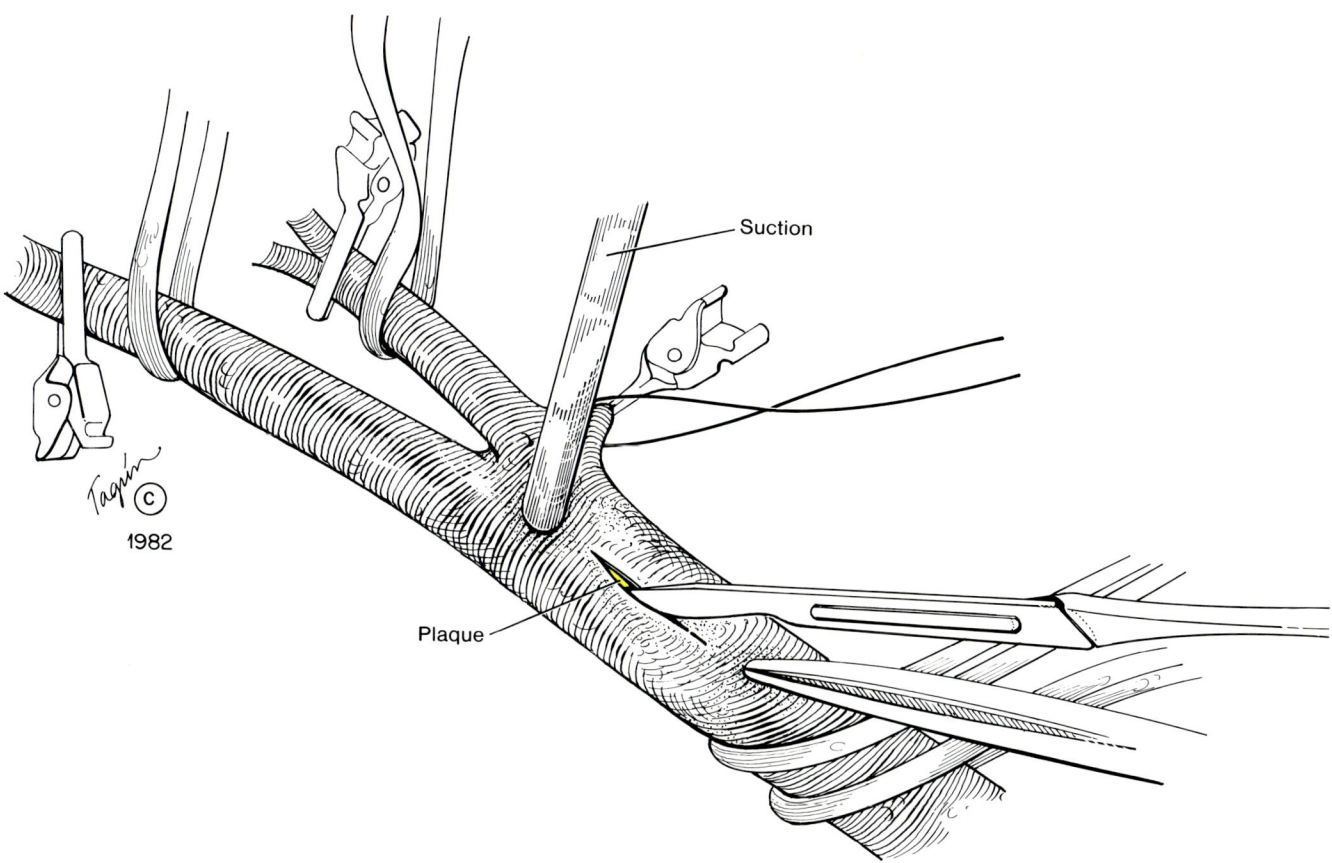

Figure 2.11. Carotid endarterectomy. The arteriotomy incision starts on the distal common carotid artery. It is carried down to but not through the atheromatous plaque. Suction is ready and a forceps steadies the vessel.

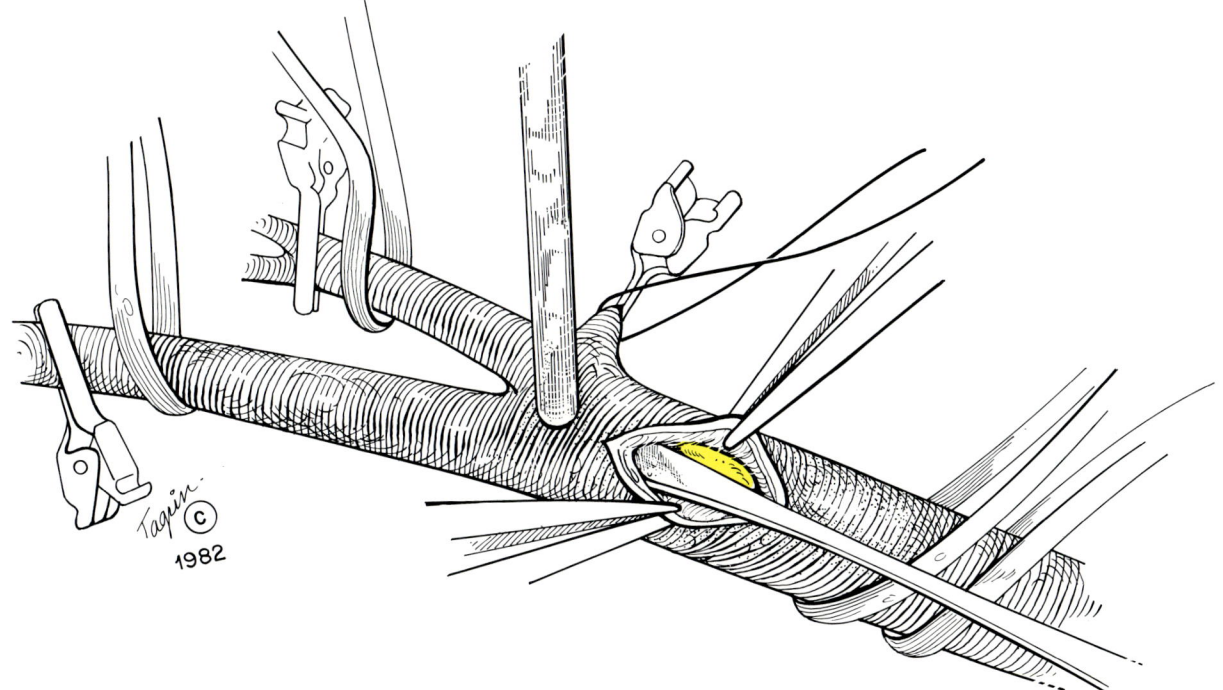

Figure 2.12. Carotid endarterectomy. The plaque is being separated from the anterior wall of the artery by a no. 4 Penfield dissector.

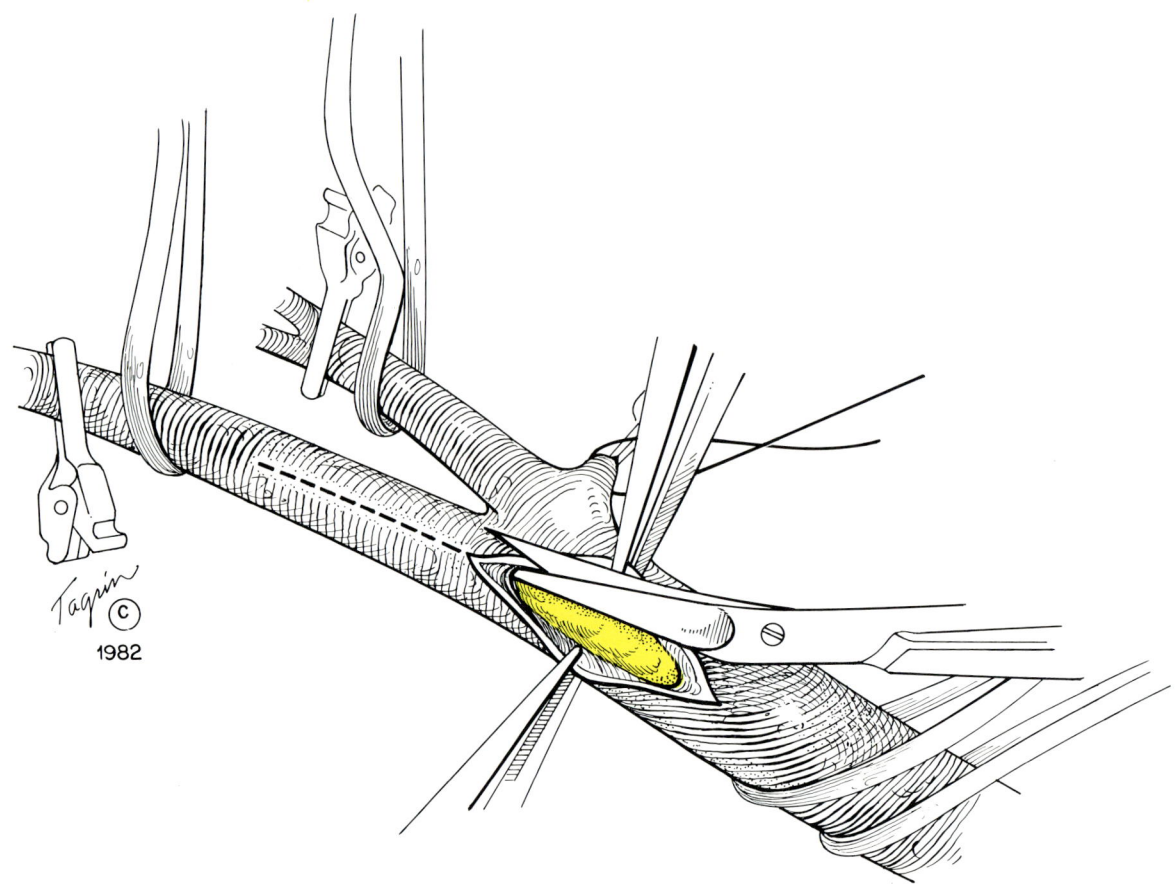

Figure 2.13. Carotid endarterectomy. The arteriotomy is extended distally using a Potts scissors.

of normal thickness and firmly adherent to the media. Occasionally, a very thin sheet of atheromatous material may extend distally in the internal carotid artery but does not cause stenosis.

The area of the endarterectomy is irrigated with heparinized saline and inspected with the help of the headlight and magnification. There are almost always some loose fragments adherent to the wall which are picked up with a fine forceps or baby intestinal clamp and removed by peeling them in a circumferential fashion. A final inspection is made of the distal end of the endarterectomy in the internal and external carotid arteries, visualizing the area directly using a headlight and fine suction.

Before closure a decision is made regarding the use of a patch graft (see page 51). The arteriotomy is closed without a patch unless the artery is small.

The arteriotomy is closed with continuous 5-0 Prolene sutures beginning one at each end of the arteriotomy (Fig. 2.18). It is important that the sutures be placed just inside the cut edge and not more than a millimeter apart. Magnification helps in placing these small sutures. The arteriotomy on the internal carotid artery is progressively closed beginning distally and when the level of the bifurcation is reached the lumen is checked and gently dilated with a clamp. A second suture is then used to close the arteriotomy beginning at the proximal end on the common carotid artery. Just before the sutures are tied, back flow is allowed from both the external and internal carotid arteries so that air and any debris are flushed out of the area of the endarterectomy (Fig. 2.19). If the back flow is poor, the arteriotomy is reopened and the problem corrected. In this situation there may be an intimal flap or narrowing at the distal end of the suture line. When the closure is completed, a rubber dam is placed over the suture line and held with gentle pressure on a sponge. Blood flow is allowed first into the external carotid artery to wash out any further residual debris and then into the internal carotid artery. Bleeding from the suture line is usually not a problem and is easily controlled by gentle pressure on the rubber dam. One should not be in any hurry to close small areas of leak from the suture line because most will stop with gentle pressure and patience. Rarely, an area of persistent bleeding requires control by bringing across a flap of periarterial tissue or utilizing a small piece of muscle. Unless the hemorrhage persists, one should avoid placing additional sutures into the arteriotomy incision.

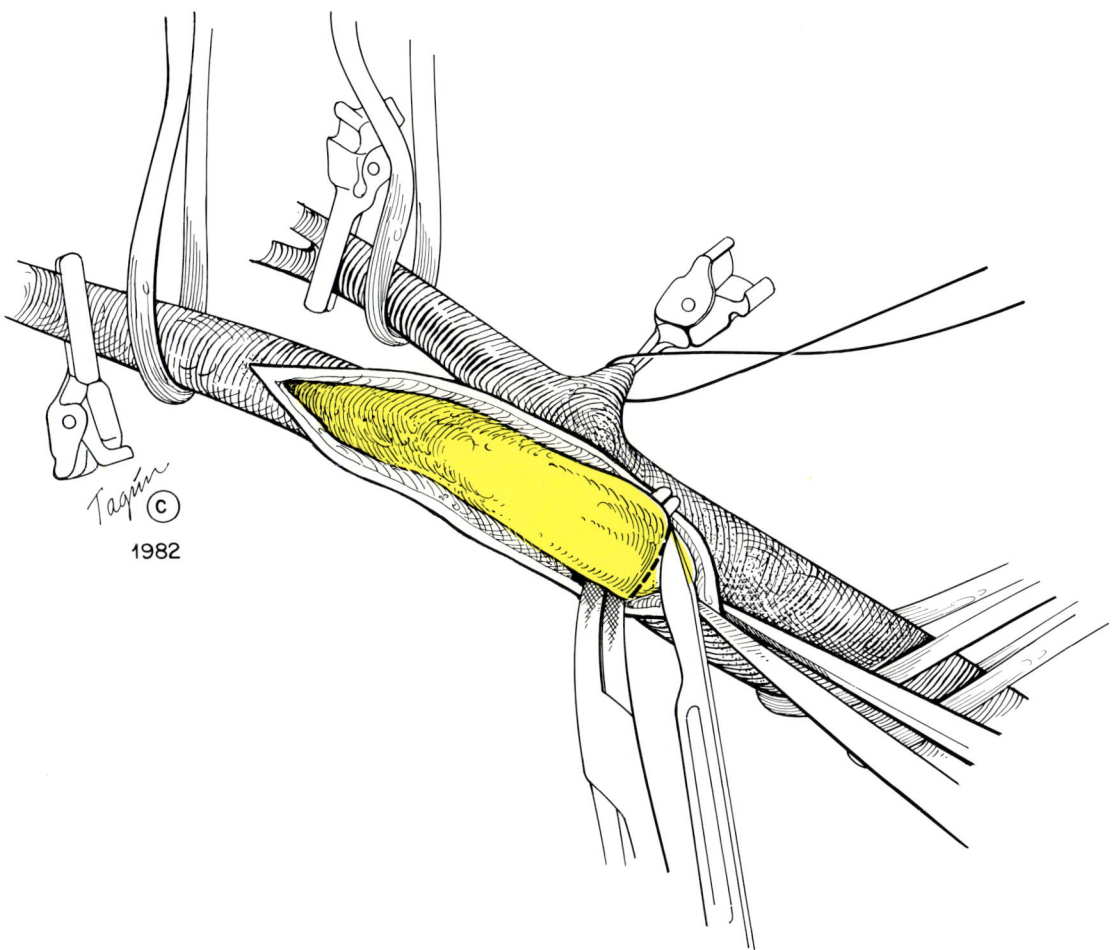

Figure 2.14. Carotid endarterectomy. A right angle clamp has been placed around the atheromatous plaque at the proximal end of the arteriotomy. The plaque is being cut off sharply with a no. 15 knife blade.

Once flow has been reestablished, the arteries are gently palpated. If there is a thrill in the internal carotid artery, the clamps are replaced and the artery reopened to correct the problem. If one is concerned about narrowing of the internal carotid lumen, a patch can be used. We use either a GORE-TEX patch or a vein graft, using the saphenous vein from the ankle. If there is a thrill in the external carotid artery, the vessel is inspected through a separate incision made on the proximal external carotid artery (Fig. 2.20). Usually a flap of intima is the cause of the problem.

A few surgeons have used routine intraoperative angiography (54, 58) or intraoperative Doppler studies for selection of patients for operative angiography (74, 97). We have not used these studies routinely but have used intraoperative angiography in patients operated for complete internal carotid artery occlusion when there is a question about the status of the artery.

At this point a decision must be made regarding reversal of the heparin. There may be some advantage to not reversing the heparin inasmuch as this may protect against thrombus formation, particularly during the first hours after the closure (82). Therefore, if hemostasis is complete, no protamine is given. If hemostasis remains a problem a partial reversal of the heparin using 20–30 mg of protamine sulfate usually solves the problem.

When hemostasis has been obtained, the operative wound is irrigated with a bacitracin solution. The platysma and subcutaneous tissue are then closed with absorbable suture material and the skin with a continuous 5-0 nylon. The authors usually do not use a drain. Some surgeons prefer to leave a drain deep to the platysma for 12–24 hours. This should be done when anticoagulation is being continued in the immediate postoperative period. The authors prefer to use a medium Hemovac for the drain. Prophylactic antibiotics, which are routinely started before the surgical incision, are continued until the drain is removed.

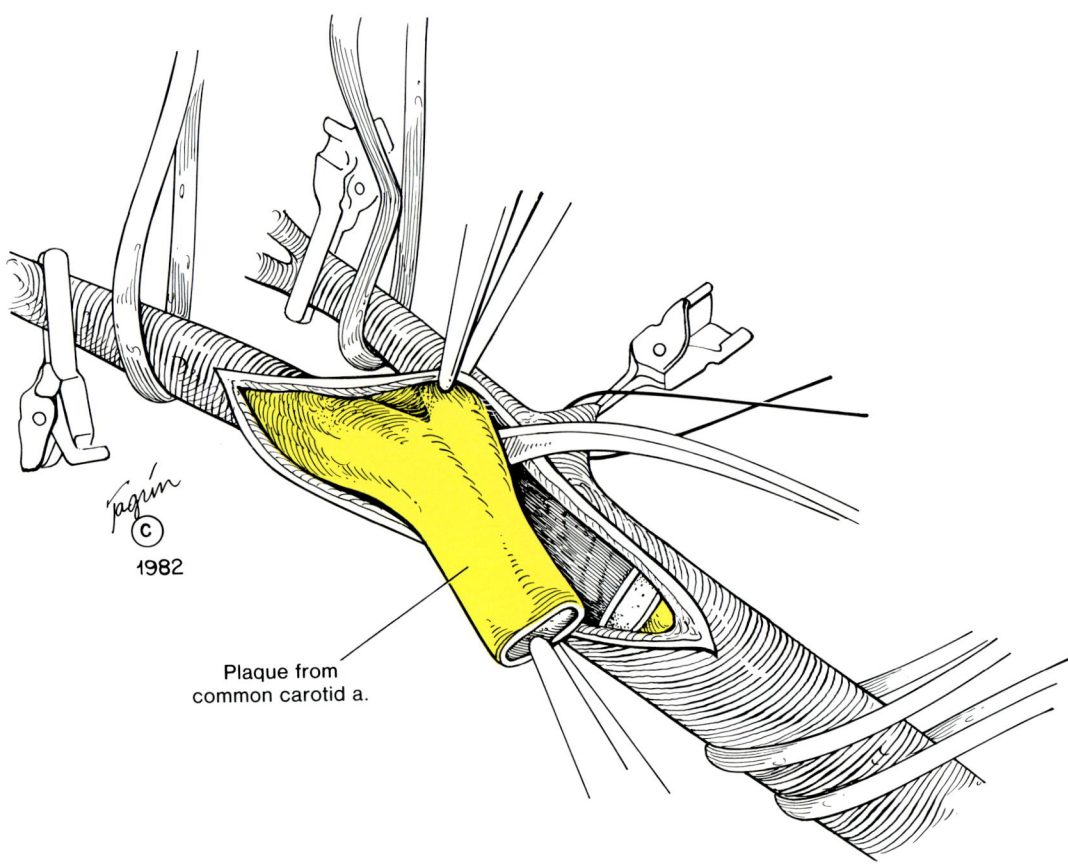

Figure 2.15. Carotid endarterectomy. The plaque has been separated from the outer wall of the common carotid artery and is now being removed from the origin of the external carotid artery.

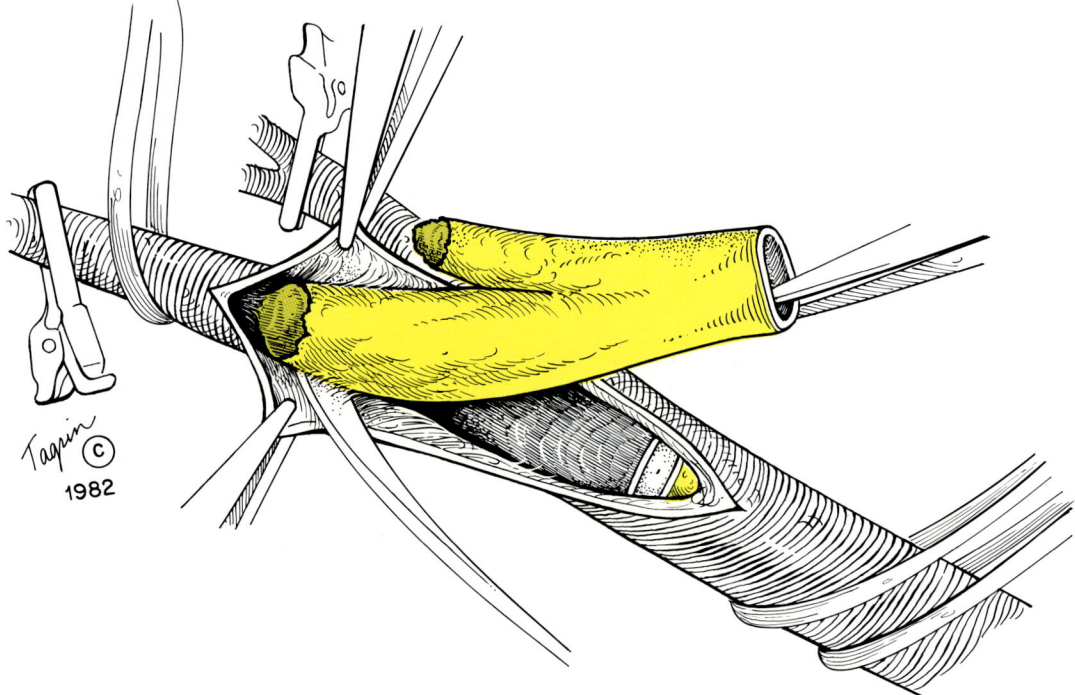

Figure 2.16. Carotid endarterectomy. The plaque is being removed from the internal carotid artery. Often the plaque may extend several millimeters farther distally on the posterior wall of the internal carotid artery.

Carotid Endarterectomy

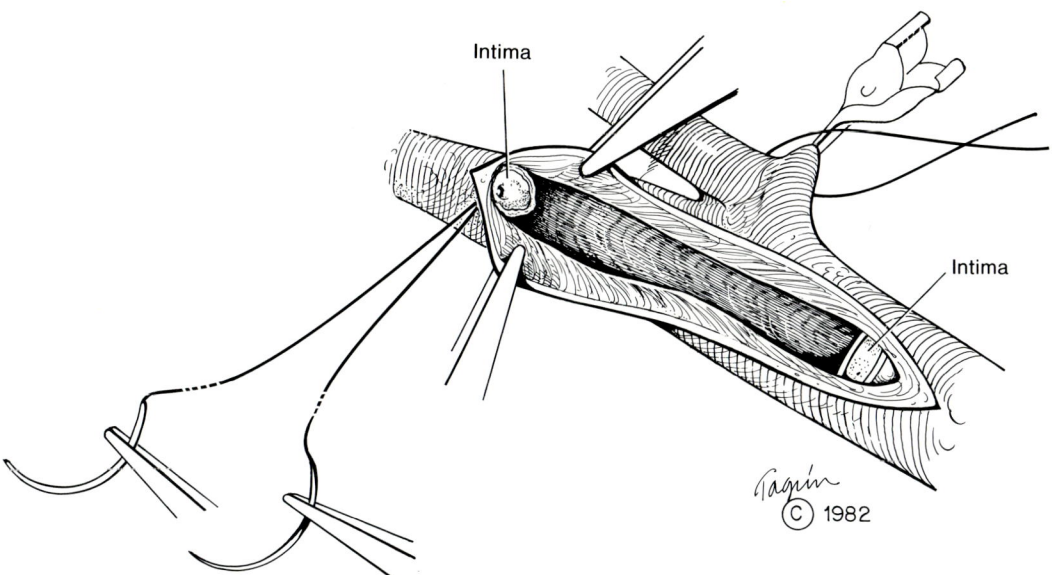

Figure 2.17. Carotid endarterectomy. Placement of sutures to tack down the distal intimal flap on the rare occasion when it is needed. The needles are put through the wall close together in an axial relationship to each other to avoid constricting the lumen.

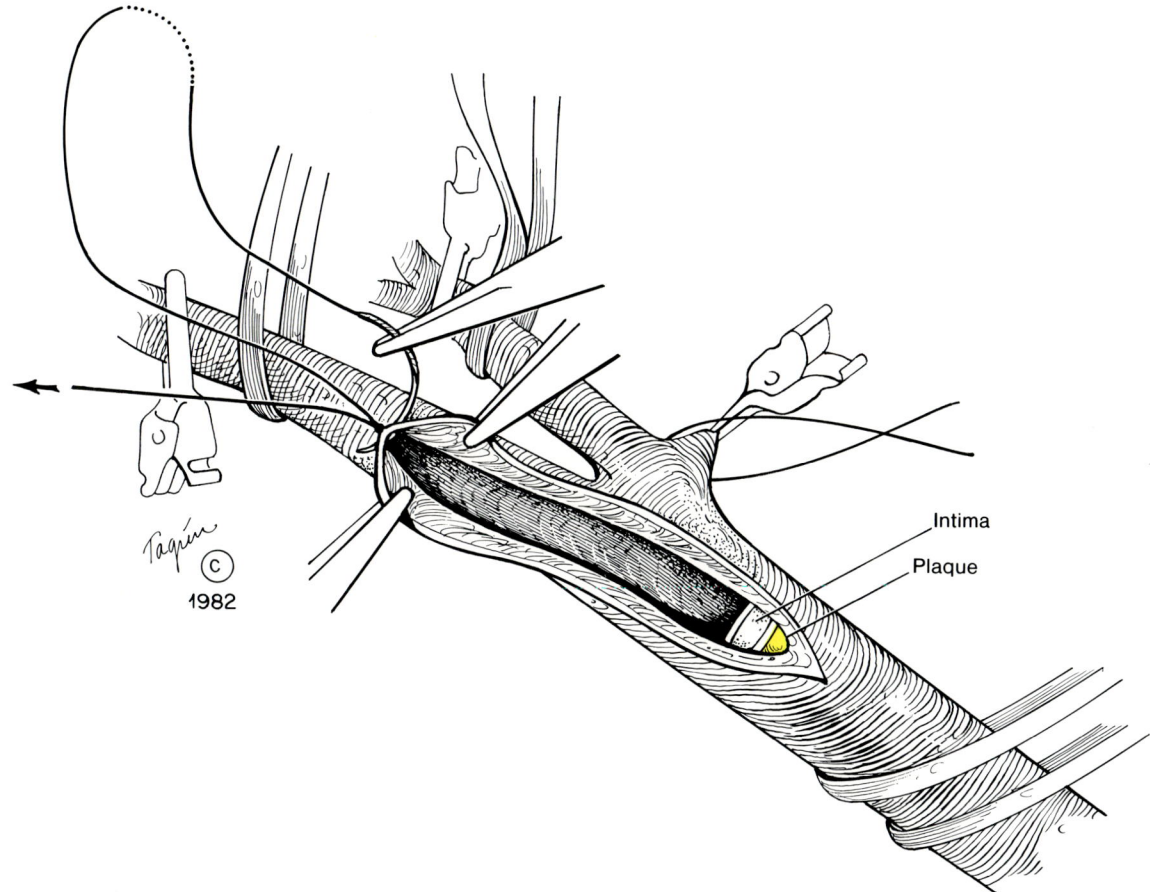

Figure 2.18. Carotid endarterectomy. Closure of the arteriotomy is started at the distal end. Care is taken to place the sutures so that there is no narrowing of the lumen.

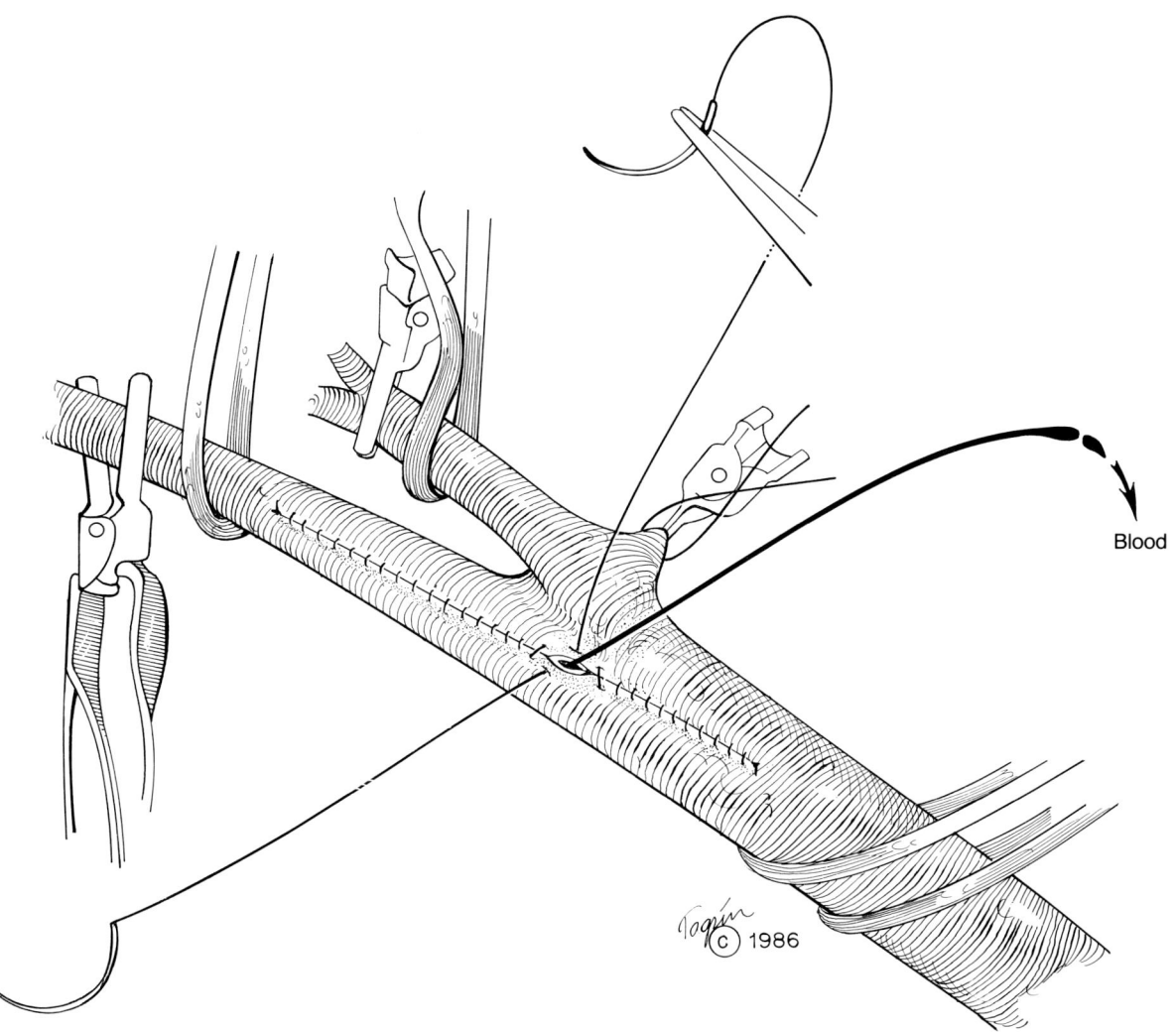

Figure 2.19. Carotid endarterectomy. Just before completing closure of the arterial incision, backflow is allowed first from the external then the internal carotid artery.

SPECIAL TECHNICAL PROBLEMS

Use of a Shunt

The authors use Argyle carotid shunt catheters. The advantage of these sterile polyethylene catheters is that the surgeon has four sizes (8, 10, 12, 14 French) immediately available which are the correct length (15 cm) and have smooth ends. A suture is tied around the midportion of the catheter to serve as a marker, to be sure the tube has not slipped, and to help with the removal of the shunt. Other types of shunts have been described (30, 46, 79).

If there is a severe change in the EEG after arterial clamps and clips are placed, a rapid arteriotomy incision is made including the plaque, starting a few millimeters more proximally on the common carotid artery than one would normally start, and extending the incision a few millimeters more distally on the internal carotid artery (Fig. 2.21). The shunt tube is first passed distally into the internal carotid artery visualizing the intima so that a flap is not dissected by the tip of the catheter. A tourniquet gently snugs the arterial wall around the shunt. The shunt is checked to be certain there is satisfactory backflow of blood. The catheter is temporarily occluded and then passed proximally into the common carotid artery and the tourniquet is tightened (Fig. 2.22). The clamp is removed from the shunt catheter. The catheter usually remains outside the lumen at this point (Fig. 2.23). The plaque can then be dissected and removed. The proximal end of the plaque can be cut around the shunt with Potts scissors. The shunt tube is then placed in the arterial lumen. Often the distal catheter must be temporarily removed (with cross-clamping) to complete removal of the plaque. To avoid an intimal flap the surgeon must not let the shunt interfere with meticulous endarterectomy. Approximately two-thirds of the arteriotomy incision is then closed in the usual fashion with a continuous suture

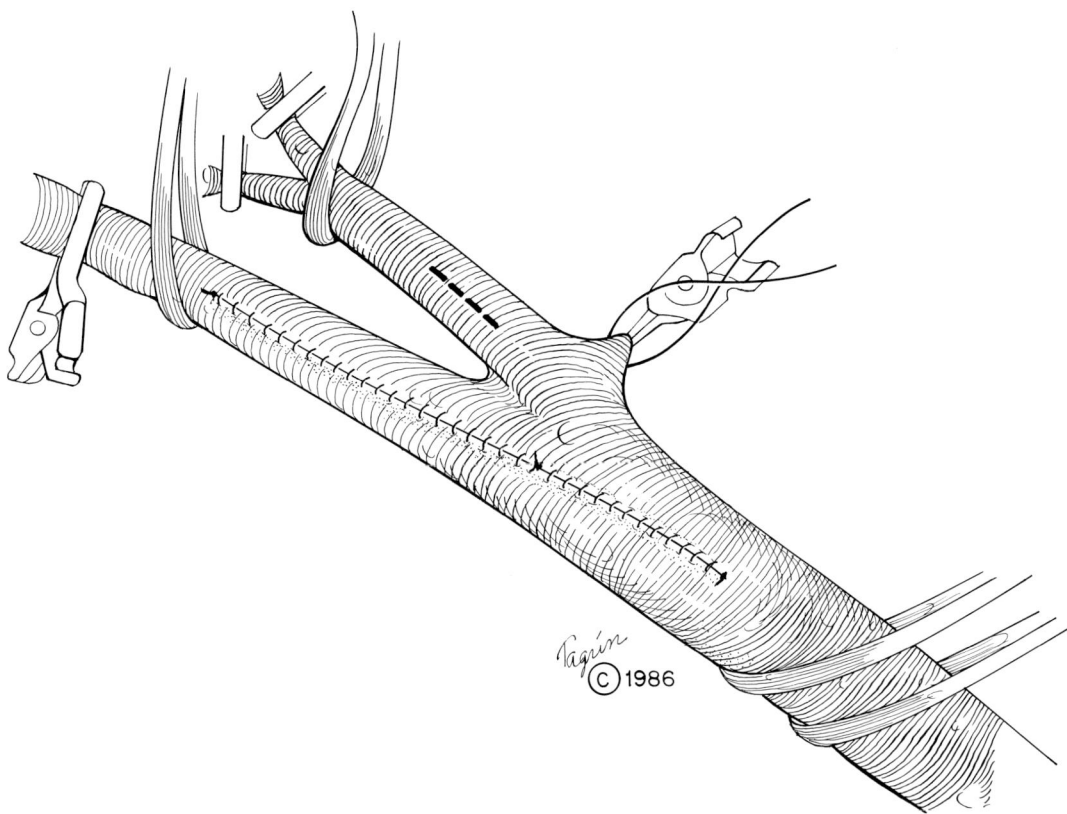

Figure 2.20. Carotid endarterectomy. If there is a thrill or reduced pulse in the external carotid artery the branches are dissected, separately occluded, and an incision made to look for a flap of intima or retained piece of atheroma.

beginning on the internal carotid artery. A second suture is then started at the proximal end of the arteriotomy on the common carotid artery and is sutured distally to within 2 mm of the previously placed suture. The catheter is then clamped and removed. Sometimes this is facilitated by utilizing two fine clamps and cutting the catheter between them. As the catheter is removed, bleeding is controlled initially with a tourniquet and then occluding clamps are placed on the common and internal carotid arteries. The closure of the arteriotomy is then completed, the sutures are tied, and the remainder of the operation is done as previously described.

An alternative method can be used when the EEG changes are not immediate or are not very severe. This consists of proceeding first with careful removal of the plaque, which usually takes only 5–10 minutes and then placing the shunt once the surgeon has ascertained that the distal lumen of the internal carotid artery is perfectly clean. After the shunt is in place, the surgeon can proceed leisurely to remove any residual bits of plaque from the common and the external carotid artery and then close the arteriotomy without unwarranted haste as described before. This method has the advantage of minimizing the risk of embolization or intimal dissection from placing the shunt before the plaque has been removed from the internal carotid artery. There is considerable evidence to suggest that the 5 or 10 minutes required to remove the plaque are unlikely to result in a permanent ischemic deficit (7, 63)

Insertion of a Patch Graft

With the routine use of magnification (loupes) for the endarterectomy, the authors have found that in most cases the arterial incision can be closed with a continuous 5-0 Prolene running suture. When the internal carotid artery appears to be too small for satisfactory closure or it appears that closure will compromise the lumen, there is no hesitation in using a patch graft. In most patients with recurrent stenosis, a patch graft is used because of scar formation in the wall of the artery. Some surgeons use a patch routinely (82). In one report early postoperative intravenous digital subtraction angiograms suggested that use of a saphenous vein patch graft was superior to primary closure of the arteriotomy (56) and in another report recurrent internal carotid artery stenosis was less common when routine patch graft was used (80). However, in the experience of the authors, postoperative noninvasive studies show excellent results from primary closure.

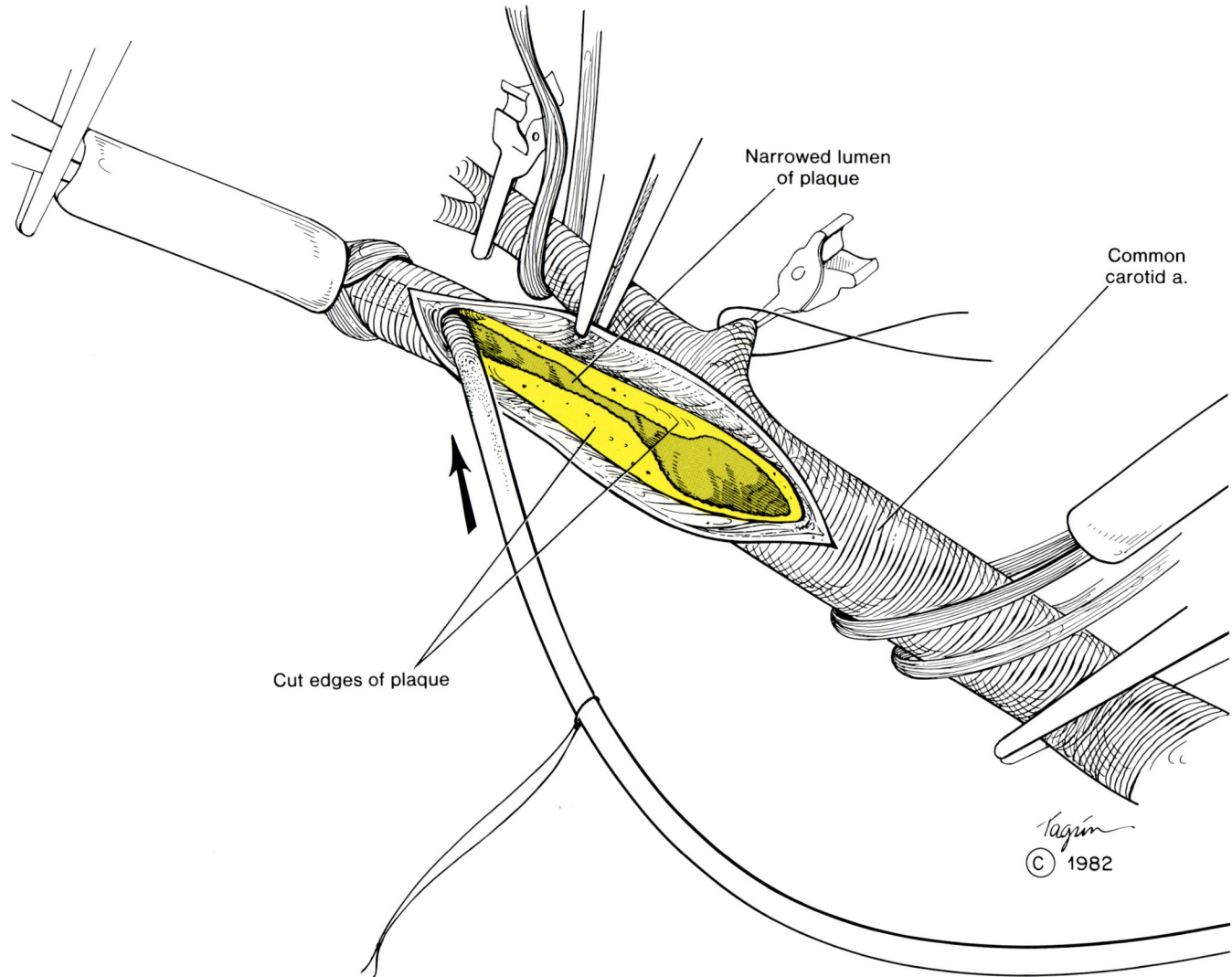

Figure 2.21. Carotid endarterectomy: placement of a shunt. The shunt is first passed distally into the internal carotid artery.

The patch graft can be made from either a saphenous vein taken from the ankle, GORE-TEX, or a preclotted knitted Dacron patch. We usually use one of the latter two for convenience and to save saphenous veins for possible future vascular surgery. The patch is cut to fit the arteriotomy as illustrated (Fig. 2.24). The graft is usually about 6 mm in width in the central portion and tapers to a blunt point at each end. A double-armed suture of 5-0 Prolene is used at each end. One arm of the suture is placed at the distal tip of the graft from outer to inner surface and then carefully placed at the distal end of the arteriotomy from inside the lumen to the outer wall. The other arm of the suture is placed in a similar fashion very close to the first and the suture is tied with two throws. The final length of the graft is then determined and another double-armed suture is placed in a similar fashion in the proximal end of the graft (Fig. 2.25).

One of the sutures is then used for a continuous closure on each side of the graft (Fig. 2.26). Just before completing the closure, backflow is allowed as is done in the usual endarterectomy closure.

Stenosis at C2 Level

Occasionally, the carotid bifurcation will be quite high in the neck or the stenosis will be localized at the C2 level (Fig. 2.27). This finding does not preclude carotid endarterectomy.

By using the full upper extent of the incision as outlined, staying on the sternocleidomastoid muscle beneath the parotid gland and following the plane between the internal jugular vein laterally and the hypoglossal nerve medially, the internal carotid artery can be exposed to the C1 level well above the stenosis. It may be necessary to divide the occipital artery and retract or at times even divide the posterior

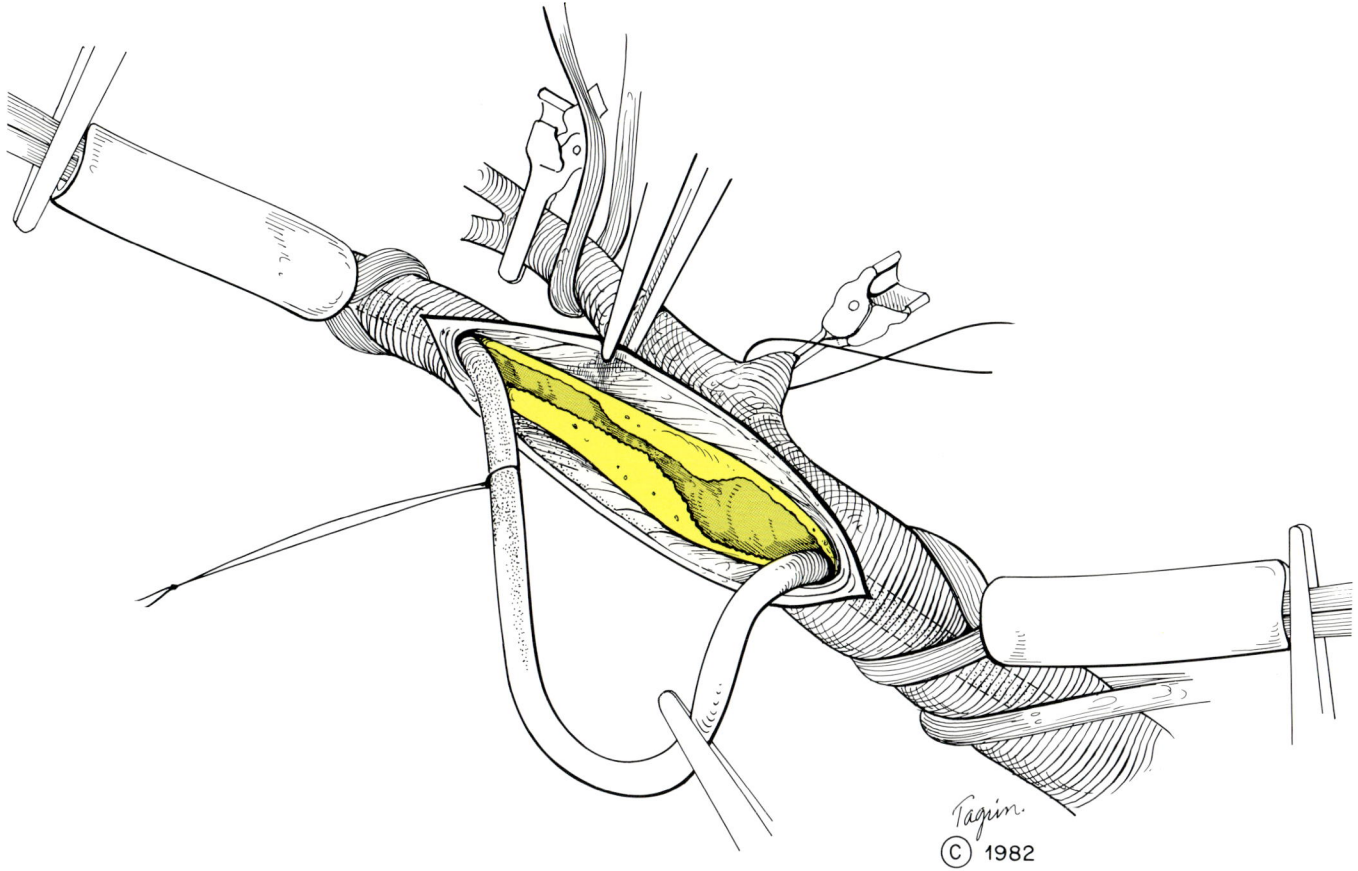

Figure 2.22. Carotid endarterectomy: placement of a shunt. The proximal portion of the shunt has been placed in the common carotid artery.

belly of the digastric muscle. We have not found it necessary to use a mandibular osteotomy (2) or mandibular subluxation (28).

Abnormal Arterial Anatomy

In a small number of patients there may be a significant loop of the extracranial internal carotid artery distal to the stenosis (Fig 2.28A and B). Care must be taken in dissection of these loops because postoperative kinking can occur with occlusion and resultant infarction (63). We try to leave the loop adherent to the posterior periarterial tissue to avoid this problem. Usually, one will need to dissect the artery distal to the loop to place the controlling tape because the atheroma may extend right up to the proximal part of the curve (Fig. 2.29). Should the loop become mobile, it may be held in place by periarterial sutures or a place made for it. In one patient, a large loop was positioned in a plane dissected under the internal jugular vein.

Unusual arterial anatomy may be found. In three patients in the authors' series, a branch arose from the internal carotid artery approximately 1.0 cm distal to its origin. This was likely a persistent hypoglossal artery. The vessel was occluded by atheromatous plaque and was not seen on the angiogram. A large ascending pharyngeal artery may arise from the anterior part of the bifurcation. In one patient, a superior thyroid artery originated from the lateral aspect of the common carotid artery and passed medially across the bifurcation (Fig. 2.30). The internal carotid artery arose medially and then turned beneath the external carotid artery to assume a more normal lateral position.

In some patients with severe carotid stenosis, the distal internal carotid artery is quite small in diameter due to reduced intravascular pressure. This has been described as the "slim" sign on the angiogram (Fig. 1.2) (55). The artery tends to dilate almost immediately when normal pressure is restored. It should not be mechanically dilated. Sometimes a patch graft is needed, but often with the use of magnification the arteriotomy can be closed primarily.

Complete Internal Carotid Artery Occlusion

When the angiogram indicates complete internal carotid artery occlusion, changes in the operative ap-

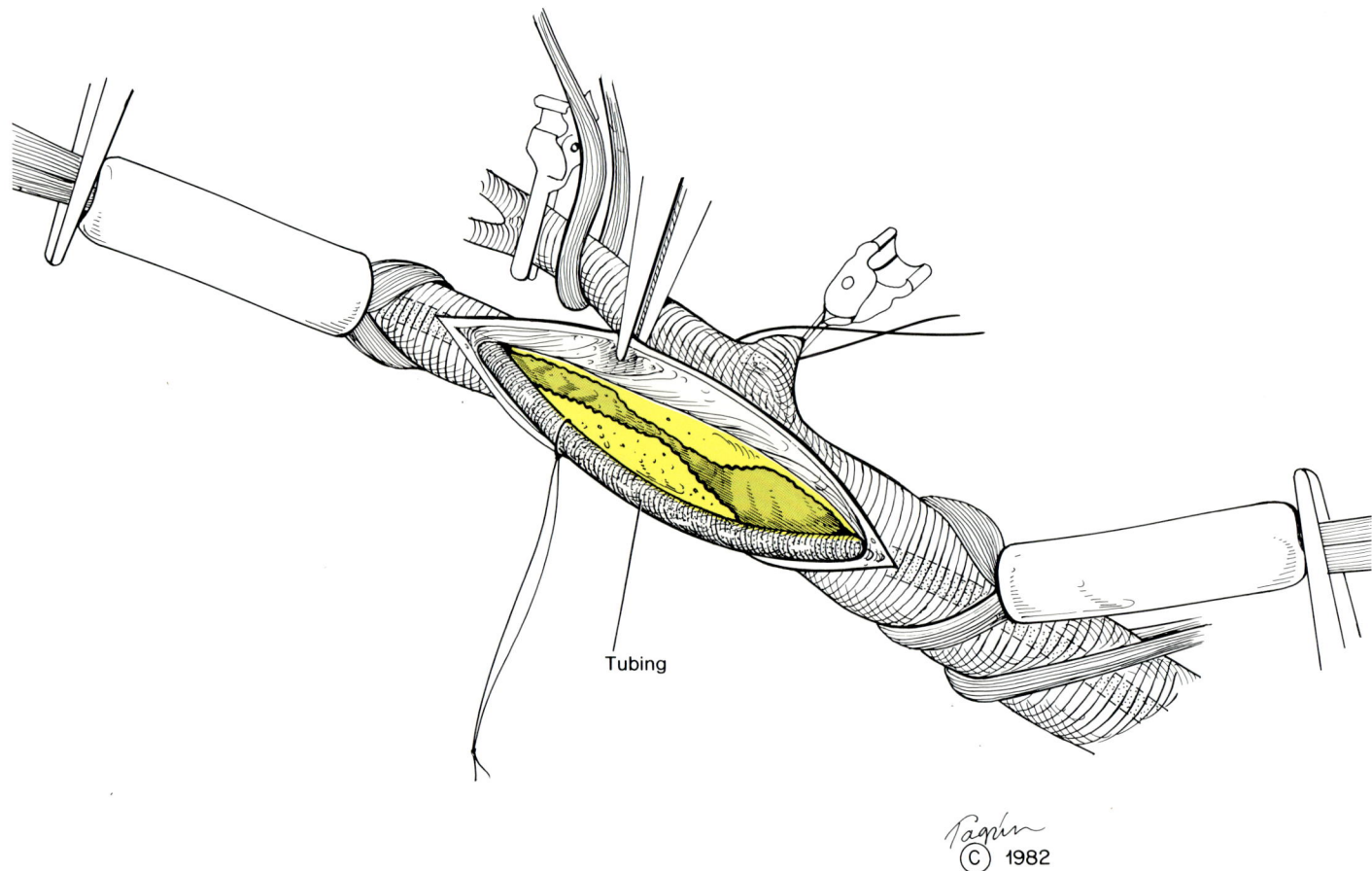

Figure 2.23. Carotid endarterectomy: placement of a shunt. The shunt tube has been positioned so that the endarterectomy can be done.

proach may be indicated. If the operation is being done as an emergency for acute neurologic deficit, every effort is made to expedite the surgery. Great care is taken to avoid hypotension.

An incision is made on the internal carotid artery distal to the plaque without occluding the common and external carotid arteries (Fig. 2.31). In the majority of patients a thrombus will be found, but in some the lumen of the internal carotid artery will be open distal to the atheromatous plaque (41). If the thrombus can be removed and backflow established, the endarterectomy is done as described. In some patients with complete occlusion of the internal carotid artery, the external carotid artery may supply significant collateral flow to the brain and a common external carotid artery shunt is used. If there is a long-standing occlusion, the internal carotid artery may be a firm fibrous cord and no further procedures are indicated.

Certain techniques may help in opening the completely occluded artery. If a thrombus is encountered in the internal carotid artery, an effort is made to withdraw it gradually with forceps using a hand-over-hand technique. Thrombi as long as 20 cm have been removed (Fig. 2.32). If this technique fails, a smooth-ended suction catheter is introduced into the internal carotid artery lumen until resistance is felt. Suction is then applied and this may withdraw the thrombus. If this method fails, a Fogerty no. 3 catheter is passed gently as far as the base of the skull, inflated, and withdrawn (34). Care is required to avoid injuring the distal internal carotid artery with subsequent development of a carotid-cavernous fistula (16). Measurements on the angiogram from the internal carotid artery origin to the base of the skull may help in determining the safe length of catheter which may be inserted. A single lateral intraoperative angiogram with 10 cc of Renograffin 70 via an Argyle shunt catheter is recommended to document restoration of flow without intimal flap or distal thrombus. When flow is reestablished, anticoagulation should be continued in the postoperative period (52). If good backflow from the internal carotid artery cannot be achieved or the artery is occluded, the origin of the internal carotid artery is oversewn to give a smooth lumen (Fig. 2.33).

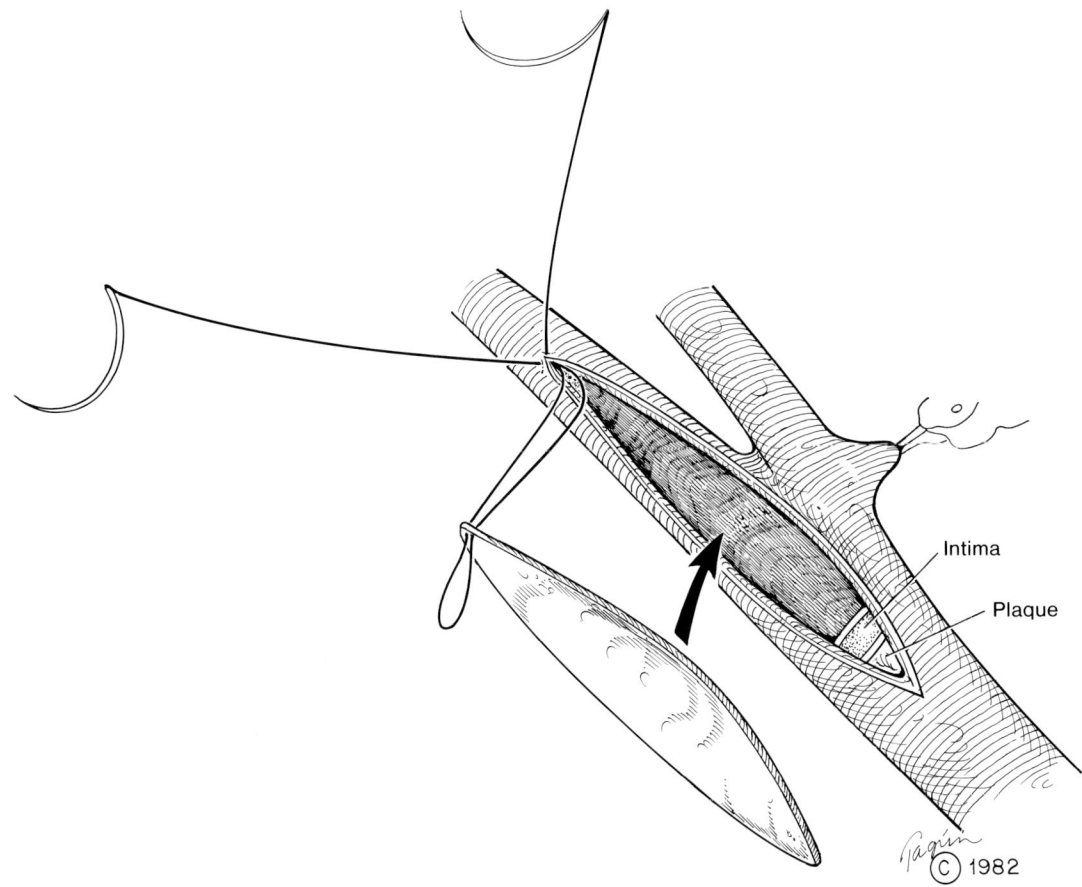

Figure 2.24. Carotid endarterectomy. Insertion of patch graft.

External Carotid Stenosis

If it is thought that external carotid artery stenosis is the cause of symptoms and the occluded internal carotid artery cannot be opened, an incision is made on the common carotid artery and extended onto the external carotid artery (36, 39, 75). Endarterectomy, including the proximal internal carotid artery, should be done in the usual fashion being sure to obliterate the origin of the internal carotid artery. The origin of the internal carotid artery is oversewn with double-armed 3-0 Prolene mattress sutures. Complete dissection of the bifurcation and use of a hemostat are helpful in placement of these sutures (53, 75) (Fig. 2.33). If the external carotid collateral is crucial for cerebral circulation, a shunt may be needed. Removal of the external carotid artery stenosis in association with the endarterectomy for internal carotid artery stenosis may require a separate incision in the external carotid artery (48).

When a proximal stump in the internal carotid artery is thought to be the source of the embolus, the operative procedure is an endarterectomy of the carotid bifurcation to include the distal common and proximal external carotid arteries. Exclusion of the stump of the proximal internal carotid artery is done by oversewing the origin of the artery to give a smooth lumen (4, 38) (Fig. 2.33). In one report of 17 patients, patch graft angioplasty was used (5), but usually this is unnecessary.

Percutaneous transluminal angioplasty was reported to be successful in 9 of 10 patients with external carotid artery stenosis in whom the internal carotid artery was occluded (92). The procedure was done in preparation for an extracranial to intracranial bypass graft.

Common Carotid Artery Stenosis and Occlusion

Occlusion of the common carotid artery is usually due to one of two atheromatous lesions. The plaque either involves the distal common carotid artery and/or both the external and internal carotid artery with development of a retrograde thrombus, or the atheromatous plaque is located at the origin of the common carotid artery and antegrade thrombus develops. The former circumstance is more common.

The problem should be initially approached as one

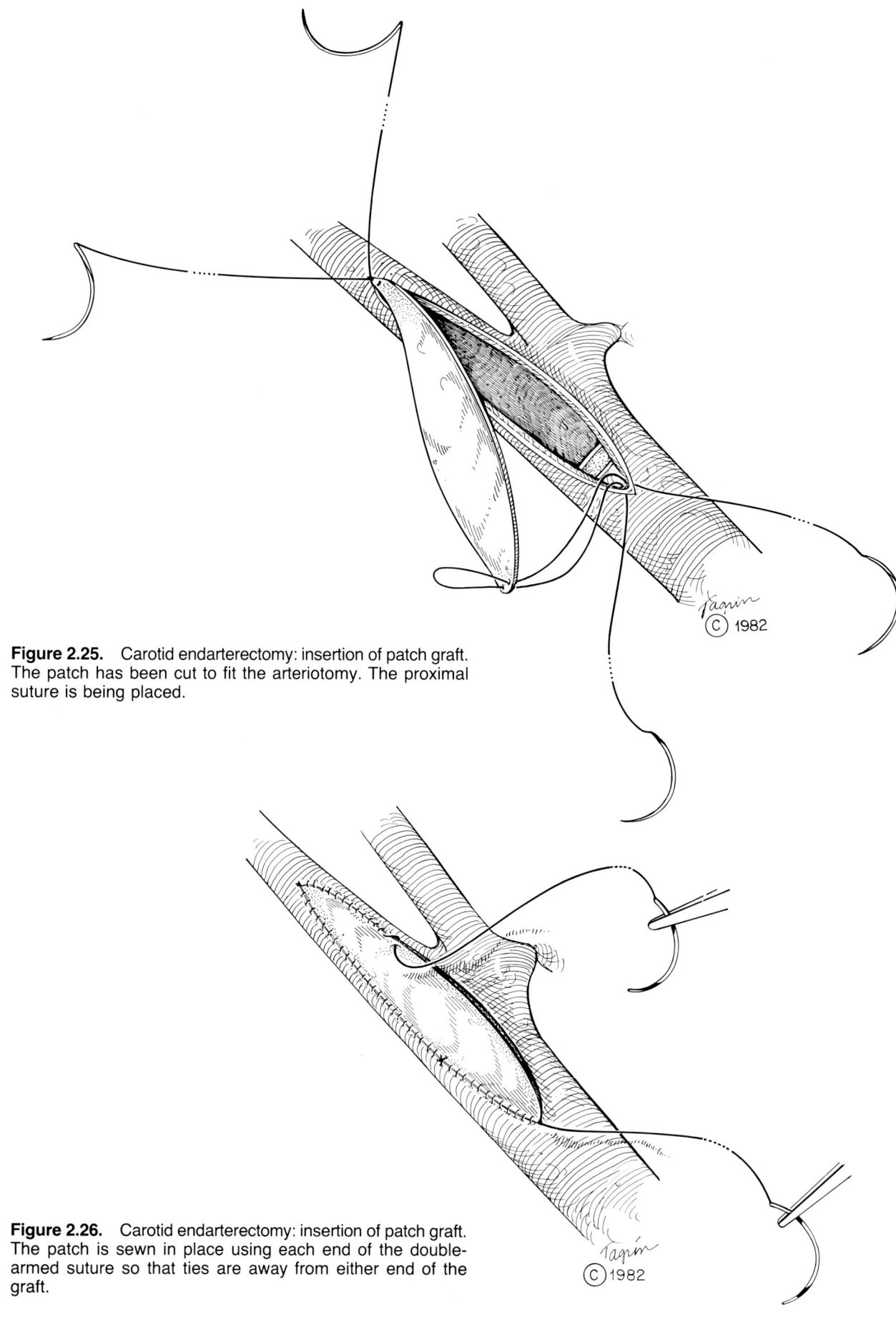

Figure 2.25. Carotid endarterectomy: insertion of patch graft. The patch has been cut to fit the arteriotomy. The proximal suture is being placed.

Figure 2.26. Carotid endarterectomy: insertion of patch graft. The patch is sewn in place using each end of the double-armed suture so that ties are away from either end of the graft.

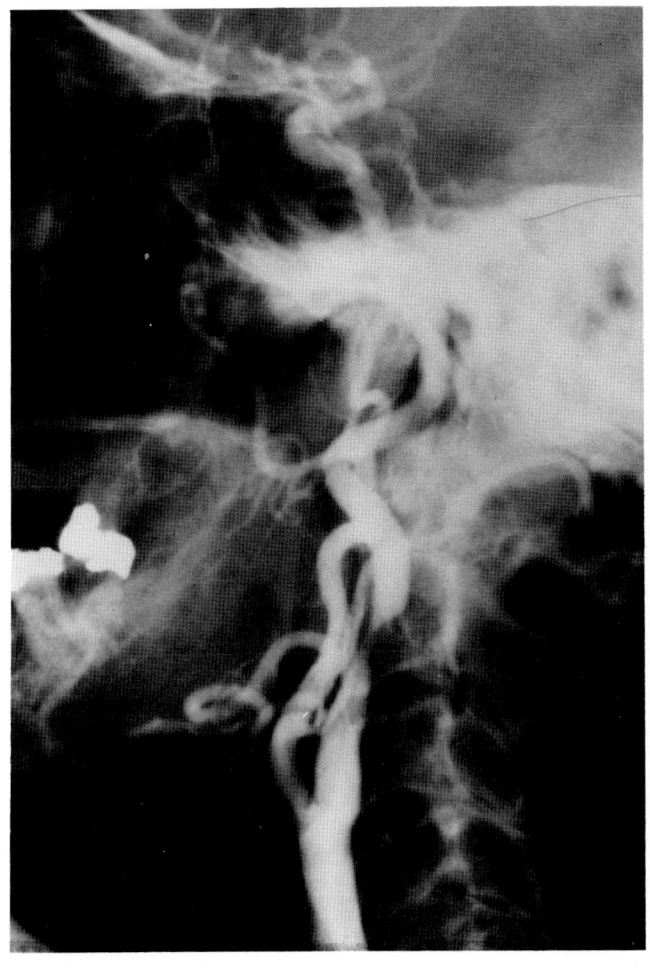

Figure 2.27. Internal carotid artery stenosis localized at the C2 level. Occasionally, atherosclerosis can cause localized stenosis 3–4 cm distal to the bifurcation. The finding of a lesion at the C2 level does not preclude surgery. Good exposure can be obtained by following the techniques outlined.

would for a carotid endarterectomy. If inspection of the distal common carotid artery and bifurcation region reveals significant atheromatous plaque, this plaque is removed, and if this appears to be the site of the occlusion with retrograde thrombus, a thrombectomy is attempted. Careful dissection identifies the plane between the organized thrombus and the arterial intima. The thrombus is divided and a smooth, large endarterectomy stripper is passed over the thrombus in the plane between the thrombus and the intima. The stripper is advanced down the lumen and if there is no significant proximal atherosclerosis, the thrombus will be freed and the thrombotic core pushed out by the head of arterial pressure. A Fogarty catheter may then be used to be sure the lumen is clean. The closure then follows the procedure described for carotid bifurcation endarterectomy, being sure to allow flow first up the external carotid artery. On rare occasions, the occlusion will involve only the distal common carotid artery (Fig. 1.26)

If the initial exploration of the carotid bifurcation reveals a thrombus in the common carotid artery without significant atheromatous occlusion in the region of the carotid bifurcation, there is likely to be atheromatous occlusion at the origin of the common carotid artery. This occurs more frequently on the left side. At this point partial thrombectomy is done. The common carotid artery is occluded to exclude the proximal thrombus. If it is deemed advisable to restore circulation to this artery, a bypass graft is done from the subclavian artery, from a point distal to the vertebral artery, to the common carotid artery (68). Although only a small number of cases have been reported, this procedure seems preferable to doing a sternotomy and trying to reconstruct the origin of the common carotid artery.

Occasionally, symptomatic stenosis may involve the midportion of the common carotid artery (Fig. 1.25). Usually, this is treated with endarterectomy. Two patients have been reported where catheter dilatation of a proximal common carotid stenosis was combined with a distal bifurcation endarterectomy (9, 51). There were no complications.

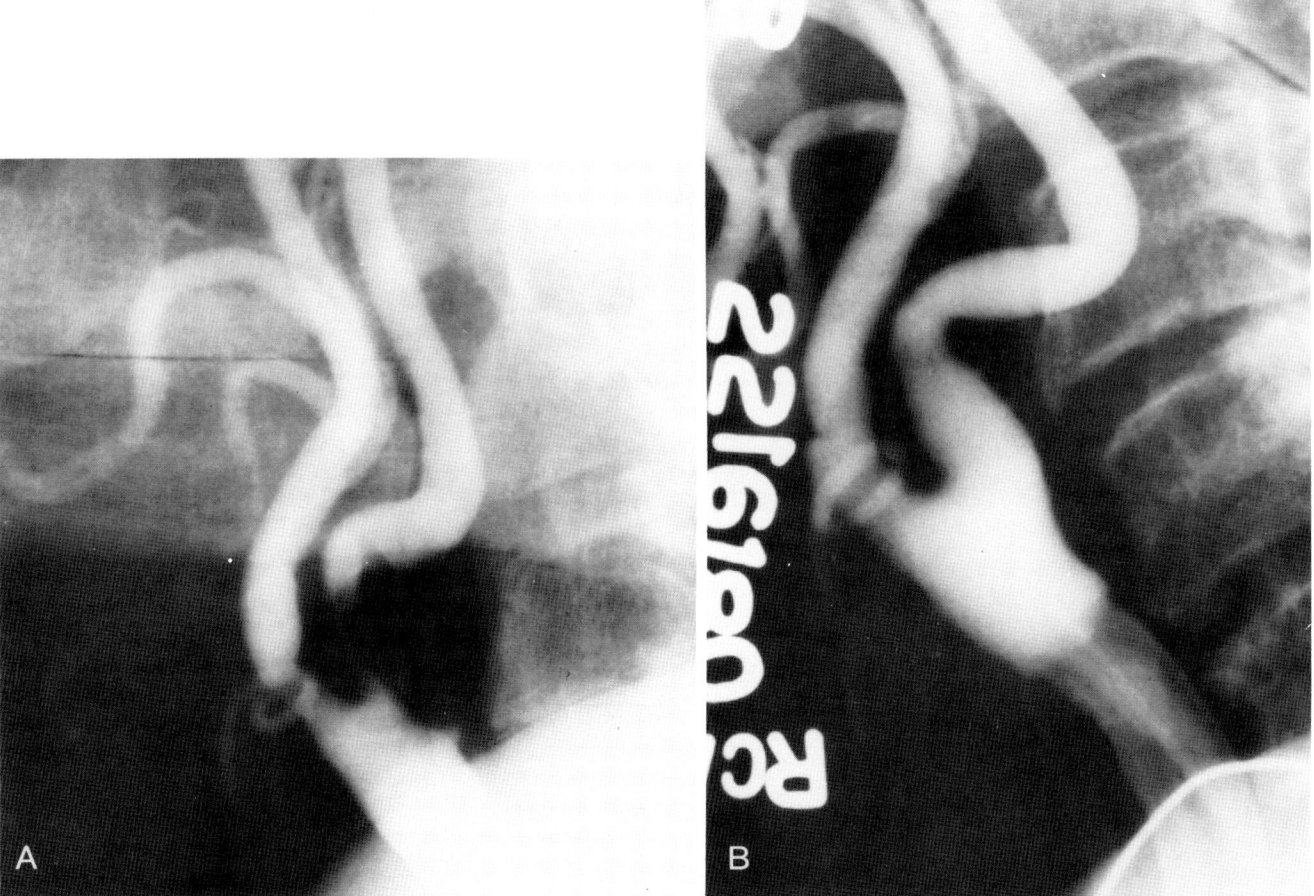

Figure 2.28. Loop in the internal carotid artery. **A**, Angiogram of bifurcation shows such severe stenosis at the origin of the internal carotid artery that only a minute thread of dye can be seen. A prominent loop in the internal carotid artery is also apparent and atheroma extends beyond the first curve. **B**, Postoperative angiogram showing restoration of normal lumen. There is slight narrowing at the proximal loop.

Extrinsic Compression of the Internal Carotid Artery

A rare case of extrinsic compression due to a hypertrophied digastric muscle and fascial band causing positional transient ischemic attacks (TIAs) has been documented by angiography (22). Symptoms were relieved by division of the muscle and the band.

POSTOPERATIVE MANAGEMENT

Medical Therapy

After completion of surgery, the patient's vital signs and neurologic functions are monitored carefully in an intensive care unit. Systolic blood pressure is generally maintained in the range of 110–150 mm Hg with efforts to avoid both hypotension and hypertension. If hypotension develops, the ECG is checked. Mild hypotension will usually respond to administration of fluid or colloid. The phenylephrine drip is available if needed. If the hypotension does not immediately respond to volume replacement, a CVP monitor is inserted. If the CVP is maintained in the range of 5–10 cm with judicious utilization of fluid, this problem will generally resolve (85). On occasion, bradycardia may develop, and administration of atropine may be necessary. Bradycardia and hypotension may be the result of increased pressure waves reaching the carotid sinus receptors after removal of the plaque (85). The blood pressure and pulse usually return to normal level within a few hours.

Control of postoperative hypertension is also important and there is a significant incidence of this problem (10, 90). In one series, the incidence of neurologic morbidity was higher in those patients with severe hypertension (90). Patients who develop postoperative systolic readings which are persistently maintained above 170 mm Hg require treatment with rapid-acting intravenous antihypertensive medication. We have utilized either sodium nitroprusside or nitroglycerin infusions until long-acting antihypertensive medications such as propranolol or hy-

Carotid Endarterectomy

Figure 2.29. Loop in the internal carotid artery: operative exposure. When a significant loop is present in the internal carotid artery beyond the stenosis, that portion of the artery distal to the loop must be exposed and care taken not to disturb any more of the artery than is necessary.

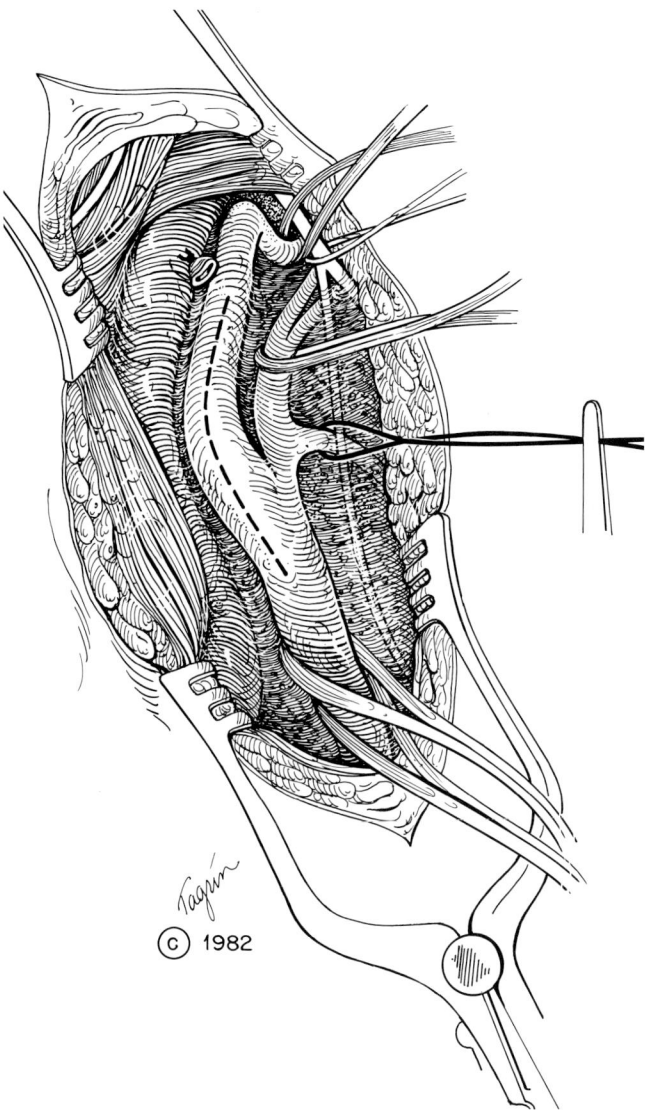

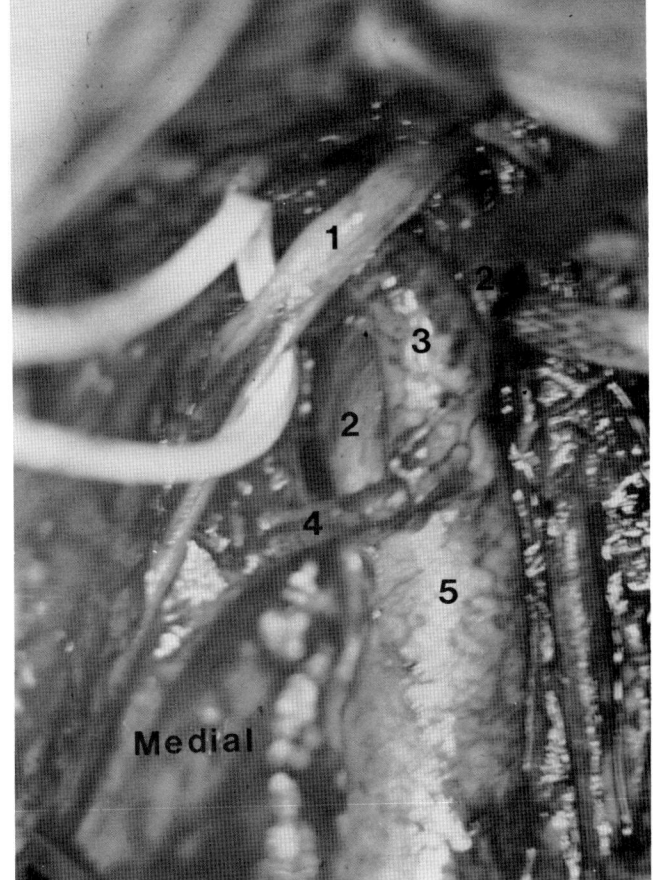

Figure 2.30. Unusual anatomy in region of the left carotid bifurcation. There is reversal of the normal origin of the internal and external carotid arteries. **1**, Hypoglossal and descendens hypoglossal nerves. **2**, Internal carotid artery arising medially and then passing behind. **3**, The external carotid artery which originates laterally and then turns medially. **4**, Superior thyroid artery arising from lateral wall of **5**, the distal common carotid artery, and then passing across the bifurcation to go medially. (From Ojemann RG, Crowell RM, Roberson GH, Fisher CM: Surgical treatment of extracranial carotid occlusive disease. In: *Clinical Neurosurgery.* Baltimore, Williams & Wilkins, 1974, vol 22, chap 14.)

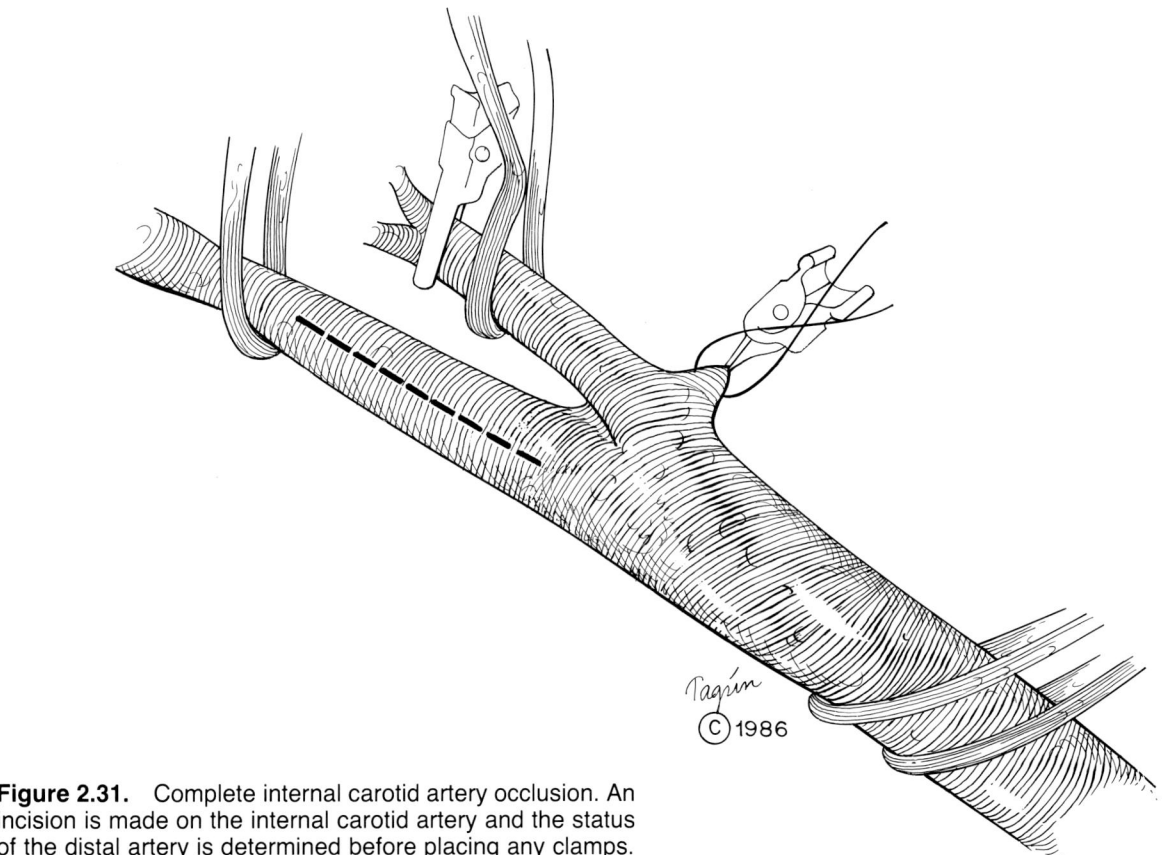

Figure 2.31. Complete internal carotid artery occlusion. An incision is made on the internal carotid artery and the status of the distal artery is determined before placing any clamps.

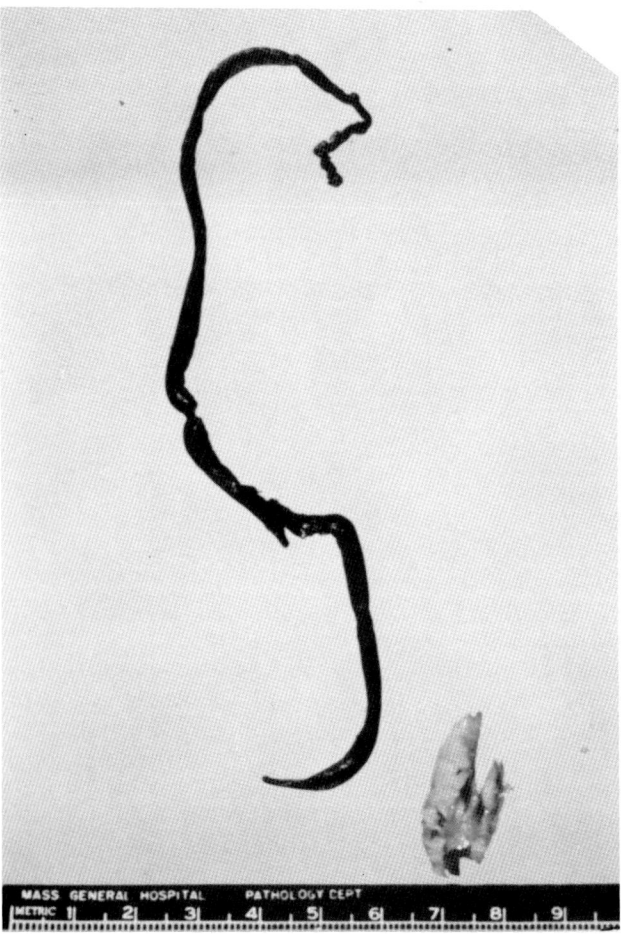

Figure 2.32. Removal of thrombus from internal carotid artery. Angiography showed a complete occlusion of the internal carotid artery. By carefully withdrawing the thrombus using forceps and with the help of back pressure from the collateral circulation, this long thrombus was removed and flow reestablished. (Courtesy of Dr. Charles Poletti).

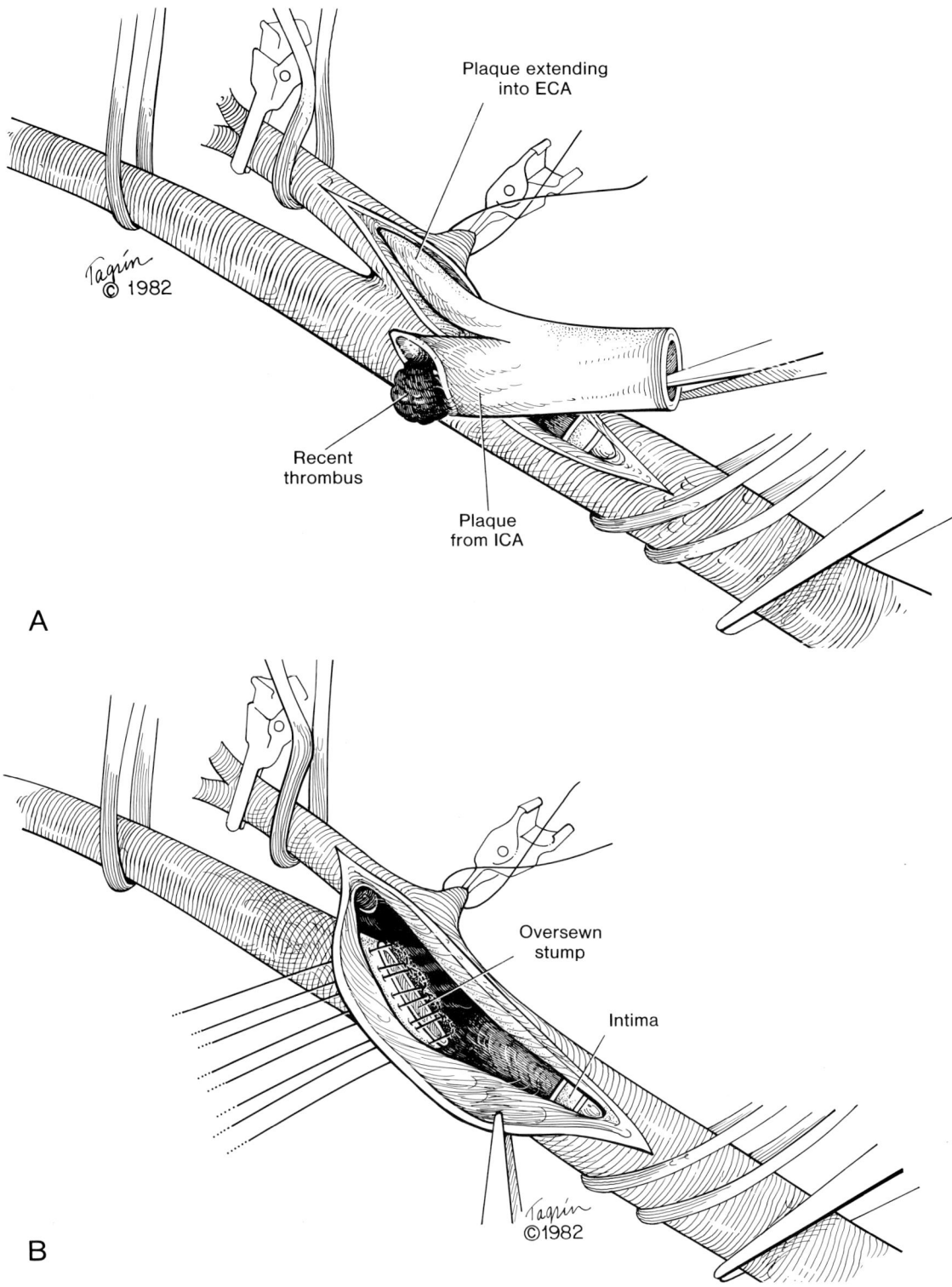

Figure 2.33. Endarterectomy for stump embolus. **A**, Endarterectomy is performed by making the arteriotomy incision onto the external carotid artery and removing a portion of the thrombus from the proximal internal carotid artery. **B**, Interrupted mattress sutures are placed across the origin of the internal carotid artery to obliterate the stump and give a smooth internal lumen. **C**, Closure is completed as shown. **D**, Operative specimen showing the thrombus in the stump of the internal carotid artery projecting into the lumen of the common carotid artery.

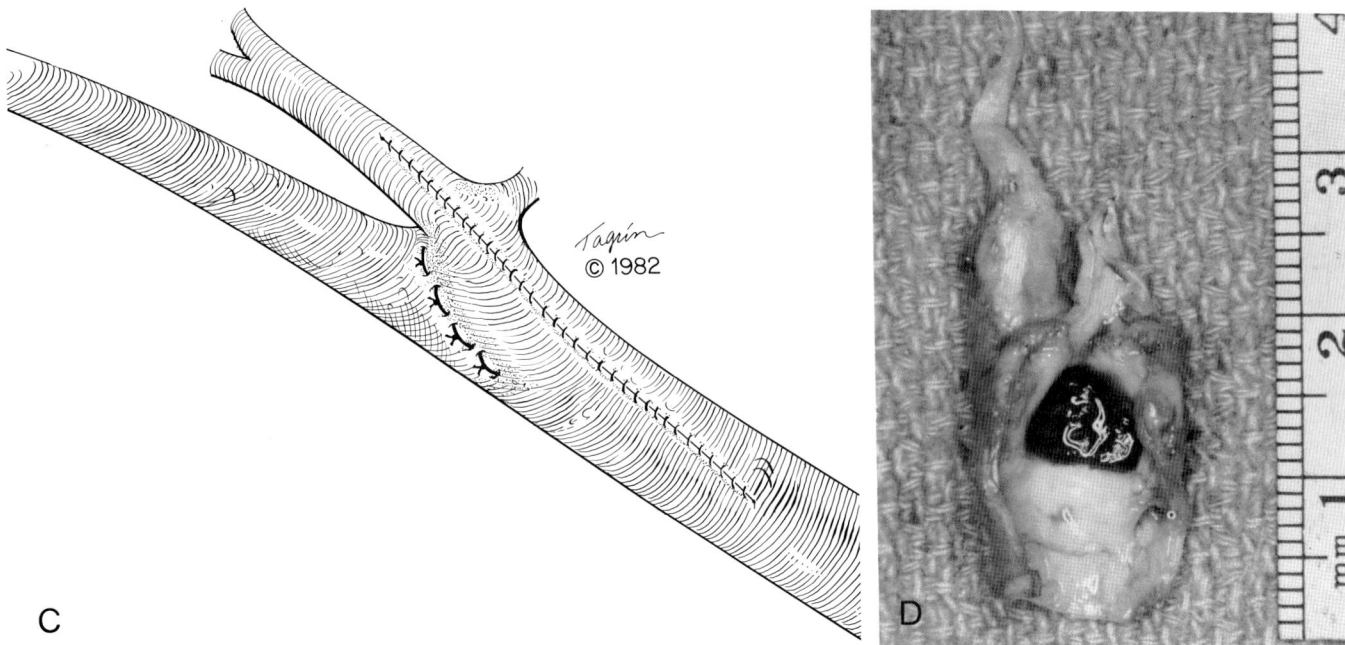

Figure 2.33 C and D.

dralazine become effective. We have encountered intracerebral hemorrhage with postoperative hypertension, as previously reported, but with the careful control of postoperative blood pressure, this complication has been rare (10,63).

Intravenous nitroglycerin is also used to control ECG changes. Subinguinal nitroglycerin is given for angina. Myocardial infarction is the most important systemic complication and accounts for the majority of the early postoperative deaths (35).

Generally, anticoagulation has not been utilized except when dissection was difficult, the endarterectomy plane seemed roughened, the plaque was particularly long, or a complete occlusion had been reopened. Heparin is used in a dose of 500 units/hr for the first few hours, then is adjusted to keep the PTT at about 50–60 seconds. A special circumstance where anticoagulation should probably be continued occurs when the patient has an asymptomatic middle cerebral artery stenosis or a severe contralateral internal carotid artery stenosis. In one patient, occlusion of a previously asymptomatic opposite middle cerebral artery stenosis led to a neurologic deficit.

In the late postoperative period, the management of risk factors is emphasized. This program aims to halt the progression of generalized atherosclerosis and prevent recurrence of carotid stenosis. If indicated, an attempt is made to reduce weight. Hypertension diabetes mellitus and hypertriglyceridemia or hypercholesterolemia are treated. In almost all cases, antiplatelet medication is given and is usually resumed the morning after surgery. The authors usually prescribe aspirin 300 mg daily.

Angiography

Postoperative angiography usually is not done. Reports of angiography in the early postoperative period have documented a number of abnormal findings including intimal flaps, roughness, stenosis, forceps marks, corrugation, filling defects, dilatation, and occlusion of the superior thyroid, external carotid or internal carotid arteries (17). However, many of the arteries showing an irregular wall will become smooth in later angiograms, and in general the endarterectomized arteries remain patent and smooth for many years (73).

Using digital subtraction angiography 262 arteries in 214 patients were studied after carotid endarterectomy during the same hospital admission (37). The internal carotid artery was normal in 94%, had a nonsignificant deficit at the distal end of the arteriotomy in 3.5%, had a stenosis over 30% in 0.8%, and was occluded in 1.9%. The external carotid artery was normal in 93% and was occluded in 4.7%. In another study of 99 arteries in 86 consecutive patients done 1 week after operation, the internal carotid artery was patent in 100% and the external carotid artery in 97% (80). Two years later 79 vessels were studied with digital subtraction angiography showing one asymptomatic occlusion and one symptomatic restenosis. Three external carotid occlusions were associated with severe stroke.

Early angiography has been reserved for those patients who have unexplained neurologic deficit in the postoperative period or who have a postoperative bruit that is found on noninvasive studies to be hemodynamically significant (see "Complications").

When angiography is done months to years after the carotid endarterectomy because of recurrent neurologic symptoms in the territory of the operated artery, recurrent stenosis is usually found. When patients are studied because of neurologic symptoms in the territory of another intracranial vessel or for other reasons, most of the operated internal carotid arteries are patent and smooth with a few showing only minor irregularities (Figs. 1.18 and 2.28B). Occasionally, external carotid stenosis or occlusion is found (Fig. 2.34).

POSTOPERATIVE COMPLICATIONS

Neurologic

Cerebral Ischemia

The EEG electrodes are left on the patient until he or she awakens in the recovery room. If a neurologic deficit is found as the patient awakens and significant EEG change has occurred, the patient is returned immediately for exploration of the artery. If the deficit is present with no change in the EEG, the patient is immediately investigated with noninvasive carotid studies and if normal, a CT scan to look for hemorrhage. If this is normal, angiography is done (Fig. 2.35) (44). If there is any question about the status of the operated artery, it is reexplored. If studies show the endarterectomy site is normal, blood volume and blood pressure are maintained and a decision is made regarding anticoagulation.

If the patient develops a severe neurologic deficit after initial good recovery, this change may mean occlusion at the site of the operation. The patient should be taken immediately to the operating room to ascertain the status of the artery. An intraoperative angiogram may be used if the artery appears to be normal. The usual reason for postoperative carotid occlusion is a residual plaque or intimal flap, but occasionally the problem may be associated with an unrecognized hypercoaguable state.

When a neurologic deficit develops several days after surgery it may be due to a postoperative hemorrhage or intracranial embolus. Noninvasive carotid studies and a CT scan are the first diagnostic procedures followed by angiography if needed.

If the neurologic deficit is mild and nonprogressive, the noninvasive carotid tests are done, but usu-

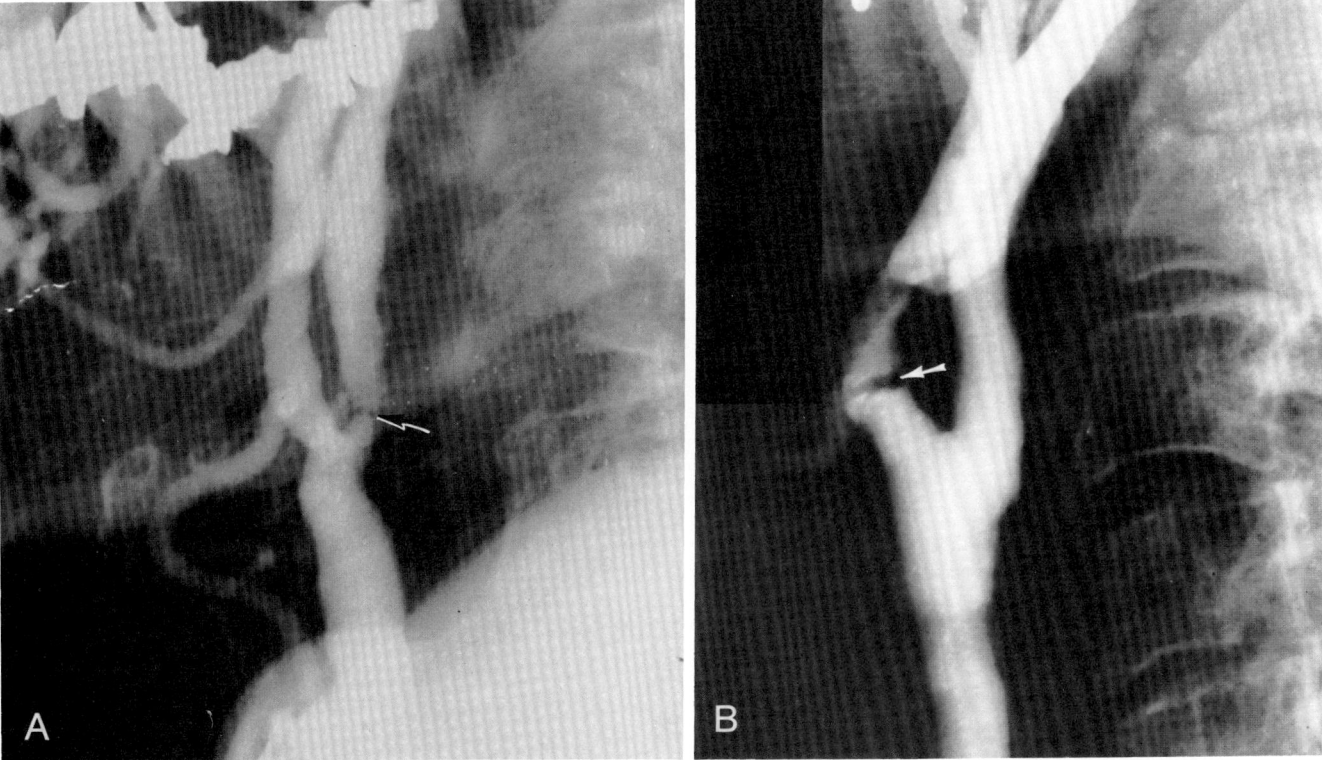

Figure 2.34. Postoperative angiography. **A**, Preoperative angiogram showing stenosis in the proximal internal carotid artery (*arrow*). **B**, Angiogram 2 years later. The internal carotid artery is smooth and has a normal caliber. A sharply localized narrowing is seen in the external carotid artery (*arrow*). Comment: The patient was studied for symptoms in the opposite carotid artery. The slight widening in the common carotid artery where the plaque was cut off is normal. The external carotid artery lesion is probably due to a flap of atheroma and intima left at the time of the endarterectomy.

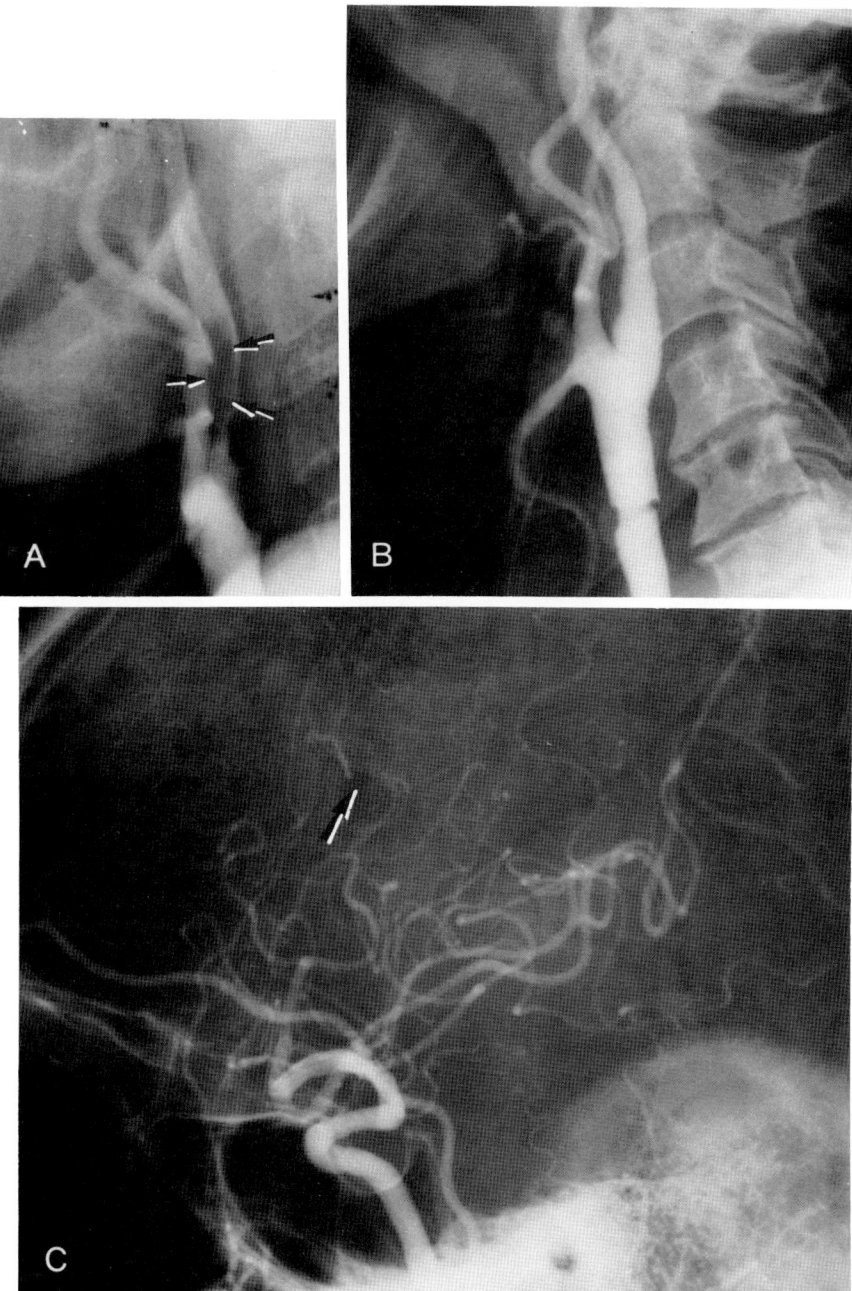

Figure 2.35. Emergency operation for intraluminal thrombus: intraoperative cerebral embolization. **A**, Preoperative left carotid angiogram. There is severe stenosis and, in addition, the irregular distal shadow (*arrows*) in the internal carotid artery suggests an intraluminal thrombus which was found at surgery. There is also reduced flow in the internal carotid artery as shown by reduced density of dye compared to the external carotid artery. **B**, Postoperative angiogram showing restoration of normal internal carotid artery. There is slight constriction at the proximal end of the endarterectomy which is not significant. **C**, Postoperative lateral angiogram of head showing embolus in a distal middle cerebral branch (*arrow*). After heparinization, the patient recovered to a mild deficit. Comment: In spite of careful dissection, occasionally an embolus will be dislodged and cause a postoperative neurologic deficit.

ally no abnormality is found. In such patients it is assumed that an embolus is the cause. These patients usually make a good recovery (71).

Transient Ischemia Attacks

A small number of patients will have one or more TIAs in the postoperative period (66). Usually it is a single attack, but if there are more than one they usually occur within the first 10–14 days after surgery. This symptom does not usually signify a serious problem in the operated artery. None of our patients who experienced this problem went on to have a stroke.

Noninvasive studies are done to ascertain whether there is a hemodynamic lesion. A significant abnormal finding would lead to an angiogram. In our experience, most patients will not have evidence of significant hemodynamic stenosis. They are treated with antiplatelet or anticoagulant therapy. If TIAs persist, angiography is indicated and will usually demonstrate a lesion that needs reoperation (73).

Intracerebral Hemorrhage

Early in the authors' series, a typical hypertensive hemorrhage occurred in the basal ganglia 4 days after surgery when blood pressure was 200/100 mm Hg (63). Since that time, careful control of postoperative hypertension has reduced the incidence of this complication. However, even with mild elevation in blood pressure, a hemorrhage may occasionally occur and it has been seen on rare occasion without any recorded rise in blood pressure (Figs. 2.36 and 2.37). In a report of one such patient with severe carotid stenosis and a fatal postoperative intracerebral hemorrhage, the pathologic findings suggested relative hyperperfusion of a cerebral hemisphere in which autoregulation had been lost because of chronic hypoperfusion (6). In one series of five hemorrhages the complication developed 5–7 days after surgery (86) and in the authors' experience, hemorrhage has not occurred before the fourth postoperative day.

Seizure

On rare occasion a seizure may occur. Presumably this is related to an embolus occluding a small cortical artery (95) but a postoperative hyperperfusion syndrome has also been suggested (82). Appropriate anticonvulsant treatment is given.

Headache

In the postoperative period, the patient may complain of significant unilateral headache in the retrobulbar, frontal, or temporal region. Blood pressure is usually normal and the pain is not like that noted in the face, jaw, or neck with internal carotid artery dissection. The symptom responds to mild analgesics and usually subsides in a few days. No serious se-

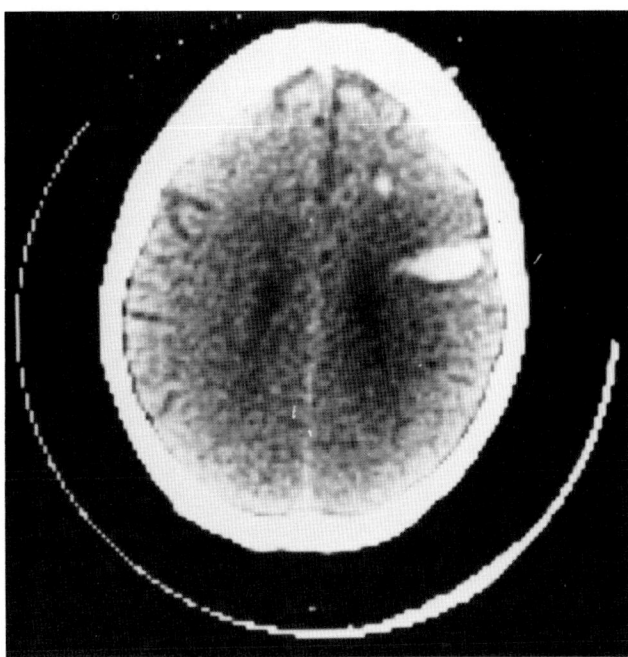

Figure 2.36. Small intracerebral hemorrhage after carotid endarterectomy. This 60-year-old man had a 6-month history of right transient monocular blindness and a 3-week history of episodes of left hemiparesis. The neurologic examination was normal. A right carotid bruit was present. Right carotid endarterectomy was done. His course was uncomplicated with systolic blood pressure ranging 140–160 mm. Five days after operation, he developed sudden headache, thickness of speech, and mild left facial and left upper extremity weakness. CT scan shows the small subcortical hemorrhage. Noninvasive carotid studies were normal. He made a full recovery.

quelae have been related to this symptom in our patients.

In a report of 50 patients (57 endarterectomies), 24 had postoperative headaches encompassing the entire spectrum of vascular headaches: nonspecific diffuse headaches, severe hemicranias, cluster headaches, chronic paroxysmal hemicranias, and carotodynia (60). The frequency and severity of headaches in the authors' series was much less.

Nerve Injury

Greater Auricular Nerve. This nerve is often encountered at the upper end of the incision deep to the platysma muscle. Injury leads to numbness over the mastoid region and the ear lobe. Care is taken in the dissection to preserve this nerve because some patients find the altered sensation on the ear lobe quite annoying. Symptoms usually subside over several months.

Facial Nerve (Mandibular Branch). If the incision is carried too near the angle of the jaw or retraction is too vigorous, the mandibular branch of the

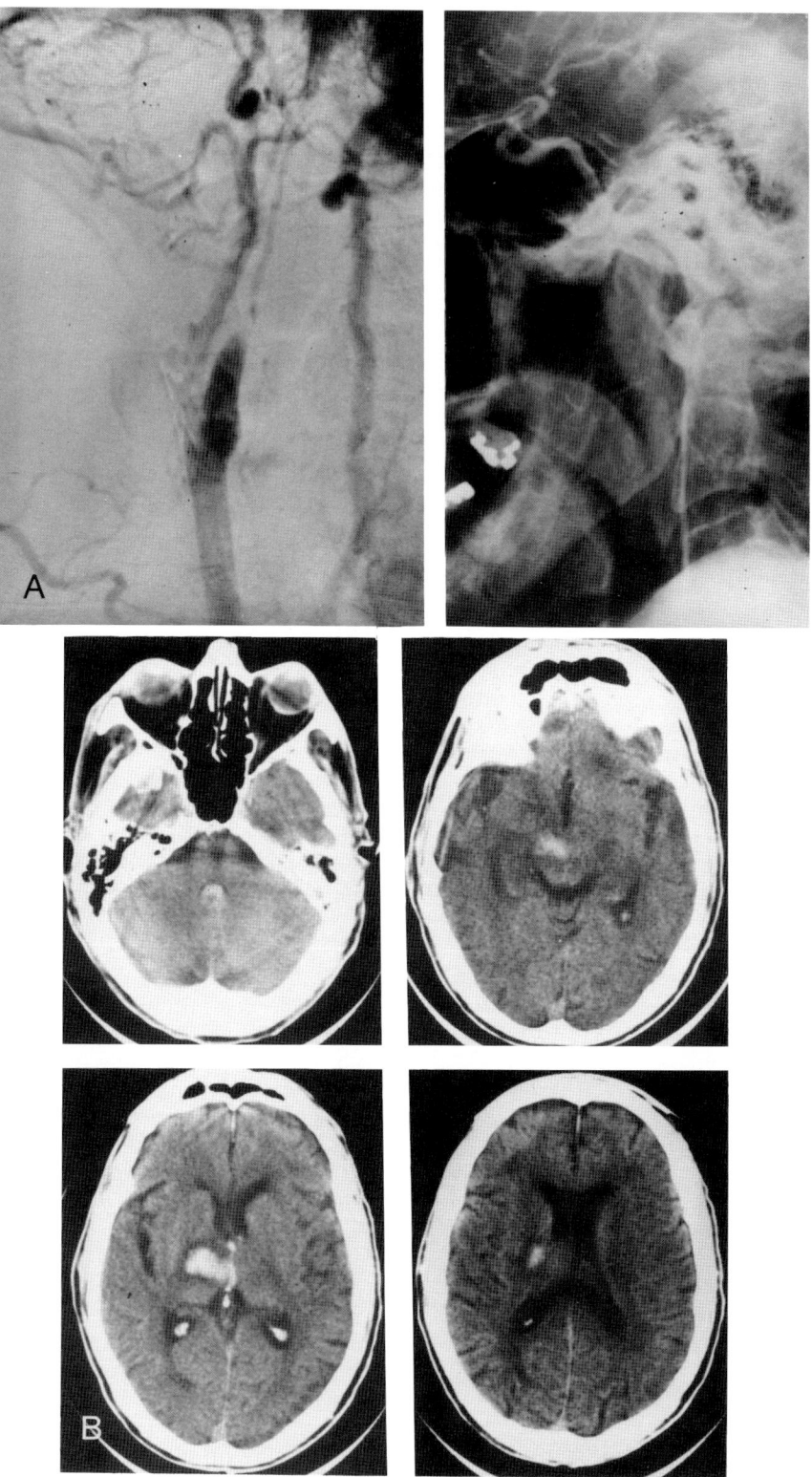

Figure 2.37. Thalamic hemorrhage 4 days after carotid endarterectomy. **A,** Note the severe stenosis and evidence of hypoperfusion. The patient had the sudden onset of a neurologic deficit with normal blood pressure. Because the deficit was mild and it occurred on the fourth postoperative day the CT scan (**B**) was the first diagnostic test. He made a full recovery.

facial nerve can be injured causing weakness of the lower lip. This is an annoying problem which causes a cosmetic change and may make the patient drool from the corner of the mouth. Spontaneous recovery almost always occurs (38). We have avoided this problem by curving the incision away from the angle of the jaw toward the mastoid process (Fig. 2.3A) and by being careful with placement of the self-retaining retractors.

Recurrent Laryngeal Nerve. Injury to the vagus or recurrent laryngeal nerve with vocal cord paresis has been reported to occur in about 1% of patients undergoing carotid endarterectomy (63, 86, 96). Traction or pressure on the nerve is the usual cause. As noted in the discussion of operative technique, the vagus nerve can lie on the anterior surface of the common carotid artery and may be encountered early in the dissection. Another area where the nerve is susceptible to injury is in dissection of the internal carotid artery where it may closely adhere to the artery. Direct injury to the recurrent laryngeal nerve may occur if the retraction blades are placed too deeply in the medial aspect of the incision. On rare occasions, a branch will come off the vagus nerve high in the neck and either run separately or join the descendens hypoglossi nerve. This branch must be saved.

In about 1% of the population a nonrecurrent laryngeal nerve arises from the vagus nerve near the carotid bifurcation and crosses posterior to the common carotid artery to enter the larynx. This anomaly is more frequent on the right side and is usually associated with an anomalous retroesophageal subclavian artery (40).

There is little that can be done about the loss of vocal cord function, although Teflon injections and other procedures may be of some palliative value. A majority of patients will show spontaneous recovery within a year (38). The problem is particularly crucial if bilateral operations are planned. If it is essential to do the opposite carotid endarterectomy after this complication, appropriate planning for tracheotomy is necessary should a bilateral weakness develop.

Superior Laryngeal Nerve. Dissection posterior to the carotid bifurcation may injure the superior laryngeal nerve. Trauma to this nerve may cause some relaxation of the ipsilateral vocal cord manifested by easy fatigability of the voice and impairment in phonation at a high pitch. Fortunately, the injury is usually asymptomatic. In one report where injury of the nerve was found on examination, four of five patients had no symptoms (38).

Accessory Nerve. Injury to the accessory nerve is a rare complication of carotid endarterectomy (84). The nerve is usually not visualized during the operation. Retraction or dissection along the upper anterior border of the sternocleidomastoid muscle when exposing a high carotid bifurcation may be the cause of the injury.

Hypoglossal Nerve. This complication is generally avoided by following the steps outlined in "Operative Technique." When it does occur, it is usually due to excessive traction on the nerve. Nothing need be done. Usually there are no symptoms. Most of the patients will have a spontaneous recovery within a few months (38, 86).

Wound Infection

The incidence of wound infection has been less than 1% in our series. Most infections have been superficial and are due to *Staphylococcus aureus*. They respond to the usual measures of opening the incision, irrigation, and antibiotics and allowing the wound to close secondarily. If the infection is deep, an angiogram should be done to check for a false aneurysm.

Wound Hematoma

Some patients will have significant swelling of the wound. This may be due to either hematoma or a lymph collection. If there is no problem with the airway, nothing need be done. The swelling will gradually subside over a few weeks. However, if the trachea is shifted and the airway is becoming compromised, the patient should be reintubated in the operating room under controlled circumstances and the wound reopened under general anesthesia.

False Aneurysm

The authors have not encountered this problem, but it has been reported (18). The diagnosis should be considered when a patient develops a late wound infection or has evidence of what appears to be a persistent hematoma or swelling in the neck. The recommended treatment is excision of the aneurysm with repair of the wall of the artery using a saphenous vein graft.

THE PATHOLOGY OF CAROTID ENDARTERECTOMY SPECIMENS

In 1975, Dr. C. Miller Fisher reported on the detailed pathologic examination of 40 endarterectomy specimens (63). Subsequently 141 sets of serial sections (1000–3000 sections, 8–10 microns in thickness for each specimen) were examined (27). The clinical categories were as follows:

Multiple hemispheric TIAs	34
Multiple episodes of transient monocular blindness	23
Asymptomatic	33
Prolonged or persistent neurologic deficit	51
TIAs followed by deficit	23
Sudden deficit without prior TIAs	28

The results of the pathologic evaluation of the TIA, transient monocular blindness, and asymptomatic patients are recorded in Table 2.1. The atherosclerotic plaque accumulated predominantly on the posterior wall of the artery with the remaining lumen lying adjacent to the carina. The residual lumen was 1 mm or less in 33 of 34 TIA cases (98%) and 19 of 21 transient monocular blindness cases (90%) (no data available in two) and in two of the three exceptions the lumen was oval or concentric in shape with the narrow axis 0.5 mm. In the asymptomatic group only 5 of 30 had a residual lumen diameter of 1 mm or less.

Mural thrombus was found on the plaque in 26 of 34 with hemispheric TIAs (77%), 22 of 23 with transient monocular blindness (96%), and 7 of 33 asymptomatic patients (21%) (Fig. 2.38). It is widely speculated that fragments of mural thrombus break away and cause TIAs. This sounds plausible enough but in the TIA group, 8 of 33 cases did not have a mural thrombus, and in the asymptomatic group 7 of 32 had a mural thrombus but did not have TIAs. Furthermore, in five TIA cases the mural thrombi were 1 mm or less in diameter, a size that would not block a main division of the middle cerebral artery had the entire thrombus broken away. In some instances, the mural thrombus was only slightly raised and appeared to merge indistinguishably with the underlying wall, a position from which it might not be easily dislodged. On the other hand, in the asymptomatic group, two of the mural thrombi were large and pedunculated yet symptomatic embolism failed to occur. Mural thrombi were composed predominantly of fibrin and in only 20% of the positive cases were platelet clumps prominent. The clumps were usually tiny and judged to be harmless had they become dislodged. The time interval between the last clinical event and endarterectomy did not account for the difference in the incidence of mural thrombi. In 31 of 33 cases in the TIA group the interval between the last spell and surgery was less than 4 weeks. The comparable figure for the transient monocular

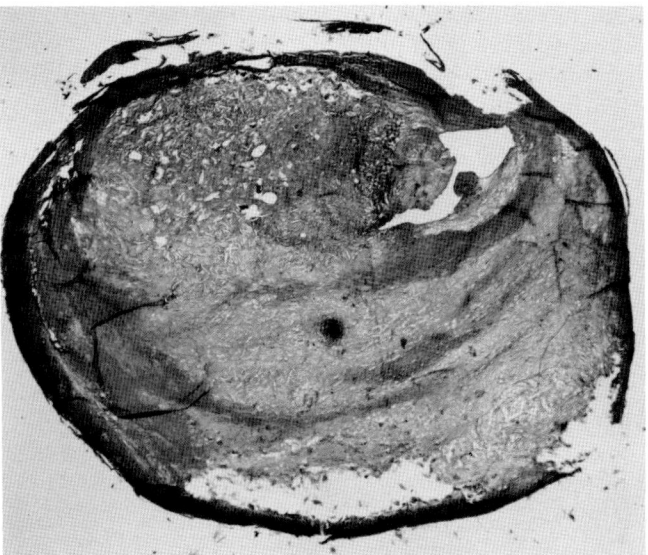

Figure 2.38. Mural thrombus. Cross-section of endarterectomy specimen, PTAH stain. At the point of maximum narrowing, a small mural thrombus is projecting into the lumen. This is the usual location when a mural thrombus is found.

blindness group was 20 of 23. In the two cases with the longest interval between symptoms and surgery (more than 7 weeks) both had mural thrombus. Of the eight TIA cases without mural thrombus two had ulcerations but neither crater contained mural thrombus.

Ulceration could not be correlated with specific clinical events. In 12 a cul-de-sac type of large outpouching was found which had been interpreted as a large ulceration on the angiogram. In seven the sac was smooth-lined and free of thrombolytic material while in five the sac was lined by a film of fibrin-platelet thrombin (Fig. 2.39).

In the previous study 60% of 35 symptomatic pa-

Table 2.1.
Pathological Finding in Patients with TIAs, TMBs, or No Symptoms

	Hemispheric TIAs	TMBs	Asymptomatic
No. of Cases	34	23	33
Residual Lumen (Diameter)			
1 mm or less	33 (98%)	19 (90%)	5 (15%)
1–2 mm	1 (2 × .5 mm)	0	8
2–3 mm	0	1 (3 × 5 mm)	15
3 mm	0	1	5
No information	0	2	0
Mural Thrombus	26 (77%)	22 (96%)	7 (21%)
Ulceration[a]	8 (24%)	13 (57%)	9 (27%)
ICA	6	10	8
CCA	2	3	1
Intraplaque Hemorrhage	13 (39%)	15 (65%)	6 (19%)
Cul-de-sacs	5	2	5

[a] Abbreviations: TMB = transient momocular blindness; ICA = internal carotid artery; CCA = common carotid artery.

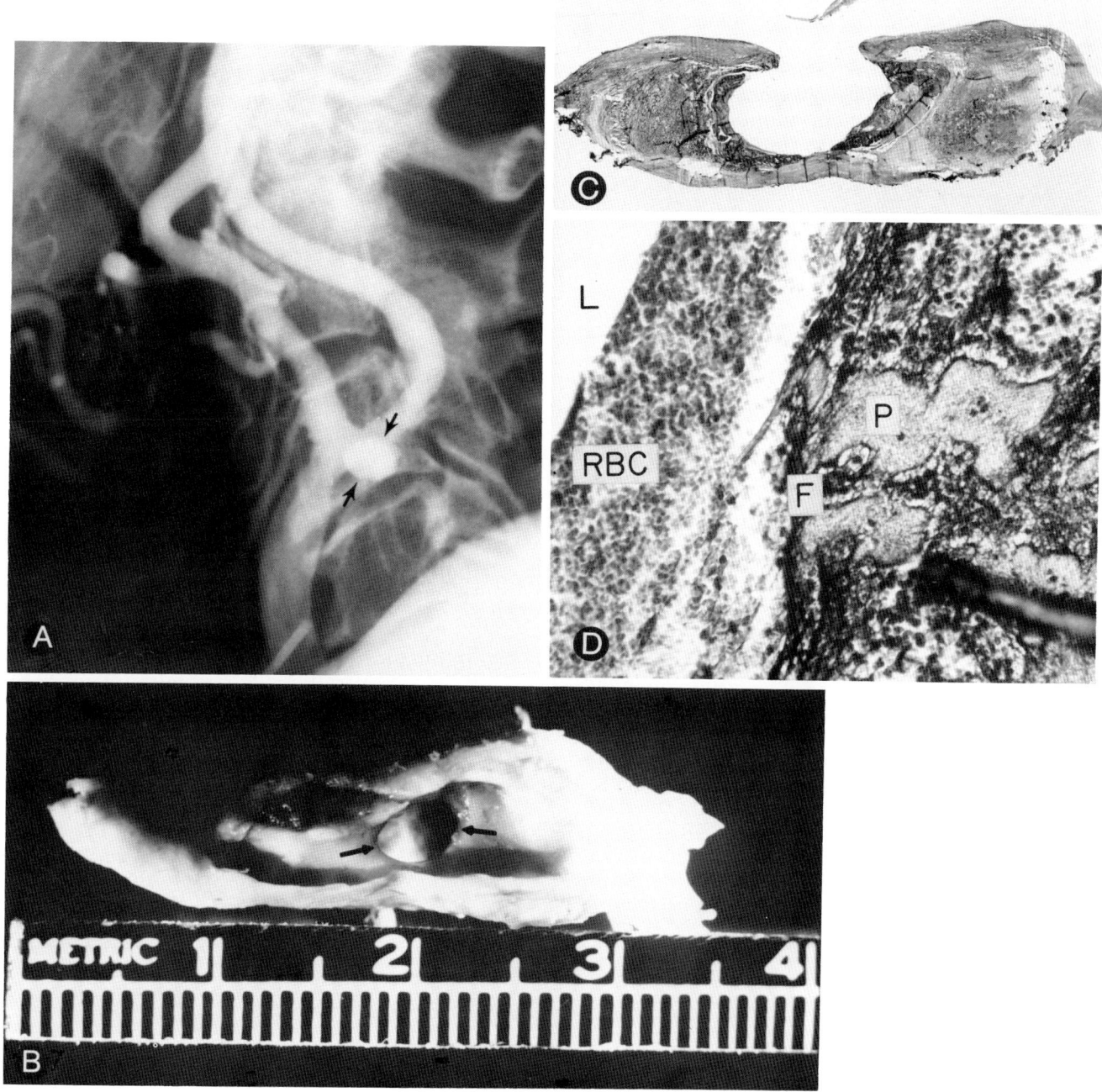

Figure 2.39. Ulcerated plaque. **A**, Left carotid angiogram showing a large, round ulcer crater (*arrows*) within a plaque at the origin of the internal carotid artery. **B**, The endarterectomy specimen was removed intact and opened longitudinally, demonstrating a large undermining cavity in the plaque (*arrows*). **C**, Microscopic section of plaque demonstrating large undermining cavitation. **D**, Wall of ulcer showing fibrin (*F*), platelet material (*P*), and red blood cells (*RBC*) at surface adjacent to lumen (*L*). (From Ojemann RG, Crowell RM, Roberson GH, Fisher CM: Surgical treatment of extracranial carotid occlusive disease. In: *Clinical Neurosurgery*. Baltimore, Williams & Wilkins, 1974, vol 22, chap 14).

tients had hemorrhage into the plaque and in 20% of the 35 it seemed to add to the mass of occluding tissue (63). In this study the incidence of intraplaque hemorrhage was 65% in the transient monocular blindness group, 39% in the TIA patients, and 19% in the asymptomatic cases (27). A higher incidence of hemorrhage into plaques from symptomatic compared to asymptomatic patients was also noted in another report (43). In the TIA, transient monocular blindness, and asymptomatic groups only one patient had a hemorrhage that was large enough to compromise the lumen. The hemorrhage seemed to start from the surface where blood penetrated from the lumen to form a small dissection.

In Table 2.2 are the results from those patients with neurologic deficits that lasted more than 24 hours. In 37 of the 51 patients a complete occlusion was seen microscopically but 15 of these had an angiogram 1 or 2 days before which showed a stenosis of 1 mm or less. It is possible that the thrombus progressed but the more likely explanation is that the systemic blood pressure had maintained a channel of blood flow which closed off under the condition of surgery and pathologic preparation. Most of the 47 occluded or severely stenotic cases showed the importance of the mural thrombus; in some it comprised approximately 75% of the residual lumen. In 11 patients hemorrhage had occurred into the plaque which in two instances significantly contributed to narrowing of the lumen.

From an overall evaluation of the results it was concluded that as the lumen narrows blood flow becomes compromised until a precarious hemodynamic insufficiency occurs. The mural thrombus contributes to the obstruction, but gives rise to neither TIAs nor serious embolism and is the early stage of the final occluding thrombus. The presence of a mural thrombus becomes significant when the residual lumen diameter is 1 mm or less. Ulceration is only rarely associated with major clinical events but occasionally is the source of emboli causing minor reversible strokes or prolonged reversible ischemic deficits.

RECURRENT STENOSIS

Incidence and Pathology

Recurrent stenosis occurs in a small percentage of patients who have had carotid endarterectomy. The earlier reports on the incidence of restenosis studied only symptomatic patients (9). In one such study recurrent stenosis within 24 months was found in 3.6% of 361 operations with a range of 5–24 months (13). Noninvasive studies done during the first 2 years after carotid endarterectomy report an incidence of stenosis of greater than 70% or occlusion in up to 10% of the patients but less than half have symptoms (1, 32, 49, 72). No clear relationship has been identified between the usual risk factors for atherosclerosis and recurrent stenosis (9).

There seem to be three groups of patients in which this problem arises:

1. Patients in whom surgical technique has contributed to the problem (29). This includes:
   a. Failure to remove the distal tongue of the plaque
   b. Narrowing of the lumen during the arteriotomy closure
   c. Damage to the intima by vascular clamps
2. Patients who have a tendency to excess scar formation
3. Patients in whom a combination of fibrosis, recurrent atherosclerosis, and at times, associated thrombus formation develops

Symptomatic stenosis may recur within a few months of the operation. This usually relates to one of the problems in surgical technique or to the thickened fibrosis of the arterial wall which is grossly and histologically distinct from the typical atherosclerotic plaque. Some of these stenoses may regress. In a report using noninvasive serial studies on 22 patients with early stenosis, 12 persisted, 9 regressed, and one became occluded (98).

The pathologic processes found with recurrent stenosis have been summarized (9, 12, 67, 77). Myointimal hyperplasia is usually found if the recurrence

Table 2.2
Pathological Findings in the Group with Persistent or Prolonged Deficit

	No.	Mural Thrombosis	Ulceration	Hemorrhage	Cul-de-sac
Lumen occluded by angiography and at pathology	22	22	0	0	0
Lumen extremely stenotic by angiography, occluded at pathology	15	15	0	0	0
Residual lumen 1 mm or less	10	7	4	2	2
Residual lumen 1 mm	4	0	2	0	2

is within 2 years of the initial operation. Later the most likely finding is friable degenerating atherosclerosis often associated with thrombus. The presence of intraplaque thrombus may not be correlated with symptoms (12). In some patients there is localized scarring at the proximal or distal end of the endarterectomy.

In the authors' series, recurrent symptomatic stenosis usually came to attention because of TIAs. The interval between operation and symptoms ranged 1–6 years. The patient with the earliest lesion had thickening of the entire arterial wall due primarily to fibrosis with no evidence of atheroma over a longitudinal distance of 3–4 cm. She had a tendency for keloid formation in other scars. Other findings in patients who had operations within 3 years of the original surgery included a fibrous weblike diaphragm at the proximal end of the endarterectomy with thickened intima and little atheroma, and a thin layer of multiple plaques of atheroma in a thickened, scarred intima with a small associated thrombus. Patients seen 3 years after operation had an atheromatous deposit in the thickened, scarred intima causing various degrees of narrowing often associated with a superimposed thrombus. In two cases of recurrent symptomatic stenosis seen approximately 4 years after operation, angiography showed a narrow, shelf-like obstruction (Fig. 2.40). Microscopic examination disclosed unusually abundant local fibrous connective tissue proliferation projecting into the lumen. Fatty deposition was relatively minor. An occasional patient will develop restenosis more than once (Fig. 2.41).

Technical Points

The operation is often difficult because of the dense periarterial scar and the fibrosis of the vessel wall.

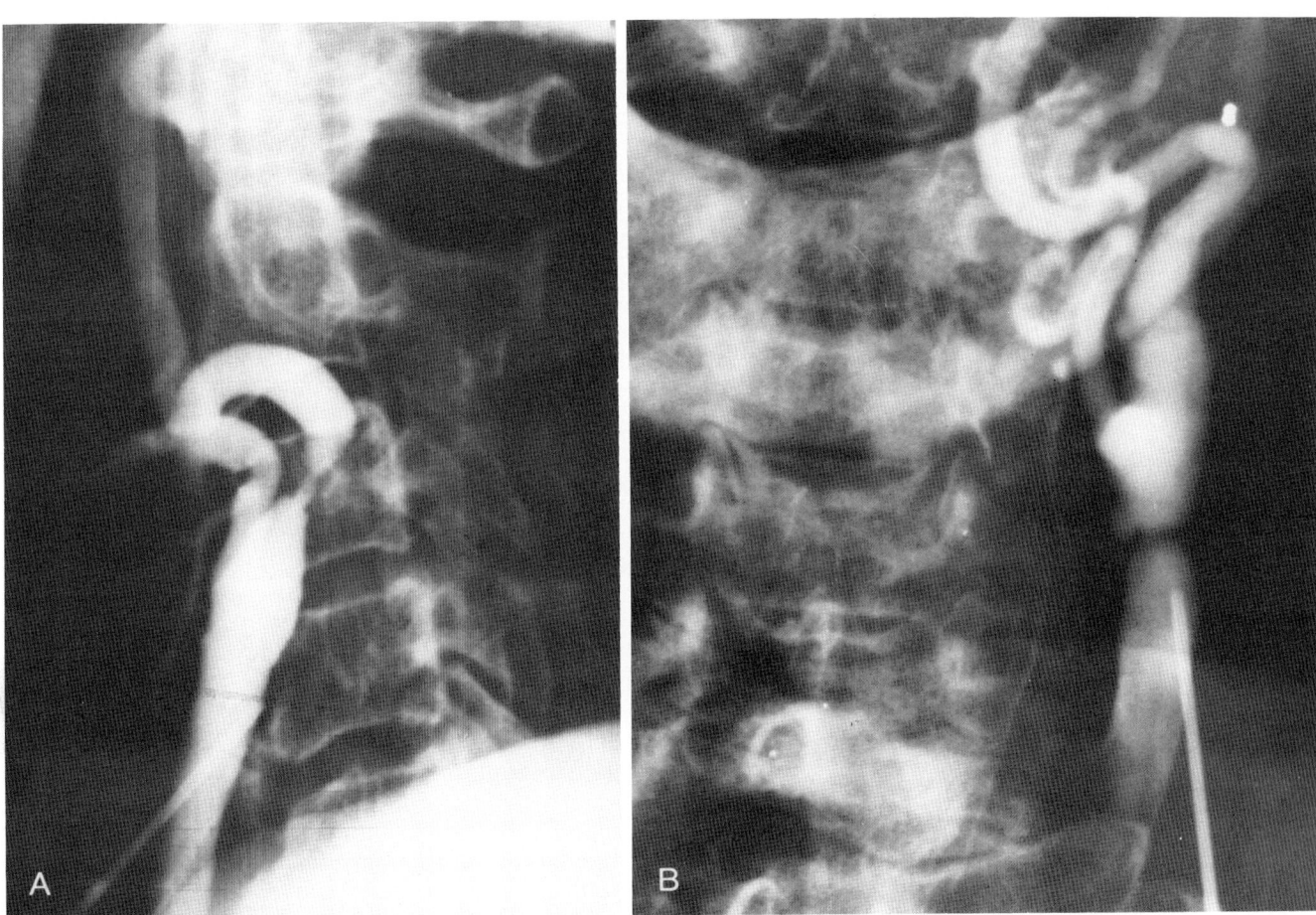

Figure 2.40. Restenosis by fibrous web. **A,** Initial angiogram shows stenosis at the origin of the internal carotid artery. There is also a prominent loop in the proximal internal carotid artery. **B,** Angiogram 4 years later shows normal internal carotid artery but a web at site of the proximal edge of the endarterectomy. Comment: Patient presented with recurrent TIAs. A localized area of thickened intima with fibrosis was found at operation. (From Ojemann RG, Crowell RM, Roberson GH, Fisher CM: Surgical treatment of extracranial carotid occlusive disease. In: *Clinical Neurosurgery.* Baltimore, Williams & Wilkins, 1974, vol 22, chap 14.)

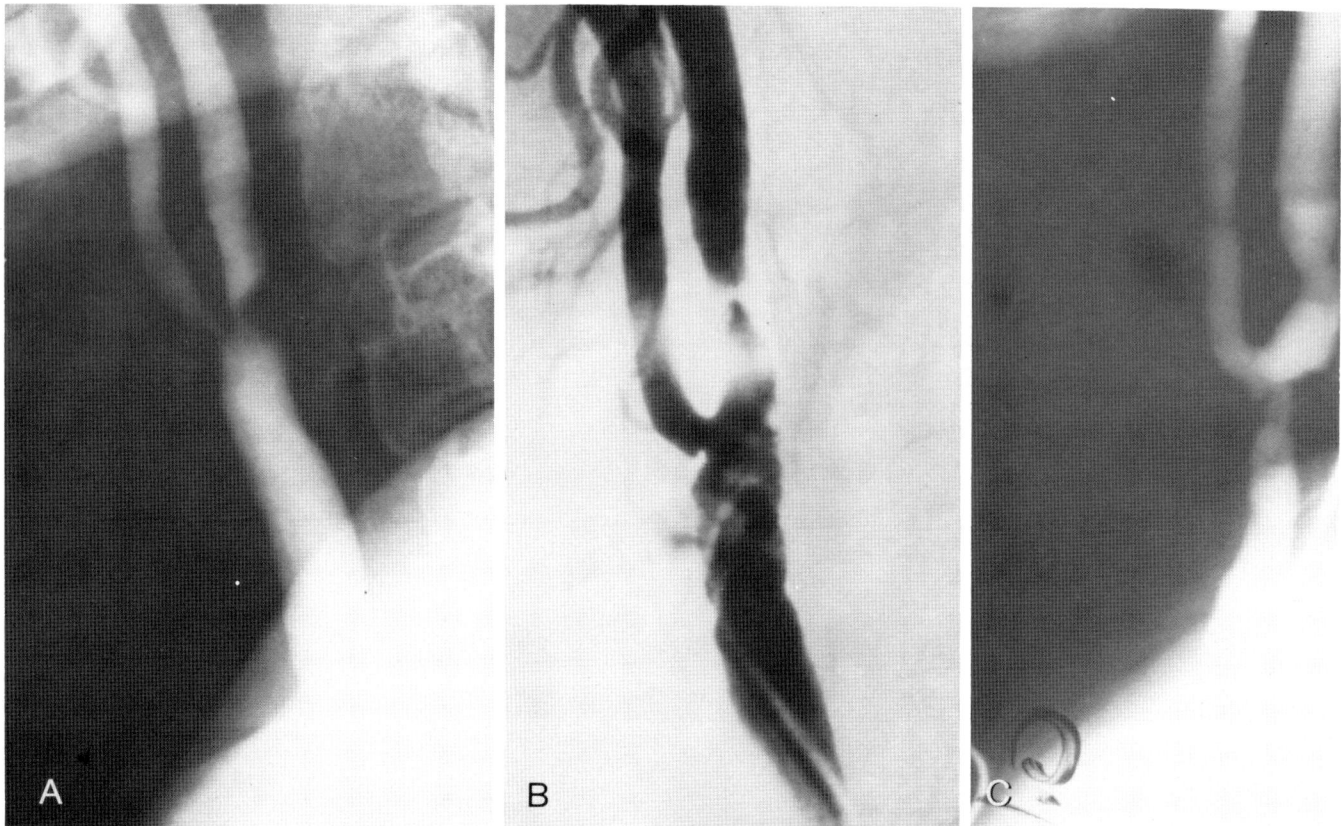

Figure 2.41. Restenosis after carotid endarterectomy. Left carotid angiograms. **A**, Patient presented with transient monocular blindness and transient hemispheric attack (tingling right hand). Angiogram shows severe stenosis at origin of left internal carotid artery. Carotid endarterectomy was done with satisfactory postoperative course. **B**, 6 years later, transient hemispheric attack followed by transient monocular blindness. Severe stenosis at distal end of endarterectomy. Carotid endarterectomy done. The plaque in the common carotid artery was fibrotic with irregular islands of atheromatous plaque. More marked atheroma was present in the internal carotid artery with an associated thrombus. Primary closure done without a patch. **C**, 3 years after the second operation, transient hemispheric attack (numbness and tingling right upper extremity). The angiogram now shows narrowing and irregularity in the distal common carotid artery and slight narrowing in the internal carotid. Carotid endarterectomy done. The plaque consisted of fibrous tissue with endothelium, but in the distal common carotid artery extending to the origin of the external and internal carotid arteries was a collar of yellowish atheromatous tissue measuring approximately 1.0 cm in longitudinal dimension and encircling the inner lumen of the vessel. At the distal end of this material at the origin of the internal carotid artery was a small thrombus. In the external and internal carotid arteries was found only scar tissue with endothelium. Because of the fibrous tissue and narrowed caliber of the artery, a Dacron patch graft was placed. Postoperative course was satisfactory.

Great care is required to avoid injury to the internal jugular vein, vagus, and hypoglossal nerves. The thickened intima is often densely adherent to the outer arterial wall, particularly in the region of the previous suture line. It is, therefore, usually wise to make a new incision to start the arteriotomy. It is also more difficult to get a "clean" removal in the distal internal carotid artery.

In patients with myointimal hyperplasia all that may be necessary is a patch graft without endarterectomy (67). In other patients, an endarterectomy is done and the arteriotomy is closed with a patch graft. It has been suggested that occasionally an interposition vein graft is necessary (67).

Transluminal Angioplasty

This procedure has been used in a few patients to dilate residual or recurrent stenosis when it was thought the pathology was fibrous myointimal hyperplasia (61, 89). There is concern about the possibility of embolic complications and the procedure should probably be used only when there is a serious medical or technical contraindication to repeat operation.

REFERENCES

1. Baker WH, Hayes AC, Mahler D, Littooy FN: Durability of carotid endarterectomy. Surgery 94:112–115, 1983.

2. Balagura S, Carter JB, Gossett DL: Surgical approach to the high subcranial internal carotid artery. *Neurosurgery* 16:402–405, 1985.
3. Barnes RW, Marszalek PB: Asymptomatic carotid disease in the cardiovascular surgical patient: Is prophylactic endarterectomy necessary? *Stroke* 12:497–500, 1981.
4. Barnett HJM, Peerless SJ, Kaufmann JCE: "Stump" of internal carotid artery: A source for further cerebral embolic ischemia. *Stroke* 9:448–456, 1978.
5. Barnett HJM, Peerless SJ, Sutherland GR: The stump syndrome. In Smith RR (ed): *Stroke and the Extracranial Vessels*. New York, Raven Press, 1984, pp 219–225.
6. Bernstein M, Fleming JF, Deck JH: Cerebral hyperperfusion after carotid endarterectomy: A cause of cerebral hemorrhage. *Neurosurgery* 15:50–56, 1984.
7. Bland JE, Lazar ML: Carotid endarterectomy without shunt. *Neurosurgery* 8:153–157, 1981.
8. Callow AD: An overview of the stroke problem in the carotid territory. *Am J Surg* 140:181–191, 1980.
9. Callow AD: Restenosis after carotid artery surgery. *Int Surg* 69:247–255, 1984.
10. Caplan LR, Skillman J, Ojemann R, Fields WS: Intracerebral hemorrhage following carotid endarterectomy: A hypertensive complication? *Stroke* 9:457–460, 1978.
11. Chiappa KH, Burke SR, Young RR: Results of electroencephalographic monitoring during 367 carotid endarterectomies. Use of a dedicated minicomputer. *Stroke* 10:381–388, 1979.
12. Clagett GP, Robinowitz M, Youkey JR, Fisher DF Jr, Fry RE, Myers SI, Lee EL, Collins GJ Jr, Virmani R: Morphogenesis and clinicopathologic characteristics of recurrent carotid disease. *J Vasc Surg* 3:10–23, 1986.
13. Cossman D, Callow AD, Stein A, Matsumoto G: Early restenosis after carotid endarterectomy. *Arch Surg* 113:275–278, 1978.
14. Crowell RM, Ojemann RG: Extracrannial cerebrovascular disease. In Hoff JT (ed): *Practice of Surgery*. Philadelphia, Harper & Row, 1981, Chap 28.
15. Crowell RM, Ojemann RG, Lee RS, deBros F, Sundaram P: Carotid endarterectomy in high risk patients with cardiopulmonary disease. *Stroke* 12:123, 1981.
16. Davie JC, Richardson R: Distal internal carotid thromboembolectomy using a Fogarty catheter in total occlusion. *J Neurosurg* 27:171–177, 1967.
17. Diaz EG, Patel S, Boulos R, Metha B, Ausman JI: Early angiographic changes after carotid endarterectomy. *Neurosurgery* 10:151–161, 1982.
18. Ehrenfeld WK, Hays RJ: False aneurysm after carotid endarterectomy. *Arch Surg* 104:288–291, 1972.
19. Emery RW, Cohn LH, Whittemore AD, Mannick JA, Couch NP, Collins JJ Jr: Coexistent carotid and coronary artery disease. *Arch Surg* 118:1035–1039, 1983.
20. Ennix CL Jr, Lawrie GM, Morris GC Jr, Crawford ES, Howell JF, Reardon MJ, Weatherford SC: Improved results of carotid endarterectomy in patients with symptomatic coronary disease: An analysis of 1546 consecutive carotid operations. *Stroke* 10:122–125, 1979.
21. Ercius MS, Chandler WF, Ford JW, Swanson DP, Burke JC: Effect of different aspirin doses on arterial thrombosis after canine carotid endarterectomy: A scanning electron microscope and indium-lll-labeled platelet study. *Neurosurgery* 14:198–203, 1984.
22. Etheredge SN, Effeney DJ, Ehrefeld WK: Symptomatic extrinsic compression of the cervical carotid artery. *Arch Neurol* 41:672–673, 1984.
23. Ferguson GG: Carotid endarterectomy. To shunt or not to shunt? *Arch Neurol* 43:615–617, 1986.
24. Ferguson GG: Intraoperative monitoring and internal shunts: Are they necessary in carotid endarterectomy? *Stroke* 13:287–289, 1982.
25. Ferguson GG, Gamache FW, Blume WT, Farrar JK: Monitoring during carotid endarterectomy. Further evidence that an internal shunt is not necessary. *Neurosurgery* 7:285, 1980.
26. Findlay JM, Lougheed WM, Gentili F, Walker PM, Glynn MFX, Houle S: Effect of perioperative platelet inhibition on postcarotid endarterectomy mural thrombus formation. Results of a prospective randomized controlled trial using aspirin and dipyridomole in humans. *J Neurosurg* 63:693–698, 1985.
27. Fisher CM, Ojemann RG: A clinico-pathologic study of carotid endarterectomy plaques. *Rev Neurol (Paris)* 142:573–589, 1986.
28. Fisher DF Jr, Clagett GP, Parker JL, Fry RE, Poor MR, Finn RA, Brink BE, Fry WJ: Mandibular subluxation for high carotid exposure. *J Vasc Surg* 1:727–733, 1984.
29. French BN, Rewcastle NB: Recurrent stenosis at site of carotid endarterectomy. *Stroke* 8:597–605, 1977.
30. Furui T, Hasuo M: Indwellling double-balloon shunt for carotid endarterectomy. Technical note. *J Neurosurg* 60:861–863, 1984.
31. Giannotta SL, Dicks RE III, Kindt GW: Carotid endarterectomy: Technical improvements. *Neurosurgery* 7:309–312, 1980.
32. Glover JL, Bendrick PJ, Dilley RS, Jackson VP, Reilly MK, Dalsing MC, Robison RJ: Restenosis following carotid endarterectomy. Evaluation by duplex ultrasonography. *Arch Surg* 120:678–684, 1985.
33. Green RM, Messick WJ, Ricotta JJ, Charleton MH, Satran R, McBride MM, DeWeese JA: Benefits, shortcomings and costs of EEG monitoring. *Ann Surg* 201:785–792, 1985.
34. Hafner LD, Tew JM: Surgical management of the totally occluded internal carotid artery: A ten-year study. *Surgery* 80:710–717, 1981.
35. Heros RC, Grundy BL: Ischemic cerebrovascular disease. In Katz J, Matjasko J (eds): *Clinical Controversies in Neuroanesthesia and Neurosurgery*. New York, Grune & Stratton, 1986, pp 1–76.
36. Hertzer NR: External carotid endarterectomy. *Surg Gynecol Obstet* 153:186–190, 1981.
37. Hertzer NR, Beven EG, Modic MT, O'Hara PJ, Vogt DP, Weinstein MA: Early patency of the carotid artery after endarterectomy. Digital subtraction angiography after two hundred sixty-two operations. *Surgery* 92:1049–1057, 1982.
38. Hertzer NR, Feldman BJ, Beven EG, Tucker HM: A prospective study of the incidence of injury to the cranial nerves during carotid endarterectomy. *Surg Gynecol Obstet* 151:781–784, 1980.
39. Hodosh RM, Boone SC: Neurological manifestations of external carotid artery disease. *Clin Neurosurg* 28:384–406, 1981.
40. Hollingshead WH: *The Head and Neck Anatomy for Surgeons*, ed 2. New York, Harper & Row, 1968, vol 1.
41. Hugenholtz H, Elgie RG: Carotid thromboendarterectomy: A reappraisal. Criteria for patient selection. *J Neurosurg* 53:776–783, 1980.
42. Imparato AM, Ramirez AR, Riles T, Mintzer R: Cerebral protection in carotid surgery. *Arch Surg* 117:1073–1078, 1982.
43. Imparato AM, Riles TS, Mintzer R, Baumann FG: The importance of hemorrhage in relationship between gross morphologic characteristics and cerebral symptoms in 376 carotid artery plaques. *Ann Surg* 197:195–203, 1983.
44. Imparato AM, Riles TS, Ramirez AA, Lamparello PJ: Early complications of carotid surgery. *Int Surg* 69:223–229, 1984.
45. Ivey TD, Strandness E, Williams DB, Langlois Y, Misbach GA, Kruse PP: Management of patients with carotid bruit undergoing cardiopulmonary bypass. *J Thorac Cardiovasc Surg* 87:183–189, 1984.
46. Javid H: Intraluminal shunting during carotid endarterectomy. In Bergan JJ, Yao JT (eds): *Cerebrovascular Insufficiency*. New York, Grune & Stratton, 1983, pp 309–325.
47. Jones EL, Craver JM, Michalik RA, Murphy DA, Guyton RA, Bone DK, Hatcher CR, Reichwald NA: Combined carotid and coronary operations. When are they necessary? *J Thorac Cardiovasc Surg* 87:7–16, 1984.

48. Karmody AM, Shah DM, Monoco VJ, Leather RP: On surgical reconstruction of the external carotid artery. *Am J Surg* 136:176–180, 1978.
49. Kartchner MM, McRae LP: The clinical use of oculoplethysmography and carotid phonoangiography. In Baker WH (ed): *Diagnosis and Treatment of Carotid Artery Disease.* Mount Kisco, NY, Futura, 1979.
50. Kelly JJ, Callow AD, O'Donnell TF, McBride K, Ehrneberg B, Korwin S, Welch H, Gembarowicz RM: Failure of carotid stump pressure. Its incidence as a predictor for a temporary shunt during carotid endarterectomy. *Arch Surg* 114:1361–1366, 1979.
51. Kerber CW, Cromwell LD, Loehden OL: Catheter dilatation of proximal carotid stenosis during distal bifurcation endarterectomy. *Am J Neurorad* 1:348–349, 1980.
52. Kusunoki T, Rowed DW, Tator CH, Lougheed WM: Thromboendarterectomy for total occlusion of the internal carotid artery: A reappraisal of risks, success rate and potential benefits. *Stroke* 9:34–38, 1978.
53. Lamberth WC: External carotid endarterectomy: Indications, operative technique and results. *Surgery* 93:57–63, 1983.
54. Larson JR, Gaspar MR, Movius JH, Rosenthal JJ, Bell DD, Lemire GC: Intraoperative arteriography in cerebrovascular disease. In Bergan JJ, Yao JT (eds): *Cerebrovascular Insufficiency.* New York, Grune & Stratton, 1983, pp 353–365.
55. Lippman HH, Sundt TM Jr, Holman CB: The poststenotic carotid slim sign; spurious internal carotid hypoplasia. *Mayo Clin Proc* 45:762–767, 1970.
56. Little JR, Bryerton BS, Furlan AJ: Saphenous vein patch grafts in carotid endarterectomy. *J Neurosurg* 61:743–747, 1984.
57. Matsumoto GH, Baker JD, Watson CW, Gleucklich D, Callow AD: Electroencephalographic surveillance as a means of extending operability in high risk carotid endarterectomy. *Stroke* 7:554–559, 1976.
58. McCready RA, Finelli JF, Hyde GL: A technique for intraoperative arteriography following carotid endarterectomy. *Surg Gynecol Obstet* 160:367–368, 1985.
59. McKay RD, Sundt TM Jr, Michenfelder JD, Gronert GA, Messick JM, Sharbrough FW, Piepgras DG: Internal carotid artery stump pressure and cerebral blood flow during carotid endarterectomy. Modification by halothane, enflurone and innover. *Anesthesiology* 45:390–399, 1976.
60. Messert B, Black JA: Cluster headache, hemicrania and other head pains: Morbidity of carotid endarterectomy *Stroke* 9:559–562, 1978.
61. Numaguchi Y, Puyau FA, Provenza LJ, Richardson DE: Percutaneous transluminal angioplasty of the carotid artery. Its application to post-surgical stenosis. *Neuroradiology* 26:527–530, 1984.
62. Ojemann RG: Extracranial carotid artery atherosclerosis. In Wilkin RH, Rengachary SS (eds): *Neurosurgery.* New York, McGraw-Hill, 1985, vol 2, pp 1236–1247.
63. Ojemann RG, Crowell RM, Roberson GH, Fisher CM: Surgical treatment of extracranial carotid occlusive disease. *Clin Neurosurg* 22:214–263, 1975.
64. Ojemann RG, Heros RC: Carotid endarterectomy. To shunt or not to shunt? *Arch Neurol* 43:617–618, 1986.
65. Ott DA, Cooley DA, Chapa L, Coelho A: Carotid endarterectomy without temporary intraluminal shunt. *Ann Surg* 191:708–714, 1980.
66. Owens ML, Atkinson JB, Wilson SE: Recurrent transient ischemic attacks after carotid endarterectomy. *Arch Surg* 115:482–486, 1980.
67. Piepgras DG, Sundt TM, Marsh WR, Mussman LA, Fode NC: Recurrent carotid stenosis. Results and complications of 57 operations. *Ann Surg* 203:205–213, 1986.
68. Podore PC, Rob CG, DeWeese JA, Green RM: Chronic common carotid occlusion. *Stroke* 12:98–100, 1981.
69. Rice PL, Pifarre R, Sullivan HJ, Montoya A, Bakhos M: Experience with simultaneous myocardial revascularization and carotid endarterectomy. *J Thorac Cardiovasc Surg* 79:922–925, 1980.
70. Ricotta JJ, Charleton MH, DeWeese JA: Determining criteria for shunt placement during carotid endarterectomy. EEG versus back pressure. *Ann Surg* 198:642–645, 1983.
71. Rosenthal D, Zerchner WD, Lamis PA, Stanton PE Jr: Neurologic deficit after carotid endarterectomy: Pathogenesis and management. *Surgery* 94:776–780, 1983.
72. Salvian A, Baker JD, Machleder HI, Busuttil RW, Baker WF, Moore WS: Cause and non-invasive detection of restenosis after carotid endarterectomy. *Am J Surg* 146:29–34, 1983.
73. Schutz H, Fleming JFR, Awerbuck B: Arteriographic assessment of carotid endarterectomy. *Ann Surg* 171:509–521, 1970.
74. Seifert KB, Blackshear WM Jr: Continuous wave Doppler in the intraoperative assessment of carotid endarterectomy. *J Vasc Surg* 2:817–820, 1985.
75. Sekkar LN, Heros RC, Wolfson SK, Segal RC, Dujovny M: External carotid endarterectomy for cerebral and ocular ischemia. *Vasc Surg* 16:185–203, 1982.
76. Sharbrough FW, Messick JM Jr, Sundt TM Jr: Correlation of continuous electroencephalograms with cerebral blood flow measurements during carotid endarterectomy. *Stroke* 4:674–683, 1973.
77. Stoney R, String T: Recurrent carotid stenosis. *Surgery* 80:705–710, 1976.
78. Sundt TM Jr: The ischemic tolerance of neural tissue and the need for monitoring and selective shunting during carotid endarterectomy. *Stroke* 14:93–98, 1983.
79. Sundt TM Jr, Ebersold MJ, Sharbrough FW, Piepgras DG, Marsh WR, Messick JM Jr: The risk-benefit ratio of intraoperative shunting during carotid endarterectomy. *Ann Surg* 203:196–204, 1986.
80. Sundt TM Jr, Houser OW, Fode NC, Whisnant JP: Correlation of postoperative and two-year follow-up angiography with neurological function in 99 carotid endarterectomies in 86 consecutive patients. *Ann Surg* 203:90–100, 1986.
81. Sundt TM Jr, Sandok BA, Whisnant JP: Carotid endarterectomy. Complications and preoperative assessment of risk. *Mayo Clin Proc* 50:301–306, 1975.
82. Sundt TM Jr, Sharbrough FW, Piepgras DG, Kearns TP, Messick JM Jr, O'Fallon WM: Correlation of cerebral blood flow and electroencephalographic changes during carotid endarterectomy. With results of surgery and hemodynamics of cerebral ischemia. *Mayo Clinic Proc* 56:533–543, 1981.
83. Sundt TM Jr, Sharbrough FW, Trautmann JC, Gronert GA: Monitoring techniques for carotid endarterectomy. *Clin Neurosurg* 22:199–213, 1975.
84. Swann KW, Heros RC: Accessory nerve palsy following carotid endarterectomy. Report of two cases. *J Neurosurg* 63:630–632, 1985.
85. Tarlov E, Schmidek H, Scott RM, Wepsic JG, Ojemann RG: Reflex hypotension following carotid endarterectomy: Mechanism and management. *J Neurosurg* 39:323–327, 1973.
86. Theodotou B, Mahaley MS Jr: Injury of the peripheral cranial nerve during carotid endarterectomy. *Stroke* 16:894–895, 1985.
87. Thompson JE: Protection of the brain during carotid endarterectomy. I. Routine shunting. *Anesthesiol Clin* 22:129–135, 1984.
88. Thompson JE: *Surgery for Cerebrovascular Insufficiency, Stroke: With Special Emphasis on Carotid Endarterectomy.* Springfield, IL, Charles C Thomas, 1968.
89. Tievsky AL, Druy EM, Mardia JG: Transluminal angioplasty in postsurgical stenosis of the extracranial carotid artery. *AJNR* 4:800–802, 1983.
90. Towne JB, Bernhard VM: The relationship of postoperative hypertension to complications following carotid endarterectomy surgery. *Surgery* 88:575–580, 1980.
91. Turnipseed WD, Berkoff HA, Belzer FO: Postoperative stroke in cardiac and peripheral vascular disease. *Ann Surg* 192:365–368, 1980.
92. Vitek JJ, Morawetz RB: Percutaneous transluminal angioplasty of the external carotid artery: Preliminary report. *AJNR* 3:541–546, 1982.

93. Whittemore AD: Carotid endarterectomy. An alternative approach. Arch Surg 115:940–942, 1980.
94. Whittemore AD, Kauffman JL, Kohler TR, Mannick JA: Routine electroencephalographic (EEG) monitoring during carotid endarterectomy. Ann Surg 197:707–713, 1983.
95. Wilkinson JT, Adams HP Jr, Wright CB: Convulsions after carotid endarterectomy. JAMA 244:1827–1828, 1980.
96. Wylie EJ, Ehrenfeld WK: *Extracranial Occlusive Cerebrovascular Disease: Diagnosis and Management.* Philadelphia, WB Saunders, 1970.
97. Zierler RE, Bandyk DF, Thiele BL: Intraoperative assessment of carotid endarterectomy. J. Vasc Surg 1:73-83, 1984.
98. Zierler RE, Bandyk DF, Thiele BL, Strandness E Jr: Carotid artery stenosis following endarterectomy. Arch Surg 117:1408–1415, 1982.

3

Asymptomatic Carotid Bruit and Stenosis

ASYMPTOMATIC CAROTID BRUIT

Etiology

Increased awareness that stroke might be preventable has led, on routine physical examination, to the frequent finding of an asymptomatic bruit over the lateral neck. While such bruits often reflect turbulent blood flow in the proximal internal carotid artery due to localized atherosclerosis causing stenosis, they may be heard over apparently normal arteries and may be associated with several other pathological conditions (4, 18) (Table 3.1).

The turbulent blood flow due to atherosclerosis is related to the flow rate in the most stenotic segment, which in turn is related to the residual lumen diameter and length of the stenosis (30). For a bruit to occur, there must be more than 70% reduction in the cross-section area of the lumen of the artery; the diameter must, therefore, be reduced more than 50% (7). Because of the difficulty in estimating the percentage diameter reduction from angiographic films, it is more practical and reliable to estimate the residual lumen diameter in millimeters (see Fig. 1.1). Bruits generally occur when the residual diameter is 2 mm or less, but when the residual lumen diameter falls below 1 mm, the bruit often diminishes in intensity (30).

Natural History

Population-based studies of patients with asymptomatic bruits but with neither noninvasive nor angiographic studies report a low risk for stroke (4, 12, 23, 33, 40, 49). In a summary of reports of such patients in which noninvasive or angiographic studies were used, the incidence of finding significant stenosis is in the range of 20–60%, and the incidence of a stroke is in the range of 2–6%/year (40).

Evaluation

Bruits associated with internal carotid artery stenosis are usually localized in the midcervical region and are not heard in the low neck or chest. The higher the pitch of the bruit, the tighter the stenosis (13). High-pitched bruits extending into diastole are particularly important because they usually indicate tightly stenotic lesions with a residual lumen diameter of less than 2 mm.

When the presence of an asymptomatic bruit in the region of the carotid bifurcation is established, noninvasive ultrasound studies are ordered (Fig. 3.1) (see also Chapter 1). When a severe, hemodynamically significant internal carotid artery stenosis is suggested (lumen diameter less than 1.5 mm), angiography is usually indicated. With further development of increasingly sensitive noninvasive techniques, these studies may eventually give all the information needed.

ASYMPTOMATIC CAROTID STENOSIS

Natural History

An important issue that has not been settled is the risk of stroke in a patient with carotid atherosclerosis who is asymptomatic with or without a bruit. Fortunately, some patients have warning transient ischemic attacks (TIAs) that precede a stroke, but review of a number of reports indicates that stroke will develop without warning in 2–19% of asymptomatic patients (40). This problem may be complicated by several factors, including associated ulceration or intraplaque hemorrhage, varying rate of change or even arrest of the atherosclerosis, different configurations of the stenosis, and the variability of the collateral circulation (2, 4, 25).

Table 3.1.
Differential Diagnosis of Cervical Bruit

Internal carotid artery stenosis
External carotid artery stenosis
Internal carotid artery dissection
Internal carotid artery kink
Fibromuscular dysplasia
Subclavian or innominate artery stenosis
Radiated cardiac murmur
High flow state
    Intracranial arteriovenous malformation
    Carotid cavernous fistula
    Hyperthyroidism
Venous hum

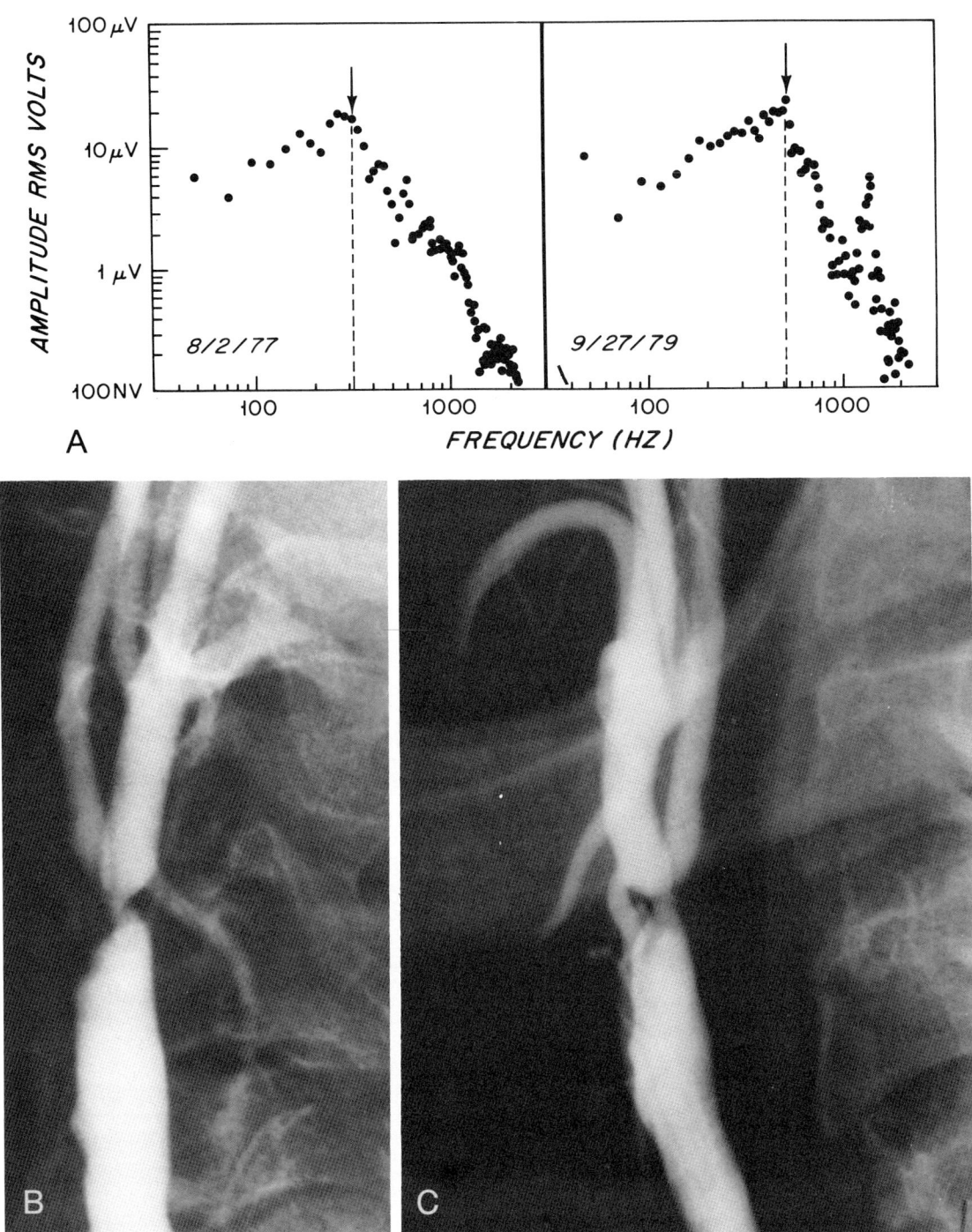

Figure 3.1. Asymptomatic bruit studied by phonoangiography. **A**, the phonoangiogram shows the sound spectrum of a left carotid bifurcation bruit with a break frequency of approximately 230 Hz. The calculated residual lumen diameter is 1.5 mm. The phonoangiogram 25 months later shows a break frequency of 510 Hz consistent with a residual lumen diameter of 1 mm. (Courtesy of Dr. Philip Kistler, MGH). **B** and **C**, The left carotid angiogram (AP and lateral) taken at the time of the second phonoangiogram in **A** shows a stenotic lesion of the left carotid bifurcation, but the residual lumen diameter is difficult to assess. **D**, Cross-section of the plaque removed at operation, at the point of maximal stenosis, from the patient shown in **A** and **B**. Note that the residual lumen diameter is 1 mm.

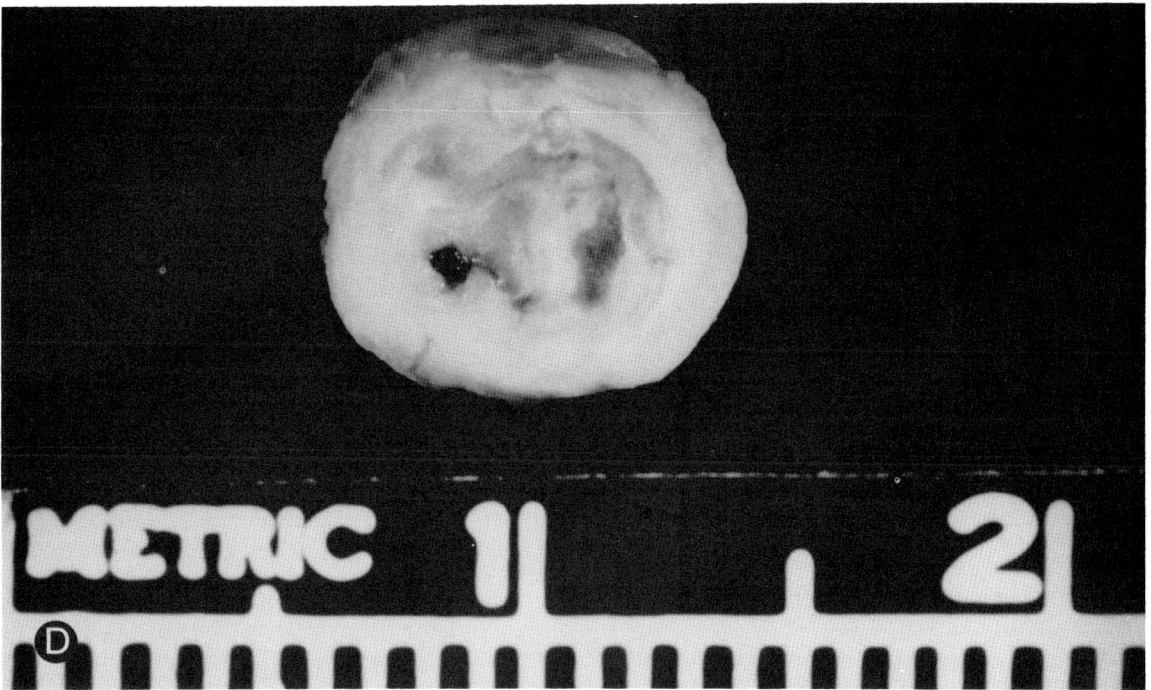

Figure 3.1D.

Several series of patients have been reported in which asymptomatic stenosis has been diagnosed and followed by noninvasive tests (10, 11, 15, 20, 40, 42). In summary, these reports indicate that there is a low risk of stroke, less than 2%/year, unless the stenosis is severe; most strokes are preceded by TIAs; the incidence of TIAs and stroke is greater when the stenosis is over 75–80%; and a small percentage of patients will have a progressive increase in stenosis.

In series of selected patients with asymptomatic stenosis documented by angiography, the stroke rate has varied 0.9%–4.5%/year (24, 45). In a summary of reports of patients with asymptomatic stenosis contralateral to a symptomatic lesion, there was a low incidence of stroke (4, 40). When there is an asymptomatic ulceration, the incidence of stroke is low (22, 31), except when there is a deep irregular ulcer (14, 36).

When the stenosis becomes hemodynamically significant (1.5 mm or less), one should be more concerned (33). In a report of noninvasive studies, it was found that 13 of 78 patients with such lesions developed stroke in a 2-year follow-up period for an average stroke rate of 8.3%/year (27), and in another report, stenosis greater than 90% was associated with a stroke rate of 1.3%/year without warning TIAs and with a stroke rate of 4.2%/year when TIAs developed (5).

Indications for Treatment

Reliable guidelines for management of asymptomatic carotid stenosis have not been established. Consequently, controversies exist as to the value of antiplatelet or anticoagulant therapy and the indications for carotid endarterectomy (40, 50). Evidence has been presented that antiplatelet therapy in patients with TIAs may diminish the subsequent frequency of stroke, at least for males (3). Anticoagulant with coumadin has long been utilized to prevent stroke, but its efficacy in patients with TIAs has not been proven (2).

Several authors have recommended carotid endarterectomy for patients with asymptomatic stenosis (18, 26, 33, 37, 45, 46). It must be pointed out that, to date, statistical evidence has not been presented that shows carotid endarterectomy improves the eventual outcome for patients with asymptomatic carotid stenosis. Included among the reports of surgical treatment of asymptomatic patients are those by Thompson et al (45) (two strokes in 167 operations for asymptomatic bruit (1.2%)) and Moore et al (36) (no complications in 78 operations for asymptomatic carotid ulcer). In the experience of Ojemann et al, no complications were noted in 41 operations (37). A few of their patients had demonstrated progressive stenosis on serial noninvasive studies. In all cases the residual carotid lumen was 1.5 mm or less on angiography. The authors have not been convinced that patients with carotid stenosis with a residual lumen greater than 1.5 mm are at a greater risk for having a stroke and, therefore, have not offered endarterectomy to this category of patient. It has been suggested that endarterectomy can be recommended for asymptomatic carotid stenosis only if the complication range is less than 1% (18). It has been emphasized that the complication rate can be minimized when the operator is experienced, carries out the procedure frequently, and utilizes standard meticulous technique (40, 41). In addition, careful perioperative medical management, particularly in regard to the cardiac status and control of hypertension in the postoperative period, has been shown to minimize risk (7, 8, 36, 39, 44).

Other authors have suggested that patients with asymptomatic carotid stenosis be followed until the appearance of TIAs (50). The patient then is in a category where the risk of possible cerebral infarction is very likely greater than the risk of surgery, and this leaves a large group of patients at risk who do not have warning attacks before the stroke (19, 39). The management of asymptomatic carotid stenosis may be critical in reducing stroke (35).

At the present time, the authors of this text recommend angiography in those medically stable patients with an asymptomatic carotid bruit who have a severe hemodynamically significant lesion or show definite evidence of progression of the stenosis on noninvasive studies (Fig. 3.1). This usually means the residual lumen diameter is 1.5 mm or less. Angiography usually confirms this finding, and surgery is recommended. Others have made similar recommendations (33, 40). If the noninvasive tests indicate the lesion is not hemodynamically significant, it is recommended the patient be followed and the noninvasive tests be repeated in 4–6 months.

In patients undergoing carotid endarterectomy who are found to have asymptomatic contralateral carotid stenosis, the authors follow the same guidelines (i.e., consider prophylactic contralateral endarterectomy only when the residual lumen is less than 1.5 mm). When contralateral endarterectomy is elected, the operation is usually delayed for at least a week after the initial procedure or longer if there is significant neck swelling or suggestion of cranial nerve dysfunction (i.e., dysphasia, dysphonia).

Another question to consider is whether there is an increased risk of stroke in patients with asymptomatic carotid occlusive disease who are to have major surgery. In reviewing the significance of the presence of an asymptomatic carotid bruit in patients undergoing major vascular operative procedures, a total of 1082 patients in three reported series were studied (9, 17, 46). The perioperative stroke rate was 1%, and none of the 167 patients (15.4%) with an asymptomatic carotid bruit suffered a postoperative stroke. Other reports based on noninvasive studies concluded there was no direct relationship between the presence of a carotid bruit, the severity of carotid disease, and the incidence of perioperative stroke (1, 4, 47). In a controlled prospective study, no increased risk in patients with asymptomatic carotid stenosis undergoing major surgery was noted (43). These results suggest that prophylactic carotid endarterectomy may not be indicated in this group of patients.

However, in a series of 234 patients undergoing major cardiovascular surgery the stroke risk without flow-reducing carotid occlusive disease was 1%, and when noninvasive carotid studies showed an internal carotid artery stenosis of 60% or more, there was a 17% incidence of stroke (29). Therefore, the authors of this text believe that a patient with a clinically suspicious carotid bruit who is planning to undergo a major surgical procedure should have noninvasive carotid studies. If the studies suggest a hemodynamically significant lesion, angiography should be considered and prophylactic carotid endarterectomy should be recommended if the residual lumen is less than 1.5 mm. This is especially appropriate if the planned major operation carries a high likelihood of intraoperative hypotension (50).

A special problem is presented by the patient with severe coronary artery disease who is a candidate for coronary bypass surgery and has an asymptomatic bruit or known carotid stenosis. In a large series, symptomatic coronary artery disease increased the operative mortality for carotid endarterectomy from 1.5% to 18.2% (16). On the other hand, the incidence of stroke in patients with asymptomatic carotid artery stenosis undergoing cardiac surgery is increased to 14.9–19% from a risk of infarction of 2–5% in the general population of patients undergoing such procedures (6, 28). With recognition of the special risks associated with combined carotid-coronary disease, what guidelines can then be recommended for these patients? It appears that the presence of preinfarction angina, left main coronary artery disease, triple-vessel disease, and elevated diastolic pressure that impairs ventricular function are strong predictors of cardiac failure or infarction after general anesthesia unless myocardial function is improved (21, 48). Therefore, the presence of any of these factors indicates that a coronary bypass should either precede or be combined with carotid endarterectomy. Most authors agree that when the carotid stenosis is severe, both procedures ought to be carried out simultaneously in a combined procedure, with endarterectomy usually being performed just prior to the coronary bypass (34, 38, 48). The authors of this text agree with Lord that if the carotid stenosis is not severe (less than 70% or 2 mm), coronary bypass can be performed with relative safety and the carotid stenosis can be followed and corrected later if it becomes more severe or symptomatic (32). These recommendations imply that the patient with an asymptomatic carotid bruit who is being considered for coronary bypass surgery should have noninvasive studies prior to the operation, and if the studies suggest severe stenosis, an angiogram is in order.

REFERENCES

1. Barnes RW, Marszalek PB: Asymptomatic carotid disease in the cardiovascular surgical patient: Is prophylatic endarterectomy necessary? *Stroke* 12:497–500, 1981.
2. Barnett HJM: Progress towards stroke prevention. *Neurology* 30:1212–1225, 1980.
3. Barnett HJM, et al: A randomized trial of aspirin and sulfinpyrazone in threatened stroke. The Canadian Cooperative Study Group. *N Engl J Med* 299:53–59, 1978.
4. Barnett HJM, Mohr JP, Yatsu FM: Asymptomatic carotid bruit or stenosis. In Barnett HJM, Mohr JP, Stein BM, Yatsu FM (eds): *Stroke*. New York, Churchill Livingstone, 1986, pp 1207–1219.
5. Bogousslavsky J, Despland PA, Regli F: Asymptomatic tight stenosis of the internal carotid artery: Long-term prognosis. *Neurology* 36:861–863, 1986.
6. Brener, BJ, Brief DK, Alpert J. Goldenkranz RJ, Parsonnet V, Feldman S, Giclchinsky I, Abel RM, Hochberg M, Hussain M: A four year experience with preoperative noninvasive carotid evaluation of two thousand twenty-six patients undergoing cardiac surgery. *J Vasc Surg* 1:326–338, 1984.
7. Brewster DC, Schlaen HH, Raines JK, Abbott WM, Darling RC: Rational management of the asymptomatic carotid bruit. *Arch Surg* 113:927–930, 1978.
8. Caplan LR, Skillman J, Ojemann R, Fields WS: Intracerebral hemorrhage following carotid endarterectomy: A hypertensive complication? *Stroke* 9:457–460, 1978.
9. Carney WI, Stewart WB, DePinto DJ, Mucha SJ, Roberts B: Carotid bruit as a risk in aortoiliac reconstruction. *Surgery* 81:567–570, 1977.
10. Chambers BR, Norris JW: The case against surgery for asymptomatic carotid stenosis. *Stroke* 15:964–967, 1984.
11. Colgan MP, Kingston W, Shanik DG: Asymptomatic carotid stenosis: Is prophylactic endarterectomy justifiable? *Br J Surg* 72:313–314, 1985.
12. Crowell RM, Ojemann RG, Kistler JP: Asymptomatic Carotid Bruit. In Thompson RA, Green JR (eds): *Controversies in Neurology*. New York, Raven Press, 1983, pp 101–115.
13. David TE, Humphries AW, Young JR, Beven EG: A correlation of neck bruits and atherosclerotic carotid arteries. *Arch Surg* 107:729–731, 1973.
14. Dixon S, Pais SO, Raviola C, Gomes A, Machelder HI, Baker JO, Busuttil RW, Baker WF, Moore WS: Natural history of nonstenotic, asymptomatic ulcerative lesions of the carotid artery. A further analysis. *Arch Surg* 117:1493–1498, 1982.
15. Durwand QJ, Ferguson GG, Barr HW: The natural history of asymptomatic carotid bifurcation plaques. *Stroke* 13:459–464, 1982.
16. Ennix CL Jr, Lawrie GM, Morris GC Jr, Crawford ES, Howell JF, Reardon MJ, Weatherford SC: Improved results of carotid endarterectomy in patients with symptomatic coronary disease: An analysis of 1,546 consecutive carotid operations. *Stroke* 10:122–125, 1979.
17. Evans WE, Cooperman M: The significance of asymptomatic unilateral carotid bruits in preoperative patients. *Surgery* 83:521–522, 1978.
18. Fields WS: The asymptomatic carotid bruit—operate or not? *Stroke* 9:269–271, 1978.
19. Fisher CM: The natural history of carotid occlusion. In Austin GM (ed): *Microneurosurgical Anastomoses for Cerebral Ischemia*. Springfield, IL, Charles C Thomas, 1976, pp 194–201.
20. Ford CS, Frye JL, Toole JF, Lefkowitz D:L Asymptomatic carotid bruit and stenosis. A prospective follow-up study. *Arch Neurol* 43:219–222, 1986.
21. Gilman S: Cerebral disorders after open heart operations. *N Engl J Med* 272:489–498, 1965.
22. Harward TR, Kroener JM, Wickbom IG, Bernstein EF: Natural history of asymptomatic ulcerative plaques of the carotid bifurcation. *Am J Surg* 146:208–212, 1983.
23. Heyman A, Wilkinson W, Heyden S, Helms MJ, Bartel AG, Karp HR, Tyroler HA, Hames CG: Risk of stroke in asymptomatic persons with cervical arterial bruits—a population study in Evans County, Georgia. *N Engl Med* 303:838–841, 1980.
24. Humphries AW, Young JR, Santilli PH, Beven EG, deWolfe VG: Unoperated, asymptomatic significant internal carotid artery stenosis: A review of 182 instances. *Surgery* 80:695–698, 1976.
25. Javid H, Ostermiller WE, Hengesh JW, Dye WS, Hunter JA, Najafi H, Julian OC: Natural history of carotid bifurcation atheroma. *Surgery* 67:80–86, 1970.
26. Javid H, Ostermiller WE, Hengesh JW, Dye WS, Hunter JA, Najafi H, Julian OC: Carotid endarterectomy for asymptomatic patients. *Arch Surg* 102:389–391, 1971.
27. Kartchner MM, McRae LP: Noninvasive evaluation and management of the "asymptomatic" carotid bruit. *Surgery* 82:840–847, 1977.
28. Kartchner MM, McRae LP: The clinical use of oculoplethysmography and carotid phonoangiography. In Baker WH (ed): *Diagnosis and Treatment of Carotid Artery Disease*. Mt Kisco, NY, Futura, 1979, pp 55–81.
29. Kartchner MM, McRae LP: Carotid occlusive disease as a risk factor in major cardiovascular surgery. *Arch Surg* 117:1086–1088, 1982.
30. Kistler JP, Lees RS, Friedman J, Pessin M, Mohr JP, Roberson GH, Ojemann RG: The bruit of carotid stenosis versus radiated basal heart murmurs. Differentiation by phonoangiography. *Circulation* 57:975–981, 1978.
31. Kroener JM, Dorn PL, Shoor PM, Wickbom IG, Bernstein EF: Prognosis of asymptomatic ulcerating carotid lesions: *Arch Surg* 115:1387–1392, 1980.
32. Lord RSA: Asymptomatic lesions. In Lord RSA (ed): *Cerebral Vascular Disease*. St Louis, CV Mosby, 1986, pp 403–435.
33. Martin NA, Hadley MN, Spetzler RF, Carter LP: Management of asymptomatic carotid atherosclerosis. *Neurosurgery* 18:505–513, 1986.
34. McCollum CH, Garcia-Rinaldi R, Graham JM, DeBakey ME: Myocardial revascularization prior to subsequent major surgery in patients with coronary artery disease. *Surgery* 81:302–304, 1977.
35. Mohr JP: Transient ischemic attacks and the prevention of strokes. *N Engl J Med* 299:93–95, 1978.
36. Moore WS, Malone JM, Boren C, Roon AJ, Goldston J: Asymptomatic ulcerative lesions of the carotid artery—natural history and effect of surgical therapy compared. *Stroke* 10:96, 1979.
37. Ojemann RG, Crowell RM, Roberson GH, Fisher CM: Surgical treatment of extracranial carotid occlusive disease. *Clin Neurosurg* 22:214–263, 1975.
38. Okies JE, MacMannus Q, Starr A: Myocardial revascularization and carotid endarterectomy: A combined approach. *Ann Thorac Surg* 23:560–563, 1977.
39. Pessin MS, Hinton RC, Davis KR, Duncan GW, Roberson GH, Ackerman RH, Mohr JP: Mechanisms of acute carotid stroke. *Ann Neurol* 6:245–252, 1979.
40. Quifiones-Baldrich WJ, Moore WS: Asymptomatic carotid stenosis. Rationale for management. *Arch Neurol* 42:378–382, 1985.
41. Robertson JT, Watridge CB: The surgical management of extracranial and intracranial occlusive disease. *Med Clin North Am* 63:681–693, 1979.
42. Roederer GO, Langlois YE, Lusiani L, Jager KA, Primozich JF, Lawrence RI, Phillips DJ, Strandness DE Jr: Natural history of carotid artery disease on the side contralateral to endarterectomy. *J Vasc Surg* 1:62–72, 1984.
43. Ropper A: Carotid bruit and the risk of stroke in elective surgery. *N Engl J Med* 307:1388–1390, 1982.
44. Sundt TM Jr, Sandok BA, Whisnant JP: Carotid endarterectomy: Complications and preoperative assessment of risk. *Mayo Clin Proc* 50:301–306, 1975.

45. Thompson JE, Patman RD, Talkington CM: Asymptomatic carotid bruit: Long-term outcome of patients having endarterectomy compared with unoperated controls. Ann Surg 188:308–316, 1978.
46. Treiman RL, Foran RF, Shore EH, Levin PM: Carotid bruit: Significance in patients undergoing an abdominal aortic operation. Arch Surg 106:803–805, 1973.
47. Turnipseed WD, Berkoff HA, Beizer FO: Postoperative stroke in cardiac and peripheral vascular disease. Ann Surg 192:365–368, 1980.
48. Urschel HC Jr: Management of concomitant coronary and carotid artery obstructive disease. Cleve Clin Q 45:128–129, 1978.
49. Wolf PA, Kannel WB, McNamara PM, Dawber TR: Asymptomatic carotid bruits and risk of stroke: The Framingham Study. Stroke 10:96, 1979.
50. Yatsu FM, Fields WS: Asymptomatic carotid bruit. Stenosis or ulceration, a conservative approach. Arch Neurol 42:383–385, 1985.

4

Extracranial to Middle Cerebral Artery Bypass Graft

INDICATIONS FOR SURGERY

The extracranial to intracranial (EC-IC) artery bypass graft was developed to revascularize the brain in patients with cerebrovascular occlusive disease not amenable to direct surgery. Superficial temporal artery to middle cerebral artery anastomosis was first performed by Donaghy and Yasargil in 1967 using microsurgical techniques (11, 48, 49). Refinements in technique have included the use of interrupted sutures for greater precision (33), use of the angular branch of the middle cerebral artery for maximum flow (6), and linear incision over the superficial temporal artery to avoid scalp flap necrosis. Interposition of a saphenous vein segment ("short vein graft") between the superficial temporal artery and a middle cerebral artery branch has been recommended to provide high flow revascularization (27).

Since EC-IC bypass often improves collateral circulation distal to an inaccessible occlusive lesion (30), it is reasonable to expect that the procedure might protect against future ischemic infarction. However, bypass also carries risk of stroke or death, and the procedure might enhance passage of emboli via the external carotid artery or increase the chance of proximal occlusion by diminishing the pressure gradient across a stenosis.

Speculative debate regarding rationales for and against EC-IC bypass has been reduced sharply by the emergence of data from a controlled study (46, 47). The Extracranial-Intracranial Bypass Study assessed in controlled, randomized fashion the impact of EC-IC bypass on stroke and death in patients with middle cerebral artery stenosis or occlusion or internal carotid artery stenosis at or above C2 or occlusion and either transient ischemic attack(s) (TIAs) or minor completed stroke(s) in the carotid artery distributions within 3 months of being studied. In the study 1495 patients from 71 centers were randomly allocated to best medical therapy (including antiaggregant therapy) or medical therapy plus EC-IC bypass. Follow-up averaged 55.8 months without loss of a single case. Technical proficiency was high in that 96% of bypasses were angiographically patent, and risk of major stroke or death was about 3%.

The major conclusion of the study was that EC-IC bypass did not reduce the risk of ischemic stroke in the groups studied, nor did any subgroup enjoy benefit from surgery. In fact, the group of patients with middle cerebral artery stenosis and internal carotid artery siphon stenosis had statistically superior results with medical treatment. In view of the results of this excellent study, it is difficult to recommend bypass using the same all-inclusive criteria used in the EC-IC Bypass Study (12).

However, the EC-IC Bypass Study did not study several categories of patients with occlusive cerebrovascular disease. These include patients with low perfusion syndromes, ischemic ocular syndromes, moyamoya disease, and the use of the procedure in conjunction with aneurysm and tumor surgery. Further investigation will be needed to define the place of bypass surgery in these special groups. Since basal arterial occlusive disease (including moyamoya cases) causes substantial neurologic complications, EC-IC bypass has been recommended for these patients (1, 25, 31). There may be a role for bypass in patients with internal carotid artery or middle cerebral artery stenosis with TIA or stroke despite maximum medical therapy. The role of bypass remains uncertain for amaurosis fugax with internal carotid artery occlusion (26), chronic cerebral ischemia (20, 21), and dementia due to multiple cerebrovascular occlusions (13).

Moreover, there still may be a selected subgroup of patients, who could be defined physiologically, who may benefit from this procedure (16). Studies of regional cerebral blood flow (CBF) and metabolism (oxygen extraction fraction) may help in defining the indications for bypass (17, 30, 37). A careful investigation will be needed to establish a role for bypass in these cases.

The use of emergency EC-IC bypass graft has been assessed and the reports indicate variable results (7, 9, 10). In most reported cases the conditions have been far from ideal with a long delay between onset of symptoms and surgery or the presence of middle cerebral artery occlusion with blockage of the origin of the lenticulostriate branches.

Bypass graft seems helpful in preventing ischemia

when planned internal carotid artery occlusion is done for a giant internal carotid artery aneurysm in the presence of poor collateral supply (2, 15, 40, 42, 47). Since some patients tolerate carotid occlusion without bypass, the precise role of bypass in this setting has not yet been fully defined. Cerebral blood flow studies may help in these cases (24) (see Chapter 20). In exceptional cases of basal tumor with high operative risk of middle cerebral artery compromise, an initial EC-IC bypass can protect against ischemia. The role of EC-IC bypass in cerebrovascular occlusive disease of the posterior circulation is also yet to be defined (4, 22, 34, 43) (see Chapter 5).

PREOPERATIVE EVALUATION

The preoperative medical evaluation is similar to that described for carotid endarterectomy. The keystone for planning a bypass operation is three-vessel angiography to delineate cerebrovascular occlusions, collateral circulation, and potential bypass vessels. Delayed films in some cases may show reconstitution of the carotid siphon with reflux to the upper cervical internal carotid artery, a sign that suggests the carotid occlusion may be opened surgically. Multiple filling defects in middle cerebral artery branches suggest embolic occlusions that probably cannot be helped by EC-IC bypass. Poor collateral circulation to a symptomatic hemisphere suggests a hemodynamic mechanism. Careful study of the angiogram usually permits identification of the best vessels for anastomosis. Failure to opacify middle cerebral artery branches by collateral routes need not imply lack of a suitable recipient branch for the operation. The larger superficial temporal artery branch, usually the frontal, is selected, and when this is less than 1 mm in diameter, the occipital artery may be chosen instead. In the setting of a tiny superficial temporal artery and a proximally branching occipital artery, a short vein graft may be interposed between the superficial temporal artery or the occipital artery and the middle cerebral artery recipient branch. Studies of regional cerebral blood flow and metabolism may help to establish the indications for revascularization (17, 30, 37).

If the patient is on heparin, this is stopped at least 8 hours prior to operation. Many patients are on aspirin. Some surgeons prefer to stop these drugs several days before operation. However, others prefer to maintain antiplatelet therapy through the operative period. This does increase the risk of intraoperative oozing, which may require platelet transfusion for hemostasis. Antihypertensive medication is maintained. Diphenylhydantoin is begun the day before surgery to ensure prophylactic blood levels of this anticonvulsant medication in the immediate postoperative period.

ANESTHESIA

Premedication is kept to a minimum. The patient's legs are wrapped with Ace bandages. General endotracheal anesthesia is used with controlled ventilation to maintain the arterial pCO_2 in the range of 35–40 torr. Precordial electrodes provide continuous electrocardiographic monitoring. Arterial blood pressure is monitored continuously with a radial artery catheter. Infusions of colloid, phenylephrine, or nitroprusside maintain blood pressure in the normal range for the individual patient during induction and surgery. An antibiotic is administered prior to incision and for 24 hours postoperatively.

OPERATIVE TECHNIQUE

Positioning

Prior to the induction of anesthesia, the operative area is shaved and the superficial temporal artery course marked with a marking pen because the pulse may be harder to delineate after induction. Sometimes a Doppler probe may be needed to trace the vessel. The patient lies supine with the head turned to the opposite side. The table is flexed slightly to bring the head above heart level. A small roll serves to elevate the shoulder on the operative side. The head is flexed and held in the three-point skeletal fixation headrest (Mayfield-Kees). The operating table may need to be tilted with the "side" adjustment to bring the temporal squama parallel to the floor.

Instruments

Several microsurgical instruments are essential for this operation. A no. 5 Dumont jeweler's forceps adapted for bipolar coagulation is needed for precise hemostasis near bypass vessels. A similar forceps and a Heifetz curved scissors serve well to prepare the small arteries for anastomosis. Kleinert-Kees miniature clips are ideal for temporary occlusion of cortical arteries with minimal trauma. A 10-mm straight Heifetz clip is satisfactory for temporary occlusion of the superficial temporal artery origin. Miniature Gelpi retractors are helpful in maintaining satisfactory exposure. A curved Heifetz microscissors is used to fashion the cortical arteriotomy. Fine Silastic tubing (0.025 inch outside diameter) can be useful as a middle cerebral artery stent during surgery. The anastomosis is performed with a curved 8-inch Rhoton needle holder and 9-0 or 10-0 monofilament nylon suture on a BV-6 needle (Ethicon).

Exposure

Before preparation of the scalp, the superficial temporal artery course is scratched into the skin over the previous pen marking. The position of the middle cerebral artery recipient branch is determined from the angiogram and is likewise marked. When a pterional or other approach to an intracranial aneurysm or tumor may be needed in conjunction with a bypass, a modified flap as shown in Figure 4.1 may provide exposure for all contemplated surgical procedures. Although one might anticipate ischemia at the tips of the flaps, the authors have not experienced this problem.

When a craniotomy is made, the authors prefer to turn the scalp and bone flaps under loupes and headlight illumination. Care is taken to avoid injury to the superficial temporal artery, which is meticulously dissected with a mosquito hemostat. The larger branch, usually the frontal, is preserved for anastomosis, and the smaller is ligated and divided. The temporalis muscle is exposed by reflecting three scalp flaps (Fig. 4.2A). The temporalis incision is planned to permit compression-free routing of the graft to the middle cerebral artery branch for anastomosis. The craniotomy is made over a point 6 cm above the external auditory meatus to optimize chances for a large middle cerebral artery branch being exposed (Fig. 4.2B). Once the dura is opened, the microscope is swung into the field.

When no other intracranial surgery is contemplated, the authors prefer linear incisions in contrast to a scalp flap (Fig. 4.3A–D). Linear incisions permit rapid superficial temporal artery preparation and avoid some scalp necrosis that may occur with a flap. One or two linear incisions may be needed, depending on the superficial temporal artery branch selected and occasionally on the middle cerebral artery branch chosen. Most frequently, the frontal branch of the superficial temporal artery and the angular branch of the middle cerebral artery are the largest and thus the best arteries available for anastomosis (Fig. 4.3A). The angular branch may be used with safety even on the dominant hemisphere. Occasionally, the posterior branch of the superficial temporal artery (Fig. 4.3B) or a frontal branch of the middle cerebral artery will be selected for bypass (Fig. 4.3C).

When a cutdown technique is used, the initial incision is made over the superficial temporal artery with the microscope at 10× (Fig. 4.4). The surgeon's arms are supported on either side. The initial incision with a no. 15 blade is made over the distal superficial temporal artery down to the subcutaneous fat to avoid injury to the superficial temporal artery trunk. Then the surgeon elevates the scalp tissue with Adson forceps, and the plane just superficial to the superficial temporal artery is developed with Metzenbaum scissors (Fig. 4.4A). When the proper plane is chosen, the superficial temporal artery is readily exposed over an 8–10-cm length.

Superficial Temporal Artery Preparation

For the flap technique, the superficial temporal artery is identified just deep to the galea. Often an appropriate branch can be traced tetrograde from the scalp incision. The superficial temporal artery is isolated by sharp dissection down to fat and hair foi-

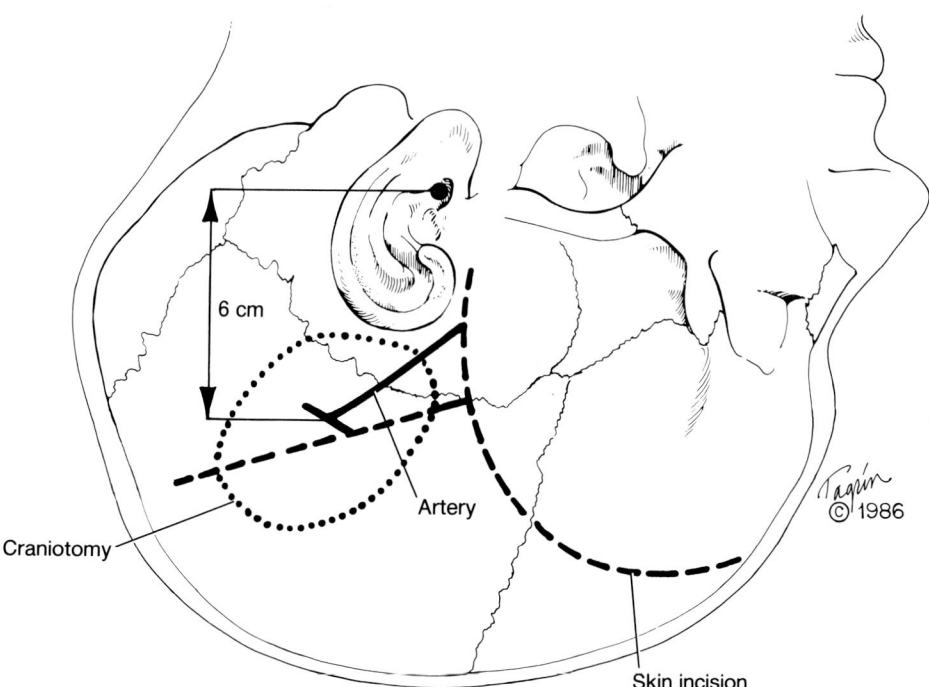

Figure 4.1. Scalp incisions for a combined EC-IC bypass graft and pterional approach to an intracranial lesion.

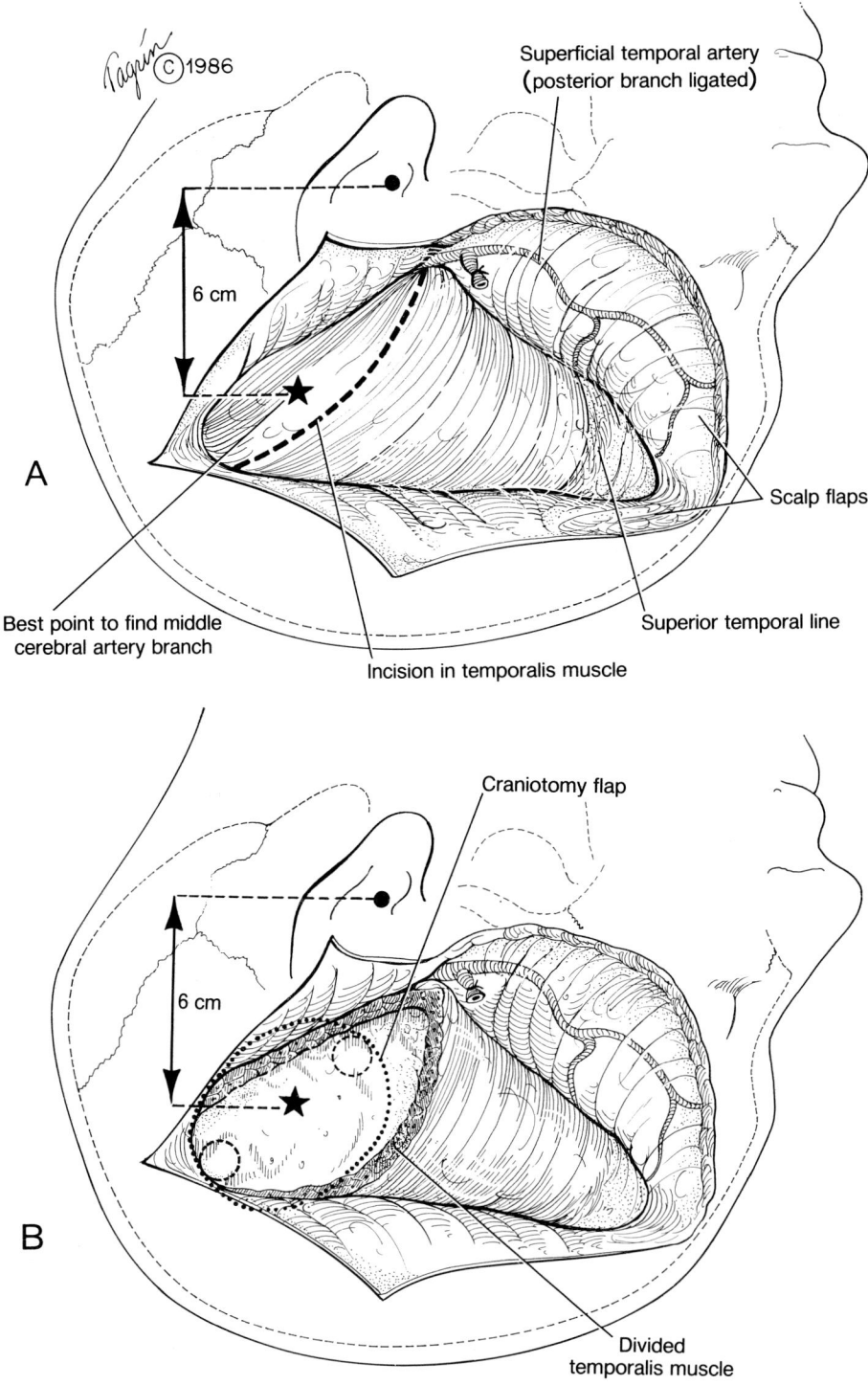

Figure 4.2. **A**, Scalp flaps and temporalis muscle incision for combined EC-IC bypass graft and pterional approach to an intracranial lesion. **B**, Craniotomy flap for EC-IC bypass graft with pterional approach for an intracranial lesion.

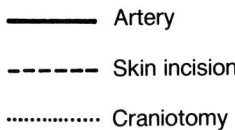

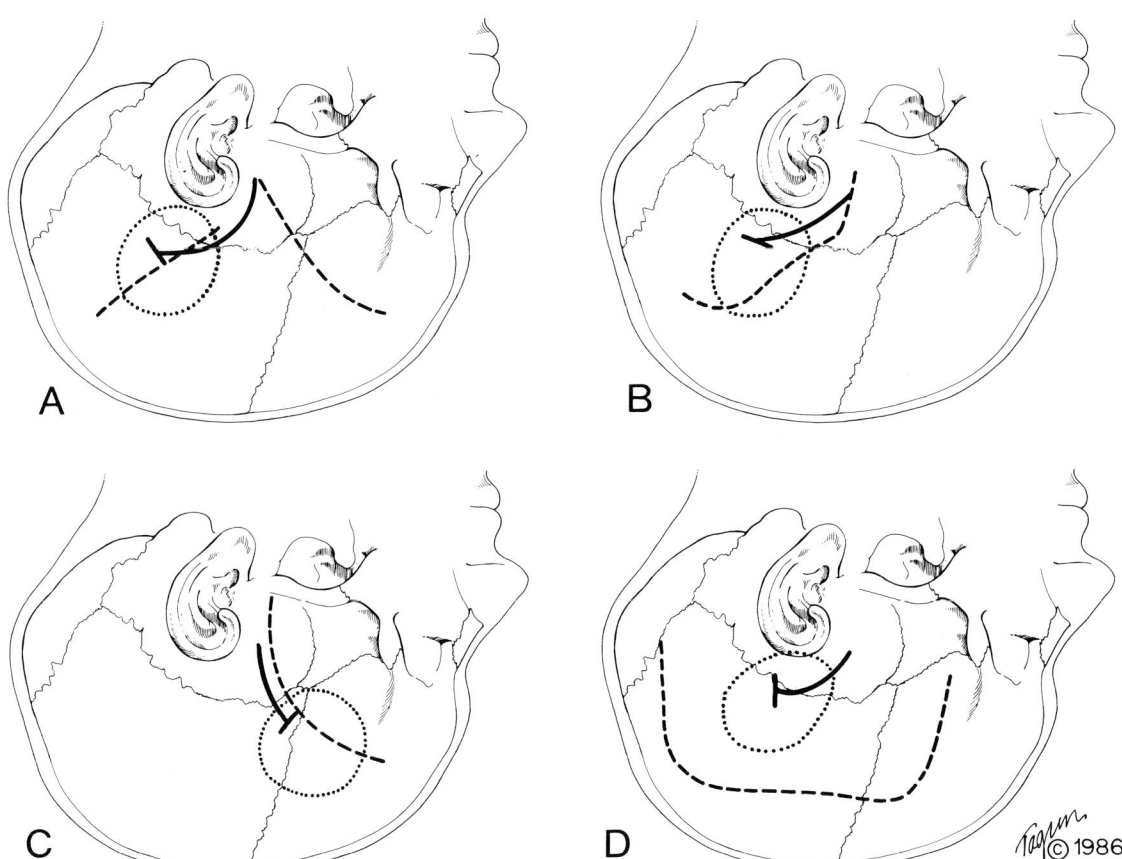

Figure 4.3. Scalp incisions. Several different approaches are used, depending on the suitability of donor and recipient vessels and on possible need for other intracranial surgery. **A**, Two linear "cutdown" incisions. This is the most commonly used approach. It permits quick access to the largest arteries, usually the frontal branch of superficial temporal artery and angular branch of middle cerebral artery, and avoids scalp edge necrosis. **B**, Single posterior "cutdown" incision. A useful approach if the parietal branch of the superficial temporal artery is larger. **C**, Single anterior "cutdown" incision. Uncommon, but can be used if the frontal branch of the middle cerebral artery is selected. **D**, Horseshoe flap which may be helpful if the status of superficial temporal artery and middle cerebral artery branches is uncertain since it gives a wide field to search out the best vessels. Be sure to keep the base of the devascularized flap broad to avoid skin edge necrosis.

licles where a plane is established superficial to the vessel. Some adventitia is left in place. Small bleeders are coagulated with bipolar cautery away from the superficial temporal artery. Branches larger than 0.5 mm are divided between 6-0 silk ligatures. To facilitate this dissection, the surgeon uses a knife and forceps and the assistant uses a sucker and bipolar cautery. When a cutdown technique is used (Fig. 4.2), small scalp flaps are elevated on either side of the superficial temporal artery (Fig. 4.4A and B). The adventitia is incised with a no. 15 knife blade approximately 2 mm to each side of the superficial temporal artery down to the temporalis fascia. A few spreading movements with the Metzenbaum scissors develop a plane between the superficial temporal artery and the temporalis fascia, thus completing isolation of the vessel (Fig. 4.4C). After exposure of the middle cerebral artery recipient branch (described below), the superficial temporal artery is cut to a satisfactory length. This is usually 8 cm and includes a bit of extra length to facilitate suturing of the back wall. The artery is then occluded with a Heifetz clip

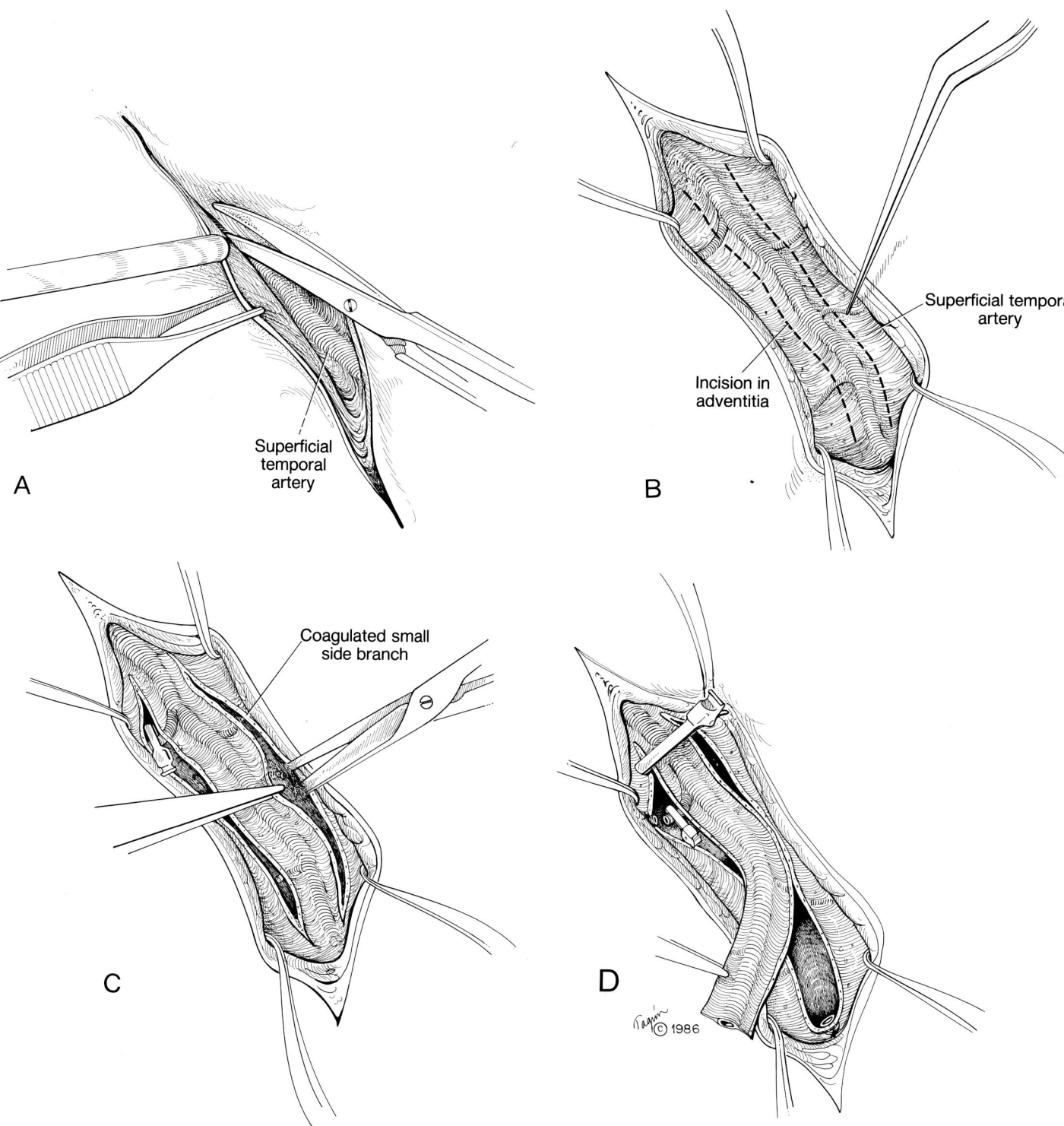

Figure 4.4. "Cutdown" technique for superficial temporal artery (*STA*). **A,** After the skin has been incised superficially with a no. 15 blade it is elevated from the artery with forceps. Metzenbaum scissors cut adventitia and overlying soft tissues. **B,** Exposure of the superficial temporal artery. After the incision is completed, miniature Gelpi retractors are placed. Small side branches are coagulated with bipolar cautery; large ones are divided between 6–0 ligatures. **C,** Isolation of the superficial temporal artery. With a no. 15 blade, the adventitia is incised down to temporalis fascia. Scissors develop the plane between the vessel and deep fascia. The largest proximal side branch is clipped and preserved with adequate length to receive an irrigation catheter. **D,** Preparation of superficial temporal artery. After checking to be sure the length is adequate, the artery is clipped proximally, cross-cut distally, and irrigated with heparinized saline.

and is divided (Fig. 4.4D). Heparinized saline is flushed into the superficial temporal artery via a no. 20 Medicut catheter. This irrigation flushes out blood and helps to identify bleeders for coagulation. When a large proximal side branch is available, an irrigation catheter may be tied into the branch to permit intermittent superficial temporal artery irrigation during anastomosis and bypass pressure measurement after its completion (Fig. 4.5). Superficial temporal artery irrigation with saline serves to clear bits of clot and to identify gaps that require additional sutures.

The tip of the superficial temporal artery is freed of adventitia over a 1-cm length and then beveled in a fishmouth fashion to maximize the anastomotic

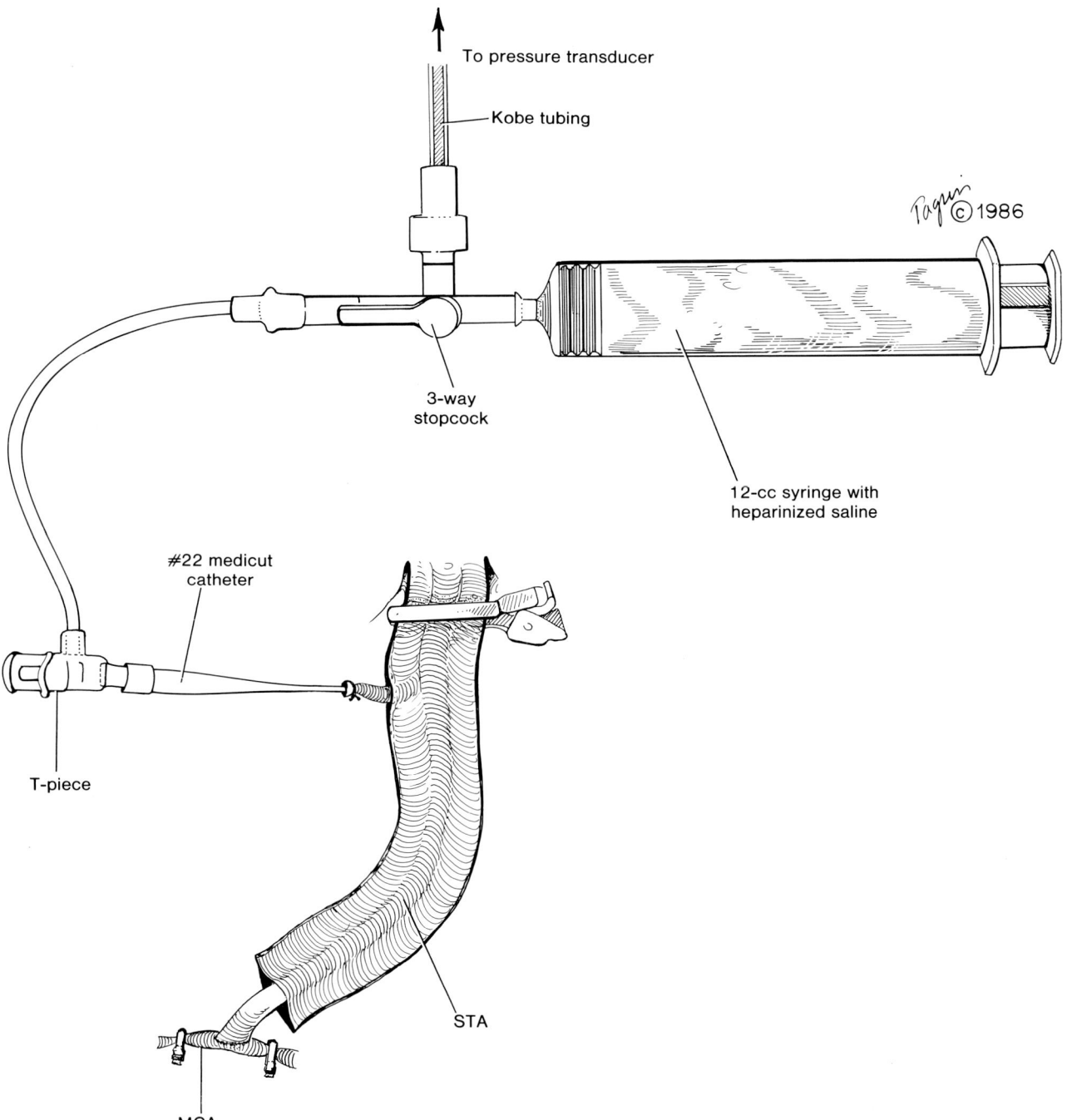

Figure 4.5. Side catheter into graft. Cannulation of a large proximal branch permits frequent irrigation with heparinized saline. Suture line leaks may be identified before restoring blood flow. The side catheter may also be used to measure pressure in the superficial temporal artery (*STA*) or in the middle cerebral artery (*MCA*).

opening (Fig. 4.6). If the intima should separate from the muscularis, a second cut a few millimeters proximally is necessary. The artery is again flushed with heparinized saline.

In some patients, the superficial temporal artery segment must be led from one incision to another. A tunnel is prepared by blunt dissection between the galea and temporalis fascia. The superficial temporal artery tip is pulled through the tunnel with a terminal silk tie. Twists and kinks in the superficial temporal artery segment are carefully avoided.

Middle Cerebral Artery Preparation

Generally the angular branch of the middle cerebral artery is used, lying about 6 cm rostral to the external auditory canal. When the frontal superficial temporal artery is used, the angular branch is exposed through a separate incision (Fig. 4.3A). Temporalis muscle is opened with a cutting cautery, which also can be used to elevate the periosteum. When a frontal branch of the middle cerebral artery is to be used, incision and exposure in this area are performed as shown in Figure 4.3C.

A small craniotomy flap, about 7 cm in diameter, is fashioned over the recipient artery with a power drill and craniotome (Fig. 4.7). The authors have found this method faster and safer than either craniectomy or trephine. Bone edges are waxed and the dura is opened in a cruciate fashion. Additional bone may be removed (especially inferiorly) if no suitable recipient branch is identified. When a suitable vessel is exposed, three drill holes are made in the bone edge for eventual bone flap replacement, and dural to pericranial sutures are placed.

Employing 25× magnification, the arachnoid next to the middle cerebral artery is cut with microscissors. Tiny side branches may be coagulated with the bipolar cautery on low power and cut as needed to prepare a 1-cm length of artery (Fig. 4.8). One or two larger side branches can be preserved by using temporary clips. A strip of rubber dam is placed under the middle cerebral artery to protect cortex (Fig. 4.9A).

Final preparation of the middle cerebral artery is achieved at 25× magnification with the prepared superficial temporal artery tip in full view. Kleinert-Kees clips are placed on the middle cerebral artery branch at least 10 mm apart. A slender oval arteriotomy, the same length as the superficial temporal artery tip width, is made in the middle cerebral artery with one or two snips of the microscissors (Fig. 4.9B and C). The vessel is irrigated with heparinized saline. At times it is helpful to insert a stent of fine silastic tubing into the vessel.

Anastomosis

It is preferable but not essential to position the superficial temporal artery tip against the middle cerebral artery opening with the tip aimed backward toward the middle cerebral artery origin to promote flow throughout the middle cerebral artery territory. A needle holder and jeweler's forceps are used to place interrupted 9-0 or 10-0 nylon sutures in each corner (Fig. 4.10). Forceps are used primarily as a counter pressor during suturing, and the vessel wall is handled as little and as gently as possible. Squeez-

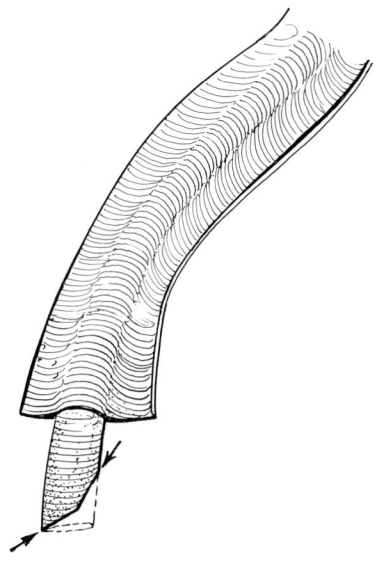

Figure 4.6. Preparation of the superficial temporal artery tip. The distal tip is freed of adventitia and fish-mouthed for maximum ostium. The authors find two snips with straight microscissors effective. The lumen is checked for an intimal flap.

Extracranial to Middle Cerebral Artery Bypass Graft

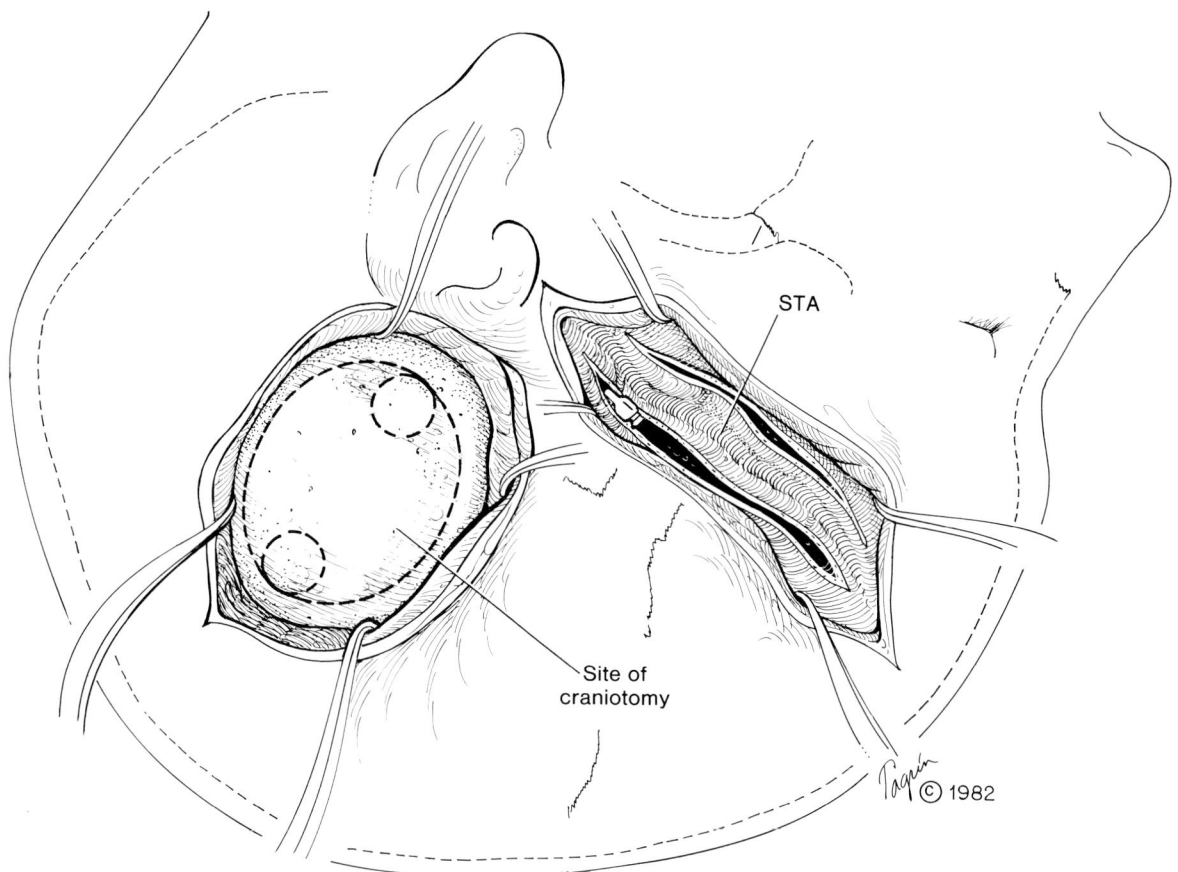

Figure 4.7. Craniotomy with "cutdown" technique. The posterior wound in deepened by cutting cauterization down to bone. A small craniotomy is fashioned with the drill and craniotome. The anterior burr hole will serve to pass the graft. The exposure must be low enough to demonstrate temporal branches. *STA*, superficial temporal artery.

ing the intima is particularly avoided. An additional 6–10 interrupted sutures are placed in the front wall (Fig. 4.11), and these are tied down after all have been placed to give maximum accuracy. Bites are a bit larger on the superficial temporal artery side to promote slight eversion and intima-to-intima apposition. Sutures must accurately include superficial temporal artery intima, which may be thickened and separated from the muscularis. In-to-out passage of the needle through the superficial temporal artery is recommended when an intimal flap threatens. Sutures are placed slightly closer together near the corner where leaks are more common. Keeping the area dry facilitates suture handling. Keeping the needle in view on the rubber dam minimizes time lost in searching. Some surgeons advocate using a running suture technique routinely, but in the authors' experience interrupted stitches have provided superior precision and maximum ostial width.

The superficial temporal artery is reflected aside to reveal the back wall of the anastomosis. The front wall suture line is inspected from inside to confirm accurate suture placement. Then, 6–10 interrupted sutures are used to complete the back wall (Fig. 4.12). Before the last two sutures are tied, the stent tube is gently removed and the three vascular limbs are opened briefly to check flow and expel air (Fig. 4.13). Final sutures are tied down.

The distal middle cerebral artery clip is removed first and then the proximal. Utilizing 25× magnification, the suture line is inspected for leaks. A major area of leak requires a stitch; suture line ooze will stop without additional sutures. The rubber dam is folded over the suture line and a cottonoid provides pressure for 1–2 minutes. In some cases, a collar of Gelfoam may secure suture line hemostasis. Finally, the superficial temporal artery clip is removed. One may measure graft pressures when a suitable side branch of superficial temporal artery has been cannulated. Graft flow may also be estimated with an electromagnetic flow probe, but great care must be exercised to avoid injury to the superficial temporal artery by the flow probe. Graft patency may also be assessed with real time Doppler ultrasonography.

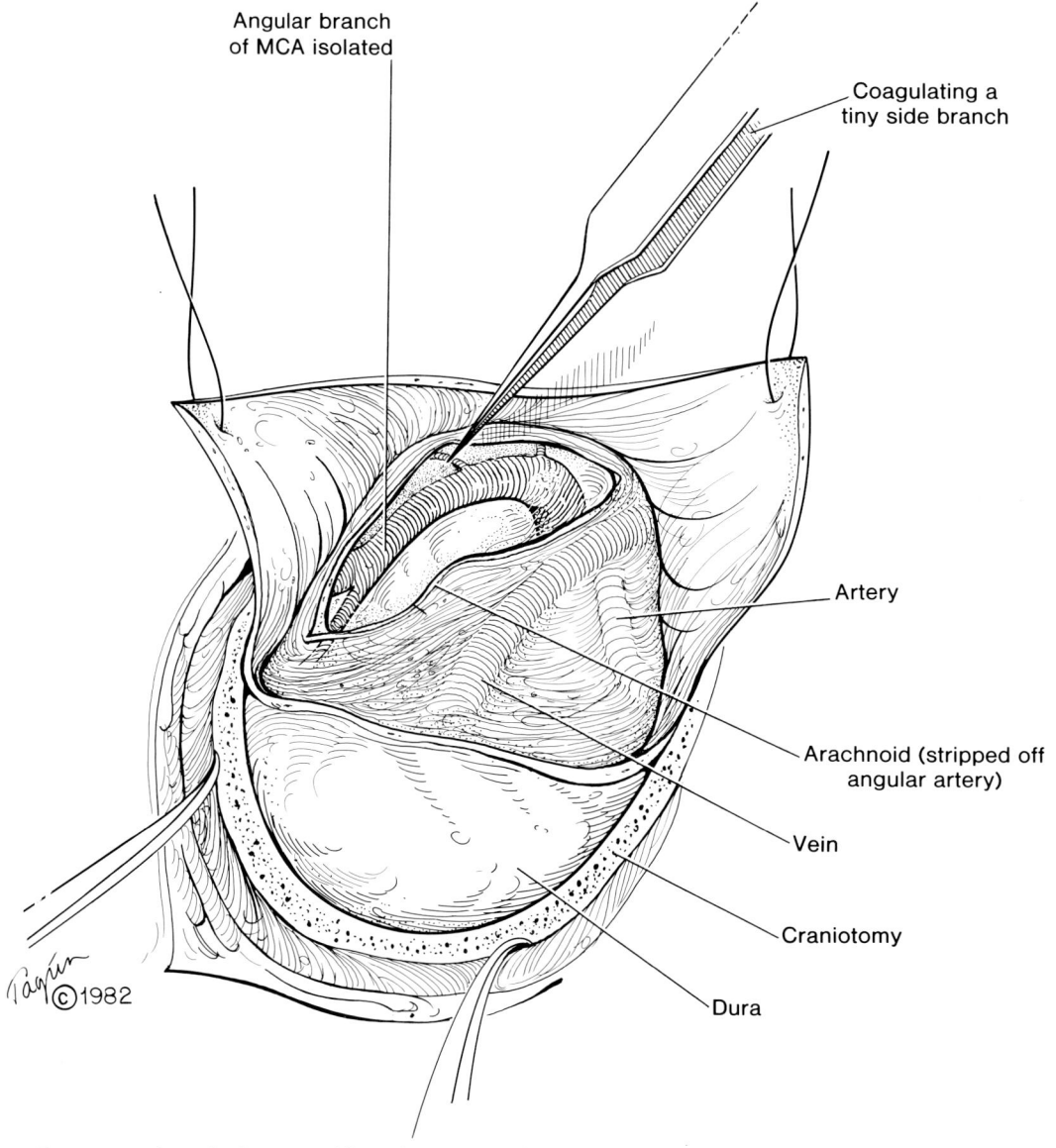

Figure 4.8. Exposure of cortical artery. After placement of dural-pericranial tenting sutures, the dura is opened enough to expose a suitable recipient artery. Under 25×, arachnoid over the vessel is opened sharply. To obtain a 10-mm segment for anastomosis, one or two tiny side branches may be coagulated and cut. *MCA*, middle cerebral artery.

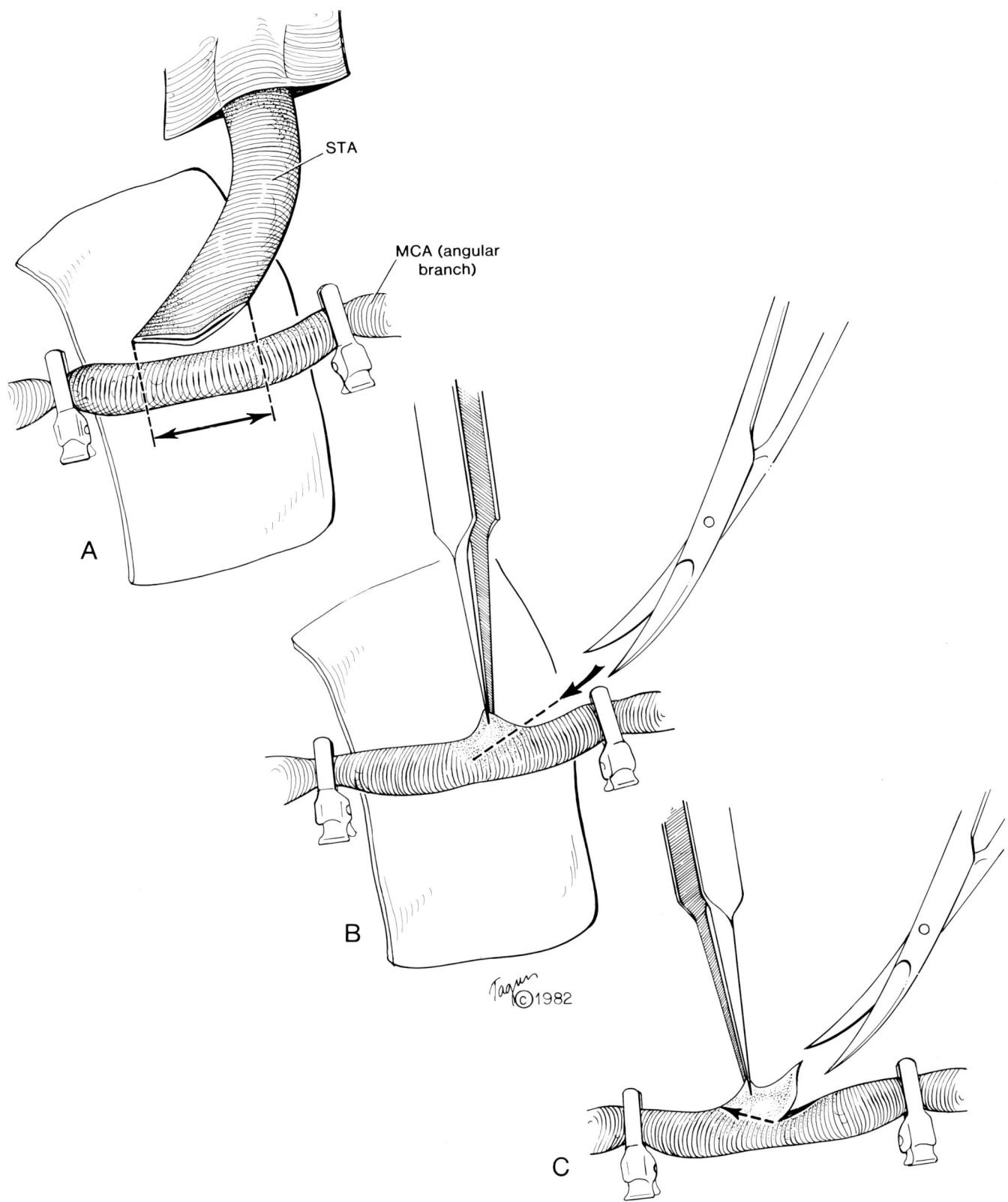

Figure 4.9. Preparation of middle cerebral artery (*MCA*). A rubber dam is slipped under the vessel to protect the brain. Kleinert-Kees clips are placed (**A**). With the corresponding superficial temporal artery (*STA*) ostium adjacent, the middle cerebral artery ostium is cut with curved microscissors (**B**). No. 5 jeweler's forceps are used to elevate the segment for excision, and two snips provide a smooth edge (**C**). The authors prefer an ostium about half as wide as the vessel with a length that is 2½ times the vessel width.

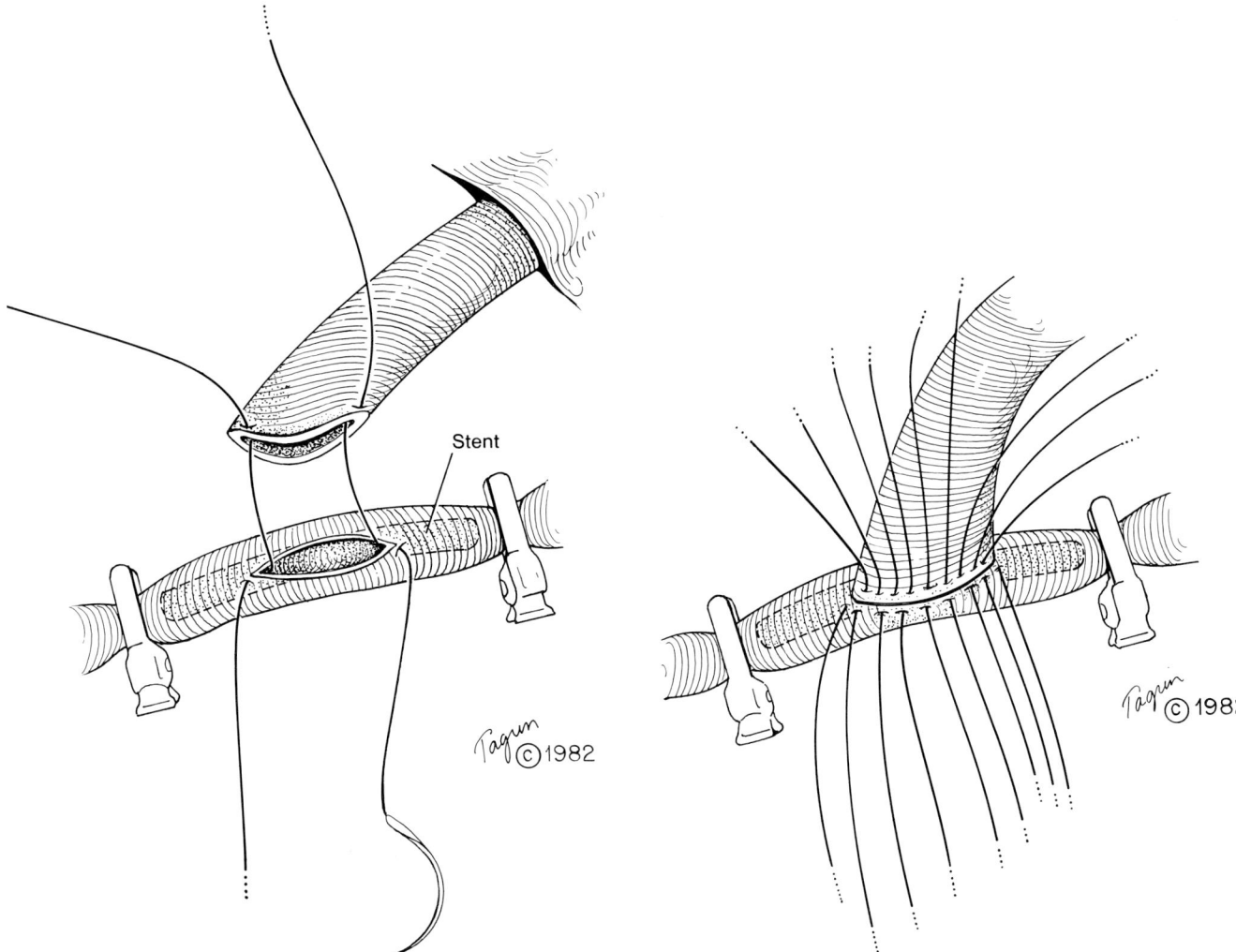

Figure 4.10. Corner stitches. 9-0 monofilament nylon is used. The distal tip is sutured first. If there is a tendency to an intimal flap in the superficial temporal artery, an in-to-out suture on this vessel is safest. If there is a discrepancy between wall lengths, it should be corrected prior to anchoring the second corner. After corner stitches are in, a fine Silastic stent is introduced to prevent injury to the back wall.

Figure 4.11. Front wall sutures. These are laid in separately without tying until all are placed. Bites are slightly thicker on the superficial temporal artery. Sutures are slightly closer together near the corners where it is most apt to leak. About seven sutures will be needed between the corner stitches.

Closure

The dura is loosely approximated with 4-0 sutures. A Gelfoam pledget covers the exposed dura and surrounds the distal superficial temporal artery segment. After the graft is routed smoothly and without kinking, the bone flap is trimmed with rongeurs to avoid contact with the superficial temporal artery and is then wired in place (Fig. 4.14). The temporalis muscle and fascia are approximated as separate layers with interrupted 3-0 coated Vicryl. Great care is taken to avoid compression of the graft. The wound is irrigated with Bacitracin solution and closed with 3-0 interrupted coated Vicryl to the galea and continuous nylon to the skin. When scalp edge viability is in question, closure using interrupted 5-0 nylon without tension offers the best chance of avoiding necrosis. A small dressing is applied together with a warning sign against pressure and a mark to indicate the point to check for pulse in the superficial temporal artery.

POSTOPERATIVE MANAGEMENT AND COMPLICATIONS

Blood pressure is carefully monitored with the aid of a radial artery catheter and is maintained in the

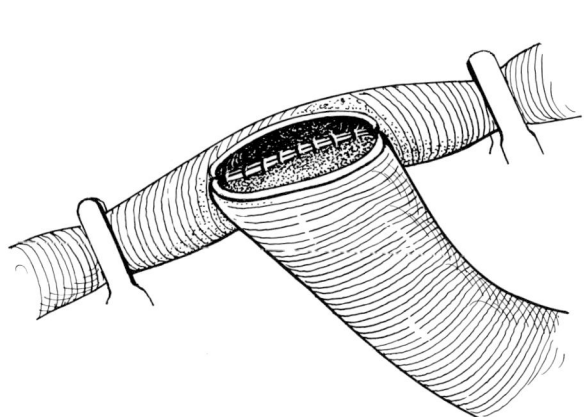

Figure 4.12. Back wall sutures. The front wall is checked from the interior to correct problems. Back wall sutures are placed just like the front wall sutures.

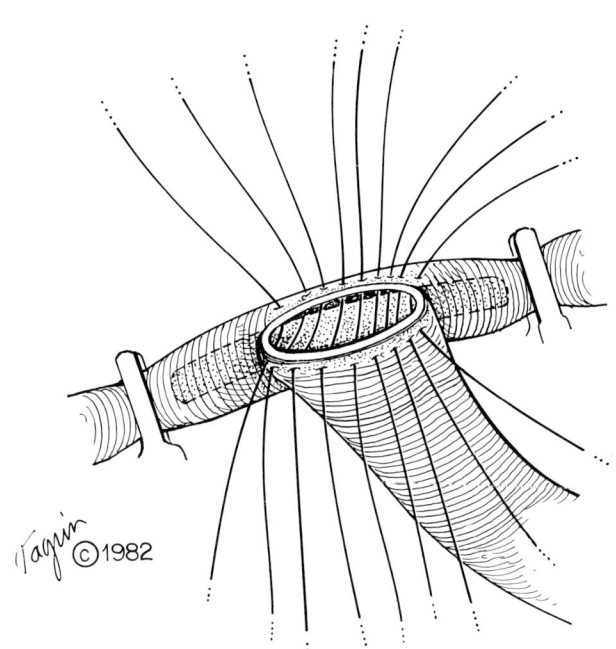

Figure 4.13. Stent removal. After all back wall sutures are placed (but not tied), the stent is gently removed.

normal range of the individual patient with infusions of colloid, pressors, or nitroprusside. Patients are gradually mobilized after 24 hours and blood pressure is controlled with oral agents as needed. Diphenylhydantoin is used and aspirin is continued indefinitely. Careful management of risk factors is planned. In the uncomplicated patient, angiography is performed about 1 week after operation to assess patency (Fig. 4.15).

If the patient is not doing well in the immediate postoperative period, a CT scan is performed; if this does not clarify the problem angiography is done.

Major complications of this procedure include intraoperative graft thrombosis, graft thrombosis with either acute or late stroke, subdural hematoma, and intracerebral hemorrhage (8, 18, 32, 47, 48). Less serious complications include transient neurologic worsening, wound infection, seizures, scalp edge necrosis, and myocardial ischemia.

Blue-black discoloration of the graft suggests intraoperative thrombosis. To confirm this fact, a suture or two must be removed. If clot is encountered and removed, a search is made for a technical error, such as an intimal flap or narrowing. Although efforts at correction are usually futile, the authors have, on one occasion, been able to reestablish flow and achieve angiographic patency.

Delayed strokes can occur despite a functioning bypass graft. This can be due to occlusion of a previously markedly stenotic intracranial internal carotid artery (14, 32).

Occasionally, a patient will continue to have TIAs following a bypass procedure. This may indicate that the mechanism of ischemia is other than that postulated preoperatively. For example, following internal carotid artery occlusion, the mechanism of TIAs may be external carotid artery stenosis or distal stump embolization rather than a hemodynamic problem and, therefore, a bypass could be ineffectual. Alternatively, the bypass may be occluded, providing no additional collateral circulation to the brain. Another possibility is the inducement of occlusion in a previously stenotic internal carotid artery. In order to evaluate the precise mechanism and symptomatology in this situation, cerebral angiography is required. In one of the authors' patients, episodes of numbness in the left face, presumably related to severe distal internal carotid artery stenosis, persisted following superficial temporal artery-middle cerebral artery bypass. Cerebral angiography confirmed continued patency of the stenotic vessel and good filling of the bypass graft into the middle cerebral artery circulation. The patient was treated with aspirin and Persantine, but the episodes persisted. Approximately 1 year later, the patient suffered a moderate right cerebral hemisphere stroke, which cleared to a mild deficit. Cerebral angiography at that time disclosed occlusion of the internal carotid artery with newly enhanced filling of the middle cerebral artery territory via the graft. An appropriate cerebral infarction was demonstrated on CT scan. Therefore, if TIAs persist after bypass graft and antiplatelet ther-

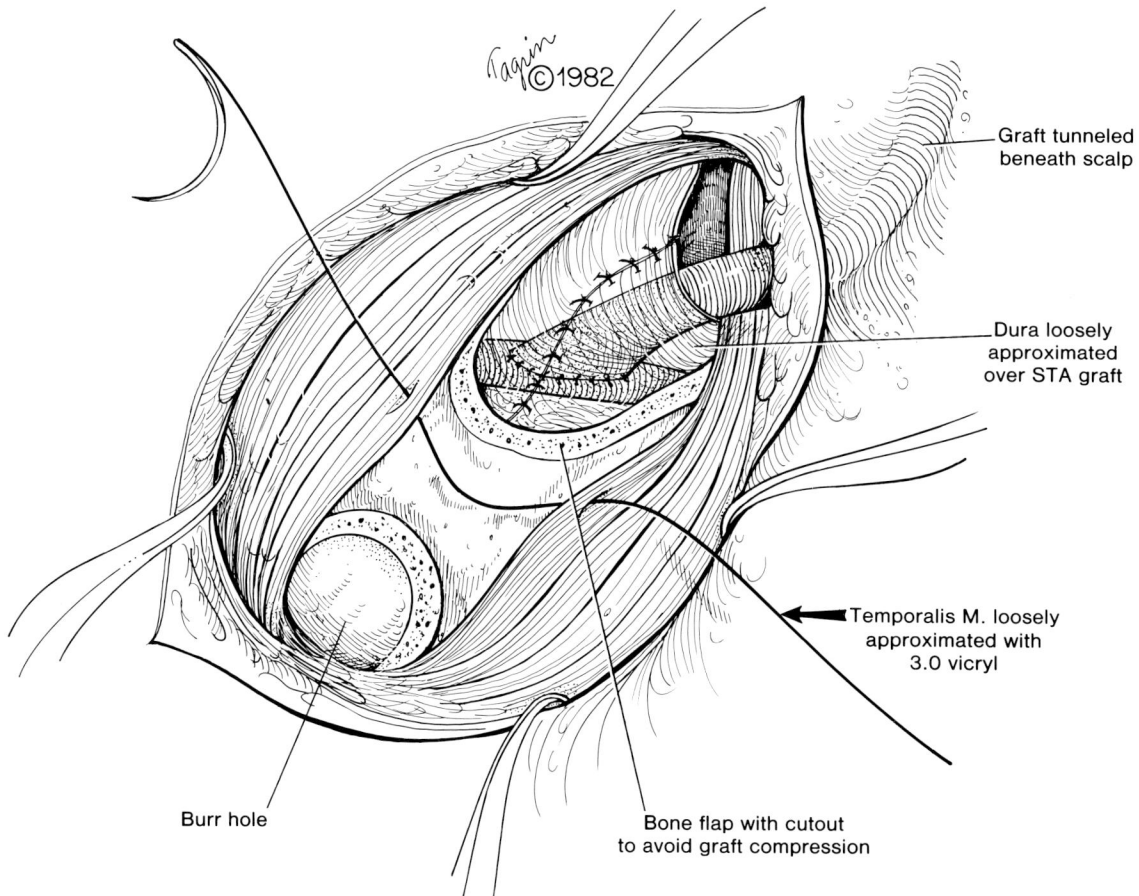

Figure 4.14. Closure. The graft is routed without kink or compression. The dura is loosely approximated without compression of the graft. The bone flap is replaced, with a cutout to avoid touching the graft. Muscle and fascia are brought together loosely with the graft piercing these as anteriorly as possible. STA, superficial temporal artery.

apy, coumadin therapy should be strongly considered.

Experience with five patients who suffered temporary, reversible neurologic deterioration after EC-IC bypass was reported (19). No satisfactory explanation could be found; all had patent grafts and none had a proximal occlusion, subdural hematoma, or evidence of seizures. It was speculated that hyperperfusion of chronically ischemic brain tissue and shifts in the watershed region resulting from the new flow pattern may have been responsible for the temporary deficits.

RESULTS

The authors' initial experience with 50 grafts in 45 patients has been reported (8). Patency was high (92%), serious complications were infrequent (4%), and there were no deaths directly attributable to surgery. Subsequent to that report they performed another 52 bypasses. The results have not been carefully analyzed, but there have been one death and one serious stroke as a result of the operation. Similar results have been reported by others (5, 6, 11, 33, 35, 44, 45, 48, 49).

ALTERNATIVE PROCEDURES

Short Vein Graft

Little et al have reported good results after interposition of a saphenous vein segment between the superficial temporal artery and a cortical branch of the middle cerebral artery (27) (Fig. 4.16). The vein segment of 5–10 cm is irrigated with herapin and aligned so that subsequent flow occurs in the direction of the valves. The ends of the vein graft are freed of adventitia to facilitate suturing. An end-to-side anastomosis of the vein to the cortical artery is carried out using continuous 9-0 nylon for the back wall and interrupted 10-0 nylon for the front wall. A temporary clip across the vein graft near the anastomosis then permits removal of temporary clips from the cortical recipient artery. Full heparinization is carried out to prevent thrombosis at the cortical anas-

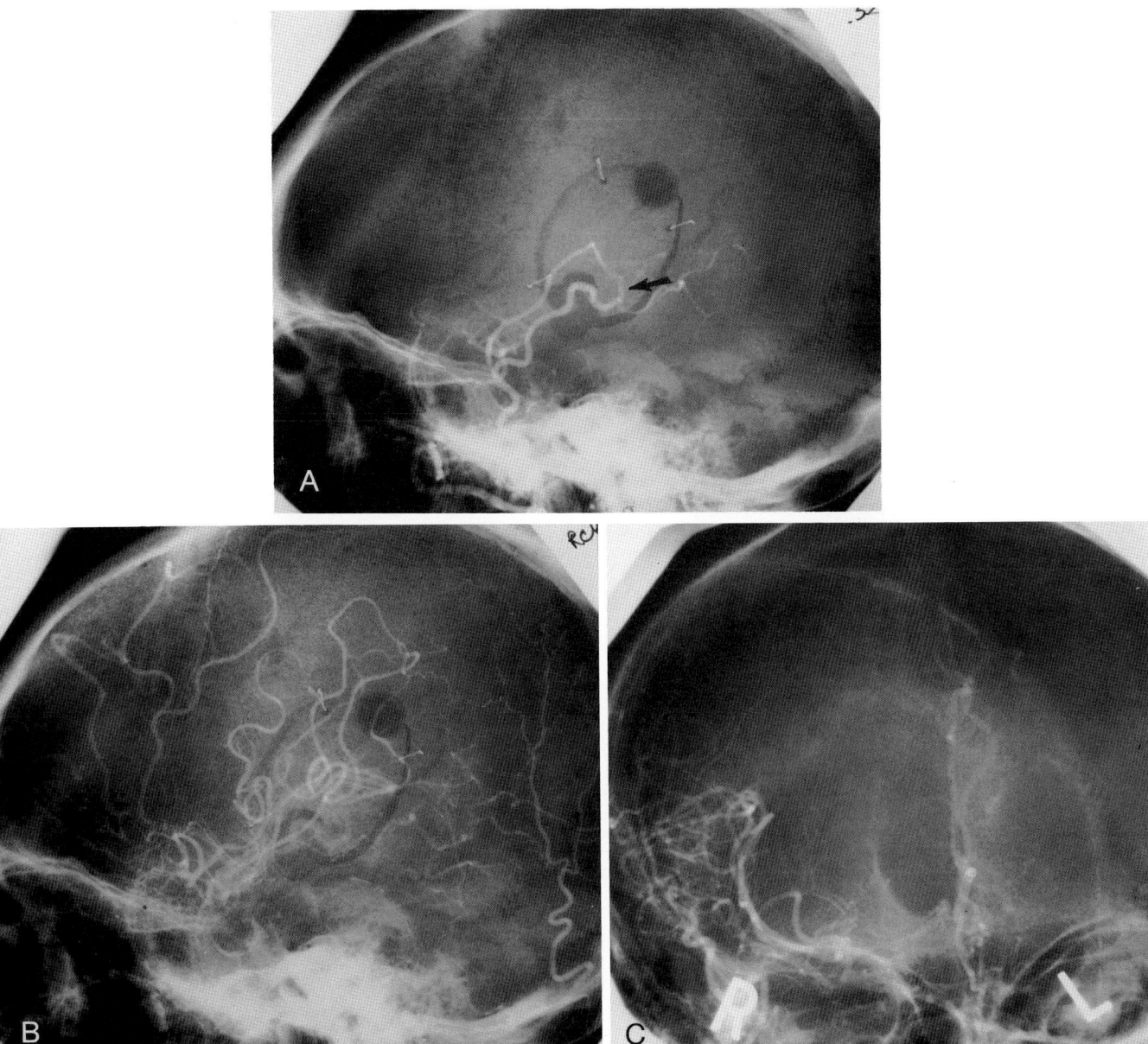

Figure 4.15. Bypass for multiple occlusions and dementia. Preoperative angiography showed left vertebral and bilateral carotid occlusions. Postoperative left carotid angiogram shows: **A**, patent bypass (*arrow*); **B**, widespread filling to left middle cerebral artery branches; and **C**, some contralateral anterior cerebral artery filling from graft. After surgery, spells ceased and mentation improved.

tomosis. An end-to-side anastomosis of the vein to the superficial temporal artery trunk above the zygoma is accomplished in similar fashion. After opening all clamps, heparin is reversed with protamine sulfate. In 19 cases, angiography demonstrated a 90% patency rate, and no patient experienced recurrent TIAs. CBF studies suggested a substantial increment in collateral circulation.

Long Vein Grafts

To provide immediate high flow revascularization, free vein grafts have been interposed between an artery in the neck and a recipient artery intracranially. Subclavian, common carotid, and external carotid arteries have served as donor arteries; supraclinoid internal carotid artery, middle cerebral artery divi-

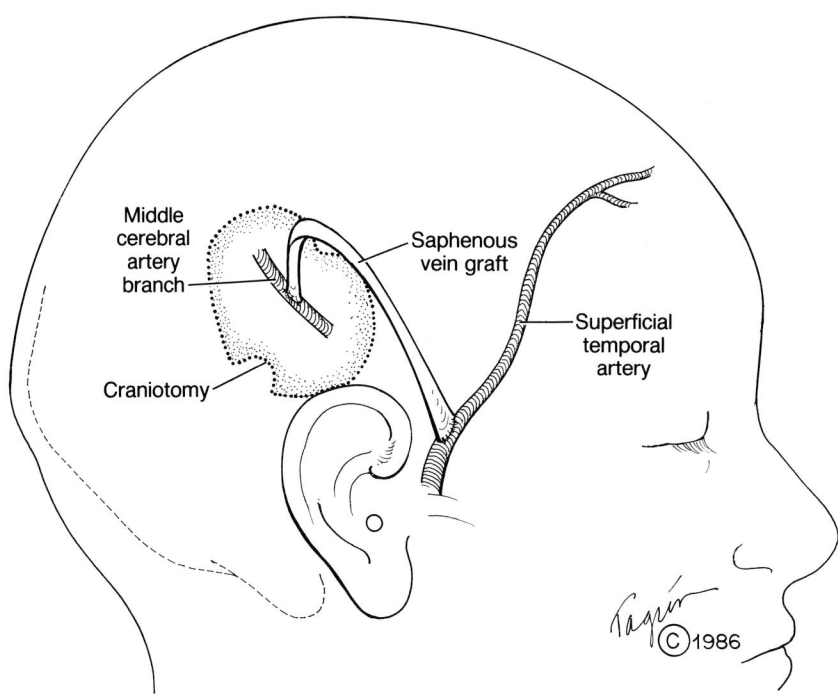

Figure 4.16. Short vein graft. Linear incisions provide exposure. The saphenous vein segment just below the knee is about 5 mm in diameter.

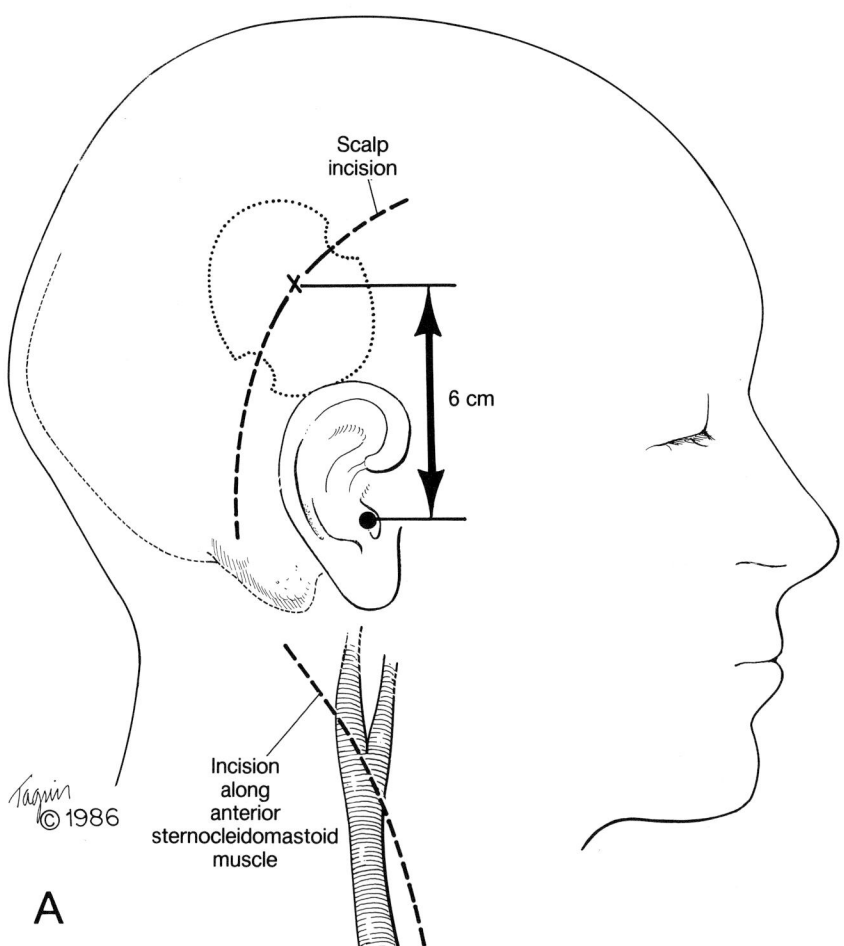

Figure 4.17. Common carotid artery to middle cerebral artery long vein graft. **A,** Outline of incisions used for the neck and cranial exposures. **B** and **C,** Details of the distal and proximal anastomosis. **D,** final position of the vein graft.

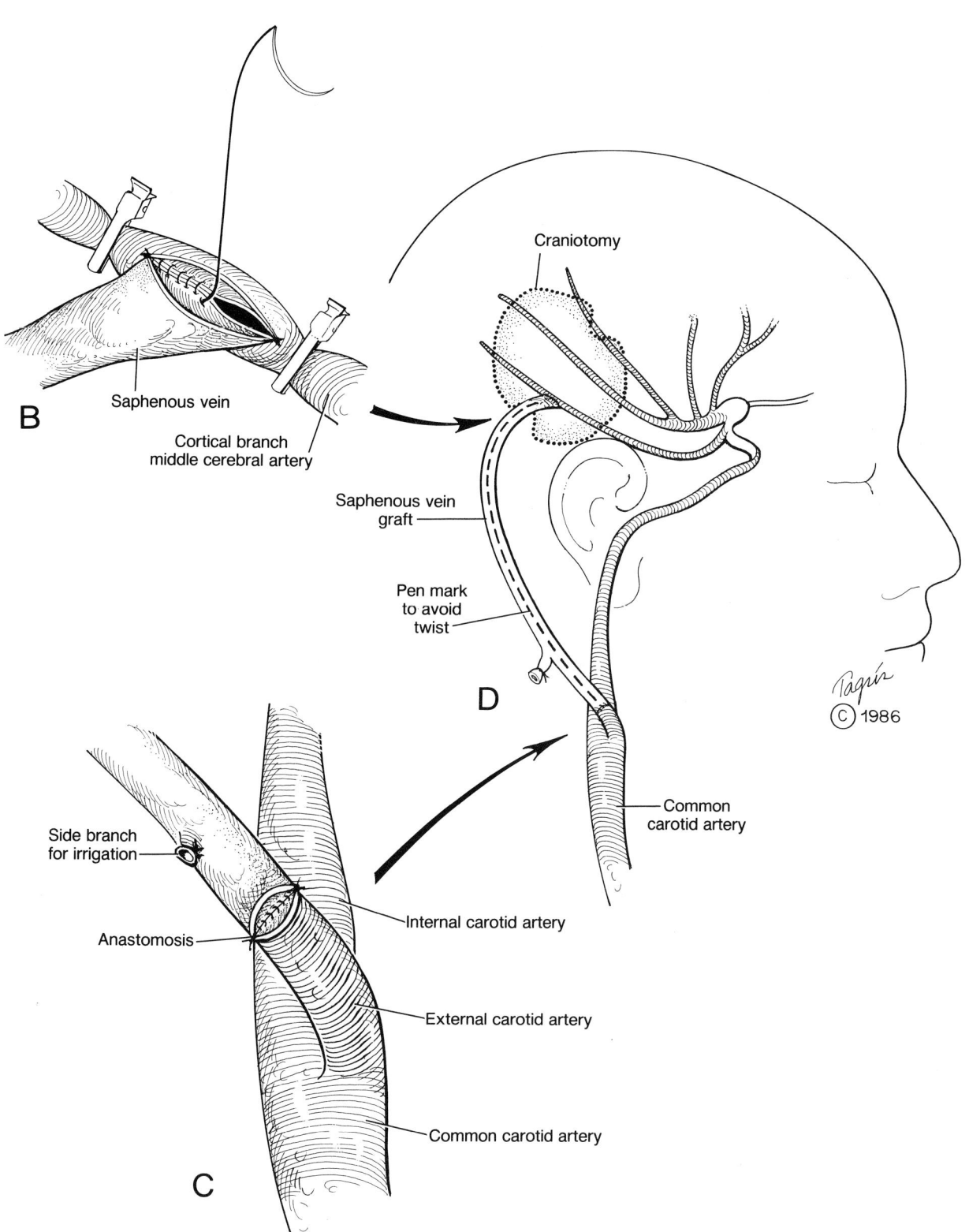

Figure 4.17 B–D.

sions within the sylvian fissure, and cortical middle cerebral artery branches have been used as recipient arteries (23, 36, 39, 41, 43). Reports indicate good patency rates with low complication rates, but indications have not been clearly established.

When immediate high flow is needed or suitable scalp vessels are lacking, the authors have performed saphenous vein interposition grafts between the external carotid artery and cortical branches of the middle cerebral artery. Two teams of surgeons work simultaneously, one to prepare the carotid arteries and perform the craniotomy, the other to harvest the saphenous vein (about 12 cm ending at the constriction near the knee). The end-to-end proximal anastomosis is done under the operating microscope with 7-0 nylon interrupted sutures. Full heparinization is done during cross-clamping; after the proximal anastomosis is completed, a Heifetz clip is applied to the vein near the anastomosis and carotid clamps are removed. The vein is routed through a drilled channel in the occipital bone to the craniotomy site. This must be done carefully to avoid compression or redundancy (Fig. 4.17). An alternative is to tunnel the vein anterior to the ear deep to the zygoma. A pen marking made with the saphenous vein in its original site helps to avoid a twist in the final site. A side branch near the proximal anastomosis is useful for irrigation through the graft. The distal vein ostium, which should be about 3–4 mm in diameter, is sutured with 9-0 monofilament nylon. A running suture technique may be useful, especially for the back wall. Intermittent irrigation through a side branch helps to clear clots and identify leakage sites. Protamine sulfate serves to reverse heparinization. Care must be taken to avoid postoperative hypertension, which can lead to hemorrhage. Dramatic angiographic filling can be achieved with long grafting (Fig. 4.18).

Other Procedures

When the superficial temporal artery is inadequate, the occipital artery may sometimes be used (38). The angiogram shows whether this vessel is adequate; in some cases the artery is small or bifurcates early into small distal branches. Palpation and Doppler probe permit marking of the artery's course. Direct cutdown on the occipital artery provides the best exposure. Careful sharp dissection is needed to free the vessel from surrounding dense adhesions. Exposure and preparation of the middle cerebral artery branch and anastomosis are completed as in superficial temporal artery-middle cerebral artery bypass.

Ordinarily, the middle meningeal artery is too small to be useful for revascularization. Occasionally, the artery may be large enough for grafting when it is enlarged due to the presence of a meningioma (29).

When no suitable recipient vessel can be identified, the superficial temporal artery may be laid directly on the cortex (4). This approach has recently been adapted for moya moya disease (28). The pedicle of the uninterrupted superficial temporal artery is inserted through a strip craniectomy to be sewn to the cut edges of dura mater. Striking superficial temporal artery-middle cerebral artery anastomoses have been shown angiographically. The procedure has several advantages: it can be done quickly in small children, the cranial defect is small, and the superficial temporal artery remains intact with small risk of thrombosis.

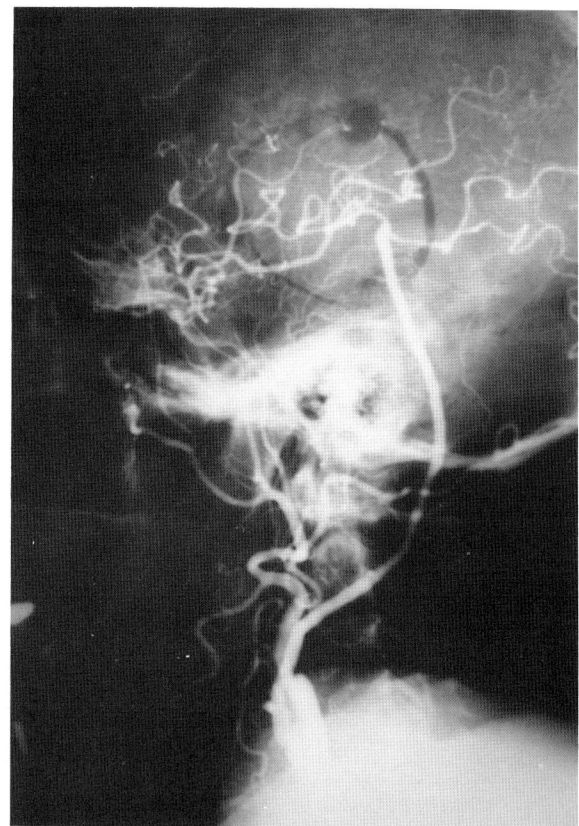

Figure 4.18. Long vein graft from external carotid artery to middle cerebral artery branch.

REFERENCES

1. Amine AR, Moody RA, Meeks W: Bilateral temporal-middle cerebral artery anastomosis for moyamoya syndrome. Surg Neurol 8:3–6, 1977.
2. Ammerman BJ, Smith DR: Giant fusiform middle cerebral aneurysm: Successful treatment utilizing microvascular bypass. Surg Neurol 7:255–257, 1977.
3. Ausman JI, Diaz FG, delos Reyes RA, Pearce JE, Shrontz CE: Extracranial-intracranial anastomoses in the posterior circulation. In Berguer R, Bauer BB (eds): Vertebrobasilar Arterial Occlusive Disease. New York, Raven Press, 1984, pp 313–319.
4. Ausman JI, Moore J, Chou SN: Spontaneous cerebral revascularization in a patient with STA-MCA anastomosis. J Neurosurg 44:84–87, 1976.
5. Chater N, Mani J, Tonnemacher K: Superficial temporal artery bypass for cerebrovascular occlusive disease. Cal Med 119:9–13, 1973.
6. Chater N, Popp J: Microsurgical vascular bypass for occlusive cerebrovascular disease: Review of 100 cases. Surg Neurol 6:115–118, 1976.
7. Crowell RM: Emergency STA-MCA bypass for acute focal cerebral ischemia. In Schmidek P, et al (eds): Microneurosurgical Anastomoses for Cerebral Ischemia. Berlin, Springer-Verlag, 1977.
8. Crowell RM: Direct brain revascularization. In Schmidek H, Sweet WH (eds): Current Techniques of Operative Neurosurgery. New York, Grune & Stratton, 1978.
9. Crowell RM, Olsson Y: Effect of extracranial-intracranial vascular bypass graft on experimental acute stroke in dogs. J Neurosurg 38:26–31, 1973.
10. Diaz, FG, Ausman JL, Mehta B, Dujovny M, delos Reyes RA, Pearce J, Patel S: Acute cerebral revascularization. J Neurosurg 63:200–209, 1985.
11. Donaghy RMP, Yasargil MG: Microvascular Surgery. Stuttgart, Georg Thieme Verlag, 1967.
12. Editorial. Extracranial to intracranial bypass and the prevention of stroke. Lancet 2:1401–1402, 1985.
13. Ferguson GG, Peerless SJ: Extracranial-intracranial arterial bypass in the treatment of dementia and multiple extracranial arterial occlusion. Presented at the twenty-sixth annual meeting of the Congress of Neurological Surgeons, New Orleans, 1976.
14. Furlan AJ, Little JR, Dohn DF: Arterial occlusion following anastomosis of the superficial temporal artery to middle cerebral artery. Stroke 11:91–95, 1980.
15. Gelber BR, Sundt TM Jr: Treatment of intracavernous and giant carotid aneurysms by combined internal carotid ligation and extra- to intracranial bypass. J Neurosurg 52:1–10, 1980.
16. Gibbs JM, Wise RJS, Leenders KL, Jones T: Evaluation of cerebral perfusion in patients with carotid artery occlusion. Lancet 1:310–314, 1984.
17. Grubb RL, Ratcheson RA, Raichle ME, Klieboth AB, Gado MH: Regional cerebral blood flow and oxygen utilization in superficial temporal-middle cerebral artery anastomosis patients. J Neurosurg 50:733–741, 1979.
18. Heros RC, Nelson PB: Intracerebral hemorrhage after microsurgical cerebral revascularization. Neurosurgery 6:371–375, 1980.
19. Heros RC, Scott RM, Kistler JP, Ackerman RH, Conner ES: Temporary neurologic deterioration after EC-IC bypass. Neurosurgery 15:178–185, 1984.
20. Holbach KH, Wassmann HW, Hoheluchter KL: Reversibility of the chronic post-stroke state. Stroke 7:296–300, 1976.
21. Holbach KH, Wassmann HW, Hoheluchter KL, Jain KK: Differentiation between reversible and irreversible post-stroke changes in brain tissue: Its relevance for cerebrovascular surgery. Surg Neurol 7:325–331, 1977.
22. Hopkins LM, Budny JL, Spetzler RF: Revascularization of the rostral brain stem. Neurosurgery 10:364–369, 1982.
23. Iwabuchi T, Kudo T, Hatanaka M, Oda N, Maeda S: Vein graft bypass in treatment of giant aneurysm. Surg Neurol 12:463–466, 1979.
24. Jafar J, Tan W: Technical note: CBF measurement and detachable balloon for planned carotid occlusion. In press.
25. Karasawa J, Kikuchi H, Furuse S, Kawamura J, Sakaki T: Treatment of moyamoya disease with STA-MCA anastomosis. J Neurosurg 49:679–688, 1978.
26. Kearns TP, Siekert RG, Sundt TM Jr: The ocular aspects of bypass surgery of the carotid artery. Mayo Clin Proc 54:3–11, 1979.
27. Little JR, Furlan AJ, Bryerton B: Short vein grafts for cerebral revascularization. J Neurosurg 59:384–388, 1983.
28. Matsushima Y, Fukai N, Tanaka K, Tsuruoka S, Inaba Y, Aoyagi M, Ohno K: A new surgical treatment of moya disease in children: A preliminary report. Surg Neurol 15:313–320, 1980.
29. Miller CF II, Spetzler RF, Kopaniky DJ: Middle meningeal to middle cerebral arterial bypass for cerebral revascularization. Case report. J Neurosurg 50:802–804, 1979.
30. Powers WJ, Martin WR, Herscovitch P, Raichle ME, Grubb RL Jr: Extracranial-intracranial bypass surgery: Hemodynamic and metabolic effects. Neurology 34:1168–1174, 1984.
31. Quest DO, Correll JW: Basal arterial occlusive disease. Neurosurgery 17:937–941, 1985.
32. Reichman OH: Complications of cerebral revascularization. Clin Neurosurg 23:318–335, 1976.
33. Reichman OH, Davis DO, Roberts TS, Satovick RM: Anastomosis between STA and Cortical branch of MCA for the treatment of occlusive cerebrovascular disease. In Mérei FT (ed): Reconstructive Surgery of Brain Arteries. Budapest, Akademiai Kiado, 1974.
34. Roski RA, Spetzler RF, Hopkins LN: Occipital artery to posterior inferior cerebellar artery bypass for vertebrobasilar ischemia. Neurosurgery 10:44–49, 1982.
35. Samson DS, Boone S: Extracranial-intracranial (EC-IC) arterial bypass: Past performance and current concepts. Neurosurgery 3:79–86, 1978.
36. Samson DS, Gerwertz BL, Beyer CW Jr, Hodosh RM: Saphenous vein interposition grafts in the microsurgical treatment of cerebral ischemia. Arch Surg 116:1578–1582, 1981.
37. Schmiedek P, Gratzl O, Spetzler R, Steinhoff H, Enzenbach R, Brendel W, Marguth F: Selection of patients for extra-intracranial arterial bypass surgery based on CBF measurements J Neurosurg 44:303–312, 1976.
38. Spetzler RF, Chater N: Occipital artery-middle cerebral artery anastomosis for cerebral artery occlusive disease. Surg Neurol 2:235–238, 1974.
39. Spetzler RF, Rhodes RS, Roski RA, Likavec MJ: Subclavian to middle cerebral artery saphenous vein bypass graft. J Neurosurg 53:465–469, 1980.
40. Spetzler RF, Shuster H, Roski RA: Elective extracranial-intracranial arterial bypass in the treatment of inoperable giant internal carotid artery aneurysms. J Neurosurg 53:22–27, 1980.
41. Story JL, Brown WE Jr, Eidelberg E, Arom KV, Stewart JR: Cerebral revascularization: Common carotid to distal middle cerebral artery bypass. Neursurgery 2:131–135, 1978.
42. Sundt TM, Piepgras DG: Surgical approach to giant intracranial aneurysms: Operative experience with 80 cases. J Neurosurg 52:731–742, 1979.

43. Sundt TM Jr, Piepgras DG, Houser OW, Campbell JK: Interposition saphenous vein grafts for advanced occlusive disease and large aneurysms in the posterior circulation. *J Neurosurg* 56:205–215, 1982.
44. Sundt TM Jr, Siekart RG, Piepgras DG, Sharbrough FW, Houser OW: Bypass surgery for vascular disease of the carotid system. *Mayo Clin Proc* 51:677–692, 1976.
45. Tew JM Jr: Reconstructive vascular surgery for prevention of stroke. *Clin Neurosurg* 22:264–280, 1975.
46. The EC-IC Bypass Study Group: The International Cooperative Study of Extracranial/Intracranial Arterial Anastomosis (EC/IC Bypass Study): Methodology and entry characteristics. *Stroke* 16:397–405, 1985.
47. The EC-IC Bypass Study Group: Failure of extracranial-intracranial arterial bypass to reduce the risk of ischemic stroke. Results of an international randomized trial. *N Engl J Med* 313:1191–1200, 1985.
48. Yasargil MG: *Microsurgery Applied to Neurosurgery*. Stuttgart, Georg Thieme Verlag, 1968.
49. Yasargil MG, Krayenbunl HA, Jacobson JH: Microneurosurgical arterial reconstruction. *Surgery* 67:221–233, 1970.

5

Atherosclerosis of the Vertebrobasilar Circulation: Evaluation, Management, and Operative Procedures

VERTEBROBASILAR ISCHEMIA

Clinical Syndromes

Symptoms of vertebrobasilar insufficiency and infarction are usually due to atherosclerotic occlusive disease within the intracranial vertebral artery, the basilar artery, or its branches (14, 16, 17). Most patients with stenosis or occlusion at the origin of one vertebral artery do not have symptoms. The likelihood of infarction depends on the location of obstructive disease and the adequacy of collateral circulation (Table 5.1).

When transient symptoms of vertebrobasilar ischemia are associated with stenosis of the extracranial vertebral artery, the patients usually do not go on to have infarction (17, 26, 40). This is probably due to the extensive collateral circulation that develops into the distal extracranial vertebral artery. Such patients are at high risk for fatal myocardial infarction (40).

Extracranial stenosis or occlusion of one vertebral artery is somewhat more likely to be symptomatic if the other vertebral artery is also severely stenotic or occluded due to atheroma, congenital hypoplasia, or absence (Fig. 5.1). Because collateral circulation from deep muscular branches and the circle of Willis is so rich, even bilateral extracranial vertebral artery occlusion is often present without infarction (22). However, in many cases collateral circulation is inadequate, and symptoms of brain stem ischemia ensue. For this group a high rate of fatal infarction has been reported (15). It is this group that might be best suited to surgical revascularization (4). Rarely, compression of the vertebral artery by an osteophyte associated with cervical spondylosis may cause symptoms (5). Vertebrobasilar ischemic symptoms secondary to carotid occlusive disease are discussed in Chapter 1 (8, 43, 56).

Intracranial vertebrobasilar occlusive disease is more likely to cause infarction. This is because deep muscular collateral circulation to the distal vertebral artery is excluded. Basilar artery stenosis (Fig. 5.2) may cause infarction by hemodynamic insufficiency to distal runoff or obstruction of perforating branches. When there is only one vertebral artery, the remaining "basilarized" vertebral artery may cause severe ischemia if it has intracranial narrowing. When basilar thrombosis occurs, it may cause acute or gradual brain stem infarction, which is often debilitating or fatal. On the other hand, if the segment of thrombosis is short and the distal collateral supply via the circle of Willis good, then the patient may have surprisingly little deficit or none at all, and the outlook to escape further neurologic deterioration is good, provided early propagation of thrombosis can be averted by anticoagulation (13).

The clinical picture is diverse, depending on the sites of occlusion and ischemia. Recognizable syndromes have been reviewed by Caplan (14) (Table 5.2). Dizziness, diplopia, dysarthria, and weakness or numbness in part or all of one or both sides of the body are the most common symptoms. Other manifestations include headache, staggering, veering to one side, blurred vision, partial or complete blindness, ptosis, dysphagia, confusion, syncope, memory lapse, and transient global amnesia (19, 21).

Evaluation

Noninvasive vascular studies are of little help. Doppler imaging can, at times, demonstrate proximal vertebral stenosis or occlusion, but this does not give the necessary information about the intracranial circulation. Brain stem auditory evoked responses are reported to be helpful in some cases (6, 48). The computed tomography scan or magnetic resonance image may provide information as to where infarction has occurred, but these are of little value in the patient with transient ischemic symptoms (11, 34). Blood flow studies remain difficult or are of limited help for posterior fossa ischemia (35, 58). Angiography is needed to define precisely the sites of vascular compromise and the extent of collateral

Table 5.1.
Indications for Vertebrobasilar Revascularization[a]

Site of Obstruction	Risk of Stroke	Indication for Revascularization	Procedure
Subclavian stenosis	Low	?	Angioplasty Carotid-subclavian bypass
Extracranial VA	Low	?	VA replantation VA endarterectomy
Bilateral extracranial VA	Low	±	Occipital–PICA bypass
Intracranial VA	Moderate	±	VA endarterectomy Occipital–PICA bypass ECA–vein–PCA bypass
Bilateral intracranial VA	Very high	+ +	Occipital–PICA bypass ECA–vein–PCA bypass
Basilar stenosis	High	?	ECA–vein–PCA bypass
Basilar occlusion	High acutely Low if stable	?	ECA–vein–PCA bypass

[a] VA, vertebral artery; ECA, external carotid artery; PCA, posterior cerebral artery; PICA, posterior inferior cerebellar artery.

circulation. Complications are rare in experienced hands (24). In complete angiography, one must visualize the aortic arch and subclavian arteries, both vertebral arteries outside and inside the cranium, the basilar artery, as well as both carotid circulations. Selective vertebral injections give the most detailed studies. However, the risk is a bit higher, and with smaller vessels, discretion may dictate a subclavian injection. Intraarterial digital subtraction angiography may be utilized to minimize the volume of injected contrast media while maintaining good clarity in the pictures. Occasionally, an aneurysm may be disclosed as the etiology of transient ischemic attacks (TIAs) (52).

Management

Most patients with vertebrobasilar ischemia respond to anticoagulation with heparin and then coumadin. Maintenance of blood pressure is often crucial (18), and sometimes all that is necessary is to reduce the dosage of antihypertensive medication. The rare patient who continues to have symptoms and has a precarious circulation should be evaluated for surgery. Several surgical procedures have been used to improve vertebrobasilar circulation: extracranial and intradural vertebral endarterectomy, vertebral artery transposition, subclavian and innominate endarterectomy, various bypass procedures, and transluminal angioplasty. The authors believe that further experience will probably confirm occasionally useful roles for long vein grafting to the posterior cerebral artery for bilateral vertebral occlusive disease and occipital artery–posterior inferior cerebellar artery bypass for some patients with distal vertebral artery pathology. Rarely, revascularization of the anterior circulation may relieve ischemic symptoms related to generalized cerebrovascular occlusive disease (39) (Fig. 5.2).

SUBCLAVIAN STEAL

Clinical Syndrome

A subclavian steal occurs when blood flows retrograde down the vertebral artery and into the distal subclavian artery. In most patients the cause is atherosclerosis with stenosis or occlusion of the subclavian or innominate artery proximal to the origin of the vertebral artery. Occasionally, subclavian steal may develop after Blalock-Taussig anastomosis for correction of tetralogy of Fallot (36).

In many patients the subclavian steal is asymptomatic, being found at the time of angiography for another problem. When the steal is symptomatic, most patients complain of vertebrobasilar neurologic symptoms, and a small number have symptoms of brachial ischemia. Production of neurologic symptoms by exercising the affected arm has been frequent in some series but rare in others (9).

On examination, there is usually a bruit over the subclavian artery. The brachial blood pressure is significantly lower on the affected side. Noninvasive studies indicate the degree of flow reduction in the upper extremity. Angiography requires study of both subclavian arteries and the carotid circulation. Late films are needed to see the retrograde flow down the vertebral artery and into the subclavian artery (Fig. 5.3A and B).

Management

Most patients do not require treatment because there are few if any symptoms, but occasionally a surgical

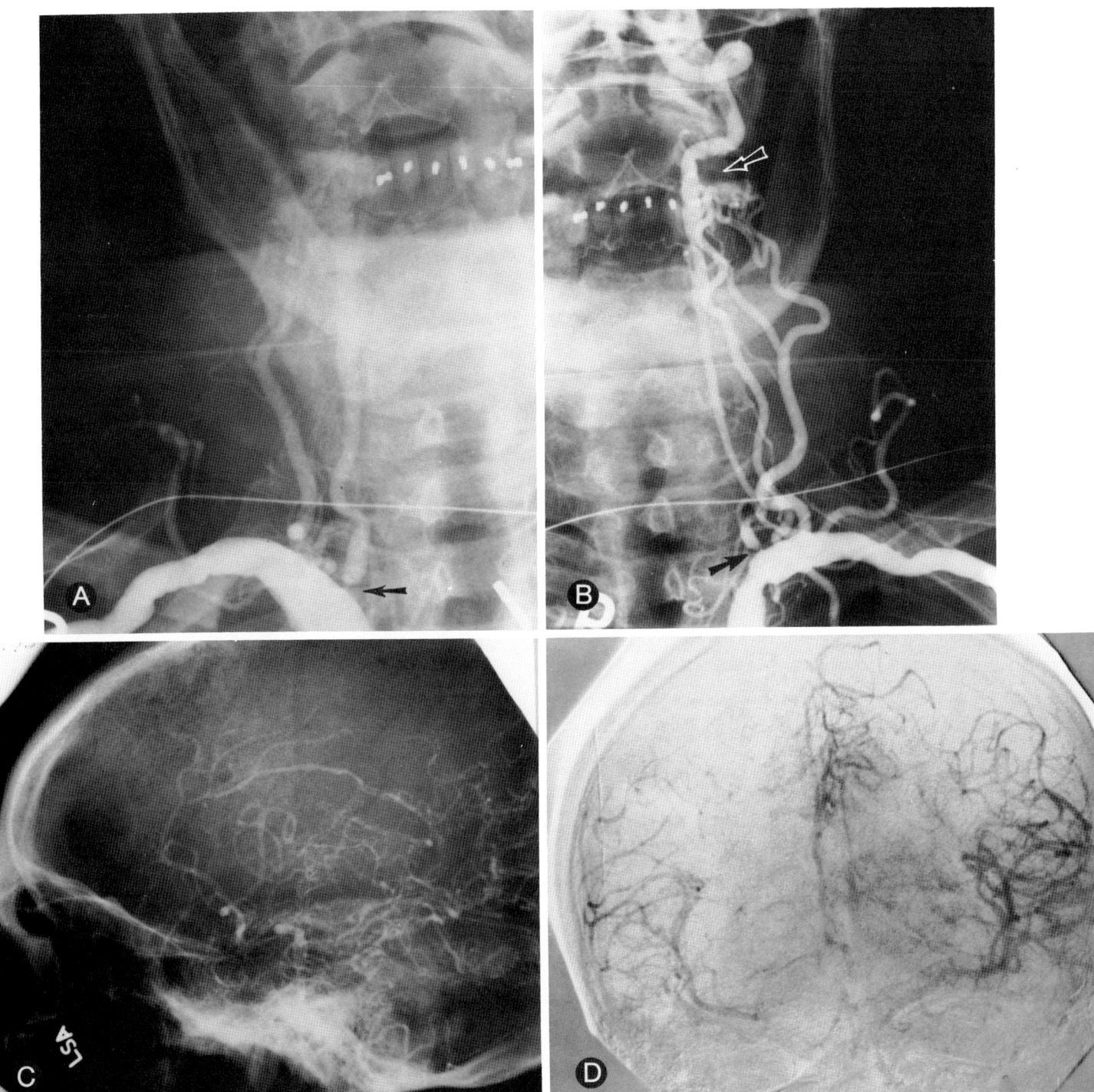

Figure 5.1. Vertebral artery stenosis. **A**, Right subclavian angiogram showing severe stenosis (*arrow*) at the origin of the vertebral artery. The carotid artery is occluded. **B**, Left subclavian angiogram showing severe stenosis (*closed arrow*) at the origin of the vertebral artery with narrowing of the proximal lumen, indicating reduced pressure. Note that the normal caliber of the distal vertebral artery is restored by collateral circulation (*open arrow*). **C** and **D**, Intracranial views show that the entire circulation depends on the marginal flow in the vertebral arteries. Unilateral stenosis at the origin of the vertebral artery is usually asymptomatic. However, when other arterial supply to the brain is occluded, the stenosis may be significant. Complete angiography in this patient confirmed bilateral carotid occlusion. Ischemic episodes ceased and mentation improved after right superficial temporal–middle cerebral artery bypass graft.

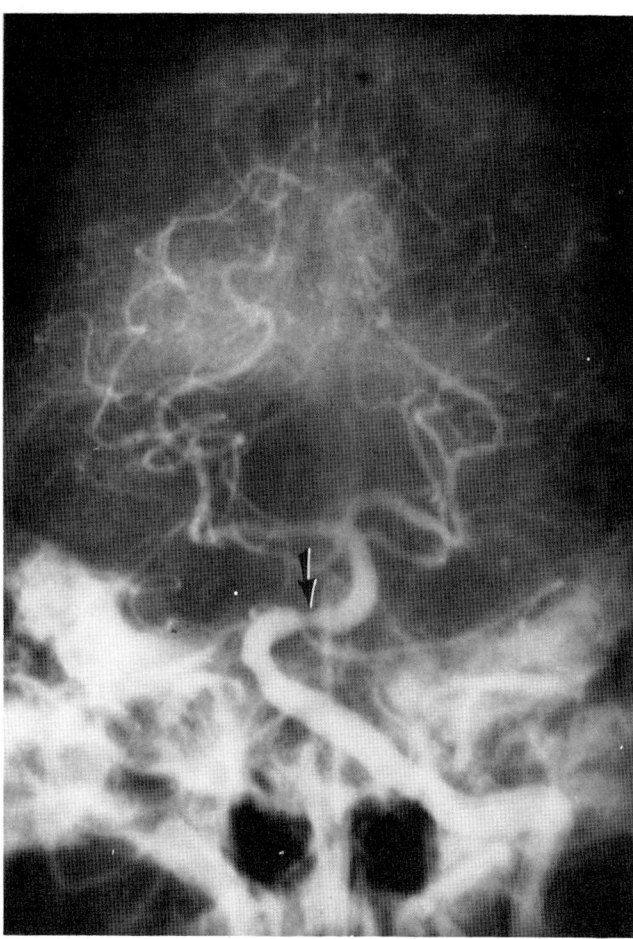

Figure 5.2. Basilar artery stenosis. Vertebral angiogram showing stenosis in the proximal basilar artery (*arrow*). The patient presented with TIAs. This is a common site for atherosclerosis to occur. At the present time, anticoagulation is the best treatment.

Table 5.2.
Clinical Patterns of Vertebrobasilar Ischemia[a]

Anatomical Site	Vessel Affected	Deficits
Left medial pontine infarction	Left basilar branch occlusion	1. Diplopia 2. Left sixth nerve palsy 3. Decreased position sense in right hand 4. Right hemiparesis
Left lateral medullary infarction	Left vertebral occlusion	1. Decreased pain and temperature in left face, right limbs 2. Nystagmus 3. Hoarseness 4. Left arm, leg ataxia 5. Left Horner's syndrome
Left cerebellar infarction	Left vertebral occlusion	1. Inability to walk 2. Vomiting 3. Ataxia of left limbs
Occipital lobe and thalamic infarction	Top of basilar embolus	1. Cortical blindness 2. Small, poorly reactive pupils 3. One or both eyes deviated down and in 4. Sleepiness
Left pontine lacunar infarction	Left penetrating vessel occlusion	1. Right arm, leg ataxia 2. Increased reflexes right limbs 3. Right extensor plantar reflex
Right and left pontine infarction	Basilar occlusion	1. Quadriparesis 2. Extensor plantar reflexes 3. Dysarthria 4. Dysphagia

[a] Modified from Caplan LR: Vertebrobasilar disease: Time for a new strategy. Stroke 12:111–114, 1981.

procedure is indicated. Several operations have been used, including bypass graft from the ipsilateral common carotid artery to the subclavian artery distal to the site of the obstruction and vertebral artery transposition. When surgery was first done for subclavian artery stenosis or occlusion, a transthoracic approach for either endarterectomy or bypass graft from the aorta was done, but there was significant morbidity and mortality (59). The preferred operation has been extrathoracic bypass graft from the common carotid artery to the subclavian artery distal to the stenosis (59).

Some surgeons have favored subclavian endarterectomy if it can be done through a supraclavicular approach (60). Vertebral artery transposition has been proposed when vertebrobasilar ischemia is more prominent than the brachial ischemic symptoms (25). Bohmfalk et al reviewed the literature and concluded that vertebral to common carotid artery transposition had the advantage of establishing a more certain antegrade flow in the vertebral artery than the carotid to subclavian bypass (9, 10).

Percutaneous angioplasty has successfully enlarged subclavian stenosis and reversed subclavian steal (37). The procedure has low risk and should be tried as the first step in management of symptomatic subclavian steal syndrome. Only rarely will open surgery be indicated.

VERTEBRAL ARTERY STENOSIS OR OCCLUSION DUE TO NECK MOVEMENT OR MANIPULATION

Occlusive disease in the vertebral artery may occasionally be associated with symptoms of dizziness or syncope when turning the head into a certain po-

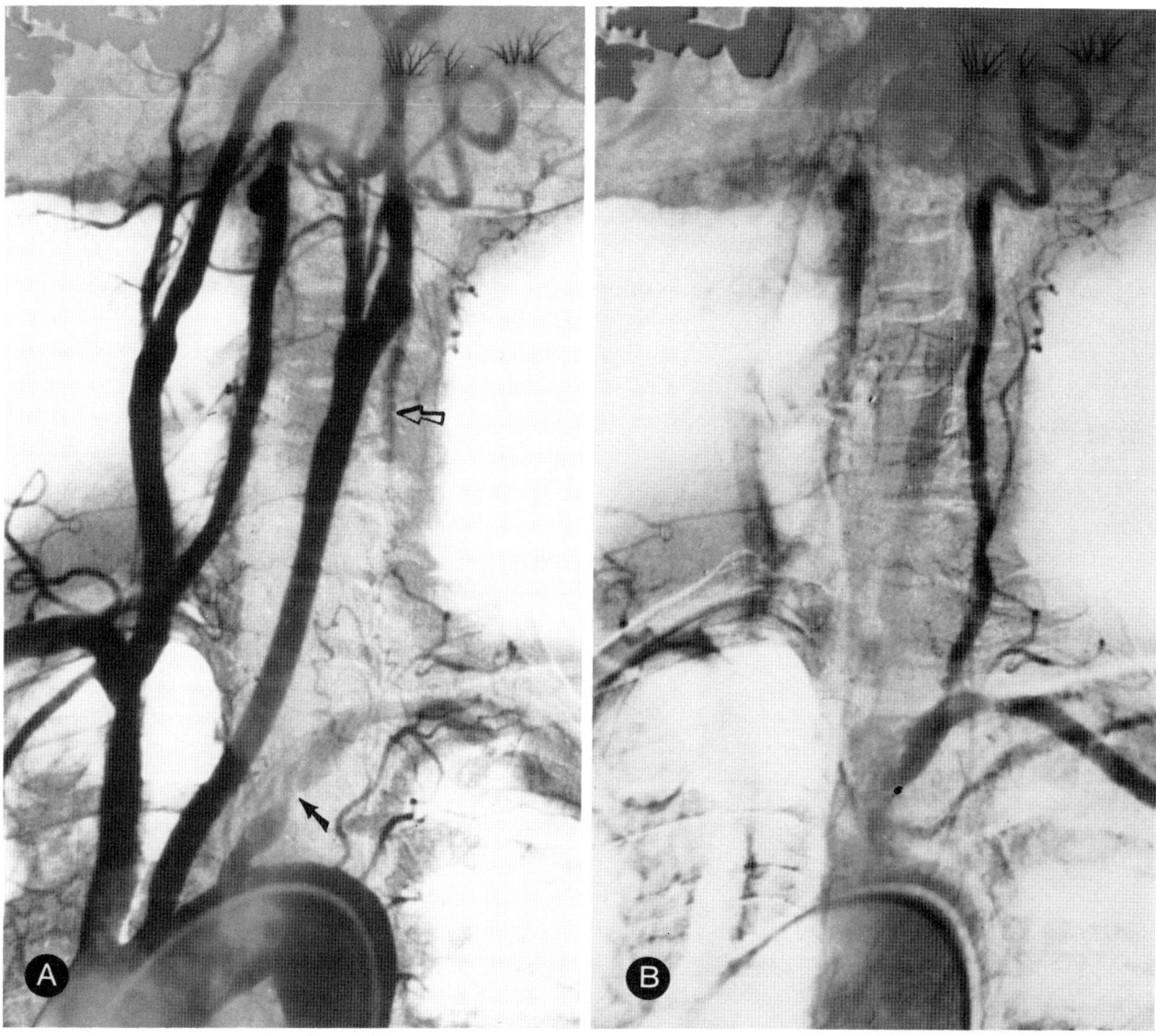

Figure 5.3. Subclavian steal. **A**, Arch angiogram showing severe stenosis in the proximal left subclavian artery (*closed arrow*), no antegrade filling of the vertebral artery, and beginning retrograde flow down the vertebral artery (*open arrow*). **B**, Later film showing retrograde flow down the vertebral artery and denser opacification of the distal subclavian artery.

sition. Angiography usually reveals absence, occlusion, or hypoplasia of one vertebral artery at the C1–C2 level when the head is turned. The vertebral artery is relatively fixed in the transverse foramen between C1 and C2 and between the exit from the foramen at C1 and the atlanto-occipital membrane (45). Since much of the rotation and tilting of the head occurs at C1–C2, the remaining patent vertebral artery may be temporarily occluded with these movements (51). Most patients avoid the positions causing symptoms, and no treatment is needed. On rare occasion a fusion may be necessary, particularly if there is occipital or lateral instability (20).

A problem caused by head and neck manipulation therapy is injury to the vertebral artery where it is fixed at C1–C2 (45, 49, 51). Injury to the intima leads to subintimal dissection, which may cause stenosis or occlusion, and thrombus formation, which is a source of distal embolus. Occasionally, the problem may be bilateral, and in some cases spontaneous dissection without antecedent trauma has been reported (27) (see Chapter 7). Transient ischemic symptoms or stroke may occur either immediately or several days later. Angiography usually shows narrowing or occlusion of the vertebral artery at the C1–C2 level. There may also be an associated pseudoaneurysm. When vertebrobasilar ischemic symptoms or a mild stroke is due to this cause, anticoagulation with heparin followed by coumadin is indicated (30). Rarely, surgical treatment with a bypass graft may be needed.

Direct repair has been proposed, but indications are yet to be defined (1).

OPERATIVE PROCEDURES

Cervical Exposure of the Subclavian and Vertebral Arteries

The supraclavicular exposure can be used for most right vertebral and subclavian operations, some left vertebral and subclavian operations, and transpositions of the vertebral artery. Many operations on the left subclavian artery, on the left vertebral artery when it originates proximally, and on the innominate artery require a median sternotomy or transthoracic approach.

A supraclavicular incision is made centered over the clavicular head of the sternocleidomastoid muscle (Fig. 5.4). The platysma is incised and the clavicular head of the sternocleidomastoid muscle is divided. The scalene fat pad is entered and the omohyoid muscle is divided or retracted superiorly. This exposes the anterior scalene muscle, phrenic nerve, and internal jugular vein (Fig. 5.5). The phrenic nerve is mobilized and retracted with a soft rubber tape. The anterior scalene muscle is divided, bringing into view the subclavian artery and brachial plexus.

The subclavian artery is mobilized proximal and distal to the origin of the vertebral artery (Fig. 5.6). On the left side, the thoracic duct is identified and spared. If it is injured, it should be ligated. The vertebral veins may need to be divided. Appropriate tapes are placed as indicated for proximal and distal control of the subclavian artery and around the vertebral artery. Separate control of the thyrocervical trunk and internal mammary artery may be necessary.

Vertebral Artery Endarterectomy

Vertebral artery endarterectomy is considered for atherosclerotic occlusive disease that involves the origin of the vertebral artery. The technique of the operation has been described (61). The vertebral artery is a much more fragile vessel than the carotid artery, and when surgery is performed on this vessel, extra care must be exercised. Direct incision into the proximal vertebral artery for endarterectomy is usually not indicated. The preferred approach is to perform the endarterectomy via a trans-subclavian artery incision. We have not seen a patient in whom this operation was indicated, but the exposure is illustrated (Fig. 5.7).

In a report from one center, 36 patients had vertebral endarterectomy (46, 60). Twenty were done on the right side by a supraclavicular cervical approach, and two also required a median sternotomy. Only 6 of the 14 on the left side could be done by the cervical approach because of the low level of the vertebral

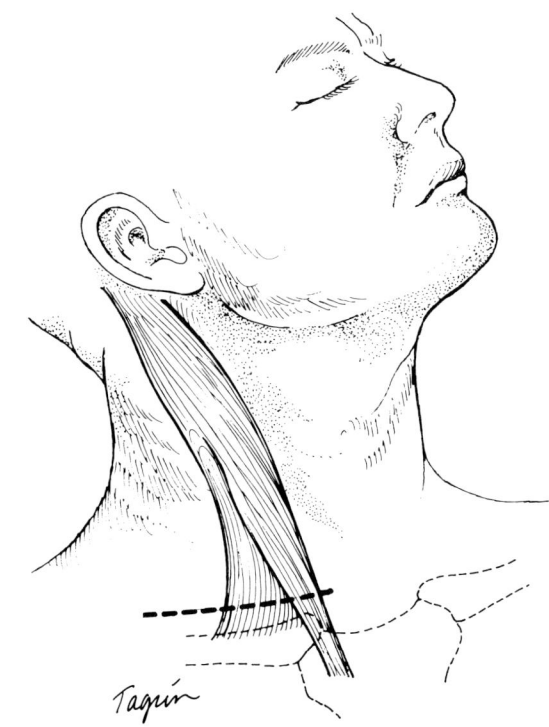

Figure 5.4. Exposure of vertebral and subclavian arteries. The supraclavicular incision is outlined.

artery origin. In the other eight, a transthoracic approach was used. If the patient was a poor risk for a thoracotomy and the origin of the left vertebral artery could not be reached by the cervical approach, the vertebral artery was replanted into the subclavian or common carotid artery. In the last 26 operations no new neurologic deficits occurred. Complications included occlusion of the vertebral artery with no symptoms, a lymphocele, and a myocardial infarction. In another report, 58 patients who had some type of unilateral vertebral artery reconstruction for presumed brain stem symptoms (syncope was the most common) or combined cerebral and brain stem symptoms after any flow-obstructing lesion in the carotid artery had been corrected had an average stroke rate over a 14-year period of only 1%/year (32).

Intradural endarterectomy of the vertebral artery in the segment from the entrance to the dura to its disappearance under the brain stem has been reported (2). The patient had TIAs that were refractory to anticoagulation. There was a satisfactory postoperative course and angiographic documentation of an open artery.

Percutaneous transluminal angioplasty has been attempted in five patients with stenosis at the origin of the vertebral artery (42). In four patients the procedure was successful, with relief of symptoms and no complications.

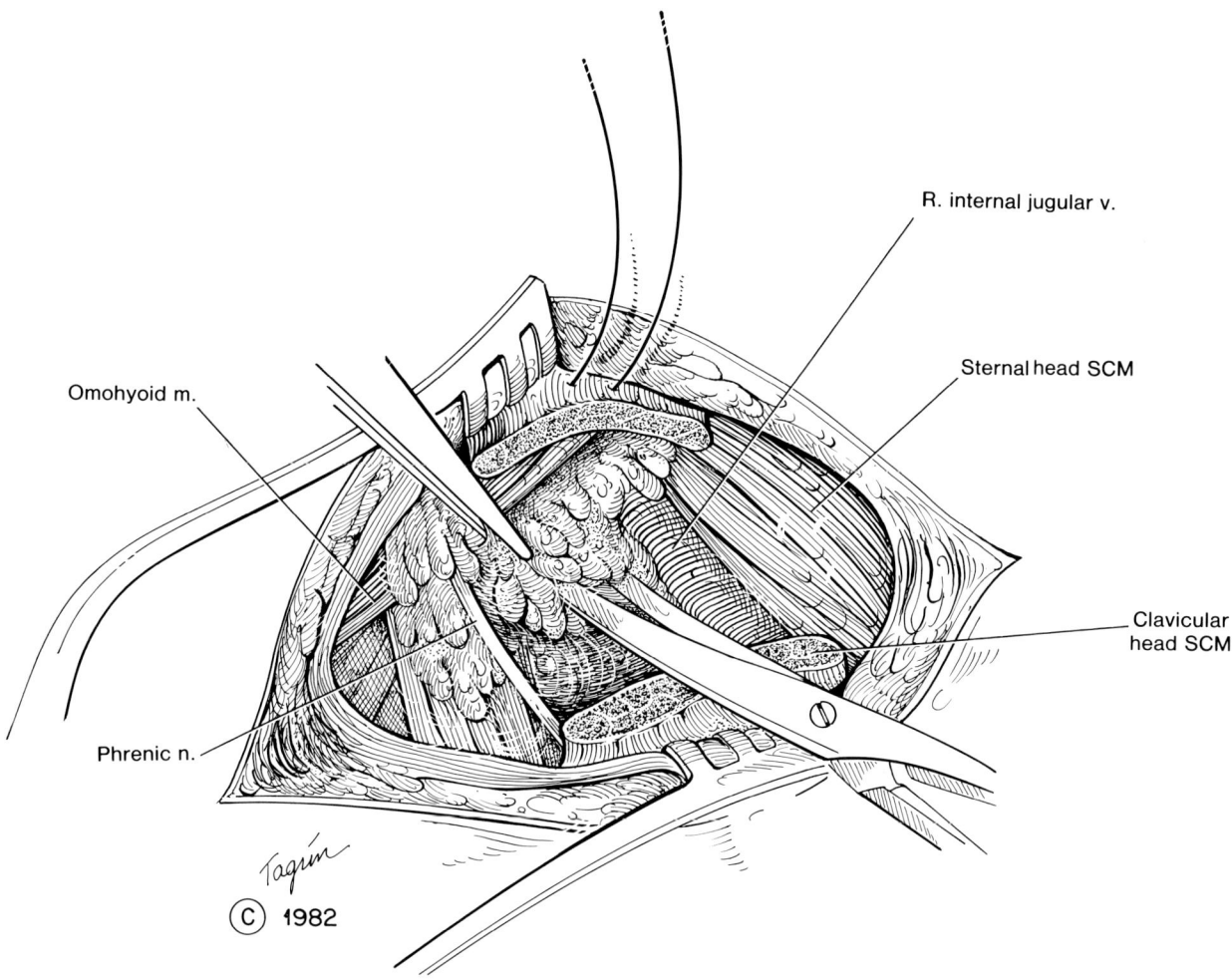

Figure 5.5. Exposure of vertebral and subclavian arteries. The clavicular head of the sternocleidomastoid (*SCM*) muscle has been divided. Adipose tissue and lymph nodes are being dissected to expose the internal jugular vein, anterior scalene muscle, and phrenic nerve.

Subclavian and Innominate Artery Endarterectomy

The approach for subclavian endarterectomy is described in Figures 5.4–5.6. In one report, a cervical incision was used in all 29 patients with right subclavian stenosis. However, this could be done in only 14 of 43 patients where the stenosis was on the left; the others required a left thoracotomy (60). In another report, 13 of 14 patients who had subclavian endarterectomy for either neurologic or arm symptoms remained free of symptoms over an average period of 53 months (29).

In a report of 33 patients with cerebral symptoms related to innominate stenosis, the surgical approach was through a median sternotomy (60). In 28 patients an endarterectomy was performed, while in five patients a bypass graft from the side of the aorta was required. All patients were relieved of their symptoms.

The treatment of innominate artery stenosis by intraoperative transluminal angioplasty in one patient has been reported, with a good result (38). In another report, two patients with subclavian steal syndrome due to left subclavian stenosis were treated with percutaneous transluminal angioplasty, with relief of symptoms (41). The procedure was performed by using systemic heparinization, and then daily aspirin was given.

Vertebral Artery Transposition

The technique for the transposition of the vertebral to the common carotid artery has been outlined by Bohmfalk et al (9, 10). The method is also described by Galbraith and McDowell (28) and Wylie and Ehrenfeld (61) and has been amplified by Fein (25). The procedure should not be used when there is significant common carotid artery atheroma (9, 25). Vertebral artery transposition to another site on the

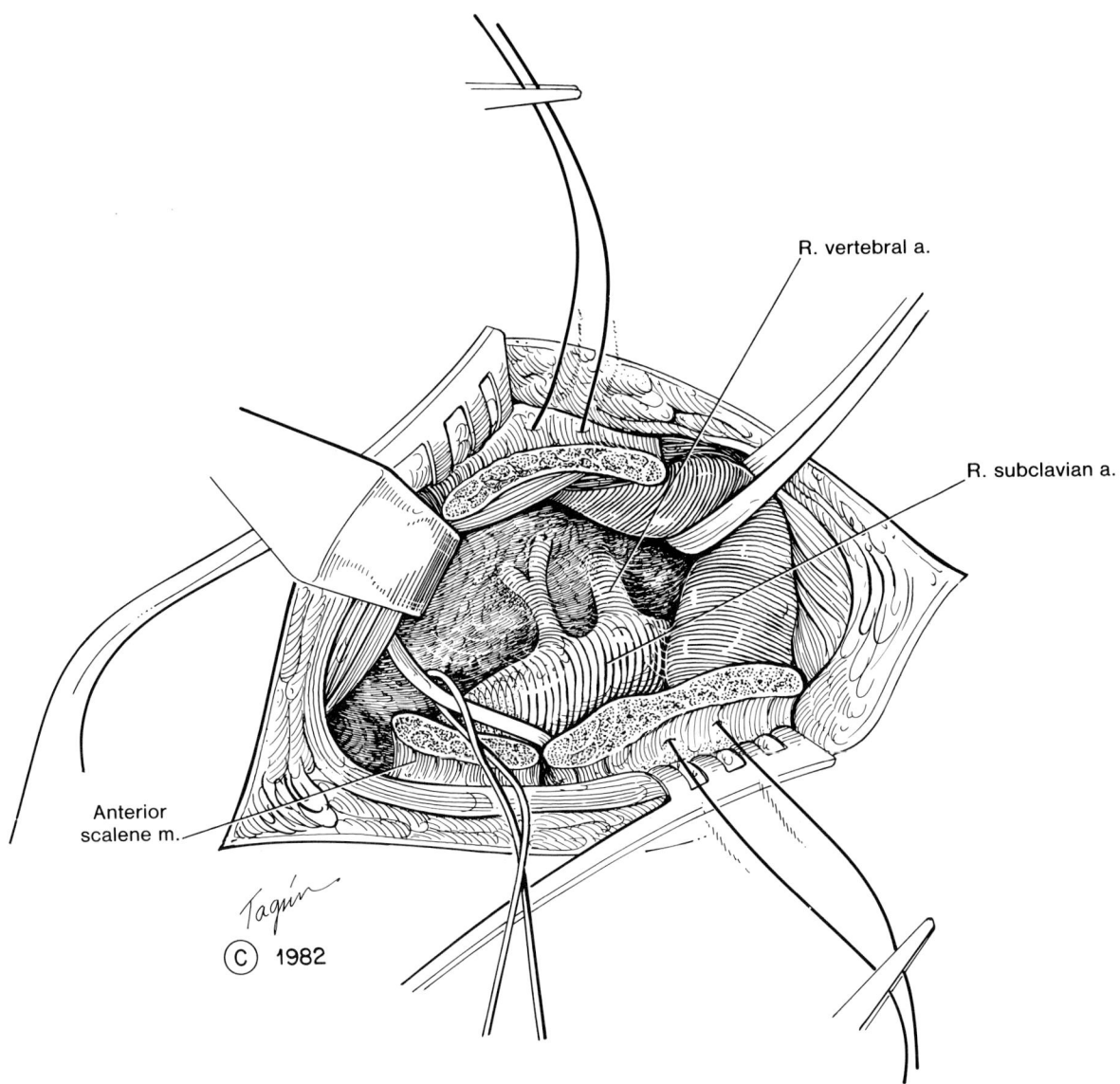

Figure 5.6. Exposure of vertebral and subclavian arteries. The anterior scalene muscle has been divided and the arteries brought into view.

subclavian artery (7, 60) and use of a subclavian to vertebral artery vein bypass (50) have been reported in a few patients. An external carotid artery to midcervical vertebral artery end-to-side anastomosis and an external carotid artery to distal cervical vertebral artery end-to-end anastomosis have also been reported (44).

The operative exposure combines features of the carotid and subclavian artery approaches that have been described. A parasternocleidomastoid incision is made that curves laterally across the insertion of the sternocleidomastoid muscle in the supraclavicular region. The platysma is incised. The sternocleidomastoid fascia is opened, and dissection along the border of the muscle exposes the carotid artery as described in Chapter 2. Two tapes are placed around the proximal common carotid artery, the carotid bifurcation is exposed, and tapes are placed around the external and internal carotid arteries.

The medial two-thirds of the sternocleidomastoid muscle is divided near its attachment to the clavicle and sternum (Figs. 5.5 and 5.6). The scalene fat pad is entered, and the anterior scalene muscle, phrenic nerve, and internal jugular vein are identified. The phrenic nerve is mobilized and retracted. The anterior scalene muscle is divided near its origin from the first rib, bringing into view the subclavian artery and brachial plexus. If the operation is being done on the right side, the vertebral origin is found by dissecting along the superior surface of the subcla-

Atherosclerosis of the Vertebrobasilar Circulation

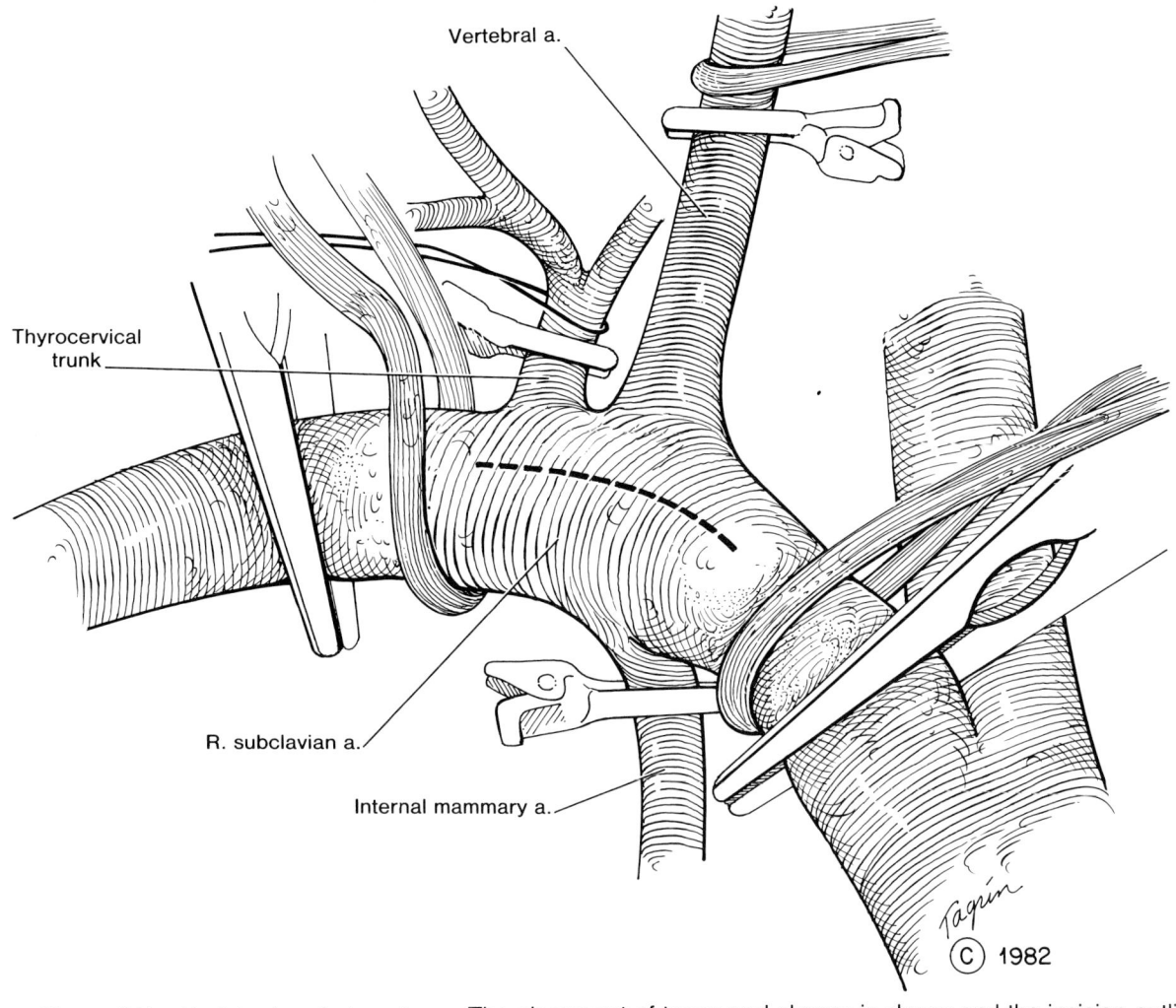

Figure 5.7. Vertebral endarterectomy. The placement of tapes and clamps is shown and the incision outlined.

vian artery. On the left side the dissection is carried behind the subclavian vein along the subclavian artery medially. Care is taken to protect the thoracic duct, which inserts on the lateral aspects of the junction between the left internal jugular and subclavian veins. If this duct is injured, it should be ligated. The vertebral artery is then followed from its origin to the transverse process at C6. The patient is heparinized, and blood pressure is elevated as indicated. If the operation is being done for subclavian steal, the brachial blood pressures are checked with temporary occlusion of the vertebral artery.

The proximal vertebral artery is then suture ligated, and a temporary aneurysm clip is used to occlude the distal portion of the vertebral artery (Fig. 5.8). The common carotid artery is temporarily occluded while monitoring the electroencephalogram (EEG). An oval arteriotomy is done in the lateral wall of the common carotid artery. A temporary shunt can be placed as indicated by EEG changes. Under mag-

nification, an end-to-side anastomosis is done with a running 5-0 or 6-0 Prolene suture. The internal carotid artery is then temporarily occluded, the clamps are removed, blood flow is allowed up the external carotid artery, and then full circulation is reestablished.

In one report, this operation was associated with five excellent results and one good result in patients with vertebral stenosis and two excellent results in patients with subclavian steal (25). The only neurologic complication was a persistent Horner's syndrome in one patient. Another report indicated a similarly low risk (23). Interposition of a venous graft between the common carotid artery and extracranial vertebral artery has been done (12).

Carotid–Subclavian Artery Graft

This procedure is best performed through a supraclavicular approach (Fig. 5.4). The subclavian artery is exposed as described. In order to expose the com-

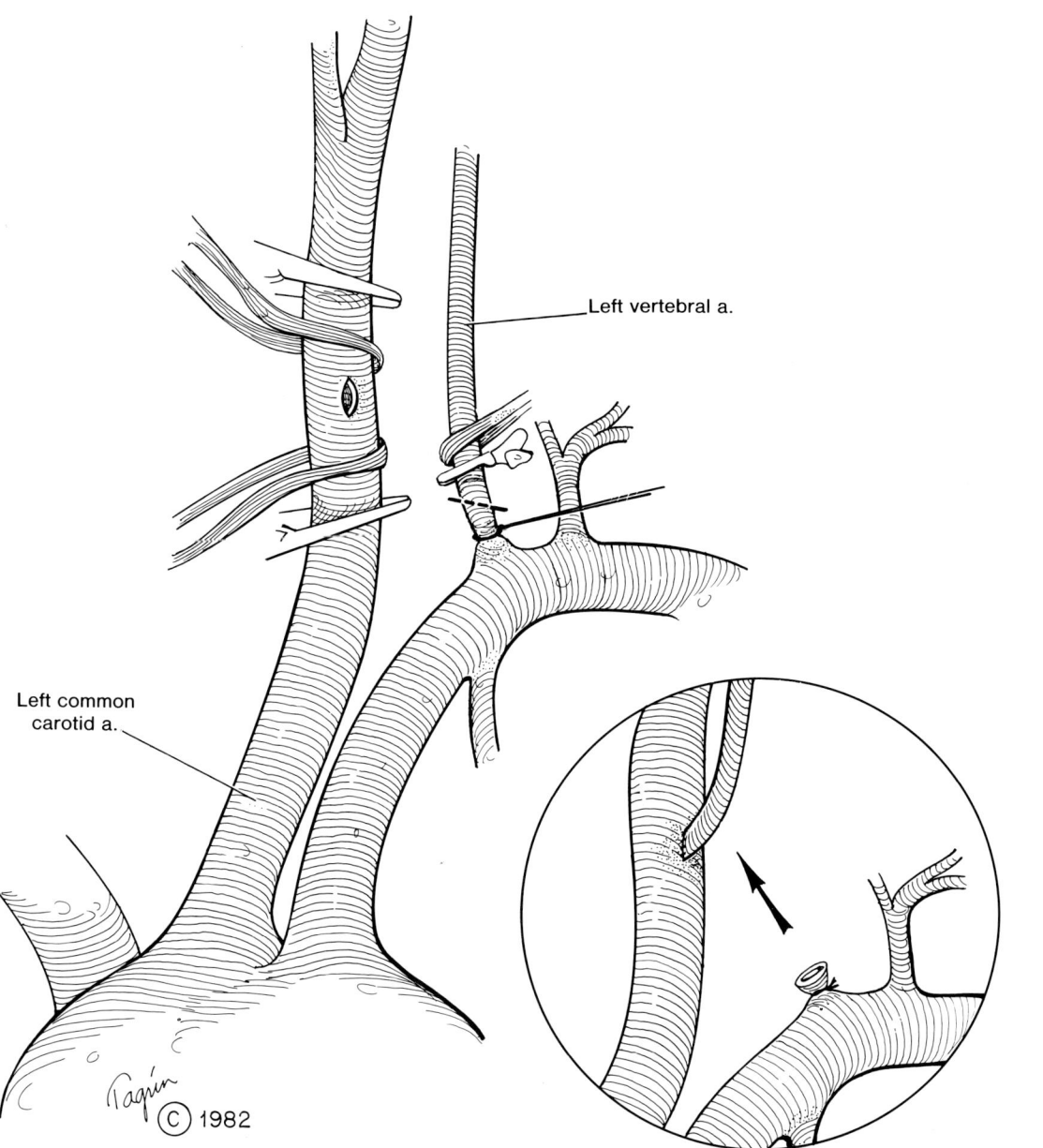

Figure 5.8. Vertebral artery transposition. The illustration shows a left side exposure. See text for details of operation.

mon carotid artery, the posterior border of the sternocleidomastoid muscle is divided and the carotid sheath is opened. Tapes are placed on the common carotid artery. An 8-mm GORE-TEX graft or a saphenous vein segment can be used for the bypass graft. The patient is given 7000 units of intravenous heparin. Blood pressure is elevated and the EEG monitored. Two clamps are placed on the common carotid artery, and an arteriotomy is made. The graft is beveled and sutured end-to-side to the common carotid artery (Fig. 5.9). Flow is then allowed into the graft, which is clamped in its proximal portion, and carotid artery blood flow is restored. The distal end of the graft is then brought to the side of the subclavian artery, and an end-to-side anastomosis is done. Clamps are removed and flow is restored. The incision is then closed in layers. In some cases when symptoms have not been relieved, studies have shown that antegrade flow has not been reestablished in the vertebral artery (9).

In a series of 57 carotid–subclavian bypass operations, there was no mortality or new neurologic problems (59). Two patients had to have further surgery because of an infected graft, and one had a thoracic duct fistula that closed spontaneously. Follow-up from 3 months to 16 years revealed no new neurologic or arm symptoms.

Occipital Artery–Posterior Inferior Cerebellar Artery Bypass

The technical feasibility and relative safety of occipital to posterior inferior cerebellar artery bypass have been established (33, 47, 54, 55, 57). Impressive angiographic filling of the vertebrobasilar circulation following this operation has been demonstrated. However, the clinical indications for this procedure are not yet well defined.

General anesthesia is required, with strict attention paid to maintenance of normal blood pressure throughout the procedure. The lateral position seems to provide adequate exposure and avoid the danger of cerebral ischemia inherent in the sitting position. A modified hockey-stick incision, rising high in the midline above the inion, provides adequate length for the occipital artery and access to the caudal posterior inferior cerebellar artery loop (Fig. 5.10). To avoid scalp edge necrosis, no clamps are placed on the flap edge. The occipital artery, which is invested in dense fascia, must be freed up by meticulous sharp microdissection. A suboccipital craniectomy, with removal of the posterior rim of the foramen magnum and a hemilaminectomy of C1, allows exposure of the cerebellar tonsils. The caudal loop of the posterior inferior cerebellar artery, which is localized angiographically, is dissected free of arachnoid and supported by a sling of rubber dam stitched to extracranial soft tissues.

The anastomosis is completed much like a superficial temporal–middle cerebral artery bypass graft. The tip of the occipital artery is cleared of adventitia and beveled. A clip is placed on the caudal loop of the posterior inferior cerebellar artery, an oval window is excised, and a small stent is inserted. Anastomosis is done with interrupted 10-0 monofilament nylon sutures. The occipital artery is beveled back toward the posterior inferior cerebellar artery origin in order to promote vertebrobasilar perfusion. During closure of the wound, one must be careful to avoid graft compression.

In a report on 22 patients, it was noted that the primary problem with the operative procedure was marginal neurologic status prior to operation, leading to respiratory complications from preoperative impairment of the cranial nerves (55). Only two patients had a permanent increase in neurologic deficits (unilateral hearing loss and homonymous hemianopia). The same general complications noted with superficial temporal–middle cerebral artery grafts were also encountered with this procedure. Occipital artery to extradural vertebral artery anastomosis has been described (31).

External Carotid–Saphenous Vein–Posterior Cerebral Artery Bypass

This procedure provides a high blood flow to the distal basilar artery. Experience has shown that patency is high and morbidity acceptable (56). The procedure should be considered for vertebrobasilar TIAs associated with bilateral intracranial vertebral occlusive disease, especially when terminal vertebral obstruction prevents occipital to posterior inferior cerebellar artery bypass. It may also be of value for patients with severe proximal basilar stenosis or occlusion and in cases of planned basilar occlusion for giant aneurysms (see Chapter 20).

Under general anesthesia, the patient is positioned supine, with a roll placed under the shoulder and with the head turned fully and held in the three-point head holder. The sitting position is avoided, and great care is taken throughout surgery to maintain normal to slightly elevated blood pressure in an effort to avoid vertebrobasilar ischemia and infarction (12). The temporal and cervical regions are prepared and draped in a single field. The medial thigh and calf (the left is more convenient) are shaved, prepared, and draped. Two teams of surgeons simultaneously expose the carotid bifurcation and harvest the saphenous vein.

The saphenous vein is removed beginning 1 cm anterior to the medial malleolus. It is convenient to dissect adventitia from the vein and to cut the skin with Metzenbaum scissors. The vessel is followed to its narrowing at the knee, a narrowing that helps to minimize the discrepancy in diameter with the pos-

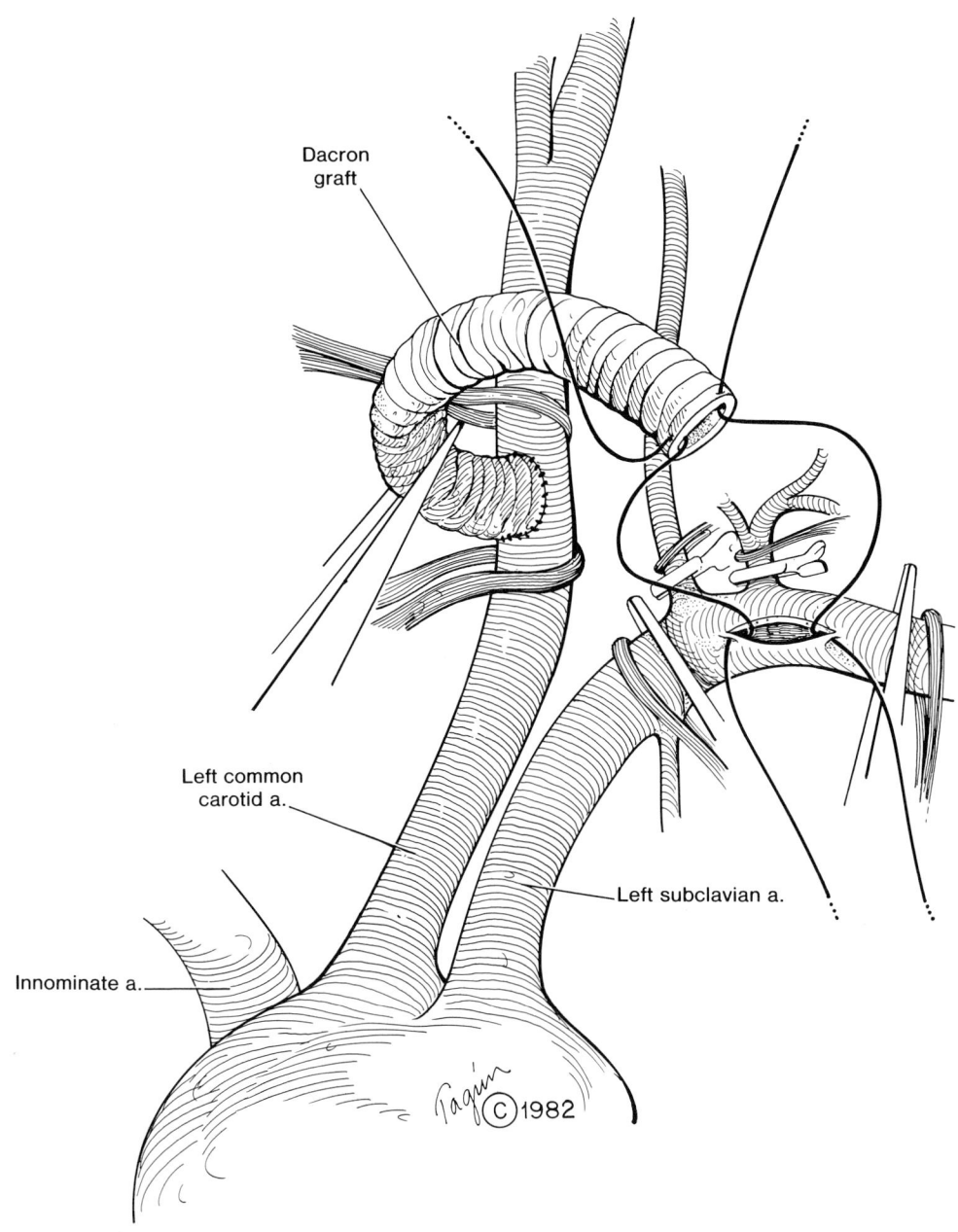

Figure 5.9. Carotid–subclavian artery graft. A Dacron or GORE-TEX graft may be used. An end-to-side anastomosis has been done on the common carotid artery. The anastomosis to the subclavian artery has been started.

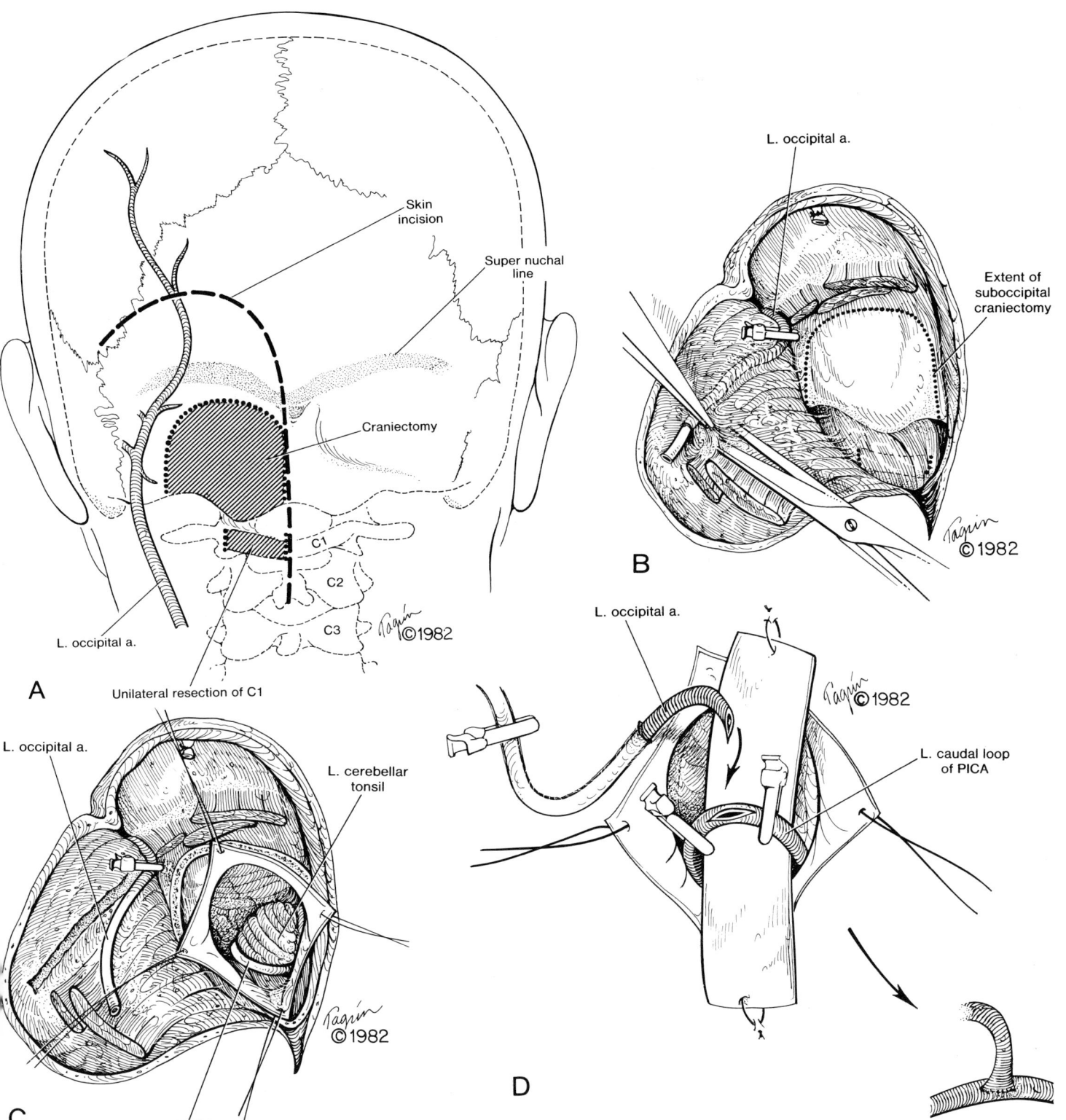

Figure 5.10. Occipital artery–posterior inferior cerebellar artery (*PICA*) bypass. **A**, Initial exposure. Hockey-stick incision is carried well above the superior nuchal line to assure adequate length for the occipital artery segment. The bony removal includes the posterior rim of foramen magnum and hemilaminectomy of C1. **B**, Preparation of occipital artery. The vessel is followed from the skin edge proximally through the muscle layers to the mastoid. Relatively little adventitia remains attached to the vessel. **C**, Exposure of posterior inferior cerebellar artery. After craniectomy and C1 hemilaminectomy, the dura is opened in a cruciate fashion to expose the cerebellar tonsil and caudal loop of posterior inferior cerebellar artery. The vessel may be followed laterally to the area of maximum diameter. **D**, Anastomosis. Posterior inferior cerebellar artery is gently lifted off the tonsil with a rubber dam, which is sutured to dura. The occipital artery is freed of adventitia distally and a fish-mouthed beveled ostium is prepared. After clipping the posterior inferior cerebellar artery with Kleinert-Kees clips, an arteriotomy is performed. End-to-side anastomosis is carried out with interrupted 10-0 monofilament nylon sutures.

terior cerebral artery. Side branches are divided between 4-0 silk ligatures, and at least one prominent branch near the ankle is saved long enough so that it can be used for later irrigation. In situ, the vessel's superficial aspect is marked with a marking pen or a long silk string sutured intermittently through the adventitia to help avoid twists in final positioning. Patency is maintained until the vessel is cut, removed, and immediately irrigated antegrade with heparinized saline. Vigorous high-pressure irrigation, which could expand the graft and exaggerate diameter discrepancy, is avoided. The graft is placed in heparinized saline until anastomosis.

While the saphenous vein is being harvested, the carotid bifurcation is exposed (see Chapter 2). Since the head is turned more than usual, the surgeon should be prepared to dissect deeper beneath the sternocleidomastoid muscle. A complete freeing of the external carotid artery is needed about 3 cm above its origin. The common carotid, external, and internal carotid arteries are controlled with tapes.

Through a linear ("tic") incision or a "horseshoe" temporal flap, a small temporal craniotomy such as is used in exposure of a basilar bifurcation aneurysm is fashioned (see Chapter 18). In order to slacken the brain for retraction, mannitol is administered (100 gm IV), and spinal fluid is withdrawn via the previously placed spinal subarachnoid catheter. The temporal lobe is gently elevated with a self-retaining retractor to expose the posterior cerebral artery lateral to the brain stem. Using a Kelly clamp, a tunnel is made from the cranial to the cervical incision by routing superficial to the zygoma, with care taken to avoid the branches of the facial nerve.

The saphenous vein graft is pulled from the cervical wound through the subcutaneous tunnel to the cranial wound by a 0-silk tied to the narrowed rostral end, with care taken to avoid twisting. This end is brought close to the posterior cerebral artery to judge appropriate graft length. The cervical end is crosscut at 90°; the valves are avoided. A side branch is catheterized with a 20-gauge Medicut catheter for intermittent irrigation with heparinized saline.

For the proximal anastomosis, 7000 units of heparin are given intravenously prior to cross-clamping the external carotid artery. At a convenient point, usually just before the first major bifurcation, the vessel is cross-cut at 90°. If there is substantial atheroma, a limited endarterectomy is warranted. Under the operating microscope, an end-to-end anastomosis is performed between the external carotid artery and the saphenous vein graft (see Fig. 4.17 for details of the technique). The authors prefer interrupted 6-0 Prolene, about six stitches on each side, without need for a stent. On one occasion, a diagonal cut of the vessels was used to minimize diameter discrepancy, but this is usually not a problem.

Length is checked and the distal graft is cross-cut at 90°. It is important to avoid too much redundancy.

During the distal anastomosis, intermittent irrigation through the side branch serves to clear small clots, identify leaks, and clear the field. Under the microscope, the posterior cerebral artery lateral to the brain stem is dissected free over at least 1 cm. It is usually possible to preserve all side branches. The vessel is cross-clamped with Sugita temporary clips. With the graft in the field as a guide, an arteriotomy of the posterior cerebral artery is made with a no. 11 blade. The anastomosis is fashioned with interrupted 9-0 nylon, about six stitches for each side, with a small Silastic stent (see Chapter 4 for details of the technique). Completion of the back wall is aided by deviation of the graft with a cottonoid toward the temporal lobe. Before the last stitch is tied, posterior cerebral artery flow is checked and brief flow through the graft is permitted to blow out debris and air. The final stitch is tied, and all clips are removed, thus establishing graft flow. At this point and after surgery, blood pressure is carefully kept in the range normal for the individual patient. Protamine sulfate is given (70 mg IV) to reverse heparin effect. Wounds are closed in routine fashion, with care taken to avoid compression of the graft.

An alternative technique, which the authors have come to prefer, is to perform the distal anastomosis first, after the vein has been tunneled but before the proximal anastomosis. This allows the surgeon to perform the distal anastomosis with sufficient "slack" so as to be able to move the vein around for the difficult back wall anastomosis. The "slack" is then removed by pulling the vein from proximally to the precise length. The easier proximal anastomosis can then be done. Proceeding in this manner, one may avoid leaving too much redundancy, which can lead to kinking as the vein stretches when flow is reestablished.

Experience with four such grafts has been encouraging. All patients had very severe bilateral intracranial vertebral disease. Two patients with disabling frequent TIAs have had no further TIAs. One patient, with two prior infarctions and multiple TIAs due to bilateral vertebral occlusion, has had occasional minor TIAs but no infarction during 3 years of follow-up. A patient with bilateral vertebral occlusion and multiple cerebral and cerebellar infarcts suffered progressive stepwise decline despite anticoagulants. The authors performed bypass reluctantly and found organized thrombus in the posterior cerebral artery, removal of which led to fairly good proximal backflow without distal backflow. They ligated the posterior cerebral artery distal to the completed anastomosis to avoid propagation of clot. The patient improved promptly after surgery only to revert to his former status when the graft occluded 3 days later, likely due to the preexisting intraluminal thrombus. The other three grafts remain patent 1–3 years postoperatively. Equally satisfactory technical results have been achieved in patients with giant basilar aneurysms, but one of these patients died of rupture of the aneurysm the night after completion of the external carotid to posterior cerebral artery vein graft (see Chapter 20).

Anastomosis to Superior Cerebellar Artery

Superficial temporal to proximal superior cerebellar artery anastomosis has been reported (23). Sundt et al have been concerned about the volume of flow achieved in this anastomosis (53). For occlusive disease in the proximal posterior cerebral or distal basilar artery, they have used a side-to-side anastomosis of the posterior cerebral and superior cerebellar arteries.

Removal of Foreign Body from Vertebral Artery

One patient was seen because the end of a guide wire, used during angiography, had broken off and lodged in the vertebral artery at the C2–C3 level just before the first turn in the artery (Fig. 5.11). An angiogram showed the artery to be open. The patient had syncopal attacks.

An incision was made paralleling the midportion of the sternocleidomastoid muscle. The posterior border of the sternocleidomastoid muscle was retracted medially, and the nerve roots of the upper brachial plexus were identified. The paravertebral muscles were separated from the anterior aspect of the transverse processes of C3 and C4; the level had been identified by x-ray. The anterior portions of the transverse processes of C3 and a portion of C4 were removed. By using the air drill with a diamond burr, bone was also removed from the medial and lateral aspects of the vertebral artery canal. Bleeding from epidural veins was controlled with bipolar coagulation. Tapes were placed around the vertebral artery at the superior and inferior margins of the exposure. Blood pressure was maintained above 150 mm Hg. A small arteriotomy was made in the artery, and the foreign body removed. A single suture closed the opening. The postoperative course was uncomplicated.

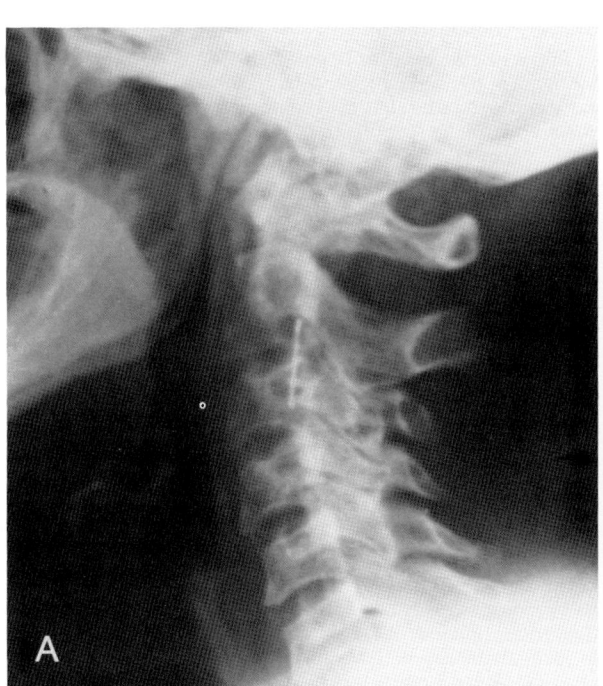
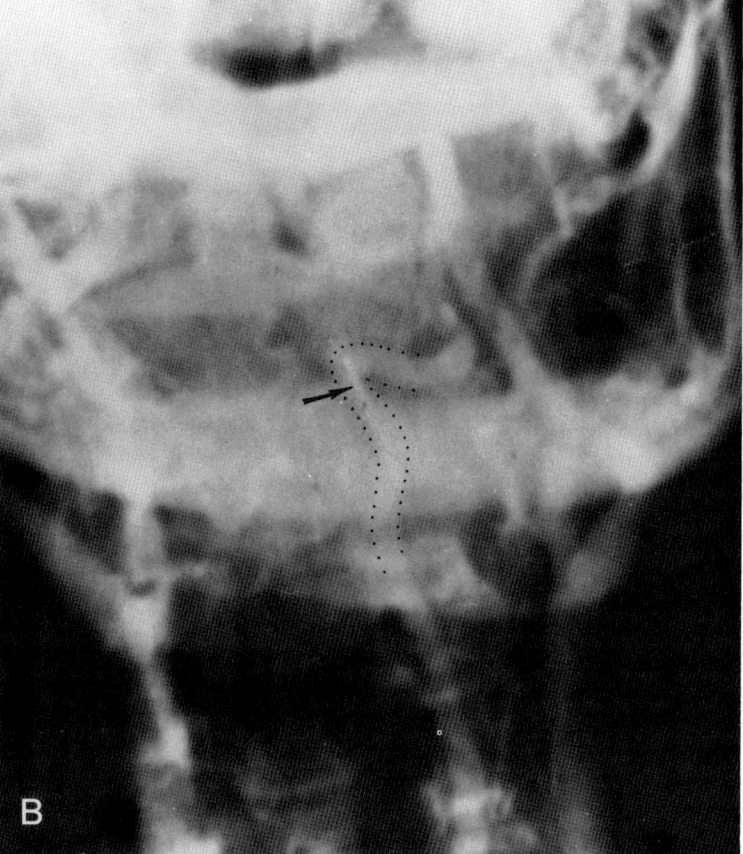

Figure 5.11. Foreign body in vertebral artery. **A**, Lateral x-ray of neck showing the end of a guide wire at C2–C3. **B**, Anteroposterior arch angiogram showing the wire (*arrow*) to be lodged at the first turn in the vertebral artery (*outlined with dots*).

REFERENCES

1. Alexander JJ, Glagov S, Zarins CK: Repair of a vertebral artery dissection. Case report *J Neurosurg* 64:662–665, 1985.
2. Allen GJ, Cohen RJ, Preziosi TJ: Microsurgical endarterectomy of the intracranial vertebral artery for vertebrobasilar transient ischemic attacks. *Neurosurgery* 8:56–59, 1981.
3. Ausman JI, Diaz FG, de los Reyes RA, Pak H, Patel S, Boulos R: Superficial temporal to proximal superior cerebellar artery anastomosis for basilar artery stenosis. *Neurosurgery* 9:56–59, 1981.
4. Ausman JI, Diaz FG, de los Reyes RA, Pearce JE, Shrontz CE: Extracranial-intracranial anastomoses in the posterior circulation. In Berner R, Bauer RB (eds): *Vertebrobasilar Arterial Occlusive Disease*. New York, Raven Press, 1984, pp 313–319.
5. Bakay L, Leslie EV: Surgical treatment of vertebral artery insufficiency caused by cervical spondylosis. *J Neurosurg* 23:596–602, 1965.
6. Baldy-Monlimr M, Rondovin G, Touchon J: Brain stem auditory-evoked potentials in the assessment of the transient ischemic attacks of the arterial vertebrobasilar system. *Monogr Neurol Sci* 11:216–221, 1984.
7. Bergnen R, Bauer RB: Vertebral artery reconstruction. A successful technique in selected patients. *Ann Surg* 193:441–447, 1981.
8. Bogousslavsky J, Regli F: Vertebrobasilar transient ischemic attacks in internal carotid artery occlusion or tight stenosis. *Arch Neurol* 42:64–68, 1985.
9. Bohmfalk GL, Story JL, Brown WE Jr, Marlin AE: Subclavian steal syndrome. Part 1. Proximal vertebral to common carotid artery transposition in three patients and historical review. *J Neurosurg* 51:628–640, 1979.
10. Bohmfalk GL, Story JL, Brown WE Jr, Marlin AE: Subclavian steal syndrome. Part 2. Intraoperative vertebral artery blood flow measurement. *J Neurosurg* 51:641–643, 1979.
11. Bonafe A, Manelfe C, Scotto B, Pradere MY, Rascol A: Role of computed tomography in vertebrobasilar ischemia. *Neuroradiology* 27:484–493, 1985.
12. Camp PE: Carotid to distal vertebral artery bypass for vertebrobasilar ischemia. Case report. *J Neurosurg* 60:187–189, 1984.
13. Caplan LR: Occlusion of the vertebral or basilar artery. Follow-up analysis of some patients with benign outcomes. *Stroke* 10:277–282, 1979.
14. Caplan LR: Vertebrobasilar disease: Time for a new strategy. *Stroke* 12:111–114, 1981.
15. Caplan LR: Bilateral distal vertebral artery occlusion. *Neurology* 33:552–558, 1983.
16. Caplan LR: Vertebrobasilar transient ischemic attacks. *Arch Neurol* 42:839–840, 1985.
17. Caplan LR: Vertebrobasilar occlusive disease. In Barnett HJM, Mohr JP, Stein BM, Yatsu FM (eds): *Stroke*. New York, Churchill Livingstone, 1986, pp 549–619.
18. Caplan LR, Sergan S: Positional cerebral ischemia. *J Neurol Neurosurg Psychiatry* 39:385–391, 1976.
19. Cattaino G, Querin F, Pomes A, Piazza P: Transient global amnesia. *Acta Neurol Scand* 70:385–390, 1984.
20. Coria F, Rebollo M, Quintana F, Polo JM, Berciano J: Occipitoatlantal instability and vertebrobasilar ischemia: Case report. *Neurology* 32:303–305, 1982.
21. Crowell GF, Stump DA, Biller J, McHenry LC Jr, Toole JF: The transient global amnesia-migraine connection. *Arch Neurol* 41:75–79, 1984.
22. Drake CG: Ligation of the vertebral (unilateral or bilateral) or basilar artery in the treatment of large intracranial aneurysm. *J Neurosurg* 43:255–274, 1975.
23. Edwards WH, Mulherin JL Jr: The surgical approach to significant stenosis of vertebral and subclavian arteries. *Surgery* 87:20–28, 1980.
24. Faught E, Trader SD, Hanna GR: Cerebral complications of angiography for transient ischemia and stroke: Prediction of risk. *Neurology* 29:4–15, 1979.
25. Fein JM: Vertebral artery transposition for vertebral basilar insufficiency. Presented at the 1981 meeting of the American Association of Neurological Surgeons, Boston, MA.
26. Fisher CM: Occlusion of the vertebral arteries. *Arch Neurol* 22:13–19, 1970.
27. Fisher, CM, Ojemann RG, Roberson G: Spontaneous dissection of cervicocerebral arteries. *Can J Neurol Sci* 5:9–19, 1978.
28. Galbraith JG, McDowell HA Jr: Stroke and occlusive cerebrovascular disease. Review and surgical results in 265 cases. *J Med Assoc Ala* 38:1107–1111, 1969.
29. Gerety RL, Andrus CH, May AG, Rob CG, Green R, DeWesse JA: Surgical treatment of occlusive subclavian artery disease. *Circulation* 64:228–230, 1981.
30. Goldstein SJ: Dissecting hematoma of the cervical vertebral artery. Case report. *J Neurosurg* 56:451–454, 1982.
31. Hadley MN, Spetzler RF, Masferrer R, Martin NA, Carter LP: Occipital artery to extradural vertebral artery bypass procedure. Case report. *J Neurosurg* 63:622–625, 1985.
32. Imparato A, Riles T, Kim GE, Mintzer R: Vertebral artery reconstruction. *Stroke* 12:125, 1981.
33. Khodadad G, Singh RS, Olinger CP: Possible prevention of brain stem stroke by microvascular anastomosis in the vertebrobasilar system. *Stroke* 8:316–321, 1977.
34. Kistler JP, Buonanno FS, DeWitt LD, Daris KR, Brady TJ, Fisher CM: Vertebral-basilar posterior cerebral territory stroke-delineation by proton nuclear magnetic resonance imaging. *Stroke* 15:417–426, 1984.
35. Koga H, Austin G: Regional cerebral blood flow in patients with vertebrobasilar disease. *Surg Neurol* 18:466–472, 1982.
36. Kurlan R, Krall RL, DeWeese JA: Vertebrobasilar ischemia after total repair of tetralogy of Fallot. *Stroke* 15:359–362, 1984.
37. Lowman BG, Queral LA, Holbrook WA: The correction of cerebrovascular insufficiency by transluminal dilatation: A preliminary report. *Ann Surg* 49:621–624, 1983.
38. Lowman BG, Queral LA, Holbrook WA, Estes JT, Bayly B: The treatment of innominate artery stenosis by intraoperative transluminal angioplasty. *Surgery* 89:565–568, 1981.
39. McNamara JO, Heyman A, Silver D, Mandel ME: The value of carotid endarterectomy in treating transient cerebral ischemia of the posterior circulation. *Neurology* 27:682–684, 1977.
40. Monfarrij NA, Little JR, Furlan AJ, Williams G, Marzewski DJ: Vertebral artery stenosis: Long-term follow-up. *Stroke* 15:260–263, 1984.
41. Moore T, Russell MT, Parent A, Parker L, Smith R: Nonsurgical treatment of "subclavian steal syndrome" with percutaneous transluminal angioplasty. *Neurosurgery* 9:466, 1981.
42. Motarjeme A, Keifer JW, Zuska AJ: Percutaneous transluminal angioplasty of the vertebral arteries. *Radiology* 139:715–717, 1981.
43. Pinkerton JA Jr, Davidson KC, Hibbard BZ: Primitive hypoglossal artery and carotid endarterectomy. *Stroke* 11:658–660, 1980.
44. Pritz MB, Chandler WF, Kindt GW: Vertebral artery disease: Radiological evaluation, medical management and microsurgical treatment. *Neurosurgery* 9:524–530, 1981.
45. Robertson JT: Neck manipulation as a cause of stroke. *Stroke* 12:1, 1981.
46. Roon AJ, Ehrenfeld WK, Cooke PB, Wylie EJ: Vertebral artery reconstruction. *Am J Surg* 138;29–36, 1979.
47. Roski RA, Spetzler RF, Hopkins LN: Occipital artery to posterior-inferior cerebellar artery bypass for vertebrobasilar ischemia. *Neurosurgery* 10:44–49, 1982.
48. Rossi L, Amantini A, Bindi A, Paznini P, Arnetoli G, Zappoli R: Electrophysiological investigations of the brain stem in vertebrobasilar reversible attacks. *Eur Neurol* 22:371–379, 1983.

49. Schellhas KP, Latchaw RE, Wendling LR, Gold LHA: Vertebrobasilar injuries following cervical manipulation. *JAMA* 244:1450–1453, 1980.
50. Senter HJ, Bittar SM, Long ET: Revascularization of the extracranial vertebral artery at any level without cross-clamping. *J Neurosurg* 62:334–335, 1985.
51. Sherman DG, Hart RG, Easton JD: Abrupt change in head position and cerebral infarction. *Stroke* 12:2–6, 1981.
52. Steinberger A, Ganti SR, McMurtry JG III, Hilal SK: Transient neurological deficits secondary to saccular vertebrobasilar aneurysms. Report of two cases. *J Neurosurg* 60:410–413, 1984.
53. Sundt TM Jr, Campbell JK, Houser OW: Transposition anastomosis between the posterior cerebral and superior cerebellar arteries. *J Neurosurg* 55:967–970, 1981.
54. Sundt TM Jr, Piepgras DG: Occipital to posterior inferior cerebellar artery by-pass surgery. *J Neurosurg* 48:916–928, 1978.
55. Sundt TM Jr, Piepgras DG: By-pass surgery for vertebral artery occlusive disease: Technique and complications. *Clin Neurosurg* 26:346–352, 1979.
56. Sundt TM Jr, Piepgras DG, Houser W, Campbell JK: Interposition saphenous vein grafts for advanced occlusive disease and large aneurysms in the posterior circulation. *J Neurosurg* 56:205–215, 1982.
57. Sundt TM Jr, Whisnant JP, Piepgras DG, Campbell JK, Holman CB: Intracranial bypass grafts for vertebral-basilar ischemia. *Mayo Clin Proc* 53:12–18, 1978.
58. Taki W, Handa H, Higa T, Tanada S, Fukuyama H, Fujita T, Yonekawa Y, Kameyamal M, Toriuska K: Distribution of the blood flow supplied by the vertebral artery in humans as assessed by emission CT. *Stroke* 15:469–474, 1984.
59. Thompson BW, Read RC, Campbell GS: Operative correction of obstructed subclavian or innominate arteries. *South Med J* 71:1366–1369, 1978.
60. Wylie EJ, Effeney DJ: Surgery of the aortic arch branches and vertebral arteries. *Surg Clin North Am* 59:669–680, 1979.
61. Wylie EJ, Ehrenfeld WK: *Extracranial Occlusive Cerebrovascular Disease: Diagnosis and Management.* Philadelphia, WB Saunders, 1970.

6

Fibromuscular Dysplasia of the Internal Carotid Artery

PATHOGENESIS

Fibromuscular dysplasia was first observed in the renal artery. In the head and neck, the most common area of involvement is one or both distal extracranial internal carotid arteries. Other arteries that can be affected include the common carotid, external carotid, vertebral, and large intracranial arteries (11). The etiology is unknown. Several reports have suggested the possibility of a hormonal influence because of a marked female preponderance, but this has not been proven. Inheritance as a dominant trait with reduced penetrance in males has also been suggested (11).

Three types of pathological change have been described (3). The most common change primarily involves the media. There are multiple small saccular dilatations due to areas of destruction and fragmentation of the media, alternating with rings of fibrous and muscular hyperplasia. This type predominately affects females. The second type, occurring in a small percentage of cases, is associated with an increase in the fibrous elements of the intima, producing concentric narrowing of the lumen. This type affects both sexes. The third type of pathological finding is a periadventitial fibroplasia which is quite rare.

CLINICAL PRESENTATION

The diagnosis of fibromuscular dysplasia is not usually made until angiography is performed. In two reported series, the incidence of fibromuscular dysplasia was 0.6% in 13,955 and 0.53% in 6,100 cerebral angiograms (3, 16). The symptoms that led to angiography in several series of patients found to have fibromuscular dysplasia are summarized in Table 6.1. It is apparent that many of these patients had symptoms related to problems other than fibromuscular dysplasia. Several of the patients with transient ischemic attacks (TIAs) and infarction had significant atherosclerosis which probably accounted for the symptoms. In the majority of patients, fibromuscular dysplasia is an incidental finding. Probably only a small number of these patients had focal cerebral ischemia due to reduced flow or emboli associated with fibromuscular dysplasia in the internal carotid artery. On rare occasion, an acute stroke may have been associated with development of a thrombus in an area of fibromuscular dysplasia in the internal carotid artery (1). A few patients will have a bruit that is disturbing enough to warrant angiography. Other symptoms that may relate to fibromuscular dysplasia include headache, facial pain, dizziness, tinnitus, seizure, and syncope (12, 16, 17, 19, 21).

The age at the time of diagnosis and sex incidence are summarized in Table 6.2. The vast majority of patients were women with symptoms occurring in the fourth, fifth, and sixth decades.

The natural history of the disease has not been fully defined, but most patients seem to have a benign course (3, 21). The results presented in Table 6.3 suggest that fibromuscular dysplasia is often an incidental finding with a low incidence of subsequent cerebral ischemia during long-term follow-up (3). In fact, 2 of the 3 patients with ischemic events were affected in the territory of an artery other than the one involved with fibromuscular dysplasia. Seven of the 13 patients with focal cerebral ischemia were treated. Five had atherosclerosis which may have been the cause of the symptoms. In another series, 1 of 17 patients was operated on; the remaining 16 patients were followed for 1–9 years (average, 3.8) (20). Fourteen showed no evidence of progression of fibromuscular dysplasia, while 2 patients with significant atherosclerotic disease had strokes. Four had received aspirin, 3 anticoagulants, and the others no specific therapy.

ANGIOGRAPHY

The typical angiographic finding is an area of alternating zones of widening and narrowing of the arterial lumen (Fig. 6.1A and B). This has been described as a "string of beads" appearance. It was seen in 80% of the angiograms in two series of 25 patients (14, 18) and in 31 of 32 patients in another series (16). The next most common finding is a tubular stenosis. Other angiographic findings include a diverticulum, a web at the carotid bifurcation, and dissection (12, 14, 16, 18, 23). In the patient with the typical angiographic findings, the area of involvement begins at the level of the first to third cervical

Table 6.1.
Symptoms That Led to Angiography in Patients Found to Have Fibromuscular Dysplasia

Reference	Total No. of Patients	No. of Patients with the Following Symptoms						
		Focal TIA	Ischemia or Infarction	Subarachnoid Hemorrhage	Signs of Mass Lesion	Asymptomatic Bruit Alone	Nonfocal Neurologic Symptoms	Other
17	15	1	2	3	1	3	4	1
14	25	8	6	9	0	0	2	0
3	79	6	7	10	29	8	3	16
16	32	9	9	5	0	2	4	3
21	17	7	2	0	0	0	8	0
11	37	4	3	21	4	0	2	3
22	30	9	3	1	4	5	5	7
19	49	14	3	3	0	11	10	8

Table 6.2.
Age and Sex Distribution from Reports of Patients with Fibromuscular Dysplasia

Reference	No. of Patients	Sex		Age Range (yr)
		Male	Female	
17	15	0	15	(21–79) (avg., 51)
14	25	5	20	(4–71) (avg., 45)
5	86	3	83	(27–83) (mean, 58)
2	18	0	18	(40–83) (mean, 60)
3	82	8	74	(18–76) (mean, 58)
16	32	0	32	(34–70) (avg., 57)
18	25	6	19	(30–70) (avg., 58)
21	17	0	17	(34–74) (mean, 58)
11	37	7	30	(24–70) (mean, 48)
22	30	7	23	(20–73) (mean, 59)
25	49	1	48	(29–82) (mean, 58)

Table 6.3.
Subsequent Cerebral Ischemic Events in Patients with Fibromuscular Dysplasia[a]

Reason for Angiogram	No. of Patients with Fibromuscular Dysplasia	Average Follow-up (mo)	Subsequent Cerebral Ischemic Events
Intracranial mass lesion	29	50	3
Aneurysm	10	52	0
Other nonischemic disorders	27	80	0
Focal cerebral ischemia	13	75	0

[a] From Corrin LS, Sandok BA, Houser OW: Cerebral ischemic events in patients with carotid artery fibromuscular dysplasia. *Archives of Neurology* 38:616–618, 1981.

vertebrae and extends distally for one or more centimeters (14, 16, 17). Rarely is the first 2.0–3.0 cm of the internal carotid artery involved. Intracranial involvement is also rare. None was reported in a series of 82 patients (3), and 4 were reported in a series of 25 patients (14); and in 1 of 17 patients the intracavernous portion of the internal carotid artery was involved (21). The incidence of bilateral internal carotid artery involvement was 37% in one series (3), 86% in another series (16), and 44% in the summary of the 109 cases reported up to 1974 (7).

Fibromuscular dysplasia has been associated with spontaneous dissection, intracranial aneurysm, carotid cavernous fistula, embolism, and reduced flow in the artery distal to the pathology (3). In the 109 cases reported up to 1974, 23 had aneurysms; a high incidence of associated aneurysm has also been a finding in other series (7, 11, 12, 19, 22). Associated atherosclerosis has been seen in several patients.

A small number of patients have had repeat angiograms. In one report, 2 of 6 patients showed progression of the lesion (16). In one of these patients, recurrent embolic infarctions led to repeat angiography 2 years later, which showed enlargement of the septum at the carotid bifurcation with an associated thrombus. Recurrent symptoms stopped after the septum was excised. In the second patient, angiography for evaluation of diffuse headache was performed 4 years later and revealed progression of bilateral fibromuscular dysplasia. Dilatation resulted in relief of the headaches. In the other 4 patients, angiograms 1.5–7 years after the initial study showed no change. Other reports described 12 patients with follow-up angiography ranging from 2 months to 6 years (16, 21). Progression of the lesion was seen in 3 patients.

TREATMENT

Since fibromuscular dysplasia is often an incidental angiographic finding and there is a low incidence of subsequent cerebral ischemia events, many patients do not require any treatment. When there are neurologic symptoms, medical therapy with anticoagulation or antiplatelet drugs is recommended. In the rare case in which this treatment is not effective or there is evidence of a significant hemodynamic or progressive lesion, surgery may be indicated.

The preferred surgical treatment for most cases has been the use of graduated internal dilatation (2, 6,

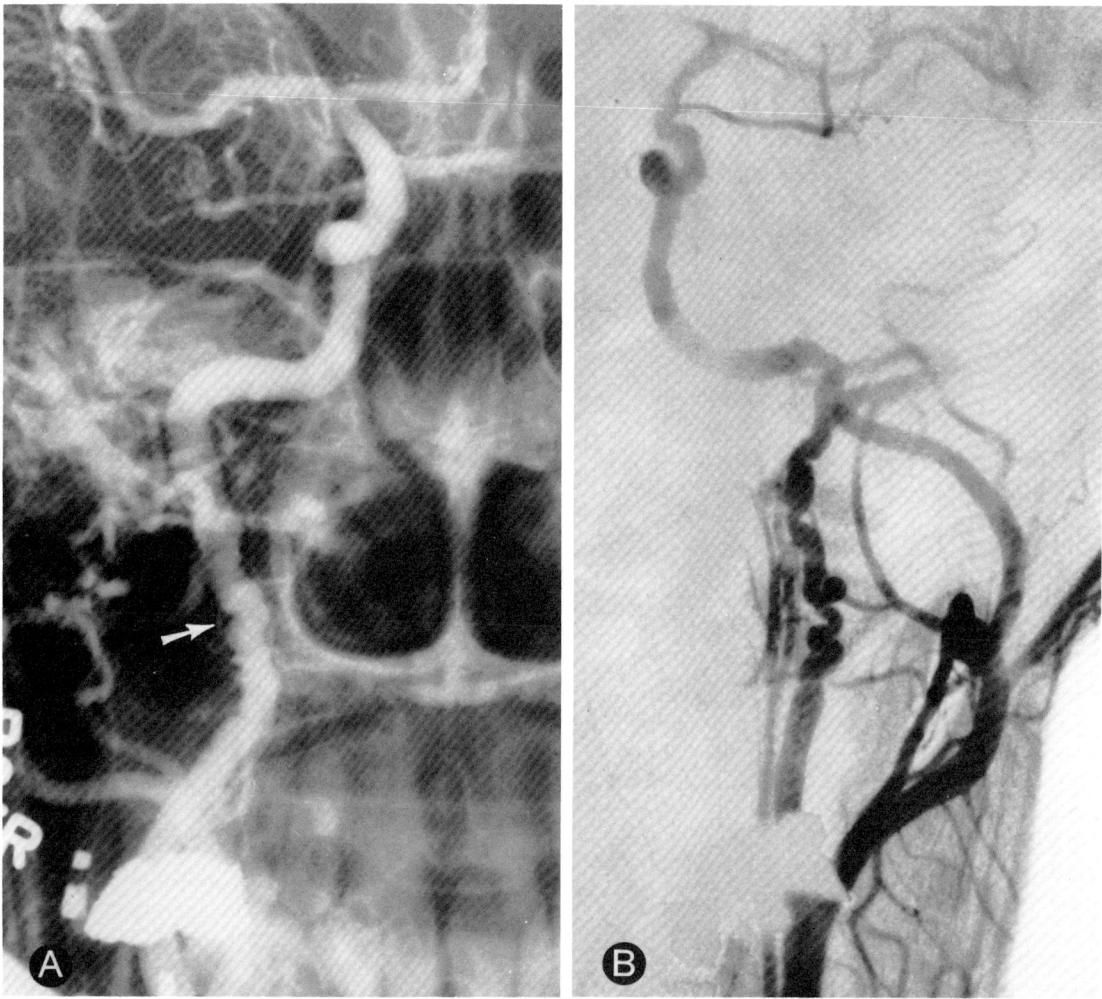

Figure 6.1. Typical angiographic appearances of fibromuscular dysplasia in the distal aspect of the extracranial internal carotid artery. **A**, Note the "corregated" or "string of beads" appearance (*arrow*). **B**, Subtraction study in another patient showing tortuosity, as well as segmental constrictions.

17, 18, 23). The exposure for this operation is the same as that utilized for a carotid endarterectomy. The principle of treatment is to dilate the stenotic segment (6, 18). Common duct dilators (Bakes) are used. After the exposure is completed, appropriate tapes are placed and the patient is heparinized. The common and external carotid arteries are clamped and the internal carotid artery is controlled with a tourniquet. A small arteriotomy is made in the distal common carotid artery. The dilators are passed into the internal carotid artery, usually beginning with one of 3.0 mm or less and progressing in 0.5-mm increments to one of 5.0 mm. The wall of the internal carotid artery may be thin, so care is taken as the dilator encounters resistance at the intraluminal septa. As the dilator is passed through the septum, a distinct give is felt. This procedure is continued until the base of the skull is reached. After each dilatation, the artery is allowed to "backbleed" for a few seconds.

When the dilatation is complete, the arteriotomy is closed with a continuous 5-0 Prolene suture. Heparin is not reversed, and antiplatelet therapy is started in the immediate postoperative period.

This procedure has been associated with a very low risk. In a series of 19 patients treated by dilatation and followed for 2–12 years (mean, 7.3 years), there was no operative morbidity or mortality and there were only two late recurrences of mild symptoms (18). In another report of 101 patients who had 150 arteries dilated, there were no deaths, 3 patients suffered strokes in the early postoperative period, and 9 patients exhibited TIAs (6). Long-term follow-up of up to 17 years revealed a very low incidence of recurrence. Other reports also record good results with dilatation (2, 6, 17).

Patients with symptomatic fibromuscular dysplasia have done well following excision of a septum, resection of the area of pathology, endarterectomy for atherosclerosis, and combined dilatation and endarterectomy (5, 16). Occasionally, a patient has been treated with an extracranial to intracranial bypass graft (3, 20, 21). In one patient, a saphenous vein graft was placed from the carotid bifurcation to the distal extracranial internal carotid artery (24). When a web is present at the carotid bifurcation, endarterectomy is an effective treatment (23).

The treatment for fibromuscular dysplasia of the internal carotid artery by dilatation with percutaneous transluminal angioplasty and a balloon dilating catheter has been described (4, 9, 10, 13). The basis for the treatment is the splitting of the intima, and to a lesser extent the media, to allow an increase in luminal diameter. Small fissures of the arterial wall may be demonstrated after angioplasty (4, 10). The reported advantages of this method of therapy include continuous fluoroscopic control of the procedure, the ability to treat multiple areas of disease, the radial application of dilatation forces, and the avoidance of general anesthesia (4, 15). The major disadvantage is the risk of embolism, since backbleeding cannot be done after the dilatation, as is done when metal dilators are used at open operation, to clean out any debris. In most of the reported patients, no complications have been noted and symptoms are usually relieved, but the follow-up intervals have been relatively short (4). In one patient, a neurologic complication, probably due to dissection, was associated with the procedure (10).

Transluminal balloon angioplasty has also been performed under fluoroscopic control after direct exposure of the carotid artery in the neck (8, 15). The authors believe this is a safer procedure than the percutaneous method because backbleeding can be done after the dilatation and an intimal flap can be dealt with, should it develop. No complications have been reported in a small group of patients.

REFERENCES

1. Balaji MR, DeWeese JA: Fibromuscular dysplasia of the internal carotid artery: Its occurrence with acute stroke and its surgical reversal. Arch Surg 115:984–986, 1980.
2. Collins GJ, Rich NM, Clagett GP, Spebar MJ, Salander JM: Fibromuscular dysplasia of the internal carotid arteries. Ann Surg 194:89–96, 1981.
3. Corrin LS, Sandok BA, Houser OW: Cerebral ischemic events in patients with carotid artery fibromuscular dysplasia. Arch Neurol 38:616–618, 1981.
4. Dublin AB, Baltaxe HA, Cobb CA III: Percutaneous transluminal carotid angioplasty in fibromuscular dysplasia. J Neurosurg 59:162–165, 1983.
5. Effeney DJ, Ehrenfeld WK, Stoney RJ, Wylie EJ: Why operate on carotid fibromuscular dysplasia? Arch Surg 115:1261–1267, 1980.
6. Effeney DJ, Krupski WC, Stoney RJ, Ehrenfeld WK: Fibromuscular dysplasia of the carotid artery. Aust NZ J Surg 53:527–531, 1983.
7. Frens DB, Petajan JH, Anderson R, Deblanc HJ: Fibromuscular dysplasia of the posterior cerebral artery; report of a case and review of the literature. Stroke 5:161–166, 1974.
8. Garrido E, Montoya J: Transluminal dilatation of internal carotid artery in fibromuscular dysplasia. A preliminary report. Surg Neurol 16:469–471, 1981.
9. Hasso AN, Bird CR, Zinke DE, Thompson JR: Fibromuscular dysplasia of the internal carotid artery. Percutaneous transluminal angioplasty. AJNR 2:175–180, 1981.
10. Jooma R, Bradshaw JR, Griffith HB: Intimal dissection following percutaneous transluminal carotid angioplasty for fibromuscular disease. Neuroradiology 27:181–182, 1985.
11. Mettinger KL: Fibromuscular dysplasia and the brain. II. Current concepts of the disease. Stroke 13:53–58, 1982.
12. Mettinger KL, Erickson K: Fibromuscular dysplasia and the brain. Observations on angiographic, clinical and genetic characteristics. Stroke 13:46–52, 1982.
13. Mullen S, Duda EE, Patronas NJ: Some examples of balloon technology in neurosurgery. J Neurosurg 52:321–329, 1980.
14. Osborn AG, Anderson RE: Angiographic spectrum of cervical and intracranial fibromuscular dysplasia. Stroke 8:617–626, 1977.
15. Smith DC, Smith LL, Hasso AN: Fibromuscular dysplasia of the internal carotid artery treated by operative transluminal balloon angioplasty. Radiology 155:645–648, 1985.
16. So EL, Toole JF, Dalal P, Moody DM: Cephalic fibromuscular dysplasia in 32 patients. Arch Neurol 38:619–622, 1981.
17. Stanley JC, Fry WJ, Seeger JF, Hoffman GL, Gabrielsen TO: Extracranial internal carotid and vertebral artery fibrodysplasia. Arch Surg 109:215–222, 1974.
18. Starr DS, Lawrie GM, Morris GC Jr: Fibromuscular disease of carotid arteries: Long term results of graduated internal dilatation. Stroke 12:196–199, 1981.
19. Stewart MT, Moritz MW, Smith RB III, Fulenwider JT, Perdue GD: The natural history of carotid fibromuscular dysplasia. J Vasc Surg 2:305–310, 1986.
20. Sundt TM Jr, Siekert RG, Piepgras DG, Sharbough FW, Houser OW: Bypass surgery for vascular disease of the carotid system. Mayo Clin Proc 51:677–692, 1976.
21. Wells RP, Smith RR: Fibromuscular dysplasia of the internal carotid artery. A long term follow-up. Neurosurgery 10:39–43, 1982.
22. Wesen CA, Elliott BM: Fibromuscular dysplasia of the carotid arteries. Am J Surg 151:448–451, 1986.
23. Wirth FP, Miller WA, Russell AP: Atypical fibromuscular hyperplasia. J Neurosurg 54:685–689, 1981.
24. Young PH, Smith KR Jr, Crafts DC, Barner HB: Traumatic occlusion in fibromuscular dysplasia of the carotid artery. Surg Neurol 16:432–437, 1981.

7
Dissection of Internal Carotid, Vertebral, and Intracranial Arteries

Dissection in the wall of the carotid, vertebral, or intracranial artery causing narrowing or occlusion of the arterial lumen or acting as a source of emboli is an established cause of cerebral ischemia (1–57). Often there is associated aneurysmal dilatation. The dissection develops when blood penetrates an intimal defect and strips the intima from the media. The etiology of the dissection is either spontaneous or traumatic. The term "spontaneous" indicates that no obvious precipitating injury was recognized, although a history of minimal trauma may be obtained in some patients. Traumatic causes include nonpenetrating injury to the head and neck, direct injury to the vessel, and angiography.

SPONTANEOUS DISSECTION OF INTERNAL CAROTID ARTERY

Pathogenesis

Dissection of the internal carotid artery begins at two sites of predilection: just distal to the origin and between C2 and the base of the skull. The possible relationship of congenital defects in the wall of the artery, of cystic medial necrosis, and of fibromuscular hyperplasia to the cause of the dissection has been discussed (14, 19, 22, 47). Hypertension does not seem to be an important factor.

In seven of the first 11 reported cases, the involved internal carotid artery as well as the opposite carotid and aorta were said to show cystic medial necrosis (14). However, this was not found in the detailed pathologic study of a specimen the authors removed at surgery (44). In that case, the wall of the artery showed no underlying intrinsic disease, but the muscle and elastic tissue had an irregular disorganized arrangement rather than the usual laminar pattern. In another report, examination of four arteries removed at operation showed dissection occurring in the outer layers of the media, decrease in the smooth muscle cells and elastic tissue, and degeneration and fragmentation of the internal elastic membrane (12). In some patients the dissection seemed to have occurred in apparently normal arteries (51). Fibromuscular dysplasia has been associated with several reported cases of dissection (10, 12, 14, 16, 22, 34, 36, 41, 47).

In spontaneous dissection, even when obvious external trauma is not a factor, it is possible that other factors relate to the onset (22). In three cases, symptoms began during a period of heavy coughing (14). Minor falls may be significant, as noted in the report of a patient who, while skiing, developed acute dissection of both internal carotid arteries, of the right vertebral artery at the level of the second vertebra, and of the left vertebral artery at the sixth cervical vertebra (47). The relationship of head rotation to injury of the internal carotid artery is discussed in the section on traumatic dissections.

It is likely that intracranial emboli from the area of the carotid dissection may be a primary cause of symptoms in many cases. This has been demonstrated in cases of both spontaneous and traumatic dissection (4, 15, 41, 47).

Clinical Manifestations

The average age of patients with dissection is in the forties (14, 19, 22, 34, 41). Both sexes are affected. The vast majority of patients present with unilateral headache and a few have neck pain (12, 13). Occasionally, focal cerebral ischemia, amaurosis fugax or syncope may be the first symptom (41).

The hallmark of dissection is the head pain localized to the forehead, orbit, and adjacent regions (13). The neck pain is usually localized to the region of the mastoid and upper carotid artery along the sternocleidomastoid muscle. In only a few patients is there tenderness over the carotid artery. The pain is often abrupt in onset and frequently severe. In some it is steady, and in others, throbbing. It may be continuous or intermittent. The pain is presumably due to the direct effect of the arterial dissection on pain receptors within the wall of the artery (40).

A history of severe unilateral headache and/or neck pain of abrupt onset followed by transient ischemic attacks (TIAs) or neurologic deficit is highly suggestive of the diagnosis, and the finding of oculosympathetic palsy (myosis and ptosis) adds further support to this impression (13, 14, 19, 34, 41). Oculosympathetic palsy is found in a little more than 50% of the patients and is due to involvement of the sympathetic fibers that accompany the internal carotid artery. A subjective bruit or pulsatile tinnitus is also a frequent complaint.

In the early reports of spontaneous dissection a high incidence of severe neurologic deficits was reported (44). However, with increasing recognition of the problem it has been found that many patients have only TIAs or no neurologic symptoms and have a benign clinical course (14, 15, 41). Most of those who have a stroke make a good recovery (14, 42).

Radiographic Findings

The diagnosis is usually established by angiography except where complete occlusion has occurred. Intracranial emboli may be seen. In some patients the diagnosis has been made with high resolution computed tomography (CT) scanning with intravenous contrast (33). Two patients had a thrombosed carotid dissection demonstrated by magnetic resonance imaging scan (18).

The angiographic profiles seen with carotid dissection are illustrated in Figure 7.1. Characteristic findings include:

A. The "string sign," a long irregular narrowing beginning above the carotid bifurcation in the neck and extending throughout much of the extracranial course of the internal carotid artery with restitution of a normal lumen usually at the entrance of the bony carotid canal (Figs. 7.2A and 7.3A and B) (44).

B. A proximal internal carotid pouch (1, 12, 14, 17, 44).

C. A distal internal carotid pouch occurring between C2 and the base of the skull associated with an adjacent area of narrowing of the internal carotid artery (Fig. 7.4A–D) (1, 12, 14, 17, 44).

D. A distal internal carotid pouch without narrowing of the internal carotid artery (Fig. 7.5A and B).

E. A double lumen occasionally has been reported, but the authors have not seen this (16, 41).

F. A complete occlusion that has no diagnostic feature. However, a gradually tapering occlusion beginning 2 cm or more distal to the bifurcation, without evidence of atherosclerosis in the area of the bifurcation, is suggestive of the diagnosis when correlated with the typical history.

In the authors' report of a single case of spontaneous carotid dissection, it was noted that the long stenotic segment of the cervical internal carotid artery (the string sign) might be a reliable indication of carotid dissection (Fig. 7.1A) (44). Subsequently, 22 cases of dissection of the cervicocerebral arteries were reported, and in 16 patients, angiography demonstrated a long narrow column of contrast material (14). In another report, 11 of 19 patients showed this finding (12). The string sign is the result of the dissecting hemorrhage compressing the natural lumen.

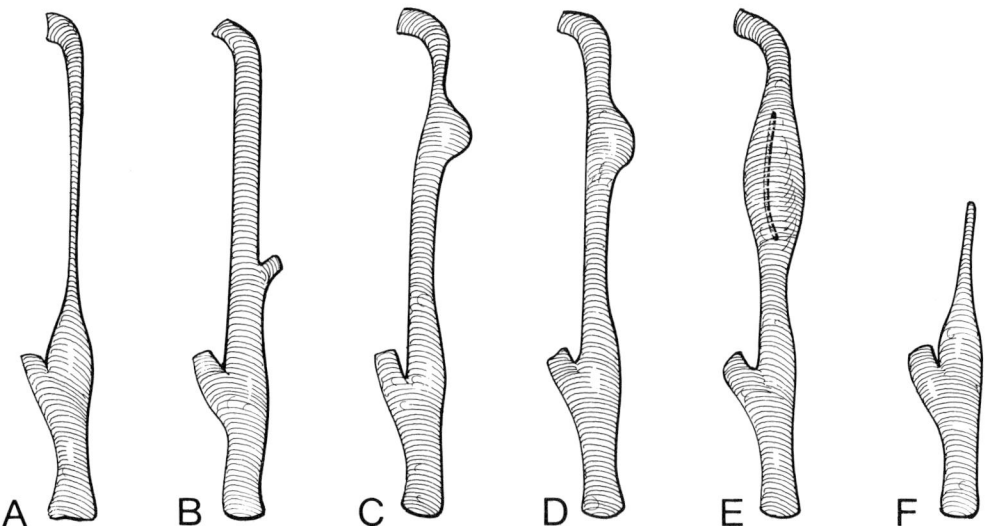

Figure 7.1. Angiographic profiles seen with internal carotid dissection. **A,** Characteristic "string sign." The extracranial internal carotid artery is narrowed from above the bifurcation to the base of the skull. **B,** Proximal internal carotid pouch. This may be evidence of a previous dissection that has healed. **C,** Distal extracranial internal carotid pouch with narrowing of the adjacent lumen—another characteristic finding. **D,** Distal extracranial pouch alone. This may occur acutely but can also remain indefinitely after the dissection heals. **E,** Double lumen, which is very rare. **F,** Complete occlusion. There is no characteristic feature.

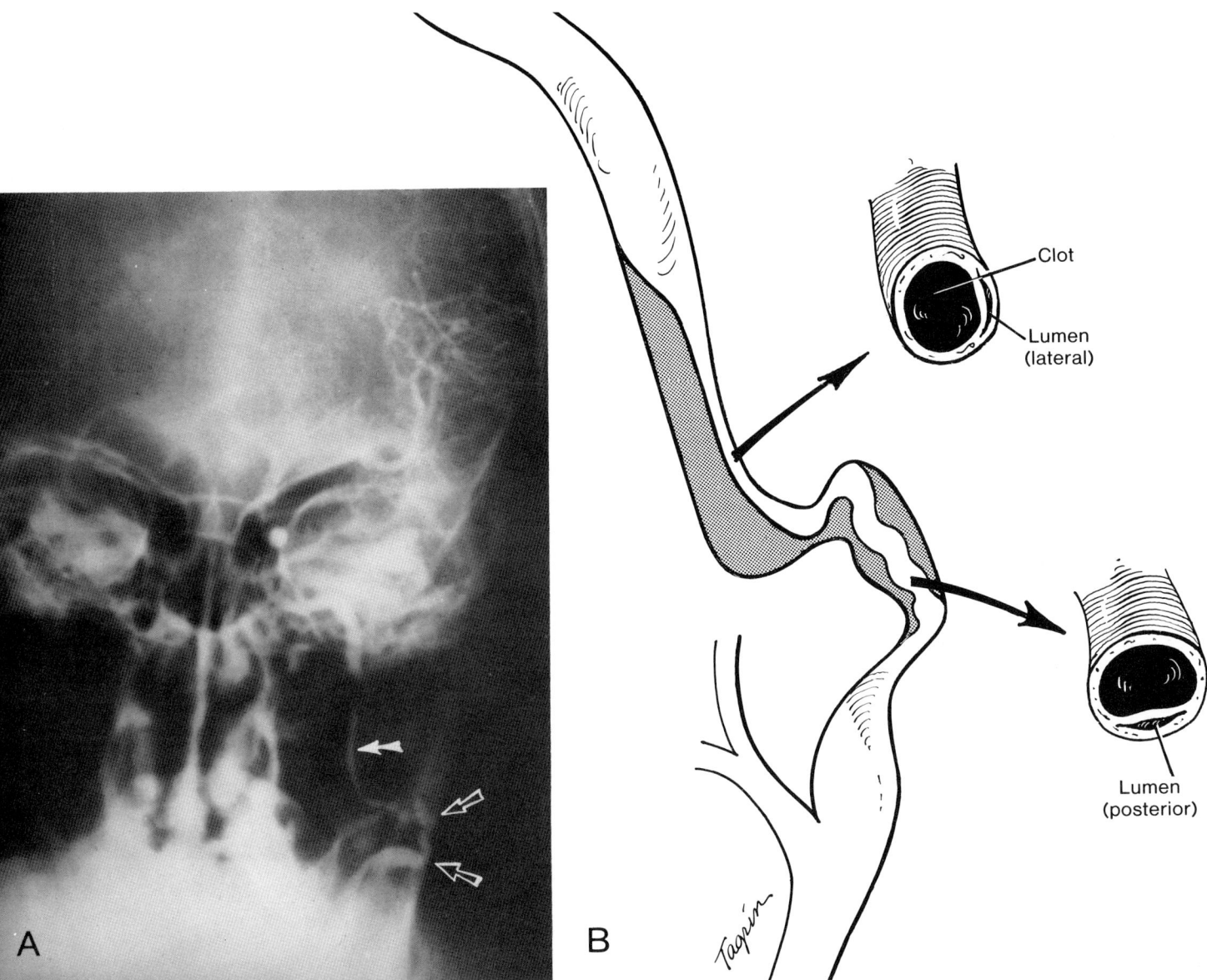

Figure 7.2. Typical angiographic finding (string sign), pathology, and surgical treatment. This 41-year-old man was well until 2 days before admission when he suddenly felt weak and noted transient blurring of vision in the left eye. He was well until the next day when he developed a right hemiparesis, which improved. On the morning of admission, he awakened with a right hemiplegia and aphasia. **A**, This anteroposterior angiogram led to the original designation of the string sign (44). The long area of narrowing in the internal carotid artery (*solid arrow*) is highly suggestive of the diagnosis. In this patient there was also an abnormally narrowed and kinked segment in the proximal internal carotid artery (*open arrows*). **B**, The nature of the pathology found at operation is shown. The internal carotid artery was dilated and had a bluish color throughout its length. **C**, Diagram of operative procedure performed. The proximal part of the dissection and the narrowed kinked segment were resected. A Fogarty catheter was inserted, inflated, and retracted, removing the dissection clot and elevated intima. A Dacron graft was sewn into place. (From Ojemann RG, Fisher CM, Rich JC: Spontaneous dissecting aneurysm of the internal carotid artery. *Stroke* 3:434–440, 1972, by permission of the American Heart Association, Inc.)

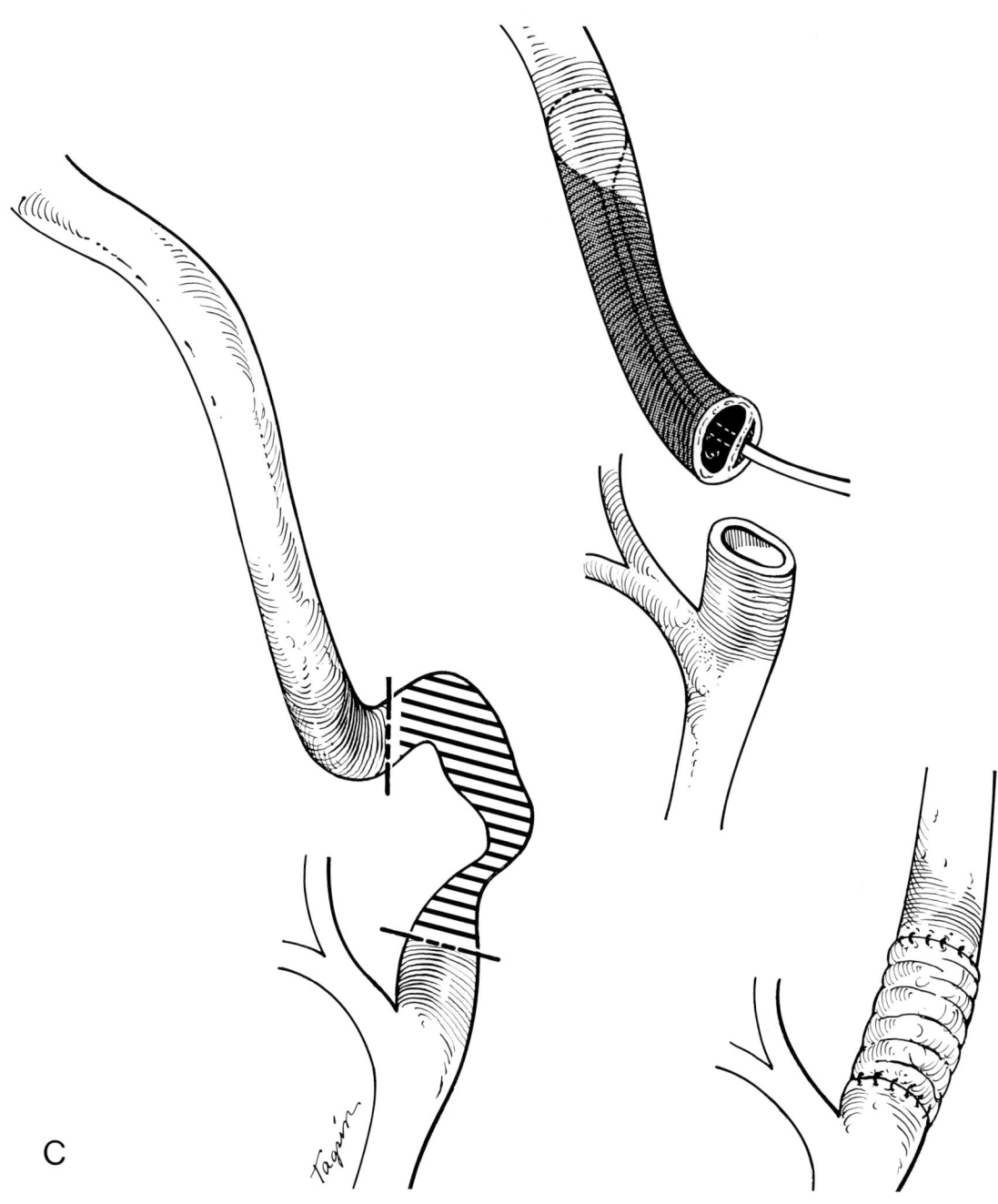

C

It differs markedly from the short usual stenotic lesion of atherosclerosis and rarely occurs with other types of occlusive cerebrovascular disease, such as fibromuscular dysplasia, arteritis, moya moya disease, and vasospasm (14). These long dissections often extend to the base of the skull where there is usually an abrupt change to a normal lumen (Figs. 7.2, 7.3A, 7.4A and B, and 7.6). This helps to differentiate the patient with the thin column of dye seen with a tight stenosis. Occasionally the dissection may involve only the petrous portion of the artery (Fig. 7.3B) (17).

Another distinctive angiographic finding in carotid dissection is a localized aneurysmal sac or outpouching on the cervical portion of the internal carotid artery between C2 and the base of the skull (Figs. 7.4 and 7.5B). The case reported by Hardin and Snodgrass (21) was proved at surgery and that of Bostrom and Liliequist (5) at autopsy. Similar pouches in the distal internal carotid artery have been described fre-

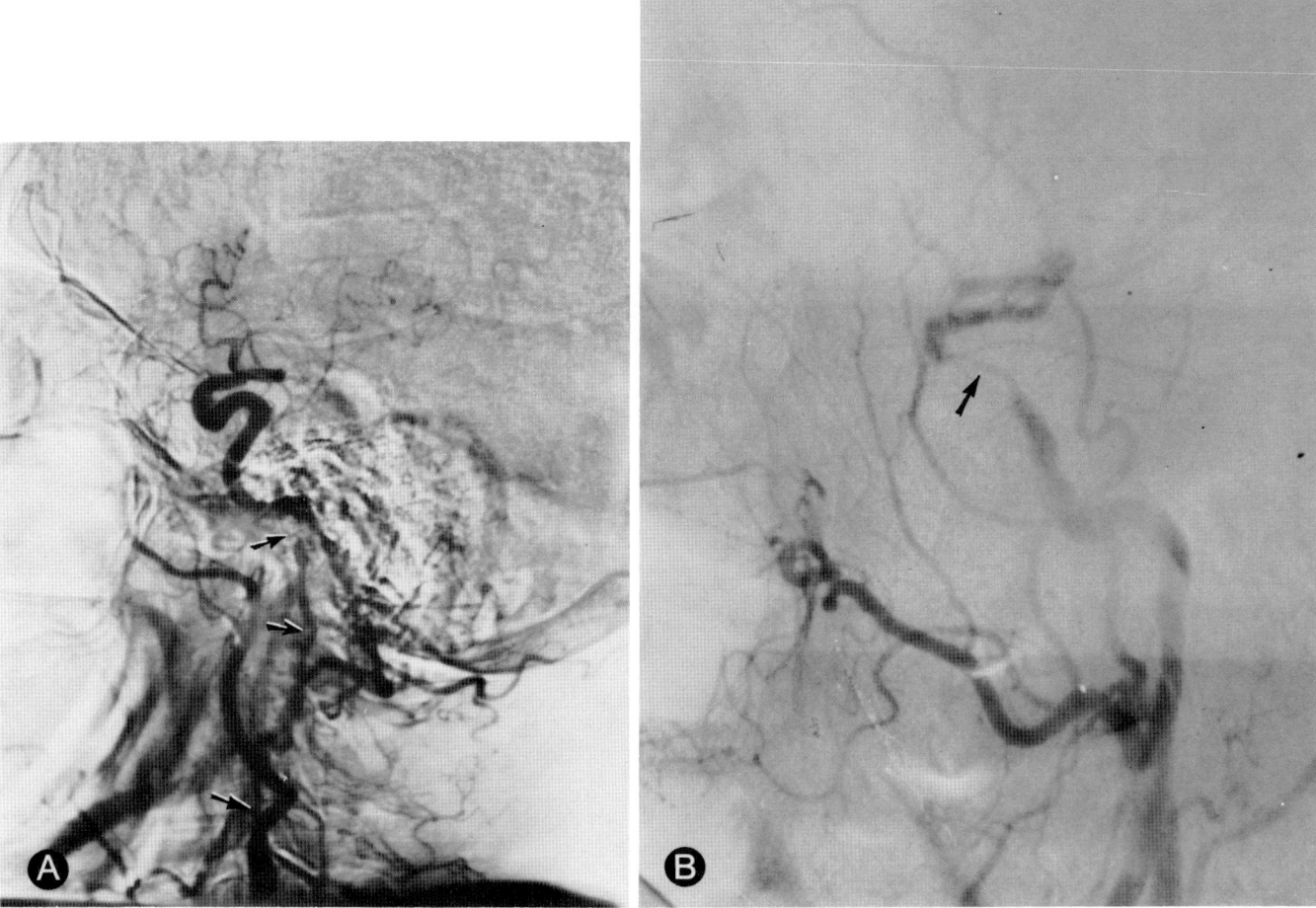

Figure 7.3. Other examples of the string sign. **A**, The internal carotid artery (*arrows*) is narrowed from its origin to the base of the skull where it abruptly widens to a normal lumen. **B**, Localized string sign in the petrous portion of the internal carotid artery (*arrow*). A presumptive diagnosis of dissection was made, since this artery subsequently developed a normal caliber.

quently in traumatic carotid dissection, and it is possible that this finding means the lesion was, in fact, traumatic in origin (52, 53).

Fisher et al, in their case 7, describe another angiographic finding in a patient who had serial angiograms (14). When first studied because of recent transient TIAs, there was a typical carotid string sign 7 cm long. The patient was treated with anticoagulation. Eight days later another angiogram revealed that the residual lumen had widened slightly. A third angiogram 7 months later showed full restoration of the lumen. At the site of the proximal end of the previous narrowing, there was an oval-shaped sac or pouch measuring 10 × 4 mm. In some patients the small sac in the midcervical portion of the internal carotid artery may be seen with narrowing of the artery (41).

In some cases, the internal carotid artery has become totally occluded. In these patients, the occlusion usually begins 2 cm or more distal to the origin of the internal carotid artery with a gradual taper of the vessel proximal to the occlusion. There is usually no evidence of atheroma in the cases studied at operation or autopsy. However, this type of carotid occlusion is not distinctive, since intracranial occlusion of the distal internal carotid artery from any cause may be associated with retrograde thrombus extending into the neck and giving the same angiographic picture.

Bilateral dissection may occur with symptoms related only to one side, and in a rare patient there may also be an associated vertebral dissection (22, 36, 41). In a small percentage of patients, changes of fibromuscular dysplasia have been noted (10, 12, 14, 16, 22, 34, 36, 41).

In a report of follow-up angiography after anticoagulation, antiplatelet drugs, or no treatment, in 23 dissections of the internal carotid artery that were

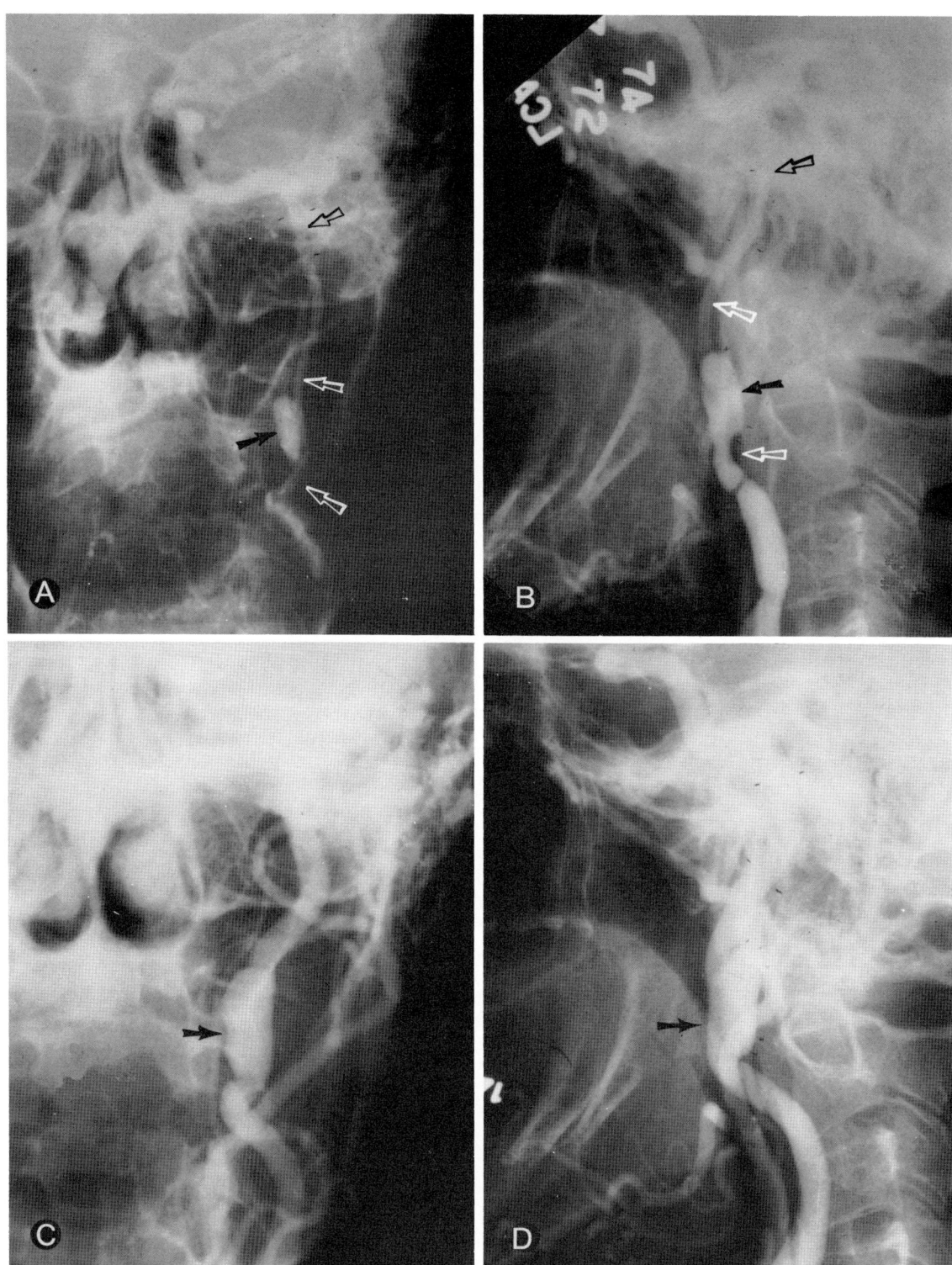

Figure 7.4. Typical angiographic finding (distal internal carotid pouch and narrowed artery). **A** and **B**, Anteroposterior and lateral carotid angiograms showing narrowing of the internal carotid artery (*open arrows*) and an aneurysmal sac (*closed arrows*) in the proximal part of the dissection. This study was done 8 days after starting heparin. On the original angiogram, the dissection was seen but not the sac. **C** and **D**, 7 months later the lumen has returned to normal size. The localized pouch persists (*closed arrows*). Comment: This 45-year-old man had a subarachnoid hemorrhage 6 years before admission. Angiography showed three aneurysms on the right side and two on the left. A right common carotid ligation had been done. One week before admission, while ill with the flu, he developed headache above the left eye and side of the head and pain on the side of the nose. Intermittent shining scintillations in the left visual field were noted. From the onset of the headache it was noted that the left upper lid drooped slightly and the left pupil was smaller. He could feel a pulsation deep in the left ear. On the day of admission there was a 15-minute episode of numbness of the right fingers, slurred speech, and sagging of the face. On examination, left oculosympathetic palsy was the only abnormal neurologic finding.

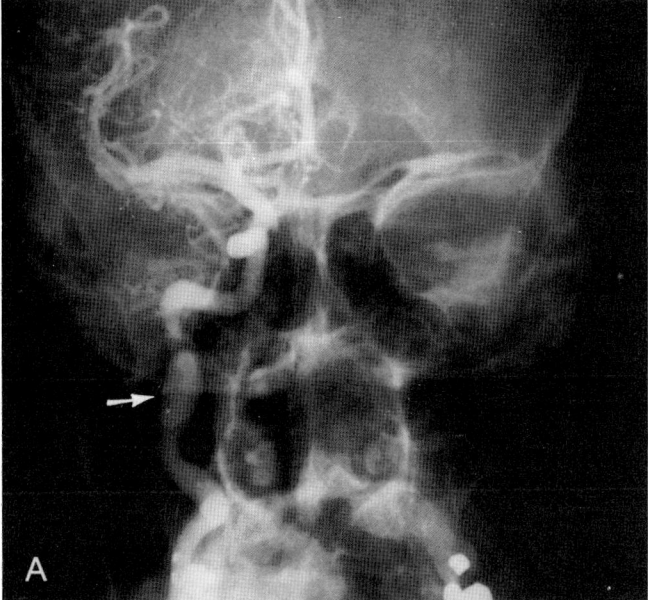
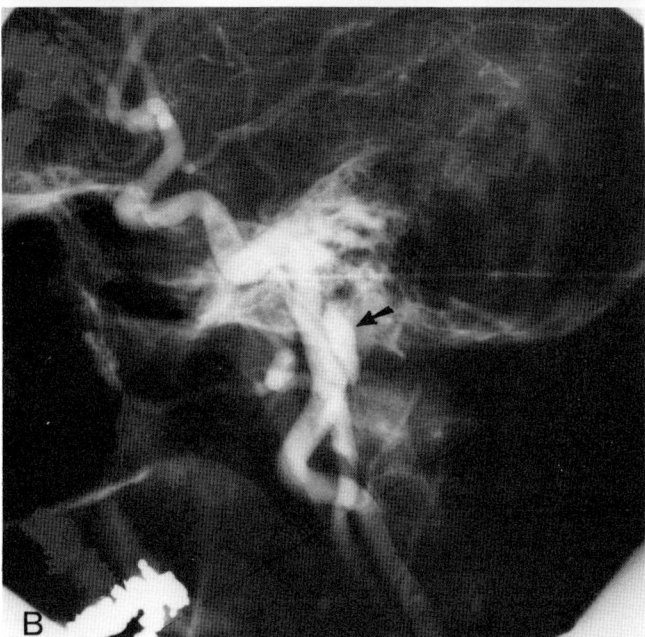

Figure 7.5. Typical angiographic finding (distal internal carotid pouch). **A** and **B**, Left carotid angiogram showing a sac protruding posteriorly (*closed arrows*) from the internal carotid artery between C1 and the base of the skull. The lumen of the internal carotid artery is slightly narrowed. Comment: A 46-year-old woman had an acute upper respiratory infection with a severe cough. She developed a superficial pain on the left side of the head with superimposed jabs of severe pain. The scalp was sensitive. At the same time, a pulsating sound was noted in the left ear. A deep left neck pain developed. She noted that the left eye was half closed due to a drooping of the upper lid. A left miosis was found. Angiography 1 year later showed the sac to be about the same size, but the arterial lumen no longer narrowed. The bruit disappeared after 5 months. The head pain persisted intermittently. The neck pain subsided after 2 months but then recurred 8 months later. No symptoms have returned over a period of 28 months.

open the stenosis resolved in 12 arteries, was improved in eight, was unchanged in one, and occlusion had developed in two with no symptoms (41). In the same report there were 11 aneurysms: six diminished in size, two were not seen, and three were unchanged. Improvement at the time of follow-up angiography has also been seen by others (15, 34, 36). In a few patients with apparent total occlusion, the artery will be open on follow-up angiography.

Treatment

The initial treatment of most patients with internal carotid dissection should be anticoagulation to prevent embolization. Satisfactory recovery of several patients treated with heparin and then coumadin has been reported (14, 15, 22, 24, 34, 36, 37, 44). One patient was treated for 5 months with continuous intravenous heparin using an implantable infusion device (9). The ideal duration of heparinization has not been established. Probably heparin should be used for at least 2 weeks. Thereafter, coumadin seems to be effective in preventing recurrent symptoms. Coumadin should be used for at least 3 months. Angiography has documented the resolution of the lesion in several cases. Even if the angiogram still shows some narrowing of the lumen, treatment probably does not need to be continued beyond this point. Antiplatelet drugs have also been used with no recurrence of symptoms (41, 46).

If symptoms progress or recur in spite of medical treatment, surgical therapy should be considered. In addition, the patient who has an acute progression or fluctuating neurologic deficit and evidence of diminished flow probably is a candidate for direct carotid surgery. At operation, the diameter of the internal carotid artery is enlarged and the vessel has a bluish appearance. This finding is characteristic for a dissection.

Surgical treatments that have been used for this problem include endarterectomy, resection and insertion of a graft, use of a balloon catheter, carotid ligation, and superficial temporal artery-middle cerebral artery bypass graft. In three cases, the dissected area was resected and a vein graft inserted (12). Osteotomy of the mandible has been used to aid this exposure, but this is probably not necessary (2, 21, 55). Removal of the dissected intima and subintimal thrombus has also been done by arteriotomy and primary closure without a patch (7, 49). Postoperative angiography was reported to show good restoration of flow. In some patients the vessel wall may be thin and difficult to suture.

The use of a balloon catheter to remove the dissected intima has been described in one case (Fig. 7.2C) (44). A second patient who presented with a fluctuating neurologic deficit was treated in a similar manner (Fig. 7.6A–D). In two other cases this technique was reported (12). In one, the postoperative

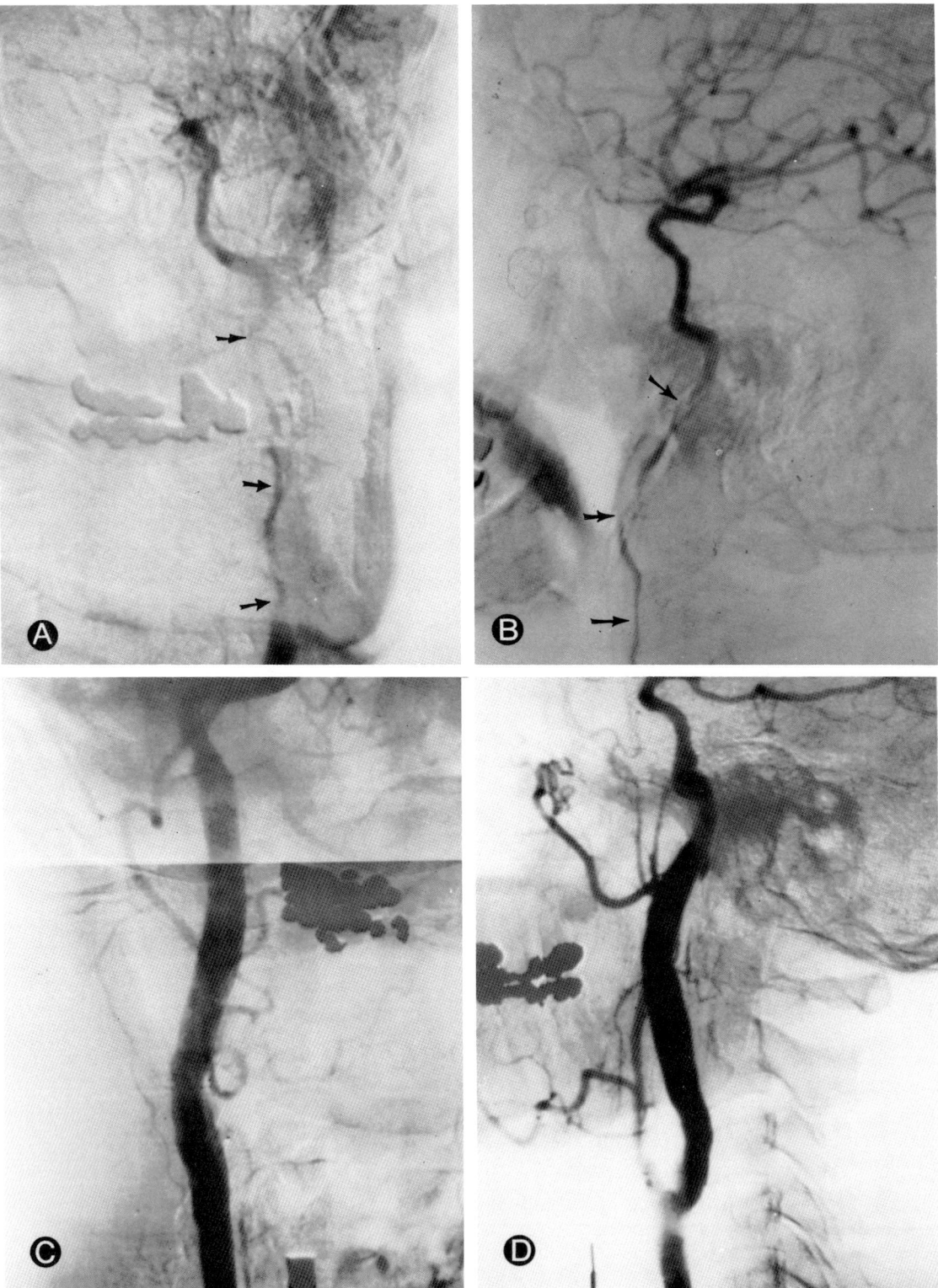

Figure 7.6. Acute neurologic syndrome with dissection of internal carotid artery: surgical treatment. This 45-year-old woman presented with a fluctuating neurologic deficit. Transient neurologic disability occurred in spite of heparin. Surgery was performed immediately. Full recovery occurred. **A** and **B**, Anteroposterior and lateral carotid angiograms showing string sign in internal carotid artery (*arrows*). At operation the internal carotid artery was enlarged and the wall had a typical bluish appearance. An arteriotomy was made in the proximal internal carotid artery and a Fogarty catheter inserted in the true lumen. The dissected intima and the clot were removed. There were no further neurologic symptoms after the operation. **C** and **D**, Postoperative angiograms showing restoration of an enlarged widely patent internal carotid artery lumen.

angiogram was normal, but in the other, a ragged appearance on the intraoperative angiogram and high stump pressure led to internal carotid artery ligation. In another patient from the same report, the carotid artery was ligated when the dissection could not be removed. No complications were noted.

Bypass surgery, with anastomosis of the superficial temporal artery to a middle cerebral artery branch, has been used in six patients with severely compromised cerebral circulation (40, 41), with encouraging results. It was noted on follow-up angiography 3–6 months later that all of these patients showed complete or partial resolution of the angiographic abnormality.

Long-term follow-up has shown resolution of headache in more than 95% of the patients, oculosympathetic paresis in 33%, and subjective bruits in 80% (41). Most patients make an excellent recovery and do not have recurrent symptoms. The persistence of an aneurysmal pouch does not usually seem to be associated with any long-term problems. However, in one patient neurologic symptoms developed related to a thrombus in an aneurysm and surgical excision was done (22). The authors had one patient with recurrent embolism from a distal pouch where occlusion of the pouch by a detachable balloon was done with maintenance of a normal internal carotid artery lumen. Spontaneous development of a total occlusion has been noted without symptoms, but in one report a complete occlusion was associated with a serious neurologic deficit (4).

SPONTANEOUS DISSECTION OF INTRACRANIAL ARTERIES

Pathogenesis

Dissection has been reported to involve all major intracranial arteries. This problem has been summarized in 1971 (29, 50), in 1977 (56), in 1979 (1), and in 1983 (22).

The middle cerebral artery has been the most frequently reported site of intracranial involvement (29, 50, 56). The internal carotid and basilar arteries are also common sites, and there are reports of involvement of the vertebral, posterior cerebral, and anterior cerebral arteries (1).

Examination of the wall of the artery shows the dissection with associated thrombus to be either circumferential or eccentric. It is usually between the intima and media, but may be located within either of these layers (1, 25, 56).

Discussion of the pathogenesis includes consideration of trauma, congenital medial defects, atherosclerotic changes in the wall, fibromuscular dysplasia, arteritis, infection, and homocystinuria (1, 17, 25, 28, 56). Cystic medial necrosis has rarely been found (1). The possible association with migraine has been raised (1, 50). Usually, a definite cause cannot be conclusively demonstrated. In the pathologic examination of a case of middle cerebral dissection, there was splitting, fraying, disintegration, and irregular thickening of the elastic lamina, but similar, although less severe, changes were seen in two other patients without dissection (8). In the detailed pathologic examination of a case of middle cerebral dissection, no specific cause could be found (25).

Trauma as a possible cause of dissection of intracranial vessels is discussed in the next section. As with internal carotid dissection, the possible relationship with minor trauma is uncertain.

Clinical Manifestations, Diagnosis, and Treatment

The onset of symptoms is most common in young adults (1, 29, 50). The age of reported patients has ranged from 6 months to 69 years (1). The majority of patients were between 15–35 (29). Several reports of spontaneous middle cerebral dissection have included a number of patients younger than 20 years of age (8, 14, 25, 28). No sex predominance has been noted.

Unusually frequent and severe headache is a prominent symptom (51). A detailed analysis of reports of intracranial dissection containing sufficient data revealed that 19 of 20 patients had headache, often severe, with localization to the side of the involved artery in supratentorial dissections (56).

The onset of neurologic symptoms is variable, but there is often an acute event with sudden loss of consciousness, a severe neurologic deficit due to infarction, or subarachnoid hemorrhage (29, 56). One patient with a dissection of the basilar artery had symptoms from compression of the pyramidal tracts and chronic subarachnoid hemorrhage before developing severe infarction (1). In another patient, an intracerebral hematoma followed rupture of the vessel, and three other reports of such cases have been noted (29).

Angiography usually shows either a narrowed or occluded artery (1). The unusual segmental narrowing (string sign) has been seen in the vertebral, middle, and posterior cerebral arteries (14, 25, 29). A double lumen has been demonstrated (26).

It is clear that intracranial dissection is a very serious condition, frequently leading to severe stroke and death (20). A likely reason for this is that the dissection involves a long segment of a major intracranial artery causing impairment of distal flow and occlusion of perforating arteries. The place of anticoagulant therapy has not been established (22).

TRAUMATIC DISSECTION OF INTERNAL CAROTID ARTERY

Pathogenesis

Dissection of the internal carotid artery and its branches can occur following nonpenetrating injury to the head and neck, direct injury to the artery, and carotid angiography (22, 30, 52, 53, 57). Nonpenetrating injury to the head and neck may cause an intimal tear in the cervical carotid vessels. The tear may lead to the development of a localized dissection or aneurysmal outpouching (8, 21). Thrombus may be the source of cerebral emboli, and occlusion of the artery may develop (8). The most likely mechanism for production of this tear is the sudden severe stretch of the internal carotid artery over the upper cervical spine when the neck is hyperextended and laterally flexed to the opposite side (8, 21, 57). It may also be caused by a direct blow to the artery (3) and by direct compression between the angle of the mandible and upper cervical vertebrae (57).

The cases of intracranial dissection where trauma has been suggested have followed closed head injury without fracture (25). Surgical trauma to the internal carotid artery during tonsillectomy and to the middle cerebral artery after ligation of an aneurysm have also been reported as causes of dissection (52, 53).

Clinical Manifestations and Diagnosis

Traumatic dissection can produce the same picture as spontaneous dissection. The patient may present with a head injury with the initial diagnosis of cerebral concussion or contusion.

The interval between the trauma and onset of symptoms is variable. In the majority of patients with internal carotid artery dissection, symptoms occur

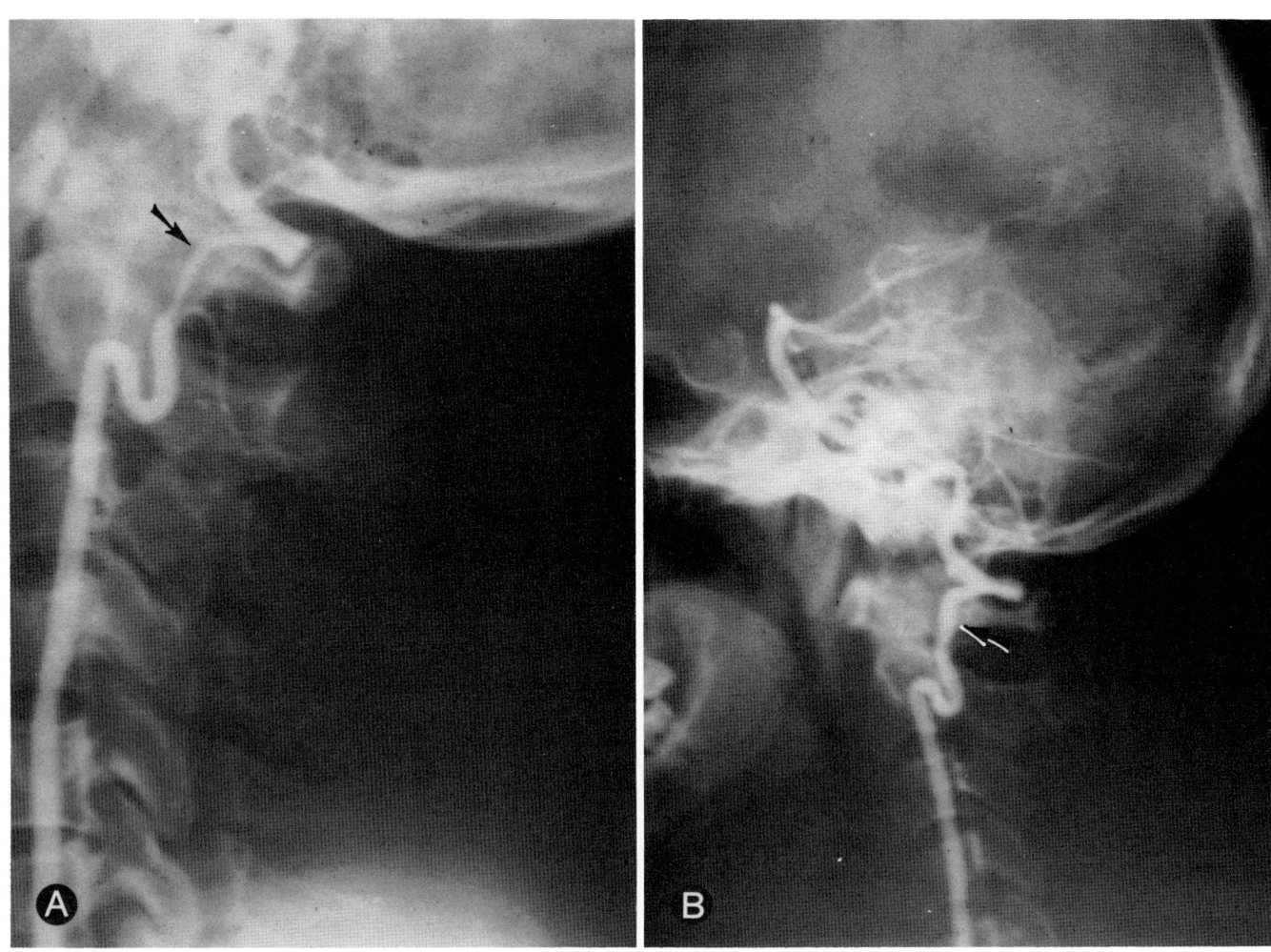

Figure 7.7. Dissection of the vertebral artery. **A**, Lateral vertebral angiogram shows dissection at the C1 level. **B**, Lateral vertebral angiogram taken 3 weeks later. A normal lumen is restored. No specific treatment had been given. Comment: This 35-year-old man was vigorously spanking his son when he felt something snap on the right side of the upper neck posteriorly. He immediately felt weak and lost his equilibrium. There was dysarthria, burning of the eyes, headache extending from the back of the head forward to behind the eye, numbness of both upper extremities and the right leg, dysphagia, and incoordination of the right extremities. He was unable to sit because of the balance problem. Examination showed a right lateral medullary syndrome. The signs and symptoms cleared over 2 weeks.

within 24 hours of the trauma (3). However, long, symptom-free intervals may occur. In a report of six patients, three developed rapid deterioration in neurologic status within 3 hours, one had the onset of symptoms in 8 days, another developed a TIA 2 weeks after an accident, and the last patient was well until 1 year after recovery from a serious head injury when he developed a stroke due to an embolus from the area of dissection and aneurysmal formation (52). In another report of six patients, four developed symptoms immediately but in two the onset was 2–3 months after the trauma (57).

Symptoms in patients with intracranial dissection may be acute or delayed (1). In a review of the reported cases of posttraumatic middle cerebral occlusion, including those where dissection had been demonstrated at autopsy, the interval between trauma and onset of symptoms varied from a few hours to several days (26).

When a patient with a history of trauma develops neurologic symptoms and the CT scan does not clarify the causes, angiography is needed to help establish a diagnosis. It is also imperative that adequate views of both the head and neck be obtained. This is particularly true in the patient with a major focal deficit and normal CT scan.

When nonpenetrating trauma to the head and neck causes arterial injury, the most common angiographic finding is internal carotid occlusion 1–3 cm above the bifurcation (53). However, in some patients an intimal tear leads to development of a dissection. The angiographic abnormalities are the same as described for spontaneous dissection: localized narrowing of the upper cervical carotid artery or aneurysmal outpouching between C2 and the base of the skull (52, 57). Intracranial emboli have been demonstrated in several patients.

Treatment

The natural history of the illness is unknown. However, the results in one report suggest that the problem may be, like spontaneous dissection, a more benign process than originally thought (52). All six patients in that report were treated medically and had an uncomplicated course. Anticoagulation was used when emboli were demonstrated, and there was no complication from this therapy. However, caution and careful judgment must be exercised in anticoagulating patients with significant head injury. Follow-up angiograms were done in four of the six patients and showed that none of the dissections progressed to complete occlusion; one had disappeared, in three the ipsilateral false aneurysm had enlarged, and in three an aneurysmal outpouching in the opposite, asymptomatic, internal carotid artery was seen that had not been demonstrated on the initial angiographic study. These aneurysmal sacs may remain unchanged for several years, or they may spontaneously thrombose (52, 53). In both circumstances, the patient has usually remained asymptomatic.

VERTEBRAL ARTERY DISSECTION

Dissection of the vertebral artery may occur alone or in combination with internal carotid artery dissection (4, 14, 22, 27, 41, 47). It has been reported as a spontaneous event (27, 41) or after apparent trauma (47). Probably the most common cause of vertebral dissection is chiropractic manipulation (hyperextension) of the neck (11, 23, 35, 38, 39, 42, 48). In a review of this subject, Heros found close to 50 cases of such an occurrence (23). The usual manifestation is vertebrobasilar ischemia in the form of acute stroke, frequently involving the lateral medullary region (Wallenberg's syndrome) or delayed ischemic events. Sometimes cerebellar infarction requiring prompt surgical decompression has resulted. The patient documented in Figure 7.7 recovered with no specific treatment, but anticoagulant therapy would seem to be the best recommendation based on reports in the literature and the experience with internal carotid artery dissection (22).

REFERENCES

1. Alexander CB, Burger PC, Goree JA: Dissecting aneurysms of the basilar artery in two patients. *Stroke* 10:294–298, 1979.
2. Balagura S, Carter JB, Gossett DL: Surgical approach to the high subcranial internal carotid artery. *Neurosurgery* 16:402–405, 1985.
3. Bergquist BJ, Boone SC, Whaley RA: Traumatic dissection of the internal carotid artery treated by ECIC anastomosis. *Stroke* 12:73–76, 1981.
4. Bladin PF: Dissecting aneurysm of carotid and vertebral arteries. *Vasc Surg* 8:203–223, 1974.
5. Bostrom K, Liliequist B: Primary dissecting aneurysm of the extracranial part of the internal carotid and vertebral arteries. *Neurology* 17:179–186, 1967.
6. Brown OL, Armitage JL: Spontaneous dissecting aneurysms of the cervical internal carotid artery: Two case reports and a survey of the literature. *AJR* 118:648–653, 1973.
7. Burklund CW: Spontaneous dissecting aneurysm of the cervical carotid artery: A report of surgical treatment in two patients. *Johns Hopkins Med J* 126:154–159, 1970.
8. Chang V, Rewcastle NB, Harwood-Nash DCF, Norman MD: Bilateral dissecting aneurysms of the intracranial internal carotid arteries in an 8-year-old boy. *Neurology* 25:573–579, 1975.
9. Chapleau CE, Robertson JT: Spontaneous cervical carotid artery dissection: Outpatient treatment with continuous heparin infusion using a totally implantable infusion device. *Neurosurgery* 8:83–87, 1981.
10. Collins GJ, Rich NM, Clagett GP, Speban MJ, Salander JM: Fibromuscular dysplasia of the internal carotid artery. *Ann Surg* 194:89–96, 1981.
11. Easton JD, Sherman DG: Cervical manipulation and stroke. *Stroke* 8:594–597, 1977.
12. Ehrenfeld WK, Wylie EJ: Spontaneous dissection of the internal carotid artery. *Arch Surg* 111:1294–1301, 1976.
13. Fisher CM: The headache and pain of spontaneous carotid dissection. *Headache* 22:60–65, 1985.
14. Fisher CM, Ojemann RG, Roberson GH: Spontaneous dissection of cervico-cerebral arteries. *Can J Neurol Sci* 5:9–19, 1978.

15. Friedman WA, Day AL, Quisling RG, Sypert GW, Rhoton AL Jr: Cervical carotid dissecting aneurysms. Neurosurgery 7:207–214, 1980.
16. Garcia-Merino JA, Gutierrez JA, Lopez-Lozano JJ, Marquez M, Lopez F, Liano H: Double lumen dissecting aneurysms of the internal carotid artery in fibromuscular dysplasia: Case report. Stroke 14:815–818, 1983.
17. Giedki H, Kriebel J, Sindermann F: Dissecting aneurysm of the petrous portion of the internal carotid artery. Case report and review of previous cases. Neuroradiology 10:121–124, 1975.
18. Goldberg HI, Grossman RI, Gomori JM, Ashbury AK, Bilaniuk LT, Zimmerman RA: Cervical internal carotid artery dissecting hemorrhage: Diagnosis using MRI. Radiology 138:157–161, 1986.
19. Greiner AL: Spontaneous dissecting aneurysms of the cervical internal carotid artery. Stroke 7:6, 1976.
20. Grosman H, Fornasier VL, Bonder D, Livingston KE, Platts ME: Dissecting aneurysm of the cerebral arteries. J Neurosurg 53:693–697, 1980.
21. Hardin CA, Snodgrass RG: Dissecting aneurysm of internal carotid artery treated by fenestration and graft. Surgery 55:207–209, 1964.
22. Hart RG, Easton JD: Dissections of cervical and cerebral arteries. Neurol Clin 1:155–182, 1983.
23. Heros RC: Cerebellar infarction resulting from traumatic occlusion of a vertebral artery. Case report. J Neurosurg 51:111–113, 1979.
24. Heros RC, Davis KR: Complex lesions of the cervical carotid artery. In Smith RR (ed): Stroke and the Extracranial Vessels. New York, Raven Press, 1984, pp 333–344.
25. Hochberg FH, Bean CS, Fisher CM, Roberson GH: Stroke in a 16-year-old girl secondary to terminal carotid dissection. Neurology 25:725–729, 1975.
26. Hollin SA, Sukoff MH, Silverstein A, Gross SW: Post-traumatic middle cerebral artery occlusion. J Neurosurg 25:526–535, 1966.
27. Hugeholtz H, Pokrupa R, Montpetit VJA, Nelson R, Richard MT: Spontaneous dissecting aneurysm of the extracranial vertebral artery. Neurosurgery 10:96–100, 1982.
28. Johnson AC, Graves VB, Pfaff JP Jr: Dissecting aneurysm of intracranial arteries. Surg Neurol 7:49–51, 1977.
29. Kunze S, Schiefer W: Angiographic demonstration of a dissecting aneurysm of the middle cerebral artery. Neuroradiology 2:201–206, 1971.
30. Lai MD, Hoffman HB, Adamkiewicz JJ: Dissecting aneurysm of internal carotid artery after non-penetrating neck injury. Case report. Acta Radiol 5:290–295, 1966.
31. Liliequist B: The roentgenologic appearance of spontaneous dissecting aneurysm of the cervical internal carotid artery: Report of a case. Vasc Surg 2:223–226, 1968.
32. Lloyd J, Bahnson HT: Bilateral dissecting aneurysms of the internal carotid arteries. Am J Surg 122:549–551, 1971.
33. Lubbers DJ, Tomsick TA: CT demonstration of spontaneous internal carotid artery dissection. J Neurosurg 63:792–793, 1985.
34. Luken MG, Ascherl GF Jr, Correll JW, Hilal SK: Spontaneous dissecting aneurysms of the extracranial internal carotid artery. Clin Neurosurg 26:353–375, 1979.
35. Lyness SS, Wagman AD: Neurological deficit following cervical manipulation. Surg Neurol 2:121–124, 1974.
36. Mas JL, Goeau C, Bousser MG, Chivas J, Verret JM, Touboul PJ: Spontaneous dissecting aneurysms of the internal carotid and vertebral arteries—two case reports. Stroke 16:125–129, 1985.
37. McNeill DH Jr, Dreisbach J, Marsden RJ: Spontaneous dissection of the internal carotid artery. Arch Neurol 37:54–55, 1980.
38. Mehalic T, Farhat SM: Vertebral artery injury from chiropractic manipulation of the neck. Surg Neurol 2:125–129, 1974.
39. Miller RG, Burton R: Stroke following chiropractic manipulation of the spine. JAMA 229:189–190, 1974.
40. Mokri B, Sundt TM Jr, Houser OW: Spontaneous internal carotid dissection, hemicrania and Horner's syndrome. Arch Neurol 36:677–680, 1979.
41. Mokri B, Sundt TM Jr, Houser W, Piepgras DG: Spontaneous dissection of the cervical internal carotid artery. Ann Neurol 19:126–138, 1986.
42. Mueller S, Sahs AL: Brain stem dysfunction related to cervical manipulation. Report of three cases. Neurology 26:547–550, 1976.
43. New PFJ, Momose KJ: Traumatic dissection of the internal carotid artery of the atlantoxial level, secondary to non-penetrating injury. Radiology 93:41–49, 1969.
44. Ojemann RG, Fisher CM, Rich JC: Spontaneous dissecting aneurysm of internal carotid artery. Stroke 3:434–440, 1972.
45. Pilz P, Hartjes HJ: Fibromuscular dysplasia and multiple dissecting aneurysms of intracranial arteries. A further cause of moyamoya syndrome. Stroke 7:393–398, 1976.
46. Pozzati E, Gaist G, Poppi M: Resolution of occlusion in spontaneously dissected carotid arteries. J Neurosurg 56:857–860, 1982.
47. Ringel SP, Harrison SH, Norenberg MD Austin JH: Fibromuscular dysplasia: Multiple "spontaneous" dissecting aneurysms of the major cervical arteries. Ann Neurol 1:301–304, 1977.
48. Robertson JT: Neck manipulation as a cause of stroke. Stroke 12:1, 1981.
49. Roome NS Jr, Aberfeld DC: Spontaneous dissecting aneurysm of the internal carotid artery. Arch Neurol 34;251–252, 1977.
50. Sato O, Bascom JF, Logothetis J: Intracranial dissecting aneurysm. Case report. J Neurosurg 35:483–487, 1971.
51. Scott GE, Neubuerger KT, Denst J: Dissecting aneurysms of intracranial arteries. Neurology 10:22–27, 1960.
52. Stringer WL, Kelly DL: Traumatic dissection of the extracranial internal carotid artery. Neurosurgery 6:123–130, 1980.
53. Sullivan HG, Vines FS, Becker DP: Sequelae of indirect internal carotid injury. Radiology 109:91–98, 1973.
54. Thapedia IM, Ashenhurst EM, Rozdilsky B: Spontaneous dissecting aneurysm of the internal carotid artery in the neck: report of a case and review of the literature. Arch neurol 23:549–554, 1970.
55. Wyle EF, Ehrenfeld WK: Extracranial Occlusive Cerebrovascular Disease. Philadelphia, WB Saunders, 1970, pp 48, 192.
56. Yonas H, Agamanolis D, Takaoka Y, White RJ: Dissecting intracranial aneurysms. Surg Neurol 8:407–415, 1977.
57. Zelenock GB, Kazmers A, Whitehouse WM Jr, Graham LM, Erlandson EE, Cronenwett JI, Lindenauer SM, Stanley JC: Extracranial internal carotid artery dissections: Noniatrogenic traumatic lesions. Arch Surg 177:425–432, 1982.

8
Embolism

GENERAL FEATURES OF ETIOLOGY, PRESENTATION, AND DIAGNOSIS

The clinical presentation of a patient with embolic occlusion in the cerebral circulation is usually the abrupt onset of a neurologic deficit, most commonly occurring during waking hours without headache or preceding transient ischemic attacks (TIAs). The deficit is usually maximal at onset without further progression or fluctuation. The usual source of the embolus is a thrombus within the heart (1, 2). The most common type of heart disease to be associated with embolism is chronic atrial fibrillation due to atherosclerosis, rheumatic heart disease, or other less common diseases. The patient with intermittent atrial fibrillation is at particularly high risk for embolism. The source of the embolus is usually a thrombus deposited within the atrial appendage. The second most frequent source of cerebral emboli is a mural thrombus deposited on the damaged endocardium overlying an area of myocardial infarction. Emboli can also arise from atrial thrombosis associated with severe mitral stenosis without atrial fibrillation. The problem can also develop as a complication of cardiac surgery.

Usually, the embolus from the heart is small enough so that it does not block a major extracranial artery but becomes arrested at an intracranial bifurcation. On occasion, however, the internal carotid artery or vertebral artery may be blocked. If the embolus does not promptly break up or collateral circulation is inadequate, ishemic infarction occurs. A hemorrhagic infarction usually means an embolic cause, but nonhemorrhagic infarction can also occur. Any region of the brain may be affected, but the territory of the middle cerebral artery is most frequently involved.

Emboli from a thrombus that has formed on an ulcerated or stenotic atheromatous plaque of the aorta or carotid artery can cause cerebral symptoms as noted in Chapter 1. In many patients these fragments are not large enough to occlude major arteries and, therefore, do not have surgical implications. However, a large enough thrombus can form and then be dislodged from the common carotid artery bifurcation in the neck to result in occlusion of the main trunk of the middle cerebral artery. This occurs almost exclusively in patients with very severe stenosis or complete occlusion of the internal carotid artery with formation of a fresh clot that then propagates or dislodges. Some of these patients have preceding TIAs or are already evolving a cerebral infarct, and the final embolic occlusion of the middle cerebral artery is the last event on a course of stepwise deterioration.

When the embolus enters the vertebral artery, it most often goes into one of the posterior cerebral arteries, causing a homonymous hemianopia and, particularly when the left side is involved, a state frequently described as "confusion" by the patient. When the patient is carefully examined, it is usually found that this "confusion" is caused by a decrease in recent memory with consequent disorientation. This syndrome is probably due to damage to the medial aspect of the temporal lobe. In some instances, the embolus can lodge either transiently or permanently in the distal vertebral artery, resulting in occlusion of the origin of the posterior inferior cerebellar artery with a resulting lateral medullary (Wallenberg) infarction or cerebellar infarction. As discussed in Chapter 9, the latter has very significant surgical implications (4, 8). In one report, 22% of cerebellar infarctions were reported to be due to emboli (8).

The diagnosis is usually based on the history. When a large embolus blocks the internal carotid artery or the stem of the middle cerebral artery, a severe neurologic deficit is usually produced; when this is suspected, emergency angiography may be indicated. The problems in evaluating and treating these patients are difficult. Since the occlusion is sudden, there is little or no chance for collateral circulation to develop to help protect the brain. Therefore, diagnosis must be made and treatment started promptly. In some patients, the embolus will break up and spontaneous recovery will follow. The patient with embolus is at risk for recurrent embolism. Therefore, anticoagulant therapy must be considered. The advisability of delaying anticoagulation for several days to avoid the risk of hemorrhage into an area of infarction has been discussed (1). If the computed tomography (CT) scan does not show hemorrhage into the infarct, heparin may be started and then followed in several days by coumadin. Alternatively, coumadin may be started from the beginning, since this will not result in full anticoagulation for several days at a time when the risk of hemorrhagic infarction may be less. The question of whether to start the patient on anticoagulants also has to be influenced by whether an intracranial surgical procedure, such as middle cerebral artery embolectomy, is contemplated. If the latter is the case, anticoagulation may need to be deferred for several days. It should be pointed out that when the embolic event occurs in the setting of bacterial endocarditis, most clinicians advise against anticoagulation because of the high frequency of hemorrhagic complications associated with this condition.

Of the nonsurgical measures that can be considered to improve circulation to marginally perfused areas of the brain, the most promising is hemodilution, particularly isovolemic hemodilution (see Chapter 2). This can be achieved by repeated phlebotomy with colloid replacement to bring the hematocrit down to what appears to be the ideal level of 30–35% (6).

CAROTID ARTERY EMBOLUS

The clinical features are the same as those described previously for carotid occlusive disease. Usually the onset of the stroke is sudden, without warning, and with the almost immediate development of severe hemiplegia. When the embolus is large enough to block the internal carotid artery, it will usually lodge at the common carotid artery bifurcation and obstruct both the external and internal carotid arteries (Fig. 8.1). Therefore, loss of superficial temporal pulse in the clinical setting described should make the physician suspicious of an embolus. This is particularly true if there is a history of heart disease or atrial fibrillation. In this setting, immediate exploration of the common carotid artery bifurcation should be considered.

If the diagnosis is suspected but the characteristic clinical syndrome is not present, angiography is done. At the same time, hemodilution is started and blood pressure increased to promote maximum collateral circulation. The guidelines for surgical treatment are similar to those described for treating acute carotid occlusion when a thrombus forms on an atheromatous plaque (Chapter 1.) The surgical exposure is the same as outlined for carotid endarterectomy (Chapter 2).

MIDDLE CEREBRAL ARTERY EMBOLUS

Most intracranial emboli lodge in distal arterial branches, but occasionally the proximal middle cerebral artery may be occluded by an embolus. The technical feasibility of middle cerebral artery embolectomy has been clearly established, and satisfactory patency rates may be obtained (3, 5). Unfortunately, the process of cerebral infarction in

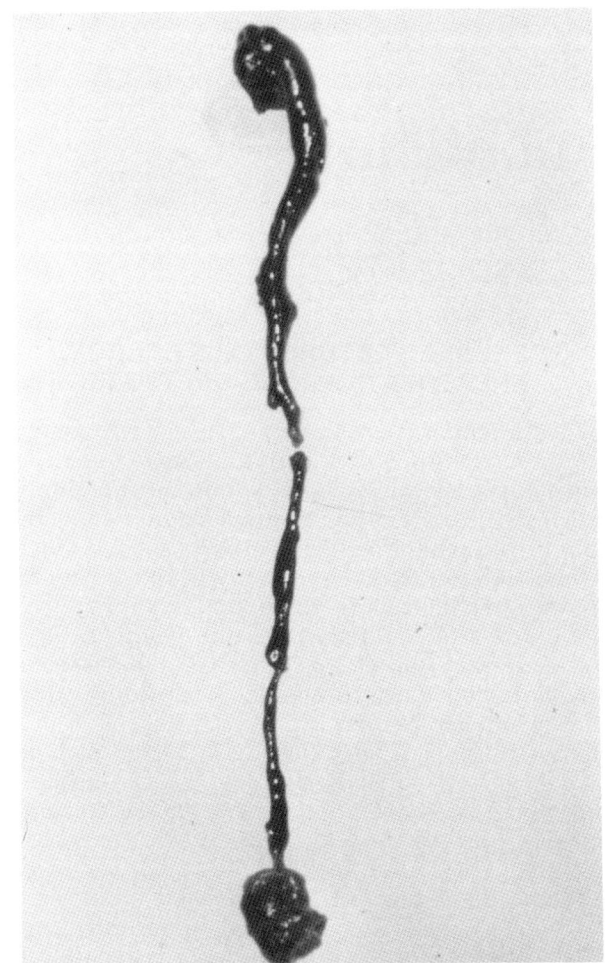

Figure 8.1. Occlusion of common carotid bifurcation by embolus from the heart. This 41-year-old man with a history of a myocardial infarction had the sudden onset of hemiplegia. Examination also disclosed an absent superficial temporal pulse. Immediate operation removed an organized thrombus at the carotid bifurcation (at bottom of picture) and a fresh thrombus in the internal carotid artery. Good backflow followed. The patient recovered with a moderate residual neurologic deficit.

most cases proceeds to irreversibility before the surgeon can restore blood flow. Early diagnosis and effective drug therapy to prolong the period of reversibility will be needed to make this procedure widely useful.

At the present time, only an occasional patient will be a candidate for this procedure. The most common presentation is a young patient, already in the hospital for evaluation of a cardiac problem, with sudden onset of hemiplegia that is promptly diagnosed. An alternative setting is that of a patient who is undergoing cerebral angiography for any reason and who suddenly develops a neurological deficit with subsequent angiographic demonstration of an occlusion of the middle cerebral artery. In these patients, immediate treatment with colloid infusions to expand the intravascular volume, moderate hypertension, and, if their sensorium is impaired, immediate intubation and barbiturate treatment are indicated to try to protect the brain until surgical revascularization can be achieved. Emergency angiography is necessary in those patients in whom the diagnosis has been made strictly on the clinical basis. Surgery can be proposed reasonably only where the obstruction is localized to the M1 segment and proximal middle cerebral artery divisions. The ideal candidates are those with good distal collateral filling of the middle cerebral artery territory (5).

A frontotemporal craniotomy should be performed rapidly. If the cortex shows marked pallor, swelling, and petechial hemorrhages, irreversible infarction has occurred and embolectomy will not be helpful and could be harmful. If the brain appears less damaged, one should rapidly split the sylvian fissure and expose the middle cerebral artery trunk in its entirety. Careful inspection of the middle cerebral artery and its bifurcation will identify the site of the embolus, which will appear dark purple. Considerable care should be taken not to dislodge the embolus at this stage. Temporary clips are placed first distal then proximal to the occlusion and microclips are placed at the origin of the largest perforating vessels. An arteriotomy is made directly over the embolus (Fig. 8.2). Ordinarily, this can be very short, about 2 mm on the M1 segment. Separate arteriotomies may be necessary on the main middle cerebral artery divisions if the embolus extends into these divisions and cannot be removed completely through the arteriotomy on the main trunk. The embolus is removed with forceps or a fine sucker. At this point usually brisk bleeding will be encountered from perforating vessels. Unless at least the largest of these have been temporarily occluded, this backbleeding can be bothersome enough to make it very difficult to close the arteriotomy properly. In most cases, no effort should be made to remove atheroma from the middle cere-

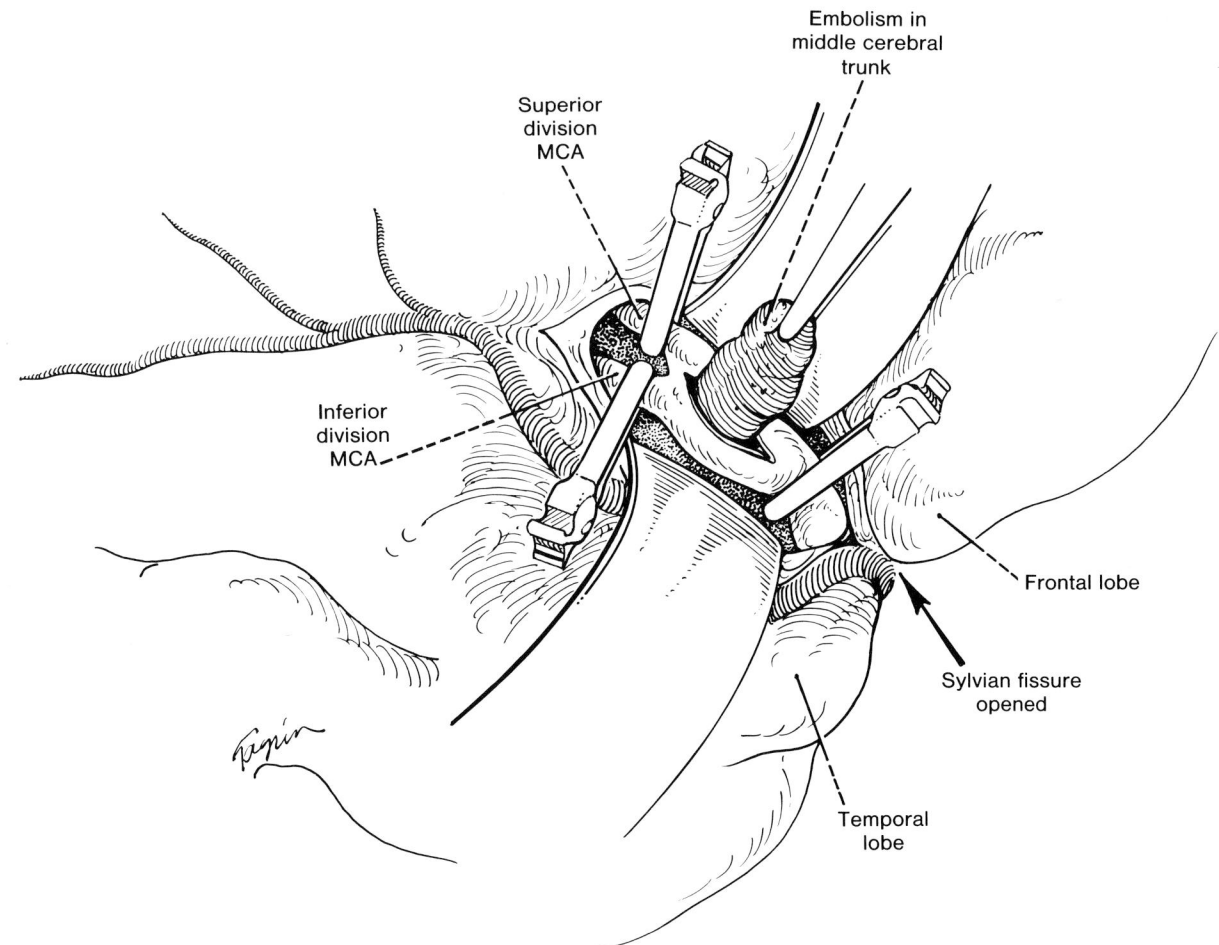

Figure 8.2. Middle cerebral artery (*MCA*) embolectomy. Exposure of right middle cerebral artery in the sylvian fissure and removal of an embolus from the M1 segment.

bral artery if such is encountered. The lumen is irrigated with heparinized saline, and backflow is checked briefly by opening the clips. The arteriotomy is then closed with running 7-0 or 8-0 monofilament nylon. A patch graft is generally not necessary. In case of brain swelling, the bone flap may be left out, and barbiturate coma may be maintained for another 24–72 hours. Blood pressure should be maintained in the high normal range. Postoperative angiography and CT scan can document impact of therapy.

The authors have performed four middle cerebral artery embolectomies for naturally occurring embolism. An additional patient was operated after an embolus to the middle cerebral artery was documented during angiography when the patient developed a sudden hemiplegia and aphasia. At surgery the cerebral artery looked normal and, therefore, the authors assumed that the embolus had lysed and passed distally. This patient made a full recovery over the next several days. Of the four patients who did undergo an embolectomy, two improved beyond what could have been expected from the natural course of the disease. One remained unchanged, and the last patient died of a pulmonary embolus 1 week after surgery after having improved slightly during the immediate postoperative period. Postoperative angiography documented patency of the middle cerebral artery in the two patients who improved (Fig. 8.3).

Another patient was operated to remove a latex balloon that had embolized to the middle cerebral artery (7). This patient had a balloon detached in the internal carotid artery to occlude this vessel as treatment for an unclippable giant aneurysm. Shortly after detachment of the balloon, the patient became hemiplegic, and at that point angiography documented occlusion of the main trunk of the middle cerebral artery by the dislodged balloon. A craniotomy was performed rapidly and the balloon was removed from the middle cerebral artery by the technique described. The neurologic deficit resolved completely over the next 24 hours and postoperative angiography demonstrated a normal appearance of the middle cerebral artery.

In 1976, the results in 35 cases of intracranial arteriotomy for embolus or thrombosis, reported in the English literature, were summarized (3). In 18 of 37 operated vessels, postoperative angiography demonstrated patency. There was no definite evidence to indicate any difference in the outcome between those with open or occluded arteries. It was concluded that the best surgical candidate is a young person, in good general medical condition, in whom the occlusion has occurred within a few hours of surgery.

In 1985, the Mayo Clinic summarized their experience with 20 cases of emergency middle cerebral artery embolectomy (5): 35% had a good or excellent result, clearly better than what could be expected from the natural history of their disease; 35% had a fair result, which could not be definitely said to have been better than what could have been expected from their disease; and 30% did poorly or died. Patients with associated ipsilateral internal carotid artery occlusion did poorly, probably because of their limited potential for collateral circulation. The best predictor of a good outcome was the preoperative angiographic finding of rich leptomeningeal collateral circulation to the middle cerebral artery territory from the anterior and posterior cerebral artery territories (Fig. 8.3). Interestingly, there were three patients in this series who had good collateral circulation preoperatively who did well even when operated as late as 12, 14, and 18 hours after the onset of the neurologic deficit.

REFERENCES

1. Adams RD, Victor M: *Principles of Neurology*. New York, McGraw-Hill, 1977, pp 530-534.
2. Fisher CM, Dalal PM, Adams RD: Cerebrovascular disease and stroke syndrome. In Harrison TR (ed): *Principles of Internal Medicine*. New York, McGraw-Hill, 1962.
3. Garrido E, Stein BM: Middle cerebral artery embolectomy. *J Neurosurg* 44:517-521, 1976.
4. Heros RC: Cerebellar hemorrhage and infarction. *Stroke* 13:106–109, 1982.
5. Meyer FB, Piepgras DG, Sundt TM Jr, Yanagihara T: Emergency embolectomy for acute occlusion of the middle cerebral artery. *J Neurosurg* 62:639–647, 1985.
6. Strand T, Asplund K, Eriksson S, Hagg E, Lithner F, Wester PO: A ranomized controlled trial of hemodilution therapy in acute ischemic stroke. *Stroke* 15:980-989, 1984.
7. Swann KW, Heros RC, Debrun GM: Middle cerebral artery embolism by a detachable balloon. Management by microsurgical embolectomy. Case report. *J Neurosurg* 64:309-312, 1986.
8. Sypert GW, Alvord EC Jr: Cerebellar infarction: A clinicopathological study. *Arch Neurol* 32:357-363, 1975.

Figure 8.3. Middle cerebral artery embolectomy. Four days after coronary artery bypass and infarctectomy, a 42-year-old man suffered sudden aphasia and right hemiplegia. **A** and **B**, Immediate left carotid angiography documented middle cerebral artery stem occlusion. **C**, Good retrograde filling of distal middle cerebral artery branches back to the bifurcation (*arrows*). Embolectomy restored flow about 7 hours after onset of deficit. **D** and **E**, Postoperative angiography documented patency. *Arrow* indicates where embolus was removed at middle cerebral artery bifurcation. There is some narrowing at that point. **F**, CT shows the infarction. The patient recovered to a mild right hemiparesis with normal language.

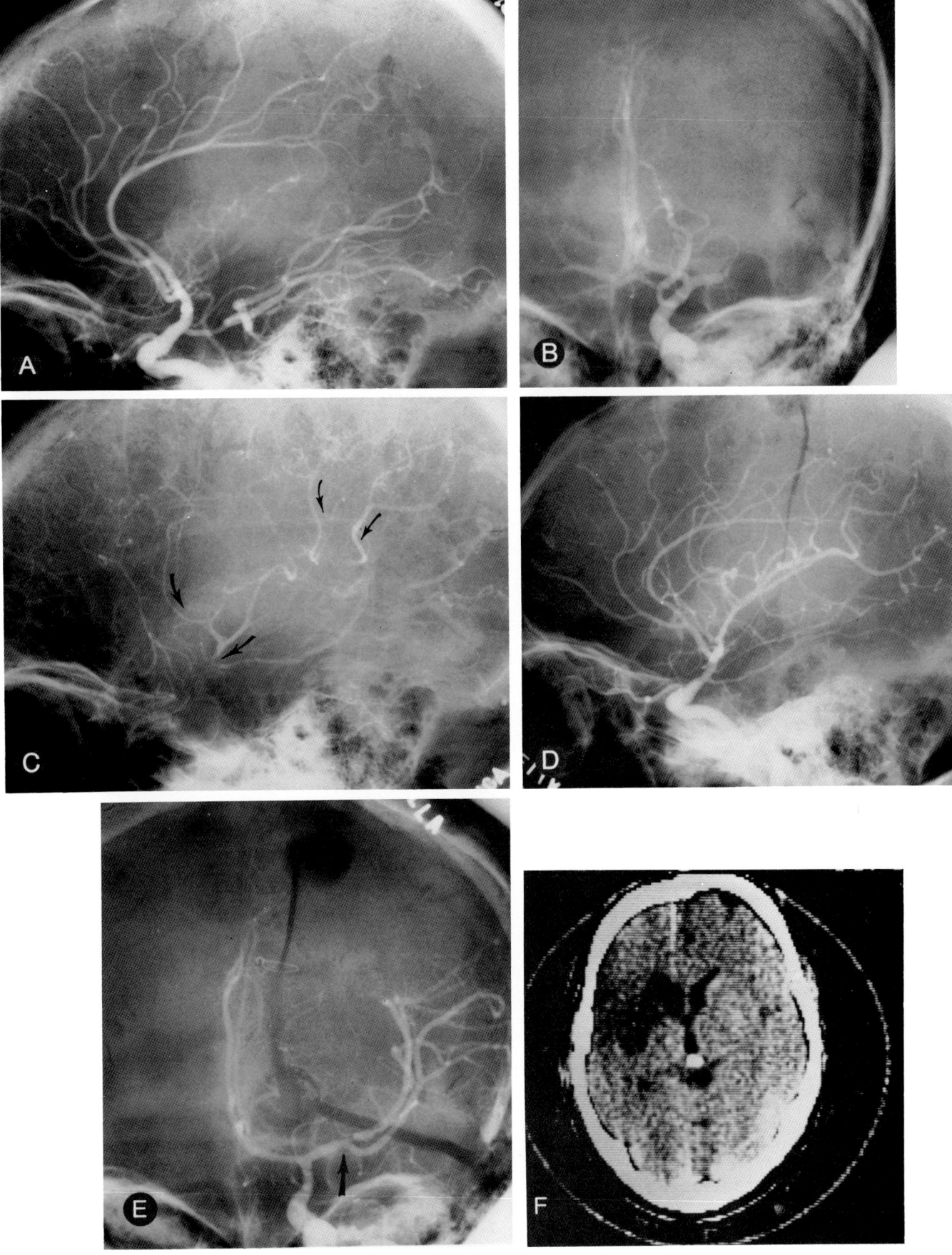

9

Cerebral and Cerebellar Infarction

Irreversible damage to brain tissue due to lack of blood is called infarction or ischemic necrosis. Brain infarcts vary greatly in size and in the amount of hemorrhage within the area. Some infarcts are pale and devoid of blood, while others show varying degrees of extravasation of blood from small vessels in the infarcted area. The latter are usually associated with embolism (see Chapter 8).

The computed tomography (CT) or the magnetic resonance imaging (MRI) scan defines the extent of the infarction. Details regarding the use of these tests in patients with infarction are presented in Chapter 1.

Most patients with infarction will be alert, with a neurologic deficit associated with the area of infarction. Treatment is directed to the cause of the infarction. Occasionally, symptoms due to swelling and edema will develop, but this condition usually responds to medical treatment. In a few very carefully selected patients, surgery to provide decompression may be required because the swollen infarcted brain tissue does not respond to medical therapy.

CEREBRAL INFARCTION

When acute massive ischemic cerebral infarction with progressive signs of brain stem compression fails to respond to medical therapy, treatment with hemicraniectomy, opening of the dura and, in some patients, resection of necrotic tissue may be indicated (9, 11, 12, 17). A dural graft is sewn in place, or Gelfoam is placed over the opening to protect the brain. The authors of this text have performed this operation in two patients with relief of pressure and eventual recovery of function.

In one report, three patients with acute massive multilobular ischemic infarction with uncal herniation who were unresponsive to medical therapy were treated with hemicraniectomy and opening of the dura (12). All three patients survived, although a severe fixed neurologic deficit persisted in two. The factors that influenced undertaking this surgery were the relatively young age of the patients, involvement of the nondominant hemisphere, lack of systemic illness, and the positive attitude of the family toward the operation.

CEREBELLAR INFARCTION

Etiology

The swollen infarcted cerebellar hemisphere may also cause brain stem compression, resulting in the need for neurosurgical treatment, often on an urgent basis. In the majority of patients, the infarction is in the posteroinferior half of the cerebellar hemisphere in the region supplied by the ipsilateral vertebral and posterior inferior cerebellar arteries (6, 16). Occasionally, an infarct is found in the region of the superior cerebellar artery (7, 13, 16).

Atherosclerotic occlusion with associated thrombosis is the most common cause of arterial occlusions. Embolism was implicated as the cause in 22% of the patients in one report (16). The problem has also been seen with traumatic occlusion of the vertebral artery, as has, for example, occurred as a result of neck manipulation (5).

Clinical Presentation and Diagnosis

The onset is usually sudden. The early symptoms are rotatory dizziness, nausea and vomiting, and inability to stand or walk unaided (1, 6, 10, 14). Initially, these symptoms may mimic a benign labyrinthine disorder (2).

In early stages, examination may reveal nystagmus, usually horizontal and rapid in the direction of gaze, truncal ataxia, dysarthria, and stiff neck. Hypertension is present in about half the patients. As the cerebellar infarction progresses, drowsiness and confusion are noted. Ocular abnormalities are common with findings of an ipsilateral abducent nerve paresis or a gaze palsy, with deviation of the eyes to the opposite side.

This type of gaze palsy differs from that encountered with supratentorial lesions, in that it will not correct itself either with the doll's head maneuver or with caloric stimulation. Bilateral extensor plantar responses are often noted. Peripheral facial palsy is commonly seen at this stage. Of note is the absence of significant hemiparesis until very late in the course of the illness when the patient becomes unresponsive with small sluggishly reactive pupils and reflex posturing. At least half these patients stabilize and improve without proceeding to later stages of deterioration. However, progression to decerebrate posturing with stupor or coma and other evidence of severe brain stem compression can occur, often fairly rapidly, even in a patient who appears to be relatively stable.

Any patient suspected of having a posterior fossa mass lesion should have an immediate CT scan. Cerebellar hemorrhage may not be differentiated from infarction on the basis of clinical features only. Emergency CT scanning can be used to locate the lesion, establish the pathology, and document the degree of hydrocephalus (Fig. 9.1). It must be remembered that the low-density lesion in the cerebellum may not develop for some hours to a few days, and therefore, the initial CT scan may be inconclusive and serial scans may be of help. Nonvisualization or displacement of the fourth ventricle, indicating a cerebellar mass effect, may be the only clue and, when seen in the patient with the classical clinical syndrome, should lead to the proper diagnosis. In some cases, contrast enhancement will show the lesion. A recent report has suggested than MRI is more accurate than CT in detecting cerebellar infarction, particularly during the first 24 hours when the CT scan is likely to be negative (15). Also, because of the lack of bone artifact, MRI is probably more accurate than CT in documenting the extent of the cerebellar infarction and any associated brain stem involvement. One problem may be that many of these patients are too ill to hold still for a satisfactory MRI scan.

In a report on cerebellar infarction documented by CT scan, 6 of 21 patients had progressive deterioration of consciousness, signs of brain stem compression, and the appearance of hydrocephalus on the CT scan (14). In 15, the course was uncomplicated, and gradual improvement occurred. In another report, about half the patients improved spontaneously (3).

Treatment

If the patient is alert and the neurologic status is stable or improving, medical treatment with steroids and/or mannitol is initiated. If there is a decreasing level of consciousness due to brain stem compression when the patient is first evaluated, immediate surgical treatment for removal of the infarcted cerebellar tissue is usually indicated. In one report, the presence of hydrocephalus was used as an important factor in deciding about surgery (13).

However, the authors of this text have seen patients who developed serious signs of brain stem compression in the absence of significant hydrocephalus. As one would expect, cerebellar infarction from occlusion of the distal vertebral artery or the posterior inferior cerebellar artery may be accompanied by a lateral medullary infarct (Wallenberg's syndrome) (6). Since in this syndrome there are intrinsic brain stem signs such as dysphagia, dysarthria, a Horner's sign, and crossed sensory loss from infarction of the lateral medulla, it is important not to confuse these signs, which are usually present in the awake patient when first seen, from later-developing signs of extrinsic brain stem compression from cerebellar swelling. The latter, already described, are more ominous, are usually associated with a decreased level of consciousness, and require surgical decompression (6).

The operation is usually carried out with the patient in the prone position; a midline incision is normally used and a craniectomy that includes removal of the midline bone and posterior rim of the foramen magnum as well as bone over the involved cerebellar hemisphere is performed. The dural opening exposes

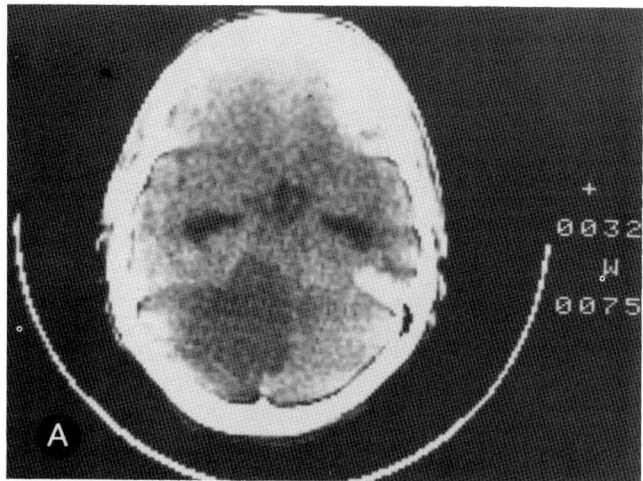

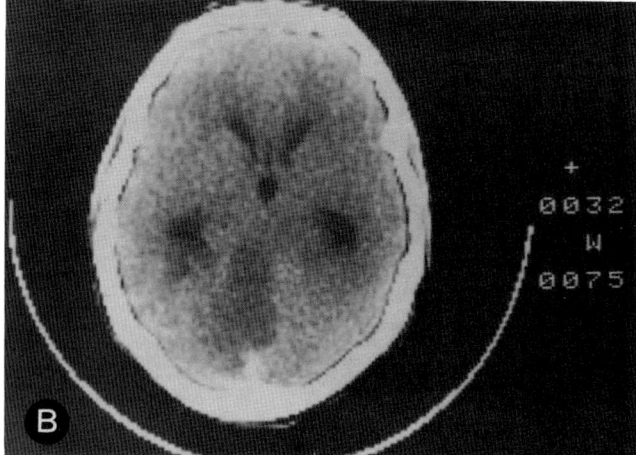

Figure 9.1. CT scan of cerebellar infarction. **A**, Large infarct of the cerebellum causing brain stem compression. Note that the low density seems to be sharply demarcated and involves most of the cerebellar hemisphere. **B**, The infarct extends superiorly, and there is evidence of hydrocephalus (confirmed on higher scans) with enlarged temporal horns and a dilated third ventricle. Comment: The patient developed increasing signs of brain stem compression that did not respond to medical treatment. Full recovery followed resection of the lateral cerebellum.

the cerebellar hemisphere and extends across the midline and over the cerebellar tonsils, which is necessary to relieve pressure on the lower brain stem from tonsillar herniation. The resection includes at least the lateral half of the cerebellar hemisphere with removal of all the grossly pale, nonviable cerebellar tissue that frequently extrudes itself after dural opening. To give a full decompression, the dura is closed by using a graft of pericranial tissue from the occipital region. A satisfactory alternative approach is the lateral "park bench" position. To avoid the risk of hypotension, the patient should not be placed in the sitting position.

The role of ventricular drainage in the treatment of these patients is controversial (6). In the rare patient who deteriorates acutely and is found to have significant hydrocephalus by CT scan, ventricular decompression can give the surgeon enough time to take the patient to the operating room for the definitive decompression by suboccipital craniectomy. Also, the rare patient who has no sign of brain stem compression but has a decreased level of consciousness that can be attributed to hydrocephalus can be managed satisfactorily with an external ventricular drain, which may need to be converted to a permanent shunt after a few days (8, 12). Certainly, if the patient does not improve with ventricular drainage or if signs of brain stem compression develop subsequently, a suboccipital decompression must be carried out. The authors of this text believe that whenever specific signs of brain stem compression such as forced eye deviation, ipsilateral facial paralysis, small and sluggishly reactive pupils, or reflex posturing develop, a prompt decompression of the posterior fossa is in order, since ventricular drainage will not relieve the pressure upon the brain stem and may actually worsen the patient by allowing upward herniation of the crowded posterior fossa contents (6).

In a review summarizing reports of 55 patients who developed signs of brian stem compression due to cerebellar infarction, it was found that 5 of 18 treated surgically and 31 of 37 not treated surgically died (2). In other reports it was concluded that medical treatment of large cerebellar infarcts was associated with an 80% mortality rate, while with surgery this figure dropped to 40% (4); and in 51 patients who had rapid worsening of signs of brain stem compression, it was found that 28 of 37 (76%) patients who were operated on survived, while only 1 of 14 (7%) patients who were not operated on lived (14). It was concluded that to be effective, surgical treatment must be initiated as soon as possible after consciousness begins to deteriorate.

REFERENCES

1. Duncan GW, Parker SW, Fisher CM: Acute cerebellar infarction in the PICA territory. Arch Neurol 32:364–368, 1975.
2. Feeley MP: Cerebellar infarction. Neurosurgery 4:7–11, 1979.
3. George B, Cophignon J, George C, Lougnon J: Surgical aspects of cerebellar infarction. Based upon a series of 79 cases. Neurochirurgie 24:83–88, 1978.
4. Greenberg J, Skubick D, Shenkin H: Acute hydrocephalus in cerebellar infarct and hemorrhage. Neurology 29:409–413, 1979.
5. Heros RC: Cerebellar infarction resulting from traumatic occlusion of a vertebral artery. Case report. J Neurosurg 51:111–113, 1979.
6. Heros RC: Cerebellar hemorrhage and infarction. Curr Concepts Cerebrovasc Dis 16:17–22, 1981.
7. Ho SU, Kim KS, Berenberg RA, Ho HT: Cerebellar infarction: A clinical and CT study. Surg Neurol 16:350–352, 1981.
8. Horwitz NH, Ludolph C: Acute obstructive hydrocephalus caused by cerebellar infarction. Treatment alternatives. Surg Neurol 20:13–19, 1983.
9. Ivamoto HS, Numoto M, Donaghy RMP: Surgical decompression for cerebral and cerebellar infarcts. Stroke 5:365–369, 1974.
10. Lehrich JR, Winkler GF, Ojemann RG: Cerebellar infarction with brain stem compression. Diagnosis and surgical treatment. Arch Neurol 22:490–498, 1970.
11. Rengachary SS: Surgery for acute brain infarcation with mass effect. In Wilkins RH, Rengachary SS (eds): Neurosurgery. New York, McGraw-Hill, 1985, vol 2 pp 1267–1271.
12. Rengachary SS, Batnitzky S, Morantz RA, Arjunan K, Jeffries B: Hemicraniectomy for acute massive cerebral infarction. Neurosurgery 8:321–328, 1981.
13. Sayama I, Sakotani AY, Yasui N, Ito Z, Kobayashi T, Nakajimak K: Cerebellar infarction: Early predication to the operative indication of posterior fossa decompression. Brain Nerve (Tokyo) 33:801–810, 1981.
14. Scotti G, Spinnler H, Sterzi R, Vallar G: Cerebellar softening. Ann Neurol 8:133–140, 1980.
15. Simmons Z, Biller J, Adams HP Jr, Dunn V, Jacoby CG: Cerebellar infarction: Comparison of computed tomography and magnetic resonance imaging. Ann Neurol 19:291–293, 1986.
16. Sypert GW, Alvord EC Jr: Cerebellar infarction. A clinicopathological study. Arch Neurol 32:357–363, 1975.
17. Young PH, Smith KR Jr, Dunn RC: Surgical decompression after cerebral hemispheric stroke: Indications and patient selection. South Med J 75:473–475, 1982.

Section 2 INTRACRANIAL ANEURYSMS, ARTERIOVENOUS MALFORMATIONS, AND BRAIN HEMORRHAGE

10

Intracranial Aneurysms and Subarachnoid Hemorrhage: Incidence, Pathology, Clinical Features, and Perioperative Management

PREVALENCE

Intracranial aneurysms and subarachnoid hemorrhage are common problems. The prevalence of intracranial aneurysms at autopsy is reported to be between 2–5% (13, 40, 78, 80). It is estimated that 400,000 Americans harbor an unruptured cerebral aneurysm. In North America the incidence of subarachnoid hemorrhage from a ruptured aneurysm is approximately 12/100,000 (76). In the United States there are approximately 25,000 new cases of ruptured intracranial aneurysms each year. About 50% of these patients die or become permanently disabled as a result of the initial hemorrhage and another 25–35% die of a later hemorrhage if left untreated (36). Disappointingly, the toll in death and disability from rupture of an intracranial aneurysm has not changed substantially in the past 30 years, in spite of many technologic advances in the radiologic diagnosis as well as in the medical and surgical treatment of this disease (72).

The prevalence of aneurysm in the population is correlated with age; the peak incidence is in the sixth decade of life, while aneurysms are rare in childhood and adolescence. A slight tendency toward female preponderance is characteristic (57, 82).

ETIOLOGY

Despite controversy spanning several decades, the etiology of intracranial aneurysms remains unknown. Table 10.1 summarizes congenital and acquired factors that have been implicated in the cause of the typical "berry" type of intracranial aneurysm (78). Medial defects, as well as defects in the elastic lamina, can be routinely found at autopsy in certain locations, such as arterial bifurcations or "forks" and at presumed sites of involution of fetal vessels. Because these defects are found routinely at autopsies of individuals without aneurysms, there must be other factors that play a role in the production of aneurysms. Inasmuch as aneurysms in infancy and childhood are uncommon, it is likely that acquired factors interact to produce aneurysms in the aforementioned areas of congenital arterial weakness (78, 81).

Typical berry aneurysms can also be found in patients with diseases that produce defects in vascular walls, including Ehlers-Danlos syndrome, Marfan's syndrome, and pseudoxanthoma elasticum. In addition, intracranial aneurysms occur with unexpected frequency and at an earlier age in patients with coarctation or hypoplasia of the aorta, polycystic kidneys, and fibromuscular dysplasia. Furthermore, in some cases, intracranial aneurysms can be said to be "familial," and several families have been reported in which many immediate relatives harbor intracranial aneurysms (10, 30, 31, 33).

Occasionally, aneurysms may be caused by trauma (11, 29), infection (see Chapter 21), tumor (20), or atherosclerosis (34). Infectious aneurysms, due to either bacterial or fungal infection, look very much like berry aneurysms on angiography except that they tend to occur in more peripheral locations and are frequently multiple (see Chapter 21). Tumor emboli, particularly from atrial myxomas, occasionally can invade and destroy the wall of cerebral arteries and result in an aneurysm (20).

Fusiform aneurysms may occur in the anterior and posterior circulations. Some of these lesions are atherosclerotic in origin. In some cases, the muscularis and elastic laminae are defective. Multiple vessels may be involved with dolichoectatic changes. Such lesions may also be associated with berry aneurysms. Gradual accretion of mural thrombus is not uncommon, and rupture can also occur. Hypertension is usual in these patients.

PATHOLOGY

Intracranial aneurysms arise at specific sites in the cerebral circulation (17). Approximately 80% occur in the anterior circulation (17). Most aneurysms of the anterior circulation are located on the anterior

Table 10.1.
Factors Involved in the Origin of Aneurysms

Congenital factors
   Medial defects
   Elastic defects
   Origin of small vessels
   Failure of branch involution

Acquired factors
   Elastic degeneration
   Inflammation
   Atherosclerosis
   Hypertension
   Hemodynamic effects

communicating, internal carotid, and middle cerebral arteries. Except for aneurysms in the region of the genu of the pericallosal artery, aneurysms arising on the distal branches of these vessels are almost always bacterial in origin. Aneurysms in the posterior circulation are most common at the apex of the basilar artery and at the origin of the posterior inferior cerebellar artery. The reported incidence of multiple intracranial aneurysms ranges from 12–31% and of bilateral aneurysms, particularly in mirror locations, 9–19% (98). In patients with intracranial aneurysms, 1.1% are reported to have associated intracranial arteriovenous malformations (71). In this situation the aneurysm is usually, but not always, located on one of the major feeding arteries to the malformation (98).

Gross examination of aneurysms indicates that they usually originate from the bifurcations of major proximal intracranial arteries (Fig. 10.1A and B) (17, 85). Most of these lesions have a definable neck amenable to surgical clipping. There are practically never any branches arising from the dome of an aneurysm. Occasionally branches that arise from the neck of the aneurysm are so densely adherent to the dome of the aneurysm that they appear actually to arise from that area and high magnification is required to confirm that indeed the branch arises from the neck region. In large aneurysms, the base of the aneurysmal complex expands to such a degree that the major branches originate from the expanded neck at a distance of several millimeters from the parent vessel. These aneurysms are not amenable to simple surgical clipping without previous aneurysmorrhaphy. Aneurysms can be classified according to their size: <15 mm in diameter (small), 15–25 mm (large), and >25 mm (giant).

Histopathologic examination reveals thinning of the entire arterial wall with absence of internal elastic lamina (Fig. 10.1C). The location of this attenuation corresponds to medial defects that appear at branch points in normal arteries (82, 83). When the aneurysm ruptures, bleeding is stopped by tissue pressure and the formation of a fibrin-platelet plug at the site of rupture (27).

PREVENTION

Because the etiology of intracranial berry aneurysms is not clearly understood, there is no effective means of preventing their occurrence. Until more is known about how aneurysms develop, we have to be content with preventing their rupture (78). Once an intracranial aneurysm is detected, surgery effectively and safely prevents hemorrhage (24). With the exception of giant aneurysms and aneurysms located in difficult areas, such as the basilar bifurcation, unruptured aneurysms can be treated with low surgical morbidity and mortality (24, 77). With the current widespread use of the computed tomography (CT) scan, more asymptomatic intracranial aneurysms are being detected. This number will increase as more sophisticated scanners with greater resolution become available. With the latest generation of CT scanners, most aneurysms larger than 5–7 mm may be detected (21). In addition to CT scanning, intravenous digital subtraction angiography is becoming increasingly sophisticated and more capable of detecting some intracranial aneurysms (55). A report discussing the use of an electronic stethoscope to detect unruptured aneurysms and arteriovenous malformations suggests that this apparatus, when refined, may become a useful tool for routine noninvasive detection of aneurysms (79). Magnetic resonance imaging can also detect intracranial aneurysms without risk. Presently, individuals at high risk of harboring aneurysms should be studied at least with one of these noninvasive techiques. Such individuals include the members of families in which more than one immediately related person is known to have an intracranial aneurysm and patients with diseases that predispose to the formation of intracranial aneurysms.

The most important impact in prevention of aneurysmal hemorrhage will be made by increasing awareness in the medical community of warning signs of aneurysmal rupture. Almost 40% of major ruptures are preceded by warning symptoms (48). Table 10.2 lists the warning signs of subarachnoid hemorrhage. As indicated in the table, these signs can usually be attributed to aneurysmal expansion, a minor hemorrhage from the aneurysm, or ischemia resulting from embolism from an intraaneurysmal clot or, rarely, from occlusion of a major vessel by aneurysmal expansion or direct compression of brain tissue. The patient presenting with localized retro-orbital pain and a third nerve palsy, particularly if the pupil is involved, is likely to harbor an intracranial aneurysm. All physicians need to know, however, that such a patient presents a major neurologic emergency. It has been well established that when aneu-

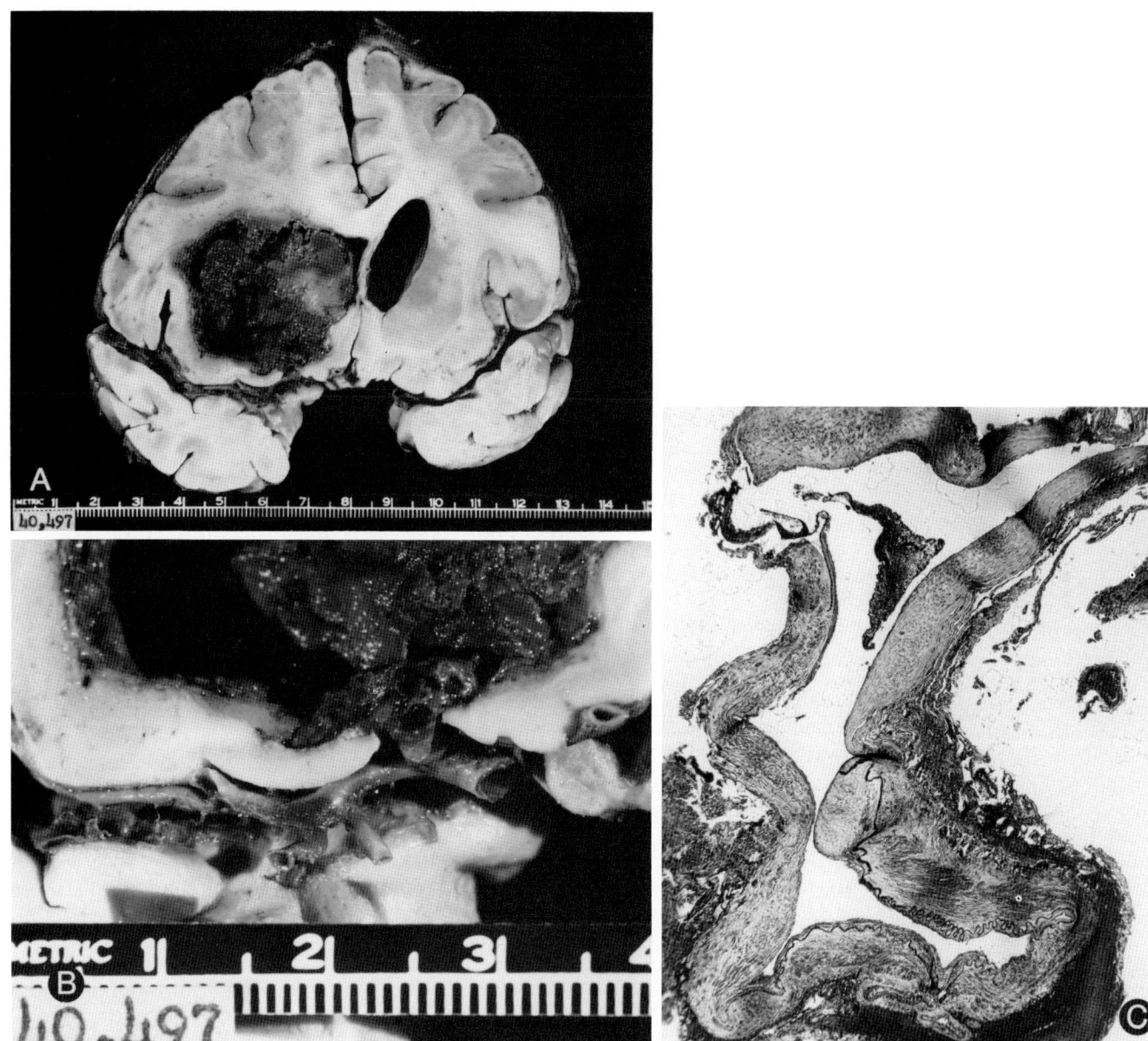

Figure 10.1. Ruptured internal carotid artery bifurcation aneurysm. **A**, Intracerebral hemorrhage. Patient expired from intracranial mass effect with shift of midline structures. **B**, Closer view shows aneurysm projecting superiorly into the hematoma. There is a well-defined neck. **C**, Microscopic section of aneurysm shows the parent artery (*bottom*) with thick muscular walls and elastic laminae. The aneurysm (*above*) has absent elastica and rupture point at upper left.

rysm expansion results in the acute development of a cranial nerve palsy, the risk of a major hemorrhage over the next week or two is extremely high and, therefore, prompt neuroradiologic investigation and surgical treatment are imperative (36, 91).

The patient complaining of an isolated severe headache without other symptoms presents a difficult diagnostic problem. In almost 20% of patients with a major subarachnoid hemorrhage, a history of a severe headache within the 2–3 weeks prior to the major rupture can be obtained. Clearly it is impractical to investigate radiologically every patient with a headache. If the patient is intact and does not have papilledema, spinal puncture should be performed to rule out subarachnoid hemorrhage.

CLINICAL DIAGNOSIS

When a major subarachnoid hemorrhage has occured, the attack is usually heralded by severe headache of precipitous onset or by sudden, transient loss

Table 10.2.
Warning Signs of Subarachnoid Hemorrhage[a]

Aneurysmal expansion
   Localized head pain
   Cranial nerve palsies
   Visual defects

"Minor leaks"
   Severe headache of sudden onset
   Nausea
   Neck pain
   Back pain
   Photophobia
   Lethargy

Ischemia
   Transcient ischemic attacks
   Focal neurologic deficit

[a]Modified from Waga S, Ohtsubo K, Handa H: Warning signs in intracranial aneurysms. Surg Neurol 3:15–20, 1975.

of consciousness followed by headache. The headache is usually described as "the most severe of my life," "explosive," "bursting," and so on. At the onset, the headache may be localized to the occipital or the subfrontal region, but it soon becomes generalized. Meningeal signs, such as nuchal rigidity and photophobia, often develop within 4–8 hours after the onset of subarachnoid hemorrhage. It is important to know that these signs may be absent if the patient is seen soon after the hemorrhage. Subhyaloid hemorrhages are virtually pathognomonic of subarachnoid hemorrhage when seen in a patient with severe headache of sudden onset (36).

The diagnosis of subarachnoid hemorrhage may be difficult when the patient presents in coma or with major focal neurologic deficits. In the alert patient who presents with major focal neurologic deficits, an ischemic cerebrovascular event and an intracerebral hemorrhage are common. Occasionally, however, an intracranial aneurysm will rupture into the brain parenchyma and the patient will present with major focal neurologic deficits. When this occurs as a result of centrally located aneurysms, the patient is unlikely to be awake. With middle cerebral aneurysms, however, bleeding into the temporal lobe is common and the patient may be wide awake with major focal deficits. Less commonly, this can occur with anterior communicating aneurysms that bleed into a frontal lobe. The history of severe headache of sudden onset will be of paramount importance in the diagnosis of a subarachnoid hemorrhage; for comatose patients, such history must be obtained from others (34).

Giant cerebral aneurysms may present as mass lesions. These lesions, arising most frequently from the middle cerebral and internal carotid arteries, may give rise to slow and progressive hemiparesis and dysphasia. The less common giant aneurysms of the posterior circulation can present with symptoms mimicking a posterior fossa mass (see Chapter 20).

In order to develop a common language to describe the clinical condition of patients with subarachnoid hemorrhage, several classifications have been developed. Most commonly used are the grading systems developed by Botterell et al (12) and by Hunt and Hess (42). Both of these systems emphasize the mental status of the patient (Tables 10.3 and 10.4). The main difference is that Hunt and Hess distinguish, among patients with normal mental status, those with meningismus (grade 2) and those without such signs (grade 1). This difference is important as a prognostic factor, since meningeal irritation means a serious subarachnoid hemorrhage with increased risk of vasospasm, hydrocephalus, increased intracranial pressure, etc. Thus, the authors prefer to use the Hunt and Hess classification and will do so throughout this book. Note also that drowsiness appears in the Hunt and Hess classification as grade 3 and in the Botterell et al system as grade 2; obviously, the two systems must be clearly distinguished to avoid confusion on this important prognostic sign. A useful modification of this classification is the addition of a separate grade (1A) to denote patients who are stable neurologically, with a normal mental status, and without signs of active meningeal irritation, but who have a fixed neurologic deficit. Experience shows that these patients can be operated with as low a risk of inducing new neurologic deficits as patients in grade 1. To compare results between different series of patients it is useful to have this separate grade because these patients will not be intact after surgery and should not be "lumped" with patients who were intact. Another suggestion that may be useful for prognostication and for deciding whether and when to operate is to add a grade to a patient with a serious medical condition, such as severe hypertension or heart disease. The authors find the latter modification difficult to use clinically and, therefore, use the classification solely in reference to the neurologic status.

Table 10.3.
Assessment of Patients with Subarachnoid Hemorrhage (Botterell et al (12))

Grade 1	Conscious ± signs of subarachnoid blood
Grade 2	Drowsy without significant deficit
Grade 3	Drowsy with a neurologic deficit
Grade 4	Deteriorating with major neurologic deficit
Grade 5	Moribund with extensor rigidity and failing vital signs.

Table 10.4.
Assessment of Patients with Subarachnoid Hemorrhage (Hunt and Hess (42))

Grade 1	Asymptomatic, or minimal headache and slight nuchal rigidity
Grade 2	Moderate to severe headache, nuchal rigidity, no neurologic deficit other than cranial nerve palsy
Grade 3	Drowsiness, confusion, or mild focal deficit
Grade 4	Stupor, moderate to severe hemiparesis, possibly early decerebrate rigidity and vegetative disturbances
Grade 5	Deep coma, decerebrate rigidity, moribund appearance

MEDICAL EVALUATION

When admitted, every patient with subarachnoid hemorrhage should have an electrocardiogram, bleeding studies (prothrombin time, partial thromboplastin time, platelet count, and bleeding time), serum electrolytes, and serum osmolarity. Noninvasive vascular evaluation of the lower extremities (plethysmography) may be used to screen for deep vein thrombosis, which may occur in patients treated with ϵ-aminocaproic acid. In patients with electrocardiographic abnormalities or where induced hypotension is planned during surgery, cardiac consultation is indicated.

RADIOLOGIC DIAGNOSIS

A plain CT scan with modern equipment will establish the diagnosis of subarachnoid hemorrhage in 90–95% of the cases (21, 22). It is important to do the CT scan initially without contrast in order to ascertain the presence of subarachnoid hemorrhage. A contrast study can also be done; sometimes this reveals the site of the aneurysm. A CT scan is valuable in indicating the severity of the hemorrhage, a sign of great prognostic significance (22, 25, 26, 49). The amount of blood in the basal subarachnoid space is the most important factor in predicting the future risk and severity of vasospasm. The CT scan is also diagnostic for other complications of subarachnoid hemorrhage, including intracerebral hematoma, subdural hematoma, and hydrocephalus.

Angiography remains the definitive diagnostic study in patients with intracranial aneurysms. There is no consensus on the optimal time for angiography. In the instances in which early surgery is not a consideration, the clinician may still choose to perform an early angiogram to establish the diagnosis and the anatomy of the aneurysm. It is well known that vasospasm will almost never be present in an angiogram done within the first 2–3 days after subarachnoid hemorrhage, so this is an optimal time to visualize the vascular anatomy thoroughly. Another reason for early angiography is to guide use of ϵ-aminocaproic acid, which is not recommended for patients with arteriovenous malformations or for those without demonstrable aneurysm. Regardless of whether one plans an early or late operation, in cases of ruptured middle cerebral aneurysms with an intratemporal hematoma, early angiography is preferable. Even if one intends to delay surgery in these cases, it may be necessary to perform an emergency, unplanned operation, since these patients sometimes deteriorate abruptly. In such instances there may not be time for angiography at the time of the acute deterioration, and the surgeon may regret not having had an angiogram that defines the arterial anatomy because it is preferable to clip the aneurysm when the hematoma is evacuated (36). Alternatively, in those cases where late surgery is planned, surgeons have reasoned that an angiogram immediately before surgery is needed so that operation can be delayed if severe angiographic vasospasm is found. Under these circumstances, an early angiogram may be considered unnecessary (22). Because angiography provides definitive diagnosis and guides medical and surgical management, the authors perform this test early in most patients after diagnosis of subarachnoid hemorrhage.

Angiography should demonstrate the aneurysmal sac and neck and their relation to parent arteries (Fig. 10.2) (3, 4, 24). Satisfactory visualization will often require oblique and base views. To exclude an arterial loop, the aneurysm should be demonstrated in at least two projections. To assure visualization of the anterior communicating artery complex, compression of one carotid artery may be used during injection of the contralateral carotid artery. This technique may also be necessary in order to demonstrate the adequacy of collateral circulation in cases of giant aneurysms where carotid artery ligation may be a therapeutic consideration. In cases of large basilar aneurysms where basilar ligation may be a consideration, the Allcock maneuver, which consists of compressing each carotid artery while the vertebral artery is injected with contrast, should be done in order to ascertain the size of the posterior communicating arteries (see Chapter 20). To exclude multiple aneurysms one requires either four-vessel angiography or three-vessel angiography with reflux into the contralateral vertebral artery to the level of the origin of the posterior inferior cerebellar artery. Three-vessel angiography is not sufficient in those cases in which the pattern of hemorrhage on the CT scan suggests that there may be a peripheral posterior inferior cerebellar aneurysm. In these cases, each vertebral artery must be injected, since it is rarely possible to achieve complete visualization of one posterior inferior cerebellar artery by injection of the contralateral vertebral artery. Subtraction techniques are

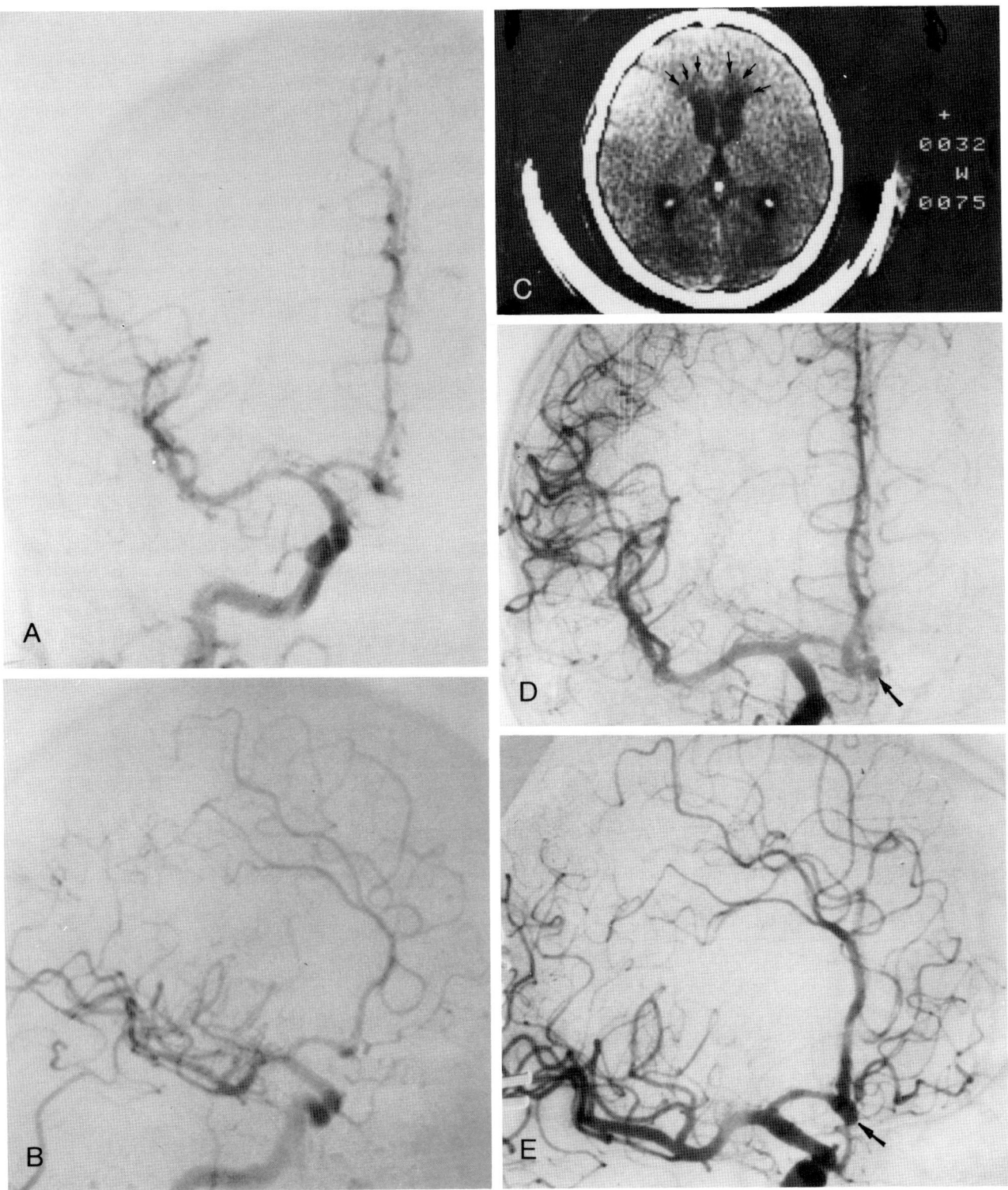

Figure 10.2. Repeat angiography discloses anterior communicating aneurysm. **A** and **B**, Right carotid angiogram performed 2 days after subarachnoid hemorrhage shows no definite aneurysm or spasm even with an oblique view to show the anterior communicating complex. Left carotid angiogram was normal. **C**, CT scan 1 week after subarachnoid hemorrhage shows low density anterior to ventricles (*arrows*) suggesting infarction due to anterior cerebral spasm. **D** and **E**, Repeat right carotid angiogram 3 weeks after subarachnoid hemorrhage shows anterior communicating aneurysm (*arrow*).

frequently very useful in delineating the vascular anatomy near the base of the skull. Some surgeons find stereoscopic views or angiotomography particularly helpful, but the present authors have had no substantial experience with these techniques.

If vasospasm is present, it is helpful to grade it according to the diameter of the residual arterial lumen: 0 = no narrowing, + = slight narrowing + + = about 1 mm in diameter, + + + = about 0.5 mm with indistinct outline, and + + + + = less than 0.5 mm, delay in flow and visualization of collateral flow to the distal territory via leptomeningeal anastomoses. These measurements apply to proximal anterior cerebral and middle cerebral arteries; for the supraclinoid internal carotid artery the measurements are about 1 mm greater (28).

The technique of intravenous digital subtraction angiography may find a role in the evaluation of intracranial aneurysms. Some centers are using this technique as a screening procedure (55). However, digital subtraction angiography by selective arterial injection is probably a more useful technique. The authors are increasingly using this procedure because it minimizes the amount of dye injected and offers rapid and less expensive imaging of the various arterial territories. They still prefer to have standard angiograms of the particular injections that demonstrate the aneurysm in question, but the digital subtraction films of a selective arterial injection are sufficient for either purpose.

In patients with a clear-cut diagnosis of subarachnoid hemorrhage in whom the initial angiogram is negative, the authors repeat the study after 1 week (or later if there is a significant neurologic deficit), because a lesion may occasionally be disclosed (this is especially true when vasospasm is present in the initial study) (Fig. 10.2). If the second study is negative and shows no vasospasm, the patient is discharged and no further study is done unless additional symptoms appear.

When the diagnosis of subarachnoid hemorrhage seems highly likely on clinical grounds (for example, intense sudden headache during intercourse) but CT and lumbar puncture are negative, the authors have performed angiography and occasionally discovered an aneurysm.

LUMBAR PUNCTURE

With the greater availability of CT scanners, lumbar puncture is less necessary to make a diagnosis of subarachnoid hemorrhage. However, when a CT scanner is not available, it is perfectly reasonable to confirm the diagnosis of subarachnoid hemorrhage by a lumbar puncture which is safe if the patient does not have focal neurologic deficits and has no papilledema. When a CT scanner is available and the diagnosis of subarachnoid hemorrhage is suspected, it is best to do a scan first and then, if the CT scan is negative, a lumbar puncture can be safely done to verify or exclude this diagnosis. Lumbar puncture is more sensitive than CT to diagnose subarachnoid hemorrhage. If the lumbar puncture is negative, it should be repeated after 24 hours because migration of blood to the lumbar area may require some time. It is preferable to have the lumbar puncture performed by an experienced physician because the diagnosis of subarachnoid hemorrhage rests on these findings and a misinterpretation of such could occur with a traumatic tap. A similar number of red blood cells in the first and last tubes and presence of xanthochromia are important to confirm the diagnosis of subarachnoid hemorrhage.

NATURAL HISTORY

The natural history of asymptomatic, incidental, unruptured aneurysms is not well known. It has been established that they rupture at a rate of approximately 2–3%/year (100). A somewhat lower chance of rupture has been estimated by a different method involving prevalence figures and decremental life table analysis (23).

The natural history of ruptured intracranial aneurysms is much better know. Approximately 20% of the patients die before ever reaching medical attention. Of those who reach the hospital, about 30% die during the next several days or weeks as a result of the initial hemorrhage or its complications. If the aneurysm is left untreated, about one-third of the patients who recover from the initial hemorrhage will die as a consequence of recurrent bleeding during the next 6 months. Even at the end of 6 months, however, a patient who has recovered from an initial rupture continues to have about a 3%/year chance of having another major hemorrhage (7, 35, 44, 99).

Earlier data indicated that the highest peak of rebleeding occurred during the second week after aneurysmal hemorrhage (7). Data from the cooperative study on the timing of aneurysm surgery indicate that the highest peak of rebleeding occurs during the first 24 hours (46). This study has indicated that the chance of rebleeding within the first day is about 4%. After 48 hours the chance of rebleeding appears to be about 1.5%/day with a cumulative rebleeding rate of 19% by the end of 2 weeks. In this particular study the 2-week cumulative rebleeding rate was 14.5% for patients taking antifibrinolytic agents and 26.5% for those patients not treated with antifibrinolytic agents.

MANAGEMENT

General Measures

Table 10.5 lists some of the general measures that the authors use routinely in the preoperative care of patients with subarachnoid hemorrhage. Bed rest is

Table 10.5.
Medical Therapy for Aneurysmal Subarachnoid Hemorrhage

1. Bed rest in a quiet room; avoid unnecessary stimulation.
2. Fluid administration aimed to maintain normal circulating volume and normal nutrition.
3. Elastic stockings or pneumatic compression boots.
4. ϵ-aminocaproic acid (30 g/day intravenously via continuous infusion) in patients not at significant risk for vasospasm.
5. Anticonvulsants (diphenylhydantoin, 300 mg/day).
6. Stool softeners (Colace, 100 mg three times a day). A bedside commode may be allowed.
7. For agitation, phenobarbital (15-30 mg intramuscularly or orally every 3 hours) or Haldol (0.5–2 mg intravenously or intramuscularly).
8. For hypertension, hydralazine (5–20 mg intramuscularly every 3 hours) to bring the systolic pressure below 150 mm Hg without causing drowsiness. In some cases propranolol is used, and occasionally resistant hypertension requires intravenous nitroprusside for control.
9. Methylprednisolone (16–80 mg orally or intravenously every 6 hours) or equivalent to reduce cerebral swelling in symptomatic patients.
10. Cimetidine is given (300 mg orally or intravenously every 8 hours) along with antacid by mouth or gastric tube every 3 hours for patients on corticosteroid treatment.
11. Codeine for headache (30–60 mg orally or intramuscularly every 3–4 hours). Demerol can be used if necessary.

recommended. The authors prefer to allow patients to use a bedside commode rather than subject them to the stress of having to use a bedpan while lying flat in bed. The "aneurysmal precautions" have been considerably liberalized. There seems to be no particular advantage in keeping the patient in a dark room with total sensory deprivation, particularly if the patient is awake and photophobia is not a major problem. They are allowed to watch television or listen to their favorite music. Likewise, it may be more stressful for them to be totally isolated than to have the comfort of regular visits by immediate members of the family or close friends.

Proper nutrition is very important. There is no reason for awake patients with a subarachnoid hemorrhage to have anything less than a regular diet. Early attention to fluid balance is also of great importance (58). These patients tend to become dehydrated and depleted of intravascular volume with a tendency to become hyponatremic. Previously, there was an inclination to keep these patients dehydrated in an effort to reduce intracranial pressure. This still may be needed in some patients with symptoms and signs of increased intracranial pressure, but it does not appear to be necessary routinely, and indeed it may be dangerous in some patients.

The authors recommend the use of corticosteroids only in those patients with major neurologic deficits or with obvious signs of increased intracranial pressure or severe headache. Regular use of stool softeners and laxatives, as well as appropriate diet, will minimize the chances of constipation. The intelligent use of analgesics and sedatives is important to eliminate the stress of pain and at the same time prevent excessive iatrogenic drowsiness, which may affect the neurologic examination and predispose to pulmonary complications. Elastic stockings or pneumatic compression boots may be helpful in preventing thrombophlebitis.

Table 10.6 is a brief summary of some of the most important complications seen after subarachnoid hemorrhage. These will be discussed in the subsequent sections.

Seizures

The routine use of anticonvulsants may reduce the 5% incidence of early seizures in patients after subarachnoid hemorrhage (35). Having patients on anticonvulsant drugs preoperatively may also minimize the risk of postoperative seizures.

Hypertension and Blood Pressure Control

The previous tendency to treat patients with subarachnoid hemorrhage vigorously with antihypertensive agents, even though they were normotensive, has gradually been modified. The authors presently aim at a normotensive level during the preoperative period. If the patient presents with hypertension, a gradual careful lowering of the blood pressure is desired. This is best accomplished with rapidly reversible antihypertensive agents. The authors prefer nitroprusside or nitroglycerin when hypertension is severe. Hydralazine or propranolol may be used if the elevation of the blood pressure is not so marked. The use of longer acting antihypertensive agents is relatively contraindicated, because one may wish to elevate the blood pressure rather rapidly if clinical vasospasm supervenes. It is best to avoid the use of diuretic agents, since volume depletion is detrimental to patients at risk for developing vasospasm (75).

Because there is an early peak of rebleeding during the first 2 days after subarachnoid hemorrhage, it may be sensible to lower the blood pressure to moderate hypotensive levels with rapidly reversible medications during this early period, inasmuch as vasospasm is not usually present at this stage (46). After the second day, the blood pressure may be allowed to rise to normotensive levels because by then the risk of rebleeding is somewhat lower and the risk of vasospasm begins to become more significant.

Table 10.6.
Complications of Subarachnoid Hemorrhage

Complications	Clinical Features	Diagnostic Tests	Therapy
Seizures	Focal motor seizures	CT, EEG	Anticonvulsants
Hypertension	Increased blood pressure		Rapidly reversible antihypertensive medication (cautiously)
Recurrent subarachnoid hemorrhage	Recurrent headache or deterioration	CT or lumbar puncture	Aneurysm obliteration and/or ϵ-aminocaproic acid
Intracerebral hematoma	Immediate focal deficit	CT	Steroids, mannitol, consider evacuation
Increased intracranial pressure	Headache, decreased alertness	CT, ventricular puncture, subarachnoid bolt	Steroids, mannitol, hyperventilation
Cardiac problems	Arrhythmia, myocardial infarct	ECG, cardiac enzymes	Therapy of arrhythmia; therapy of myocardial infarction
Hypothalamic disturbance: syndrome of inappropriate antidiuretic hormone secretion	Neurologic deterioration	Serum and urine electrolytes, blood volume	Water restriction; volume replacement with colloid.
Hydrocephalus	Decreased alertness, increased deficit	CT	Ventricular drainage or ventriculoperitoneal shunt (delay if possible until after clipping)
Vasospasm and infarction	Delayed focal deficit	CT, angiography, cerebral blood flow	Volume replacement, with colloid, blood pressure increase with vasopressors
Vitreous hemorrhage	Blindness	Funduscopy	Observation; sometimes vitrectomy
Thrombophlebitis and pulmonary embolism	Swollen leg, chest pain	Noninvasive tests, venogram, pulmonary angiogram	Umbrella

Recurrent Hemorrhage and Antifibrinolytic Agents

Antifibrinolytic agents have been given to patients with subarachnoid hemorrhage in an effort to retard lysis of the fibrin-platelet plug responsible for sealing the aneurysmal rent and thus prevent rebleeding (61, 64). Initial uncontrolled studies showed that the rebleeding rate over a period of about 2 weeks was decreased substantially in patients in whom antifibrinolytic agents were used when compared to historical controls. Later, several large controlled studies showed substantial benefit from antifibrinolytic agents, but other studies did not show such a benefit (1, 73). The statistical power of those studies that show a benefit is greater than that of the studies not showing a benefit (32). However, it is clear that antifibrinolytic agents increase the incidence of thrombophlebitis and possibly also of pulmonary embolism when used during the preoperative period in patients on bed rest. In addition, they are responsible for less frequent complications, including allergic reactions, myoglobinuria (which rarely causes renal damage), and hematologic disorders (that rarely may lead to a generalized bleeding diathesis) (1, 61). More importantly, it has now become well established that the incidence of hydrocephalus and ischemic complications is higher in patients treated with antifibrinolytic agents (1, 47, 60). Two large studies, one uncontrolled (47) and one controlled (60), showed that, even though the incidence of rebleeding is reduced by half in patients treated with antifibrinolytic agents, the incidence of serious ischemic complications probably attributable to vasospasm is doubled. Therefore, the overall results are almost identical regardless of whether the patients are treated with antifibrinolytic agents. Based on these results and on the authors' own experience, the authors presently treat with antifibrinolytic agents only those aneurysm patients with a thin layer of blood on the early CT scan in whom vasospasm is unlikely to develop (49). The patients with thick clots in the basal cistern who usually develop vasospasm are presently not treated with antifibrinolytic agents.

Intracranial Hypertension

Intracranial hypertension occurs almost invariably to some degree after subarachnoid hemorrhage. In the uncomplicated case, intracranial hypertension does not require specific treatment. The symptoms subside spontaneously or are ameliorated by the use of corticosteroids, and the intracranial pressure gradually returns to normal by the end of the first week. When the clinical course is complicated by intracerebral hemorrhage, vasospasm, or hydrocephalus, intracranial hypertension may be so severe as to require treatment. The important point to remember about treating intracranial hypertension is that it must be done conservatively and with great care in the patient with a ruptured aneurysm that has not been clipped. Recurrent hemorrhage can be brought about by an abrupt iatrogenic decrease in intracranial pressure after lumbar puncture, following ventricular drainage or ventriculoperitoneal shunting, and even after rapid infusion of mannitol (65, 74). Withdrawal of cerebrospinal fluid can result in significant shifts of the brain, with motion of the aneurysm in relation to fixed structures, such as the tentorium. In addition, reduction of intracranial pressure increases the transmural pressure (between the interior of the aneurysm and its environment), thus increasing the chances of another rupture. When the pressure must be lowered by ventricular or lumbar cerebrospinal fluid drainage, such drainage is done gradually, and the authors are content with levels somewhat above normal.

Whether the intracranial pressure needs to be monitored constantly in patients with severe subarachnoid hemorrhage remains controversial. In patients who are awake, monitoring of the clinical symptomatology suffices. In patients in coma, one can usually presume the presence of significant intracranial hypertension if the comatose state is due to major intracerebral or intraventricular hemorrhage. In these patients the intracranial hypertension can be treated empirically without the necessity for invasive monitoring. In patients in coma as a result of ischemia from vasospasm, the intracranial pressure is usually, but not necessarily always, elevated. It may be helpful in these patients to monitor the intracranial pressure to guide therapy.

Cardiac Arrhythmias

It is well known that cardiac arrhythmias occur after subarachnoid hemorrhage (18, 38, 39). Bradycardia, tachycardia, premature atrial and ventricular contractions, and, less commonly, sinus arrest may be seen. More common are electrocardiographic changes such as short P-R intervals, peaking or inversion of T waves, prolonged Q-T intervals, and tall U waves. These changes correlate highly with plasma and urinary levels of circulating catecholamines. Similar changes can be induced in animals by injections of large doses of catecholamines. Occasionally, subendocardial infarction occurs after severe subarachnoid hemorrhage in previously healthy patients. It has become evident that these effects are directly related to an abnormal release of catecholamines induced by hypothalamic dysfunction. These patients usually have other evidence of hypothalamic problems, such as increased level of circulating cortisol, abnormal circadian rhythms, abnormal metyrapone and dexamethasone suppression tests, and a variety of electrolyte disturbances thought to be due to hypothalamic dysfunction (16, 18, 37, 96).

The cardiac arrhythmias that occur in the patient with subarachnoid hemorrhage as well as the occasional frank subendocardial ischemia, which can result in cardiac failure, must be treated in the same manner as if these problems occurred in a setting other than subarachnoid hemorrhage. α and β blockers have been used effectively and a recent subarachnoid hemorrhage in no way precludes their use. Digitalis may be necessary when there is evidence of cardiac failure. Occasionally, intravenous nitroglycerin must be used to reverse some of the overt ischemic changes (19, 68, 92, 98).

Electrolyte Imbalance

The most severe form of electrolyte imbalance seen after subarachnoid hemorrhage is hypernatremia with hyperosmolarity. This occurs only rarely, indicating a grave prognosis (53, 86). Occasionally, such hypernatremia leads to the syndrome of hyperosmolar coma, which frequently is associated with severe intracranial hypertension and can be irreversible. Treatment is difficult because attempts to treat the hypernatremia and hyperosmolarity with hypotonic solutions almost invariably lead to an exacerbation of intracranial hypertension.

Hyponatremia is frequently seen after subarachnoid hemorrhage, and, fortunately, its treatment is more effective. The incidence of hyponatremia seems to correlate with the severity of the initial subarachnoid hemorrhage (62) and the onset of the clinical symptoms of vasospasm (39). Typically, the serum sodium starts falling about the fourth day after subarachnoid hemorrhage, and, if uncorrected, severe hyponatremia will develop by the end of the first week (35, 39). In one report it was found that patients with subarachnoid hemorrhage who developed hyponatremia were more prone to develop cerebral infarction, especially when treated with fluid restriction (95). These hyponatremic patients usually have the high urinary sodium and osmolarity that one would expect to find in patients with inappropriate secretion of antidiuretic hormone. However, in contradistinction to such patients, the typical patient with subarachnoid hemorrhage and hyponatremia has a contracted intravascular volume (46, 62, 63). The decrease in intravascular volume can be due to a number of factors, including supine diuresis secondary to increased thoracic blood volume, negative nitrogen balance, decreased erythropoiesis, increased levels of catecholamines, and phlebotomy (62). It is thought that the initial event is volume depletion and excessive natriuresis, which may be stimulated by some unknown brain natriuretic substance. The contraction of the intravascular volume then leads to an "appropriate" excessive release of antidiuretic hormone, which exacerbates the hyponatremia. The logical treatment for this syndrome is not only water restriction, but also replenishment of the intravascular volume with colloid and/or blood (63).

There is still some controversy as to whether these patients fare better with a slightly lower than normal hematocrit, as is suggested by experiments in which increased regional cerebral blood flow was found to accompany dilutional hypervolemia (101, 102). Empirically, the authors aim at maintaining the hematocrit in the range of 30–35% in order to achieve what appears to be the optimal balance between the rheologic advantages of hemodilution and the decrease in oxygen delivery capacity of blood that becomes an important factor at hematocrits below 30% (101).

Hydrocephalus

Hydrocephalus after subarachnoid hemorrhage usually develops in one of three general patterns. Acute hydrocephalus can be seen immediately. The symptomatology can be very dramatic, leading to coma and decerebration. This syndrome is usually associated with intraventricular hemorrhage, which can be seen with aneurysms in almost any location but is more common with anterior communicating and basilar aneurysms. This condition must be treated by immediate ventriculostomy. Frequently, bilateral ventriculostomies need to be placed because there is a thick clot in the third ventricle that may block either or both foramina of Monro. If the hemorrhage has been severe enough, ventriculostomies usually will not function well, but in an occasional patient this maneuver will result in dramatic improvement. Other times, improvement as a result of ventricular drainage may be gradual. Ventriculostomies should not remain longer that 5–7 days because the risk of infection increases, and at that time a decision must be made as to whether to replace the ventriculostomies through a new site, proceed with an internal shunt, or omit ventricular drainage. This decision is guided by the clincial condition as well as the nature of the ventricular fluid. In general, when the fluid is still very bloody, the available shunts are incapable of handling it; therefore, another period of external ventricular drainage is advisable (34). If the patient and CT scan are unchanged upon raising the drainage bag 20 cm above the head for 24 hours, the drain may safely be removed.

A subacute form of hydrocephalus is commonly seen after subarachnoid hemorrhage. This usually develops over the first few days and almost always is communicating in nature. The authors prefer to be very conservative with these patients; the ventricles are drained or a shunt is placed only when clinical deterioration is quite significant and the patient does not respond to steroids or mannitol. The authors are hesitant to drain the ventricles because of the risk of a second hemorrhage when the ventricles are acutely decompressed, either by a shunt or by a ventricular or lumbar drain (65, 74). This subacute form of hydrocephalus frequently resolves without the need for a permanent shunt (34). When a patient deteriorates significantly (especially as regards alertness) in relation to demonstrable communicating hydrocephalus, a spinal subarachnoid catheter may be used to drain excess cerebrospinal fluid. The drainage bag is placed at head level to avoid excessive decompression.

A delayed form of hydrocephalus, sometimes with normal intracranial pressure, is also seen after subarachnoid hemorrhage (66). This usually becomes clinically manifested after the aneurysm is clipped. The patient simply fails to improve as expected and a classic syndrome of "normal pressure hydrocephalus" with dementia, sometimes with gait disturbance and occasionally with incontinence, develops. This form of normal pressure hydrocephalus often responds dramatically to a ventricular drainage procedure; when the syndrome is classic and the aneurysm has been dealt with surgically, the patient should be shunted regardless of the results of the cerebrospinal fluid flow studies, since the prognosis for improvement in these cases is favorable.

Vasospasm

Vasospasm is the most important cause of morbidity and morality in the patient who has recovered from an initial subarachnoid hemorrhage. Depending on the criteria used to define it, vasospasm can be detected on 30–70% of angiograms performed 4–12 days after subarachnoid hemorrhage from a ruptured aneurysm (93). However, only about 20–30% of patients with subarachnoid hemorrhage from a ruptured aneurysm have delayed clinical deterioration from cerebral ischemia (symptomatic vasospasm). Almost invariably, these are the patients whose angiograms show severe regional or generalized vasospasm. Of these patients, about one-half either die or are left with a serious neurologic deficit (39). Cerebral vasospasm is rarely seen, either angiographically or clinically, before the third or fourth day after subarachnoid hemorrhage. Angiographic vasospasm can sometimes persist for 3–4 weeks, but it is rare for these patients to develop symptoms if they have remained asymptomatic for the first 10–12 days after subarachnoid hemorrhage (38, 39, 93). Whether or not operation exacerbates vasospasm is very controversial. Certainly, when severe angiographic vasospasm is present and surgery is carried out during the first 10–12 days after subarachnoid hemorrhage, there is a significant incidence of postoperative morbidity as a result of vasospasm (3, 15). The authors agree that if 2 weeks have passed, patients in good preoperative conditions fare well after surgery, even in the presence of significant preoperative vasospasm (24).

The clinical syndrome of vasospasm has salient features (26, 28, 38, 39). The onset is frequently preceded by a slight increase in headache, sometimes accompanied by meningismus, as well as low-grade fever. Hyponatremia is frequently noted a day or two before the onset of symptomatic vasospasm. Most commonly there is an early disturbance of consciousness, such as confusion, disorientation, or drowsiness. Focal symptoms corresponding to the arterial territories involved usually develop after a change in sensorium, but sometimes subtle focal neurologic signs, such as pronator drift or visual hemineglect, are the first signs noted. The syndrome may progress no further and, after some fluctuations, resolve within a few days. It can progress gradually to a major focal deficit; or it can progress relentlessly, resulting in deep coma and decerebration within hours. When the anterior cerebral territory is affected, disturbances of sensorium are prominent and frontal release signs, incontinence, and akinesia are observed early and may progress to mutism. Middle cerebral arterial spasm in the dominant hemisphere leads to hemiparesis and aphasia. In the nondominant hemisphere it results in hemiparesis and anosognosia. When both middle cerebral territories or the anterior cerebral and at least one middle cerebral territory are involved, disturbances of consciousness are prominent. This is also the case when the posterior circulation is involved extensively.

The cause of vasospasm remains unknown. Vasospasm after subarachnoid hemorrhage correlates directly with the amount of blood in the subarachnoid space (25, 26, 49, 59). Furthermore, the fact that vasospasm usually develops in vessels surrounded by thick layers of blood indicates that the blood itself may be directly responsible for the spasm. How blood around these vessels leads to vasospasm is not presently known, although many theories have been proposed. Endogenous substances that have been thought to operate in the genesis of vasospasm include serotonin, catecholamines, prostaglandins, angiotensin, and hemoglobin derivatives, particularly oxyhemoglobin (5, 38, 39, 67, 88, 94, 98, 107). In addition to chemical factors, some mechanical factors, such as distortion of arachnoidal strands and compression of the vessels within the distended arachnoidal cisterns, are believed to play a role (8). Neurogenic factors may also be important. There is a rich plexus of adrenergic fibers within the adventitial layers of the pial vasculature. The dense core vesicles located in the varicosities within these nerve fibers are responsible not only for the synthesis and release of norepinephrine, but also for the reuptake of this neurotransmitter and thus for the regulation of its effect on the smooth muscle cell. After subarachnoid hemorrhage these dense core vesicles disappear and the cerebral blood vessels may then be rendered abnormally susceptible to the effect of circulating catecholamines, which are usually elevated in these patients (69, 70)

It has become increasingly clear that vasospasm, whether induced experimentally or occurring after spontaneous subarachnoid hemorrhage, can be associated with morphologic changes in the affected blood vessels, which include myonecrosis, infiltration of the media with macrophages, swelling and disruption of the intima, and subendothelial fibrosis. These changes may make the spasm relatively irreversible and unresponsive to pharmacologic manipulation (2, 14, 38, 39, 41, 87, 89). In addition, evidence from the authors' laboratory indicates that normally some of the nourishment of cerebral blood vessels that lack vasa vasorum may come directly from cerebrospinal fluid through adventitial pores. The adventitial infiltration by erythrocytes, leukocytes, and mast cells seen in vasospasm may block these pores and impair normal nourishment of these vessels (39, 54, 89, 106).

There is probably not a single cause of vasospasm. It is possible that vasoactive substances, such as serotonin, prostaglandins, and catecholamines, released from platelets within the clot in the subarachnoid space, in some way sensitize the arterial wall to the effects of certain by-products of hemoglobin degradation. These by-products take several days to appear because the lysis of red blood cells in the subarachnoid space is gradual. Another factor may be the abnormal sensitivity of these blood vessels to catecholamines. These factors may lead to a derangement of the energy processes within the membrane of the cell and intracellular organelles that permits abnormally high accumulation of sarcoplasmic calcium, thus resulting in sustained contraction. This contraction, which may begin as a reversible physiologic response, may be sufficiently protracted and severe to cause structural damage to the vessel wall, perhaps by interfering with its normal nutrition. If the patient survives, the vessels regain a normal appearance, if not function, within a few weeks (39).

There is no currently available prophylaxis against vasospasm that has been conclusively proved to be effective. There is suggestive evidence that the calcium channel blocker nimodipine may be beneficial. In a well-designed double-blind controlled study involving 125 patients, no substantial difference was found in overall outcome between patients given nimodipine and control subjects (6). There was also no significant difference in the incidence of vasospasm. However, when the causes of deterioration were analyzed in a retrospective but blinded fashion, it was found that in the control group 16 patients developed ischemic symptoms, eight of whom had a poor outcome or died; in the group treated with nimodipine, 13 patients developed ischemic symptoms, but only one of them had a permanent bad outcome (6). Two other groups have also reported satisfactory results using intravenous nimodipine after early surgery (9, 56). In another study it was found that low doses of reserpine and oral kanamycin, which reduce blood levels of serotonin and other catecholamines without substantially reducing the systemic blood pressure, were effective in preventing experimental vasospasm (104, 105). Subsequent clinical studies have suggested that this regimen is of some value in preventing symptomatic postoperative vasospasm (51, 103). Experimental studies have also demonstrated satisfactory prevention of experimental vasospasm by nitroglycerin (50, 90).

Empirically, the authors maintain an elevated intravascular volume in patients at high risk of developing vasospasm (those patients with thick blood clots on the basal cisterns on the initial CT scan). This is accomplished by giving them 3–5 units of serum albumin per day if they are young and have no history of cardiac disease. In older patients, or in patients with a history of cardiac disease, the authors use a central venous pressure line and try to maintain the central venous pressure at a level of 6–10 cm H_2O. This is done even in asymptomatic patients in an effort to prevent vasospasm; so far, the authors have a favorable clinical impression of the effectiveness of this regimen (39).

Once symptomatic vasospasm develops, the only treatment generally accepted to be effective is to increase cerebral perfusion pressure (24, 39, 45, 52, 84, 97). This can be practically accomplished by increasing the intravascular volume, artificially elevating the blood pressure, and reducing intracranial pressure. The latter can be accomplished by ventricular drainage when there is ventriculomegaly or by mannitol infusions in the absence of enlarged ventricles. Intravascular volume can be increased with infusions of crystalloid and colloid or blood. The authors aim to keep the hematocrit between 30–35% under the presumption that dilutional hypervolemia is helpful. In all patients the central venous pressure should be monitored, and in elderly patients or in patients with a history of cardiac disease, a Swan-Ganz line is essential. Digitalis may be used in patients with evidence of pulmonary vascular congestion or a deteriorating cardiac output. The blood pressure can be elevated with vasopressors. The authors have found phenylephrine and dopamine particularly helpful and safe in this respect. They use induced hypertension even in patients with unclipped aneurysms if they are deteriorating clinically. The authors do not hesitate to bring the blood pressure up to levels of approximately 180 mm Hg systolic in patients with unclipped aneurysms. During the postoperative period, the blood pressure can be increased to somewhat higher levels, because there is no danger of aneurysmal rupture once the aneurysm is clipped. If instituted early, the regimen of volume expansion and hypertension may be successful in approximately 50% of patients with symptomatic vasospasm (39, 45). Patients with a milder syndrome respond more rapidly and completely. The regimen has to be continued sometimes for several days until the patient becomes much improved or asymptomatic. At that point, the patient may be gradually weaned off hypertensive agents. Sometimes the symptoms will recur and the treatment will need to be continued for several more days. The authors have had patients on vasopressors for as long as a week. The administration of mannitol (100 g intravenously over 8 hours) may improve cerebral blood flow and neurologic function (without significant change in intracranial pressure) in patients with vasospasm and ischemia (43). However, care must be taken to replace fluid loss, usually with a colloid solution such as albumin, to prevent volume depletion.

Other Preoperative Complications

Patients with subarachnoid hemorrhage are subject to a number of preoperative complications other than those already described. Thrombophlebitis and pulmonary embolism are particularly threatening in patients receiving antifibrinolytic agents. The management of these conditions usually will involve placing an intravascular umbrella, since anticoagulation is contraindicated until the aneurysm is secured. Pulmonary and bladder infections may occur and require treatment. Drug reactions, such as a diphenylhydantoin allergy, can present as a fever of unknown etiology (34).

REFERENCES

1. Adams HP Jr: Current status of antifibrinolytic therapy for treatment of patients with aneurysmal subarachnoid hemorrhage. Stroke 16:23–27, 1981.
2. Alksne JF, Greenhoot JH: Experimental catecholamine-induced cerebral vasospasm: Myonecrosis in vessel wall. J Neurosurg 41:440–445, 1974.
3. Allcock JM, Canham PB: Angiographic study of the growth of intracranial aneurysms. J Neurosurg 45:617–621, 1976.
4. Allcock JM, Drake CG: Ruptured intracranial aneurysms—The role of arterial spasm. J Neurosurg 22:21–29, 1965.
5. Allen GS, Henderson LM, Chow NS, French LA: Cerebral arterial spasm. I. In vitro contractile activity of vasoactive agents on canine basilar and middle cerebral arteries. J Neurosurg 40:433–441, 1974.
6. Allen GS, Hyo SA, Preziosi TJ, Battye R, Boone SC, Chou SN, Kelly DL, Weir BK, Crabbe RA, Lavik PJ, Rosenbloom SB, Dorsey FC, Ingram CR, Mellits DE, Bertsch LA, Boisvert DPJ, Hundley, MB, Johnson RK, Strom JA, Transou CR: Ce-

rebral arterial spasm—controlled trial of nimodipine in patients with subarachnoid hemorrhage. *N Engl J Med* 308:619–624, 1983.
7. Alvord EC Jr, Thorn RB: Natural history of subarachnoid hemorrhage: Early prognosis. *Clin Neurosurg* 24:167–175, 1977.
8. Arutinunov AL, Baron MA, Majorova NA: The role of mechanical factors in the pathogenesis of short term and prolonged spasm of the cerebral arteries. *J Neurosurg* 40:459–472, 1974.
9. Auer LM: Acute operation and preventive nimodipine improve outcome in patients with ruptured cerebral aneurysms. *Neurosurgery* 15:57–66, 1984.
10. Bannerman RM, Ingall GB, Graf CJ: The familial incidence of intracranial aneurysms. *Neurology (NY)* 20:283–292, 1970.
11. Benoit BG, Wortzman G: Traumatic cerebral aneurysms: Clinical features and natural history. *J Neurol Neurosurg Psychiatry* 36:127–138, 1973.
12. Botterell EH, Lougheed WM, Scott JW, Vandewater SL: Hypothermia, and interruption of carotid, or carotid and vertebral circulation, in the surgical management of intracranial aneurysms. *J Neurosurg* 13:1–42, 1956.
13. Chason JL, Hindman WM: Berry aneurysms of the circle of Willis. *Neurology (NY)* 8:41–44, 1958.
14. Conway LW, McDonald LW: Structural changes of the intradural arteries following subarachnoid hemorrhage. *J Neurosurg* 37:715–723, 1972.
15. Cooper PR, Shucart WA, Tenner M, Hussain S: Preoperative arteriographic spasm and outcome from aneurysm operation. *Neurosurgery* 7:587–592, 1980.
16. Crompton MR: Hypothalamic lesions following the rupture of cerebral berry aneurysms. *Brain* 86:301–314, 1963.
17. Crompton MR: The pathology of subarachnoid hemorrhage. *J R Coll Physicians Lond* 7:235–237, 1973.
18. Cruickshank JM, Neil-Dwyer G, Brice J: Electrocardiographic changes and their prognostic significance in subarachnoid hemorrhage. *J Neurol Neurosurg Psychiatry* 37:755–759, 1974.
19. Cruickshank JM, Neil-Dwyer G, Stott AW: Possible role of catecholamines, corticosteroids, and potassium in production of electrocardiographic abnormalities associated with subarachnoid hemorrhage. *Br Heart J* 36:697–706, 1974.
20. Damasio H, Seabra-Gomes R, da Silva JP, Damasio AR, Antunes JL: Multiple cerebral aneurysms and cardiac myxoma. *Arch Neurol* 32:269–270, 1975.
21. Davis KR, Kistler JP, Heros RC, Davis JM: Neuroradiologic approach to the patient with a diagnosis of subarachnoid hemorrhage. *Radiol Clin North AM* 20:87–94, 1982.
22. Davis KR, New PFJ, Ojemann RG, Crowell RM, Morawetz RB, Roberson GH: Computed tomographic evaluation of hemorrhage secondary to intracranial aneurysm. *AJR* 127:143–153, 1976.
23. Dell S: Asymptomatic cerebral aneurysm: Assessment of its risk of rupture. *Neurosurgery* 10:162–166, 1982.
24. Drake CG: Management of cerebral aneurysm. *Stroke* 12:273–283, 1981.
25. Fisher CM, Kistler JP, Davis JM: The correlation of cerebral vasospasm and the amount of subarachnoid blood detected by computerized cranial tomography after aneurysm rupture. In Wilkins RH (ed): *Cerebral Arterial Spasm*. Baltimore, Williams & Wilkins, 1979, pp 397–408.
26. Fisher CM, Kistler JP, Davis JM: Relation of cerebral vasospasm to subarachnoid hemorrhage visualized by computerized tomographic scanning. *Neurosurgery* 6:1–9, 1980.
27. Fisher CM, Ojemann RG: Basal rupture of saccular aneurysm. A pathological case report. *J Neurosurg* 48:642–644, 1978.
28. Fisher CM, Roberson GH, Ojemann RG: Cerebral vasospasm with ruptured saccular aneurysm—the clinical manifestations. *Neurosurgery* 1:245–248, 1977.
29. Fleisher AS, Patton JM, Tindall GT: Cerebral aneurysms of traumatic origin. *Surg Neurol* 4:233–239, 1975.
30. Fox JL, Ko JP: Familial intracranial aneurysms: Six cases among 13 siblings. *J Neurosurg* 53:501–503, 1980.
31. Graf CJ: Familial intracranial aneurysms: Report of four cases. *J Neurosurg* 25:304–307, 1966.
32. Haines S: Are antifibrinolytic agents useful after subarachnoid hemorrhage? In Warlow CP, Garfield J (eds): *Dilemnas in the Management of the Neurological Patient*. London, Churchill Livingstone, 1983.
33. Hashimoto I: Familial intracranial aneurysms and cerebral vascular anomalies. *J Neurosurg* 46:419–427, 1977.
34. Heros RC: Preoperative management of the patient with a ruptured intracranial aneurysm. *Semin Neurol* 4:430–438, 1984.
35. Heros RC, Kistler JP: Intracranial arterial aneurysm—an update. *Stroke* 14:628–631, 1983.
36. Heros RC, Kistler JP: Intracranial arterial aneurysm—An update. *Stroke* 14:628–631, 1983.
37. Heros RC, Zervas NT: Subarachnoid hemorrhage. *Annu Rev Med* 34:367–375, 1983.
38. Heros RC, Zervas NT, Negoro M: Cerebral vasospasm. *Surg Neurol* 5:354–362, 1976.
39. Heros RC, Zervas NT, Varsos V: Cerebral vasospasm after subarachnoid hemorrhage: An update. *Ann Neurol* 14:599–608, 1983.
40. Housepian EM, Pool JL: A systematic analysis of intracranial aneurysms from the autopsy file of the Presbyterian Hospital, 1914 to 1956. *J Neuropathol Exp Neurol* 17:409–423, 1958.
41. Hughes JT, Schianchi PM: Cerebral artery spasm: A histological study at necropsy of the blood vessels in cases of subarachnoid hemorrhage. *J Neurosurg* 48:515–525, 1978.
42. Hunt WE, Hess RM: Surgical risk as related to time of intervention in the repair of intracranial aneurysms. *J Neurosurg* 28:14–20, 1968.
43. Jafar JJ, John LM, Mullan SF: The effect of mannitol on cerebral blood flow. *J Neurosurg* 64:754–759, 1986.
44. Jane JA, Winn HR, Richardson AE: The natural history of intracranial aneurysms: Rebleeding rates during the acute and long term period and implication for surgical management. *Clin Neurosurg* 24:176–184, 1977.
45. Kassell NF, Peerless SJ, Durward QJ, Beck DW, Drake CG, Adams HP: Treatment of ischemic deficits from vasospasm with intravascular volume expansion and induced arterial hypertension. *Neurosurgery* 11:337–343, 1982.
46. Kassell NF, Torner JC: Aneurysmal rebleeding: A preliminary report from the cooperative aneurysm study. *Neurosurgery* 13:479–481, 1983.
47. Kassell NF, Torner JC, Adams HP Jr: Antifibrinolytic therapy in the acute period following aneurysmal subarachnoid hemorrhage. Preliminary observations from the Cooperative Aneurysm Study. *J Neurosurg* 61:225–230, 1984.
48. King RB, Saba MI: Forewarnings of major subarachnoid hemorrhage due to congenital berry aneursym. *NY State J Med* 74:638–639, 1974.
49. Kistler JP, Crowell RM, Davis KR, Heros R, Ojemann RG, Zervas T, Fisher CM: The relation of cerebral vasospasm to the extent and location of subarachnoid blood visualized by CT scan: A prospective study. *Neurology* 33:424–436, 1983.
50. Kistler JP, Lees RS, Candia G, Zervas NT, Crowell RM, Ojemann RG: Intravenous nitroglycerin in experimental cerebral vasospasm: A preliminary report. *Stroke* 10:26–29, 1979.
51. Knuckey NW, Stokes BAR: Medical management of patients following a ruptured cerebral aneurysm with epsilon-aminocaproic acid, kanamycin and reserpine. *Surg Neurol* 17:181–184, 1982.
52. Kosnik EJ, Hunt WE: Postoperative hypertension in the management of patients with intracranial arterial aneurysms. *J Neurosurg* 45:148–154, 1976.
53. Landolt AM, Yasargil MG, Krayenbuhl H: Disturbances of the serum electrolytes after surgery of intracranial arterial aneurysm. *J Neurosurg* 37:210–218, 1972.

54. Liszczak TM, Varsos VG, Black PMcL, Kistler JP, Zervas NT: Cerebral arterial constriction after experimental subarachnoid hemorrhage is associated with blood components within the arterial wall. *J Neurosurg* 58:18–26, 1983.
55. Little JR, Furlan AJ, Modic MT, Bryerton B, Weinstein MA: Intravenous digital subtraction angiography: Application to cerebrovascular surgery. *Neurosurgery* 9:129–136, 1981.
56. Ljunggren B: Data presented at the annual meeting of the Congress of Neurological Surgeons, Hawaii, 1985.
57. Locksley HB: Natural history of subarachnoid hemorrhage, intracranial aneurysm and arteriovenous malformations: Based on 6368 cases in the cooperative study. Parts I and II. In Sahs AL, Perret GE, Locksley HB, Nishioka H (eds): *Intracranial Aneurysms and Subarachnoid Hemorrhage: A Cooperative Study*. Philadelphia, JB Lippincott, 1969, pp37–108.
58. Maroon JC, Nelson PB: Hypovolemia in patients with subarachnoid hemorrhage. Therapeutic implications. *Neurosurgery* 4:223–226, 1979.
59. Mizukami M, Takemae T, Tazawa T, Kawase T, Matsuzaki T: Value of computed tomography in the prediction of cerebral vasospasm after aneurysm rupture. *Neurosurgery* 7:583–586, 1980.
60. Muizelaar JP: Antifibrinolytics in subarachnoid hemorrhage: A randomized double blind placebo controlled study with 479 patients. *Stroke* 15:188–189, 1984.
61. Mullan S, Dawley J: Antifibrinolytic therapy for intracranial aneurysms. *J Neurosurg* 28:21–23, 1968.
62. Nelson PB, Seif SM, Maroon JC, Robinson AG: Hyponatremia in patients with subarachnoid hemorrhage: a study of vasopressin and blood volume. In Wilkins RH (ed): *Cerebral Arterial Spasm*. Baltimore, Williams & Wilkins, 1979, pp 654–658.
63. Nelson PB, Seif SM, Maroon JC, Robinson AG: Hyponatremia in intracranial disease: Perhaps not the syndrome of inappropriate secretion of anti-diuretic hormone (SIADH). *J Neurosurg* 55:938–941, 1981.
64. Norlen G, Thulin CA: Experiences with epsilon-amino caproic acid in neurosurgery. A preliminary report. *Neurochirurgia* 10:81–86, 1967.
65. Nornes H: The role of intracranial pressure in the arrest of hemorrhage in patients with ruptured intracranial aneurysm. *J Neurosurg* 39:226–234, 1973.
66. Ojemann RG: Normal pressure hydrocephalus. *Clin Neurosurg* 18:337–370, 1971.
67. Ozaki N, Mullan S: Possible role of the erythrocyte in causing prolonged cerebral vasospasm. *J Neurosurg* 51:773–778, 1979.
68. Peerless SJ: Pre- and postoperative management of cerebral aneurysms. *Clin Neurosurg* 26:209–231, 1979.
69. Peerless SJ, Griffiths JC: Plasma catecholamines following subarachnoid hemorrhage. *Ann R Coll Physicians Can* 5:48–49, 1972.
70. Peerless, SJ, Yasargil MG: Adrenergic innervation of the cerebral blood vessels in the rabbit. *J Neurosurg* 35:148–154, 1971.
71. Perret G, Nishioka H: Report on the cooperative study of intracranial aneurysms and subarachnoid hemorrhage. Section VI arteriovenous malformations. *J Neurosurg* 25:467–490, 1966.
72. Phillips LH, Whisnant JP, O'Fallon WM, Sundt TM Jr: Unchanging pattern of subarachnoid hemorrhage in a community. *Neurology* 30:1034–1040, 1980.
73. Ramirez-Lassepas M: Antifibrinolytic therapy in subarachnoid hemorrhage caused by ruptured intracranial aneurysms. *Neurology* 31:316–322, 1981.
74. Rosenorn J, Westergaard L, Hansen P: Mannitol-induced rebleeding from intracranial aneurysm. Case report. *J Neurosurg* 59:529–530, 1983.
75. Rosenwasser RH, Delgado TE, Buchheit WA, Freed MH: Control of hypertension and prophylaxis against vasospasm in cases of subarachnoid hemorrhage: A preliminary report. *Neurosurgery* 12:658–661, 1983.
76. Sahs AL, Nibbelink DW, Torner JC (eds): *Aneurysmal Subarachnoid Hemorrhage*. Baltimore, Urban & Schwarzenberg, 1981.
77. Samson DS, Hodosh RM, Clark WK: Surgical management of unruptured asymptomatic aneurysms. *J Neurosurg* 46:731–734, 1977.
78. Sekhar LN, Heros RC: Origin, growth and rupture of saccular aneurysms: A review. *Neurosurgery* 8:248–260, 1981.
79. Sekhar LN, Wasserman JF: Noninvasive detection of intracranial vascular lesions using an electronic stethoscope. *J Neurosurg* 60:553–559, 1984.
80. Stehbens WE: Aneurysms and anatomical variation of cerebral arteries. *Arch Pathol* 75:45–64, 1963.
81. Stehbens WE: Histopathology of cerebral aneurysms. *Arch Neurol* 8:272–285, 1963.
82. Stehbens WE: Intracranial arterial aneurysms. In: *Pathology of the Cerebral Blood Vessels*. St Louis, CV Mosby, 1972, pp 351–470.
83. Stehbens WE: Ultrastructure of aneurysms. *Arch Neurol* 32:798–807, 1975.
84. Sundt TM Jr, Kobayashi S, Fode NC, Whisnant JP: Results and complications of surgical management of 809 intracranial aneurysms in 722 cases. *J Neurosurg* 56:753–765, 1982.
85. Suzuki J, O'Hara H: Clinicopathological study of cerebral aneurysms. Origin, rupture, repair, and growth. *J Neurosurg* 48:505–514, 1978.
86. Takaku A, Shindo K, Tanaka S, Mori T, Suzuki J: Fluid and electrolyte disturbances in patients with intracranial aneurysms. *Surg Neurol* 11:349–356, 1979.
87. Tanabe Y, Sakata K, Yamata H, Ito T, Takuda M: Cerebral vasospasm and ultrastructural changes in cerebral arterial wall: An experimental study. *J Neurosurg* 49:229–238, 1978.
88. Toda N, Shimizu K, Ohta T: Mechanism of cerebral arterial contraction induced by blood constituents. *J Neurosurg* 53:312–322, 1980.
89. Varsos VG, Liszczak TM, Han DH, Kistler JP, Vielma J, Black P McL, Heros RG, Zervas NT: Delayed cerebral vasospasm is not reversible by aminophylline, nifedipine, or papaverine in a "two-hemorrhage" canine model. *J Neurosurg* 58:11–17, 1983.
90. Von Essen C, Kistler JP, Lees RS, Zervas NT: Cerebral blood flow and intracranial pressure in the dog during intravenous infusion of nitroglycerin alone and in combination with dopamine. *Stroke* 12:331–338, 1981.
91. Waga S, Ohtsubo K, Handa H: Warning signs in intracranial aneurysms. *Surg Neurol* 3:15–20, 1975.
92. Walter P, Neil-Dwyer G, Parsons V: The effect of phentolamine and propranolol in subarachnoid hemorrhage. In Wilkins RH (ed): *Cerebral Arterial Spasm: Proceedings of the Second International Workshop*. Baltimore, Williams & Wilkins, 1980, pp 584–588.
93. Weir B, Grace M, Hansen J, Rothberg C: Time course of vasospasm in man. *J Neurosurg* 48:173–178, 1978.
94. Wellum GR, Irvine TW Jr, Zervas NT: Cerebral vasoactivity of heme proteins in vitro. *J Neurosurg* 56: 777–783, 1982.
95. Wijdicks EF, Verneulen M, Hijdra A, van Gijn J: Hyponatremia and cerebral infarction in patients with ruptured intracranial aneurysms: Is fluid restriction harmful? *Ann Neurol* 17:137–140, 1985.
96. Wilkins RH: Hypothalamic dysfunction and intracranial arterial spasm. *Surg Neurol* 4:472–480, 1975.
97. Wilkins RH: Attempted prevention or treatment of intracranial arterial spasm: A survey. In Wilkins RH (ed): *Cerebral Arterial Spasm*. Baltimore, Williams & Wilkins, 1979, pp 542–555.
98. Wilkins RH: Update-subarachnoid hemorrhage and saccular intracranial aneurysm. *Surg Neurol* 15:92–101, 1981.

99. Winn HR, Richardson AE, Jane JA: The assessment of the natural history of single cerebral aneurysms that have ruptured. In Hopkins LN, Long DM (eds): *Clinical Management of Intracranial Aneurysms*. New York, Raven Press, 1982, pp 1–10.
100. Winn HR, Richardson AE, O'Brien W, Jane JA: Long-term prognosis in untreated cerebral aneurysms. II. Late morbidity and mortality. *Ann Neurol* 4:418–426, 1978.
101. Wood JH, Simeone FA, Kron RE, Litt M: Rheological aspects of experimental hypervolemic hemodilution with low molecular weight dextran: Relationships of cortical blood flow, cardiac output and intracranial pressure to fresh blood viscosity and plasma volume. *Neurosurgery* 11:739–753, 1982.
102. Wood JH, Snyder LL, Simeone FA: Failure of intravascular volume expansion without hemodilution to elevate cortical blood flow in region of experimental focal ischemia. *J Neurosurg* 56:80–91, 1982.
103. Zervas NT, Candia M, Candia G, Kido D, Pessin MS, Rosoff CB, Bacon V: Reduced incidence of cerebral ischemia following rupture of intracranial aneurysms. *Surg Neurol* 11:339–344, 1979.
104. Zervas NT, Hori H, Rosoff CB: Experimental inhibition of serotonin by antibiotic prevention of cerebral vasospasm. *J Neurosurg* 41:59–62, 1974.
105. Zervas NT, Kuwayama A, Rosoff CB, Salzman EW: Cerebral arterial spasm: Modification by inhibition of platelet function. *Arch Neurol* 28:400–404, 1973.
106. Zervas NT, Liszczak TM, Mayberg MR, Black PMcL: Cerebrospinal fluid may nourish cerebral vessels through pathways in the adventitia that may be analogous to systemic vasa vasorum. *J Neurosurg* 56:475–481, 1982.
107. Zervas NT, Wellum GR, Peterson JW: Current concepts in experimental cerebral vasospasm. In Barnett J, Paoletti P, Flamm E, Brambilla G (eds): *Cerebrovascular Diseases: New Trends in Surgical and Medical Aspects*. Amsterdam, Elsevier/North-Holland, 1981, pp 285–296.

11
Intracranial Aneurysms: General Aspects of Surgical Treatment

INDICATIONS FOR SURGERY

The most common indication for surgical treatment of an intracranial aneurysm is subarachnoid hemorrhage. The prognosis for a patient treated conservatively after a subarachnoid hemorrhage is so poor that if the patient recovers from the effects of the initial hemorrhage, surgical treatment is indicated in almost every case (9, 41–43, 46). Exceptions are the patient with poor neurologic condition without hope of recovery or the patient with a serious medical condition with unacceptably high anesthetic risk. Old age per se is no contraindication to intracranial surgery for aneurysms, since it has been shown that these operations can be carried out with acceptable morbidity and mortality, even in elderly patients, provided they are in good medical condition (9).

A second indication for surgical treatment of intracranial aneurysm is the development of neurologic signs and symptoms referable to compression of adjacent structures by the aneurysm. This development usually implies that the aneurysm has expanded recently or that a focal hemorrhage has taken place and, therefore, it is generally assumed that under these circumstances the aneurysm is more likely to hemorrhage (57). In addition, there is some urgency to treat the aneurysm so as to reverse the neurologic deficits resulting from compression. This is particularly important when the compressed structures are cranial nerves, since the chances of recovery decrease appreciably with delay in treatment.

A third indication for surgery is embolus from the aneurysm to a distal branch. The urgency of surgery is related to possible further embolic events. Whether such lesions have a greater likelihood for hemorrhage is unknown. Recovery from the embolic event is desirable prior to surgical treatment.

The fourth indication for surgical treatment is the finding of an asymptomatic intracranial aneurysm. This is a problem of increasing significance, as newer diagnostic methodologies are increasingly more capable of detecting asymptomatic aneurysms. As has been discussed in the previous chapter, asymptomatic aneurysms carry a risk of rupture that, depending on the type of analysis, appears to be between 1 and 3%/year (6, 75). Since almost all non-giant aneurysms of the anterior circulation can be obliterated with a combined surgical morbidity and mortality of less than 2 or 3%, it appears clear that any such aneurysm of significant size should be obliterated if the patient is under 60 years of age and in good medical condition (51, 52). For patients between 60 and 70 years of age, individual judgment should be exercised. However, the authors recommend surgical treatment, even in this age bracket, if the patient is in good medical condition and if from the radiographic studies it appears that, from the surgical point of view, the aneurysm is relatively straightforward. What constitutes "significant" size for an aneurysm has been the subject of some controversy. A retrospective study suggested that aneurysms less than 1 cm in diameter had a relatively good natural history with little risk of hemorrhage (74). However, it is common knowledge among aneurysm surgeons and pathologists that many aneurysms that hemorrhage are indeed between 5 and 10 mm in diameter. It is our recommendation that if the aneurysm is at least 5–7 mm in diameter, it should be obliterated (9, 45). Surgical treatment of giant aneurysms and basilar aneurysms ordinarily carries a higher morbidity; therefore, whether such aneurysms should be treated when asymptomatic is a controversial matter that requires individual judgment, with much consideration given not only to the size, configuration, and location of the aneurysm but also to the particular surgeon's experience with these lesions (see Chapter 20).

TIMING OF SURGERY

During the early years of direct intracranial surgery for aneurysms, surgeons learned that early surgery (within the first week) carried a very high morbidity and mortality. The brain was often swollen, retraction was difficult, and vasospasm, if present, seemed to be exacerbated. This realization led to the policy of deferring intracranial surgery until at least 8–10 days after subarachnoid hemorrhage (9). During the past 10 years, first in Japan, then in Europe, and finally in the United States, a gradual shift toward very early surgery (within 72 hours of subarachnoid hemorrhage) has occurred. It was argued by the initial proponents of this approach that even though early surgery might probably carry a higher morbidity, the prevention of vasospasm by washing out the subarachnoid clots and of rebleeding by clipping the aneurysm would more than compensate, so that the overall case management morbidity and mortality would be decreased by this approach. Another argument is that early surgery would also make it safer to treat vasospasm aggressively with induced hypertension and hypervolemia, since the aneurysm would already be obliterated. The results of early surgery in relatively good grade patients reported by experienced surgeons indeed compare favorably with the best statistics available when total case management morbidity and mortality are considered (32, 37, 53, 55, 69). In poor grade patients, however, it appears that the results of early surgery are not so good. In a nationwide cooperative study carried out in Japan, the mortality rate of early direct surgery in poor risk patients was 51% and 39% when surgery was carried out within the first 24 hours or within the first week, respectively (44). It has been reported that the results of early operation are worse for patients with anterior communicating artery aneurysms than for patients with aneurysms in other locations in the anterior circle of Willis (32). There is no evidence as yet available on the results of early surgery for posterior circulation aneurysms compared with aneurysms in other sites. The recently completed large uncontrolled international cooperative study on the timing of aneurysm surgery indicated that the results of early surgery are comparable overall to the results of late surgery (30). In good grade patients, there appeared to be a slight, statistically insignificant advantage in early surgery compared with late surgery. This study indicated that, as expected, early surgery reduces the incidence of rebleeding. However, vasospasm was not prevented by early surgery. The study also found that early surgery is not any more difficult and does not result in more frequent intraoperative rupture than late surgery.

At the present time, the authors consider early surgery in patients in good clinical condition (all patients in Hunt's grade 1 or 2). Angiography is performed immediately if these patients are seen within the first 2 days after a subarachnoid hemorrhage. If an accessible small or large aneurysm of the anterior circulation or of the vertebral artery is seen, early surgery is recommended. For basilar and giant aneurysms, surgery is delayed, since in these cases, brain retraction and dissection need to be more extensive. In patients who present grade 3 or worse, the authors prefer to delay surgery. This includes any patient who is drowsy or confused or has a neurologic deficit other than a cranial nerve paresis. In these patients, surgery is planned for 10–14 days after subarachnoid hemorrhage if the patient improves clinically. Angiography is performed just before the planned day for surgery, and if severe vasospasm is seen at angiography, the operation is postponed for another week, at which time the operation takes place if the patient remains in good condition. If the patient deteriorates significantly from symptomatic vasospasm, the authors wait approximately 3 weeks from the time of initial hemorrhage and then proceed with surgery if the patient is stable, even though there still may be a significant neurologic deficit.

ANESTHESIA

Premedication

The night before surgery, steroids, if not already included in the regimen, are begun. Propranolol (Inderal) is started because this agent appears to improve the stability of blood pressure control intraoperatively. The authors use 1.5 mg/kg in two divided doses, half at bedtime and half with the premedication given 90–120 minutes before surgery. For an adult, premedication often includes diazepam (10–15 mg), droperidol (5–7.5 mg), and scopolamine (0.2 mg).

Preparation

An intravenous (IV) line, preferably a large bore plastic cannula, is established in the induction room. In many patients receiving ϵ-aminocaproic acid, suitable veins are hard to identify, and rather than cause agitation by repeated venipuncture efforts, it is better to place a small gauge needle intravenously and then to establish two large bore IV routes after the patient is anesthetized. If necessary, the external jugular vein or a leg vein may be used. If no IV line can be easily established, a mask induction of anesthesia may be necessary. Prophylactic antibiotics are given after a good IV line is in place.

A catheter is introduced into the radial artery for continuous monitoring of arterial pressure. The pressure transducer is fixed at the level of the external auditory meatus. Such monitoring is particularly important during induction, when wide swings of arterial pressure may occur. Pressor and antihypertensive agents are available for infusion; phenylephrine hydrochloride (10 mg in 250 ml 5% dextrose in water) and sodium nitroprusside (50 mg in 250 ml 5% dextrose in water shielded with tinfoil) serve well for these needs.

Induction

Once all preparations are complete, a slow induction is carried out over 10 minutes or more prior to intubation. After initial preoxygenation, sodium pentobarbital is given in increments of 50–150 mg until the patient is asleep. This is often preceded by 100–300 mg of IV fentanyl. After it is certain that the airway can be maintained, pancuronium (0.1 mg/kg) is given and hyperventilation is slowly established. A twitch monitor is applied to the ulnar nerve to assess the completeness of neuromuscular blockade. An additional increment of pentobarbital is given just prior to intubation. Ideally, at this point, the blood pressure is in the range of 100 mm Hg systolic. Laryngoscopy is carried out, and the vocal cords are sprayed with a local anesthetic solution. The blood pressure response to laryngoscopy is noted; if a substantial increase in blood pressure has occurred, an additional increment of pentobarbital is administered. Finally, with the patient stable and well anesthetized, laryngoscopy for gentle endotracheal intubation is performed. The cuff of the endotracheal tube is inflated and checked for leaks.

Controlled ventilation is preferred, with arterial pCO_2 maintained in the range of 30 torr, as demonstrated by frequently sampled arterial blood gases. The arterial blood gases likewise provide a frequent check on the adequacy of oxygenation. Prior to the application of the three-point Mayfield headrest, more pentobarbital is given to prevent hypertension.

Anesthesia is maintained with 30% O_2 in N_2O along with an inhalation agent, usually isoflurane. Intermittent doses of fentanyl and pancuronium are used as needed.

Reduction of Brain Tension

As soon as the catheter is inserted in the bladder, IV furosemide (20 mg) is administered. Most patients receive 100 gm of mannitol (or 1 gm/kg IV if they are small) during the preparation and exposure. This usually gives excellent relaxation of the brain. Steroids are continued every 4 hours.

For most cases, intraoperative aspiration of cerebrospinal fluid (CSF) is helpful in reducing brain tension. In many patients, this can be accomplished by gradual removal of CSF from the basal cisterns during the initial exposure. When this method is ineffective, especially with obliteration of cisterns by blood, direct ventricular puncture may be used to drain CSF. In some patients it may be anticipated that a lumbar subarachnoid spinal catheter for drainage of CSF may be helpful. The authors use spinal drainage routinely only for basilar artery aneurysms, when the subtemporal route is to be used, and for giant aneurysms that fill the suprasellar cisterns, making it difficult to aspirate CSF. In those cases in which a catheter (22-gauge polyethylene tubing from Portex) is used, it is introduced via a Touhy needle after the induction of anesthesia. Only a small amount of fluid is allowed to escape at the time of introduction. The catheter is placed in such a fashion that upon request, further fluid may be removed by the anesthesiologist after dural incision.

Monitoring

In addition to routine monitoring of cardiovascular parameters, the authors occasionally use intraoperative electroencephalographic monitoring when prolonged but temporary vessel occlusion is anticipated. When a small pterional exposure is planned, all but two of the standard electroencephalographic leads can be applied to the scalp. The authors have found this technique only of limited usefulness. Other centers have had satisfactory experience with indirect measurement of cortical blood flow by thermal probes and by direct intraoperative recordings of somatosensory evoked responses (4, 71). The authors tried recording visual evoked potentials in cases of giant aneurysms producing compression of the optic apparatus but, due to the delay in recording, did not find this technique of practical value.

Controlled Hypertension

Over the past few years, the authors have gradually used less and less hypotension during aneurysm surgery. They have come to depend, with increasing frequency, on temporary proximal occlusion, when feasible, for large and difficult aneurysms. For smaller straightforward aneurysms, they lower the blood pressure only to a level of 90–110 mm Hg systolic, which can usually be accomplished by increasing the anesthetic administration. In cases in which the aneurysm is in a difficult location and proximal occlusion is not practical, such as some low-lying basilar artery bifurcation aneurysms, there is still a place for relatively deep hypotension. Whenever this technique is used, frequent communication between the neuroanesthesiologist and the neurosurgeon is crucial. The combination of a low concentration of isoflurane (0.2–1.5%) with narcotics and low doses of a vasodilator (nitroglycerin) in a β-blocked patient often produces ideal conditions for induced hypotension. Occasionally, sodium nitroprusside will be required to further diminish the blood pressure. Once the aneurysm is obliterated, cerebral perfusion is maximized by volume expansion with colloid. Packed cells are rarely necessary unless there has been extensive bleeding. By using a pressor, as needed, the blood pressure is elevated to about 130 mm Hg systolic.

SURGICAL TECHNIQUE

Every aspect of surgery for intracranial aneurysm is designed to minimize brain injury during obliteration of the lesion. Neuroanesthetic techniques discussed in the preceding section reduce brain tension to allow for safer exposure and to slacken the aneurysm for safer dissection. Surgical techniques aim for safe exposure and dissection through application of microsurgical principles. Retraction of 2 cm usually provides adequate exposure. With microsurgical visualization and instrumentation, the neurosurgeon can see and dissect the plane between the aneurysm and surrounding structures. These factors have led to improved results in aneurysm surgery.

Operating Room Layout

Though many layouts may be used, the authors have found the one shown in Figure 11.1 to be useful. The operating table is positioned in the center of the room. The surgeon stands or sits at the head. For a right-handed surgeon, the scrub nurse stands to the right to facilitate passing instruments. The neuroanesthetist sits at the patient's left side, with extension tubes from the patient to the anesthesia machine as needed, particularly when the head is turned to the right. The assistant usually stands to the surgeon's left. During microsurgery, a floor-mounted microscope stands just to the left of the rostral end of the operating table. The television monitor for microsurgery is attached to the wall for viewing by the scrub nurse, neuroanesthetist, and other observers. An overhead table, or attached Mayo stand, brought up to the patient's shoulder, conveniently holds the instruments.

Instrumentation

The development of microsurgery has revolutionized the surgery of intracranial aneurysms (31, 76). The use of the operating microscope provides dramatic magnification and brilliant illumination, with reduced requirements for retraction. For most aneurysms, the authors prefer 275-mm objective, variable-angle binoculars and high-eye-point 12.5× eyepieces. If the surgeon is right-handed, the stereoscopic binocular observer tube is placed on the left. A Telstil adaptor is placed on the right side of the microscope to provide a place for video monitoring and intermittent photography.

Microsurgical instrumentation has kept pace with the development of the surgical microscope. The Greenberg self-retaining retractor provides steady, minimally traumatic brain retraction (19). Its primary post is attached horizontally to the left side of the Mayfield headrest, and secondary parts and retractor arms take a low profile to avoid inadvertent bumps. Bipolar coagulating forceps permit precise hemostasis, gentle dissection with spreading motions, and shrinkage of the aneurysmal neck (35). A variety of microsurgical dissectors aid blunt dissection of arteries and aneurysms. The fine curved Rhoton dissectors (nos. 6–8) and a straight flat microdissector are particularly helpful. Fine microscissors and arachnoid knives may be used for sharp dissection of adhesions to the sac. For aneurysm surgery, it is helpful to have three suctions available. The authors use two no. 16 or 18 suctions set to low vacuum on the controlled suction unit. The third suction is a no. 1 sucker at full vacuum, to be used in case of massive aneurysm rupture.

Positioning

For aneurysm surgery, the patient is generally positioned horizontally. This posture minimizes car-

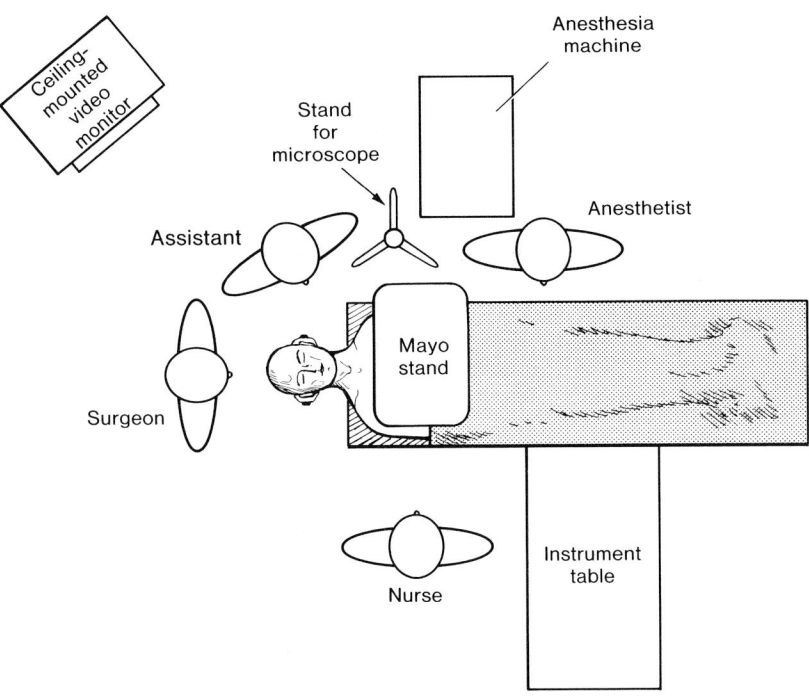

Figure 11.1. Operating room layout for most aneurysm operations performed by a right-handed surgeon.

diovascular stress and promotes cerebral perfusion, especially during induced hypotension. For most anterior circulation lesions, a supine position is best. A supine or lateral position with the head turned completely to the side is chosen for the subtemporal approach to basilar aneurysms. A lateral position with the head straight or turned slightly toward the floor ("park bench position") may be chosen for a suboccipital approach to a vertebral aneurysm. Here the knees and hips are flexed and a roll is placed under the dependent axilla. For midline posterior inferior cerebellar artery aneurysms, a prone position may be preferable. The authors almost never place the patient in the sitting position.

Several general principles govern head position. A minimal space of two fingerbreadths is maintained between the jaw and the clavicle to avoid jugular compression. The three-point Mayfield headrest provides solid fixation. For the frontotemporal or subtemporal approaches, the vertex is tilted about 15° toward the floor so the brain falls away from the base.

Turning of the head depends on the specific aneurysm site as well as the direction of the aneurysm. Figure 11.2 is a guideline for the most commonly used angles of rotation of the head for specific aneurysm sites. This angle needs to be varied from case to case, depending on the projection of the aneurysm. Most pericallosal artery aneurysms are best approached with the head in the straight position and slightly flexed (about 20° of flexion of the chin on the chest). With these aneurysms, it is easy to get lost unless the head is straight. Most ophthalmic artery aneurysms and anterior communicating aneurysms require only slight rotation of the head (30–45° to the contralateral side). With posterior communicating aneurysms, the degree of rotation depends on the direction of the aneurysm. When the aneurysm points straight laterally, only a slight degree of rotation of the head (30–45°) is necessary. However, if the aneurysm points straight posteriorly, a better profile of the aneurysm can be seen by turning the head considerably more (60–75°). This po-

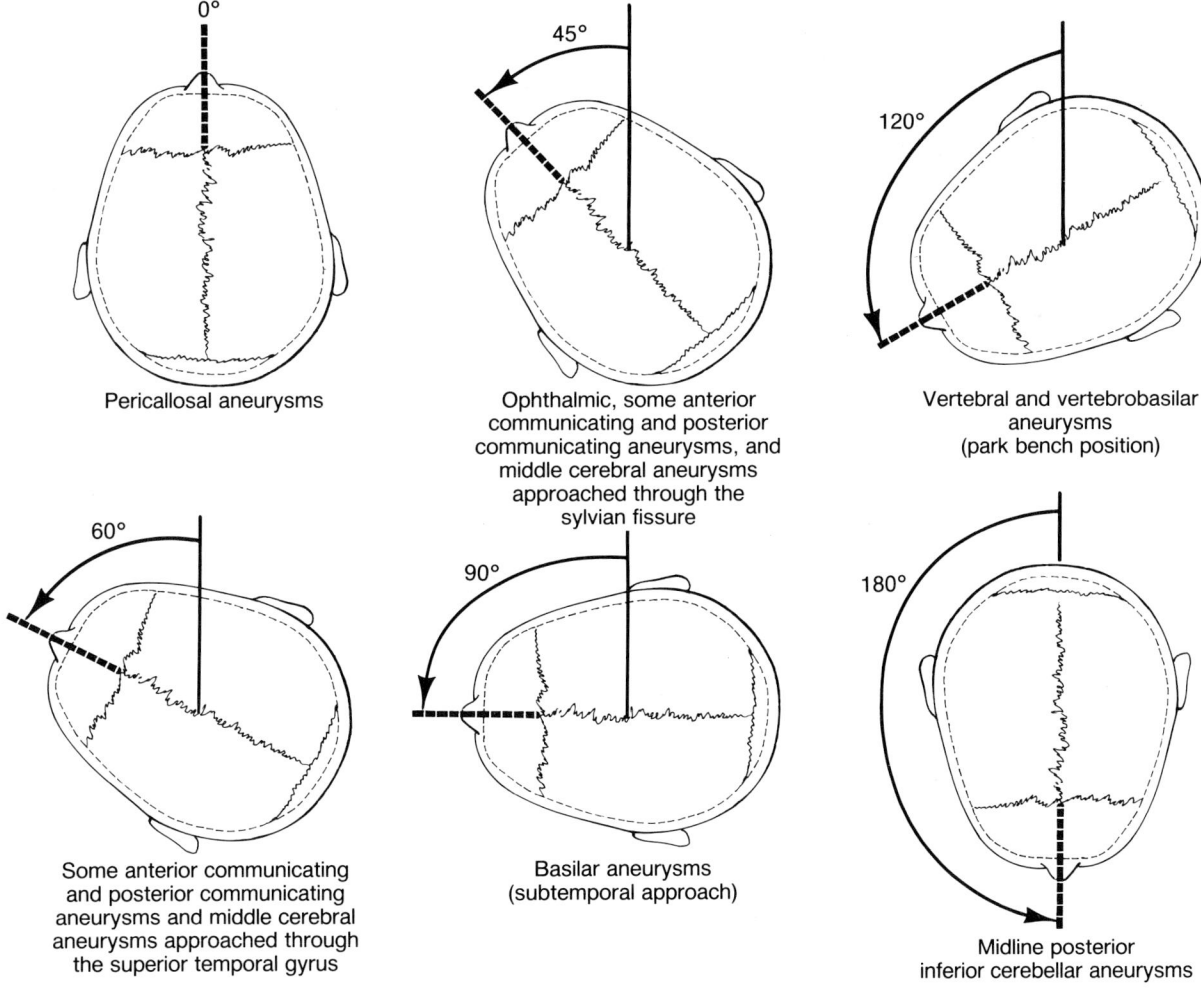

Figure 11.2. Positioning of the head for aneurysm surgery (see text).

sition is also useful for approaching middle cerebral artery aneurysms via the superior temporal gyrus (24). However, when these aneurysms are approached by opening the medial aspect of the sylvian fissure, it is better to turn the patient's head only about 30°. For basilar artery aneurysms, the authors rotate the patient's head only slightly when using the pterional approach, but if the subtemporal approach is used, the authors rotate the head to a straight lateral position (90°). For vertebral and vertebrobasilar artery aneurysms, which the authors prefer to approach via the park bench position, the patient's head is rotated toward the floor (about 30°) if the aneurysm is proximal in the vertebral artery, but if the aneurysm is deep at the vertebrobasilar junction, the authors prefer not to rotate the patient's head at all but rather to keep it in the lateral position so that a better look can be obtained of the front of the brain stem from laterally (22). For a midline posterior inferior cerebellar artery aneurysm, it is best to use a straight prone position with the patient's head straight toward the floor so as to not lose appropriate orientation to the midline.

Cranial Approaches

The flap is determined by the lesion site (Fig. 11.3). In general, smaller flaps are needed for microsurgical exposure. A pterional flap provides versatile exposure of the anterior circle of Willis (76). Exposure is excellent for aneurysms of the internal carotid, anterior communicating, and middle cerebral arteries. In some cases, basilar bifurcation aneurysms can be approached via this route. The key to this exposure is access to the floor of the anterior fossa. This access is assured by accurate placement of the key burr hole at the frontozygomatic point, a low craniotome cut anteriorly, and extensive removal of the lateral sphenoid ridge (76) (see Chapter 12). A full frontotemporal flap provides good exposure for middle cerebral aneurysms when a superior temporal gyrus approach is used (24).

A coronal flap and interhemispheric approach provide exposure for clipping azygos and pericallosal aneurysms (34). Though the nondominant right side is preferable if there is a choice, reference to the angiogram will indicate which side has the less formidable veins crossing the field. Care is needed to avoid injury to posterior frontal bridging veins and to the superior sagittal sinus, since occlusion of these structures can result in serious brain injury. Injury to the motor cortex can be avoided by positioning the flap just anterior to the coronal suture. Since the anterior burr holes are in front of the hairline, they are filled with methylmethacrylate at the conclusion of the procedure.

A small temporal bone flap, turned via a straight ("tic") incision, provides sufficient subtemporal access to a basilar tip aneurysm (8). The bony exposure should extend down to the zygoma and floor of middle fossa.

An S-shaped incision permits a lateral suboccipital craniectomy with removal of the foramen magnum and the arch of C1 for exposure of vertebral and vertebrobasilar artery aneurysms (22). The key is a lateral exposure to the vertebral artery over the arch of C1 and to the retrocondylar region at the foramen magnum. This facilitates a view into the cerebellopontine angle and around the brain stem with minimal cerebellar retraction.

A combined subtemporal-suboccipital approach is occasionally useful for exposure of the basilar trunk (29). Angiography should demonstrate a contralateral patent transverse sinus if the ipsilateral lateral sinus is to be sacrificed to widely divide the tentorium. This maneuver is rarely necessary.

Deep Exposure

The brain is slowly elevated with a hand-held retractor. Depending on the location of the aneurysm, CSF is aspirated by opening the basal cisterns or by a spinal catheter until the brain is slack enough to insert a self-retaining retractor. The authors prefer the Greenberg retractor for its stability and versatility.

Once brain retractors are placed, the microscope is wheeled into the field for magnified visualization of the small, relatively fixed field. Sometimes, retractor manipulation and arachnoid dissection will suffice for a beautiful exposure of the aneurysm. But often, a small corticectomy in silent brain serves to diminish the pressure of retraction and its attendant injury. The gyrus rectus corticectomy is well-known and recommended for almost all anterior communicating artery aneurysms. For some internal carotid artery aneurysms, particularly those at the bifurcation, deeper exposure can be obtained by opening the medial sylvian fissure. When this proves difficult, a 1-cm medial frontal corticectomy, with sparing of perforating arteries, can safely give the needed exposure. For laterally placed middle cerebral artery aneurysms, a superior temporal gyrus corticectomy gives the required view with a minimum of retraction. Sometimes, distal anterior cerebral and posterior cerebral artery aneurysms can be exposed with greater ease through a small corticectomy in the cingulate or parahippocampal gyri, respectively.

Microsurgical Dissection

The aneurysm is approached under 10–16× magnification. On parent arteries, blunt dissection is often used. A no. 16 sucker with low vacuum can provide countertraction for a Rhoton no. 6 or other fine dissector in the other hand. The side of the dissector is less likely to perforate than is the tip. A microcot-

Intracranial Aneurysms: General Aspects of Surgical Treatment

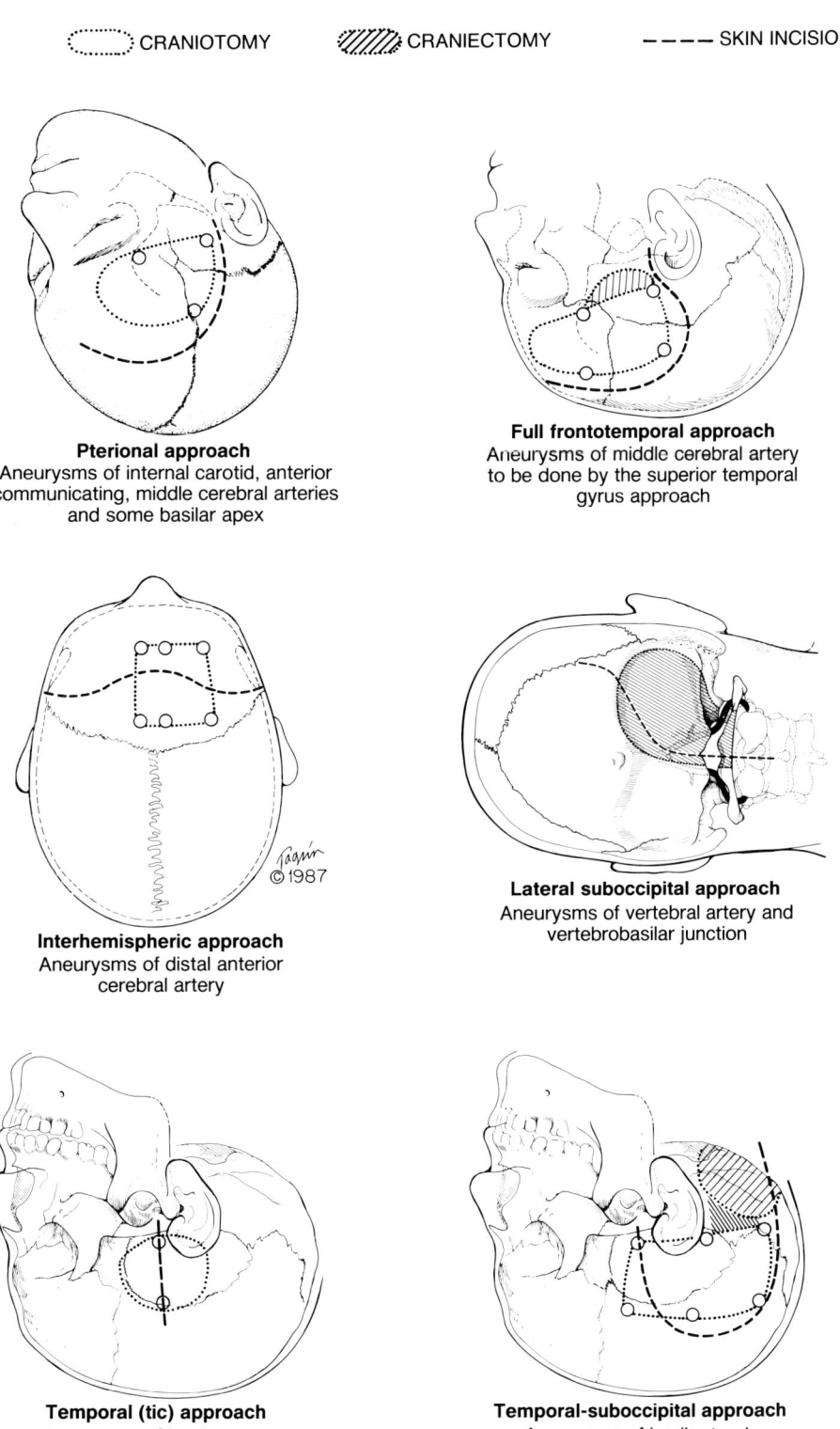

Figure 11.3. Cranial approaches for aneurysm surgery.

tonoid in the field can be used for retraction and to protect aneurysm and brain. Near the aneurysm, sharp dissection is preferred when the lesion's margins can be clearly visualized. Delicate tissue attachments are coagulated and cut with microscissors or a sharp knife. After dissecting the parent vessels, the surgeon frees the neck. A broad path must be prepared for each blade of the clip, lest the neck be torn during clipping. Mobilization of the dome may be needed to adequately prepare the neck and to facilitate sparing adherent critical vessels, particularly on anterior communicating and middle cerebral artery aneurysms. The dome of the aneurysm rarely needs to be dissected completely in cases of aneurysms at the carotid bifurcation or at the top of the basilar artery. It is a myth that the dome should never be mobilized (2). Inadequate dissection is one of the main causes of intraoperative catastrophe. When the dome is to be mobilized, it is wise to leave a layer of brain or arachnoid attached at the point of bleeding if such is obvious.

Aneurysm Clips

A host of different surgical clips may be used effectively. For many lesions, the authors have, in the past, used the Heifetz clip. This clip is held rigidly in the clip applying forceps for precision of application, and its jaws open broadly to accept even large necks. Its main disadvantage is the breadth of its blade, which may be too wide for safe insertion in a narrow aperture. It should also be noted that there have been reports of delayed fracture with the Heifetz clip (11), and its ferromagnetic properties may result in clip rotation during magnetic resonance imaging (12). Fortunately, other clips (such as Yasargil and Sugita) do not have the same danger relative to magnetic resonance imaging.

The Yasargil or the Sugita clips with their narrower blades are presently preferred by the authors. These types of clips have, in general, stronger closing force, and the design of the blades makes them less likely to slip (61). Great versatility is provided by the many different shapes and sizes, as well as by the incorporation of the Drake fenestration in some of the clips. The latter modification allows ideal clip application over a posterior cerebral artery in the case of basilar aneurysms, over the anterior cerebral arteries in cases of anterior communicating artery aneurysms, and over the internal carotid artery in cases of internal carotid aneurysms that project directly posteriorly or medially (62). In the latter, the series of Sugita clips with blades at right angles to the fenestration allow clipping of the aneurysm with the blades parallel to the internal carotid artery and the long axis of the neck of the aneurysm, which minimizes the chances of neck fracture during clip application (see Chapter 12). This particular type of clip is also very useful for fusiform aneurysms of the vertebral artery and for other unusual situations (62).

Either the straight Sugita or Yasargil clips with a Drake aperture or the classical Drake clips are very useful for "tandem" clip applications in cases of larger aneurysms (7). Because of their many different sizes, the straight Drake clips are particularly useful for aneurysms at the top of the basilar artery. In this location, the aneurysm clip must be of a precise length so as to have the blades go across the neck of the aneurysm just to, but not into, the opposite posterior cerebral artery (8). Other useful clips, with which the authors have less experience, are the MacFadden clip and the Variangle clip. It is important to have some Sundt-Kees clip-grafts available because this is the only type of clip that may be helpful in repairing tears on the parent artery (65). The recently introduced booster clips can be very useful in cases of giant and thick-walled aneurysms in which the closing force of the primary clip is insufficient to obliterate the aneurysm (66). Sugita has also developed ultralong clips that can occasionally be invaluable in the management of giant aneurysms (63).

Temporary clipping of the parent vessel and, sometimes, of all of its divisions in preparation for clipping should be considered. Initially, this technique was used almost exclusively for giant and large aneurysms when aneurysmorrhaphy was contemplated (7). Some surgeons, notably Suzuki, have advocated temporary occlusion of the parent vessel routinely even when dealing with smaller aneurysms (68). This practice in anything less than giant aneurysms had not been popular until recently. In order to prolong the safe period for temporary arterial occlusion, bolus injection of mannitol alone or combined with antioxidants and perfluorochemicals has been reported (67). It appears that even without the addition of these "protective" agents, it is safe to use temporay arterial occlusion of the internal carotid, middle cerebral, basilar or anterior cerebral arteries for periods of up to 10 or 15 minutes (9, 67, 70, 71). When possible, the authors limit the occlusion time to 5 minutes and prefer to release the clip intermittently and allow recirculation for a few minutes when longer periods of occlusion are necessary. It is important to use only especially designed low-force clips such as those by Suzuki, Sugita or Yasargil whenever temporary occlusion is undertaken. With the ordinary higher pressure permanent clips, there is a greater chance of endothelial injury (9). Whether the addition of barbiturates or other protective agents is beneficial in this situation is not clear. The authors avoid bolus injections of barbiturates for fear of lowering the blood pressure and use a bolus of mannitol (100 gm 15 minutes prior to clipping), from which there have been no ill effects.

In terms of clip appliers, the authors have become increasingly reliant on the Sano multipurpose all-angle clip applier. This particular applicator is extremely versatile and can be used both with the Yasargil and the Sugita clips. It allows for clip application at many different angles, which would be impossible with other less flexible types of applicators (54).

Obliteration of the Aneurysm

In dealing with intracranial aneurysms, it is important to keep in mind some basic anatomic principles (48). Aneurysms usually arise at a point of branching from the parent artery. This branching may be formed either by a side branch from the parent artery or by a division of the main arterial trunk into two main branches. Aneurysms arise at turns or curves in the parent arteries. These curves, by producing alterations in intravascular hemodynamics, exert unusual force on apical regions from which the aneurysms arise. Saccular aneurysms point in the direction that the blood would have gone if the curve at the aneurysm site were not present. As the aneurysm enlarges, it may encounter obstacles that may change the direction of growth, but the initial growth is usually in the direction of the maximal hemodynamic thrust in the preaneurysmal segment of the parent vessel (48).

The surgeon is well advised to approach the aneurysm with a broad array of techniques for dealing with the problem. For the great majority of aneurysms, clipping is most effective. Occasionally, an aneurysm will defy safe clipping, and reinforcement must be used. Coating of the aneurysm should be avoided, if possible, since this technique rarely results in complete protection and the adhesives may be toxic (25, 59). Furthermore, with the exception of an occasional middle cerebral artery aneurysm, it is almost never possible to expose and wrap completely an aneurysm that is too large to accept a clip (7). Various wrapping materials have been evaluated (13). Muslin wrapping appears to be more effective and less dangerous than application of adhesive (38), but complications have been reported (3).

Precise application of the clip is required. The clip is advanced gently, with axial rotational movements to reduce drag until the tips are just beyond the opposite side of the neck. Generally, it is possible to visualize one of the two blades as it advances. If significant resistance is encountered, one should stop and remove the clip. Usually, dissection with freeing of arachnoid attachments will take care of the problem. In some cases, with a paper-thin aneurysmal neck, a brief deepening of hypotension or, more frequently in later years, temporary proximal occlusion may be needed just at the time of clip application.

After clip application, one must check the adequacy of the clipping and the condition of the parent vessel and all adjacent branches. Clip tips must be visualized beyond the opposite edge of the lesion, and the entire aneurysm should be obliterated. Satisfactory clipping of the lesion can be proved by puncture of the aneurysm with a 25-gauge spinal needle. If bleeding from the aneurysm persists after the needle perforation, it must be ascertained whether the clips fail to go completely across the neck, which can usually be corrected by advancing the clip or using a larger clip. In some cases, the clip is not strong enough to obliterate the lesion, and the blades open with each systole. The latter situation usually requires placement of extra clips either in parallel or in tandem. Sundt et al have devised "booster" clips to be used over the primary clip precisely for this indication (66).

A goal of aneurysm obliteration is preservation of normal arteries, including perforating branches. Occasionally, when other options seem more risky, deliberate occlusion of an artery may be preferable. The posterior communicating artery can be sacrificed when on angiography the vertebral artery is seen to fill the posterior cerebral artery. The anterior communicating artery (but not its perforating branches) can be sacrificed unless on angiography the A_1 segment is absent. A small anterior temporal branch of the middle cerebral artery may be occluded if this is strictly necessary. Even a division of the middle cerebral artery has been unintentionally occluded without deficit, but this cannot be recommended without immediate distal bypass (72). Deliberate vertebral occlusion is suitable if the posterior inferior cerebellar artery and the contralateral vertebral artery can be preserved (7). Drake states that the P_1 or a single P_1 perforating branch can be sacrificed (7), but the authors have seen prolonged coma after such occlusions. Finally, the surgeon should be satisfied that as retractors are removed, the clip will not produce dangerous torque on the aneurysmal neck or compression of adjacent neural or vascular structures.

Bipolar cauterization of the neck of the aneurysm may be helpful in some cases (35, 76). This technique may narrow the neck for easier clipping. In addition, it may thicken the neck, eradicating dangerous thin spots in this critical area. When this maneuver is undertaken, the bipolar cautery should be set low, with prior testing of its electrocautery effect, and the blades of the forceps should pass completely across the neck of the lesion, to reduce the danger of rupture. It is best to use forceps with relatively broad-tipped blades to decrease the chance of perforation as the blades are passed across the neck. As current is turned on, the surgeon alternately applies very gentle pressure and release. Ideally, a slow coagulation with whitening and thickening of the neck is produced without charring or popping. During this time, continuous irrigation of the area of coagulation should be done to help prevent adherence to the tissue (20). In some cases, the coagulation may completely obliterate the neck of a small aneurysm. Occasionally, the authors have been able to use this technique to shape aneurysms with very broad necks or multiple lobes to permit safe clipping. The surgeon should carefully avoid current spread or excess power, for the authors have seen unwanted occlusion of nearby perforator branches.

For some aneurysms, a ligature may be helpful, particularly in lesions with a wide neck, making it difficult to define a clear area for a clip. A variety of ligature passers are available. If space is limited, a doubled, waxed 3–0 silk ligature may be placed deep to the aneurysm with fine forceps. The surgeon then reflects the lesion to the opposite side, searching for the ligature beyond the aneurysm neck and retrieving it gently with forceps. After the ligature is placed about the neck, a surgeon's knot is fashioned and gently pulled taut. The surgeon then checks the impact of this maneuver on local branches which may be kinked by the ligature. In some cases, the neck may be obliterated totally by the ligature. More often the ligature narrows the neck for subsequent clipping.

Under the microscope, an aneurysm rarely defies clipping or ligation. When it does, reinforcement with muslin may be the safest technique. The authors use a sheet of fine mesh muslin or several strips applied to cover, insofar as possible, the entire lesion. In addition, small pieces of muslin are applied to thickened areas near the neck that may escape clipping. Use of muslin where it is not necessary is not recommended, since it can result in arachnoiditis with neurologic deficit (3). In one such case, the authors used lysis of adhesions and postoperative steroids and Cytoxan which may have been useful in reversing a chiasmal syndrome.

Intraoperative Rupture

Intraoperative rupture of the aneurysm usually occurs under one of the following circumstances: when the aneurysmal dome is dissected; when the parent artery is retracted and the dome is adherent to the brain; when the brain is retracted away from the aneurysm and the aneurysm is adherent to it; while the neck is undergoing coagulation, particularly when the blades of the bipolar forceps are not passed completely around the neck; and, most commonly, when the clip is being applied. Sometimes, if the neck is incompletely dissected, the aneurysm is very tense, and the neck is very thin, a blade can actually perforate the sac. If the dome has not been completely freed up and remains adherent to the retracted adjacent brain, the neck can be fractured away from the parent vessel as the clip is being closed. Obviously, the best way to handle rupture is to prevent it. The authors believe that temporary clipping and complete dissection serve to prevent rupture in most cases.

Deliberate action is necessary in the event of aneurysmal rupture at any point during the operation. The surgeon must proceed in an orderly fashion with temporary hemostasis, precise visualization of the source of hemorrhage and its relation to critical structures, and then accurate hemostasis. Small areas of hemorrhage can be controlled with suction and a cottonoid. Very careful direction of the suction tip to the precise point of bleeding should be attempted to clear the field entirely of bleeding. Then, precise application of a bit of Surgicel or muscle, with compression with a small cottonoid for a few minutes, may seal a minor leak. If hemostasis can be obtained in this way, it is best to direct the dissection to another corner and return to the area of hemorrhage at a later time. The authors have usually been unsuccessful in their attempts to coagulate, with the bipolar forceps, an area of active bleeding from an aneurysm. More often than not these attempts have resulted in an enlargement of the tear.

In some cases, collapse of the aneurysm into a large bore (no. 7) sucker may actually facilitate complete dissection and clipping. The use of a no. 19 butterfly needle and suction to deliberately achieve aneurysmal collapse by aspiration has been advocated (15). When the closure of the clip stops bleeding but occludes an important branch, adjustment will be needed, but this dry field will afford an opportunity for precise dissection before the clip is repositioned.

Brisk bleeding requires the use of a large suction or multiple suctions. If this occurs, the anesthesiologist must be alerted to keep up with the blood loss by rapid transfusion and alter the technique to keep the blood pressure up, since blood loss can be rapid and maximum collateral circulation may be required if temporary arterial occlusion is needed. Application of a temporary clip to the dome may be helpful. If there is access to the parent vessel, temporary clipping or, if possible, complete trapping is the ideal maneuver. If a tear at the neck of an aneurysm cannot be controlled with a clip, repair with either an interrupted suture technique (10-0 nylon) or tissue adhesive may be used after temporary clipping. Blind attempts at clip placement usually result in more trouble and, at times, catastrophe and are strongly condemned. The worst reaction the surgeon can have at the time of a major rupture is to call for profound hypotension. That can also be the first reaction of the inexperienced anesthesiologist in an effort to help the surgeon by "stopping the bleeding" with hypotension. With massive hemorrhage the patient needs, more than ever, adequate perfusion pressure to maintain collateral circulation in areas distal to the point of rupture. The authors, in fact, call for the anesthesiologist to raise the blood pressure, so that temporary occlusion of the parent vessel can be used.

Closure

Irrigation is carried out with saline. All visible clots around accessible arteries are removed. Papaverine is applied to these vessels. When the brain is slack, saline may be added to fill the dead space. The dura is closed and Surgicel is placed in the epidural space for hemostasis. The bone flap is wired in place with 28-gauge stainless steel wire sutures, and the dura is apposed to the bone flap with a central suture. The operative area is irrigated with bacitracin solution. The muscle, fascia, galea, and skin are closed with appropriate sutures.

Indirect Surgery

For some lesions, particularly giant aneurysms, direct attack may be too risky (see Chapter 20). A safe treatment may be ligation of a proximal parent artery, either in the neck or in the head (36). Occlusion of the internal or common carotid artery diminishes pressure and often results in thrombosis of internal carotid artery aneurysms. A snare ligature can be used to occlude the middle cerebral or basilar arteries to thrombose aneurysms of these vessels (7). To prevent ischemic infarction, several methods for revascularization of the brain can be used prior to arterial occlusion (60) (see Chapter 4). These techniques are further elaborated in the discussion of giant aneurysms (see Chapter 20).

Other Techniques

The authors have had no firsthand experience with other unusual techniques of aneurysmal obliteration, which include stereotactic clipping (28), stereotactic (1) or direct (39) injection of wires or needles in an effort to achieve thrombosis, and obliteration by intraaneurysmal detachable balloon techniques (5, 49, 58, 78). All of these techniques, at best, must be considered experimental, and their use should be restricted to the few centers currently developing them. The results obtained with use of any of these methods cannot yet be compared with those obtained by more conventional operations. These procedures are usually being performed only for patients with aneurysms that would be otherwise very difficult to treat.

POSTOPERATIVE MANAGEMENT

Guidelines for postoperative care have been presented (14, 26, 27, 47). At the conclusion of the procedure, the patient is treated prophylactically against vasospasm if the preoperative computed tomography (CT) scan or clinical course suggest this complication is likely to occur. The central venous pressure is brought to 10 cm of water with use of colloid, if there is no cardiac contraindication. The hematocrit is maintained at 30–35%. Transfusion of packed cells is necessary only if there has been major intraoperative blood loss. The blood pressure is maintained in the range of 140–150 mm Hg systolic with volume and pressors as required. These measures are not necessary in patients with minor or no subarachnoid hemorrhage or in stable patients operated fairly late after subarachnoid hemorrhage. Medications include steroids, an antacid, and diphenylhydantoin. Elastic stockings or pneumatic compression boots are used until the patient is ambulatory, usually a day or two after surgery.

Every effort is made by the neuroanesthesia team to awaken the patient immediately after surgery to permit early clinical assessment. If this examination with the patient fully awake discloses a new substantial deficit, the surgeon should consider first whether his clip may have compromised a critical vessel, e.g., the anterior choroidal artery or a lenticulostriate perforating branch. If this appears likely, then immediate treatment for ischemia with hypertension and the use of mannitol should be instituted and strong consideration given to immediate reoperation to adjust the clip. By this tactic, the authors have successfully returned a patient with flaccid hemiplegia to a normal neurologic condition.

If unwanted arterial occlusion by the clip seems unlikely or if there is delayed neurologic deterioration, a CT scan to rule out intracranial hematoma, hydrocephalus, or cerebral edema is performed. Appropriate treatment is instituted if these conditions are found. If the CT scan fails to disclose an adequate explanation for the deterioration, angiography is performed. If significant vasospasm (grade 3+ or 4+) is seen (fig. 11.4 A–D), additional medical treatment is indicated with hypervolemia and induced hypertension (17) (see chapter 10).

Earlier in the authors' experience, postoperative angiography was used routinely to ascertain the adequacy of aneurysm obliteration and maintenance of normal vasculature (10). With increasing experience and the availability of better clips that rarely "slip," the authors have gradually abandoned routine postoperative angiography. Instead, the aneurysm is now opened or punctured at surgery to ensure adequacy of clipping. The authors still recommend postoperative angiography when the adequacy of clipping is in doubt, when the aneurysm is not opened at surgery, or when the patient awakens with or later in the course develops an unexplained neurologic deficit.

RESULTS

Results of aneurysm surgery have improved very substantially over the past 40 years. The Cooperative Study of Subarachnoid Hemorrhage and Intracranial Aneurysms recorded an overall surgical mortality rate of 36.8% for patients who had an intracranial ap-

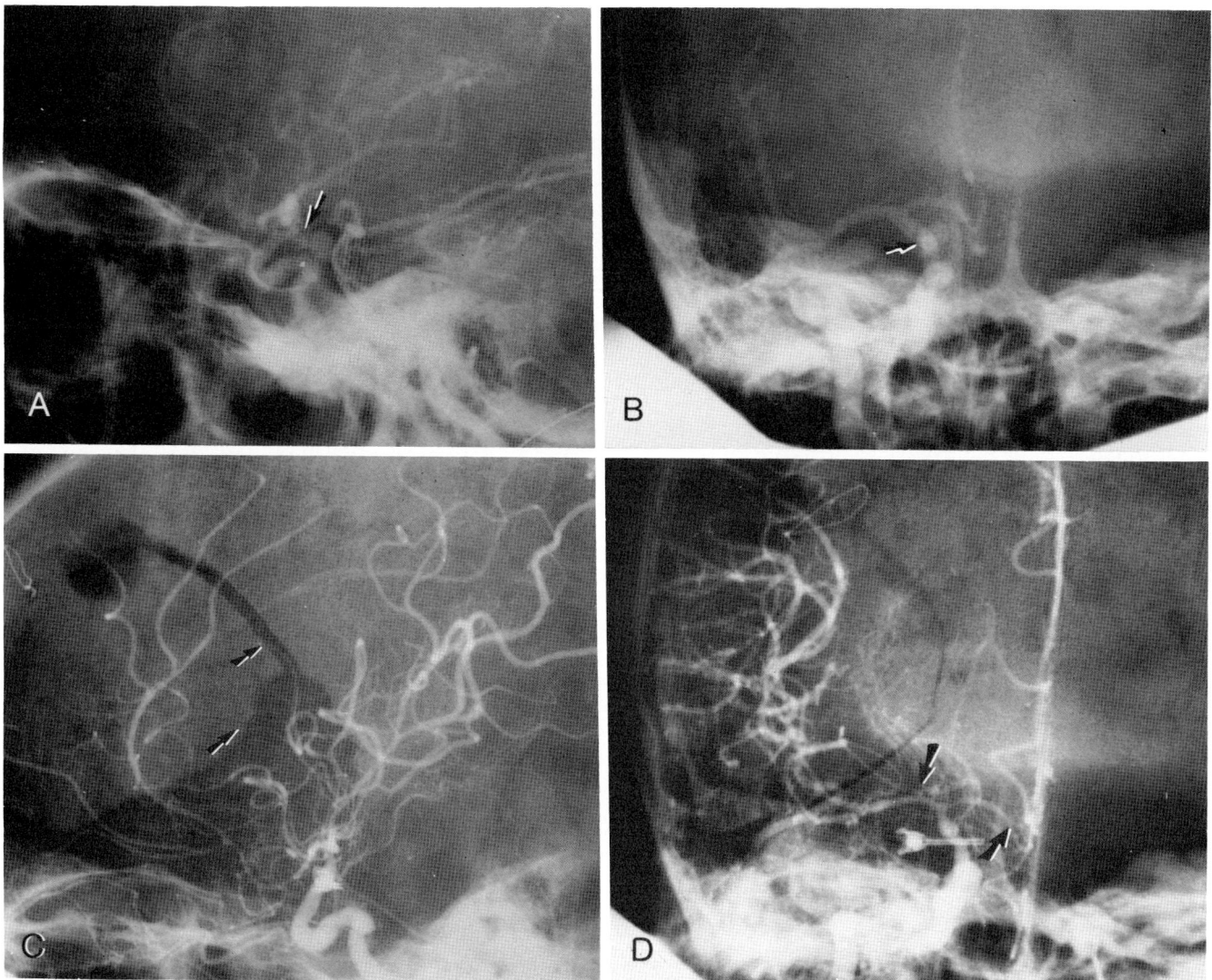

Figure 11.4. Postoperative cerebral vasospasm. **A** and **B**, right carotid angiogram shows aneurysm (*arrow*) of internal carotid-posterior communicating arteries and no spasm 8 days after subarachnoid hemorrhage. **C** and **D**, Postoperative right carotid angiogram performed 1 day after surgery and 9 days after subarachnoid hemorrhage shows obliteration of aneurysm with intense spasm of internal carotid, anterior cerebral, and middle cerebral arteries and delayed flow in the middle cerebral artery branches (*arrows*).

proach for an aneurysm of the anterior circulation (44.5% for those who had had operations performed within 14 days of subarachnoid hemorrhage and 23.3% for those who had had operations performed later) (18). Several centers now report that intracranial aneurysms can, in general, be operated on with a combined serious morbidity and mortality rate of under 10% for patients in good preoperative condition (21, 23, 64, 76). However, the results of intracranial surgery for aneurysms must be considered in relationship to the timing of the operation, since vasospasm is probably the most important cause of surgical morbidity and the risk of developing postoperative vasospasm is very low in operations carried out more than 12 or 14 days after subarachnoid hemorrhage. The problem is that, as discussed earlier, many patients are lost to rebleeding if one waits this long.

To facilitate comparisons, the term "management morbidity and mortality" has been popularized (50, 73). This refers to the results of overall management regardless of if or when surgery is carried out. When overall management results are analyzed, one realizes that the improvement in overall results are not as dramatic as the improvements in surgical results would suggest. A patient that arrives at the hospital in good condition after a subarachnoid hemorrhage still has a 20–30% chance of dying or being left with significant neurologic disability, whether operated on early or late (30, 50, 73).

In addition to the timing of surgery, other factors of paramount significance in influencing surgical results are the condition (clinical grade) of the patient preoperatively and the location and size of the aneurysm. In one large series, the serious morbidity and mortality was 6% for patients in grades 1 and 2 (Hunt's classification) and 52% for patients in grades 3 and 4 (77). Whether the results are early postoperative or late is also significant. It is clear that most patients who are not severely incapacitated after surgery improve with time, at least from the physical and neurologic points of view. In a study of 1000 aneurysm patients, it was found that 62% of the patients who were minimally to moderately incapacitated at discharge from the hospital ("fair" results) were found to have improved significantly enough to return to a "normal life" weeks to months later (77). However, caution is required in judging what a "normal life" or "good condition" means (33). A sobering study from the authors' own institution showed that even though the immediate surgical mortality and serious morbidity in 100 patients with subarachnoid hemorrhage due to a ruptured aneurysm was only 7%, only 44% of the entire group of patients had returned to their previous occupation, and 20% had returned to some lesser form of occupation 1 year after surgery, and the rest remained unemployed mostly because of less than obvious psychologic and cognitive problems such as lack of initiative, excessive fatigability, decreased capacity for concentration, etc. (50). Similar results were found in another study in which only 51% of the patients had returned to their previous full-time job or an equivalent occupation (16). Similarly disappointing results were found in another study when, in addition to purely physical and neurologic criteria, cognitive and psychosocial impairment were carefully assessed 1 year after subarachnoid hemorrhage (56). Of the initially good risk patients (grades 1 and 2), only 60% showed a good physical outcome without concomitant indication of severe cognitive dysfunction and/or psychosocial impairment. Because of the differences in results between aneurysms in different locations and between ordinary aneurysms and giant aneurysms, these results are included in the subsequent chapters on aneurysms in specific locations and on giant aneurysms.

REFERENCES

1. Alksne JF, Smith RW: Stereotaxic occlusion of 22 consecutive anterior communicating artery aneurysms. *J Neurosurg* 52:790–793, 1980.
2. Ausman J, Diaz F, Malik GM, Fielding AS, Son CS: Current management of cerebral aneurysm: Is it based on fact or myth? *Surg Neurol* 24:625–635, 1985.
3. Carney PG, Oatey PE: Muslin wrapping of aneurysm and delayed visual failure. A report of three cases. *J Clin Neuro Ophthalmol* 3:91–96, 1983.
4. Carter LP, Raudzens PA, Gaines C, Crowell RM: Somatosensory evoked potentials and cortical blood flow during craniotomy for vascular disease. *Neurosurgery* 15:22–28, 1984.
5. Debrun G, Fox AJ, Drake CG, Peerless S, Girvin J, Ferguson G: Giant unclippable aneurysm: Treatment with detachable balloons. *AJNR* 2:167–173, 1981.
6. Dell S: Asymptomatic cerebral aneurysm: Assessment of its risk of rupture. *Neurosurgery* 10:162–166, 1982.
7. Drake CG: Giant intracranial aneurysms: Experience with surgical treatment in 174 patients. *Clin Neurosurg* 26:12–95, 1979.
8. Drake CG: The treatment of aneurysms of the posterior circulation. *Clin Neurosurg* 26:96–144, 1979.
9. Drake CG: Management of cerebral aneurysm. *Stroke* 12:274–282, 1981.
10. Drake CG, Allcock JM: Postoperative angiography and the "slipped" clip. *J Neurosurg* 39:683–689, 1973.
11. Dujovny M, Kossovsky N, Kossowsky R, Haines S, Maroon JC: Heifetz clip: Failure. A metallurgical study. *J Neurosurg* 50:368–373, 1979.
12. Dujovny M, Kossovsky N, Kossowsky R, Perlin A, Segal R, Diaz FG, Ausman JI: Intracranial clips: An examination of the devices used for aneurysm surgery. *Neurosurgery* 14:257–267, 1984.
13. Ebina K, Iwabuchi T, Suzuki S: A clinico experimental study on various wrapping materials of cerebral aneurysms. *Acta Neurochir* 72:61–71, 1984.
14. Flamm ES: Parasurgical treatment of aneurysms. *Clin Neurosurg* 24:240–247, 1976.
15. Flamm ES: Suction decompression of aneurysm: technical note. *J Neurosurg* 54:275–276, 1981.
16. Fortuny LA, Prieto-Valiente L: Long-term prognosis in surgically treated intracranial aneurysms. Part 2: Morbidity. *J Neurosurg* 54:35–43, 1981.
17. Giannotta SL, McGillicuddy JE, Kindt GW: Diagnosis and treatment of postoperative cerebral vasospasm. *Surg Neurol* 8:286–290, 1977.
18. Graf CJ, Nibbelink DW: Randomized treatment study. Intracranial surgery. In Sahs AL, Nibbelink DW, Torner JC (eds): *Aneurysmal Subarachnoid Hemorrhage, Report of the Cooperative Study*. Baltimore, Urban & Schwarzenberg, 1981, pp 145–202.
19. Greenberg IM: Self-retaining retractor and handrest system for neurosurgery. *Neurosurgery* 8:205–208, 1981.
20. Greenwald R, Crowell RM, McDonald LW: Experimental evaluation of a new bipolar coagulator with minimal adhesion to tissue. *Neurosurgery* in press.
21. Guidetti B: Results of microsurgical treatment of intracranial anterior circle saccular aneurysms. In Barnett H, Paoletti P, Flamm E, Brambilla G (eds): *Cerebrovascular Diseases: New Trends in Surgical and Medical Aspects*. New York, Elsevier, 1981, pp 297–311.
22. Heros RC: Lateral suboccipital approach for vertebral and vertebrobasilar aneurysms and arteriovenous malformations. Technical note. *J Neurosurg* 64:559–562, 1986.
23. Heros RC, Kistler JP: Intracranial arterial aneurysm—an update. *Stroke* 14:628–631, 1983.
24. Heros RC, Ojemann RG, Crowell RM: Superior temporal gyrus approach to middle cerebral aneurysms. Technique and results. *Neurosurgery* 10:308–313, 1982.
25. Hood TW, Mastri AR, Chou SN: Neural and vascular tissue reaction to cyanoacrylate adhesives: A further report. *Neurosurgery* 11:363–366, 1982.
26. Hopkins LN: Postoperative management of the aneurysm patient. In Hopkins LN, Long DM (eds): *Clinical management of Intracranial Aneurysms*. New York, Raven Press, 1982, pp 295–304.
27. Hunt WE, Kosnik EJ: Timing and perioperative care in intracranial aneurysm surgery. *Clin Neurosurg* 21:79–89, 1974.

28. Kandel EI, Peresedov VV: Stereotaxic clipping of arterial aneurysms and arteriovenous malformations. J Neurosurg 46:12–23, 1977.
29. Kasdon DL, Stein BM: Combined supratentorial and infratentorial exposure for low-lying basilar aneurysms. Neurosurgery 4:422–426, 1979.
30. Kassell N: Timing of aneurysm surgery. Results of the Cooperative Study. Paper presented at the Congress of the International Federation of Neurosurgical Societies, Toronto, 1985.
31. Krayenbuhl HA, Yasargil MG, Flamm ES, Tew JM Jr: Microsurgical treatment of intracranial saccular aneurysms. J Neurosurg 37:678–686, 1972.
32. Ljunggren B, Brandt L, Kagstrom E, Sundbarg G: Results of early operations for ruptured aneurysms. J Neurosurg 54:473–479, 1981.
33. Ljunggren B, Sonneson B, Saveland H, Brandt L: Cognitive impairment and adjustment in patients without neurological deficits after aneurysmal SAH and early operation. J Neurosurg 62:673–679, 1985.
34. Lougheed WM, Marshall BM: Management of aneurysms of the anterior circulation by intracranial procedures. In Youmans JR (ed): Neurological Surgery. Philadelphia, WB Saunders, 1973, pp 731–767.
35. Malis LI: Neurosurgical photography through the microscope. Clin Neurosurg 28:233–245, 1981.
36. Miller JD, Jawad K, Jennett B: Safety of carotid ligation and its role in the management of intracranial aneurysms. J Neurol Neurosurg Psychiatry 40:64–72, 1977.
37. Mizukami M, Kawase T, Usami T, Tazawa T: Prevention of vasospasm by early operation with removal of subarachnoid blood. Neurosurgery 10:301–307, 1982.
38. Mount L, Antunes JL: Results of treatment of intracranial aneurysms by wrapping and coating. J Neurosurg 42:189–193, 1975.
39. Mullan S: Experiences with surgical thrombosis of intracranial berry aneurysms and carotid cavernous fistulas. J Neurosurg 41:657–671, 1974.
40. Nelson PB, Seif SM, Maroon JC, Robinson AG: Hypoatremia in patients with subarachnoid hemorrhage: A study of vasopressin and blood volume. In Wilkins RH (ed): Cerebral Arterial Spasm. Baltimore, Williams & Wilkins, 1979, pp 654–658.
41. Nibbelink DW, Torner JC, Henderson WG: Intracranial aneurysms and subarachnoid hemorrhage—report on a randomized treatment study. IV-A. Regulated bedrest. Stroke 8:202–218, 1977.
42. Nishioka H: Report on the cooperative study of intracranial aneurysms and subarachnoid hemorrhage. Section VII, Part I. Evaluation of the conservative management of ruptured intracranial aneurysms. J Neurosurg 25:574–600, 1966.
43. Nishioka H. Torner JC, Graf CJ, Kassell NF, Sahs AL, Goettler LC: Cooperative study of intracranial aneurysms and subarachnoid hemorrhage: A longterm prognostic study. II. Ruptured intracranial aneurysms managed conservatively. Arch Neurol 41:1142–1146, 1984.
44. Nishimoto A, Ueta K, Onbe H, et al: Nationwide co-operative study of intracranial aneurysm surgery in Japan. Stroke 16:48–52, 1985.
45. Ojemann RG: Management of the unruptured intracranial aneurysm. N Engl J Med 304:725–726, 1981.
46. Pakarinen S: Incidence, etiology, and prognosis of primary subarachnoid hemorrhage. A study based on 589 cases diagnosed in a defined urban population during a defined period. Acta Neurol Scand 43 (Suppl) 29:9–128, 1967.
47. Peerless SJ: Pre- and postoperative management of cerebral aneurysms. Clin Neurosurg 20:209–231, 1979.
48. Rhoton Al Jr: Anatomy of saccular aneurysms. Surg Neurol 14:59–66, 1980.
49. Rodomanov AP, Shcheglov VI: Intravascular occlusion of saccular aneurysm: Advances and technical standards. Neurosurgery 9:25–49, 1983.
50. Ropper AH, Zervas NT: Outcome 1 year after SAH from cerebral aneurysm. Management morbidity, mortality and functional status in 112 consecutive good-risk patients. J Neurosurg 60:909–915, 1984.
51. Salazar JL: Surgical treatment of asymptomatic and incidental intracranial aneurysms. J Neurosurg 53:20–21, 1980.
52. Samson DS, Hodosh RM, Clark WK: Surgical management of unruptured asymptomatic aneurysms. J Neurosurg 46:731–734, 1977.
53. Samson DS, Hodosh RM, Reid WR, Beyer CW, Clark WK: Risk of intracranial aneurysm surgery in the good grade patient: Early versus late operation. Neurosurgery 5:422–426, 1976.
54. Sano K: A multipurpose all-angle clip applier for aneurysm surgery. Technical note. J Neurosurg 53:260–261, 1980.
55. Sano K, Saito I: Timing and indication of surgery for ruptured intracranial aneurysms with regard to cerebral vasospasm. Acta Neurochir (Wien) 41:49–60, 1978.
56. Saveland H, Sonesson B, Ljunggren B, Brandt L, Uski T, Zygmunt S, Hindfelt B: Outcome evaluation following subarachnoid hemorrhage. J Neurosurg in press.
57. Sekhar LN, Heros RC: Origin, growth and rupture of saccular aneurysms: A review. Neurosurgery 8:248–260, 1981.
58. Serbinenko FA: Balloon catheterization and occlusion of major cerebral vessels. J Neurosurg 41:125–145, 1974.
59. Smith TW, DeGirolami U, Crowell RM: Neuropathological changes associated with the transorbital application of ethyl 2-cyano-acrylate adhesive to the basal cerebral arteries of cats. J Neurosurg 62:108–114, 1985.
60. Spetzler RF, Shuster H, Roski RA: Elective extracranial-intracranial arterial bypass in the treatment of inoperable aneurysms of the giant internal carotid artery. J Neurosurg 53:22–27, 1980.
61. Sugita K, Hirota T, Iguchi I, Mizutani T: Comparative study of the pressure of various aneurysm clips. J Neurosurg 44:723–727, 1976.
62. Sugita K, Kobayashi S, Inoue T, Banno T: New angled fenestrated clips for fusiform vertebral artery aneurysms. J Neurosurg 54:346–350, 1981.
63. Sugita K, Kobayashi S, Inoue T, Takemae T: Characteristics and use of ultra-long aneurysm clips. J Neurosurg 60:145–150, 1984.
64. Sundt TM Jr, Kobayashi S, Fode NC, et al: Results and complications of surgical management of 809 intracranial aneurysms in 722 cases. Related and unrelated to grade of patient, type of aneurysm, and timing of surgery. J Neurosurg 56:753–765, 1982.
65. Sundt TM Jr, Murphey F: Clip grafts for aneurysm and small vessel surgery. Part 3: Clinical experience in intracranial internal carotid artery aneurysms. J Neurosurg 31:59–71, 1969.
66. Sundt TM Jr, Piepgras DG, Marsh WR: Booster clips for giant and thickbased aneurysms. J Neurosurg 60:751–762, 1984.
67. Suzuki J, Fujimoto S, Mizoi K, Oba M: The protective effect of combined administration of anti-oxidants and perfluorchemicals on cerebral ischemia. Stroke 15:672–679, 1984.
68. Suzuki J, Kwak R, Okudaira Y: The safe time limit of temporary clamping of cerebral arteries in the direct surgical treatment of intracranial aneurysm under moderate hypothermia. In Suzuki J (ed): Cerebral Aneurysms Experience with 1000 Directly Operated Cases. Tokyo, Neuron Publishing, 1979, pp 325–329.
69. Suzuki J, Onuma T, Yoshimoto T: Results of early operations on cerebral aneurysms. Surg Neurol 11:407–412, 1979.
70. Symon L, Vajda J: Surgical experiences with giant intracranial aneurysms. J Neurosurg 61:1009–1028, 1984.
71. Symon L, Wang AD, Costa e Silva I, Gentili F: Perioperative use of somatosensory evoked responses in aneurysm surgery. J Neurosurg 60:269–275, 1984.
72. Umansky F, Montoya J, Dujovny F, Spetzler R, Carter P (eds): Proceedings of the VII International Symposium on Neurosurgical Anastomoses. New York, Thieme-Stratton, 1984.

73. Weir B, Aronyk K: Management mortality and the timing of surgery for supratentorial aneurysms. *J Neurosurg* 54:146–150, 1981.
74. Wiebers DO, Whisnant JP, O'Fallon WM: The natural history of unruptured intracranial aneurysm. *N Engl J Med* 304:696–698, 1981.
75. Winn HR, Richard AE, O'Brien W, Jane JA: Long-term prognosis in untreated cerebral aneurysms: II. Late morbidity and mortality. *Ann Neurol* 4:418–426, 1978.
76. Yasargil MG, Fox JL: The microsurgical approach to intracranial aneurysms. *Surg Neurol* 3:7–14, 1975.
77. Yoshimoto T, Uchida K, Kaneko U, Kayama T, Suzuki J: An analysis of follow-up results of 1000 intracranial saccular aneurysms with definitive surgical treatment. *J Neurosurg* 50:152–157, 1979.
78. Zeumer H, Bruckmann H, Adelt D, Hacke W, Ringelstein EB: Balloon embolization in the treatment of basilar aneurysm. *Acta Neurochir* 78:136–141, 1985.

12
Internal Carotid Artery Aneurysms

Approximately one-third of all intracranial aneurysms arise from the internal carotid artery (5, 11, 17, 25, 26, 30, 31). These aneurysms can be divided into those arising from the petrous segment of the internal carotid artery, the cavernous segment of the internal carotid artery, the paraclinoid region, the origin of the posterior communicating artery, the origin of the anterior choroidal artery, and from the internal carotid artery bifurcation. Those arising from the paraclinoid region of the internal carotid artery (the intradural portion of the internal carotid artery proximal to the posterior communicating artery) present special technical problems and, therefore, will be discussed separately in Chapter 13.

The general surgical approach is described below, while the clincial presentation and special surgical features at each site are considered separately.

GENERAL ASPECTS OF SURGICAL APPROACH

Positioning

The pterional (frontotemporal) craniotomy is useful for almost all aneurysms of the anterior circulation, as well as for some aneurysms of the basilar artery. Only minor variations on the position of the head and the amount of bone removed either anteriorly or posteriorly will be necessary for the different types of aneurysms. The variations in the position of the head have been described in the previous chapter; both the origin and the projection of the aneurysm are considered. For posterior communicating artery aneurysms that project laterally we turn the head only slightly, and when the aneurysm projects directly posteriorly we turn the head 60–75° in order to see the aneurysm in profile from the lateral aspect of the carotid artery. With larger aneurysms of the posterior wall of the internal carotid artery, we turn the head about 45° so as to dissect the aneurysm both laterally as well as medially and then occlude the aneurysm with a right-angle fenestrated Sugita clip applied over the internal carotid artery, leaving the artery in the fenestration. We prefer to have the patient flat in the horizontal position and with the head tilted back about 15° to facilitate frontal lobe retraction. We also tilt the head slightly towards the contralateral shoulder.

Incision and Scalp Flap

We prefer to start the incision just in front of the tragus at the level of the zygoma (Fig. 12.1). By starting the incision this far posteriorly one can usually preserve the anterior branch of the superficial temporal artery with the skin flap and prevent injury to the frontalis branch of the facial nerve. The incision is then gently curved behind the hairline medially and anteriorly to the midline at the anterior hairline. An alternative is to make a shorter incision that curves forward to a point about 1 or 1.5 cm in front of the hairline at the level of the pupil. We have not found any cosmetic difficulty with this smaller incision provided the skin in front of the hairline is closed separately with paper strips and subcuticular stitches. The incision is carried just to the muscle fascia below the superior temporal line and to the bone medially. The fascia of the muscle is then opened sharply with scissors rather than with electrocautery to prevent it from shrinking. In this manner it is possible later to

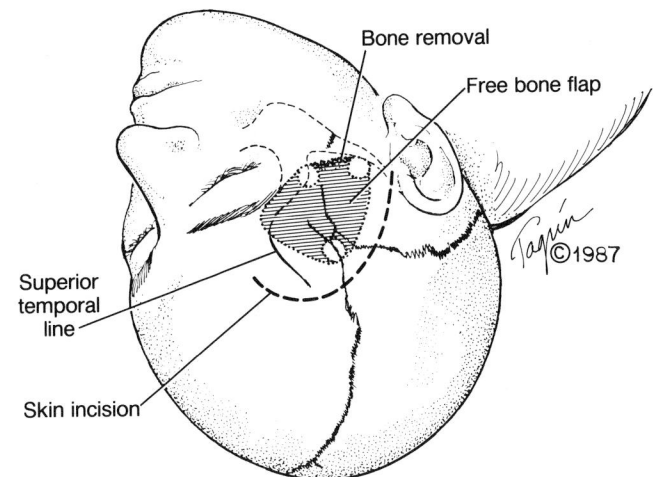

Figure 12.1. Pterional craniotomy. Head is turned 30–75° depending on projection of aneurysm. Incision is behind the hairline but may come to 1 or 1.5 cm in front of the hairline at the front end of the incision which is at the level of the pupil. After removal of the pterion and lateral sphenoid ridge, retractors are inserted to approach the optic nerve and internal carotid artery along the sphenoid wing.

close the fascia as a separate layer from the muscle, which the authors believe results in a better cosmetic effect and is less painful. The temporalis muscle is then opened along the line of the skin incision with electrocautery. The muscle and the skin are then reflected as one flap without separating the fascia from the skin. Subperiosteal dissection with a periosteal elevator or with electrocautery is used to reflect the muscle down and leave the skull exposed for a free bone flap. The muscle needs to be pulled down enough to expose the zygomatic process of the frontal bone and the frontozygomatic recess where the key burr hole must be placed in order to achieve a very low exposure. The skin flap is then folded over a sponge and held down with traction by fishhooks or strong sutures attached to rubber bands which are then held to the fixed drapes. Since the authors have been turning the muscle and skin down as one flap in the fashion just described, injury to the frontalis branch of the facial nerve has not been evident.

Bone Flap

The bone flap is relatively small, measuring approximately 6–8 cm along the base and about 5 cm in height (Fig. 12.1). Usually we use only three burr holes. The first burr hole is made at the key point behind the frontal process of the zygomatic bone, in the zygomaticofrontal recess. The second burr hole is made about 3 cm behind the first on the temporal side of the pterion. The last burr hole is made superiorly just above the superior temporal line. The dura is then separated from the bone flap using a Penfield no. 3 dissector. A power craniotome is then used to cut the bone flap. It is important to make the anterior cut along the base of the flap as low as possible, just over the supraorbital rim. This frontal cut extends for about 3 cm in front of the key hole. In cases of anterior communicating artery aneurysms or large ophthalmic aneurysms, one may wish to extend this frontal cut to about 5 cm from the key hole in order to have more generous frontal exposure. The basal frontal cut turns upward in a gentle curvilinear fashion to the superior burr hole. From the superior burr hole the cut then extends as far back in the temporal area as the skin incision allows and then it turns forward to communicate with the inferior-posterior burr hole in the temporal bone. Using a rongeur, one can then cut from each of the two inferior burr holes on either side of the pterion so as to be able to break the bone flap right at the base of the pterion. The lateral wing of the sphenoid bone at the pterion is then rongeured away.

The dura is separated from the lateral sphenoid wing and in so doing one may find bridging vessels from the bone to the dura that need to be coagulated and divided individually. Once the dura is stripped far medially, a high-speed drill is used to flatten completely the lateral aspect of the sphenoid wing to about the junction of the outer two-thirds with the inner one-third. The high-speed air drill is also useful to drill away any prominent projections from the orbital roof. In doing so one may occasionally enter the orbit, but this is not a problem if the orbital periosteum is not opened. The drill may also be used to bevel the inner table of the bone along the frontal cut in front of the key burr hole. Care must be taken not to drill the outer aspect of this bony edge because this would result in a cosmetic deformity. By the above maneuvers one obtains a very flat approach along the base which minimizes the need for retraction (31, 32). Occasionally, with the frontal cut one enters a very lateral extension of the frontal sinus. If this occurs the mucosa is stripped and the sinus is packed with bacitracin-soaked Gelfoam. The bone opening can then be covered with a flap of pericranium dissected from the back of the scalp flap and sewn to the adjacent dura.

After the bone flap has been removed, a fine drill point is used to create holes which are then used to resuture the bone flap with wires at the end and also to tent the dura up toward the bone flap with fine (4-0) Neurolon sutures. These dural tenting sutures go only through the outer layer of dura to avoid injury to underlying blood vessels, resulting in a subdural hematoma. These tenting sutures are placed at intervals of approximately 1.5–2.0 cm. The dura along the base of the flap is not tented until the time of closure, as is described later.

Initial Exposure

The dura is opened as an inferiorly based curvilinear flap of about 2–3 cm in height. The flap of dura is then tented up tightly with sutures inferiorly so as to afford a perfectly flat approach along the base. We also use some sutures to evert the superior aspect of the dural opening all around so as to avoid any dripping of blood into the field. At this point the surgeon inspects the brain to ascertain whether the frontal lobe may be safely retracted to withdraw cerebrospinal fluid for brain relaxation. If the brain is very full, the ventricle is punctured with a small ventriculostomy catheter through a small separate dural incision in the highest aspect of the bony opening. In most instances it is possible to retract the frontal lobe very gently with a handheld retractor. One then slides the retractor gradually along the edge of the sphenoid wing to identify the medial aspect of the olfactory tract which is a good guide to the location of the optic nerve (Fig. 12.2). The arachnoid around the optic nerve is then punctured for free flow of cerebrospinal fluid. With patience and minimal retraction, enough cerebrospinal fluid can usually be suctioned to allow for excellent relaxation of the frontal lobe. Upon removing the retractor, the frontal lobe

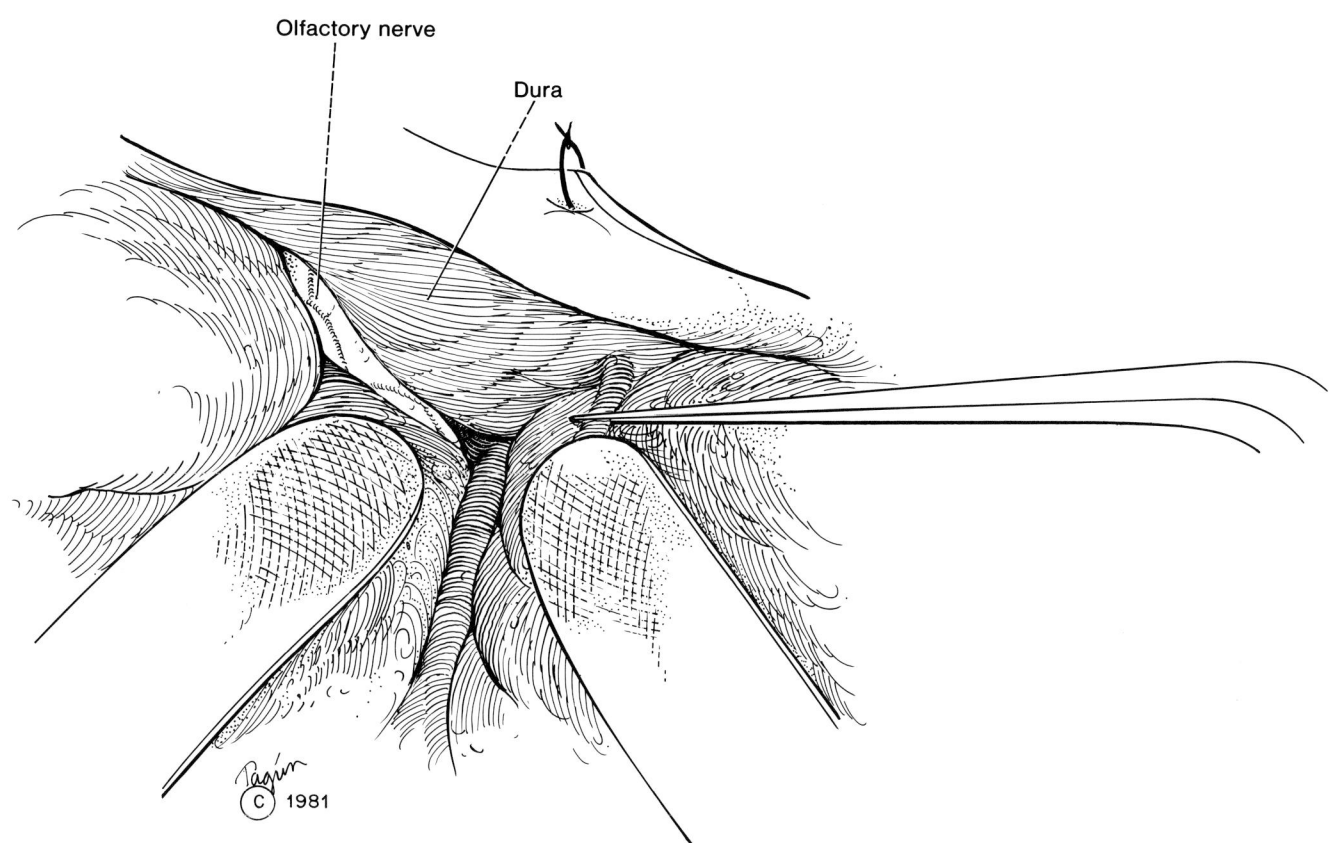

Figure 12.2. Approach to the internal carotid artery. If the lesion does not point laterally, temporal tip veins are divided to mobilize the temporal lobe. The approach is along the edge of the sphenoid wing except when the aneurysm points laterally in which case a more frontal approach is chosen to avoid early temporal lobe retraction. The convergence of the posterior end of the olfactory tract with the medial end of the sphenoid wing is the landmark for locating the optic nerve.

should stay back enough to reveal the origin of the optic nerve. In cases done acutely where there is some brain swelling, this degree of relaxation may not be achievable, at least during the initial stages.

In cases where the aneurysm is likely to be adherent to the temporal lobe, one may retract the frontal lobe from a more frontal direction to avoid any traction on the temporal lobe. In cases where temporal lobe retraction is not a concern, the tip of the temporal lobe is retracted to expose, coagulate, and divide all the draining veins (Fig. 12.2). No ill effects have been evident from this maneuver and with it one prevents bothersome venous bleeding which could occur during the critical phases of dissection. At this point one is ready to bring the microscope into the field. Microsurgical dissection is described separately for each aneurysm location.

Closure

After completion of aneurysmal clipping and inspection of the brain under the microscope to ensure complete hemostasis, one is ready for closure. The dura is closed in a watertight fashion using running 4-0 Neurolon or Prolene sutures. Before completing dural closure, a central tenting suture is placed to be brought out through two small central holes in the bone flap. In addition, approximately three tenting sutures are placed inferiorly to bring the dura up against the temporalis muscle posteriorly and the periosteum anteriorly. These sutures are placed before the dura is closed to ensure that the brain is not injured with the needle. The sutures are tied only after the dural closure is completed so that they will not pull on the dura and make it difficult to close. Alternatively, these sutures are tied first and a small graft of pericranial tissue is used to close the dura.

The bone flap is replaced and held with wire sutures through the previously placed small holes. The central dural tenting suture is then tied to bring the dura against the bone flap and prevent epidural bleeding. The muscle is closed by first using two or three sutures from the muscle to the pericranium in front of the key burr hole. This maneuver brings the muscle anteriorly, over the key burr hole, to prevent an unsightly depression in this area. The muscle mass is then closed posteriorly with several interrupted sutures (3-0 Vicryl is very satisfactory). The fascia of the muscle is then closed as a separate layer, again with interrupted 2-0 or 3-0 Vicryl sutures. The galea is closed with interrupted, inverted vertical mattress sutures (3-0 Vicryl). The skin is closed with a running nylon suture right up the hairline. Any extension of the incision into the forehead is closed with subcuticular sutures and paper strips.

INTERNAL CAROTID ARTERY—PETROUS ANEURYSMS

Presentation

Table 12.1 summarizes the important clinical aspects of these aneurysms. In general they tend to be large when detected and frequently come to the attention of the otorhinolaryngologist because the patient complains of decreased hearing, earache, or a subjective bruit referred to the ear. An occasional patient has presented with massive epistaxis or otorrhagia. On otologic examination, a retrotympanic mass may be seen and only awareness of the possibility of this diagnosis will relieve the specialist from the temptation to take a biopsy of the mass, which could result in a catastrophe. Other patients may present with diplopia from paresis of the sixth cranial nerve or with facial numbness. Rarely the patient presents with typical transient ischemic attacks (TIAs) or a stroke, usually from emboli from a partially clotted aneurysm.

These aneurysms may be spontaneous (developmental), atherosclerotic, traumatic, or infectious in origin. There is a higher incidence of the latter because of the close anatomical relationship to the middle ear (2, 19, 32).

Management

The natural history of these aneurysms is not well known since most have been symptomatic when detected and an effort at treating them has been undertaken.

Some of these aneurysms have been treated by primary resection with reconstruction of the internal carotid artery directly or by vein graft (12). In the opinion of the authors, these procedures are not generally indicated at present since the risks of stroke and cranial nerve injury are high and the alternative treatment, carotid ligation, is very effective for aneurysms in this location (19).

Whether or not an asymptomatic aneurysm of the petrous portion of the internal carotid artery should be treated is a question that cannot be answered from the data available. If the aneurysm is large and the patient healthy and likely to tolerate carotid occlusion, treatment is recommended. Otherwise the aneurysm can be followed with periodic CT scans and treated only if it grows.

Whenever the surgeon decides to attempt carotid ligation to treat an intracranial aneurysm, there are a number of options to consider. Should the internal or the common carotid artery be ligated? Should a bypass graft be done preliminarily to avoid ischemic complications? Should the occlusion be gradual or abrupt? Should the occlusion be done surgically or by detachable balloon? These options will be discussed in considerable detail in Chapter 20 which deals with giant aneurysms. The authors believe that common carotid ligation is a very effective and safe method of treatment for these aneurysms (28). Alternatively, the aneurysm can be trapped with separate detachable balloons distal and proximal to the aneurysm with or without a preliminary extracranial-intracranial (EC-IC) bypass procedure, depending on the availability of collateral circulation (19). Where the technique is well developed and considerable experience exists, the latter mode of treatment is ideal. However, it must be emphasized that even in expert hands complications such as embolism from local thrombosis or from deflation and distal migration of the balloon can occur (27).

Table 12.1.
Internal Carotid Artery—Petrous Aneurysms

Etiology
  Spontaneous
  Traumatic
  Atherosclerotic
  Infectious

Presentation
  Earache
  Decreased hearing
  Subjective bruit
  Retrotympanic mass
  Massive otorrhagia
  Diplopia (sixth nerve)
  Facial pain and numbness (fifth nerve)
  Ischemic (embolic) symptoms

Treatment
  Medical
  Direct exposure
    Clipping
    Resection and vein graft
  Common carotid ligation
    Abrupt
    Gradual
  Internal carotid ligation (clamp or ligature, balloon)
    With EC-IC bypass
    Without EC-IC bypass
  Trapping

INTERNAL CAROTID ARTERY—CAVERNOUS ANEURYSMS

Presentation

Table 12.2 summarizes the clinical features. Usually these aneurysms present with symptoms of a partial or fully developed cavernous syndrome with diplopia, retro-orbital pain, proptosis and numbness and/or facial pain from involvement of the fifth cranial nerve. In the authors' experience the most common early presenting symptom has been an isolated sixth nerve paresis. When the aneurysm ruptures it can result in a carotid cavernous fistula with the additional symptoms of pulsatile exophthalmos, chemosis, scleral injection, a bruit, and occasionally visual loss. Infrequently, TIAs or a stroke are caused by embolism. Subarachnoid hemorrhage can occur when the aneurysm is large and has eroded the covering of the cavernous sinus. Rarely massive epistaxis from erosion into the sphenoid or ethmoid sinuses can occur (3, 14, 30).

These aneurysms may be spontaneous (developmental), atherosclerotic, traumatic, or infectious due to direct extension of a sinus infection. There is a significant incidence of traumatic aneurysms because of the frequency of skull fractures through this region and the relative tethering of the internal carotid artery as it pierces the dura.

Management

The treatment options are similar to those for petrous aneurysms. The natural history of asymptomatic cavernous aneurysms is not known. The authors prefer to follow these aneurysms with periodic CT scanning unless they are very large.

Symptomatic aneurysms, even those resulting only in partial ophthalmoplegia, should be treated if the patient is in good health since the clinical course is usually progressive once symptoms develop (3, 9, 14). Direct treatment of these aneurysms by exposure of the internal carotid artery (15, 21), or by packing of the cavernous sinus (9) has been successful in a few instances but is not generally recommended because of the high risk and technical difficulties of these approaches. Metallic injection of the aneurysm with wire and needles in hopes of producing spontaneous or electrically induced thrombosis are also risky techniques that should be reserved for the few centers where these techniques are being refined (13, 20). As is the case with petrous aneurysms, common carotid ligation is an effective and safe mode of treatment (28, 29). When the aneurysm fails to thrombose after common carotid ligation, trapping by intracranial occlusion of the internal carotid artery, below the ophthalmic artery if possible, can be done. Where the technique is well developed, internal carotid artery occlusion by detachable balloon with or without preliminary EC-IC bypass may be the treatment of choice (1, 6, 7, 9, 23) (see Chapter 20). Trapping with balloons is not recommended because the distal balloon has a significant risk of occluding the origin of the ophthalmic artery and resulting in blindness.

Results

The results of treatment of internal carotid artery-cavernous aneurysms by the authors at the Massachusetts General Hospital (MGH) during the past 5 years are summarized in Table 12.3. A good result implies eventual improvement of the presenting symptoms and thrombosis of the aneurysm. The case treated by trapping had failed to thrombose initially after common carotid artery occlusion. It should be pointed out that in some of these patients the cavernous syndrome worsened initially, probably as a result of aneurysmal expansion at the time of acute thrombosis. However, all of these patients eventually improved. Those patients in whom the symptoms resolved completely ("excellent" result) have not been separated from those who improved only partially. Both of these results are grouped as "good." Similarly good results have been obtained by others using proximal carotid ligation or balloon occlusion (1, 9, 30).

INTERNAL CAROTID—POSTERIOR COMMUNICATING ARTERY ANEURYSM

Presentation

About 50% of all aneurysms of the internal carotid artery, or 25% of all intracranial aneurysms, arise in

Table 12.2.
Internal Carotid Artery—Cavernous Aneurysms

Presentation
   Diplopia
   Retro-orbital pain
   Proptosis
   Subjective bruit
   Facial numbness and/or pain
   Carotid-cavernous fistula
   Subarachnoid hemorrhage
   Epistaxis
   Cerebral or ocular ischemic symptoms

Treatment
   Conservative
   Common carotid ligation
   Internal carotid ligation (clamp or ligature, balloon)
      With EC-IC bypass
      Without EC-IC bypass
   Trapping
   Direct approach with or without cardiopulmonary bypass
   Stereotactic or direct metallic injection

Table 12.3.
Results of Treatment of Internal Carotid Artery—Cavernous Aneurysms

Mode of Treatment[a]	Number of Patients	Result Good	Result Poor	Result Dead
CCA ligation				
Gradual	1	1	0	0
Abrupt	4	4	0	0
ICA occlusion by balloon				
With EC-IC bypass	1	1	0	0
Without EC-IC bypass	1	1	0	0
Trapping	1	1	0	0
Totals	8	8	0	0

[a]CCA = common carotid artery; ICA = internal carotid artery; EC-IC = extracranial-intracranial.

relation to the origin of the posterior communicating artery (Fig. 12.3) (8, 11, 22, 30). These aneurysms usually present with subarachnoid hemorrhage or with an isolated third nerve paresis or both. The third nerve paresis is usually painful and difficult to distinguish from that occurring spontaneously in patients with diabetes, except that the pupil is usually involved when the paresis is due to an aneurysm. However, cases have been reported of pupillary sparing with third nerve palsies secondary to aneurysms (16). Therefore, pupillary sparing is not a reason for complacency and, in the authors' opinion, all these patients should be evaluated immediately with angiography.

Management

Almost all internal carotid-posterior communicating artery aneurysms are approached using a pterional craniotomy. A subtemporal exposure has been used only for incidental posterior communicating artery aneurysms when the subtemporal approach was chosen because the primary problem was a basilar tip aneurysm. Table 12.4 lists some of the important points to keep in mind in the surgical management of these aneurysms.

It is important to know from the preoperative angiogram the projection of the aneurysm. When the aneurysm projects straight laterally or superolaterally, one must be extremely careful not to use deep temporal retraction. In these cases only a self-retaining frontal retractor is used for the initial aspects of the dissection. When the aneurysm projects directly posteriorly or inferolaterally, it is safe to apply very slight gentle retraction to the temporal lobe since in these instances the aneurysm almost invariably projects beneath the tentorial edge. As a rule, most aneurysms that involve the third cranial nerve project inferior to the tentorial edge and, therefore, are not adherent to the temporal lobe, but one cannot depend on this rule. Once the self-retaining retractors are in place, one proceeds to open the arachnoid widely (Fig. 12.4). Wide opening of the arachnoid over the optic nerve, internal carotid artery, and between the frontal and temporal lobes at the medial aspect of the sylvian fissure allows for much easier retraction and also allows one to retract the frontal lobe without significant deep traction on the temporal lobe. In cases of posterior communicating artery aneurysms it is rarely necessary to open the sylvian fissure widely. The authors have not found it necessary to open the cistern over the lamina terminalis to inspect the anterior communicating complex, although this maneuver has been used routinely by others (30).

Table 12.4.
Internal Carotid—Posterior Communicating Artery Aneurysms

Position head according to projection
Avoid deep temporal retraction in laterally and superiorly projecting aneurysms
Identify and preserve posterior communicating artery (if possible)
Identify and protect third nerve
Avoid long clips with danger of occluding perforators

After wide opening of the arachnoid the authors usually begin dissection on the medial aspect of the internal carotid artery and develop the plane between the internal carotid artery and the optic nerve so as to inspect the posterior wall of the artery by retracting it laterally. Posterior communicating artery aneurysms rarely project medially and, unless the angiogram shows medial projection, it is quite safe to develop this medial plane first. If there is a thick clot over the internal carotid artery, the clot can usually be suctioned away and the more adherent deeper aspect of the clot can be gently "rolled" from medial to lateral to expose the origin of the aneurysm. In most instances the origin of the aneurysm will be clearly seen laterally. The distal aspect of the neck of the aneurysm can usually be dissected easily without a need for removal of the anterior clinoid process or the falciform edge of the petroclinoid ligament.

In order to expose the proximal aspect of the neck of the aneurysm when it is relatively proximal or when the anterior clinoid is very prominent, it may

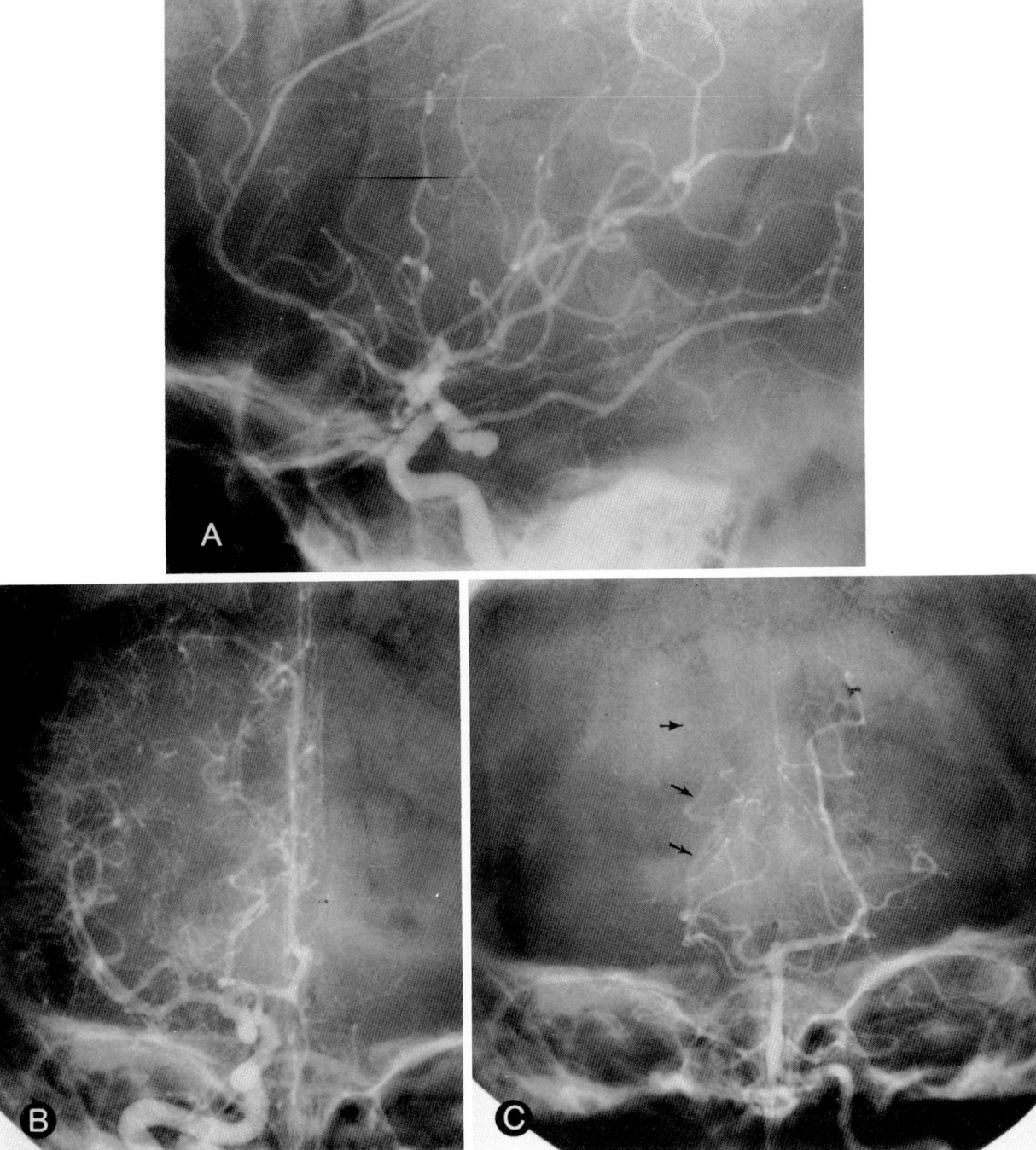

Figure 12.3. Internal carotid-posterior communicating artery aneurysm: importance of vertebral angiography. **A** and **B**, Right carotid angiogram shows large internal carotid artery aneurysm at origin of fetal-type posterior cerebral artery. No washout from posterior circulation. **C**, AP vertebral angiogram, however, shows filling of the right posterior cerebral artery (*arrows*) which is faint due to washout. There is a tiny aneurysm at the basilar apex.

be necessary to open the petroclinoid ligament (Fig. 12.5) or to drill away the anterior clinoid in a manner which will be described later (Chapter 13). To open this tough falciform ligament the authors have found it helpful to place a right angle sharp hook under the ligament at a point proximal and away from the aneurysmal dome which is frequently attached to the ligament. By applying very low monopolar current to the metal hook, the dura can be coagulated and opened simultaneously. The authors prefer to use this tech-

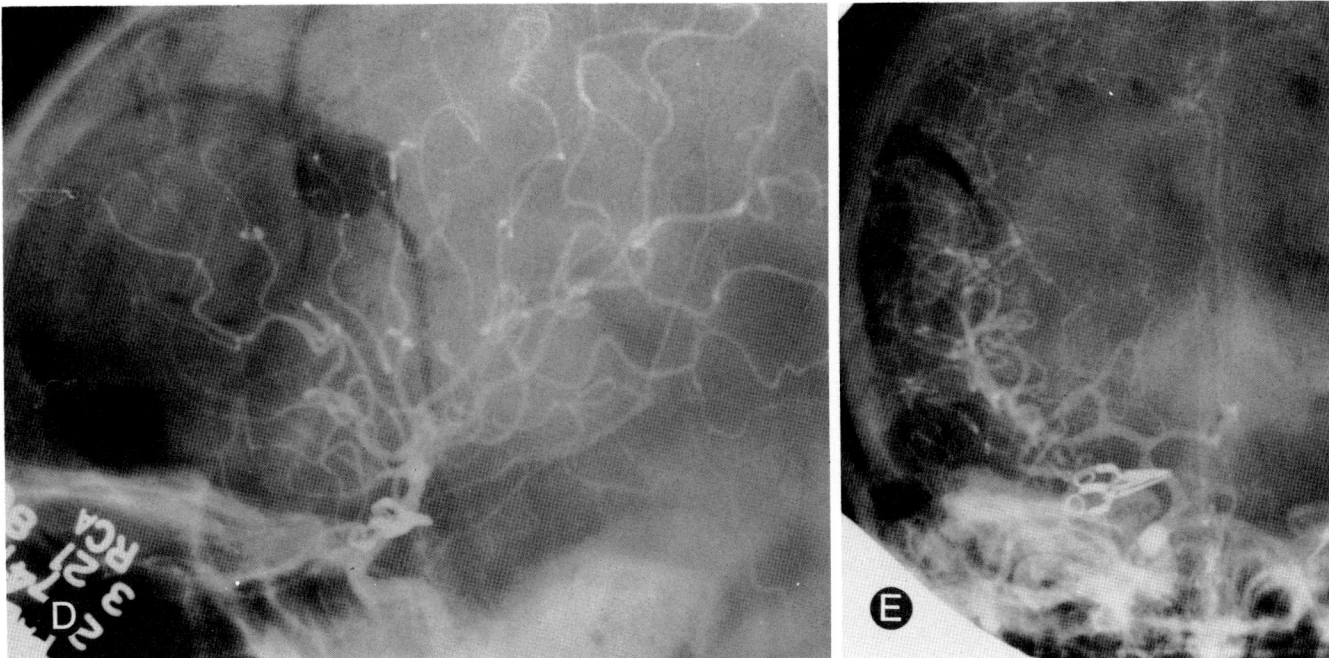

Figure 12.3. **D** and **E**, Postoperative right carotid angiograms show (a) nonfilling of the aneurysm and (b) nonfilling of the fetal posterior cerebral artery which required clipping to collapse aneurysm. Vertebral angiogram had demonstrated that this maneuver would likely be safe. The postoperative neurologic examination was normal.

nique because the dura can be quite vascular along this edge. Usually a vertical opening of only a few millimeters in this area will allow the surgeon to visualize the proximal aspect of the neck of the aneurysm. That is really all that needs to be exposed in order to define the proximal anatomy. The dome is left undisturbed.

In instances where the aneurysm projects laterally and is adherent to the temporal lobe, one must work from a more frontal angle by retracting only the frontal lobe (Fig. 12.6). Alternatively, one may carefully enter the pia-arachnoid of the temporal lobe around the aneurysm and, by subpial suction, leave a bit of brain attached to the dome, thus permitting gentle retraction of the temporal lobe. In posteriorly projecting aneurysms, as stated before, the temporal lobe can be retracted without danger.

In posterior communicating artery aneurysms the critical anatomy is restricted to the area of the neck and the dome is not dissected in order to avoid premature rupture. The anterior choroidal artery must be preserved, but this is rarely a problem except with the large aneurysms. The anterior choroidal artery, which may be multiple, is always found distal to the aneurysm on the lateral aspect of the internal carotid artery. This artery may be adherent to the dome, but its separation from the neck of the aneurysm is rarely a problem. In some cases, the anterior choroidal artery may be easier to discover by inspection of the medial aspect of the internal carotid artery (Fig. 12.7).

The posterior communicating artery, however, is a bit more difficult to dissect. This artery almost always arises in the area of the inferior aspect of the neck along the lateral surface of the internal carotid artery. The posterior communicating artery immediately turns posteromedially and this is why it is difficult to see at first glance. Frequently all that one sees is an area of slight bulge along the inferior aspect of the neck of the aneurysm. To identify the posterior communicating artery it is usually necessary to elevate gently the inferior aspect of the aneurysm as one looks from an inferotemporal angle of vision. In this manner the posterior communicating artery can usually be separated from the aneurysm and the true aneurysmal neck can be defined. In some instances it is impossible to see the artery from this lateral angle and one must then retract the internal carotid artery toward the aneurysm and identify the posterior communicating artery from medially in the angle between the optic nerve and the internal carotid artery. For this maneuver it is necessary to move the microscope so as to come from a frontal line of vision (Fig. 12.7). It is safe to retract the internal carotid artery toward the aneurysm since in this manner the aneurysm is not pulled away from its attachments at the dome. It is never advisable to retract the internal carotid artery toward the optic nerve (away from the dome of the aneurysm) because this maneuver is quite likely to bring about bleeding since the aneurysmal dome is usually attached laterally either to the pe-

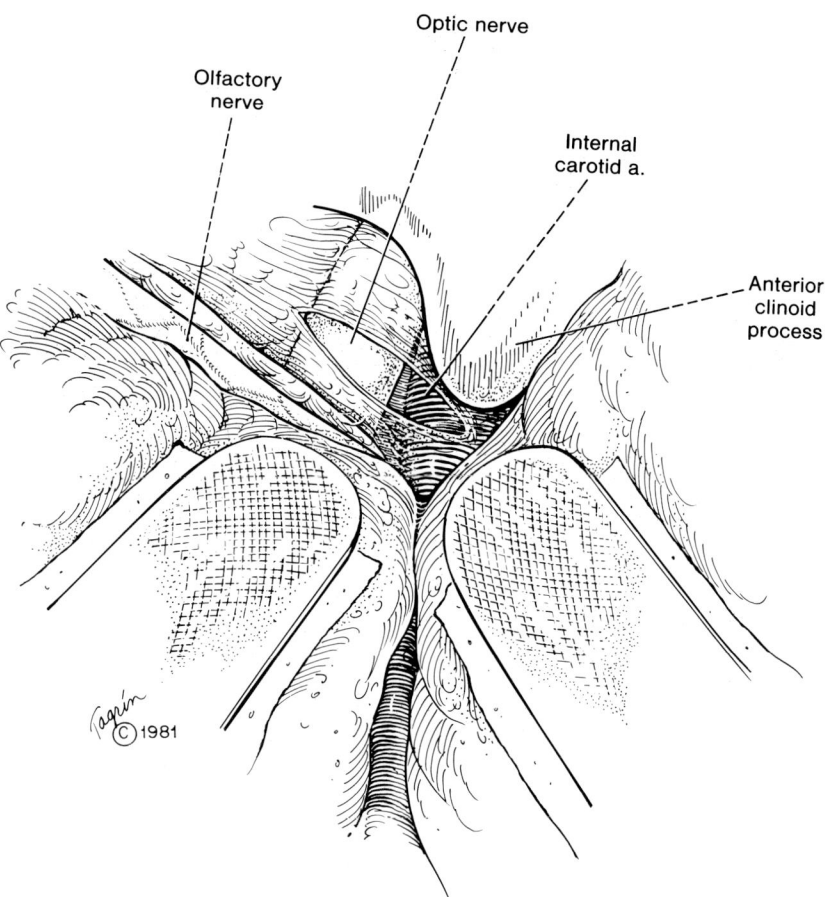

Figure 12.4. Opening arachnoid. Microscissors and a fine right-angled hook are used to open arachnoid over the optic nerve and internal carotid artery. Wide opening of the arachnoid over the optic nerve, carotid artery and between the frontal and temporal lobes permits retraction of the frontal lobe without undue traction on the temporal lobe.

troclinoid ligament, to the temporal lobe, or to the third cranial nerve. Once the inferior and the superior aspects of the aneurysmal neck are well identified and a space is created between the neck and the posterior communicating artery, the aneurysm is occluded with a clip just long enough to go around the aneurysmal neck. Excessively long clips should be avoided because there is a risk of occluding some of the perforating vessels from the posterior communicating artery that course upwards behind the internal carotid artery. Likewise with a long clip directed laterally, one may injure the third nerve.

After clipping, one must carefully inspect the distal end of the blades to ensure that neither the third nerve nor any of the perforators are included. The perforators can be checked most easily by retracting the internal carotid artery laterally and looking in the angle between the optic nerve and the internal carotid artery. Rarely, it is too difficult to separate the origin of the posterior communicating artery from the aneurysm or a tear in this area of the neck forces inclusion of the posterior communicating artery origin in the clip (Fig. 12.8). This is usually safe provided that the posterior communicating artery is not of the dominant (fetal) type, a fact that should be known beforehand from preoperative study of the angiograms. When the posterior communicating artery is included in the clip, it is important also to occlude it between the first of its perforators and the aneurysm to avoid backfilling of the aneurysm from the posterior communicating artery. In all cases posterior communicating artery perforating branches must be spared because occlusion of even a single perforant artery can cause symptomatic thalamic infarction (Fig. 12.9). Once the surgeon has checked the clip position and has confirmed that the third nerve, the perforators, the posterior communicating artery and the anterior choroidal are free and the internal carotid artery is not compromised or kinked, one is ready to puncture the aneurysm to ensure that it is indeed completely obliterated. This maneuver is recommended in all cases. The authors prefer to do this with a 25-gauge needle to avoid excessive bleeding if indeed the aneurysm is not completely obliterated.

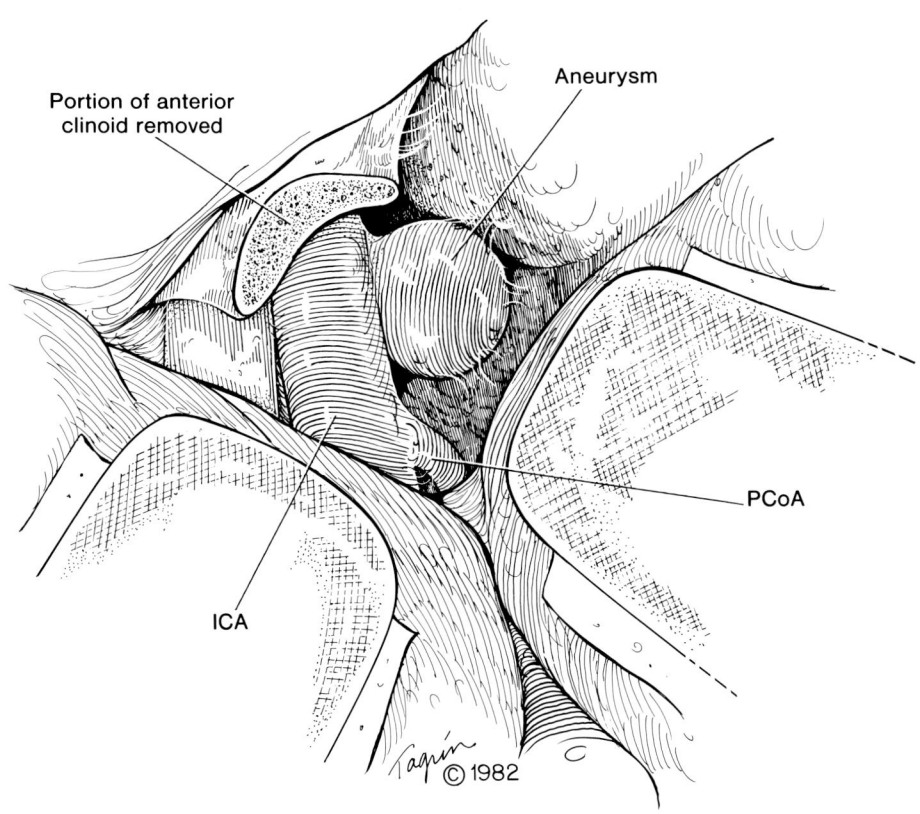

Figure 12.5. Proximal internal carotid artery aneurysm. Like a carotid ophthalmic lesion, this aneurysm may require removal of the anterior clinoid process for adequate exposure. In other instances the proximal aspect of the aneurysmal dome may be covered not by bone but by the tough, falciform petroclinoid ligament. This dural edge is frequently quite vascular and should be coagulated before dividing it which is necessary to expose the proximal aspect of the neck. A sharp hook inserted under the ligament can be used to cut it by touching the distal hook with the monopolar cautery at a very low setting.

Posteriorly projecting aneurysms present the surgeon with a slightly more difficult situation. To deal with these aneurysms the head is turned 60° so that the surgeon can see the aneurysm in profile working from the temporal side. In this fashion sometimes a curved clip can be applied to occlude the aneurysm (Fig. 12.10). In clip application perpendicular to the parent vessel, one must determine whether the internal carotid artery is kinked or narrowed at the aneurysm origin. Alternatively, a Sundt clip graft may be applied right over the internal carotid artery (Fig. 12.11). Since the Sugita fenestrated right-angle clips have been available, Sundt clips have been necessary only rarely. These particular types of Sugita clips are ideal for posteriorly projecting aneurysms (24). The aperture of the clip is at a right angle to the blades so that the clip can be applied over the internal carotid artery preserving the anterior choroidal artery. The blades then close on the back side of the artery, along the longitudinal axis of the neck. Again, care must be taken to place the clips inside the posterior communicating artery so that the artery is preserved (Fig. 12.12). With this maneuver some very large aneurysms have been clipped that, in the authors' opinion, could not have been clipped satisfactorily with any other type of clip.

In cases of larger aneurysms, it may be desirable to place the clip a bit distal to the origin of the aneurysm so that when the clip closes there will be no kinking of the internal carotid artery. It is preferable to leave a very slight portion of the neck unclipped rather than kink the artery or avulse the neck of the aneurysm by placing the clip too close to the artery (11). Before closing the clip blades, the surgeon must ensure that there is no undue traction on the aneurysm that will lead to a rupture as the blades are closed. If this is the case, some dissection along the dome will be necessary in order to free the aneurysm enough so that as the blades pull the walls of the aneurysm together it will not avulse from its attachments. A proximal temporary clip on the internal carotid artery may slacken a turgid, thin-walled neck for cauterization and clipping. In spite of this precaution, avulsion of the dome may still occur, but closure of the clip usually suffices to stop the bleeding. If the bleeding occurs from an avulsion right at the neck, temporary clips on the internal carotid artery will be needed to allow inspection and correc-

Internal Carotid Artery Aneurysms

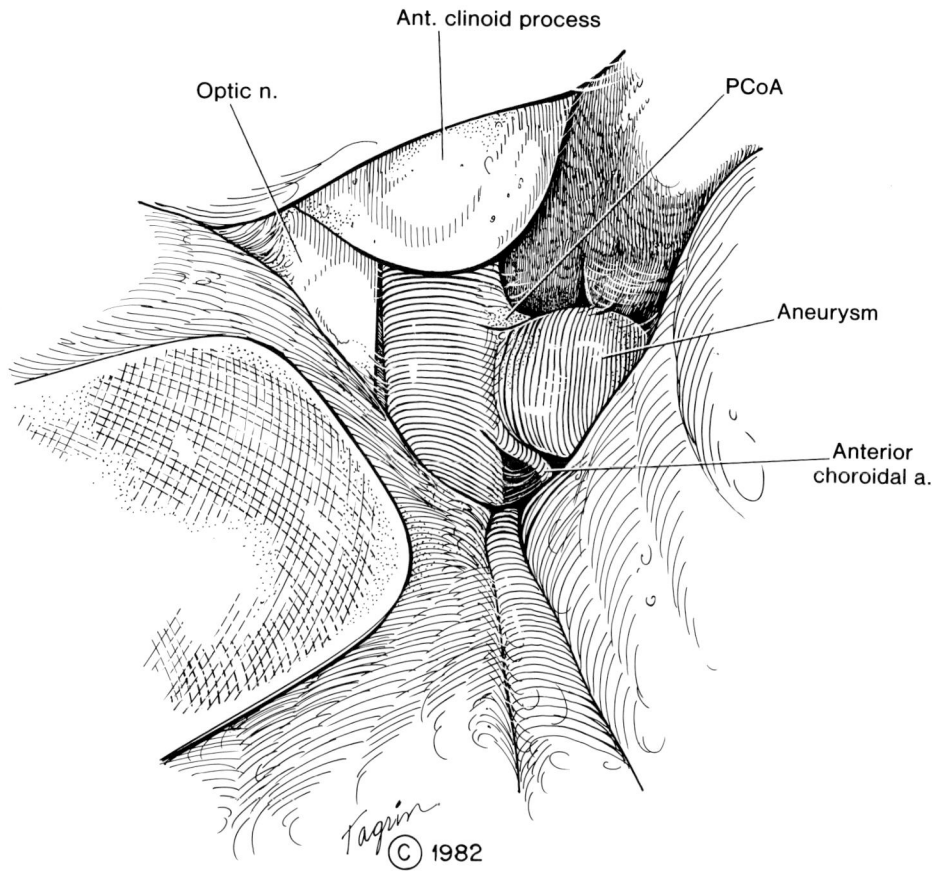

Figure 12.6. Lateral projection of internal carotid-posterior communicating artery aneurysm. The temporal lobe is not retracted. The dome is usually left adherent to the temporal lobe. The anterior choroidal artery must be spared. If the projection is inferolateral (below the tentorial edge), the aneurysmal dome is usually adherent to the third nerve and should not be mobilized to avoid further injury to that nerve.

tion of the situation. The deliberate steps recommended earlier (Chapter 11) in cases of rupture must always be kept in mind.

Results

The operative results in patients with nongiant internal carotid artery aneurysms treated by direct intracranial obliteration by the authors at the MGH during the past 10 years are given in Table 12.5. This table excludes paraclinoid aneurysms which are discussed in the next chapter. Aneurysms at the origin of the posterior communicating artery are grouped together with aneurysms at the origin of the anterior choroidal artery because of the frequent difficulty in separating these aneurysms. The majority (over 70%) of the operations were performed late (about 10–14 days) after subarachnoid hemorrhage since the authors have been operating early only during the past 2 years. Almost all of our patients were in good condition preoperatively or had a stable neurologic deficit (grades 1, 2 or 1A, Hunt).

Of the poor results, one patient was in poor preoperative condition and the rest were in good con-

Table 12.5.
Results of Surgery for Nongiant Internal Carotid Artery Aneurysm

	Good	Poor	Dead	Total
Trunk (PCoA, AChA)[a]	96	4	0	100
Bifurcation	14	1	1	16
Totals	110	5	1	116

[a]PCoA = posterior communicating artery; AChA = anterior choroidal artery.

dition but deteriorated either as a result of vasospasm or, in two instances, as a result of a technical error. Perforator occlusion lead to infarction of the basal ganglia in one patient and premature rupture with need for temporary occlusion compounded by hypotension resulted in infarction in another.

Yasargil obtained a good surgical result in 83.2% of 173 patients with internal carotid-posterior communicating artery aneurysms (30). His 5.8% mortality and 1.2% poor results were mostly among patients in poor preoperative grade. He noted full recovery of oculomotor palsy in 82.1% of the patients and partial recovery in 10.4% over a period of weeks to months.

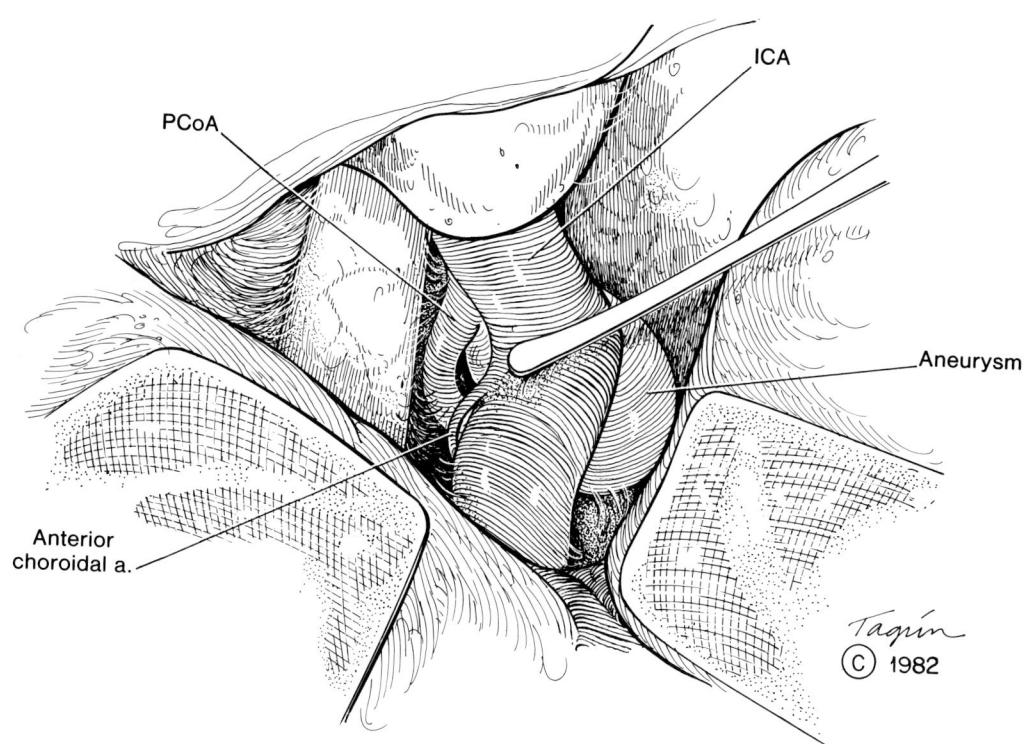

Figure 12.7. Posterior projection of internal carotid artery aneurysm. Deflection of the internal carotid artery laterally and changing the angle of vision to come from a more medial direction may expose the medial wall of the aneurysm and its relation to internal carotid artery branches.

INTERNAL CAROTID—ANTERIOR CHOROIDAL ARTERY ANEURYSMS

Presentation

Anterior choroidal artery aneurysms account for about 5–10% of all aneurysms of the internal carotid artery (30). They usually present with subarachnoid hemorrhage but on occasion there may be a third nerve palsy.

Management

Table 12.6 lists some of the key points to remember in the surgical management of these aneurysms. They project superolaterally, posterolaterally, or straight laterally and are often in intimate relationship to the medial aspect of the temporal lobe and frequently the dome is buried in the uncus. Usually the aneurysm projects above the tentorium and away from the third nerve although occasionally, when large, they can involve the third nerve.

After the standard pterional craniotomy, as described in the previous section, the internal carotid artery is approached starting the dissection medially, in the plane between the optic nerve and the internal carotid artery, since the anterior choroidal artery aneurysms usually project laterally. For these aneu-

Table 12.6.
Internal Carotid—Anterior Choroidal Artery Aneurysms

Avoid deep temporal retraction
Open medial sylvian fissure widely but carefully
Preserve anterior choroidal artery (arteries)
Avoid long clips and perforator occlusion

rysms it is almost always necessary to open the medial aspect of the sylvian fissure and expose the inferior aspects of the anterior and the middle cerebral arteries at the bifurcation. Particular care must be taken not to put excessive retraction on the medial aspect of the temporal lobe to which these aneurysms are frequently adherent. It is preferable at first to retract only the frontal lobe and to open all the arachnoidal bands of the medial sylvian fissure to avoid traction on the temporal lobe. Frequently, a bit of the medial aspect of the temporal lobe is resected, leaving some of the brain adherent to the dome of the aneurysm. With this maneuver one can then retract the temporal lobe to better expose the bifurcation and see clearly the anatomy between the distal aspect of the neck of the aneurysm and the internal carotid artery. The dissection proceeds from the internal carotid artery laterally toward the neck of the aneurysm.

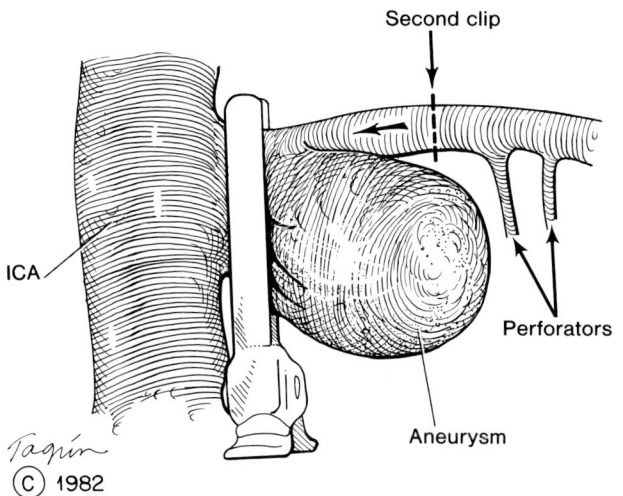

Figure 12.8. Internal carotid-posterior communicating artery aneurysm. This clip placement is only very rarely necessary because the posterior communicating artery can almost always be separated from the true neck of the aneurysm. However, in an occasional instance of rupture at the neck it may be necessary to sacrifice the origin of the posterior communicating artery. When this is done the lesion may backfill from the posterior communicating artery after clipping. A second clip to occlude the posterior communicating artery must avoid important perforator branches. Preoperative angiography indicates whether the posterior communicating artery may be sacrificed safely.

The anterior choroidal artery is the key landmark in the dissection of these aneurysms. In about 70% of patients this artery arises as a single trunk from the inferior aspect of the neck of the aneurysm (30). The artery is easier to identify than the posterior communicating artery because it runs a more lateral course and usually is readily visible from the lateral aspect of the internal carotid artery. Occasionally there are two distinct anterior choroidal arteries and rarely three or more. When there is more than one artery the aneurysm usually arises from the angle between the largest of the anterior choroidal arteries and the lateral aspect of the internal carotid artery; that is, the largest of the arteries can be found along the inferior aspect of the neck of the aneurysm on the lateral wall of the internal carotid artery. The second choroidal artery may then arise distal to the aneurysm or along the medial aspect of the wall of the aneurysm which may create a problem with the dissection. The key to the surgery of this aneurysm is to preserve the anterior choroidal artery since about 20% of patients in whom this artery is occluded develop a serious hemiparesis (4).

Usually it is easier to dissect first the inferior aspect of the neck and to define the plane between the anterior choroidal artery and the aneurysm. Since the artery usually runs laterally, there is little problem developing this plane. One must avoid medial traction on the carotid artery at all cost since this may lead to rupture of the aneurysm by pulling it away from its attachments at the dome. Once the inferior aspect of the neck is clearly defined, one must move to the distal aspect of the neck where it may be necessary to do a small amount of medial-temporal resection. The distal aspect of the neck must be defined just as thoroughly as the proximal aspect since occasionally a second choroidal artery will arise from this area and it should be preserved (Fig. 12.13). Occasionally, when the aneurysm projects quite superiorly, the recurrent artery of Huebner may pass behind the internal carotid artery in relation to the superior aspect of the aneurysm and it must also be preserved.

Once the proximal and distal aspects of the neck are defined, a clip is slowly introduced with the proximal blade passing between the anterior choroidal artery and the base of the aneurysm and the distal blade close to the aneurysm neck. Again, the authors prefer to use a clip that is just long enough to go across the neck because of the risk of a longer clip occluding some of the perforating branches from the anterior choroidal artery, posterior communicating artery or possibly even the recurrent artery of Huebner. After clipping, one must carefully inspect the anatomy to ensure that all small arteries are preserved and that there is no kinking of the anterior choroidal artery or the internal carotid artery. One must also ensure that there is not an additional anterior choroidal artery that has been included in the clip and that the recurrent artery of Huebner has not been inadvertently clipped. Once the surgeon is satisfied, the aneurysm is punctured to ensure that clipping has been complete. Closure can then proceed as previously described.

Results

With 21 internal carotid-anterior choroidal artery aneurysms Yasargil obtained good results in 76.2% (30). Of three patients who had either a poor result or died (14.3%), two were in poor condition preoperatively. The authors' results have been equally good but internal carotid-anterior choroidal artery aneurysms have not been separated from the much more common internal carotid-posterior communicating artery aneurysms (Table 12.5).

INTERNAL CAROTID ARTERY—BIFURCATION ANEURYSMS

Presentation

These aneurysms account for about 10–15% of all internal carotid artery aneurysms (18, 30). They usually present with subarachnoid hemorrhage. Occasionally the onset is a syndrome suggestive of a basal ganglia hemorrhage or infarction and the CT scan

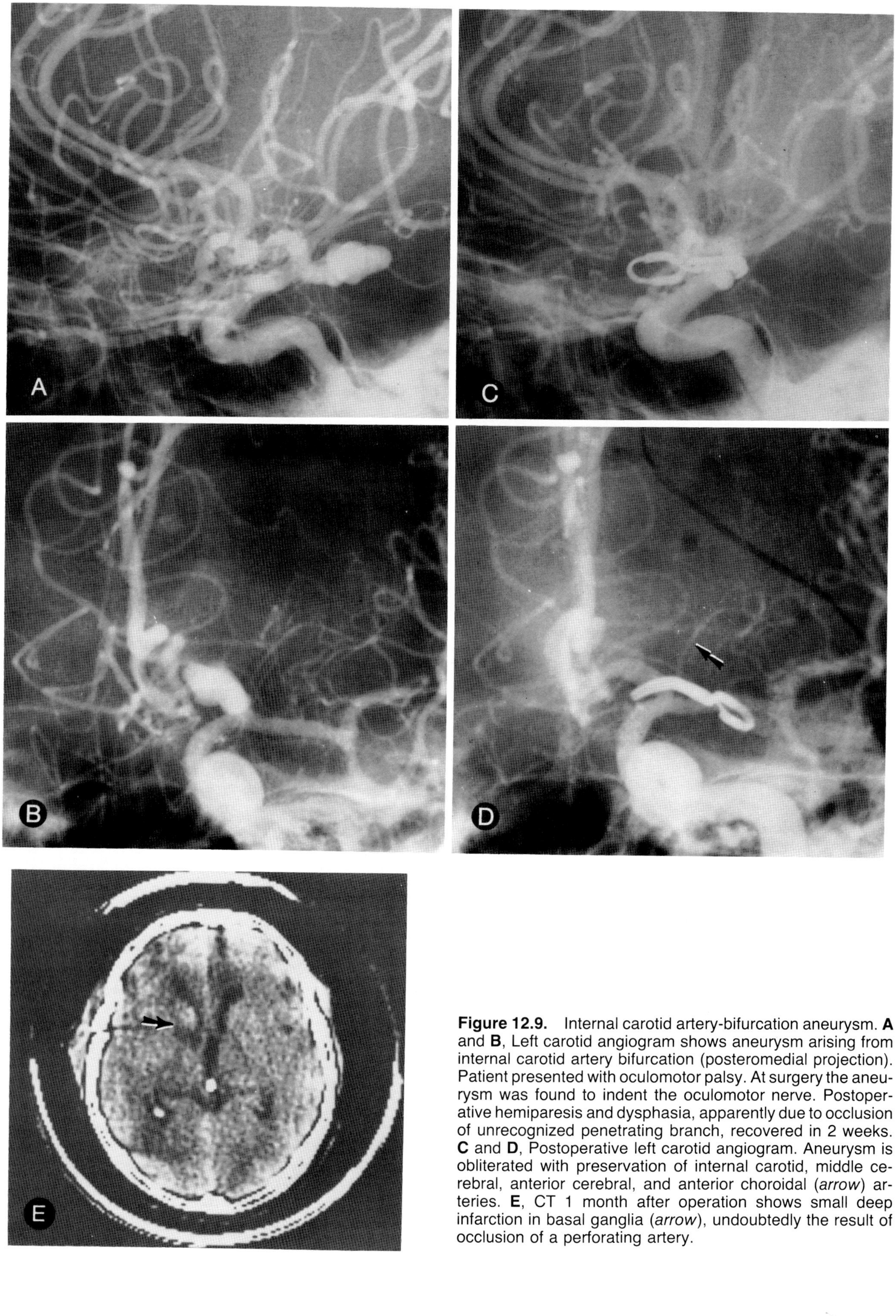

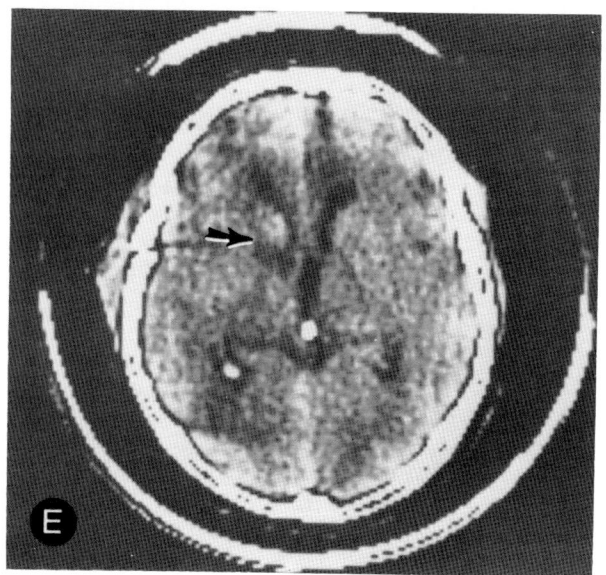

Figure 12.9. Internal carotid artery-bifurcation aneurysm. **A** and **B**, Left carotid angiogram shows aneurysm arising from internal carotid artery bifurcation (posteromedial projection). Patient presented with oculomotor palsy. At surgery the aneurysm was found to indent the oculomotor nerve. Postoperative hemiparesis and dysphasia, apparently due to occlusion of unrecognized penetrating branch, recovered in 2 weeks. **C** and **D**, Postoperative left carotid angiogram. Aneurysm is obliterated with preservation of internal carotid, middle cerebral, anterior cerebral, and anterior choroidal (*arrow*) arteries. **E**, CT 1 month after operation shows small deep infarction in basal ganglia (*arrow*), undoubtedly the result of occlusion of a perforating artery.

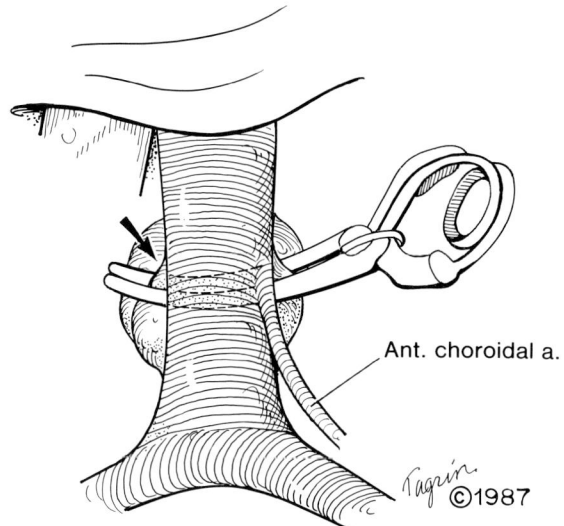

Figure 12.10. Posterior projection of internal carotid artery aneurysm. A markedly curved or right-angle clip may be effective. One must be sure this perpendicular application does not buckle the internal carotid artery causing dangerous narrowing. If a tiny dog-ear is left (*arrow*), application of muslin is indicated to prevent later enlargement.

shows what appears to be a typical ganglionic hemorrhage. This occurs because the domes of these aneurysms are frequently adherent to the orbital basal portion of the frontal lobe and, when the aneurysm bleeds, the hemorrhage can dissect directly deep into the brain parenchyma rather than into the subarachnoid space. Rarely, these patients have presented with ischemic symptoms from embolization from partial thrombosis of the aneurysm.

Management

Table 12.7 lists the important points to remember in the surgical management. Most commonly, these aneurysms project directly superiorly. Occasionally they can project posteriorly or anteriorly, depending on the curve of the internal carotid artery. Not infrequently they appear to arise in relation to either the anterior cerebral artery or the middle cerebral artery. Traditionally the surgery of these aneurysms has been more difficult than in other types of internal carotid artery aneurysms. This difficulty is related first to the fact that deep retraction is necessary for exposure and second, to the fact that the posterior aspect of these aneurysms is related to a number of very important perforating vessels.

The aneurysm dome is frequently buried in the orbital-basal aspect of the frontal lobe, and therefore, it is most satisfactory to expose the aneurysm through a small cortical resection on the frontal lobe just medial to the superficial sylvian vein that marks the medial end of the sylvian fissure (Fig. 12.14). Any crossing superficial veins in this area as well as tiny superficial arterial branches can be sacrificed. The

Table 12.7.
Internal Carotid Artery—Bifurcation Aneurysm

Open medial sylvian fissure with great care
Subpial resection frequently desirable
Identify inferior aspect of anterior cerebral artery and middle cerebral artery
Change angle of microscope to dissect the neck from the anterior cerebral artery and middle cerebral artery
Dome of aneurysm does not need to be exposed
Preserve all perforators from:
    Dorsal wall of the internal carotid artery
    Anterior choroidal
    Posterior communicating
    Origin of anterior cerebral
    Origin of middle cerebral
Identify and preserve Heubner's artery
Preserve deep veins (Rosenthal and medial sylvian)
Avoid longer than necessary clip

dissection proceeds from the proximal aspect of the internal carotid artery which is first identified. After identifying the anterior choroidal artery one gradually proceeds to expose first the inferior aspects of the anterior cerebral and the middle cerebral arteries at the bifurcation. The aneurysm neck between the anterior cerebral artery and the middle cerebral artery is then carefully dissected. Only the neck needs to be exposed and the dome can be left undisturbed, buried in the frontal lobe. To expose the neck on each side it is usually necessary to change radically the angle of vision of the microscope, coming from the far frontal side to dissect the area between the anterior cerebral artery and the aneurysm and from the temporal side to dissect between the middle cerebral artery and the aneurysm. In these aneurysms the ability to look from the frontal and the temporal side is critical (Fig. 12.15). The former is facilitated by a slightly more generous frontal exposure on the bone flap.

In cases of large aneurysms, particularly if the aneurysm is quite adherent to the anterior cerebral artery or to the middle cerebral artery, it is preferable to proceed distally with dissection of these arteries so as to have a clear space away from the aneurysm to place a temporary clip on either artery in case of rupture or to facilitate dissection. The temporary clip on the internal carotid artery usually has to be placed either proximal to the posterior communicating artery or between the posterior communicating artery and the anterior choroidal artery. It is best not to place a clip distal to the anterior choroidal artery because this clip may actually perforate the back of the aneurysm. On occasion the cistern of the lamina terminalis is opened to enable better retraction of the lateral basal frontal lobe and to identify the artery of Huebner (30). In addition, by inspecting the anterior communicating complex, one can estimate the potential for collateral circulation in case the origin of

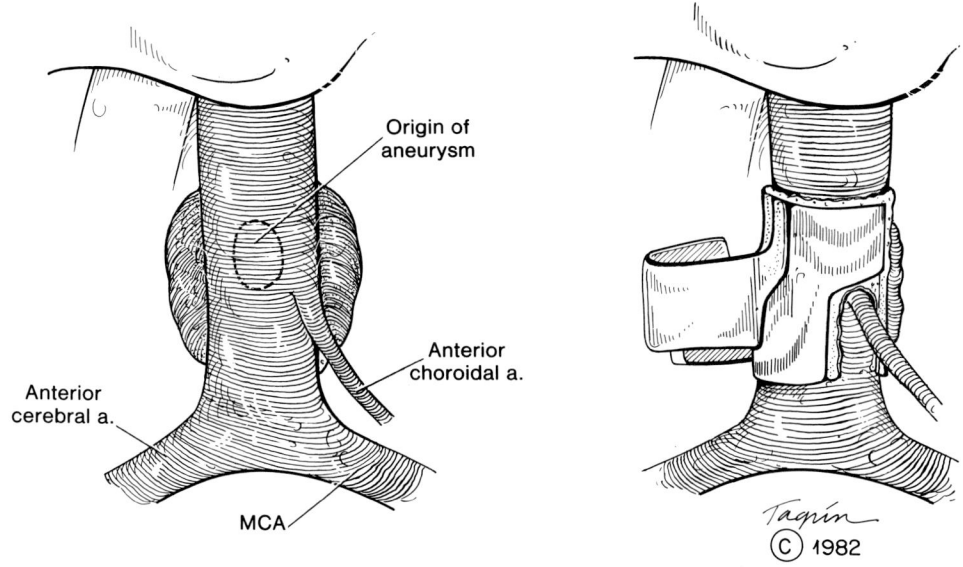

Figure 12.11. Posterior projection of internal carotid artery aneurysm. A Sundt clip-graft (with or without window) may be the answer. However, since the availability of the Sugita right-angle clips with a Drake aperture, the Sundt clip grafts are used mostly in cases of tears right at the wall of the parent vessel.

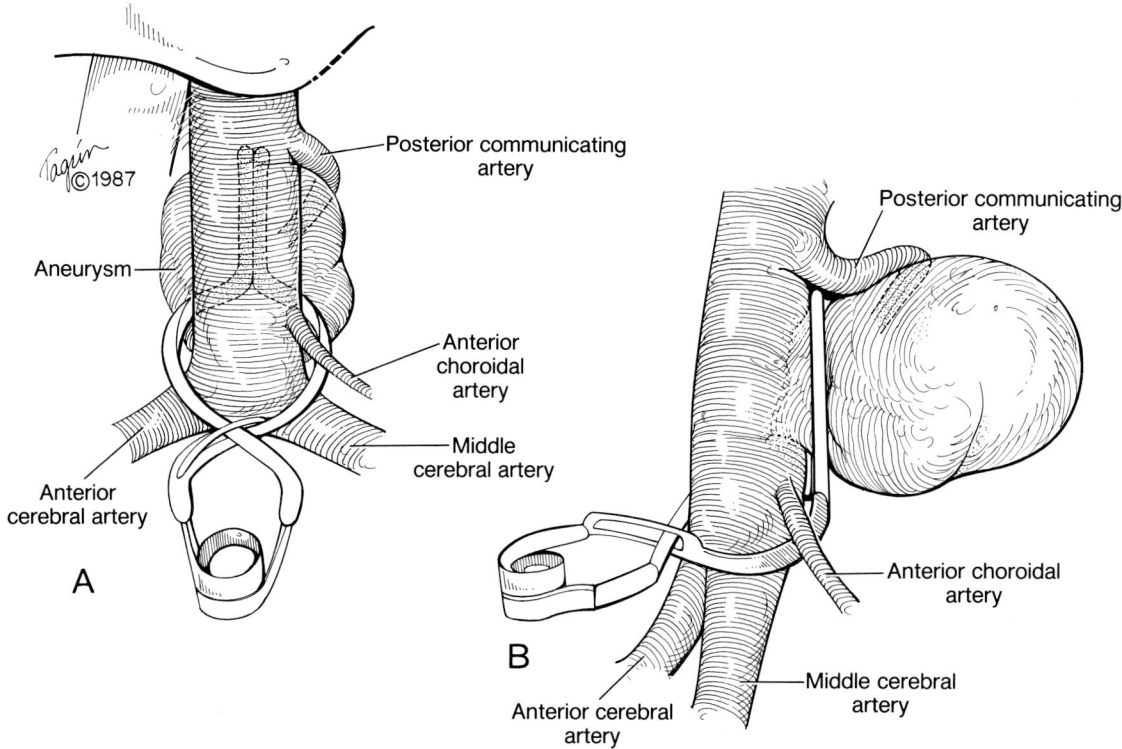

Figure 12.12. The preferable way to occlude posteriorly or posterior medially projecting aneurysms may be to apply a right-angle fenestrated Sugita clip that fits over the carotid artery and occludes the neck in the direction parallel to the axis of the parent vessel. With the fenestration, the anterior choroidal artery can be preserved. The distal clip blades are medial to the origin of the posterior communicating artery.

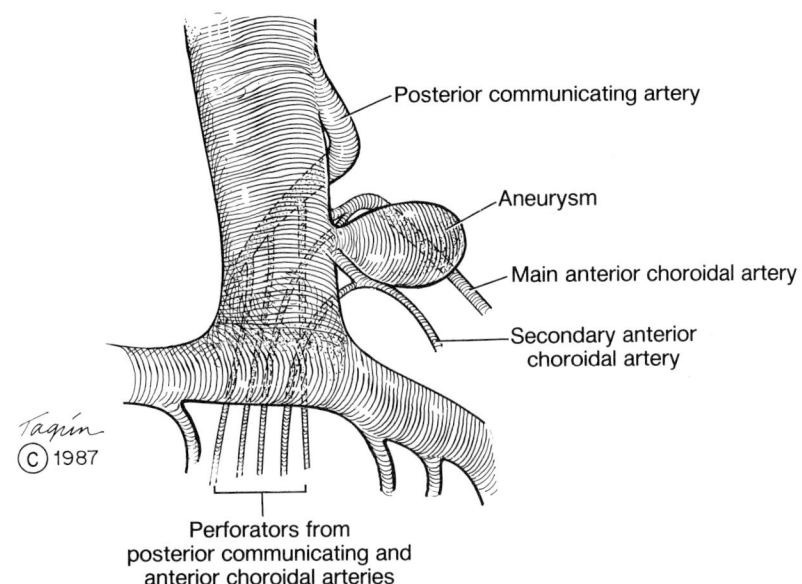

Figure 12.13. Internal carotid-anterior choroidal artery aneurysm. The anterior choroidal artery, which may be in duplicate, must be preserved. In this sketch a secondary anterior choroidal artery arises distal to the aneurysm.

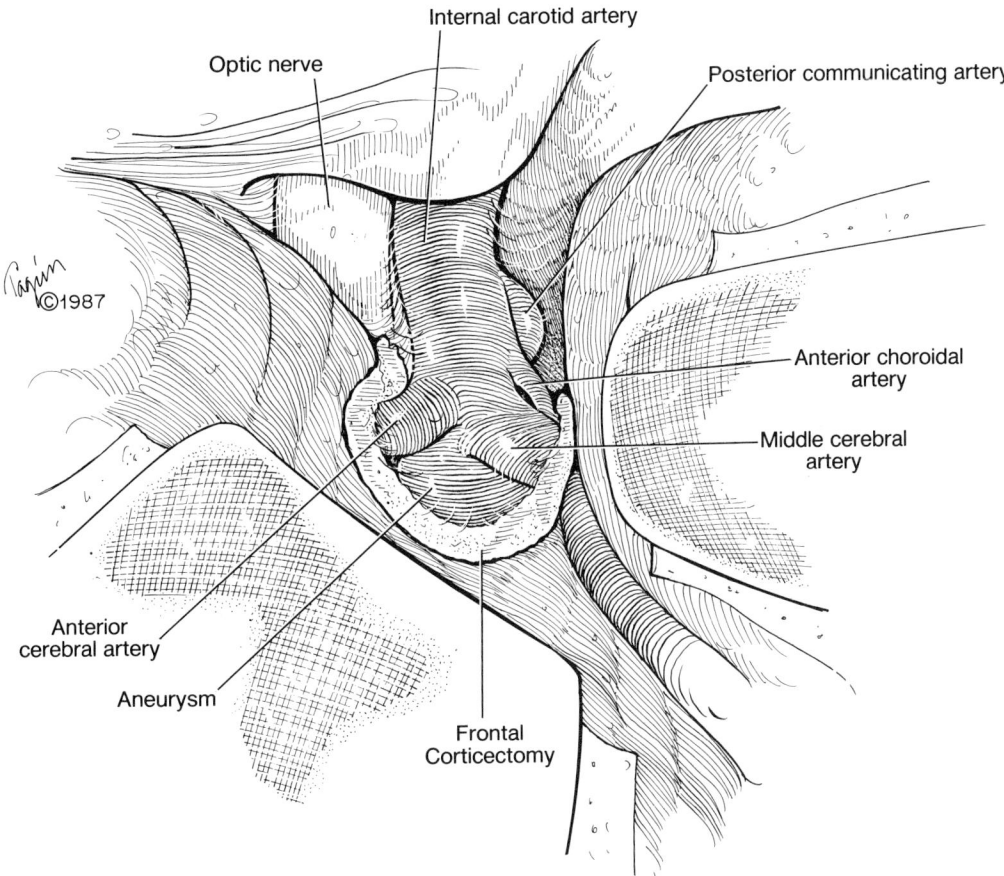

Figure 12.14. Frontal corticectomy (or opening the sylvian fissure) provides distal exposure of the origin of the anterior and middle cerebral arteries and of the base of the aneurysm.

the anterior cerebral artery must be included in the clip either as a premeditated maneuver or as a life-saving maneuver in case of rupture.

After the anterior and middle cerebral arteries are exposed and the spaces between them and the aneurysm are developed, one proceeds to retract the aneurysm to one side and then to the other as the angle of vision is changed to identify and dissect the important perforating branches away from the back of the aneurysm (Fig. 12.15). These arise near the origin of both the middle cerebral and the anterior cerebral arteries; from the anterior choroidal artery and posterior communicating artery; and, less commonly, directly from the back wall of the internal carotid artery. In addition, the recurrent artery of Huebner usually runs in the space behind the internal carotid artery bifurcation or slightly higher in relation to the posterior aspect of these aneurysms, but the course is variable and the artery may be inferior and deep to the plane of the bifurcation or it may be more superior and adherent to the dome of the aneurysm. All these arteries run in the subarachnoid cistern deep to the aneurysm. However, with microsurgical techniques, it is possible to identify and preserve all the important perforating vessels.

When the aneurysm is large, the perforating arteries may be quite adherent to the posterior wall and it may be very difficult to visualize all the important posterior anatomy without very thorough mobilization of the aneurysm. In some patients temporary clips may be needed to make the aneurysm more collapsible for safe retraction and dissection. It is not necessary to dissect all the fundus of the aneurysm and it is permissible to leave some of the perforating branches adherent to the distal aspect of the dome provided a space is created for the clip to pass beyond

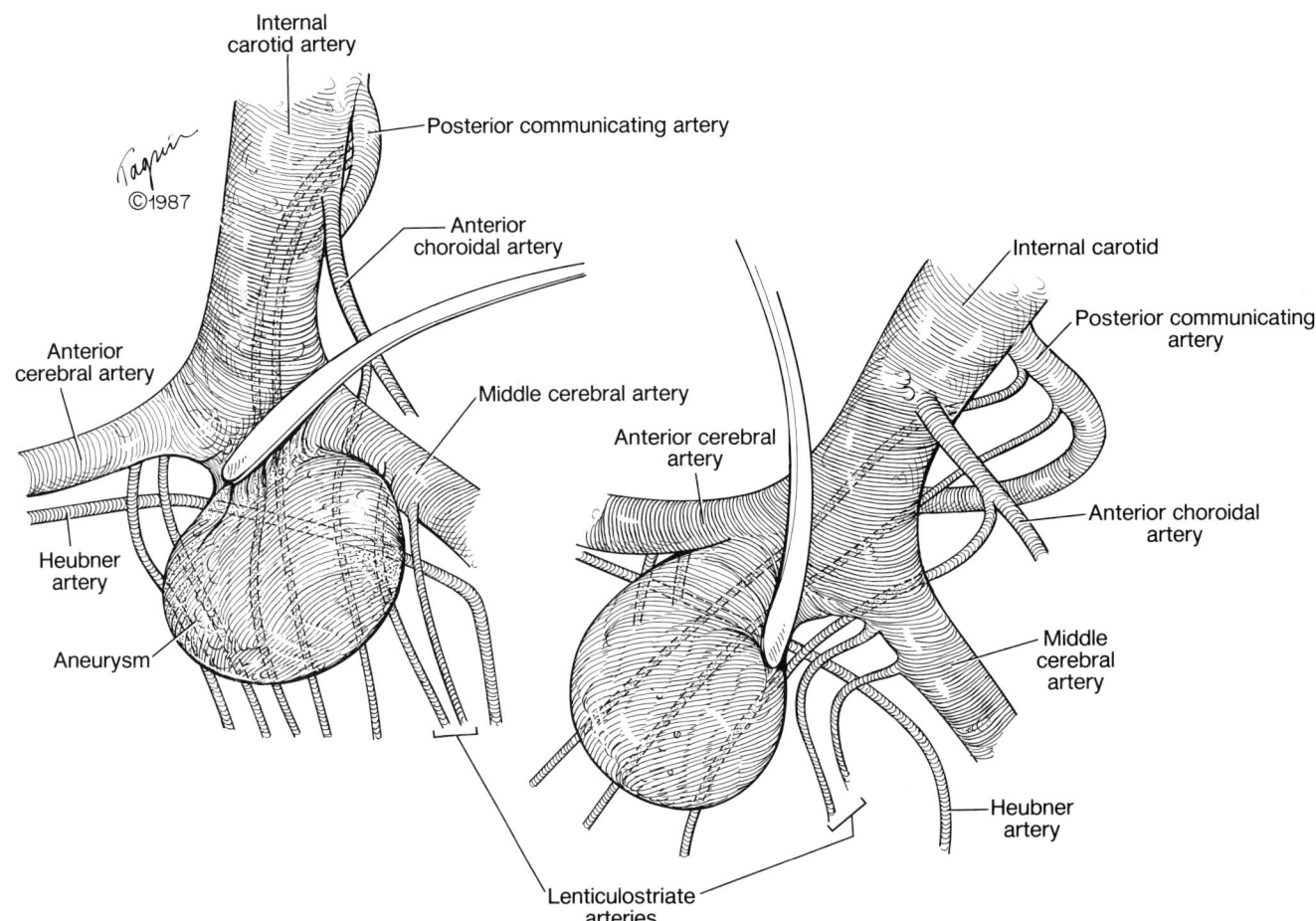

Figure 12.15. Internal carotid bifurcation aneurysm. Careful dissection of the neck ensures preservation of critical perforating branches from anterior and middle cerebral arteries as well as preservation of Heubner artery and the perforating branches of the posterior communicating artery, the anterior choroidal artery and the back wall of the carotid artery. Changing the angle of vision from the frontal side to dissect the anterior cerebral artery to the temporal side to dissect the middle cerebral artery helps in this critical aspect of the exposure.

the dome without occluding any of the perforators.

One must also be careful with the deep venous anatomy. The superficial veins can be coagulated with impunity. However, the deep sylvian vein and the basal vein of Rosenthal pass deep to these aneurysms and they can be injured, particularly with a long clip. This can create very bothersome bleeding and may necessitate coagulation of these important veins which could lead to a significant neurologic deficit.

The angle of application of the clip varies from case to case depending on the longest axis of the neck. One of the problems with these aneurysms is that it is usually impossible to see on both sides of the aneurysm as the clip is being applied. Usually the clip is applied under direct visualization on the most difficult side as the aneurysm is being retracted. Once the ipsilateral blade passes between the aneurysm and the perforating branches it may be necessary then to change the angle of vision completely by moving the microscope and then continue to advance the clip with the second blade under direct vision as one rotates the clip so that the second blade then passes between the aneurysm and the perforating branches in the other side. It is preferable once again to use a clip only long enough to go completely across the neck of the aneurysm so as to avoid injuring the deep structures. The optic tract courses deep to the aneurysm and could also be injured by the use of excessively long clips. In spite of all these precautions, one can still occasionally end up with a significant perforator injury that was not recognized at surgery (Fig. 12.9).

After the correctness of clip application is confirmed and one ensures that no perforating vessels are in the clip, the aneurysm is punctured in the usual fashion and closure is done as described.

Results

The operative results in patients with nongiant internal carotid artery bifurcation aneurysms operated by the authors at the MGH during the past 10 years are given in Table 12.5. The only death we had in this series was in a preoperative grade 3 patient who was operated on the tenth day after subarachnoid hemorrhage. Postoperatively he developed progressive vasospasm and some days later died of pulmonary embolism and a disseminated intravascular coagulopathy. In retrospect, he was operated too early after his subarachnoid hemorrhage.

Among 55 patients with internal carotid artery bifurcation aneurysms, Yasargil obtained a good result in 49 (30). The two deaths in this group occurred in patients with a poor preoperative grade. Similarly good results have been obtained by other surgeons (8, 10, 11, 25, 26).

REFERENCES

1. Berenstein A, Ransohoff J, Kupersmith M, Flamm E, Graeb D: Transvascular treatment of giant aneurysm of the cavernous carotid and vertebral arteries. Surg Neurol 21:3–12, 1984.
2. Brihaye J: Internal carotid aneurysms arising in the carotid canal. In Pia HW, Langmaid C, Zierski J (eds): Cerebral Aneurysms, Advances in Diagnosis and Therapy. Berlin, Springer-Verlag, 1979, pp 55–62.
3. Brihaye J: Intracavernous carotid aneurysms. In Pia HW, Langmaid C, Zierski J (eds): Cerebral Aneurysms, Advances in Diagnosis and Therapy. Berlin, Springer-Verlag, 1979, pp 67–88.
4. Cooper IS: Surgical occlusion of the anterior choroidal artery in Parkinsonism. Surg Gynecol Obstet 99:207–291, 1954.
5. Crompton MR: The pathology of subarachnoid hemorrhage. J R Coll Physicians Lond 7:235–237, 1973.
6. Debrun G, Fox A, Drake C, Peerless S, Girvin J, Ferguson G: Giant unclippable aneurysms: Treatment with detachable balloons. AJNR 2:167 173, 1981.
7. Debrun G, Lacour P, Caron JP, Hurth M, Comoy J, Kervel Y: Inflatable and released balloon technique—Experimentation in dog. Application in man. Neuroradiology 9:267–271, 1975.
8. Fein JM: Internal carotid posterior communicating artery aneurysms. In Fein JM, Flamm ES (eds): Cerebrovascular Surgery. Berlin, Springer-Verlag; 1985, vol III, pp 841–860.
9. Ferguson GG, Vascik JM, Drake CG, Peerless SJ, Fox AM, Vinuela F: Carotid-cavernous aneurysms: Clinical presentation and management of 78 cases. Presented at the annual meeting of the American Association of Neurological Surgeons, Atlanta, 1985.
10. Flamm ES: Aneurysms of internal carotid and anterior communicating arteries. In Wilkins RH, Rengachary SS (eds): Neurosurgery. New York, McGraw-Hill, 1985, pp 1394–1403.
11. Fox JL: Technique of aneurysm surgery. III. Internal carotid artery aneurysms. In Fox JL (ed): Intracranial Aneurysm. Berlin, Springer-Verlag, 1983, vol II, pp 949–1011.
12. Glassock ME, Smith PG, Whitaker SR, et al: Management of aneurysms of the petrous portion of the internal carotid artery by resection and primary anastomosis. Laryngoscope 93:1443–1445, 1983.
13. Hosobuchi Y: Electrothrombosis of carotid-cavernous fistulas. J Neurosurg 41:657, 1975.
14. Jefferson G: On the saccular aneurysm of the internal carotid artery in the cavernous sinus. Br Surg 26:267–302, 1938.
15. Johnston I: Direct surgical treatment of bilateral intracavernous internal carotid artery aneurysms. Case report. J Neurosurg 51:98–102, 1979.
16. Kissell JT, Burke RM, Klingele TG, Zeiger HE: Pupil-sparing oculomotor palsies with internal carotid-posterior communicating artery aneurysms. Ann Neurol 13:149–154, 1983.
17. Krayenbuhl HA, Yasargil MG, Flamm ES, Tew JM Jr: Microsurgical treatment of intracranial saccular aneurysm. J Neurosurg 37:678–686, 1972.
18. Lassman LP: Internal carotid artery bifurcation aneurysms. In Pia HW, Langmaid C, Zierski J (eds): Cerebral Aneurysms, Advances in Diagnosis and Therapy. Berlin, Springer-Verlag, 1979, pp 96–106.
19. McGrail K, Heros RC, Debrun G; Aneurysms of the ICA petrous segment treated by balloon entrapment after EC-IC bypass. J Neurosurg 65:249–252, 1986.
20. Mullan S: Experiences with surgical thrombosis of intracranial berry aneurysms and carotid cavernous fistulas. J Neurosurg 41:657–670, 1974.
21. Parkinson D: A surgical approach to the cavernous portion of the carotid artery. Anatomical studies and case report. J Neurosurg 23:474–483, 1965.
22. Pia HW: Classification of aneurysms of the internal carotid system. Acta Neurochir (Wien) 40:5, 1978.

23. Serbinenko FA: Balloon catheterization and occlusion of major cerebral vessels. *J Neurosurg* 41:125–145, 1974.
24. Sugita K, Kobayashi S, Kyoshima K, Nakagawa F: Fenestrated clips for unusual aneurysms of the carotid artery. *J Neurosurg* 57:240–246, 1982.
25. Sundt TM Jr, Whisnant JP: Subarachnoid hemorrhage from intracranial aneurysms. Surgical management and natural history of disease. *N Engl J Med* 229:116–122, 1978.
26. Suzuki J (ed): *Cerebral Aneurysms: Experiences with 1000 Directly Operated Cases.* Tokyo, Neuron, 1979.
27. Swann K, Heros RC, Debrun G, Nelson C: Inadvertent middle cerebral artery embolism by a detachable balloon: Management by embolectomy. *J Neurosurg* 64:309–312, 1986.
28. Swearingen B, Heros R: Common carotid ligation for unclippable carotid aneurysms. *J Neurosurg* in press.
29. Tindall GT, Odom GL: Treatment of intracranial aneurysms by proximal carotid ligation. *Progr Neurol Surg* 3:66–114, 1969.
30. Yasargil MG: Internal carotid artery aneurysms. In Yasargil MG: *Microsurgery.* New York, Thieme-Stratton, 1984, vol 2, pp 33-123.
31. Yasargil MG, Fox JL: The microsurgical approach to intracranial aneurysms. *Surg Neurol* 3:7–14, 1975.
32. Yasargil MG, Smith RD: Management of aneurysms of anterior circulation by intracranial procedures. In Youmans JR (ed): *Neurological Surgery,* ed 2. Philadelphia, WB Saunders, 1982, pp 1663–1696.

13
Paraclinoid Aneurysms

Aneurysms arising from the intradural portion of the internal carotid artery proximal to the posterior communicating artery usually, but not always, are related to the origin of the ophthalmic artery and for this reason are most commonly referred to as "ophthalmic aneurysms" (Fig. 13.1). However, frequently the aneurysm arises from the ventral (posterior) aspect and, rarely, from the lateral aspect of the internal carotid artery without a clear relation to the ophthalmic artery. In about 5% of the cases the aneurysm involves all of the internal carotid artery (global aneurysms) and the specific site of origin is unclear (12). For these reasons these aneurysms are referred to collectively as "paraclinoid" since what they do have in common is a radiographic and surgical relation to the anterior clinoid process. Because of the clinical features (Table 13.1) and the different surgical approach of these aneurysms, they are discussed separately from aneurysms of the internal carotid artery in other locations discussed in the previous chapter. Giant aneurysms are common in this region, but they are discussed separately (Chapter 20).

PRESENTATION

Paraclinoid aneurysms, like other intracranial aneurysms, present most frequently with subarachnoid hemorrhage. In a report of 100 patients, 39% presented with subarachnoid hemorrhage even though this particular series is somewhat biased toward large and giant aneurysms that presented with visual symptoms (7). In other series, between 50 and 70% of the patients have presented with subarachnoid hemorrhage (1, 12, 13, 17, 22). In the authors' own series, approximately 50% of the patients have presented with subarachnoid hemorrhage.

The second most common form of presentation for these aneurysms is visual loss. The visual loss is usually unilateral from involvement of the ipsilateral optic nerve. Frequently, however, on detailed examination these patients are found to have signs of chiasmal compression with bilateral temporal field defects in addition to unilateral decrease in visual acuity from compression of the ipsilateral optic nerve. Depending on the proportion of large and giant aneurysms in the different series reported, between 20 and 50% of the patients present with symptoms of compression of the visual apparatus (1, 7, 10–13, 17, 22). A much rarer form of presentation is with ischemic symptoms due to embolization from a partially thrombosed aneurysm (13).

PREOPERATIVE EVALUATION

The initial evaluation and preoperative treatment for these patients is not any different than in other patients with intracranial aneurysms with the exception that it is useful to examine the visual fields carefully in all patients with large and giant aneurysms whether or not they are complaining of visual difficulty. This preoperative documentation of the visual status is important because, in dealing with these aneurysms by a direct surgical approach, optic damage can occur from surgery.

During the angiographic evaluation of patients with large and giant aneurysms, it is important to have a good understanding of the potential for collateral circulation in case carotid occlusion is required. This evaluation should include at least a cross-compression injection of the opposite carotid artery while the ipsilateral carotid artery is temporarily occluded. In these cases it is also helpful to demonstrate angiographically the size and course of the superficial temporal artery in case an extracranial-intracranial (EC-IC) bypass procedure is contemplated.

SURGICAL MANAGEMENT

After careful study of the angiogram, the surgeon must decide whether a direct approach to the aneurysm is possible or whether such an attempt is certain to be futile. In all but massive aneurysms, it may be worthwhile to proceed with intracranial exploration because occasionally, even what appears to be a very large aneurysm can be satisfactorily clipped (Fig. 13.2A–E). In cases of massive aneurysms where there is no doubt that direct clipping is impossible, or in patients where such has been found to be the case after direct exploration, carotid occlusion should be considered. The different alternatives, special techniques, and problems related to carotid occlusion are discussed in considerable detail in Chapter 20 which deals with giant aneurysms. For now, suffice it to say that common carotid artery ligation is still an

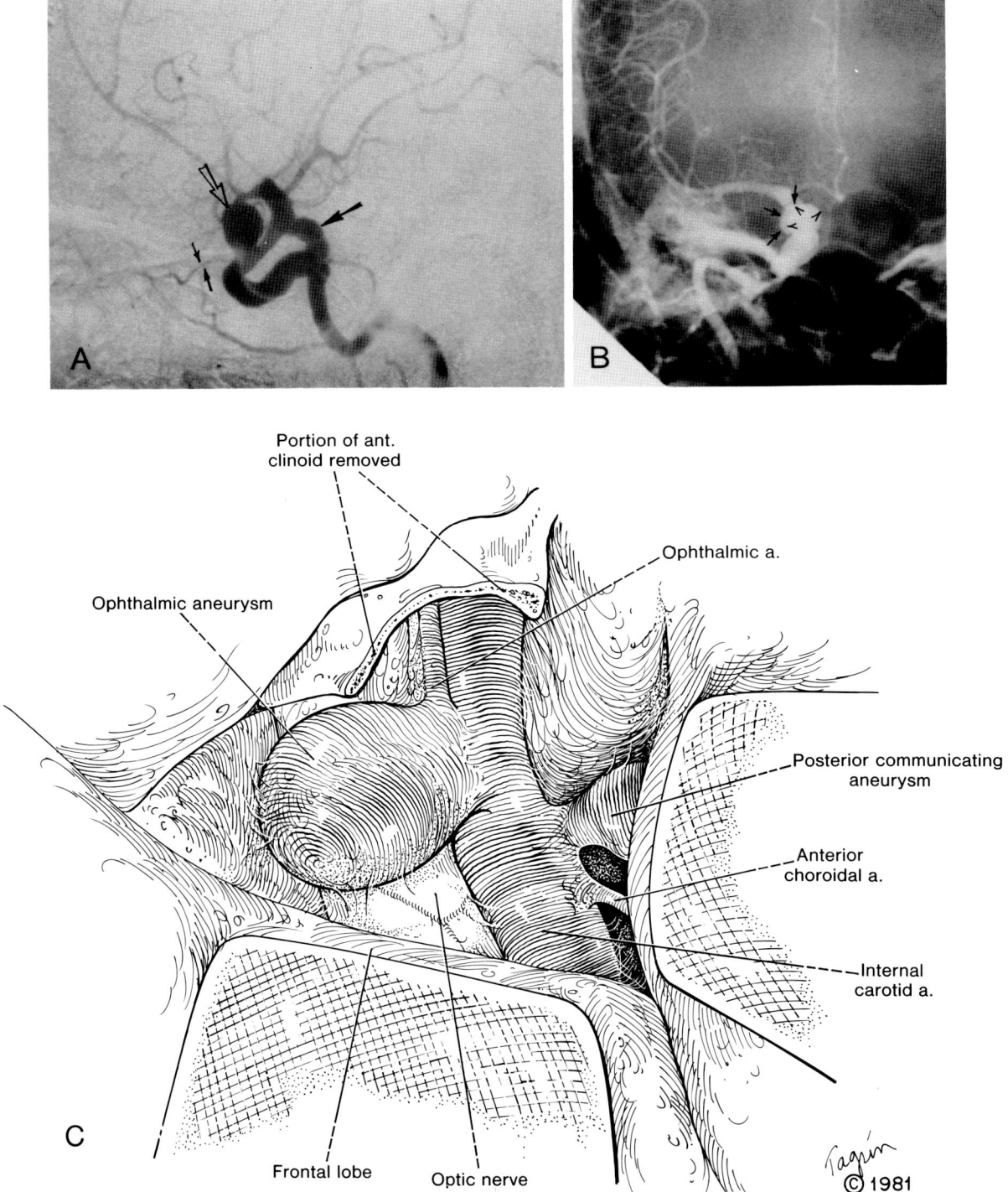

Figure 13.1. Paraclinoid aneurysm arising from internal carotid artery at origin of ophthalmic artery ("ophthalmic aneurysm") and a second aneurysm at the origin of the posterior communicating artery. **A**, Lateral right carotid angiogram shows paraclinoid aneurysm (*open arrow*), internal carotid-posterior communicating artery aneurysm (*large closed arrow*), and ophthalmic artery (*small arrows*). **B**, AP right carotid angiogram shows that the paraclinoid aneurysm (*arrowheads*) projects rostrally and internal carotid-posterior communicating artery aneurysm (*small arrows*) projects posteriorly. **C**, Illustration of intraoperative view of right pterional craniotomy. Anterior clinoid process has been removed. Both aneurysms are dissected for clipping and the ophthalmic and anterior choroidal arteries are preserved. **D** and **E**, Postoperative angiogram shows nonfilling of aneurysms and preservation of anterior choroidal artery and ophthalmic artery.

Paraclinoid Aneurysms

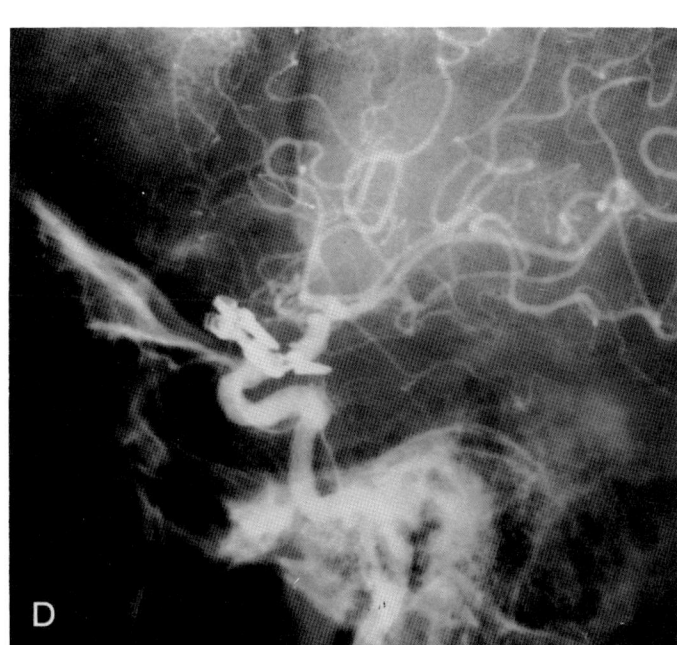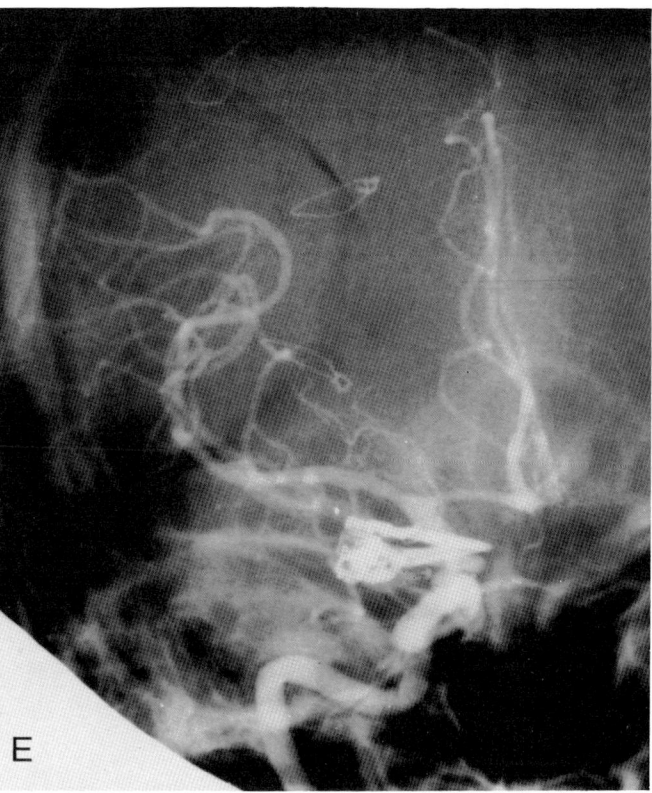

Figure 13.1 D and E.

effective mode of treatment for many of these unclippable aneurysms. Alternatively, internal carotid artery occlusion, preferably by balloon, with or without an EC-IC bypass procedure depending on the potential for collateral circulation, can be considered. Not infrequently it is necessary to trap the internal carotid artery intracranially because proximal occlusion is insufficient to result in aneurysmal thrombosis and amelioration of the symptoms of chiasmatic compression.

When a direct approach is chosen, the surgeon must initially decide whether to expose the carotid artery in the neck. This step is strongly recommended for any large or giant aneurysm. Smaller aneurysms that appear easy to clip may be approached without exposing the carotid artery in the neck. However, the authors still prefer to prepare and drape the neck in these cases so that, if at surgery it appears necessary, the carotid artery can quickly be exposed in the neck without having to redrape the patient. In some centers where the anesthesiologist has considerable experience, it is possible to depend on the anesthesiologist to achieve temporary carotid occlusion by digital compression (15). When the decision is made to expose the carotid artery in the neck, it is usually done through a 4- to 5-cm incision along one of the higher creases in the neck. This transverse incision is centered at the anterior border of the sternocleidomastoid muscle. The incision is carried sharply through the platysma, trying to avoid injury to the greater auricular nerve which runs under the fibers of the platysma and, if injured, can result in considerable numbness in the anterior auricular region. The plane anterior to the sternocleidomastoid muscle is then followed down to the carotid artery sheath. Umbilical tapes are then placed around the common, the internal, and the external carotid arteries. This precaution adds only a short time to the total operation and we have found it frequently invaluable.

Table 13.1
Paraclinoid Aneurysms—Clinical Features

Account for 5% of all intracranial aneurysms
Much more common in females than males (4:1)
Frequently associated with other aneurysms (50%)
Frequently large and giant in size (50%)
Frequently produce visual symptoms (1/3)
Frequently bilateral (7%)

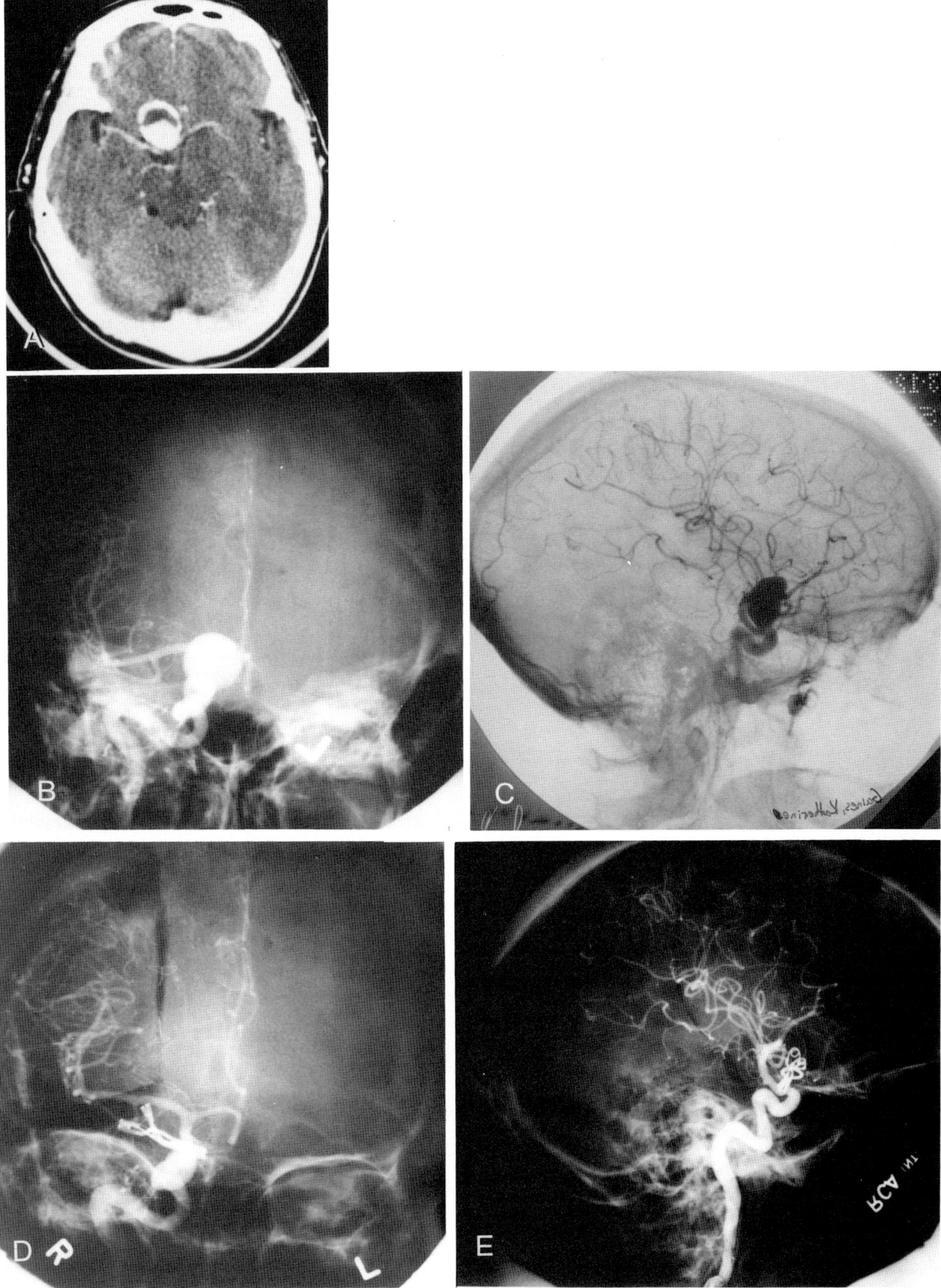

Figure 13.2. Giant paraclinoid aneurysm that appeared to be unclippable due to its size, the fact that it was partially thrombosed and had a heavily calcified neck. **A**, CT scan with contrast showing partial thrombosis in anterior aspect of aneurysm. **B** and **C**, Right carotid angiogram confirms CT scan findings. The aneurysm was explored and, after thorough drilling of the anterior clinoid and unroofing of the optic nerve, it was possible to clip the aneurysm. The neck of the aneurysm was in the paraclinoid region extending from the origin of the ophthalmic artery distally for about 1 cm. **D** and **E**, Postoperative angiogram shows that the aneurysm was satisfactorily clipped and the internal carotid artery was preserved.

A combined epi- and subdural direct approach to paraclinoid aneurysms where the proximal internal carotid artery is exposed in the distal cavernous sinus by a very thorough removal of bone in this region has been described (4). The authors have not had any experience with this technique. Like most other surgeons, the authors approach these lesions by a standard frontotemporal (pterional) craniotomy as described in detail in Chapter 12. The craniotomy is almost always ipsilateral to the aneurysm. Rarely, for a lesion which points medially or inferiorly from the internal carotid artery, contralateral craniotomy may provide satisfactory visualization of the aneurysm sac and neck (3, 23). However, the authors have always used an ipsilateral approach when dealing with a single aneurysm. For bilateral ophthalmic artery aneurysms, careful selection of the most appropriate side for craniotomy may permit direct operation on both lesions from one side.

Several authors have provided technical accounts dealing with these aneurysms (2, 3, 5, 6, 8–11, 13, 17, 22). In general, the basal frontal cut of the pterional craniotomy is extended an extra 2 or 3 cm medially so as to have better visualization and more room to work from the front. One must be very careful with the initial subfrontal retraction, particularly with the aneurysms that point superiorly since they are commonly buried in the lateral orbital gyrus of the frontal lobe. Usually gentle retraction exposes the aneurysm immediately. With large aneurysms the suprasellar cisterns may be occupied by the aneurysm and it is difficult to aspirate cerebrospinal fluid (CSF) from that area. In these cases, if a lumbar catheter has not been previously inserted, one can usually either obtain CSF by retracting the temporal lobe and opening the carotid artery cistern laterally or by directly tapping the ventricle. After relaxation is obtained and the arachnoid is opened widely, one must decide whether it is necessary to remove the anterior clinoid process and unroof the optic nerve. This step is necessary in order to expose the proximal aspect of the neck and the ophthalmic artery in almost all the large and giant aneurysms of this area. Smaller aneurysms can be frequently clipped without any further exposure or simply by opening for a few millimeters the falciform dural edge covering the optic nerve as it enters the optic canal.

Removal of the Anterior Clinoid Process

The dura overlying the clinoid process and the optic canal is removed (Fig. 13.3). The monopolar electrocautery, set at low current, is used with a coated Penfield no. 4 dissector to coagulate a semicircular path in the dura over the anterior clinoid process and optic canal. Great care must be exercised to avoid injury to the optic nerve which may lie under the dura, unprotected by bone in this area. By gently "feeling" through the dura with the instrument one can ensure that there is bone under the dura to be coagulated. No cautery should be used over dura that directly overlies the optic nerve without intervening bone. Lateral coagulation must be terminated at the edge of the cavernous sinus. This coagulated area is incised with a no. 15 knife blade. The resulting flap of dura may be conveniently elevated with a fine-angled microcurette and reflected posteriorly. This flap of dura lies over the internal carotid artery and optic nerve, thus protecting them during subsequent drilling (Fig. 13.4).

The anterior clinoid process is removed with a high-speed drill and diamond burr (Fig. 13.5). The surgeon can conveniently control this instrument with his dominant hand, resting his wrist firmly while the fine sucker is held in the field with the other hand. During controlled drilling, a fine stream of irrigation is directed onto the drill point using the combined suction irrigation system or a microirrigator is used by the assistant (12-ml syringe with a 22-gauge Medicut plastic catheter). The anterior clinoid process may be isolated by drilling its medial and lateral bony supports. Usually, one drilling spot accurately placed on either side of the process will achieve this goal. Once underlying soft tissue is encountered, drilling is redirected slightly superiorly or inferiorly until each buttress, lateral and medial, is weakened. Then a 5-0 straight bone curette is used to fracture and mobilize the resulting anterior clinoid fragment gradually (Fig. 13.6). This is accomplished with utmost care and control to avoid abrupt movement of the fragment with possible injury to nearby structures. The 5-0 curette and microcurettes are used to dissect the fragment free from underlying soft tissues. If the bony exposure seems inadequate, additional drilling may be used to widen the field of view. If space permits a fine microantrostomy punch may be used for additional bony removal (Fig. 13.7). Paranasal sinus mucosa may in some cases extend into bone in this area. If mucosa is encountered, the overlying bony opening must be carefully waxed. If bleeding from soft tissue occurs, application of tiny amounts of Surgicel or Gelfoam may be used for hemostasis. Frequently brisk venous bleeding is encountered laterally from the cavernous sinus. This can be controlled with gentle packing with Surgicel and patience. If further exposure is necessary the surgeon should proceed by gradually pushing the pack forward to stop the bleeding while more bone is removed to achieve the necessary exposure.

Dissection of the Aneurysm

Once the anterior clinoid process is removed and the proximal portion of the optic nerve is unroofed, the surgeon proceeds to open the inner layer of dura (dura propia). For this maneuver it is best to cut vertically in a direction parallel to the lateral edge of the optic nerve (Fig. 13.8). At this point the sur-

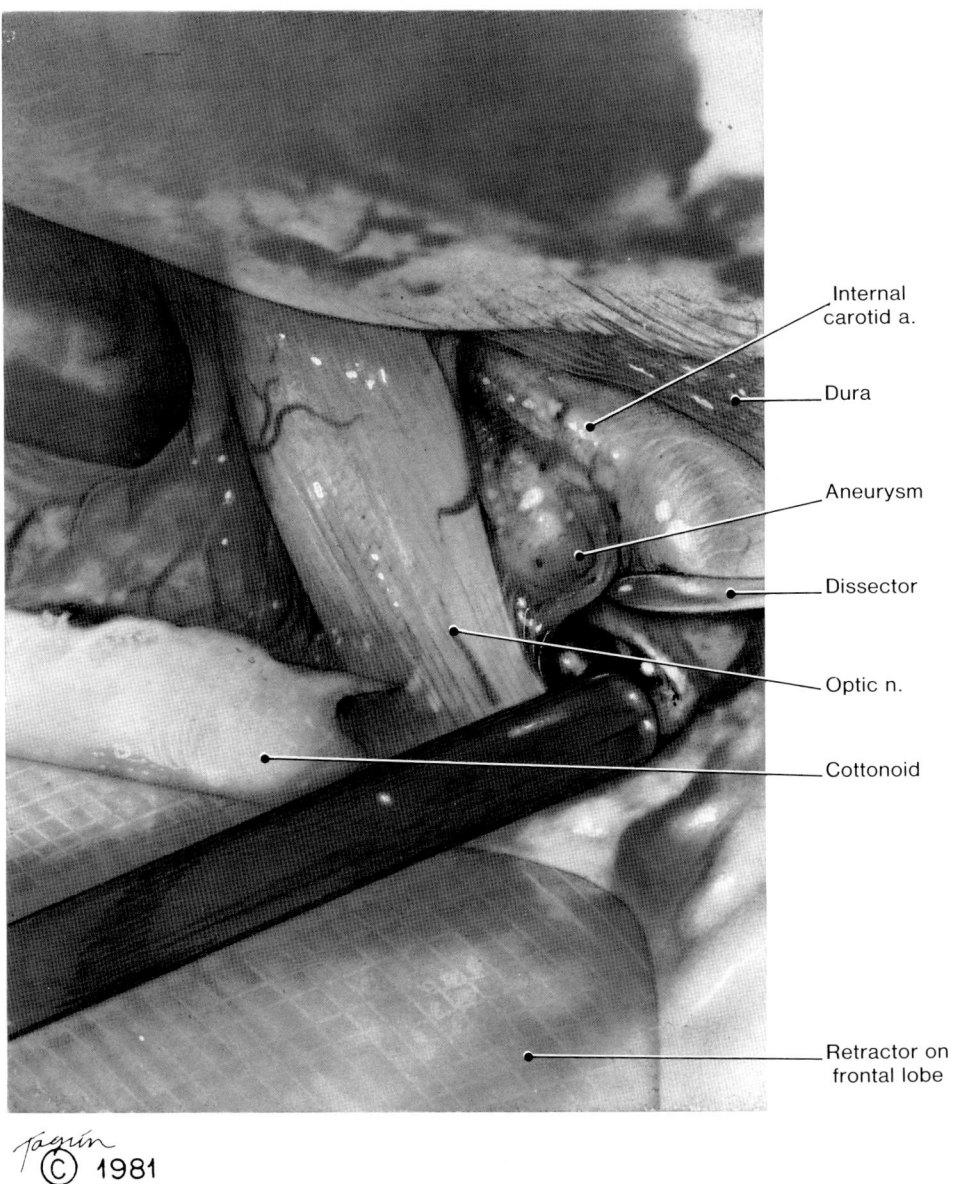

Figure 13.3. Retouched photograph of a paraclinoid aneurysm with a right pterional craniotomy. The aneurysm points medially under the optic nerve, and the proximal neck is hidden by the anterior clinoid process.

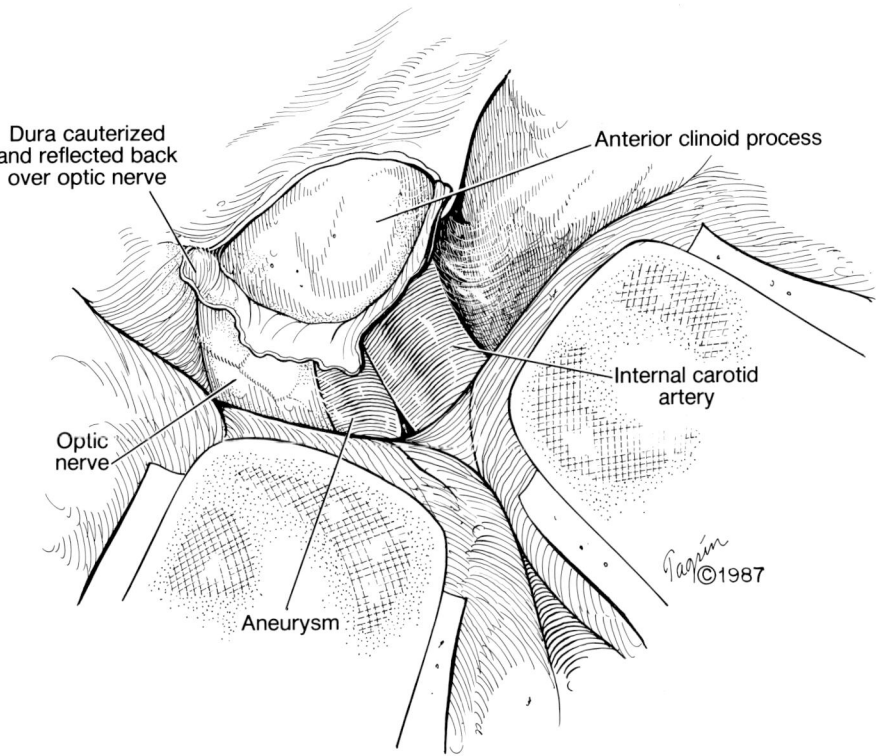

Figure 13.4. The dural flap over the clinoid process and optic canal has been reflected back to protect the internal carotid artery and optic nerve.

geon is ready to dissect the neck of the aneurysm. In most cases, definition of the distal aspect of the neck is straightforward. The posterior communicating and anterior choroidal arteries provide a distal boundary for dissection. Definition of the proximal aspect of the neck is usually a greater challenge. At this point in the procedure, because of the threat of aneurysmal rupture, the surgeon may choose to occlude the exposed internal carotid artery in the neck temporarily. The internal carotid artery is freed proximal to the aneurysm. Often a Rhoton no. 6 microdissector serves nicely for this dissection. Dense arachnoid bands may be cut sharply. Every effort should be made to visualize and spare the ophthalmic artery which usually arises from the internal carotid artery just proximal to the neck of the aneurysm. If the ophthalmic artery is not seen, the proximal neck of the aneurysm must be completely dissected and visualized prior to application of a clip (Fig. 13.9). In many cases, where the aneurysm projects superiorly, gentle deflection of the lesion posteriorly with a sucker will permit passage of a fine dissector proximal to the neck and medially as far as the optic nerve or beneath it. Gentle lateral deflection of the aneurysm may permit dissection of the medial aspect of the aneurysm from the optic nerve. Frequently, gentle deflection of the nerve medially and superiorly will be required to isolate the neck of the aneurysm. Commonly, the blunt dissector needs to be passed with great care, by "feel," in a blind manner in the space between the ophthalmic artery proximally, the aneurysmal wall distally, and the optic nerve superiorly (Fig. 13.10). Here again temporary proximal occlusion of the internal carotid artery usually softens the aneurysm sufficiently to prevent it from rupturing as the instrument is gradually insinuated along the proximal neck softly pushing the aneurysm back and lateral.

Clipping of the Aneurysm

Clipping of the smaller aneurysms in many cases can be accomplished without substantial manipulation of the sac or neck, and thus moderate hypotension (systolic pressure 80–90 mm Hg) provides adequate reduction of tension in the lesion. For most larger lesions or even for small aneurysms with very thin walls, the authors prefer to apply the clip while

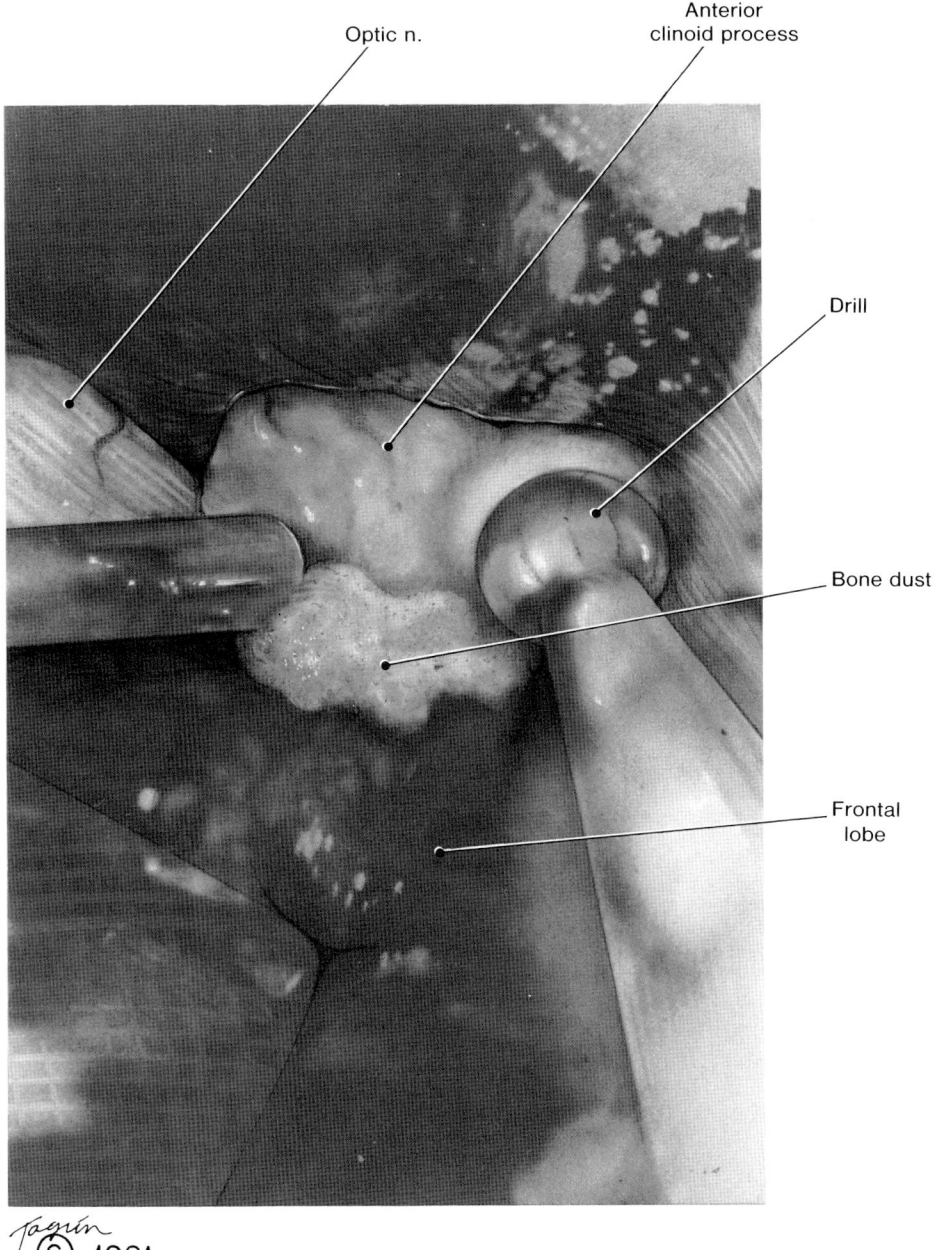

Figure 13.5. Removal of the anterior clinoid process. After the dura is incised and stripped posteriorly, the anterior clinoid process is removed by using a diamond drill.

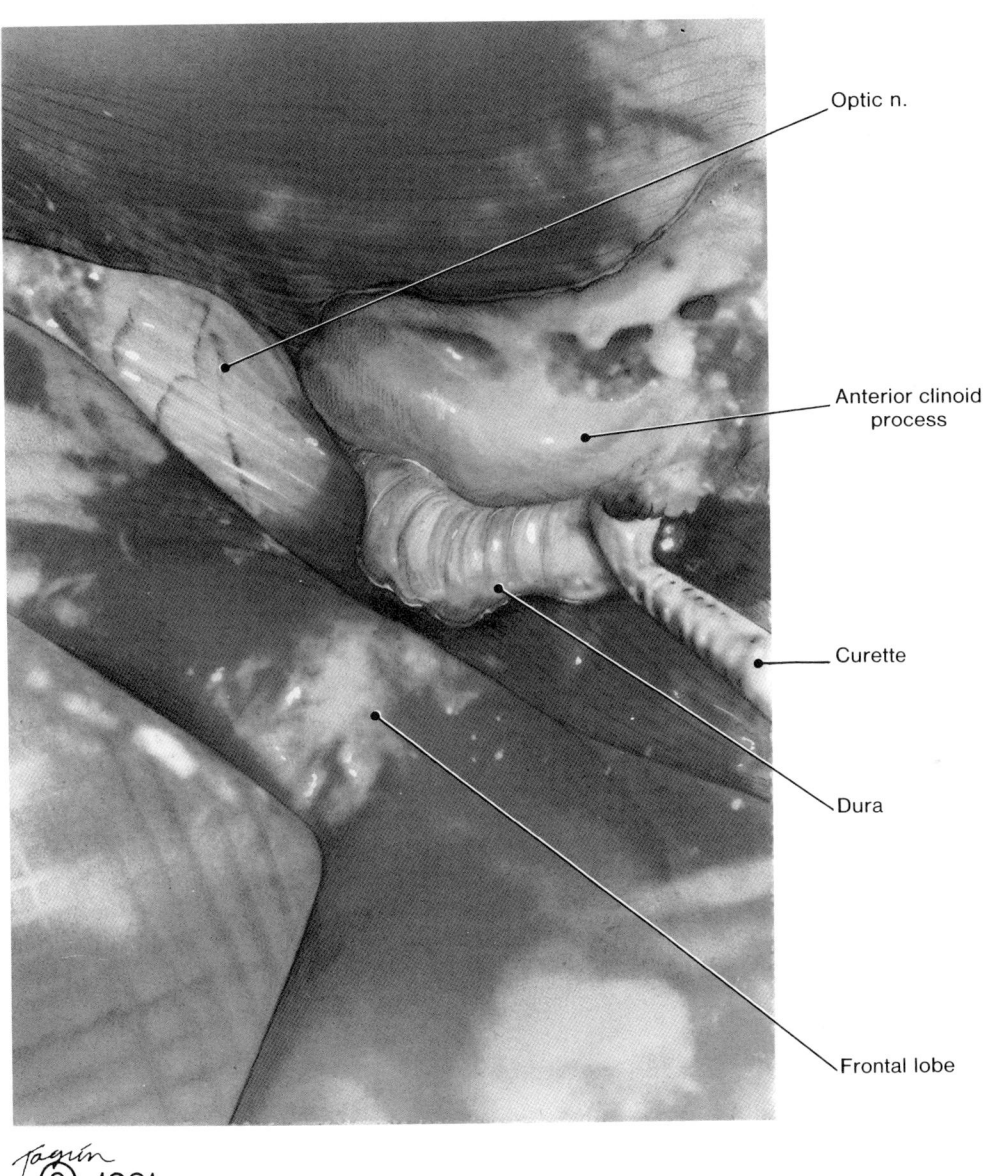

Figure 13.6. Curetting the anterior clinoid process. A 5–0 straight curette is used to gently fracture the bony fragment.

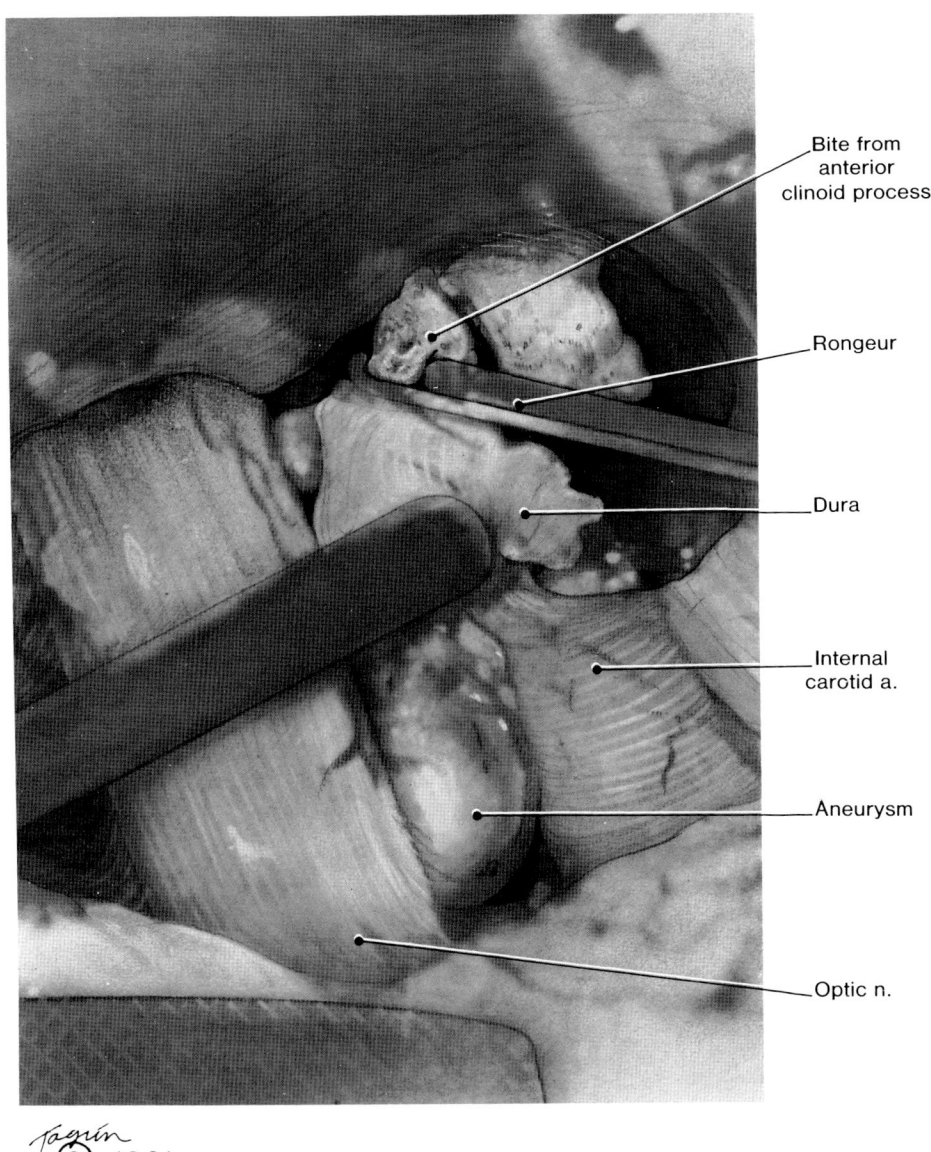

Figure 13.7. Rongeuring anterior clinoid process. A microantrostomy instrument may be used to complete the removal. Bone wax and Surgicel secure hemostasis.

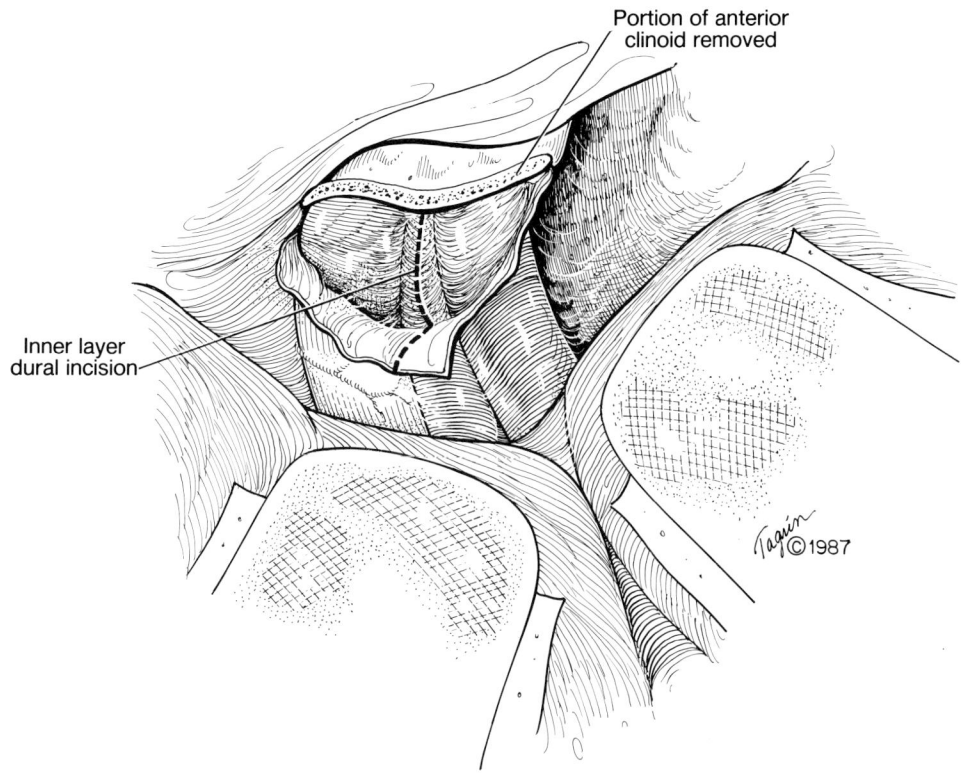

Figure 13.8. The dura proper is opened in a direction parallel to the lateral edge of the optic nerve.

the internal carotid artery is temporarily occluded in the neck. Usually a 2- to 3-minute period of temporary occlusion is all that is necessary. If this does not soften the aneurysm sufficiently another clip may be applied intracranially to the internal carotid artery proximal to the posterior communicating artery to trap the lesion completely. Very rarely it will also be necessary to occlude the external carotid artery in the neck to reduce retrograde ophthalmic artery flow. For some aneurysms, bipolar coagulation may be helpful to shrink the neck before applying a clip (Fig. 13.11). In others, especially those with a broad base, a ligature may help prepare the neck for clipping. With the very large and giant aneurysms the authors have been unable to use bipolar coagulation successfully and in these cases it is also usually impossible to pass a ligature around the neck. These problems will be discussed later when dealing with giant aneurysms (Chapter 20). As a rule, the available space between the internal carotid artery, the base of the skull, and the optic nerve dictate use of a Yasargil or Sugita clip because of their narrow blades (Fig. 13.12).

In most cases, the sac is deflected distally with a fine suction in order to visualize the neck and ophthalmic artery during clip application. If application of the clip is not satisfactory because of incomplete neck obliteration, encroachment on the optic nerve, or occlusion of the ophthalmic artery, the clip is repositioned. If this is not satisfactory, the clip is removed and a different type used. The internal carotid artery and ophthalmic artery must not be compressed or kinked, and the optic nerve should not be excessively deformed. Minor contact between the clip and nerve is common and unavoidable. When significant nerve displacement is caused by the clip, further dissection of the nerve and, at times, the chiasm may permit a gentle sloping displacement with limited infringement on the nerve. If more unroofing of the optic canal is necessary to allow gentle medial displacement of the optic nerve without having it sharply kinked as it enters the canal, the authors do not hesitate to proceed even to the point of completely unroofing all of the optic canal. Rarely, an unusual situation may be encountered where a Drake clip or a Sugita clip with a Drake aperture may be

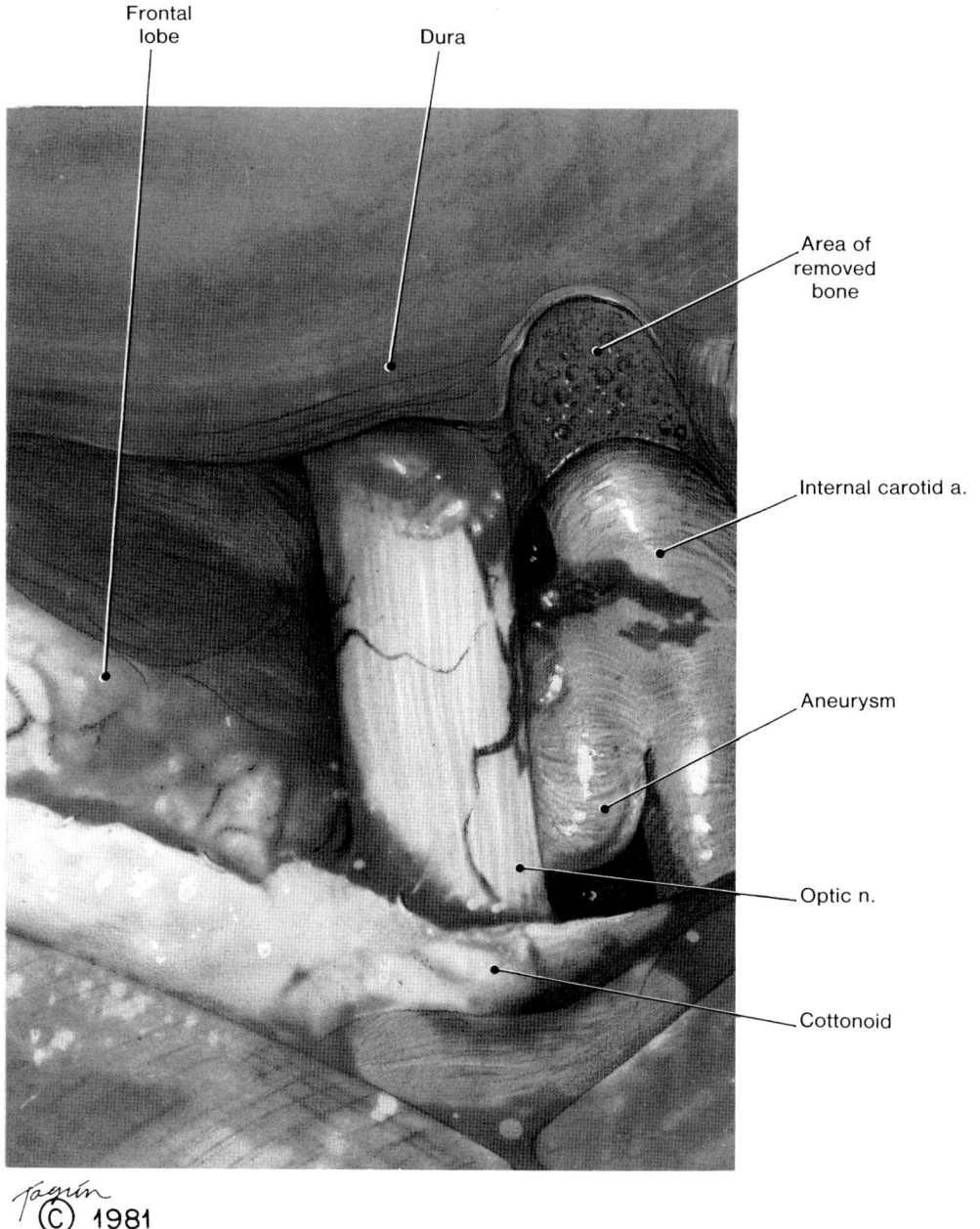

Figure 13.9. Proximal control of internal carotid artery. Removal of anterior clinoid permits dissection of proximal neck and internal carotid artery. The ophthalmic artery needs to be visualized by gentle dissection along the proximal aspect on the neck of the aneurysm.

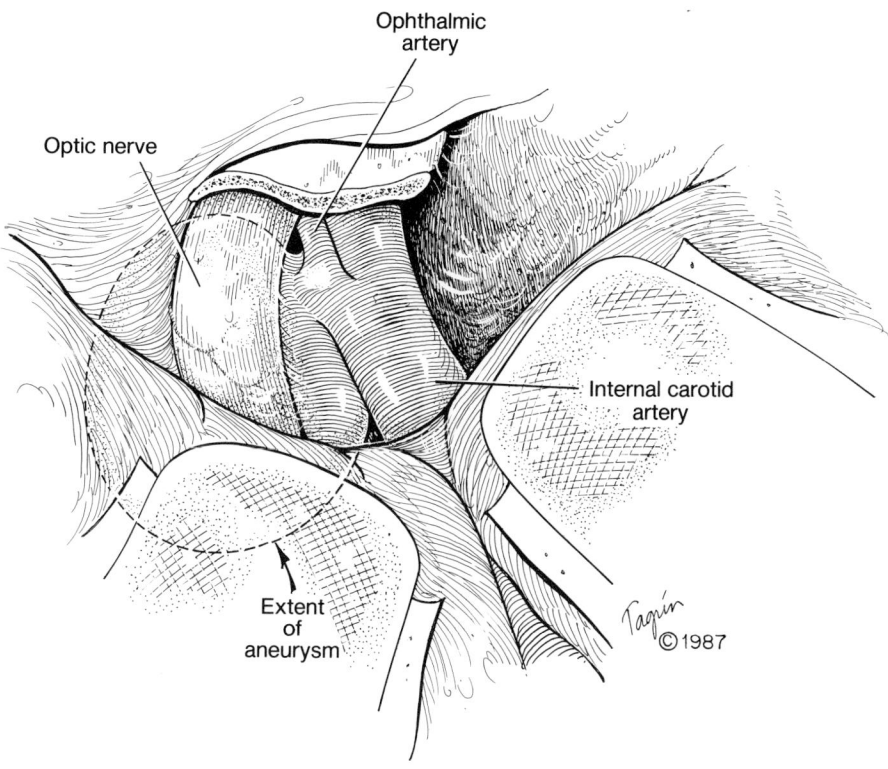

Figure 13.10. The space between the ophthalmic artery, the aneurysm, and the optic nerve which is developed to allow passage of one of the blades of the clip.

used to obliterate the lesion and preserve the optic nerve which passes through its aperature.

Clipping of a Contralateral Aneurysm

A paraclinoid aneurysm may be treated through a contralateral frontotemporal craniotomy (3, 23) (Fig. 13.13). This approach may be indicated when there are bilateral paraclinoid aneurysms or when an incidental aneurysm projects inferiorly and medially and a contralateral exposure has been done to primarily treat another aneurysm. In the exposure of a contralateral lesion, retraction will be deep. Removal of CSF via a subarachnoid catheter may be useful. Extra care must be taken to avoid tearing one or both olfactory nerves at the cribriform plate. As the frontal lobes are elevated, the arachnoid attachments to the optic nerves and chiasm are severed sharply. The contralateral proximal internal carotid artery comes into view inferior to the optic nerve. In this area, the contralateral paraclinoid aneurysm may be visualized projecting inferiorly and medially from its origin. The neck is freed and the ophthalmic artery preserved. A straight clip, just long enough to do the job, obliterates the neck. Occasionally, removal of the bony tuberculum sellae will be needed to expose the proximal aneurysm neck. Coagulation and reflection of the dura will permit drilling of the obstructing bony prominence. Usually, only a small amount of bone need be removed. Care must be taken to avoid entry into the sphenoid sinus. Careful obliteration of the opening is carried out with bone wax or fat if the sinus is entered. The authors advise reserving this contralateral exposure only for small incidental aneurysms and would urge terminating the attempt and returning at a later date through an ipsilateral craniotomy if any difficulty is encountered or if the lesion is less than optimally visualized.

Aneurysms of the Posterior or Lateral Wall of the Internal Carotid Artery

Most paraclinoid aneurysms arise distal to the ophthalmic artery in the angle between this artery and the internal carotid artery in the medial or superomedial aspect of the internal carotid artery. They can then project distally anteriorly in which case they may not involve the optic nerve and then clipping is usually more straightforward, or they may project medially, toward the pituitary fossa, under the optic nerve which is usually displaced upward and medially. About 20% of all the aneurysms related

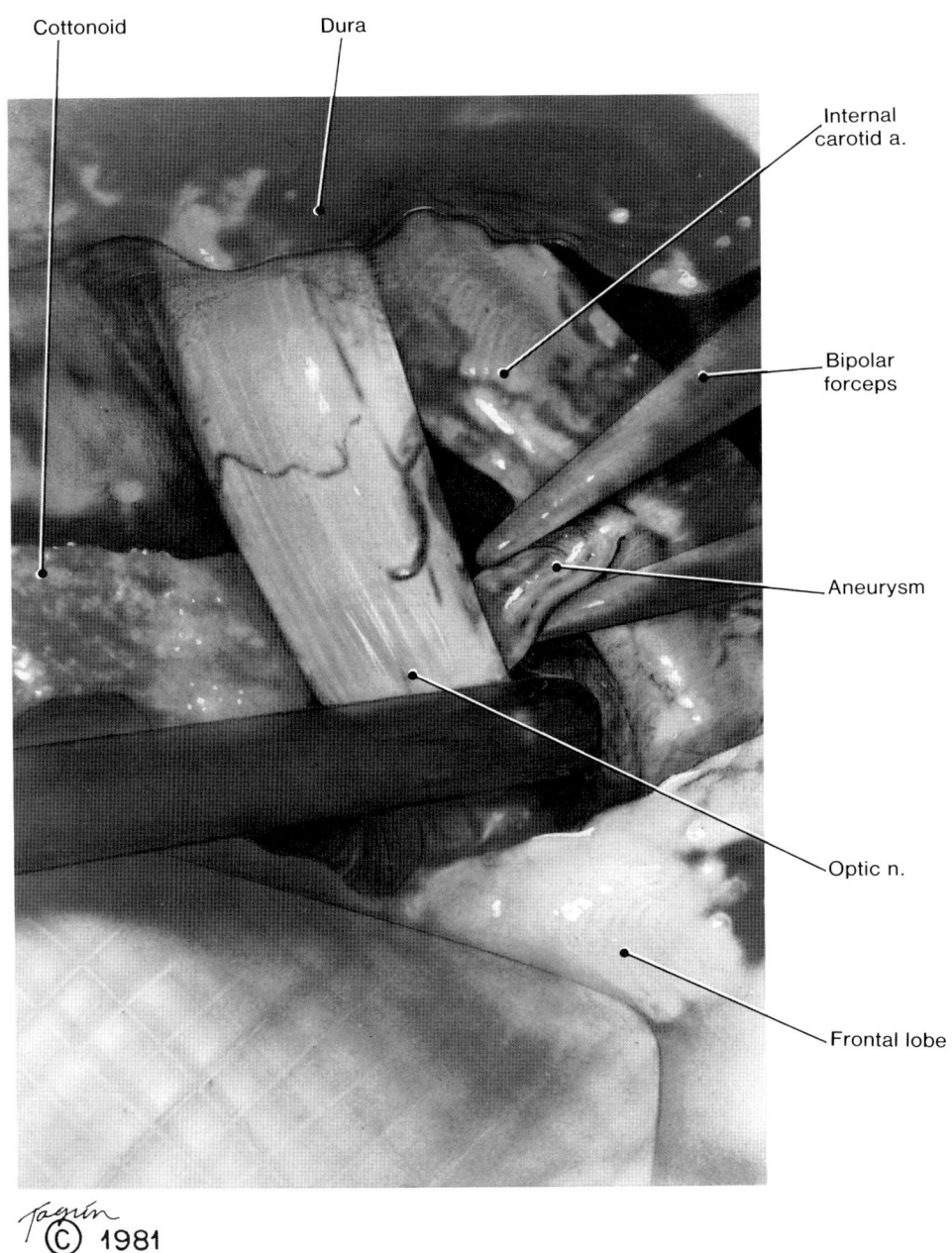

Figure 13.11. Preparation of neck of aneurysm. Gentle application of bipolar cautery at low voltage can define and toughen the neck.

Paraclinoid Aneurysms

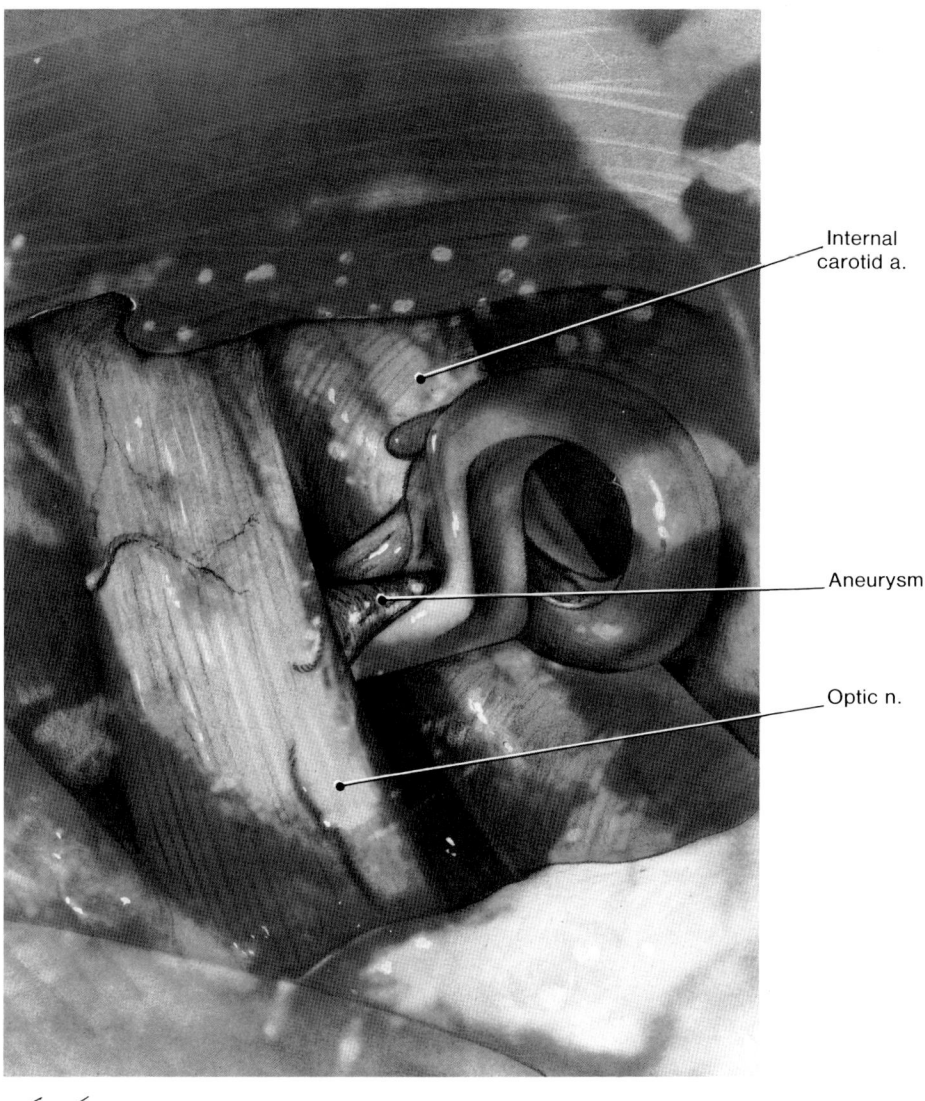

Figure 13.12. Clipping the aneurysm. Often a straight Yasargil or Sugita clip with their slender blades fits best in the narrow cleft between artery and optic nerve.

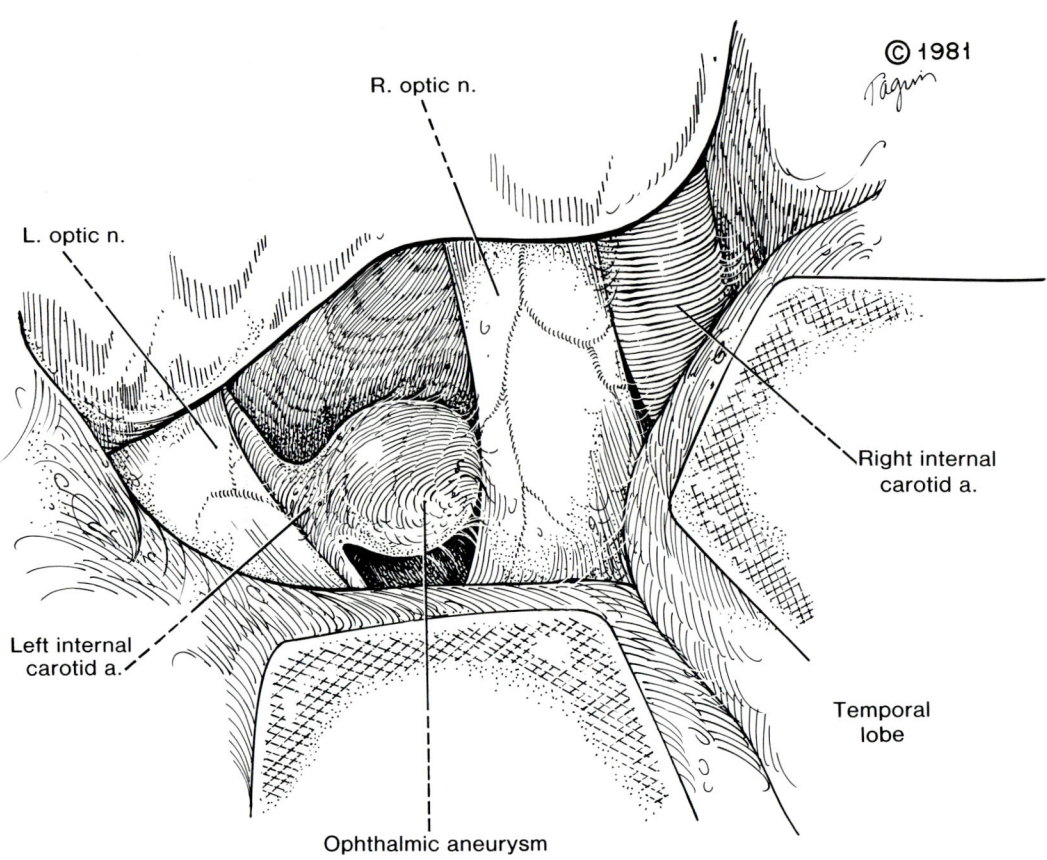

Figure 13.13. Exposure of contralateral paraclinoid aneurysm projecting inferomedially via a right pterional craniotomy.

to the opthalmic area project forward, over the anterior clinoid and away from the optic nerve and the rest project in a medial direction under the optic apparatus (subchiasmatic) (12).

Aneurysms of the posterior (ventral) and lateral wall of the internal carotid artery proximal to the posterior communicating artery have some special surgical considerations. Both of these aneurysms usually require removal of the anterior clinoid process for full exposure. Exposure is frequently even more difficult in aneurysms of the posterior wall than in those arising from the medial wall because in the former the neck is hidden by the internal carotid artery, they tend to have a very broad ill-defined neck, and they are frequently partially intracavernous (14, 20, 21). It has been suggested that on preoperative angiography a line drawn from 1 mm proximal to the takeoff of the ophthalmic artery defines the limits of the dura and, therefore, aneurysms arising distal to this line are intradural (extracavernous) (16). This landmark, though more reliable than the location of the anterior clinoid process which can be very variable, is more helpful in aneurysms related to the ophthalmic artery than in aneurysms of the ventral and lateral wall. Sometimes there is simply no way of knowing and one must, when in doubt, proceed with intracranial exploration if it appears that most of the aneurysm neck is intradural. Many of the aneurysms of the posterior wall involve all of the internal carotid artery and they may not be typical saccular aneurysm but rather may represent a form of atherosclerotic aneurysm or ectasia of the internal carotid artery (20). When large, these aneurysms may incorporate within their necks the origins of the posterior communicating and the anterior choroidal arteries.

These ventral aneurysms of the posterior wall frequently presented insurmountable problems until the development of the right-angle fenestrated Sugita clips (18). With this clip the surgeon is sometimes able to "reconstruct" the internal carotid artery even when the artery is globally distended by the aneurysm (Fig. 13.15A and B). This clip should almost always be applied under temporary proximal ligation of the exposed cervical portion of the internal carotid artery. Frequently, if space allows, a distal temporary clip to completely entrap the area of the aneurysm during clipping is desirable. The Sugita clip, which has its fenestration at a right angle from the blades, is applied over the internal carotid artery and then gently advanced into the cavernous sinus if necessary, until it is felt that it has gone completely across the neck. Again, bleeding from the cavernous sinus can be controlled with packing if it is venous. Brisk arterial bleeding usually signifies perforation of the sac by the advancing blades. In these cases one must withdraw and then reapply the clip closer to the internal carotid artery, over the presumed area of aneurysmal perforation. Sometimes persisting arterial bleeding can be controlled by forceful packing, but occasionally a permanent trapping procedure with sacrifice of the internal carotid artery may become necessary as a lifesaving maneuver. When the origin of the posterior communicating artery and the anterior choroidal artery are related to the distal aspect of the aneurysm, they can occasionally be preserved by including them in the aperture or by ingenious use of multiple clips (18, 20).

The rare laterally projecting aneurysms usually present less of a problem since at least the distal aspect of the neck can be well-defined and a clip can be applied even if part of the proximal neck is not clearly seen because it arises from the cavernous sinus. Since the internal carotid artery turns medially as one follows it from distally into the cavernous sinus, a straight clip can frequently be applied even when the distal blades protrude blindly for a short distance into the cavernous sinus provided the clip aims slightly laterally and away from the expected course of the internal carotid artery (Fig. 13.14). As the tips of the clip protrude into the sinus brisk venous bleeding is

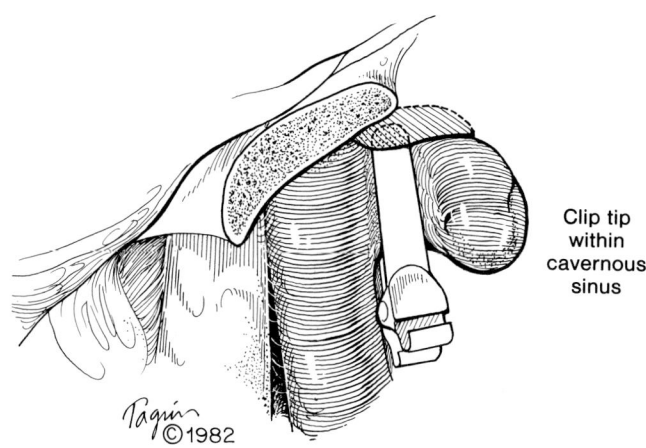

Figure 13.14. Proximal internal carotid artery aneurysm at the lateral wall partially within cavernous sinus. Anterior clinoid process may be removed for exposure. The cavernous sinus may be opened for a short distance and bleeding controlled with packing to permit clipping.

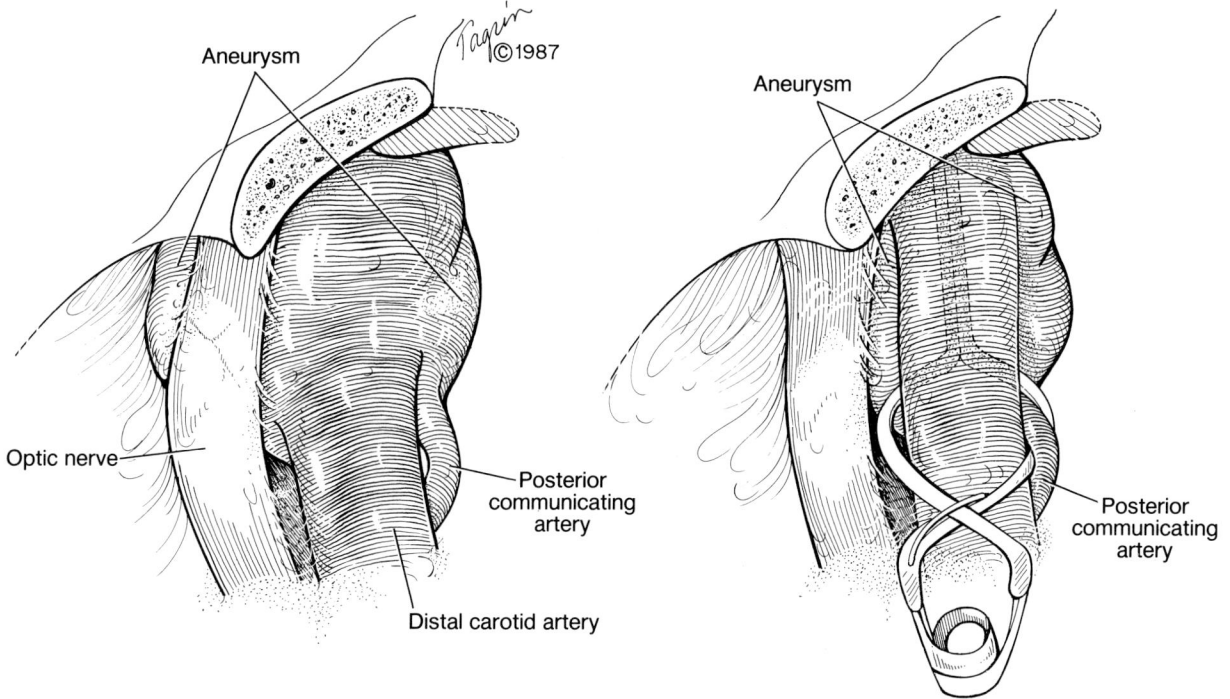

Figure 13.15. **A**, Posterior wall aneurysm displacing the already distended internal carotid artery. **B**, The aneurysm has been clipped with preservation of the internal carotid artery lumen by a right-angle fenestrated Sugita clip applied over the artery leaving it and the origin of the posterior communicating artery in the fenestration which is at right angles to the blades of the clip.

to be expected, but it can be stopped by packing with Surgicel around the blades of the clip. Here again proximal temporary occlusion of the exposed cervical portion of the internal carotid artery is invaluable in preventing perforation of the aneurysm as the tips of the clip blades are advanced.

RESULTS

Indirect operations (carotid ligation) have frequently been necessary in cases of giant aneurysms and the authors' results with these procedures will be discussed in Chapter 20. The results with direct (intracranial) operations for nongiant paraclinoid aneurysms over the past 10 years at the Massachusetts General Hospital are given in Table 13.2. All patients were in good preoperative condition and only three were operated acutely after subarachnoid hemorrhage. In the rest the operation took place generally between 10 and 15 days after subarachnoid hemorrhage. There have been no deaths in this group of patients. One bad result was in a patient who had good vision preoperatively and became totally blind in the ipsilateral eye from excessive manipulation or vascular compromise of the optic nerve at surgery. The other bad result was a patient that developed a hemiparesis as a consequence of forced, unplanned trapping of the internal carotid artery which was necessary to control bleeding at surgery. A few patients suffered slight to moderate ipsilateral visual loss as a result of surgical manipulation. They are still listed as "good" results because they are well in every other respect and the aneurysm has been obliterated.

Yasargil obtained a good result in 32 of 33 patients with ophthalmic aneurysms (20). In 21 patients with aneurysms of the ventral wall of the internal carotid artery, he obtained good results in 18. There were two deaths in patients in poor preoperative condition and with large aneurysms and one poor result in a patient with a giant aneurysm (20). Ferguson and Drake obtained good or excellent results in 86% of 70 patients treated by a direct approach for an ophthalmic aneurysm (9). There were nine deaths and one poor result in this series, but these generally occurred with very large and giant lesions or in patients in poor preoperative condition. Similarly good results have been reported by other authors (1, 10, 11, 17, 19).

REFERENCES

1. Almeida GM, Shibata MK, Bianco E: Carotid-ophthalmic aneurysms. *Surg Neurol* 5:41–45, 1976.
2. Benedetti A, Curri D: Direct attack on carotid ophthalmic and large internal carotid aneurysms. *Surg Neurol* 8:49–54, 1977.
3. Crowell RM, Ojemann RG: Surgical treatment of carotid ophthalmic aneurysms. In Schmidek HH, Sweet WH (eds): *Current Techniques in Operative Neurosurgery*. New York, Grune & Stratton, 1982, pp 869–889.
4. Dolenc VV: A combined epi- and subdural direct approach to carotid-ophthalmic artery aneurysms. *J Neurosurg* 62:667–672, 1985.
5. Drake CG: Giant intracranial aneurysms: Experience with surgical treatment in 174 patients. *Clin Neurosurg* 26:12–95, 1979.
6. Drake CG, Vanderlinden RG, Amacher AL: Carotid ophthalmic aneurysms. *J Neurosurg* 29:24–31, 1968.
8. Ferguson GG, Drake CG: Carotid-ophthalmic aneurysm: The surgical management of those cases presenting with compression of the optic nerves and chiasm alone. *Clin Neurosurg* 27:263–308, 1980.
9. Ferguson GG, Drake CG: Carotid-ophthalmic aneurysms: Visual abnormalities in 32 patients and the results of treatment. *Surg Neurol* 16:1–8, 1981.
10. Ferguson GG: Carotid-ophthalmic artery aneurysms. In Wilkins RH, Rengachary SS (eds): *Neurosurgery*. New York, McGraw-Hill, 1985, pp 1385–1393.
11. Fox JL: Technique of aneurysm surgery. III. Internal carotid artery aneurysms. In Fox JL (ed): *Intracranial Aneurysms*. Berlin, Springer-Verlag, 1983, vol II, pp 949–1011.
12. Guidetti B, Nicole S: Carotid-ophthalmic aneurysms. In Fein JM, Flamm ES (eds): *Cerebrovascular Surgery*. Berlin, Springer-Verlag, 1985, pp 805–839.
13. Heros RC, Nelson PB, Ojemann RG, Crowell RM, Debrun G: Large and giant paraclinoid aneurysms: Surgical techniques, complications and results. *Neurosurgery* 12:153–163, 1983.
14. Nutik S: Carotid paraclinoid aneurysms with intradural origin and intracavernous location. *J Neurosurg* 48:526–533, 1978.
15. Peerless SJ, Durward QJ: Comment on large and giant paraclinoid aneurysms: Surgical techniques, complications and results by Heros et al. *Neurosurgery* 12:163, 1983.
16. Punt J: Some observations on aneurysms of the proximal internal carotid artery. *J Neurosurg* 51:151–154, 1979.
17. Sengupta RP, Gryspeerdt GL, Hankinson J: Carotid-ophthalmic aneurysms. *J Neurol Neurosurg Psychiatry* 39:837–853, 1976.
18. Sugita K, Kobayashi S, Kyoshima K, Nakagawa F: Fenestrated clips for unusual aneurysms of the carotid artery. *J Neurosurg* 57:240–246, 1982.
19. Sundt TM Jr, Piepgras DG: Surgical approach to giant intracranial aneurysms: Operative experiences with 80 cases. *J Neurosurg* 51:731–742, 1979.
20. Yasargil MG: Internal carotid artery aneurysms. In Yasargil MG (ed): *Microneurosurgery*. New York, Thieme-Stratton, 1984, vol 2, pp 33–123.
21. Yasargil MG, Fox JL: The microsurgical approach to intracranial aneurysms. *Surg Neurol* 3:7–14, 1975.
22. Yasargil MG, Gasser JC, Hodosh RM, Rankin TV: Carotid-ophthalmic aneurysms: Direct microsurgical approach. *Surg Neurol* 8:155–165, 1977.
23. Yamada K, Hayakawa T, Oku Y, Maeda Y, Ushio Y, Yoshimine T, Kawai R: Contralateral pterional approach for carotid-ophthalmic aneurysm: Usefulness of high resolution metrizamide or blood computed tomographic cisternography. *Neurosurgery* 15:5–8, 1984.

Table 13.2.
Paraclinoid Aneurysms Treated by Direct Operation (Nongiant)

Results	Number
Good	24
Poor	2
Dead	0

14
Anterior Communicating Artery Aneurysms

PRESENTATION

Anterior communicating artery aneurysms represent a common and difficult problem in management. These lesions usually present with subarachnoid hemorrhage. Often the subarachnoid hemorrhage is a minor "warning leak" causing severe headache and a stiff neck, but in many patients there are significant neurologic deficits. By virtue of its location, the aneurysm may hemorrhage upward into the third ventricle and hypothalamic region. Damage in these areas may be associated with memory disturbance (particularly for recent events), abulia, inappropriate secretion of antidiuretic hormone, symptomatic hydrocephalus, or autonomic instability with unstable pulse and blood pressure (1, 17). Lateral rupture directly into the parenchyma may involve the internal capsule (21). Delayed complications are common following subarachnoid hemorrhage from these aneurysms. The most frequent problem is vasospasm, but hydrocephalus may also cause symptoms.

In a few patients, these aneurysms reach a giant size and compress visual pathways, the hypothalamus, or the internal capsule (see Chapter 20). The patient may present with progressive visual symptoms, mental disturbance, or hemiparesis.

EVALUATION

The program of evaluation and medical management is outlined in Chapter 10. The timing of angiography and surgery is discussed in Chapter 11. Angiography often requires special views to define the anatomy of the aneurysm neck (Fig. 14.1). Oblique views can throw the aneurysm neck into profile. Compression of the contralateral internal carotid artery during ipsilateral internal carotid artery injection may be needed to depict the anterior communicating artery complex, including both A_1 segments. At times a base view is helpful if other projections fail to show the lesion adequately (Fig. 14.2). When vasospasm has been present, the authors have repeated angiography up to three times to finally demonstrate an anterior communicating artery aneurysm. In a case where suspicion was high, despite negative angiography, they explored and clipped an anterior communicating artery aneurysm.

In the past the authors tended to delay surgery 10–12 days after subarachnoid hemorrhage from an anterior communicating artery aneurysm (3). This policy was based on the serious mental disturbances caused by vasospasm related to basal perforating arteries. However, recent personal experience supplements published reports of good results for anterior communicating aneurysms (8, 9, 16, 24). The present authors now proceed with early operation in grade 1 and 2 patients. For patients in grade 3 or worse, the authors continue to defer surgery for 10 days or longer.

SURGICAL TREATMENT

In the early days of aneurysm surgery results from direct operation on anterior communicating artery aneurysm were poor enough to persuade some skilled surgeons that an indirect procedure to diminish transmural pressure might offer better results (10). Such an approach may still rarely be warranted in selected high-risk cases (Chapter 20). However, for the vast majority of patients, direct microsurgical obliteration offers the best results (3, 6, 17, 18, 20, 23, 25).

Initial Exposure

The authors prefer a unilateral frontal craniotomy and gyrus rectus approach for most patients (3, 7, 23). A modified pterional craniotomy provides good exposure (see Chapter 12 and Fig. 14.2A) (26, 27). The aneurysm is usually approached from the side of the dominant feeding artery (almost always the largest A_1 segment) because this allows early control of the major efferent vessel. In addition, the aneurysm usually projects to the opposite side so that an approach from the side of the dominant A_1 segment usually brings the surgeon to the area of the aneurysmal neck (almost always between the dominant A_1 segment and the anterior communicating artery) and away from the area of rupture in the dome (4, 13). In the rare cases where both A_1 segments are of equal size and the aneurysm fills equally from both sides, the aneurysm is approached from the side opposite to where the dome seems to project or from the right side if the aneurysm projects symmetrically in the midline. The exception to this rule may be in

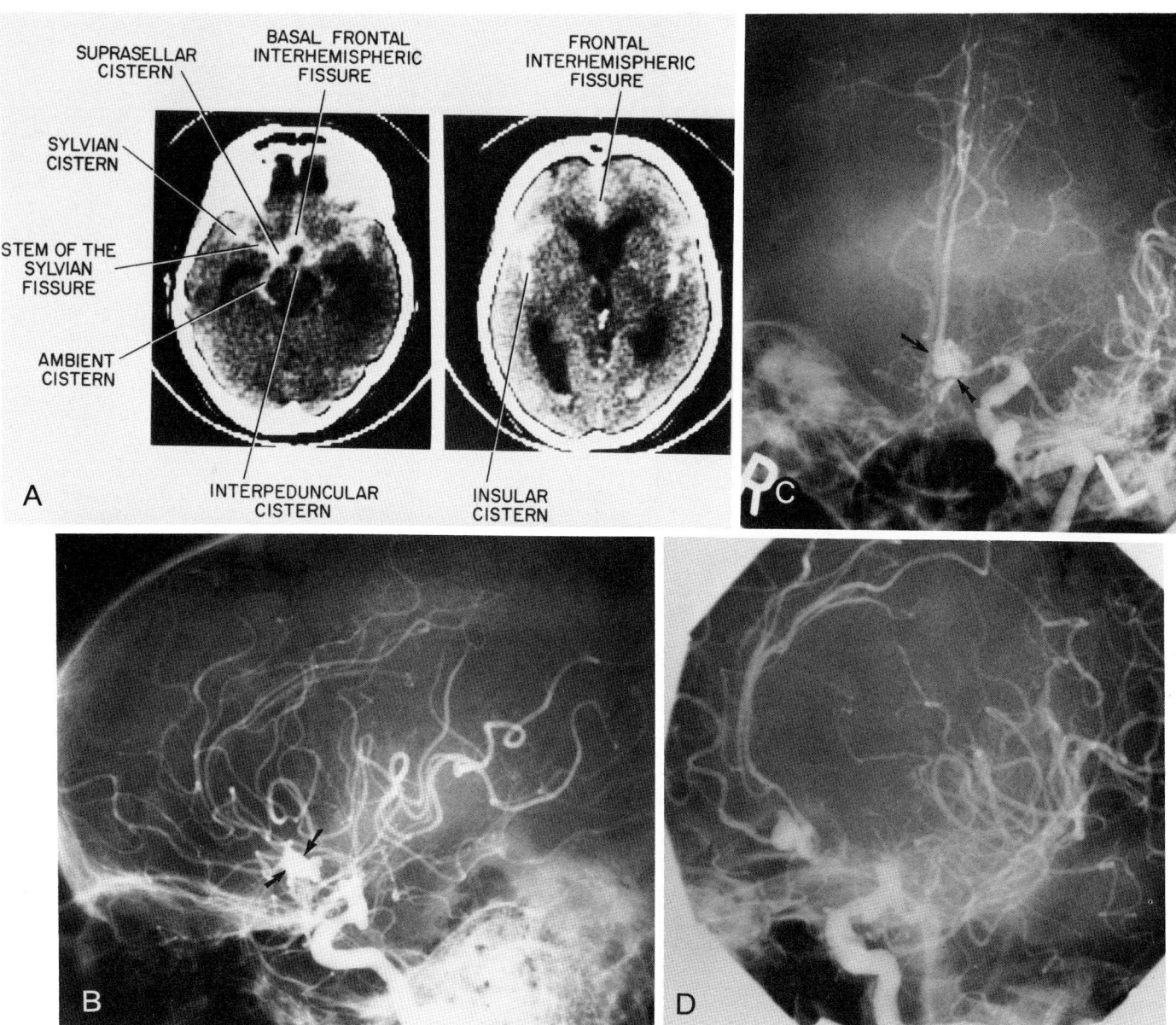

Figure 14.1. Anterior communicating artery aneurysm. CT predicts spasm. Operation delayed 2 weeks after subarachnoid hemorrhage. Drake clip encircles right A_1 segment to obliterate lesion. **A**, CT shows hematoma in basal cisterns 1 day after subarachnoid hemorrhage. Patient intact. **B–D**, Left carotid angiogram demonstrates an aneurysm arising from the junction of the left A_1 segment of the anterior cerebral and anterior communicating arteries (*arrows*). Note information about anatomy gained on the oblique view. There is grade 2 spasm of anterior and middle cerebral arteries. No filling of aneurysm on right carotid angiogram. **E**, Left carotid angiogram 8 days after subarachnoid hemorrhage shows more severe left middle cerebral artery spasm with patient confused and lethargic. Head is slightly turned so aneurysm is behind the distal internal carotid artery. Right frontal craniotomy was deferred until 16 days after subarachnoid hemorrhage. **F** and **G**, Postoperative left carotid angiogram shows Drake clip and obliteration of the aneurysm (*open arrow*). The right A_1 segment passes through the clip. No significant spasm. Patient intact.

a case of hematoma that has destroyed the basal-medial portion of one frontal lobe. If this has occurred, it may be preferable to approach the aneurysm from the side of the hematoma to avoid bilateral basofrontal damage (1). The patient's head is usually turned about 60° to the vertical to permit a direct view, but the degree of rotation may be varied depending on the anatomy of the aneurysm. To afford easy subfrontal exposure, the bone flap is taken 2 cm further medially than for internal carotid aneurysms. It is very important not to try to retract the frontal lobe until the brain is relaxed. For some cases, par-

Anterior Communicating Artery Aneurysms

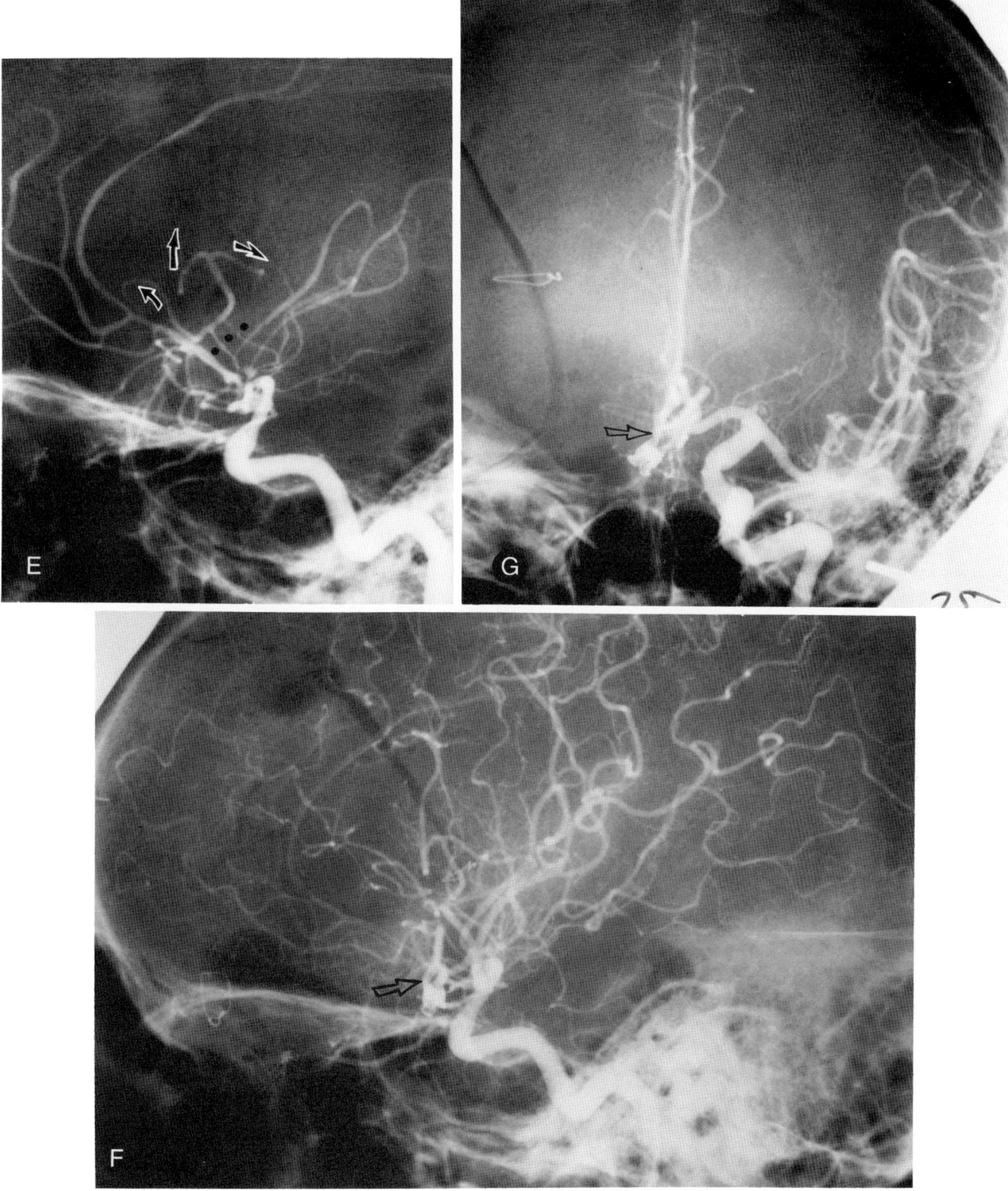

Figure 14.1E–G.

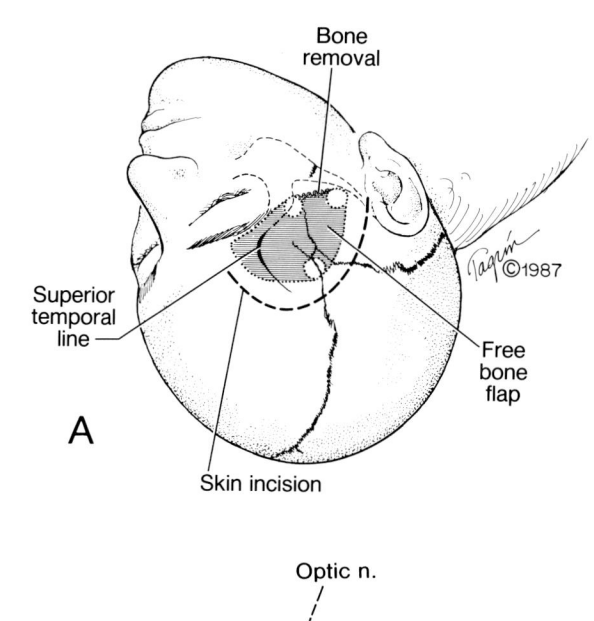

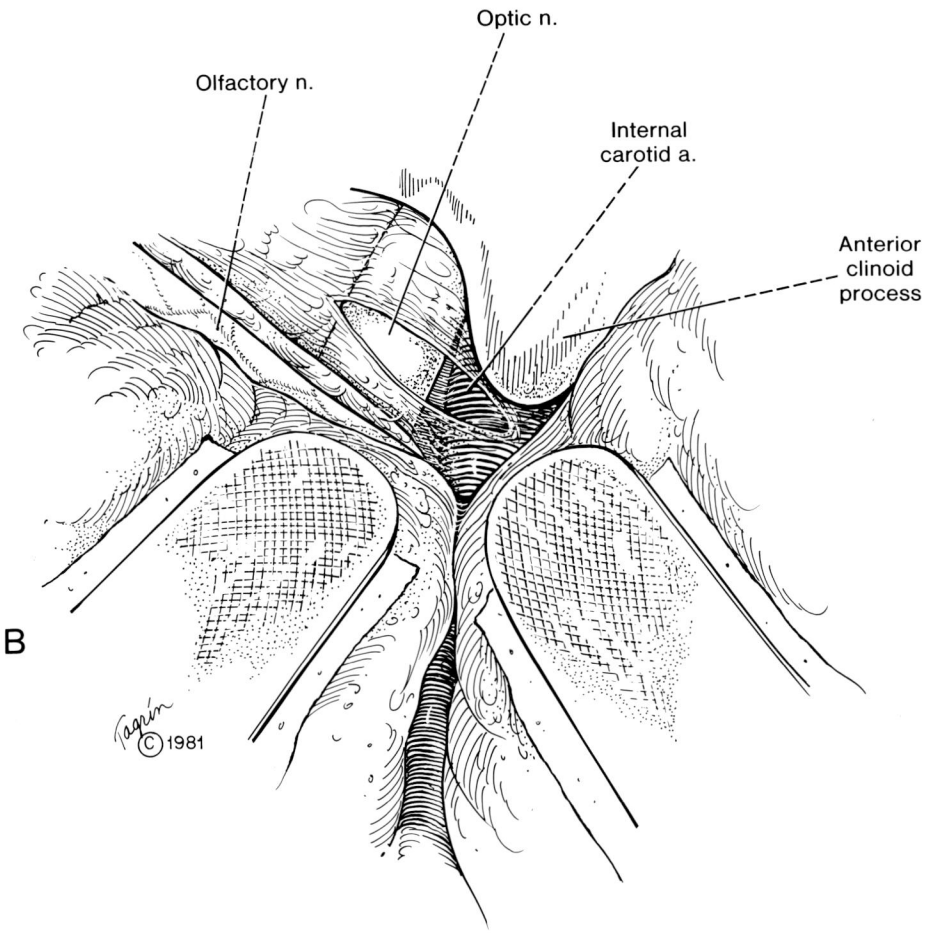

Figure 14.2. **A**, Incision and pterional craniotomy. The skin incision is just behind the hairline and the anterior branch of superficial temporal artery. The key burr hole lies just behind the zygomatic process of the frontal bone and inferior to the superior temporal line. Often three burr holes are sufficient. **B**, Elevation of frontal lobe. This is done gradually with suction removal of CSF. The olfactory tract leads back to the optic nerve. Temporal bridging veins are coagulated and cut near the cortex.

ticularly in patients operated acutely, the authors place a spinal subarachnoid catheter and remove 50–75 ml of CSF to achieve a slack brain. When a spinal catheter has not been placed and the brain is full despite efforts to remove CSF directly from the basal cisterns, they do not hesitate to puncture the frontal horn with a ventricular catheter to achieve a slack brain. This latter maneuver also may be preferable to forceable retraction of the frontal lobe to aspirate CSF in cases where the aneurysm points downward and may be adherent to the tuberculum sellae or the chiasm. In these cases frontal lobe retraction may result in avulsion of the aneurysm before the surgeon is in a position to deal with a massive rupture effectively. When the authors suspect basal adherence of the aneurysm, they try to achieve relaxation by retracting the tip of the temporal lobe and aspirating CSF from the carotid cistern rather than from the chiasmatic cistern. If this is not enough, the ventricle is punctured. A self-retaining retractor is then placed only superficially in the frontal lobe, the microscope is brought to the field, and then gentle retraction is gradually deepened after the surgeon has achieved control of at least the carotid artery. In cases of a downward projection of the aneurysm, the gyrus rectus approach, to be discussed later, is particularly recommended in order to avoid avulsion of the aneurysm by deep frontal retraction. The olfactory tract leads the surgeon to the optic nerve and internal carotid artery (Fig. 14.2B). The Greenberg self-retaining retractors are then placed.

Microsurgical Dissection

With a fine hook, the arachnoid is opened over the internal carotid artery and optic nerve (Fig. 14.2B). The surgeon further opens the cistern of the internal carotid artery holding a small suction in the nondominant hand and using the hook, microdissector, or microscissors in the dominant hand. The internal carotid artery is followed distally. In some patients, the origin of the right A_1 segment of the anterior cerebral artery can be visualized and the anterior edge of this vessel can be followed medially toward the aneurysm (Fig. 14.3). When this is the case, the aneurysm can often be exposed without a large gyrus rectus corticectomy. In most patients, however, the internal carotid artery segment is longer and the an-

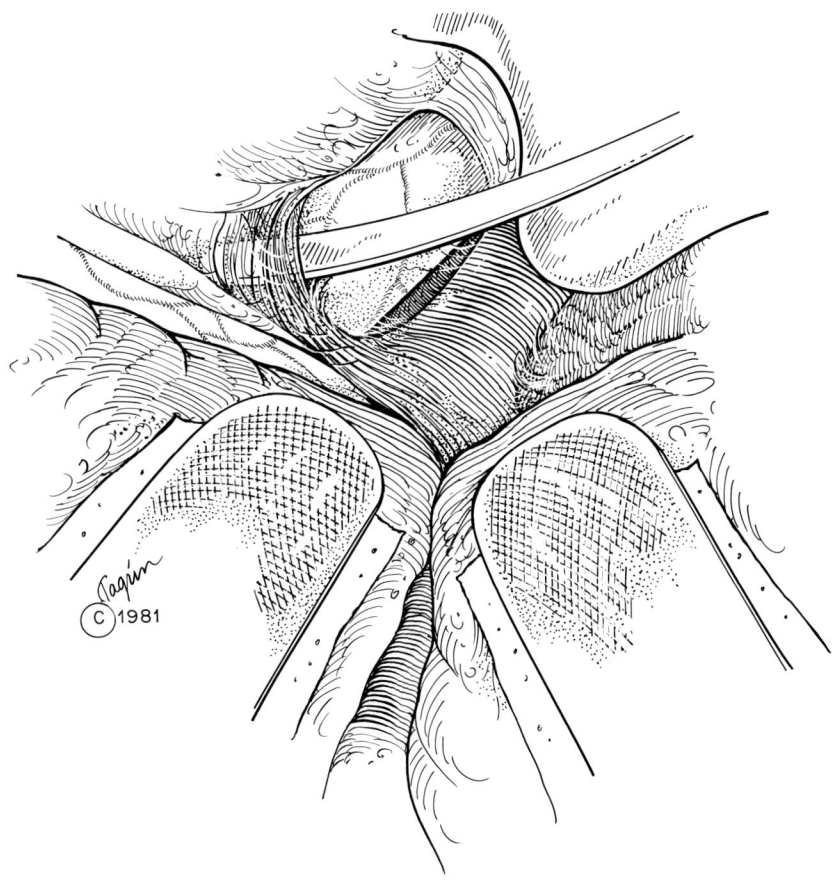

Figure 14.3. Dissection of right A_1 segment. The anterior border of the vessel is freed of arachnoid with a microdissector and microscissors.

terior cerebral artery origin higher and more posteriorly placed. In such instances, excessive frontal retraction would be needed to see the origin of the A_1 segment; inasmuch as it is not necessary to expose the entire A_1 segment, it seems wiser to proceed directly to the gyrus rectus corticectomy. A controlled suction device is helpful to provide adequate low-level suction without danger of injury to critical structures. Retraction at this point involves not only elevation of the frontal lobe and olfactory tract, but also a gentle lifting of the lobe away from the interhemispheric fissure. Only when the brain is slack can one obtain and hold this type of critical retraction. One needs to be able to look from the front by angling the scope to the left, and from behind by angling the scope to the right. It is important to have the flexibility to change the angle of vision frequently during operation.

A variable number of perforating arteries arise from the A_1 segments, proximal A_2 segment, and anterior communicating artery (11, 12, 15, 27). These arteries tend to follow a recurrent course backward to enter the anterior perforate substance. Hypothalamic arteries frequently originate from the inferior or posterior aspect of the anterior communicating artery or from the larger A_1 segment. They are often adherent to but rarely, if ever, originate from the posterior inferior wall of the aneurysm (12, 27). The recurrent artery of Heubner usually arises from the origin of the A_2 segment at or near the anterior cerebral and anterior communicating arteries and follows a course laterally either anterior or posterior to the A_1 segment to join the lenticulostriate arteries (5). Anomalous configurations of the anterior cerebral-anterior communicating artery complex are common (11–13, 27). Important normal variants include: (a) hypoplastic A_1 segment, (b) reduplicated anterior communicating arteries, and (c) persistent artery to the corpus callosum from the anterior communicating artery. Another rare but important anomaly is for both the pericallosal and the callosomarginal arteries to arise as separate vessels directly from the anterior cerebral-anterior communicating artery complex, giving the impression of essentially three different A_2 segments. One of the authors' patients with a frontal lobe hematoma in one side was devastated by inadvertent occlusion of such a "third A_2 segment," which resulted in infarction of the contralateral frontal lobe (Fig. 14.4) The authors have also seen perforating arteries and aneurysms arising from two reduplicated anterior communicating arteries in the same patient.

Keeping in mind the possible locations of these important perforating arteries, a corticectomy is made in the gyrus rectus, just medial to the olfactory tract, beginning at the level of the optic nerve and extending anteriorly for about 1.5 cm (Fig. 14.5). The gyrus is removed by suction until the pia-arachnoid over the A_1 segment and then the interhemispheric fissure are reached. This protective layer overlying the aneurysm is left intact. The arachnoid overlying the A_1 segment is opened (Fig. 14.6). Branches of this vessel, which may include Heubner's artery, must be preserved. The A_1 segment is followed distally to the anterior communicating artery and then to the origin of the ipsilateral A_2 segment. If possible, the aneurysm is avoided at this stage. Dissection proceeds by a combination of blunt dissection with a fine microdissector and microscissors cutting arachnoid after bipolar coagulation. Next, the contralateral A_2 segment is identified in the interhemispheric fissure (Fig. 14.7). The angiogram should be reviewed to determine whether the contralateral A_2 segment is anterior or posterior to its counterpart. In cases of large aneurysms in which the aneurysm projects forward, it is usually easier to identify the contralateral A_2 segment behind the aneurysm by tilting the microscope toward the ipsilateral side and pushing the base of the aneurysm forward. With aneurysms projecting directly upward or posteriorly, it may be easier to identify the contralateral A_2 segment by tilting the microscope forward and pushing the base of the aneurysm backwards. Once the opposite A_2 segment is identified, it may be followed retrograde to the A_1 segment. With a dorsally directed dome it is safer and easier to identify the opposite A_1 segment from in front of the aneurysm before seeking the deeper opposite A_2 segment. In cases of forward and downward projection of the aneurysm, the opposite A_1 segment is best identified by working behind the aneurysm without disturbing the dome. Careful scrutiny of the angiograms and knowledge of the anatomic variants guide the dissection. Almost always the aneurysm arises from the junction of the large A_1 segment and the anterior communicating artery.

As the surgeon seeks to identify the opposite segments, significant retraction of the aneurysm is often needed. This is best accomplished by leaving pia-arachnoid overlying the lesion, with retraction applied by the suction through an intervening cottonoid. One seeks to identify and free all major arterial trunks prior to working on the aneurysm. Then the aneurysm must be dissected completely, usually leaving a bit of the adherent brain in the area of the rupture. Only after complete dissection of the aneurysm can the surgeon be sure that the anatomy is understood and be in a position to decide which is the optimal way to clip the aneurysm.

Care is taken to preserve the perforating arteries. At this stage it is wise to leave in place any small potentially important arterial branches that are adherent to the dome of the lesion.

In straightforward cases, a narrow aneurysm neck can be prepared with the patient under normotension. Larger aneurysms or aneurysms with paper-thin, angry red patches near the neck will demand

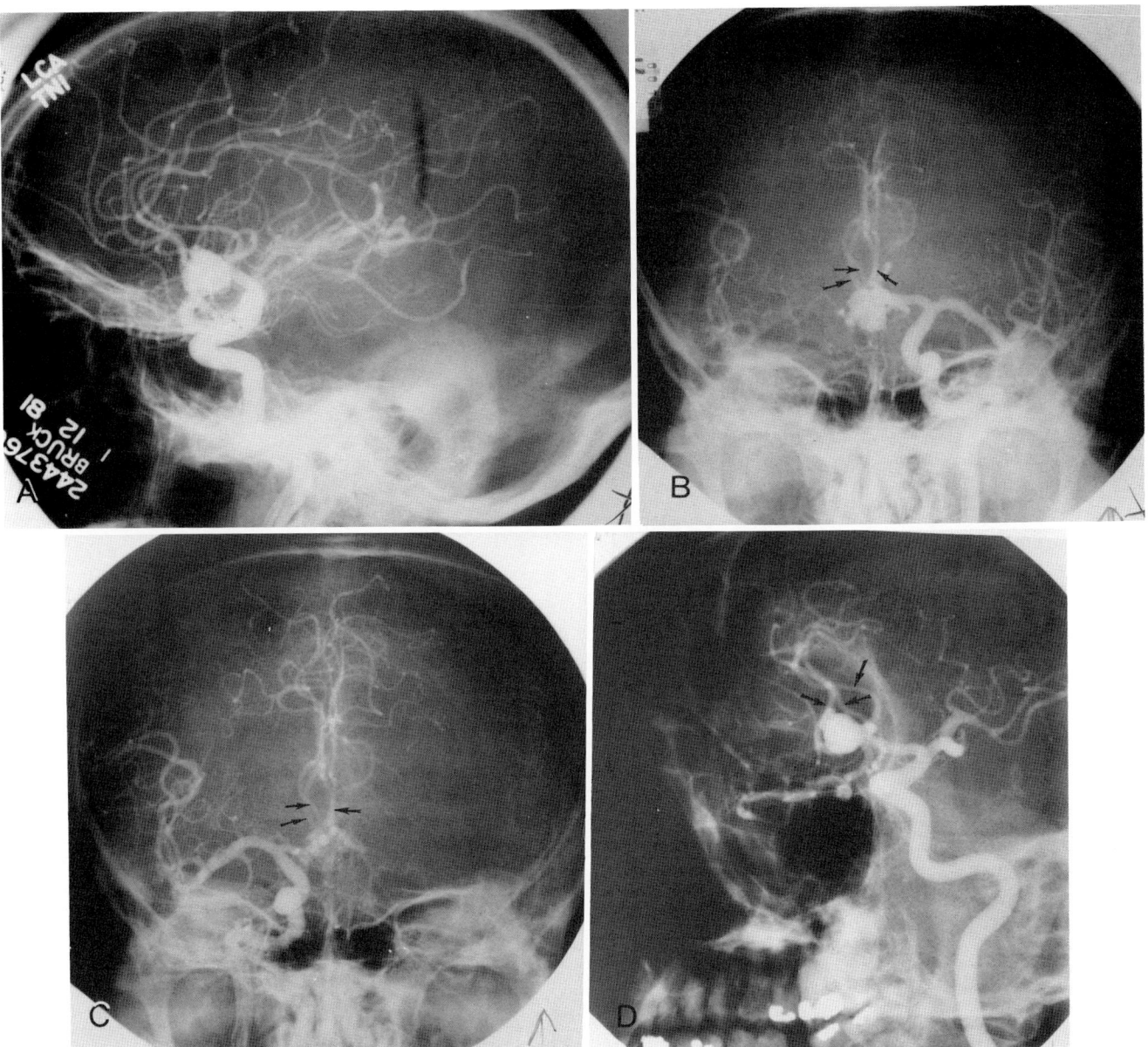

Figure 14.4. Patient with ruptured anterior communicating artery aneurysm who had a hemorrhage (moderately sized) into the left frontal lobe. **A–E**, Preoperative angiogram. The patient was operated from the left because of fear of injury to the right frontal lobe, since there was preexisting injury to the left frontal lobe from the hematoma. Clipping was unremarkable, but the patient developed a severe and irreversible memory, personality, and affect disorder. **F–H**, Postoperative angiography demonstrated absence of a third major vessel arising from the anterior communicating aneurysm complex and supplying the right frontal lobe. Retrospectively, when the preoperative anteroposterior (**B** and **C**), oblique (**D**), and base (**E**) views were reanalyzed, it became clear that there were three large vessels coming directly from the anterior communicating complex (*arrows*). In the postoperative angiogram (**F–H**) only two vessels are seen. At surgery two A_2 segments were clearly identified and preserved, but once this was done, the authors proceeded to clip the large aneurysm without dissecting it completely. Complete circumferential dissection of the aneurysm at surgery would have revealed the third "A_2" vessel and may have prevented this devastating complication.

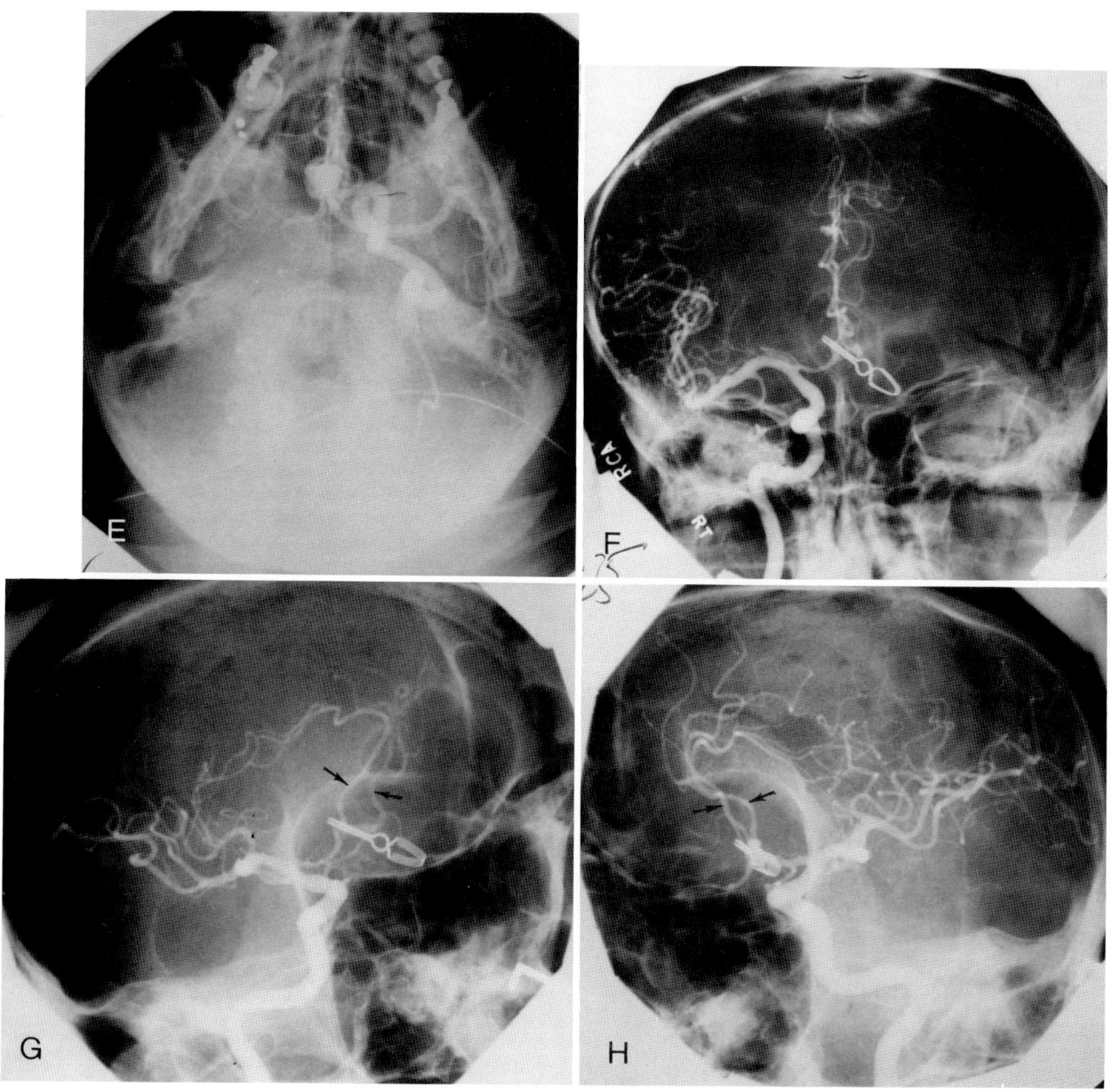

Figure 14.4 E–H.

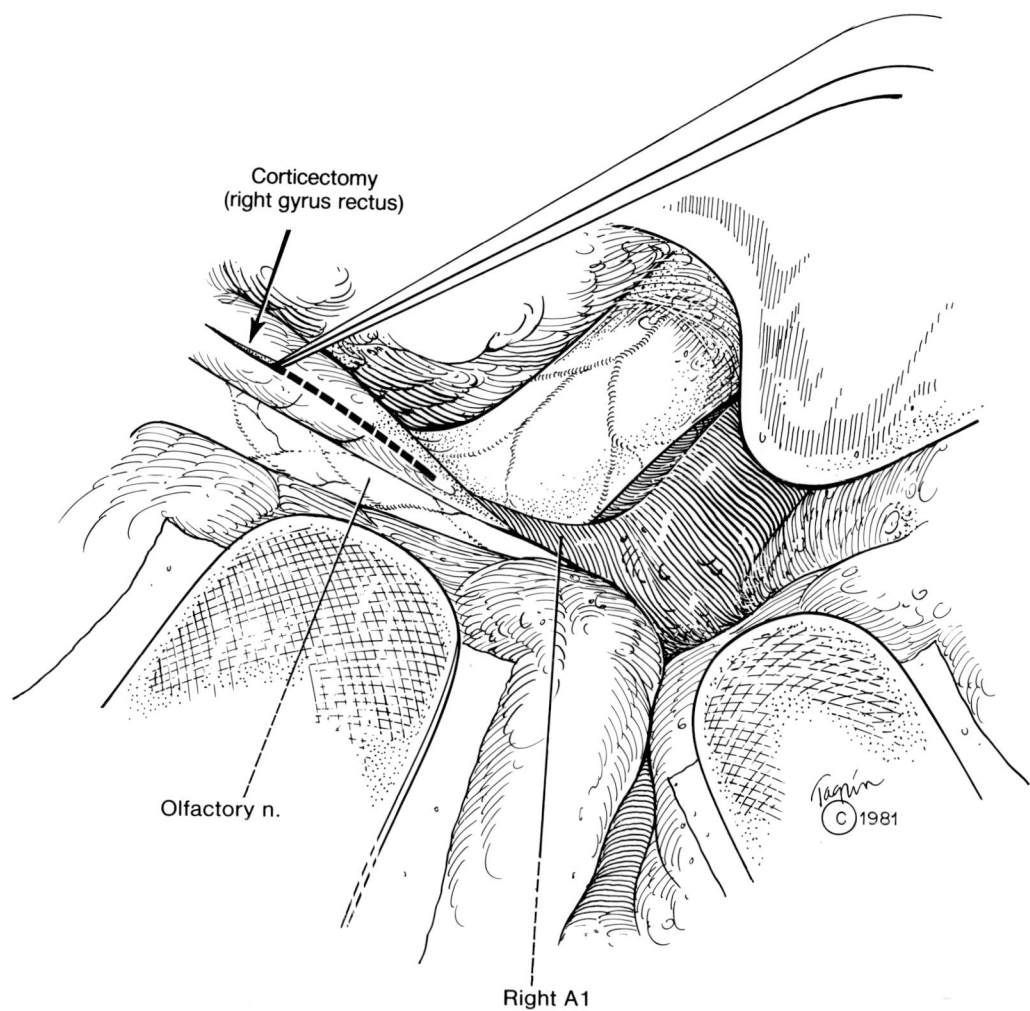

Figure 14.5. Gyrus rectus corticectomy. Bipolar cauterization and incision of pia over 1.0–1.5 cm. Care must be taken to place corticectomy over aneurysm site (usually near the level of the medial edge of optic nerve).

special adjuncts to prevent rupture. When the risk of rupture seems modest, a brief period of moderate hypotension (systolic 70 torr for 5–10 minutes) may suffice to permit safe dissection and clipping. When the danger of rupture is great, however, the authors prefer temporary clips and deliberate hypertension with mannitol protection (28) (see Chapter 11). This is preferable to uncontrolled rupture and a hasty dissection. Whatever the precautions, precise definition of the aneurysm neck is crucial.

For these maneuvers, the suction, with or without a cottonoid, is used to reflect the lesion to one side, and a fine dissector or microscissors frees the neck from adherent structures (Fig. 14.8). It is particularly important, and frequently very difficult, to define the plane of cleavage between the opposite A_2 segment and the aneurysm. When the aneurysm is approached from the side of the dominant A_1 segment, as the authors usually do, it will project to the contralateral side and will frequently be very adherent to the opposite A_2 segment right at the base of the aneurysm, giving the false appearance of a very broad neck until the plane of cleavage between the anterior communicating artery, the opposite A_2 segment, and the aneurysm is well defined. For this maneuver sharp dissection is preferable. With the microscope, it is usually possible to identify a cleavage plane right to the edge of the neck. Initially it is wise to dissect a bit up on the wall in case of a tear in the neck, which can be disastrous. It is necessary to reflect the lesion superiorly to assure preservation of the perforating branches of the anterior communicating artery. These vessels are often adherent to the ventral posterior wall of the aneurysm and must be carefully separated from it. In many cases, gentle reflection of the aneurysm anteriorly while looking over the A_2 segment will give the needed view. However, in some instances, with a posteriorly or posteroinferiorly directed lesion, reflection of the aneurysm and the ipsilateral A_2 segment superiorly will give a nice view

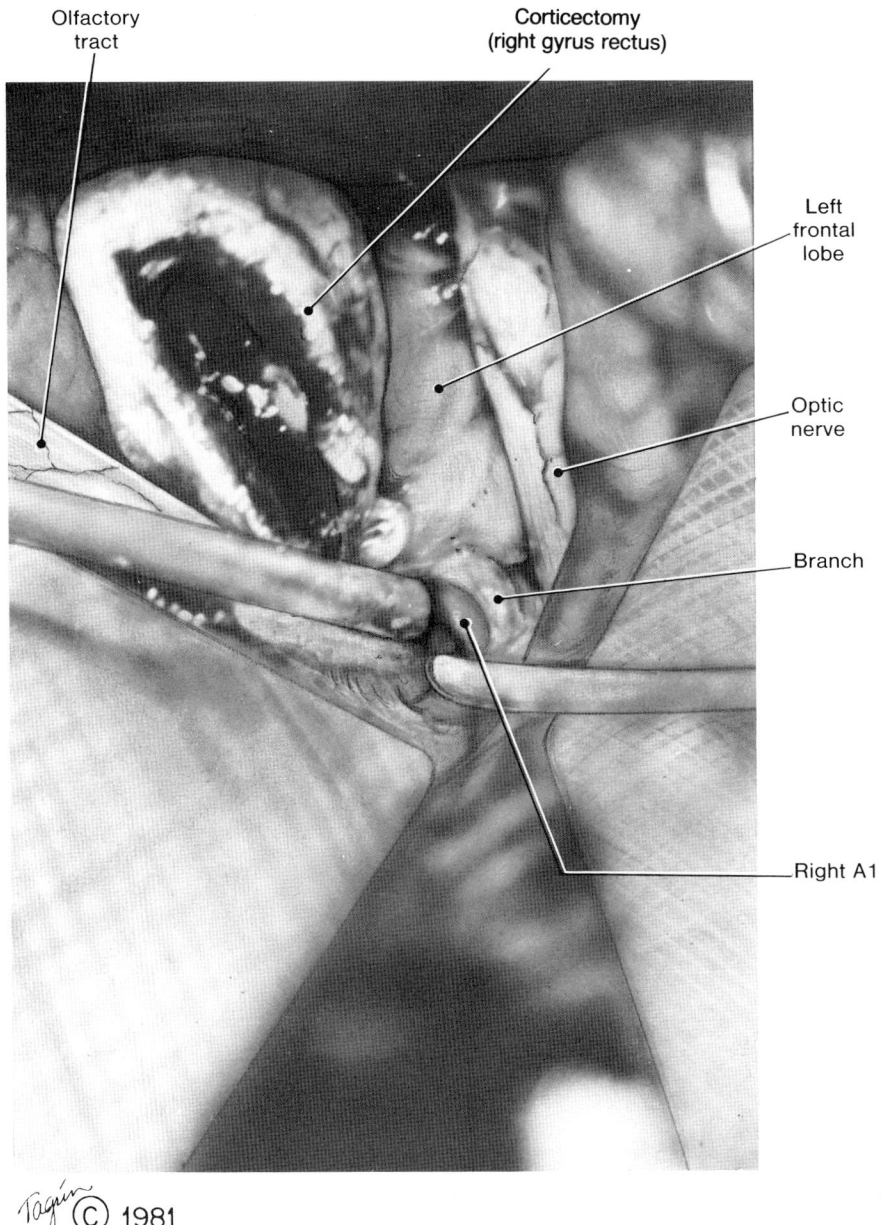

Figure 14.6. Dissection of right A_1 segment through the corticectomy. The microscope has been directed more medially. Suction and bipolar cauterization remove cortex down to interhemispheric pia-arachnoid. With a fine dissector, pia-arachnoid is removed from right A_1 segment.

of the ventral aspects of these structures and their plane of separation from the perforators (Fig. 14.9). Whatever the technique, the primary aim is to develop clear cleavage between the ventral-posterior aspect of the aneurysm and the numerous critical perforating arteries emanating from the posterior aspect of the anterior communicating artery. This is particularly important to achieve prior to clipping of the aneurysm because visualization of these perforators during application of the clip is frequently difficult or impossible. Finally, adherent arterial branches overlying the dome of the aneurysm may be dissected free. Such branches may yield to blunt dissection with a right angle hook or ball dissector. In some cases, where accurate visualization of arachnoid bands is possible, sharp dissection with scissors may be preferred. If aneurysmal rupture occurs at this point, the problem can be controlled since the aneurysm neck has been essentially completely dissected.

Obliteration of the Aneurysm

In almost all cases, an aneurysm clip is the best solution. Once the lesion is completely dissected and

Anterior Communicating Artery Aneurysms

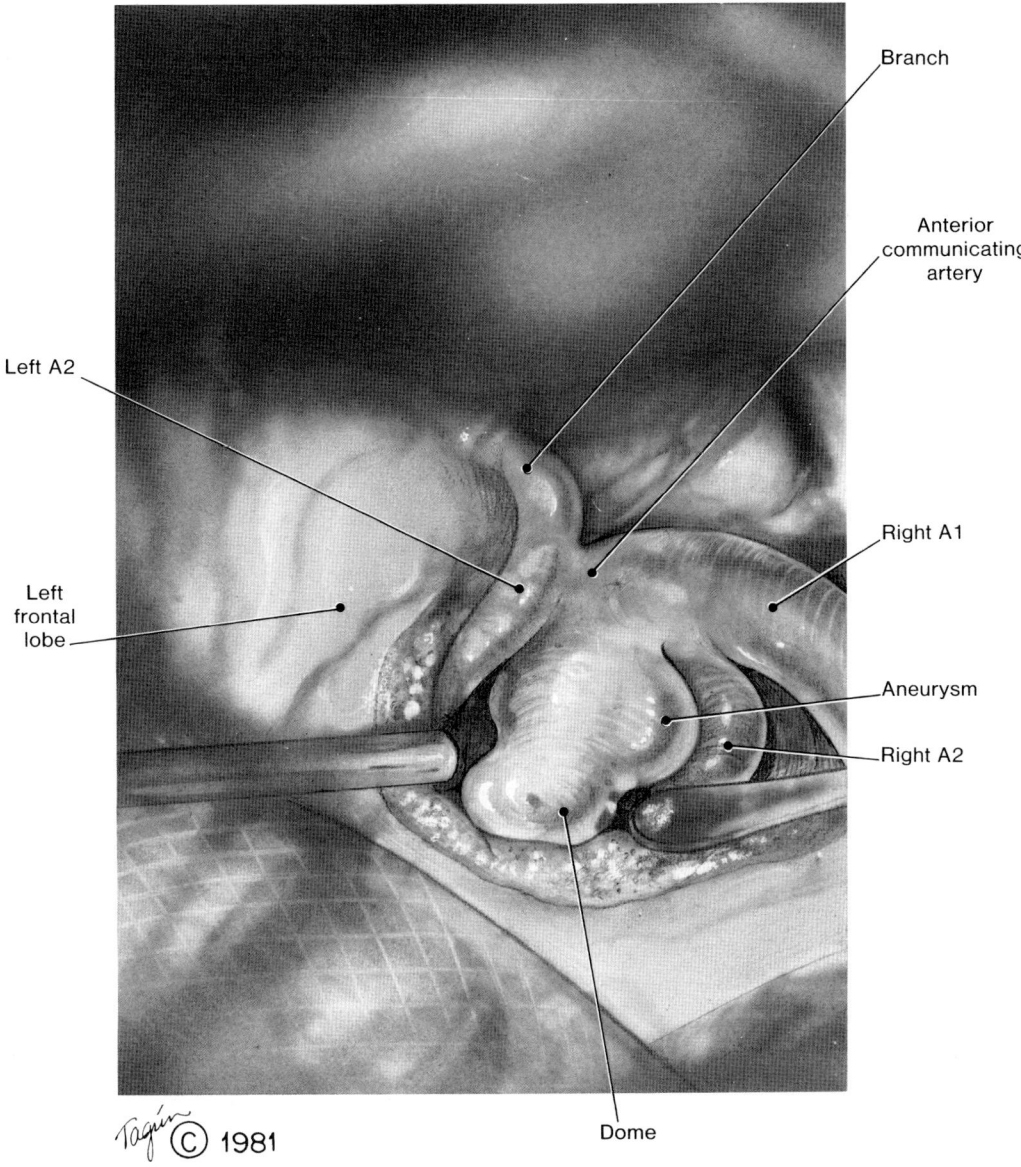

Figure 14.7. Dissection of aneurysm. Proceeding clockwise, the surgeon frees up the right A_1 and A_2 segments of the anterior cerebral arteries, then the left A_2 and A_1 segments. Finally, the aneurysm is exposed circumferentially, and the neck is completely dissected.

the relationship of its neck to surrounding critical structures (including the perforating arteries) is defined, the surgeon can determine which technique will best obliterate the lesion. The authors usually use a Sugita or Yasargil clip. A long straight clip is particularly effective for upward pointing lesions. Because of the angle of application, the Sano applier is frequently used. Sometimes a clip with a slight curve or even a very abrupt curve will be useful to occlude an aneurysm neck. Often a projecting lobe can be gathered up with the suction tip into the jaws of a clip (Fig. 14.10). Release is sometimes difficult with the Yasargil and Sugita clips and may be facilitated by distracting the handle blades of the clip applier with the third and fourth fingers placed interiorly. Occasionally an aperture clip may be needed, with the aperture enclosing either the ipsilateral A_1 or A_2 segment (Figs. 14.1 and 14.11). In an occasional patient bipolar coagulation or a preliminary ligature can be used to prepare the lesion for clipping. In some patients, the force of one clip reinforced by a booster clip may be needed to assure complete closure of a thick aneurysmal wall (19). In other patients, a combination of two clips is necessary for optimum obliteration of the aneurysm neck. In a persistent corner the authors have found that a straight clip may occasionally be nicely supplemented with a triangular Heifetz clip since the hubs of this pair do not

228 Surgical Management of Cerebrovascular Disease

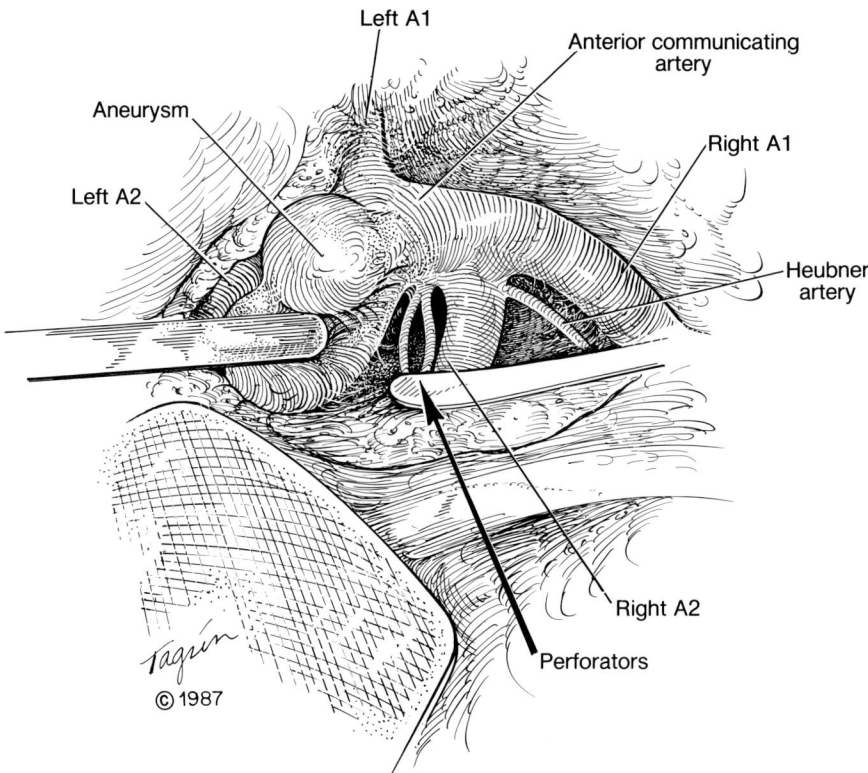

Figure 14.8. Dissection of perforating branches. These crucial vessels emerge from the anterior communicating artery and proceed posteriorly to the hypothalamus. They must be gently freed from the aneurysm and excluded from clipping. Note retraction of the aneurysm with the suction.

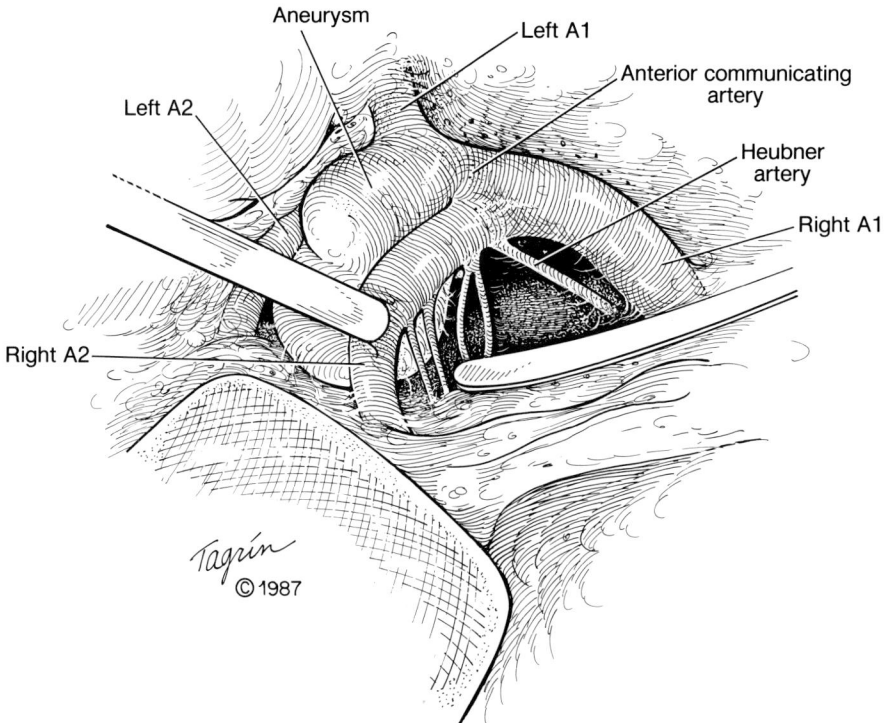

Figure 14.9. Dissection of perforating branches. For posteriorly projecting lesions, access to perforators may be facilitated by reflecting the right A_2 artery upwards with the suction tip.

Anterior Communicating Artery Aneurysms

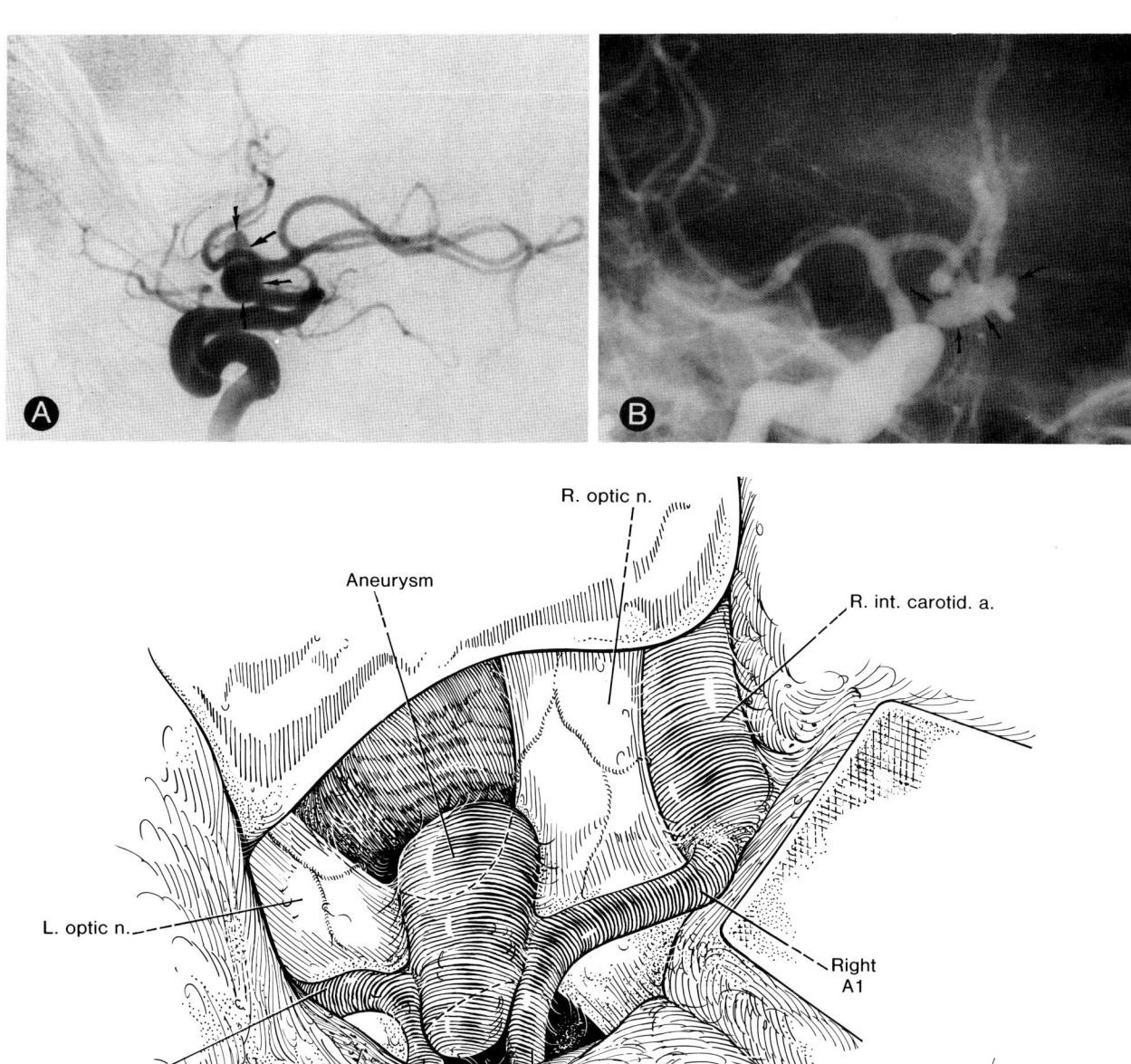

Figure 14.10. Bilobed anterior communicating artery aneurysm: adherence to optic chiasm and posterior bulge. **A** and **B**, Right carotid angiogram shows projection of aneurysm rostrally and to both sides (*arrows*). Position of lesion near tuberculum sellae suggests it may be adherent to basal structures. **C**, Intraoperative illustration shows aneurysm adherent to superior and anterior surfaces of optic chiasm. Sharp and blunt dissection isolated lesion. Perforating arteries coursing posteriorly were spared. **D**, A suction was used to gather up both bulges of the aneurysm for inclusion in a straight clip placed transversely. **E** and **F**, Postoperative right carotid angiogram shows nonfilling of aneurysm and preservation of arteries. The patient was neurologically intact.

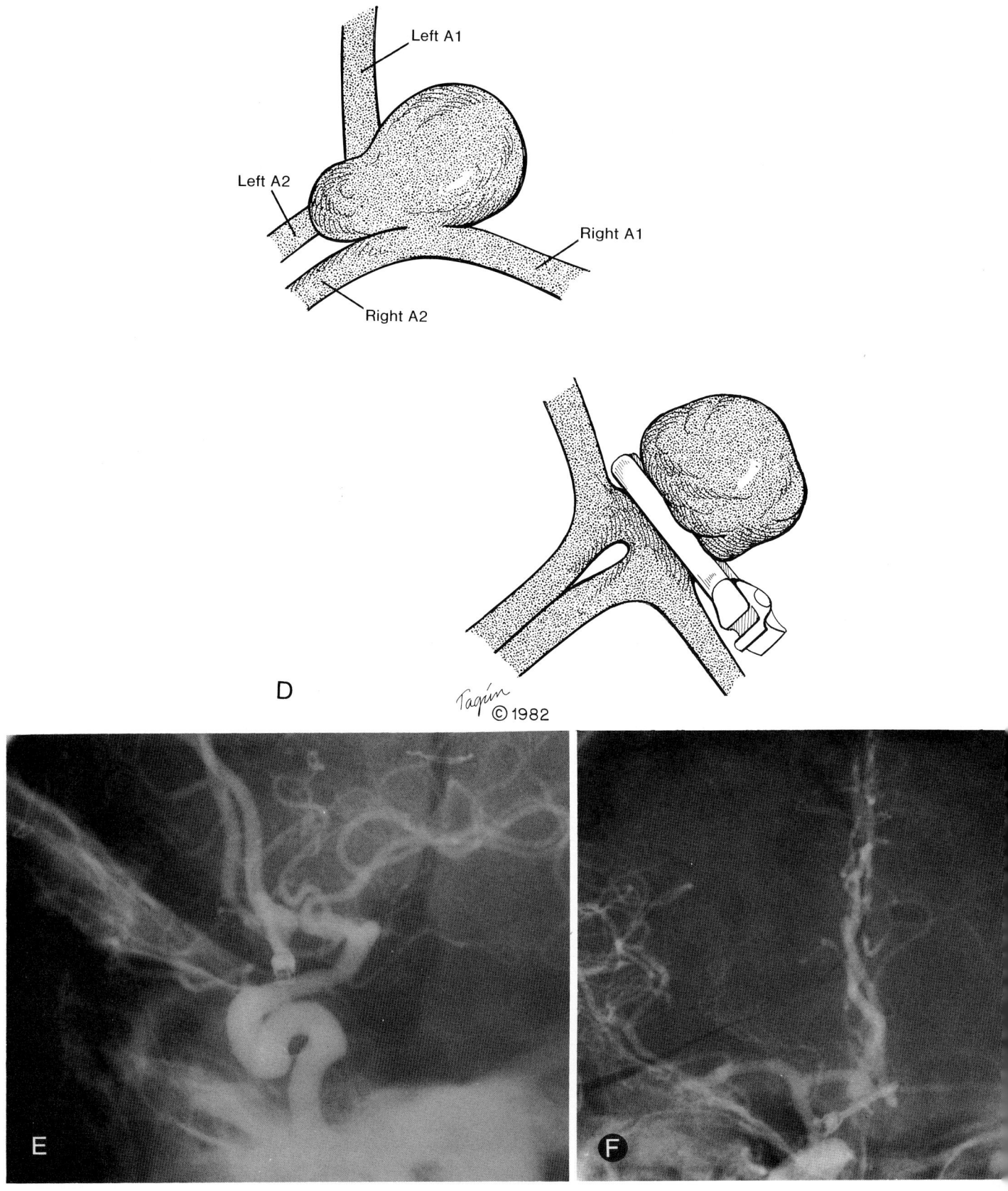

Figure 14.10D–F.

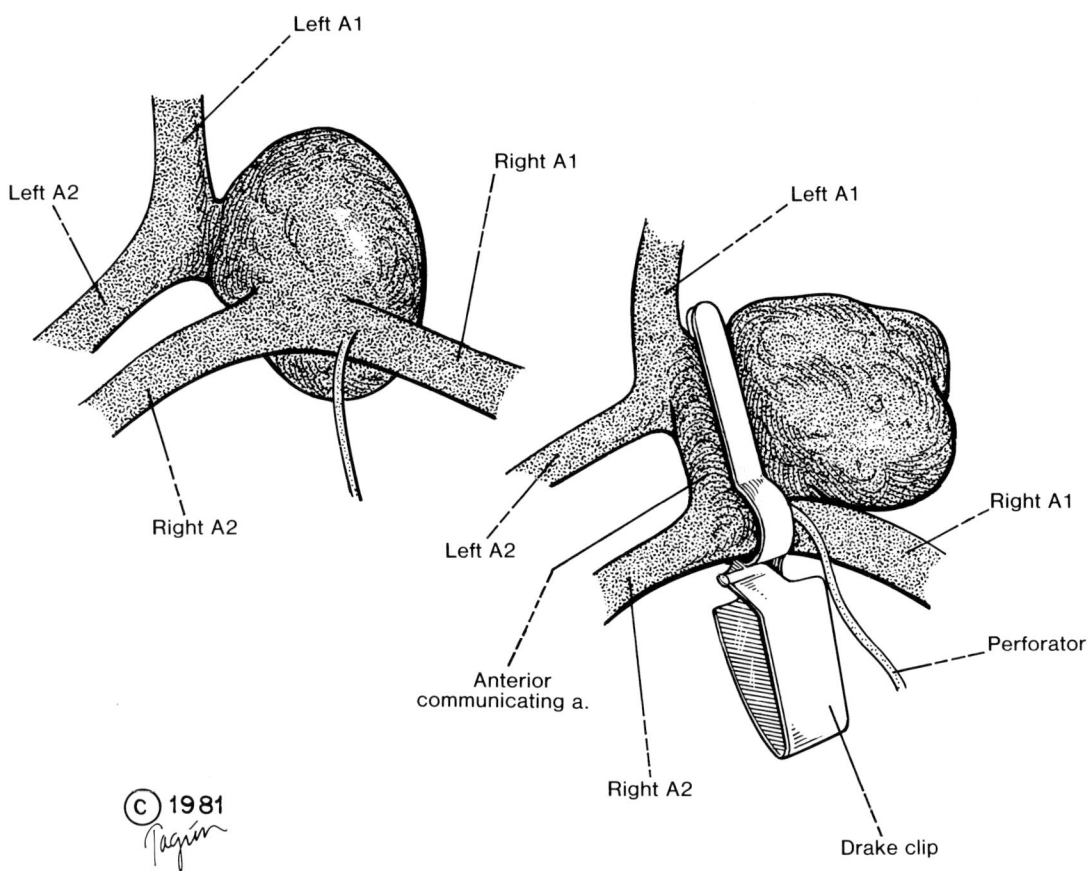

Figure 14.11. Common wall for aneurysm and right A_1 segment. Solution of problem: Drake clip spares right A_1 segment and perforating arteries. An angled Sugita fenestrated clip can also be useful for such situations.

mutually interfere. For giant anterior communicating artery aneurysms, the Drake clips (up to 24 mm) or the ultralong Sugita clips may provide the only accurate and adequate clipping (see Chapter 20).

Occasionally an aneurysm with adherent perforating arteries hidden behind major arterial trunks will defy clipping. A carefully applied ligature may offer the best solution (Fig. 14.12). This is particularly helpful when the neck of the aneurysm can be completely dissected but irregularity or bulging or dome adherence renders a standard clip blade hazardous. The authors have found ligature carriers of no assistance; however, a double, waxed 3-0 silk suture may be advanced behind the neck with a fine forceps and then retrieved with a hook beyond the far edge for tying with a surgeon's knot using two hemostats. As the ligature is tightened, the effects on adjacent vessels should be observed to avoid occlusion by kinking. Whatever the means of obliteration both anterior cerebral arteries and the anterior communicating artery with its perforating vessels must be maintained intact. If these criteria are not satisfied, obliteration will need to be adjusted to obtain a satisfactory application. If there is any question of an unclipped weak spot, a bit of muslin may be applied as reinforcement. The muslin should not touch the chiasm, however, for fear of adhesive arachnoiditis (2).

RESULTS

The authors' surgical results with anterior communicating aneurysms at the Massachusetts General Hospital during the past 10 years are given in Table 14.1. All but eight had delayed surgery. A "good" result implies a patient with a normal neurologic examination and without major psychosocial disability. It has become increasingly apparent that many such patients who appeared "normal" to the neurosurgeon in a follow-up visit 6 to 8 weeks after surgery do not, in fact, return to work or return to a less demanding job because of subtle psychosocial impairment that can be detected by sophisticated testing techniques (8, 14). Since in general the authors have not subjected their patients to such rigorous late follow-up evaluations, they no longer use the "excellent" classification and accept that some of the patients in the "good" result category may have sub-

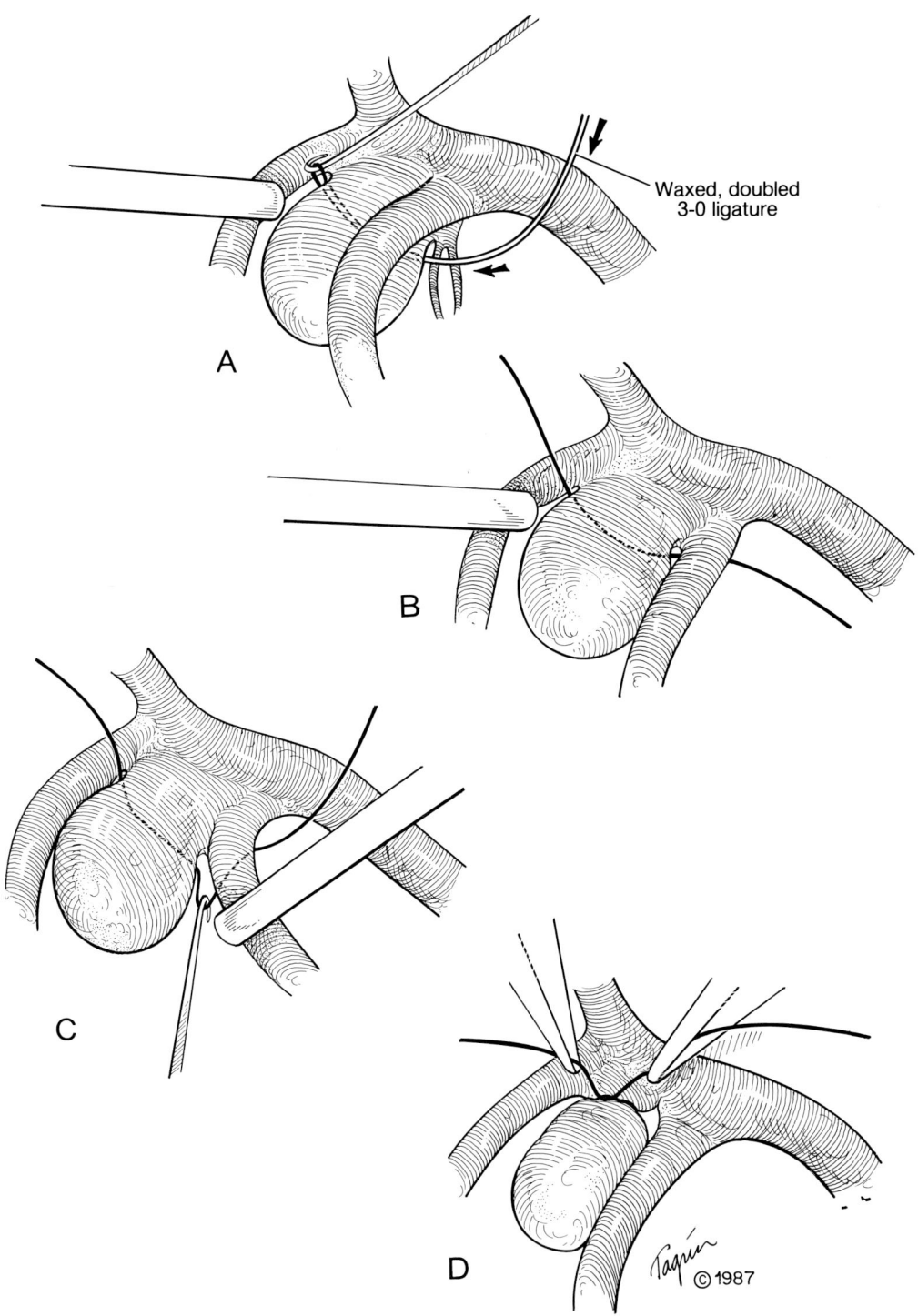

Figure 14.12. Ligature for anterior communicating artery aneurysm. **A**, Waxed, doubled 3-0 silk is advanced between perforators and posterior wall of neck, exposed by retracting right A_2. **B**, Loop of ligature is identified by deflecting aneurysm and pulled through with a microhook. **C**, The proximal ligature is then brought between the aneurysm neck and right A_2. **D**, Ligature is tied with two fine straight hemostats, using a surgeon's knot and grasping as near the knot as possible.

Table 14.1.
Results of Operation

Preoperative Grade (Hunt)	Good	Fair	Poor	Dead	Total
0, 1, and 2	83 (91.2%)	3	4	1	91
1A	0	1	2	0	3
3 and 4	5	0	5	1	11
Totals	88 (83.8%)	4 (3.8%)	11 (10.5%)	2 (1.9%)	105

tle degrees of psychologic impairment and may not have returned fully to their previous level of performance. A "fair" result implies an independent patient with minor neurologic or cognitive disability. A "poor" result refers to a patient with a moderate to major permanent disability. All the grade 3 and 4 patients in this series were operated during the earlier part of the authors' experience. Lately, they have only operated patients in good condition (grades 0, 1 or 2) or patients who are stable but have a fixed neurologic deficit as a result of either vasospasm or the initial subarachnoid hemorrhage (grade 1A). Of the three patients classified as grade 1A, one improved to a fair condition and the other two remained with a significant neurologic deficit (poor result); none was made worse by the operation.

There were two deaths in the series—one in a patient in good preoperative condition who died of a myocardial infarction after surgery. The second death occurred in a grade 4 comatose patient operated for a large intracerebral hematoma. There were four poor results in good grade patients and each deserves a comment. One patient awoke blind in the right eye and vision never returned; the authors assume this occurred as a result of inadvertent intraoperative trauma to the optic nerve or to its blood supply. The other three patients suffered significant and permanent impairment of memory, judgment, and emotional expression. They remain incapacitated and dependent although without noticeable physical impairment. In two cases the cause of the deficit has not been understood because the postoperative angiogram looked unremarkable. Intraoperative trauma to the medial basal frontal region bilaterally or, more likely, perforator occlusion is suspected as the etiology of these deficits. The third patient has already been described; he had inadvertent occlusion of a contralateral callosomarginal artery that originated directly from the anterior cerebral-anterior communicating artery complex (see Fig. 14.4).

Earlier in the authors' series late surgery (usually 10–15 days after subarachnoid hemorrhage) was the rule, but during the past 2 years they have begun to operate early on patients in good condition who are seen within the first 48 hours after their subarachnoid hemorrhage. Eight patients in this series were operated early and all have done well, but it must be emphasized that they were in good condition preoperatively and, therefore, are a selected group.

Yasargil reported in detail a series of 375 patients operated for an anterior communicating artery aneurysm (25). Good results were obtained in 87.5% of the patients, although in 11.2% there were transient deficits that resolved in time. Overall there were 9.6% poor results and deaths, but only 1.6% of these were directly attributed to the operation. Yasargil observed a postoperative "psychoorganic" syndrome with variable disturbances of consciousness, memory, concentration, and personality in 18.9% of patients who were well before surgery. However, these changes were permanent in only 1.3% of the patients. Only 11 patients in good condition were operated early (within 3 days) and all remained well. Interestingly, he found that of the anatomic factors other than size, an inferior projection of the aneurysm was associated with increased operative morbidity and mortality.

Suzuki has also achieved good or excellent results in 84% of his patients with anterior communicating artery aneurysms (6, 22). He has used a bifrontal interhemispheric approach and has described how to preserve olfaction with this approach by early dissection and protection of the olfactory bulb and tract (22). He also routinely uses temporary proximal occlusion of both A_1 segments and occasionally also of the A_2 segments. Sengupta et al also reported excellent results with these aneurysms (17). They subjected many of their patients to rigorous late psychologic testing and found little evidence of intellectual impairment, although subtle personality changes and diminished drive and interest were commonly found. Other surgeons have achieved equally good results with these aneurysms (4, 20).

REFERENCES

1. Alexander MP, Freedman M: Amnesia after anterior communicating artery aneurysm rupture. Neurology 34:752–757, 1984.
2. Carney PG, Oatey PE: Muslin wrapping of aneurysm and delayed visual failure. A report of three cases. J Clin Opthalmol 10:91–96, 1983.
3. Crowell RM, Ojemann RG: Surgical treatment of anterior communicating artery aneurysms. In Schmidek HH, Sweet WH (eds): Operative Neurosurgical Techniques. New York, Grune & Stratton, 1982, pp 829–854.
4. Flamm ES: Anterior cerebral artery aneurysm. In Fein JM, Flamm ES (eds): Cerebrovascular Surgery. New York, Springer-Verlag, 1985, vol 3, pp 879–898.
5. Gomes F, Dujovny M, Umansky F, Ausman JI, Diaz FG, Ray WJ, Mirchandi HG: Microsurgical anatomy of the recurrent artery of Heubner. J Neurosurg 60:130–139, 1984
6. Hori S, Suzuki J: Early and late results of intracranial direct surgery of anterior communicating artery aneurysms. J Neurosurg 50: 433–440, 1979.
7. Kempe LG: Operative Neurosurgery, vol 1: Cranial, Cerebral and Intracranial Vascular Disease. New York, Springer-Verlag, 1968, pp 54–74.

8. Ljunggren B, Brandt L, Sundbarg G, Saveland H, Cronqvist S, Stridbeck H: Early management of aneurysmal subarachnoid hemorrhage. *Neurosurgery* 11: 412–418, 1982
9. Ljunggren B, Saveland H, Brandt L, Zygmunt S: Early operation and overall outcome in aneurysmal subarachnoid hemorrhage. *J Neurosurg.* 62:547–551, 1985.
10. Odom GL, Tindall GT: Carotid ligation in the treatment of certain intracranial aneurysms. *Clin Neurosurg* 15:101–116, 1968.
11. Perlmutter D. Rhoton AL: Microsurgical anatomy of the anterior cerebral-anterior communicating-recurrent artery complex. *J Neurosurg.* 45:259–272, 1976
12. Rhoton AL Jr, Fujuii K, Saeki N, Perlmutter D, Zeal A: Microsurgical anatomy of intracranial aneurysm. Part I. In Hopkins LN, Long DM (eds): *Clinical Management of Intracranial Aneurysms.* New York, Raven Press, 1982, pp 201–243.
13. Rhoton AL Jr, Saeki N, Perlmutter D, Zeal A: Microsurgical anatomy of common aneurysm sites. *Clin Neurosurg* 26:248–306, 1979.
14. Ropper AH, Zervas NT: Outcome 1 year after SAH from cerebral aneurysm. Management morbidity, mortality and functional status in 112 consecutive good-risk patients. *J Neurosurg* 60:909–915, 1984.
15. Rosner SS, Rhoton AL Jr, Ono M, Barry M: Microsurgical anatomy of the anterior perforating arteries. *J Neurosurg* 61:468–485, 1984.
16. Sano K, Saito I: Timing and indication of surgery for ruptured intracranial aneurysms with regard to cerebral vasospasm. *Acta Neurochir* 41:49–60, 1978.
17. Sengupta RP, Chin JSP, Brierly H: Quality of survival following direct surgery for anterior communicating aneurysms. *J Neurosurg* 43:58–64, 1975.
18. Sugita K: *Microneurosurgery Atlas.* Berlin, Springer-Verlag, 1986.
19. Sundt TM Jr, Piepgras DG, Marsh WR: Booster clips for giant and thick-based aneurysms. *J Neurosurg* 60:751–762, 1984.
20. Sundt TM Jr, Whisnant JP: Subarachnoid hemorrhage from intracranial aneurysms. Surgical management and natural history of disease. *N Engl J Med* 299:116–122, 1978.
21. Suzuki J (ed): *Cerebral Aneurysms, Experiences with 1000 Directly Operated Cases.* Tokyo, Neuron Publishing, 1979.
22. Suzuki J, Mizoi K, Yoshimoto T: Bifrontal interhemispheric approach to aneurysms of the anterior communicating artery. *J Neurosurg* 64:183–190, 1986.
23. VanderArk GD, Kempe LG, Smith DR: Anterior communicating aneurysms: The gyrus rectus approach. *Clin Neurosurg* 21:120–133, 1974.
24. Vapalahti M, Ljunggren B, Saveland H, Hernesniemi J, Brandt L, Tapaninaho A: Early aneurysm operation and outcome in two remote Scandinavian populations. *J Neurosurg* 60:1160–1162, 1984.
25. Yasargil MG: Anterior cerebral and anterior communicating artery aneurysms. In Yasargil MG (ed): *Microneurosurgery.* New York, Thieme-Stratton, 1984.
26. Yasargil MG, Fox JL: The microsurgical approach to intracranial aneurysms. *Surg Neurol* 3:7–14, 1975.
27. Yasargil MG, Smith RD: Management of aneurysms of anterior circulation by intracranial procedures. In Youmans JR (ed): *Neurological Surgery.* Philadelphia, WB Saunders, 1982, pp 1663–1696.
28. Yoshimoto T, Suzuki J: Temporary clipping—prolongation of the time of occlusion by mannitol. In Pia HW, Langmaid C, Zierski J (eds): *Cerebral Aneurysms.* Berlin, Springer-Verlag, 1979, pp 382–392.

15
Distal Anterior Cerebral Artery Aneurysms

PRESENTATION AND EVALUATION

Because they present special surgical problems, aneurysms arising from the distal anterior cerebral artery deserve separate consideration. These aneurysms comprise 2–4.5% of all intracranial aneurysms. They generally arise near the genu of the corpus callosum, usually at the bifurcation of the pericallosal and callosomarginal arteries and rarely at the origin of the frontopolar artery (13). Anatomic variations are common in this area, including communications between the two pericallosal arteries (5, 6, 8, 12) and an azygous or single anterior cerebral artery (2, 4, 10) that may give rise to an aneurysm. For aneurysms distal to the callosomarginal origin, a diagnosis of a bacterial aneurysm must be considered (see Chapter 21). Rarely these aneurysms are familial (14).

Clinical presentation is usually with subarachnoid hemorrhage. With bleeding there is a high incidence of pyramidal signs, especially a crural predominant hemiparesis (1) or contralateral lower limb monoparesis (9). This is due to the fact that these aneurysms frequently result in intracerebral hemorrhage rather than diffuse subarachnoid hemorrhage (Fig. 15.1A and B). These aneurysms may also present with mass effect causing mental deterioration and urinary incontenence, simulating frontal lobe tumor or hydrocephalus, or a frontopolar aneurysm may cause chiasmal compression (3).

The diagnosis can rarely be suspected from the clinical picture of crural monoparesis in the setting of subarachnoid hemorrhage. The computed tomography (CT) scan, however, by showing a dense clot high in the interhemispheric fissure is frequently of help. Occasionally, the CT scan is almost pathognomonic of an aneurysm in this location when it shows a "butterfly" type of intracerebral hemorrhage in both frontal lobes (Fig. 15.1B).

It has been said that the prognosis tends to be worse for patients with these aneurysms (11, 13), but this has not been the experience of the authors. The standard program of evaluation and preoperative management is utilized for these patients (see Chapters 10 and 11). At angiography, base and oblique films generally add little to the information obtained from anteroposterior and lateral views. Surgery may be difficult because of limited interhemispheric access, problems obtaining proximal control of the arterial circulation, and the frequent finding of a broad neck containing atheroma (16).

OPERATIVE TECHNIQUE
Preparation and Positioning

Spinal drainage is a useful adjunct in these patients because of the limited exposure available in the interhemispheric fissure. As an alternative, direct ventricular puncture, which is easy to perform with the exposure required for these aneurysms, may be used to obtain the necessary relaxation. Mannitol, with or without Lasix, is administered at the time of the skin incision to promote a brisk diuresis and subsequent slackening of the brain. Moderate hyperventilation is routine. The preparation and the anesthesia technique are described in Chapter 11.

The patient is positioned with the head and neck flexed on the chest and with the orbitomeatal line about 20° above the horizontal. The head is fixed in the three-point headrest with the nose straight ahead to place the midline in a true vertical orientation. With the head in this position, interhemispheric access from the precoronal area may proceed downward to the area of the corpus callosum and the origin of the aneurysm.

Initial Exposure

The approach is via a parasagittal interhemispheric route. A subfrontal approach has proved difficult for distal exposure (9), but a bifrontal approach coming from the base upward in the interhemispheric fissure has been used successfully, particularly for the more proximally located aneurysms (17). The authors have had no experience with this approach, which has the advantage of early proximal control and which is the only approach for the rare more proximal aneurysms located beneath the genu. For the interhemispheric approach the nondominant side is chosen whenever possible.

Review of the angiogram will outline the venous drainage along the superior sagittal sinus. Occasionally, extensive bridging veins from the brain to the sagittal sinus may bar the way and suggest a domi-

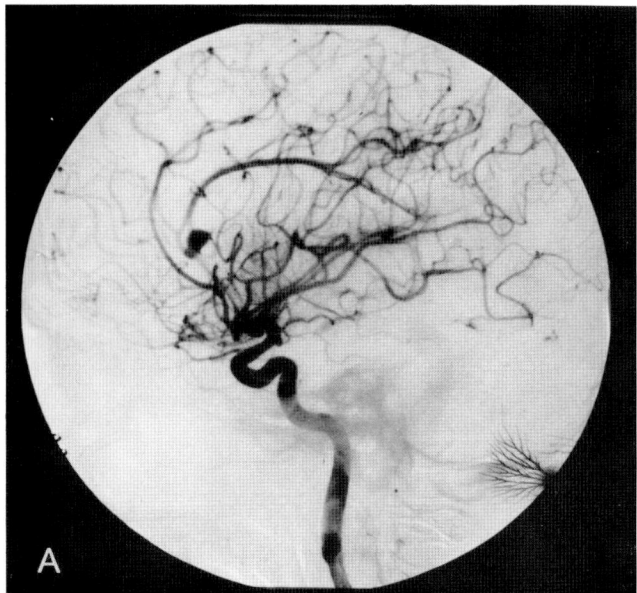
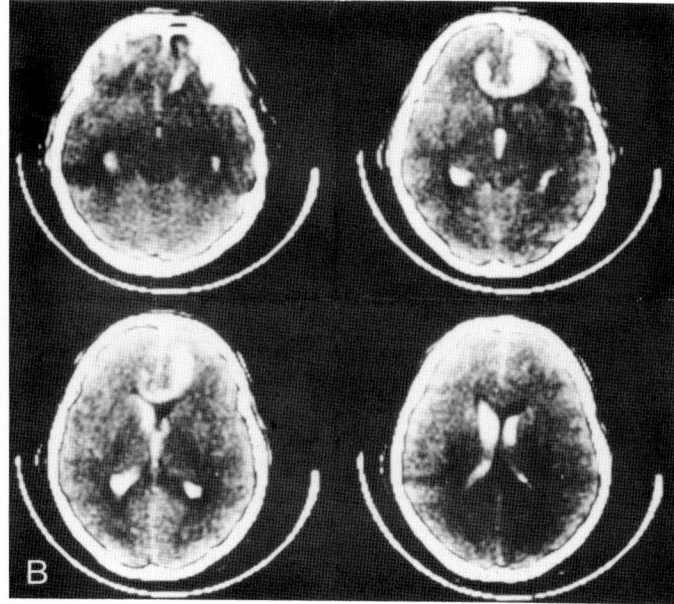

Figure 15.1. Pericallosal aneurysm. **A**, Lateral angiogram shows an aneurysm near the genu of pericallosal artery. **B**, Typical CT scan appearance of intracerebral hemorrhage from this aneurysm.

nant side approach. Veins anterior to the coronal suture can usually be divided without deficit. If the CT scan shows a hematoma in the left frontal lobe, a left parasagittal approach is usually indicated to avoid bifrontal damage.

For most lesions that lie just at or above the genu of the corpus callosum, a bicoronal incision is used. A bone flap just in front of the coronal suture and crossing the midline gives adquate exposure (Fig. 15.2A). The dura is opened with a horseshoe-shaped flap with the hinge on the midline. Precoronal bridging veins from the frontal lobe may be divided for access to the interhemispheric fissure. A large or critical bridging vein may be spared by dissecting it from the brain and retracting it aside (10). Entry into the fissure is begun gradually with retraction on the exposed hemisphere with a hand-held retractor. As cerebrospinal fluid is removed from the spinal catheter or ventricular needle, and mannitol takes its effect, the brain becomes slack. Dense adhesions of brain to falx may be taken down with electrocoagulation and sharp dissection. The dissection is deepened past the edge of the falx. A self-retaining retractor held by the Greenberg apparatus is introduced over the falx for medial retraction. Retraction on the superior sagittal sinus is avoided. The medial surface of the hemisphere is covered for protection, and lateral retraction is applied with a self-retaining, medium width retractor.

Microsurgical Dissection

The surgical operating microscope is positioned and dissection proceeds at $10\times$ or $16\times$. The exposure is gradually deepened by separating the two cingulate gyri. This can be accomplished with a no. 16 suction and microdissector. A small cottonoid in the field may be used to control minor oozing. The cottonoid may protect the brain for gentle suction retraction. In some instances, particularly when extensive subarachnoid hemorrhage has occurred, there may be dense adhesions between the surfaces of arachnoid on the two sides. In this setting, very careful blunt or sharp dissection is used. Occasionally, the interhemispheric fissure is "fused" in its depth and does not open easily with retraction. In these cases, the authors have not hesitated to proceed with subpial dissection by suctioning a bit of the cingulate gyrus on the side of the approach.

The general aim of the initial dissection is to expose the pericallosal arteries distal to the aneurysm origin. Often this effort is aided by following a callosomarginal or other branch artery down to its parent arterial trunk. Reference to the cerebral angiogram will assist in tracing the arteries to the pericallosal parent vessel.

Once the pericallosal artery is identified, it is followed retrograde toward its origin (Fig. 15.2B). Dissection in this area is particularly perilous because the aneurysm may be densely adherent to the lobes of the brain, and proximal control has not been achieved. Therefore, once the aneurysm is seen, the blood pressure is lowered slightly to help minimize chances of rupture. Obviously, a temporary clip is of no avail in this situation until proximal control is achieved. Even then it is difficult due to limited proximal access. When the aneurysm is encountered, every effort is made to avoid the dome of the lesion, with the surgeon proceeding along the side of the pericallosal artery to obtain proximal exposure of

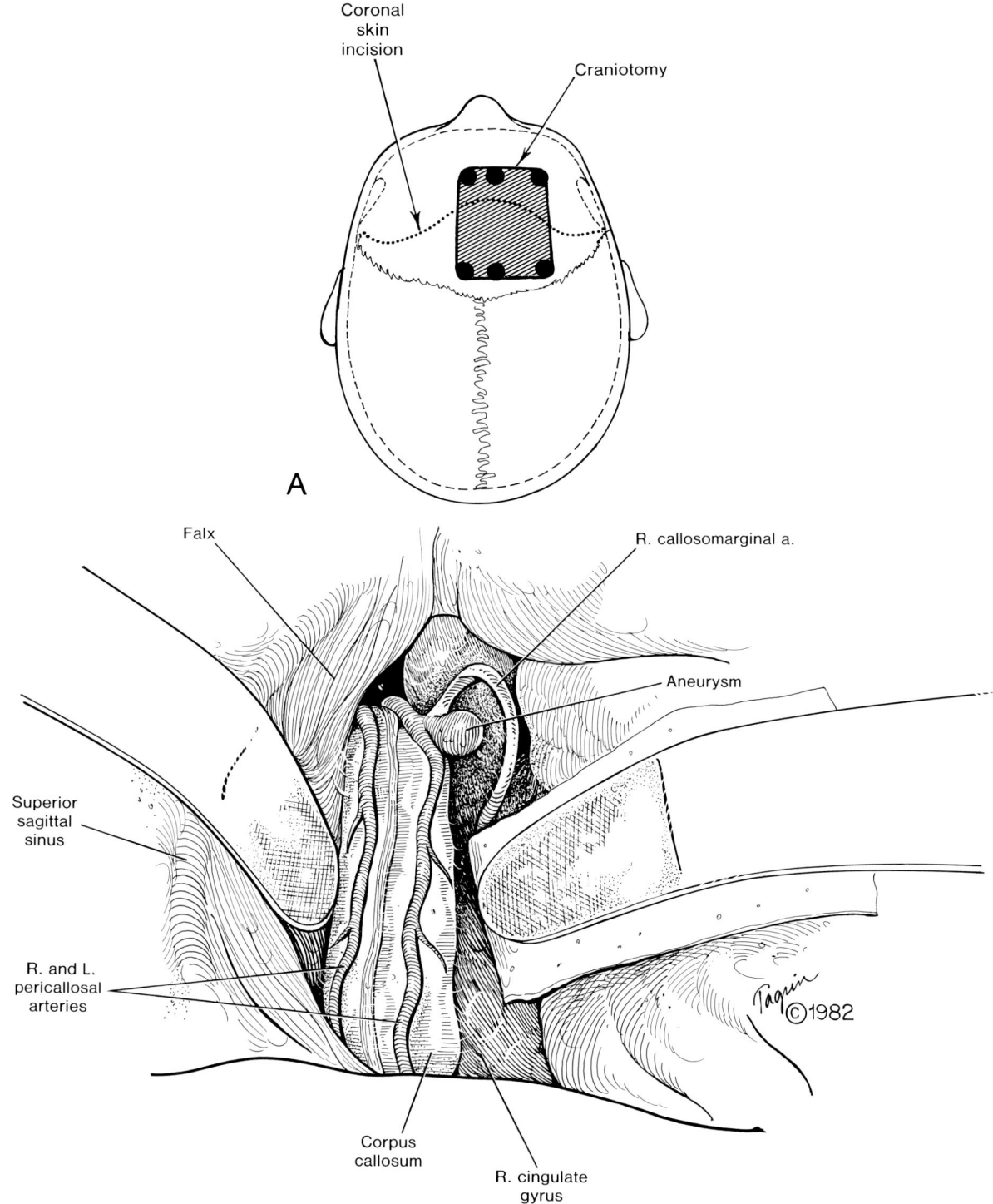

Figure 15.2. Distal anterior cerebral artery aneurysms. **A**, A coronal incision is used. The bone flap must cross the midline and extend posteriorly to just in front of the coronal suture. **B**, The pericallosal artery is identified by the midline exposure between the medial frontal lobe and the falx. The artery is followed retrograde to expose the aneurysm.

this vessel. As the dissection is deepened, the aneurysm is inspected to check the effects of hemispheric retraction.

Ordinarily, the aneurysm will arise from a carina at the origin of a branch vessel from the pericallosal artery, usually the callosomarginal. In this situation, the branch vessel is generally proximal to the aneurysm and its initial segment must also be isolated. No effort is made to dissect the neck of the aneurysm until proximal control of both the pericallosal and the branch vessel has been obtained. Once proximal control is achieved, dissection of the neck is undertaken. Ordinarily, this is accomplished with a fine microdissector or by sharp dissection of adherent portions. Suction removal of a small amount of adherent brain tissue may assist in defining the neck. Not infrequently, freeing the dome (with pia-arachnoid left attached) assists the surgeon's effort to define the neck without distortion of the aneurysm.

Obliteration of Aneurysm

Application of bipolar cautery or a ligature may be needed to narrow the neck of the aneurysm for final clipping. Since the aneurysm origin and arterial carina are approached from end on, special clipping techniques may be required. A useful approach is application of a curved clip, such as the Sugita clip, in the same axis as the parent vessel, with the curvature flush with the carina of the bifurcation (Fig. 15.3A) Alternately, a straight clip may be brought across the neck from side to side by grasping the hub at right angles to the blade (Fig. 15.3B), or a right angle clip may be used (Fig. 15.4). This may be achieved with a Sugita clip in the Sano applicator or by use of a pivot or McFadden clip. In some cases, a triangular-shaped clip from the Heifetz-Weck series may perfectly occlude the lesion. When neck dissection seems perilous, an angled fenestrated Sugita clip, encircling either the pericallosal or callosomarginal artery, can be applied with the Sano applicator.

After application of the clip, careful inspection should confirm complete occlusion of the aneurysm with sparing of the parent and branch arteries. Although pericallosal occlusion is often asymptomatic, it can cause hemiplegia and should be avoided (9). Finally, aspiration of the aneurysm dome will make certain that adequate occlusion of the neck has been accomplished.

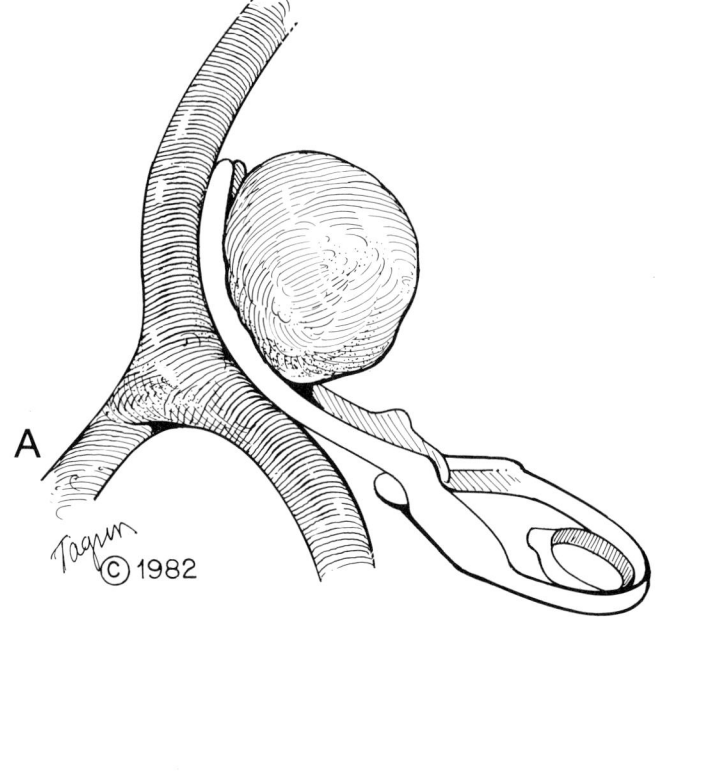
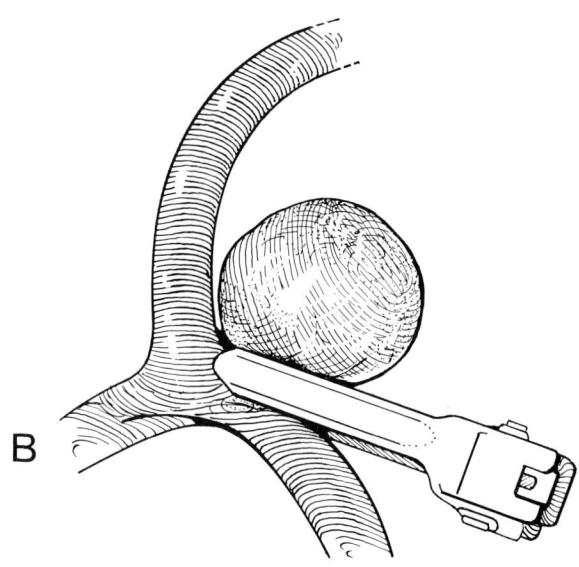

Figure 15.3. Distal anterior cerebral artery aneurysm. The aneurysm usually arises at a major arterial bifurcation. Either a curved Sugita clip (**A**) or a straight clip with the applicator at right angles to the blades (**B**) is used to obliterate these aneurysms and preserve the circulation.

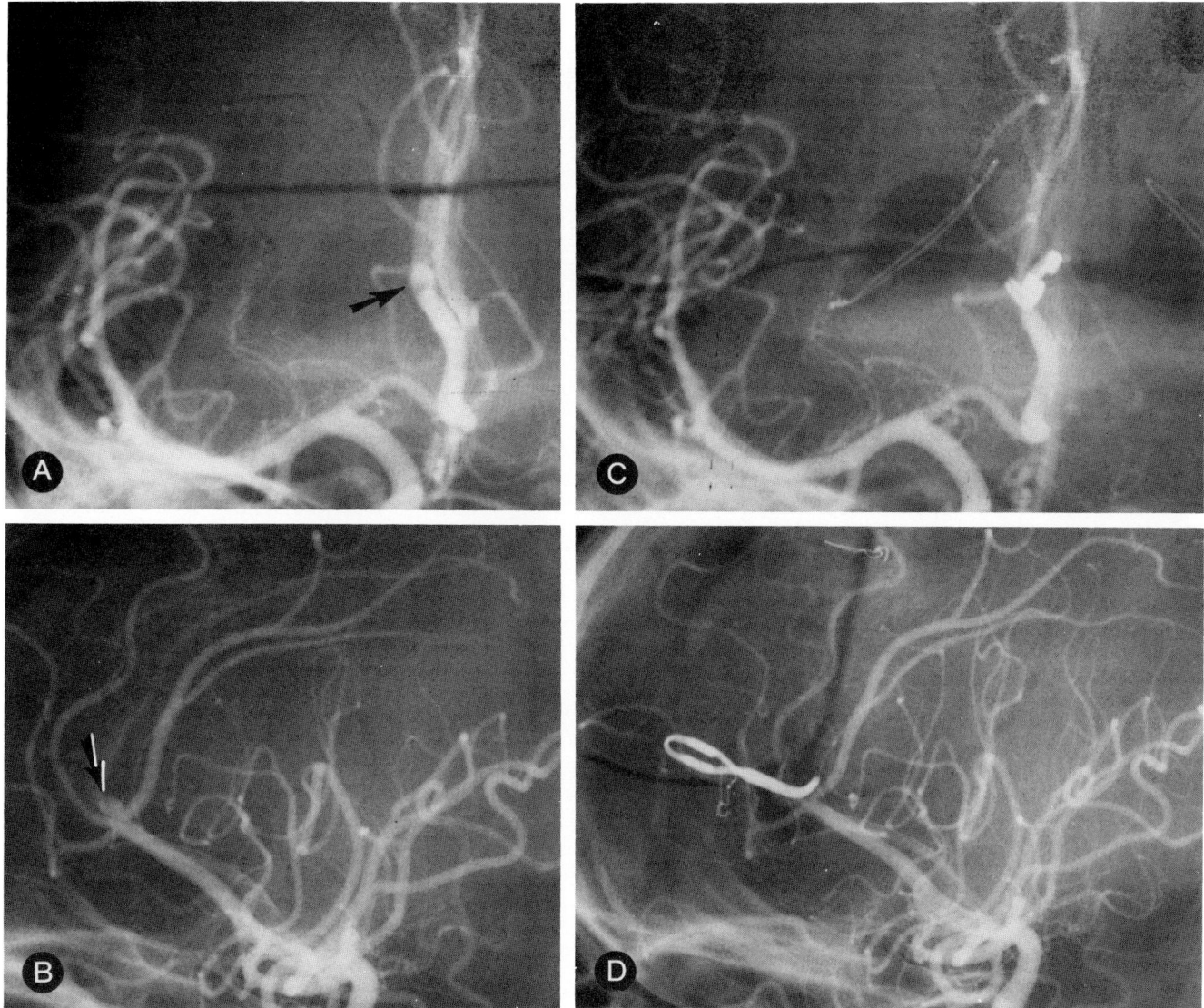

Figure 15.4. Pericallosal aneurysm. **A** and **B**, Anteroposterior and lateral angiograms 10 days after subarachnoid hemorrhage show aneurysm (*arrows*) arising from the genu of the pericallosal artery at the origin of the callosomarginal artery. There is no spasm. **C** and **D**, Postoperative angiograms. A Yasargil clip with a right angle on the end has been applied. The aneurysm is obliterated and normal arterial circulation preserved. Note the location of the bone flap. The postoperative neurologic examination was normal.

RESULTS

In the authors' small series of eight cases, complete obliteration of the aneurysm was obtained with excellent neurologic outcome. There were no complications. Four of these cases involved multiple aneurysms. In one instance, it was possible to obliterate an aneurysm of the azygous anterior cerebral A_2 segment along with a middle cerebral artery aneurysm, both approached through a large frontotemporal flap that crossed the midline. In another patient, a total of five aneurysms were clipped through a wide frontotemporal craniotomy. Other authors have also noted increased incidence of multiple aneurysms when a pericallosal aneurysm is present (12, 15, 16). A higher incidence of azygous A_2 segments has also been found with these aneurysms (7).

Several series with similarly low mortality have been reported in the literature (9, 13, 16, 17). In an earlier article, Yasargil and Carter reported a 15% morbidity and commented specifically on the difficulties encountered with these aneurysms (16), but in a later article, Yasargil reported only two poor results and one fair result in a group of 23 patients; the rest had a good result (15). Yoshumoto et al achieved similarly good result in a series of 34 patients (17).

REFERENCES

1. Becker DH, Newton TH: Distal anterior cerebral artery aneurysms. *Neurosurgery* 4:495–503, 1979.
2. Benedetti A, Curri D: Aneurysm of azygous anterior cerebral artery. *Neurochirurgia (Stuttg)* 26:56–58,1983.
3. Fleischer AS, Barrow DL: Distal anterior cerebral artery aneurysms. In Wilkins RH, Rengachary SS (eds): *Neurosurgery*, New York, McGraw-Hill, 1986, pp 1383–1385.
4. Fujimoto K, Waga S, Kojima T, Shimosaka S: Aneurysm of distal anterior cerebral artery associated with azygous anterior cerebral artery. *Acta Neurochir (Wein)* 59:65–69, 1981.
5. Hayashi M, Kobayashi H, Kawano H, Handa Y, Kabuto M: Giant aneurysms of an azygous anterior cerebral artery: Report of two cases and review of the literature. *Neurosurgery* 17:341–344, 1985.
6. Kaneko D, Morooka S, Kamio M, Sanada S: Aneurysm of peripheral cerebral arteries with developmental anomaly of the anterior cerebral artery. *No Shinkei Geka* 11:1193–1198, 1983 (English abstract).
7. Katz RS, Horoupian DS, Zingesser L: Aneurysms of azygous anterior cerebral artery. Case report. *J Neurosurg* 48:804–808, 1978.
8. Korosue K, Kuwamura K, Okuda Y, Tamaki N, Matsumoto S: Saccular aneurysm arising from a fenestrated anterior cerebral artery. *Surg Neurol* 19: 273–275, 1983.
9. Laitinen L. Snellman A: Aneurysms of the pericallosal artery. A study of 14 cases verified angiographically and treated mainly by direct surgical attack. *J Neurosurg* 17:447–458, 1960.
10. Niizuma H, Kwak R, Uchida K, Suzuki J: Aneurysms of the azygous anterior cerebral artery. *Surg Neurol* 15:225–228, 1981.
11. Nishioka H: Report on the cooperative study of intracranial aneurysms and subarachnoid hemorrhage: Section VII, Part 1. Evaluation of the conservative management of ruptured intracranial aneurysms. *J Neurosurg* 25:574–592, 1966.
12. Perlmutter D, Rhoton AL Jr: Microsurgical anatomy of the distal anterior cerebral artery. *J Neurosurg* 49:204–228, 1978.
13. Snyckers FD, Drake CG: Aneurysm of the distal anterior cerebral artery. A report of 24 verified cases. *S Afr Med J* 47:1787–1791, 1973.
14. Verdura J, Resnikoff S, Rosenthal J, Cardenas J: Familial intracranial aneurysms, with two occurring at the distal anterior cerebral artery. *Neurosurgery* 12:214–216, 1983.
15. Yasargil MG. *Microsurgery*. Stuttgart, George Thieme Verlag, 1984, pp 224–231.
16. Yasargil MG, Carter LP: Saccular aneurysms of the distal anterior cerebral artery. *J Neurosurg* 40:218–223, 1974.
17. Yoshumoto T, Uchida K, Suzuki J: Surgical treatment of distal anterior cerebral artery aneurysms. In Suzuki J (ed): *Cerebral Aneurysms*. Tokyo, Tokyo Press, 1979, pp 250–255.

16
Middle Cerebral Artery Aneurysms

CLINICAL PRESENTATION

Approximately 20% of all intracranial aneurysms occur on the middle cerebral artery with nearly 80% located at the bifurcation, 10% on the proximal trunk (M_1 segment), and the rest more peripherally, usually at a point of first branching of one of the main middle cerebral artery divisions (2, 4, 16, 22). Aneurysms occurring more peripherally than the bifurcation are usually infectious or traumatic in origin and will not be covered in this chapter.

The most common presentation for patients with middle cerebral artery aneurysms is subarachnoid hemorrhage. The second most common form of presentation is detection of an asymptomatic aneurysm on a CT scan obtained for unrelated reasons. When large enough, unruptured aneurysms of the middle cerebral artery can produce clinical symptoms from mass effect or result in temporal lobe epilepsy from compression of the medial temporal lobe. Ischemic symptoms, such as transient ischemic attacks and, rarely, major strokes, are in general very uncommon with intracranial aneurysms, but they occur more frequently with middle cerebral artery aneurysms than with aneurysms at any other location (4).

When a middle cerebral artery aneurysm ruptures, it usually results in a clinical syndrome that is indistinguishable from subarachnoid hemorrhage from an aneurysm in any other intracranial location. However, there are certain clinical characteristics that can at times favor the diagnosis of a ruptured middle cerebral artery aneurysm (7). About 60% of patients with a middle cerebral artery aneurysm have transient loss of consciousness at the time of rupture, which is a higher proportion than with aneurysms at other locations. About one-third have headache that is clearly restricted to one side of the head; this is much less common with aneurysms in any other location, and when it occurs it almost invariably occurs on the side of the aneurysm. In one series, 80% of the patients had focal neurologic deficits when they were first seen and such deficits were of definite localizing value (hemiparesis, visual field cuts, and aphasia) (7). In the authors' own experience, the incidence of focal deficits associated with ruptured middle cerebral artery aneurysms has not been as high (4). However, it still has been higher than with aneurysms in any other location. This is probably because middle cerebral artery aneurysms result in intracerebral hemorrhage more frequently than aneurysms in any other location. In one report of 156 patients with middle cerebral artery aneurysms, 49.8% presented with an intracerebral clot, whereas only 15.8% of patients with internal carotid artery aneurysms and 20.2% of patients with anterior communicating artery aneurysms presented with an intracerebral clot (11). This may also be why patients with ruptured middle cerebral artery aneurysms have a higher frequency of seizures both at the onset as well as later, compared with patients with aneurysms in other locations (7).

Radiologically, a middle cerebral artery aneurysm may be suspected when initial CT scan shows blood primarily in the area of one sylvian fissure (Fig. 16.1A). This type of hematoma extending into both the frontal and temporal lobes and bridging the sphenoid ridge is, in fact, almost pathognomonic for ruptured middle cerebral artery aneurysm.

SURGICAL MANAGEMENT

Middle cerebral artery aneurysms can be approached in three different ways:

1. By opening the sylvian fissure from medially and following the middle cerebral artery from proximal to distal until the aneurysm is encountered;
2. By entering the sylvian fissure distally through a small incision in the superior temporal gyrus with subpial dissection and identification of the distal middle cerebral artery branches, which can then be followed proximally to the aneurysm;
3. By opening the sylvian fissure peripherally and following the distal branches within the sylvian fissure proximally to the aneurysm.

Frequently the surgeon starts the operation by one of these approaches but changes to a different approach when difficulties are encountered. It is important to realize that, depending on the location of the aneurysm, one or another of these approaches may be ideal.

Medial Trans-sylvian Approach

The medial trans-sylvian is probably the approach most frequently used for middle cerebral artery aneu-

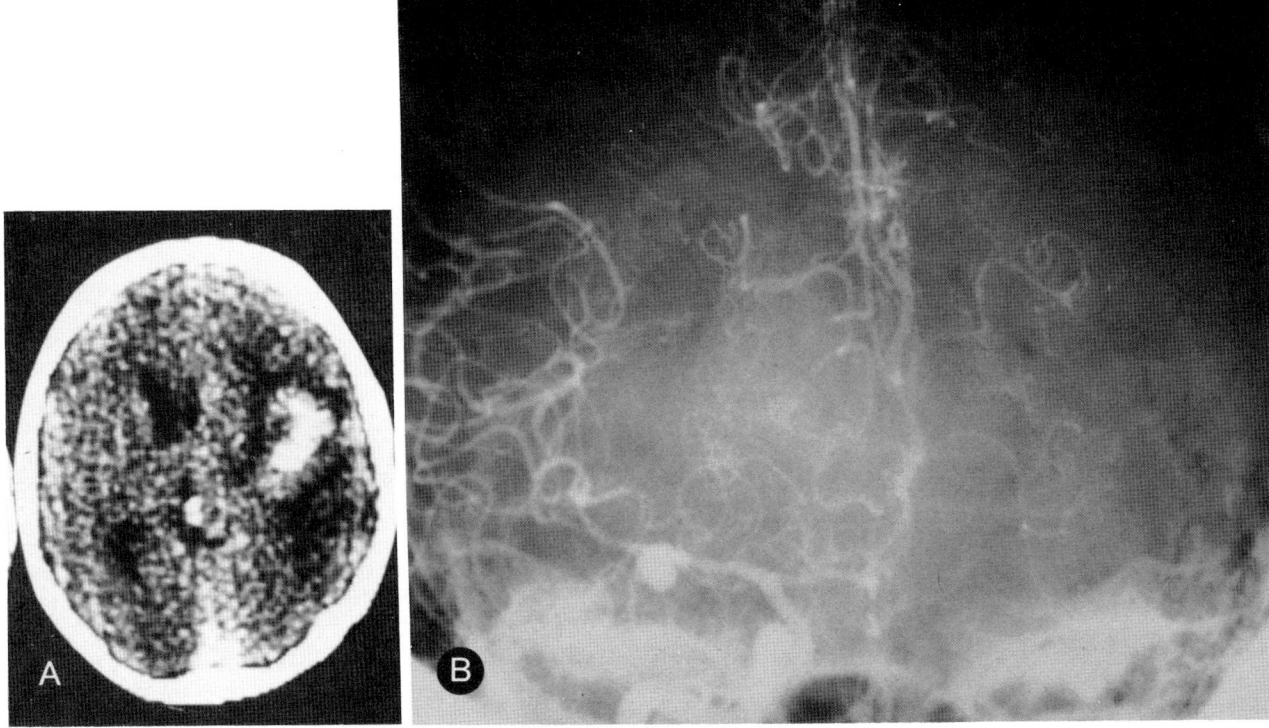

Figure 16.1. Middle cerebral artery aneurysm: evaluation. **A,** CT scan (without contrast) shows a localized hematoma in the anterior aspect of the sylvian fissure. This finding is highly suggestive of a middle cerebral artery aneurysm in a patient who presents with subarachnoid hemorrhage. **B,** The angiogram shows considerable spasm. The middle cerebral artery bifurcation and the aneurysm are much closer to the internal carotid bifurcation than those seen in Figure 16.4. This aneurysm is best approached by a medial trans-sylvian exposure, following the middle cerebral artery distally in the sylvian fissure.

rysms (7, 11, 12, 15, 16, 19, 21, 23). This approach must be used when the aneurysm is located proximally on the M_1 segment of the middle cerebral artery (Fig. 16.2) and is also preferred in cases of aneurysms at the middle cerebral artery bifurcation when the M_1 segment is short and the aneurysm is located beneath the insula (Figs. 16.1 and 16.3). This approach can also be used for more peripherally located aneurysms (Fig. 16.4). However, the authors believe that in these latter aneurysms, the amount of dissection necessary to follow the middle cerebral artery all the way from medially is unnecessary and that it is preferable to expose these aneurysms more directly by opening the fissure distally or through the superior temporal gyrus.

The initial craniotomy is identical to the basic pterional approach (see Chapter 12). The dura is opened on a flap based inferiorly in the same manner as for other aneurysms located in the medial aspect of the circle of Willis. The arachnoid is then opened widely under the microscope and the medial aspect of the sylvian fissure is identified and opened. The present authors, like others, have never hesitated to coagulate and divide the bridging veins between the frontal and temporal lobes that cross the medial aspect of the sylvian fissure (2, 22). The exact location of the fissure medially is not always apparent in cases of recent subarachnoid hemorrhage. Sometimes when the brain is swollen, this plane is not clear, and one must then identify the fissure by following the internal carotid artery as it continues into the middle cerebral artery. This may be facilitated by a small amount of subpial resection at the level of the internal carotid artery bifurcation on the frontal lobe. Once the origin of the middle cerebral artery is identified, the location of the sylvian fissure is usually more evident.

The placement of self-retaining retractors at this stage is critical. The frontal and temporal lobes must be gently retracted to put the medial aspect of the sylvian fissure under some stretch. This is best accomplished by gradually opening the tips of the retractors as dissection proceeds. It is preferable to place slightly stronger retraction on the temporal lobe, since excessive retraction of the frontal lobe can be harmful, particularly on the dominant side where it can result in expressive aphasia from pressure transmitted to Broca's area (14). The middle cerebral artery is followed along its anterior inferior aspect away from the perforating arteries. The anterior temporal branch often arises from this surface of the middle

Middle Cerebral Artery Aneurysms

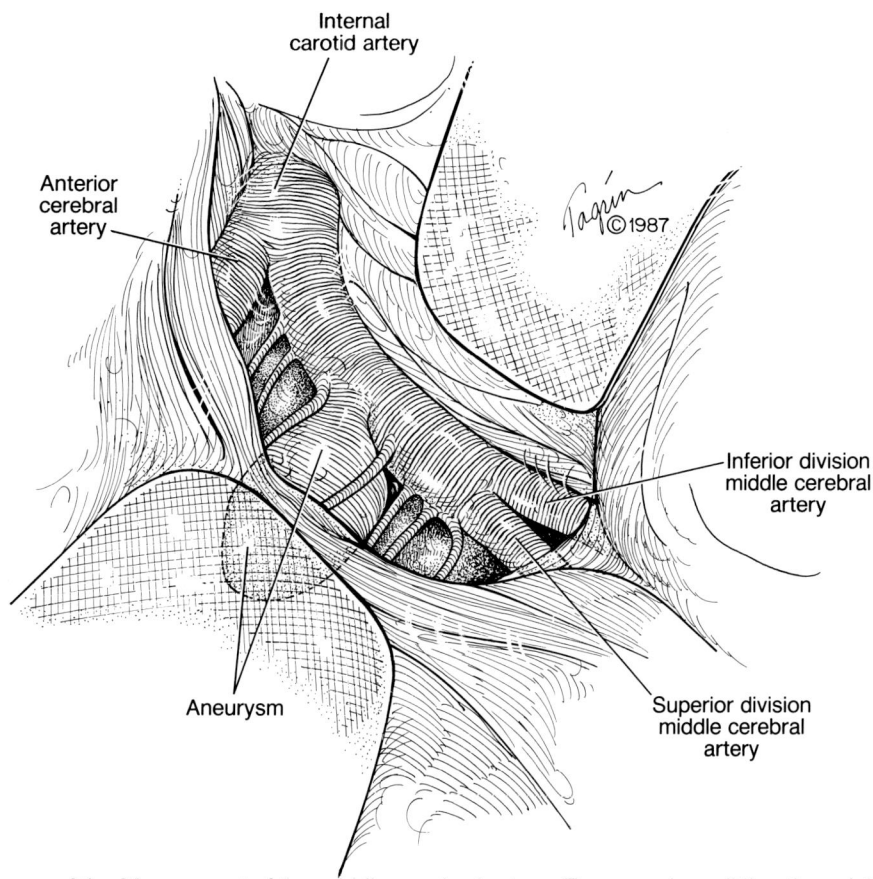

Figure 16.2. Aneurysm of the M_1 segment of the middle cerebral artery. Exposure by splitting the sylvian fissure from medially and following the middle cerebral artery distally. Note placement of retractors in the frontal and the temporal lobes opening the fissure. It is not necessary to expose the dome of the aneurysm, which is buried deep in the frontal lobe. The neck must be dissected completely, and lenticulostriate arteries must be carefully separated from the neck.

cerebral artery; therefore, care must be taken not to avulse it as one retracts the temporal lobe (22). Thick arachnoid bands that bridge the fissure must be carefully divided to allow for progressive, gradual opening of the sylvian fissure.

Aneurysms of the M_1 segment of the middle cerebral artery will usually arise from the posterosuperior surface of the middle cerebral artery in relation to lenticulostriate arteries (Fig. 16.2). The number and the configuration of these arteries are extremely variable (3, 8, 15). There is no need to estimate the relationship of the aneurysm to these lenticulostriate arteries from preoperative angiography. Many of these vessels are very fine and will not be well visualized angiographically. These aneurysms arise in relation to one or more lenticulostriate arteries. Therefore, the neck of the aneurysm must be dissected thoroughly, and the fine perforating vessels must be separated from the aneurysm at least in the area of the neck, creating a space for the blades of the clip between the perforating vessels and the neck. Fortunately, most of these aneurysms are relatively small and dissection is straightforward. Since all of the important anatomy is at the neck of the aneurysm, there is no need to dissect the entire dome of the aneurysm, which sometimes is deeply embedded into the frontal lobe and basal ganglia, particularly in the larger aneurysms. Bipolar cauterization is hazardous here because current spread can thrombose a perforating artery. It is important not to use longer-than-necessary clips so as to avoid injury to the frontal lobe. When the aneurysm is large, it may be preferable to use a temporary clip in a previously prepared segment of the middle cerebral artery that is free of perforating arteries.

For aneurysms located at the bifurcation of the middle cerebral artery, the sylvian fissure is gradually opened until the aneurysm is reached. It is useful to have prepared a small segment of the middle cerebral artery for possible temporary clipping. Preferably, this prepared segment should be distal to the major perforators. Once the aneurysm is reached, one must be careful with retraction because the aneurysm can be quite adherent to the brain and could be rup-

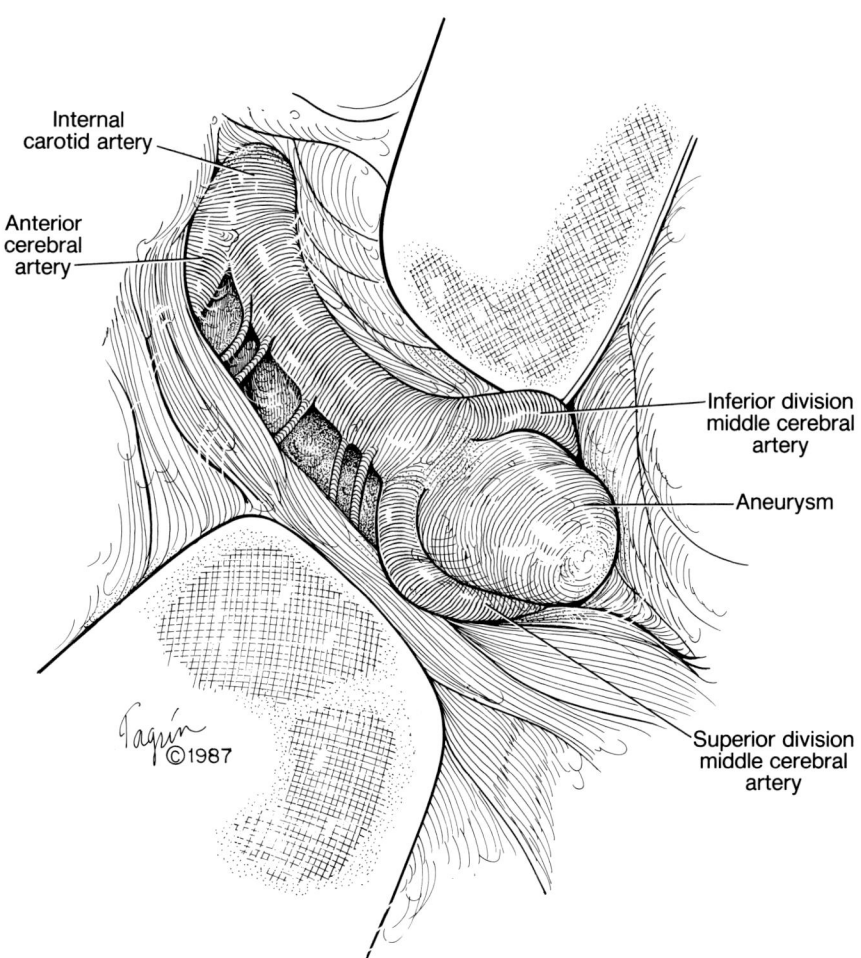

Figure 16.3. Aneurysm of the middle cerebral artery bifurcation with short M_1 segment exposed by opening the sylvian fissure medially and following the middle cerebral artery distally. At least one of the two major divisions is usually adherent to the aneurysm and may give the impression that it arises from the aneurysm itself. However, with careful dissection the divisions can be separated and a neck can be developed in all but the largest aneurysms.

tured by excessive retraction. With larger aneurysms it is not infrequent to encounter first the dome of the aneurysm as one progresses distally within the sylvian fissure. It is likewise not uncommon for these larger aneurysms to obstruct the view to the neck. When this is the case, one should stop the dissection, after a space is prepared for temporary clipping, and proceed to open the fissure distally and then come from distal to proximal until the anatomy can be well defined (22). The authors do not hesitate to resect a small amount of either temporal or frontal lobe so as to expose, by subpial dissection, the major arterial divisions. Sometimes this is preferable to forceful retraction of the brain, which could lead to rupture. With small aneurysms, the two major divisions come rapidly into view (Fig. 16.3), but this is rarely the case with larger aneurysms when they must be retracted one way or the other to see the second division. One must not be content when the two major divisions are found. Frequently, major lenticulostriate arteries arise from the origin of one or the other or both divisions, and they must be carefully spared (3, 15). In addition, an early anterior temporal branch or frontal or temporal lobe branches that may have already arisen from the M_1 segment will pass behind the aneurysm and can be included in the clip if they are not identified and carefully separated from the aneurysm. Total circumferential dissection of the base of the aneurysmal complex is always necessary in these aneurysms.

The authors have been using temporary clipping of the middle cerebral artery for all but the smaller aneurysms of the middle cerebral artery bifurcation. Often they prefer to do the entire dissection before applying the temporary clip and to restrict the period of temporary occlusion only to the 2–3 minutes required for clip placement. However, temporary clips have been used for up to 30 minutes (preferably opened

Middle Cerebral Artery Aneurysms

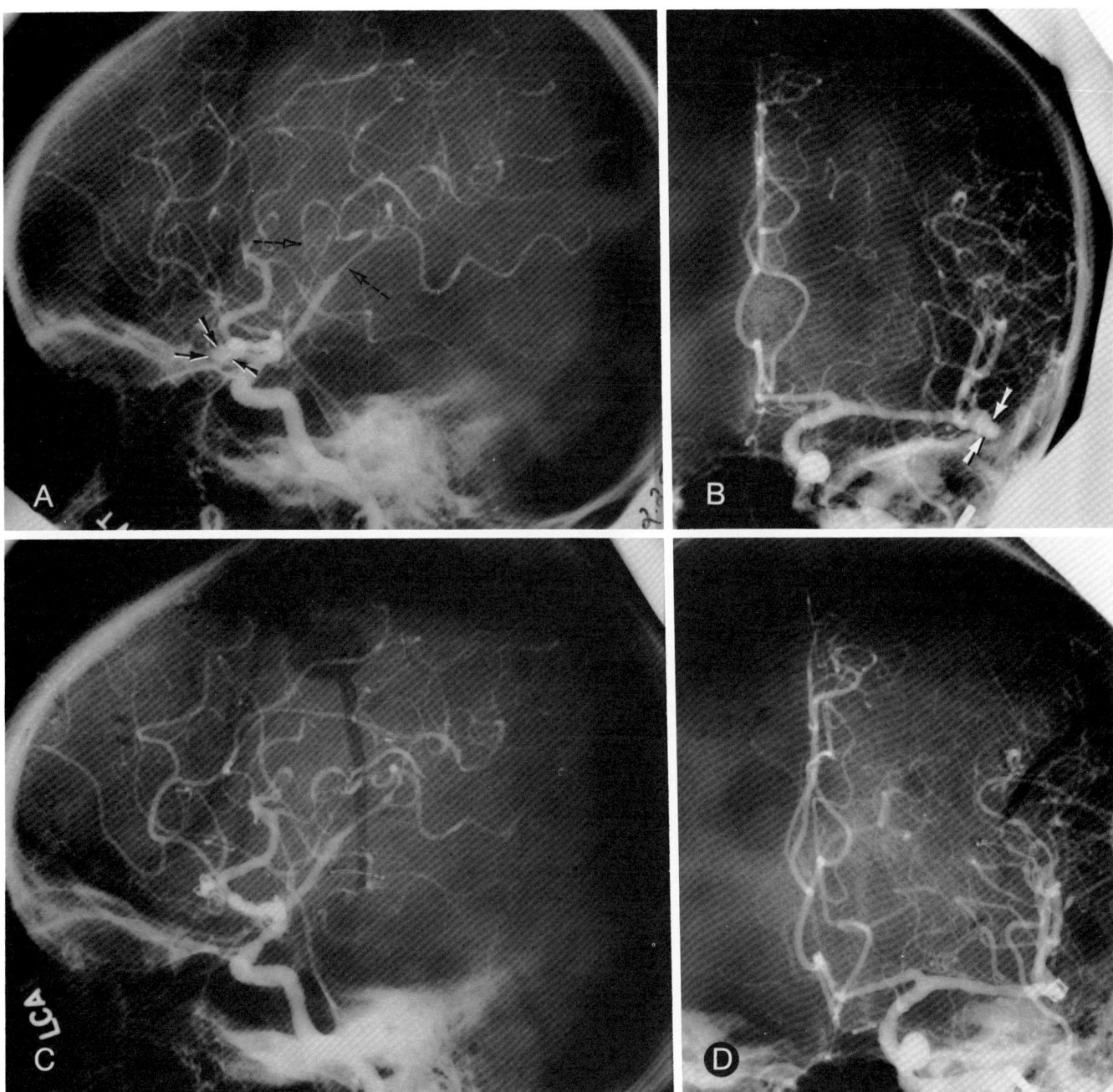

Figure 16.4. Middle cerebral artery aneurysm: clipping via superior temporal gyrus. **A** and **B**, The aneurysm projects laterally and anteriorly from the middle cerebral artery bifurcation (*closed arrows*). The location is ideally suited for a superior temporal gyrus approach or an approach directly through the fissure by opening it peripherally. Note the spasm in the distal middle cerebral artery branches (*open arrows*). **C** and **D**, Postoperative angiogram shows that the clip obliterates the aneurysm. Some spasm persists.

for 1 minute every 5 minutes), with mannitol (50 g intravenously given 15 minutes prior to clamping) used for cerebral protection and maintenance of the systemic blood pressure slightly above the normal level for that patient. Under these conditions, even complex aneurysms may be accurately dissected, aspirated, and clipped, in some cases with one or more clips used (18).

In some patients, application of a preliminary (permanent type) clip to the aneurysm neck may obliterate the lesion but also occlude or narrow critical parent vessels, resulting in an unsatisfactory clipping. This situation may be turned to advantage by completing aneurysmal dissection and collapsing the aneurysm by aspiration. Then a final clip may be applied distal to the preliminary clip, which is then removed to permit perfusion of the parent vessels. If there is still an unclipped dogear, an additional final clip may be applied, just touching the first clip, but done with care to preserve patency of the parent arteries (13, 16). When multiple clips are needed, Sugita has described use of Silastic tubing covering proximal portions of clip blades to fill the gap created when the tips cross another clip (18). Instead of this maneuver, the present authors have occasionally cut a second clip to length with wire cutters and then polished it with a high-speed drill.

Superior Temporal Gyrus Approach

The superior temporal gyrus approach was first utilized by the authors in the early 1960s after seeing the illustration by Poppen of a middle cerebral artery aneurysm exposed through an intratemporal hematoma (13). Subsequently, it was learned that the first detailed description of this technique was by Tonnis and Walter (20). Others have also used this approach (1, 9, 17). There are several advantages in using the superior temporal gyrus approach to some middle cerebral artery aneurysms. Many middle cerebral artery bifurcation aneurysms project laterally as a direct continuation of the middle cerebral artery (Fig. 16.4) or, less commonly, anteriorly, inferiorly, or superiorly (Fig. 16.5) (6, 15, 22). In these patients, the superior temporal gyrus approach allows the surgeon to expose the main trunk of the middle cerebral artery without disturbing the dome of the aneurysm by following the branches proximally to the base of the aneurysm. Vigorous retraction is avoided, and retractors are used simply to hold the exposure, which is accomplished by suctioning nonessential brain tissue. This advantage is particularly important in early operations when the brain is swollen and hyperemic or in the presence of a large intracerebral hematoma. In the latter instance, the hematoma should be suctioned only as necessary to gain exposure. The hematoma related to the dome of the aneurysm should be left undisturbed until exposure of the base of the aneurysmal complex is completed. This approach also avoids manipulation of the medial circle of Willis and of the proximal portion of the middle cerebral artery with its important dorsal perforators. The anatomy of the distal and dorsal aspects of these aneurysms, which includes the relationship of the major divisions and their branches to the neck and dome, can be most difficult to define. In almost one-half of the patients, important lateral lenticulostriate arteries arise from the major divisions shortly after their origin. These small but important vessels run back in a medial direction, usually behind the neck of the aneurysm, to enter the basal ganglia (3, 8, 15). This complex anatomy can be best defined by a circumferential exposure of the base of the aneurysm via the transtemporal approach combined with thorough removal of the pterion. This circumferential exposure also permits application of the clip from whatever angle seems best.

The superior temporal gyrus approach is not suited for aneurysms of the main trunk of the middle cerebral artery proximal to the bifurcation (Fig. 16.2), for aneurysms of the middle cerebral artery at the point of origin of an early temporal branch, or for patients with a short main trunk of the middle cerebral artery where the aneurysm arises from an early bifurcation that occurs before the genu (Fig. 16.1).

The main disadvantage of the transtemporal approach is that the base of the aneurysmal complex is encountered before proximal control of the afferent vessel is assured. However, it is almost always possible to expose enough of the middle cerebral artery before exposing the dome of the aneurysm so that a temporary clip could be applied in case of premature rupture. Another minor disadvantage of this approach is the need for a slightly larger bone flap than is required for the usual pterional approach. A theoretical disadvantage is the possibility of increasing the risk of epilepsy by the cortical resection. The authors have the impression that in their patients with middle cerebral artery aneurysms there has been an increased incidence of epilepsy, and most of these patients have been operated via the superior temporal gyrus approach. However, because many of these patients also had temporal hematomas and because others have also found that patients with middle cerebral artery aneurysms operated by other approaches had an increased incidence of epilepsy, it is difficult to know what, if any, is the contribution of the particular surgical approach to the postoperative seizures (7).

For this approach, the patient is placed in the supine position with the head turned to the opposite side nearly 70° and tilted slightly backward. In some patients, slight elevation of the ipsilateral shoulder may be necessary. All other aspects of anesthesia, use of the skeletal fixation headrest, and initial preparation and draping are as described in Chapter 11.

The incision starts at the level of the zygoma just in front of the tragus and curves slightly backward above the ear before swinging forward to the edge of the hairline about 2–3 cm lateral to the midline (Fig. 16.6). The branch of the facial nerve to the frontalis muscle and the main trunk and anterior branch of the superficial temporal artery are saved with the scalp flap. The muscle is turned down with the skin flap to allow retraction of the muscle down into the temporal region and facilitate exposure of the area of the pterion. The bone flap is then cut in the same manner as for the standard pterional approach, but

Figure 16.5. Middle cerebral artery aneurysm. **A,** CT scan (without contrast) done at the time of admission after sudden onset of headache, drowsiness, and left hemiparesis. A large hematoma is present in the medial aspect of the sylvian fissure. **B** and **C,** The angiogram shows the aneurysm pointing superiorly and slightly anteriorly. The middle cerebral artery is elevated and bowed laterally. Operation was done through a superior temporal gyrus approach. **D** and **E,** Postoperative angiograms showing the aneurysm to be clipped and relief of the mass effect.

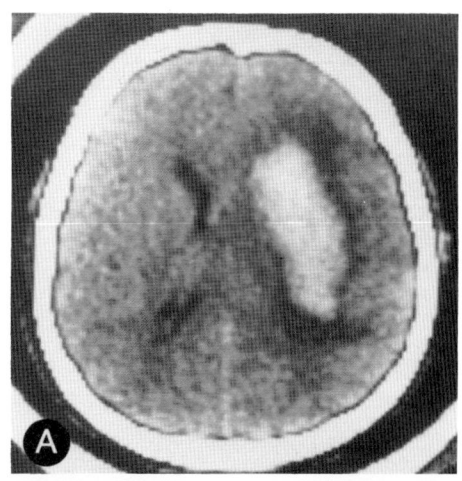

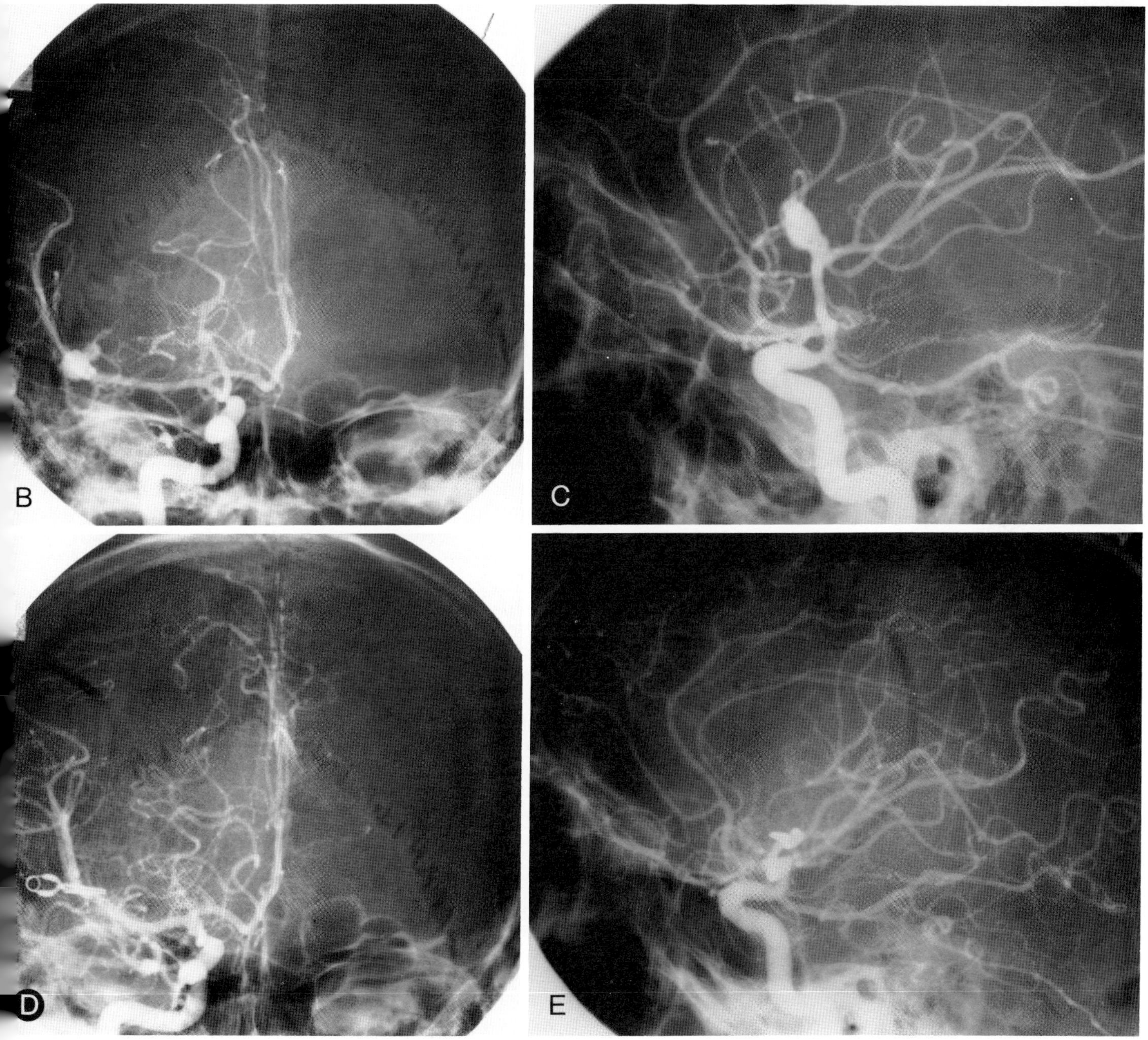

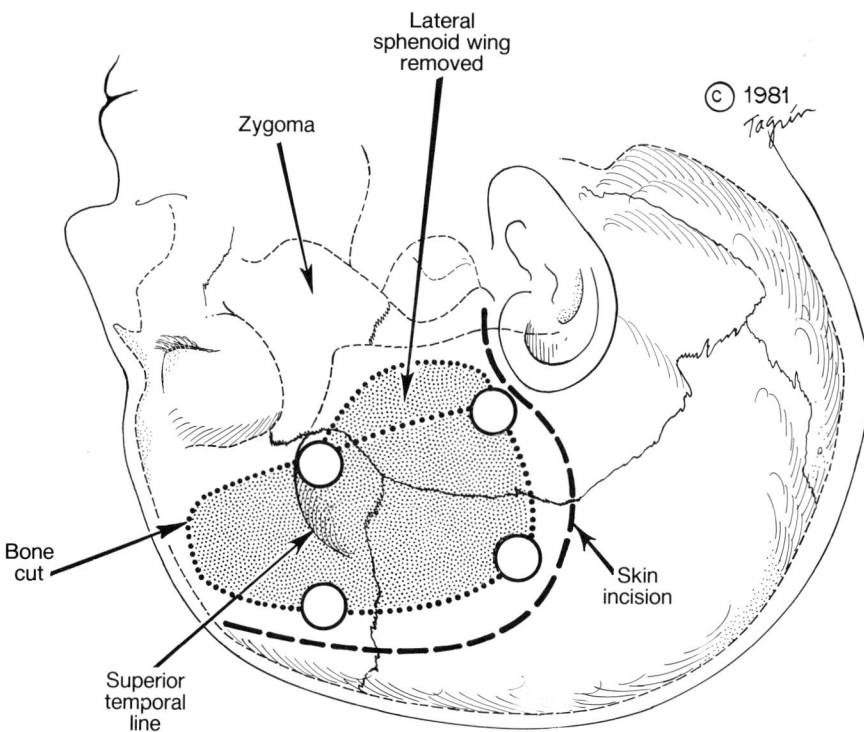

Figure 16.6. Superior temporal gyrus approach to middle cerebral artery aneurysm: incision and bone flap. Note that the incision is placed slightly more posteriorly than for the subfrontal exposure, to expose more of the anterior temporal lobe. (From Heros RC, Ojemann RG, Crowell RM: The superior temporal gyrus approach to middle cerebral aneurysms: Techniques and results. *Neurosurgery* 10:308–313, 1982.)

the cut is extended further back into the temporal bone to expose more of the temporal lobe (Fig. 16.6). The pterion and lateral aspect of the sphenoid ridge are removed in the same manner as in the pterional approach. This step is important because it exposes the anterior aspect of the sylvian fissure and allows dissection of the aneurysm and clip application from an anterolateral direction in cases where this is preferable. Without removing the pterion, the surgeon is forced to work only from behind, underneath the overhanging bone, which can be a major handicap. During this phase of the operation, the surgeon can assess brain tension. Lasix and mannitol will have been given as described in Chapter 11, and the pCO_2 will be in the low thirties. Usually these measures will reduce brain tension sufficiently.

The dura is opened over the inferior frontal region approximately 25 mm above the inferior margin of the bone opening. The incision is extended over the anterior temporal region. A perpendicular cut is then made parallel to the sylvian fissure. The flaps of dura are retracted with sutures (Fig. 16.7). If the brain still appears to be tense, one may gently retract the frontal lobe and drain cerebrospinal fluid from the medial cisterns until the brain is relaxed.

The operating microscope is then brought into place. An incision about 2–3 cm long is made in the superior temporal gyrus starting about 1 cm behind the front of the sylvian fissure in a direction parallel to the fissure (Fig. 16.7). With suction and bipolar coagulation used as needed, the incision in the superior temporal gyrus is extended medially. Self-retaining retractors are used to aid the exposure. The dissection extends into the vertical segment of the sylvian fissure over the insula. Once a major division is seen through the pia, the pia-arachnoid is opened to gain access to the subarachnoid space of the sylvian fissure. With microsurgical technique, the branches of the middle cerebral artery are followed proximally toward the aneurysm (Fig. 16.8). In many cases, subarachnoid hematoma will be adherent to these vessels and will need to be removed. Without disturbing the dome of the aneurysm, one of the two major divisions can usually be followed, on the side away from the aneurysm, to the main stem of the middle cerebral artery, which curves medially and slightly posteriorly. Only enough of the main trunk of the middle cerebral artery is exposed to allow application of a temporary clip, if needed. Once the distal part of the middle cerebral artery and the origin of the main divisions are identified, the authors usually dissect the entire aneurysmal complex, frequently leaving some adherent brain attached to the dome in the area of rupture (Fig. 16.9). Earlier in their expe-

Middle Cerebral Artery Aneurysms

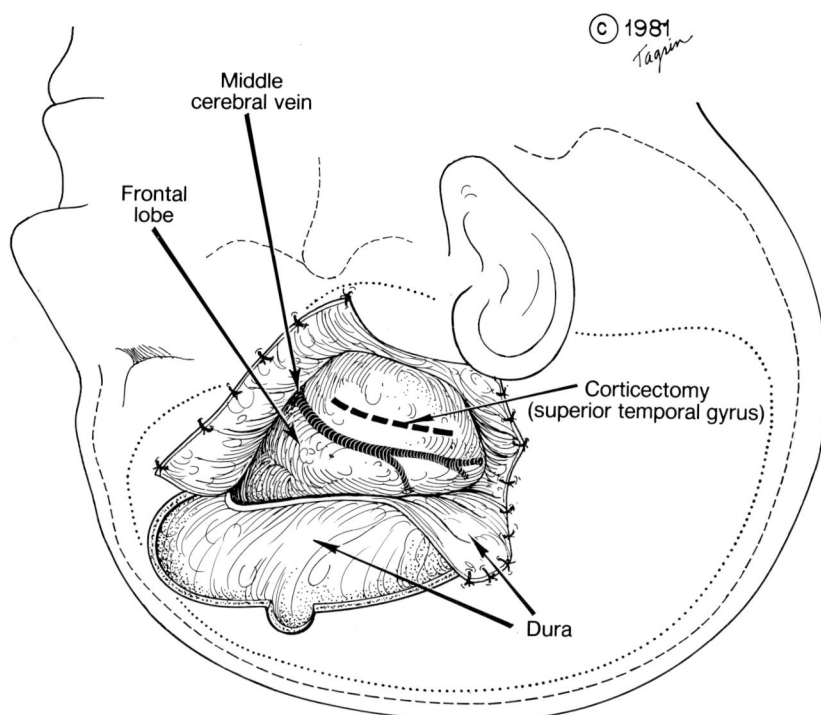

Figure 16.7. Superior temporal gyrus approach: dural opening and corticectomy. The dura has been opened to expose the superior and middle temporal gyrus of the anterior temporal lobe and the posterior inferior frontal region. The cortical incision is outlined. (From Heros RC, Ojemann RG, Crowell RM: The superior temporal gyrus approach to middle cerebral aneurysms: Techniques and results. *Neurosurgery* 10:308–313, 1982.)

rience they used moderate hypotension at this stage. This is still a satisfactory method to reduce aneurysmal tension and prevent premature rupture. However, they now prefer to use normotension and temporary occlusion of the middle cerebral artery for the final critical stages of dissection and clipping in all but the smaller aneurysms.

Complete dissection of the aneurysm allows its safe mobilization to provide full visualization of the neck. This is particularly helpful in the case of the large aneurysms, when the anatomy may not be entirely clear until all of the aneurysm is exposed. Frequently, a third major branch is encountered and must be dissected away from the neck. At least one of the divisions is usually quite adherent to the aneurysm and must be separated from it with sharp dissection to define the neck. Recurrent lenticulostriate arteries arising from the origin of the main divisions must be identified and separated from the neck. For this final preparation of the neck, the authors have sometimes found it helpful in cases of large aneurysms to retract the dome by using a microdissector, which fits nicely into one of the arms of the Greenberg self-retaining retractor. Once the neck is ready, a clip can be applied from whatever direction seems most appropriate. Frequently, they have had to replace or adjust the clip several times or have used multiple clips, especially for larger aneurysms. The clip position should be changed if there is any indication of kinking or constriction of the middle cerebral artery trunk or branches. In avoiding this constriction, a small portion of the neck may not be included in the clip. If this is the case, the region is reinforced with gauze and tissue adhesive. Should the aneurysm rupture, steps should be followed as outlined in Chapter 11.

By careful and persistent dissection under the operating microscope, the authors have found that almost all nongiant middle cerebral artery aneurysms can be clipped. This has also been the finding in other series (11, 12, 21, 22).

Lateral Trans-sylvian Approach

The third approach to middle cerebral artery aneurysm consists simply of opening the sylvian fissure peripherally and identifying the distal branches of the middle cerebral artery directly through the fissure rather than by resection of a small amount of the superior temporal gyrus (14, 22). Once the distal branches of the middle cerebral artery are found, they are followed to the aneurysm within the subarachnoid space of the sylvian fissure and the dissection proceeds exactly as outlined under the previous ap-

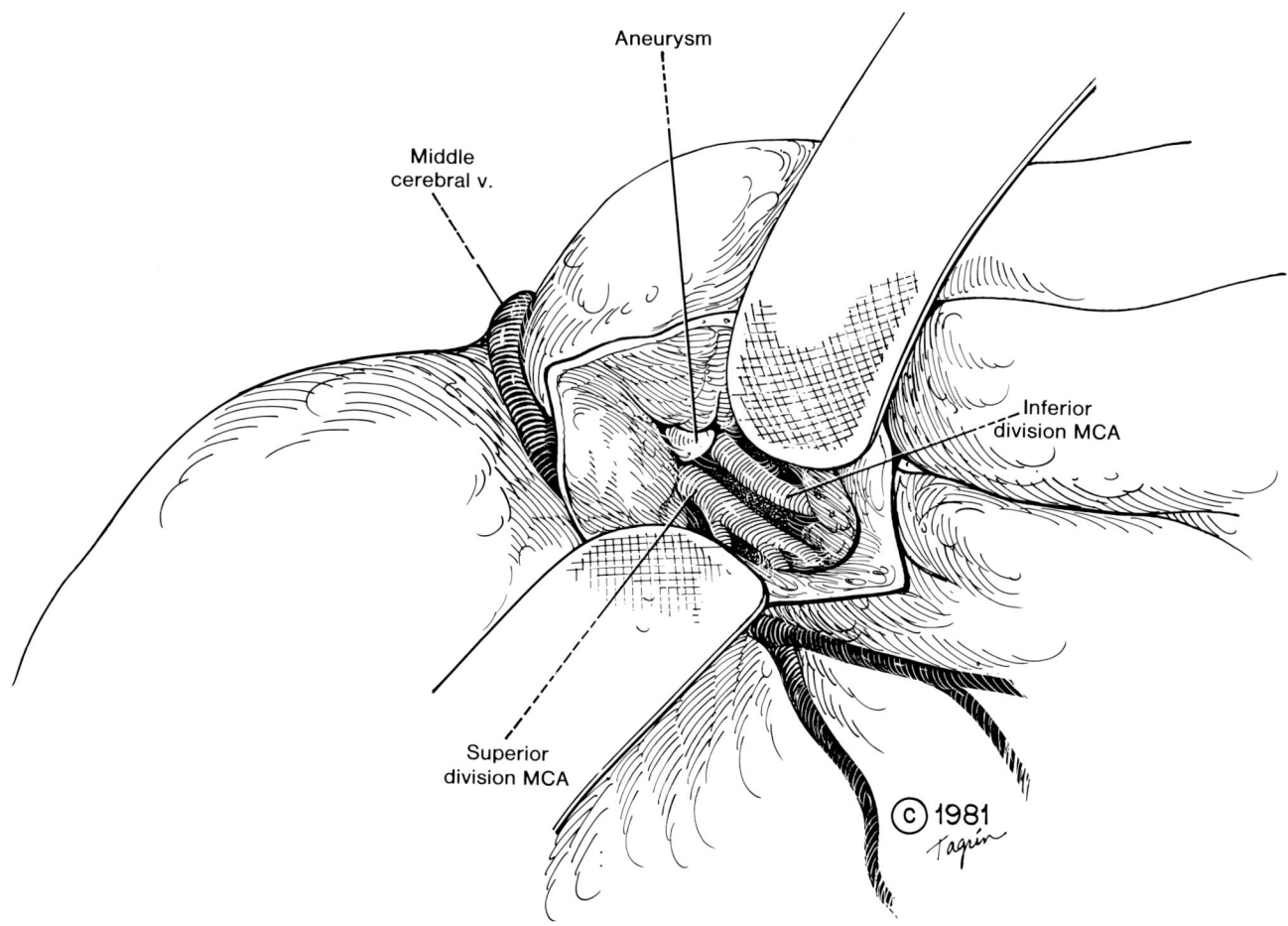

Figure 16.8. Superior temporal gyrus approach: initial exposure of aneurysm. The sylvian fissure has been entered. The middle cerebral artery (*MCA*) branches are followed anteriorly until the base of the aneurysm is exposed. (From Heros RC, Ojemann RG, Crowell RM: The superior temporal gyrus approach to middle cerebral aneurysms: Techniques and results. *Neurosurgery* 10:308–313, 1982.)

proach where the sylvian fissure is entered at a deeper level by resection of a small amount of superior temporal gyrus. The main disadvantage of this approach is the fact that proximal control is not achieved until the aneurysm is encountered.

The authors' main objection to the lateral transsylvian approach is the fact that, in cases of recent hemorrhage, it is difficult to find the plane of the sylvian fissure, particularly if there is a large hematoma within the subarachnoid space of the sylvian fissure. It is easier to identify the branches deep in the sylvian fissure through the pia-arachnoid after a small amount of brain resection in the superior temporal gyrus without having to disturb most of the clot more superficially in the fissure. By resection of a small amount of brain, less brain retraction is required. Furthermore, in working through the superior temporal gyrus, one avoids damage to the sylvian veins, which are frequently in the way when one tries to open the fissure peripherally. However, in cases where there is no recent hemorrhage and the sylvian fissure is well defined, it may be a relatively simple matter to open it peripherally, and the authors have used this approach rather than the superior temporal gyrus approach, particularly if the sylvian veins do not seem to be in the way. Another helpful maneuver that can be used when the fissure is not clearly defined is to follow a large cortical vessel centrally into the fissure until a large branch is identified (14, 22).

RESULTS

Table 16.1 illustrates the results in patients with middle cerebral artery aneurysms operated by the authors or under their supervision at the Massachusetts General Hospital during the past 10 years. In 58 of 64 who were grades 0–2, there was a good result.

This series included 17 patients with giant middle cerebral artery aneurysms. Almost all of these presented with symptoms related to mass effect rather

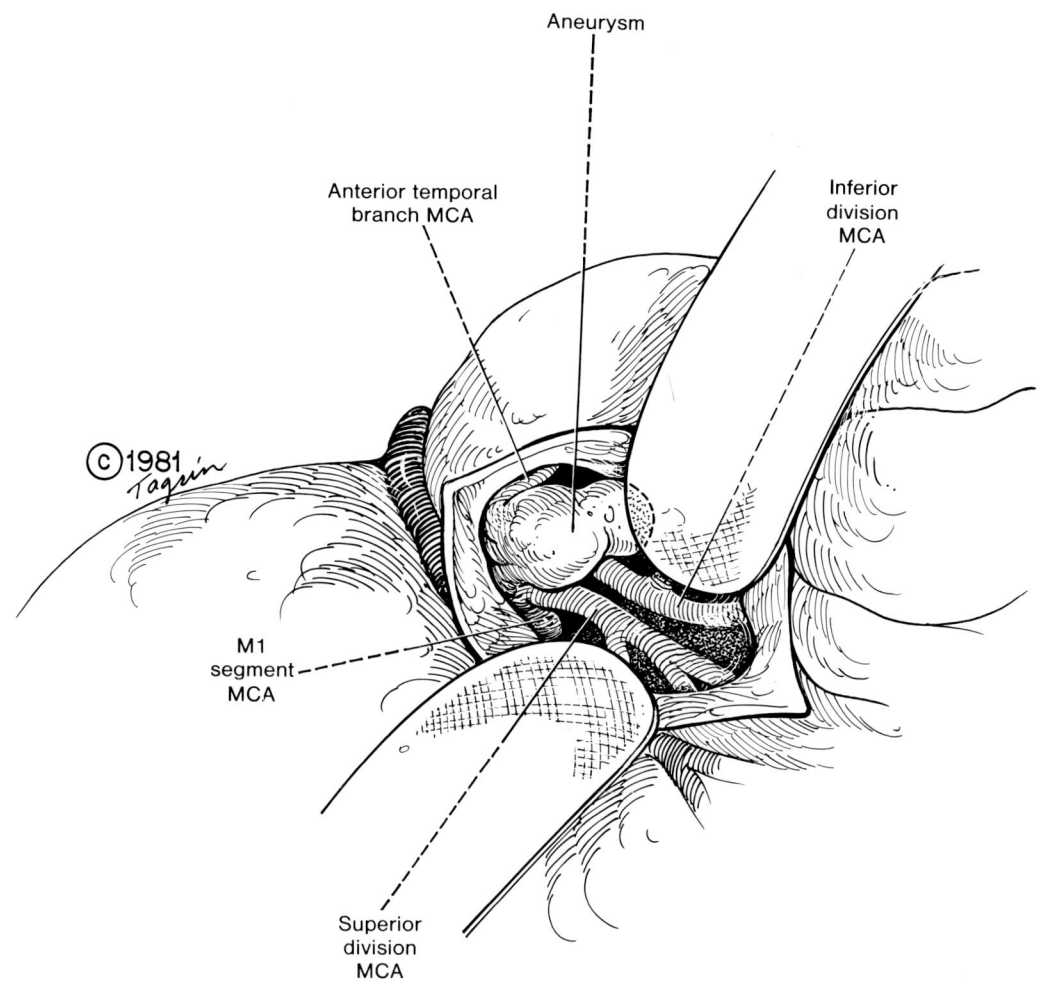

Figure 16.9. Superior temporal gyrus approach: dissection of the aneurysm. The distal M_1 segment is identified. Note its medial posterior course. The aneurysm is now dissected from middle cerebral artery (*MCA*) branches and the surrounding tissue after leaving some tissue adherent at the site of the rupture. (From Heros RC, Ojemann RG, Crowell RM: The superior temporal gyrus approach to middle cerebral aneurysms: Techniques and results. *Neurosurgery* 10:308–311, 1982.)

than subarachnoid hemorrhage. In the group of giant aneurysms, there were two poor results and two deaths. These were all in patients who had significant mass effect and edema associated with their giant aneurysms. The results in this latter group of patients were especially bad (5). Two other patients in the group with giant aneurysms were treated by bypass graft, in one case with a saphenous vein graft, and proximal middle cerebral artery occlusion. Two other giant aneurysms could not be clipped and had to be wrapped, which is not satisfactory treatment. The rest of the aneurysms could be clipped.

The fair and poor results in patients with nongiant aneurysms who were in good preoperative condition were mostly related to technical errors, usually kinking or damage to one division or, in one case, avulsion of the neck of the aneurysm with unsuccessful suturing of the tear and postoperative occlusion of the middle cerebral artery. Postoperative vasospasm accounted for a few bad results, but in general, it was not a major factor in this series because, with the exception of the operations in those patients who needed emergency evacuation of the temporal lobe hematoma (usually grades 4 and 5), most operations were performed late after subarachnoid hemorrhage. In the group of patients operated urgently, the aneurysm was always clipped at the time of the evacuation of the hematoma, a policy the authors strongly recommend.

During the past 2–3 years, the authors have begun to operate early in most patients with middle cerebral artery aneurysms who present within the first 2 days after subarachnoid hemorrhage. This group still constitutes a minority in their series, and it is too early for them to have a definite opinion as to the safety and ease of early surgery in these patients. However,

Table 16.1.
Middle Cerebral Artery Aneurysms[a]

Preoperative Grade (Hunt)	No. of Cases	Surgical Result			
		Good	Fair	Poor	Dead
0, 1, 2	64	58	3	2	1[b]
1A or 3	15	4	8	2[b]	1
4	5	1	2	1	1[b]
5	4	0	1[c]	0	3[c]
Total	88	63	14	5	6

[a]Includes 17 patients with giant middle cerebral artery aneurysms.
[b]Cases of symptomatic giant aneurysms; one (grade IV preoperatively) had herniated from mass effect.
[c]All four cases were operated on in extremis after herniation from a large temporal hematoma.

it is their preliminary impression that this is a very favorable group of patients for early surgery and that, particularly if the operation is performed through the superior temporary gyrus, early surgery can be carried out with as much ease and safety as late surgery in patients with middle cerebral artery aneurysms who are in good preoperative condition. In another report, there were 13 patients with a good result out of a group of 16 patients with middle cerebral artery aneurysms operated early (10).

Similarly satisfactory results with surgery for middle cerebral artery aneurysms have been reported (11, 12, 19). In a series of 114 patients operated mostly "late," Flamm and Fein achieved good to excellent results in 86.8% (2). Of particular note is the remarkable achievement of Yasargil who, in a group of 184 patients, had no deaths and only one poor result in the 127 patients who were grades 0, 1, or 2 preoperatively (22).

REFERENCES

1. Berger E: Targeted approach to middle cerebral artery trifurcation. *Excerpta Med Int Congr Ser* 418:199, 1977.
2. Flamm ES, Fein JM: Middle cerebral artery aneurysms. In Fein JM, Flamm ES (eds): *Cerebrovascular Surgery*. New York, Springer-Verlag, 1985, vol 3, pp 861–877.
3. Grand W: Microsurgical anatomy of the proximal middle cerebral artery and the internal carotid artery bifurcation. *Neurosurgery* 7:215–218, 1980.
4. Heros RC: Middle cerebral artery aneurysm. In Wilkins RH, Rengachary SS (eds): *Neurosurgery*. New York, McGraw-Hill, 1985, vol 2, pp 1376–1383.
5. Heros RC, Kolluri S: Giant intracranial aneurysms presenting with massive cerebral edema. *Neurosurgery* 15:572–577, 1984.
6. Heros RC, Ojemann RG, Crowell RM: The superior temporal gyrus approach to middle cerebral aneurysms: Techniques and results. *Neurosurgery* 3:308–313, 1982.
7. Hook O, Norlen G: Aneurysms of the middle cerebral artery. A report of 80 cases. *Acta Chir Scand (Suppl)* 235:1–39, 1958.
8. Jones TH, Crowell RM: Microsurgical anatomy of the middle cerebral artery stem (M_1 segment). *Neurosurgery* in press.
9. Kempe L: *Operative Neurosurgery*. New York, Springer-Verlag, 1968.
10. Ljunggren B, Brandt L, Kagstrom E: Results of early operations for ruptured aneurysms. *J Neurosurg* 54:473–479, 1981.
11. Lougheed WM, Marshall BM: Management of aneurysm of the anterior circulation by intracranial procedures. In Youmans JR (ed): *Neurosurgical Surgery*. Philadelphia, WB Saunders, 1973, vol 2, pp 742–750.
12. Peerless SJ: The surgical approach to middle cerebral and posterior communicating aneurysms. *Clin Neurosurg* 21:151–165, 1974.
13. Poppen JL: *An Atlas of Neurosurgical Techniques*. Philadelphia, WB Saunders, 1960, pp 158–161.
14. Rand RW: Microneurosurgery in cerebral aneurysms. In Rand (ed): *Microneurosurgery*, ed 2. St Louis, CV Mosby, 1978, pp 311–324.
15. Rhoton AL, Saeki N, Perlmutter D, Zeal A: Microsurgical anatomy of common aneurysm sites. *Clin Neurosurg* 26:248–306, 1979.
16. Robinson RG: Ruptured aneurysms of the middle cerebral artery. *J Neurosurg* 35:25–33, 1971.
17. Shepard RH: Operation for aneurysms of the middle cerebral artery. In Rob C, Smith R (eds): *Operative Surgery. Fundamental International Techniques*, ed 3. London, Butterworth, 1979, pp 252–257.
18. Sugita K: *Microsurgical Atlas*. New York, Springer-Verlag, 1985.
19. Suzuki J, Kodama N, Fujiwara S, Ebina T: Surgical treatment of middle cerebral artery aneurysms: From the experience of 174 cases,. In Suzuki J (ed): *Cerebral Aneurysms*. Tokyo, Tokyo Press, 1979, pp 278–283.
20. Tonnis W, Walter W: Ein neuer operativer Zugang zu den sackformigen Aneurysmen der basalen Hirngefasse. *Wien Med Wochenschr* 110:145–147, 1960.
21. Wilson CB, Spetzler RF: Operative approaches to aneurysms. *Clin Neurosurg* 26:232–247, 1979.
22. Yasargil MG: Middle cerebral artery aneurysms. In Yasargil (ed): *Microneurosurgery*. New York, Thieme-Stratton, 1984, vol 2, pp 124–164.
23. Yasargil MG, Fox L: The microsurgical approach to intracranial aneurysms. *Surg Neurol* 3:7–14, 1975.

17

Basilar Bifurcation, Posterior Cerebral, and Superior Cerebellar Artery Aneurysms

Aneurysms of the posterior circulation account for about 15% of all intracranial aneurysms. About half of these arise at the basilar bifurcation. Because of the similarity of surgical approach, aneurysms arising at the origin of the superior cerebellar artery and on the posterior cerebral artery are considered together with the distal basilar aneurysms. Basilar aneurysms occasionally originate in relation to anatomic variants such as basilar fenestrations (2). Aneurysms in relationship to the anterior inferior cerebellar artery, vertebral artery, vertebrobasilar junction, and posterior inferior cerebellar artery are considered separately because the surgical approach is generally different (Chapter 18).

BASILAR BIFURCATION ANEURYSMS

Presentation

The usual presentation is subarachnoid hemorrhage. The symptoms are almost always indistinguishable from those caused by subarachnoid hemorrhage from anterior circulation aneurysms. Abrupt loss of consciousness is somewhat more common after rupture of a posterior circulation aneurysm. On occasion, a basilar tip aneurysm may compress the adjacent third cranial nerve with resultant palsy. Large or giant aneurysms in this location can cause signs of peduncular and oculomotor nerve compression (Weber's syndrome), hydrocephalus (12), or even quadriparesis (10) (Chapter 20).

Evaluation

Computed tomography (CT) scanning can detect subarachnoid hemorrhage, and the location of the hematoma may suggest the site of bleeding. However, this can be misleading. The authors have frequently seen interpeduncular hematomas caused by posteriorly directed internal carotid-posterior communicating artery aneurysms.

Careful angiographic study is the most important investigation for basilar aneurysm. All four vessels are studied. On the angiogram a basilar tip aneurysm usually projects upward in line with the basilar artery trunk; less commonly, it may project posteriorly between the peduncles or anteriorly against the clivus. The angiogram may be misleading in several respects. A tuft of perforating arteries may appear to arise from the aneurysm, but in fact they usually originate from the distal basilar or proximal posterior cerebral arteries (P_1 segments) and sweep up and back around the dome of the aneurysm (5, 6). The P_1 segment, which may also appear to arise from the aneurysm, originates from the basilar artery, although the distal basilar artery may be widened so that the base of the aneurysm is in common with the origin of the P_1 segments. Although on the angiogram the P_1 segments may appear to be well away from the side of the aneurysm in some cases, this is often the result of a thick aneurysmal wall or mural thrombus, and most commonly P_1 segments are tightly applied to the aneurysm. When occlusion of the basilar artery is being considered in the treatment plan, the posterior communicating arteries must be visualized (5). At times, vertebral injection with concomitant carotid compression will be needed to visualize this vessel (Allcock test). If a basilar aneurysm is suspected but not shown on initial angiogram, the study should be repeated after a week or more, since delayed appearance has been documented (1).

Preoperative review of the angiographic studies is of help in directing the surgical approach. For basilar tip aneurysms, the height of the basilar bifurcation in relation to the dorsum sellae is important (15). Usually the basilar bifurcation is at or just above the posterior clinoid process and, therefore, may be exposed subtemporally with moderate temporal lobe retraction. Occasionally the bifurcation is high above the dorsum; in this situation, greater temporal lobe retraction may afford access, but a trans-sylvian (pterional) approach may be easier and safer. When the basilar apex is below the posterior clinoid process, this bony prominence will occlude the surgeon's view. Yasargil has drilled away the posterior clinoid process in this situation (21), but the present authors have preferred to use a subtemporal approach with section, as needed, of the tentorium posterior to the entry point of the trochlear nerve. For especially low-lying basilar tip aneurysms and for aneurysms of the anterior inferior cerebellar artery origin, the authors have used the combined subtemporal-suboccipital approach with tentorial section (see Chapter 18).

Surgical Management

In the absence of substantial data on early surgery for basilar aneurysms (3, 8, 17), and in view of the technical difficulties associated with these lesions, the authors have continued to defer surgery 10–12 days in grade 1 and 2 patients. Grade 3 patients are operated on at about 3 weeks, or sooner if they improve. Balloon catheter occlusion of basilar aneurysms has been reported, but this therapy has not been fully evaluated (22).

Selection of Approach

A subtemporal approach offers good exposure of most basilar bifurcation aneurysms (5, 6, 9, 18). This is done from the right side, except in some patients in whom the aneurysm points to the right or when the patient has a left oculomotor palsy or right hemiparesis, and then a left subtemporal route is selected. For high-lying basilar tip aneurysms, a trans-sylvian (pterional) approach is used in order to avoid excessive temporal lobe retraction (15, 16, 21). The perforating vessels on the posterior aspect of the aneurysm are more difficult to dissect via the pterional approach in cases of basilar tip aneurysms. When an anterior circulation aneurysm is associated, the authors turn a combined pterional-temporal bone flap to provide both avenues of access.

Subtemporal Approach

Anesthesia, Positioning and Initial Exposure. Preoperative treatment and induction of anesthesia follow the guidelines outlined in Chapter 11. The patient is placed in the lateral decubitus position. A spinal subarachnoid catheter is placed. The head is fixed in a three-point headrest with the temporal squama parallel to the floor and the vertex tilted 15° below the horizontal. A linear incision provides sufficient exposure to turn a small temporal bone flap (Fig. 17.1). It is very important to carry the bone removal with rongeur or drill right down to the temporal floor and to provide a flat broad inferior margin to the craniotomy because the surgeon needs the freedom to work initially from more posteriorly and later, as exposure of the basilar artery is gained, from a more anterior direction. The lower the craniotomy base, the less temporal retraction required. The authors prefer to expose the zygoma by subperiosteal dissection all the way from its base posteriorly to its junction with the zygomatic process of the frontal bone anteriorly to remove temporal bone right down to the level of the zygoma from its base posteriorly to its end anteriorly. For this, rather than carrying the skin incision below the zygoma, which would result in a frontalis palsy, the authors prefer to stop

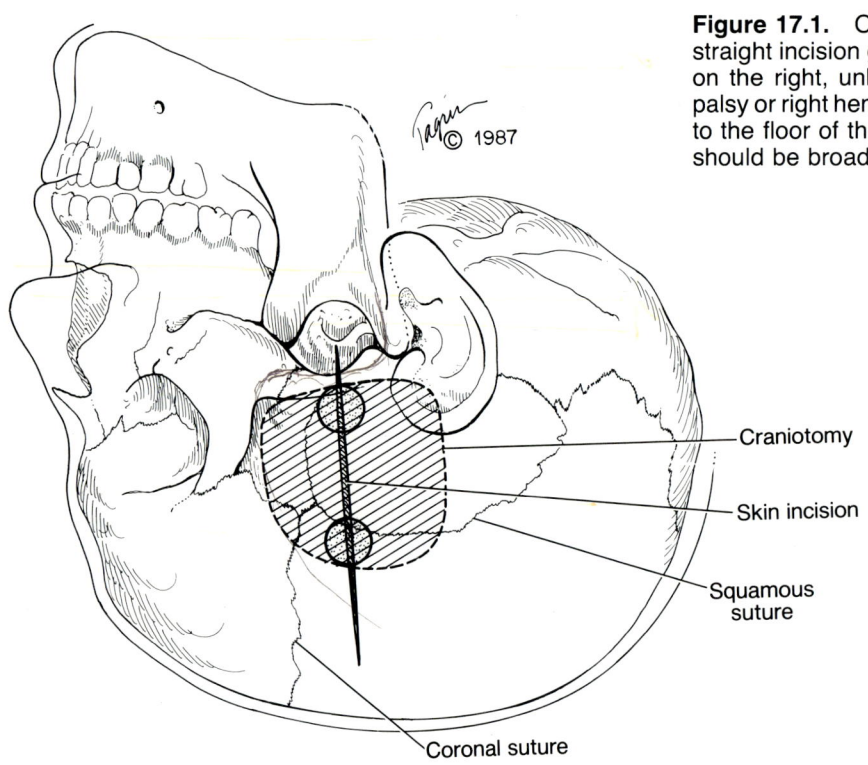

Figure 17.1. Operative technique: temporal craniotomy. A straight incision gives enough room. The approach is usually on the right, unless there is a preoperative left third nerve palsy or right hemiplegia. The craniotomy should be extended to the floor of the middle fossa. The base of the craniotomy should be broad and flat and flush with the zygoma.

the skin incision just below the midlevel of the zygoma and then retract the skin downward and hold the incision widely opened with fish hooks. Removal of the zygoma has been suggested (13), but it is usually not necessary. However, drilling away the upper portion of the zygoma may afford better exposure in cases when the temporal bone is particularly deep. Lumbar drainage, hyperventilation, and osmotic diuresis provide a slack brain.

In the past, the authors routinely used drug-induced hypotension to slacken the aneurysm during dissection to avert rupture. Nitroprusside or increased inspiratory concentration of anesthesia (isoflurane) was used to depress mean arterial pressure as low as 45–50 torr for up to 45 minutes. More recently, they have tended to use little hypotension, perhaps 90 torr systolic during the initial approach, with temporary clips applied after restoration of normotension to avert rupture during final dissection (see Chapter 11). In the case of basilar tip aneurysms, there is often just enough room to place a temporary clip across the basilar artery, usually just proximal to the superior cerebellar arteries. Sometimes, section of the tentorium behind the insertion of the fourth nerve will be needed to give room for this maneuver. When temporary clips are used, an additional infusion of mannitol (50 gm) is given 15 minutes prior to clamping, and systolic blood pressure is elevated to above normal during cross-clamping for cerebral protection.

Monitoring of brain stem auditory evoked responses has been used during basilar artery surgery (14). However, the authors have observed rostral brain stem damage despite normal brain stem auditory evoked response. Addition of somatosensory evoked responses may help to assess function of long tracts in the brain stem during this surgery. Further experience will be needed to evaluate such monitoring.

The dura is opened as an inferiorly based flap which is sutured up to provide a flat approach to the middle fossa (Fig. 17.2). Telfa or a cottonoid strip is gently introduced under the temporal lobe down to the uncus. A ⅜-inch retractor blade gently elevates the temporal lobe, exposing the free edge of the tentorium. For these maneuvers, it may become necessary to coagulate and divide bridging veins from the inferior temporal lobe to the transverse sinus. This is best done early in the exposure, under loupes and headlight, to avoid annoying bleeding. Only those veins likely to be torn are sacrificed, lest venous drainage of the lobe be compromised excessively. The vein of Labbé must be carefully preserved to avoid venous infarction. This is especially true on the dominant side where aphasia could result. Mobilization of the vein of Labbé, with preservation of its main channel, can be utilized to improve exposure in some cases, but usually this vein is situated posteriorly enough so as not to interfere with exposure. The third nerve should be visualized beneath the covering of arachnoid (Fig. 17.3). This is the central landmark for exposure. If the side of the brain stem and the fourth nerve are directly in view, or if the brain stem seems to curve and recede posteriorly, the line of sight is too far posterior. Once the retractor blade is in place, it may be fixed to the Greenberg retractor. Excessive retraction should be avoided, for it may cause temporal lobe infarction. A slack brain is the keystone to safe exposure, and this can usually be achieved with spinal drainage, hyperventilation, and diuretics.

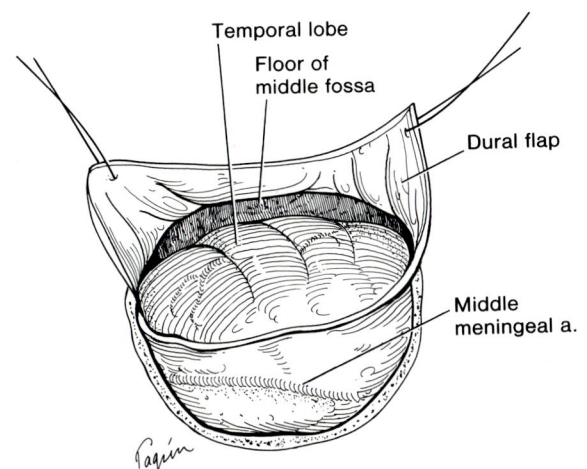

Figure 17.2. Dural opening. This is taken to the floor of the middle fossa to minimize brain retraction.

Microsurgical Dissection. With the initial exposure established, the operating microscope is moved into position. Under the microscope the retractor may be adjusted. The tip of the retractor blade should lie just on the uncus. The third nerve will rise with the temporal lobe during elevation. In cases of a high basilar bifurcation, more extensive dissection of the third nerve may be required in order to be able to work above the nerve. In most patients, however, simply working inferior to the third nerve avoids excessive manipulation and reduces the chance of third nerve palsy. A 4-0 Neurolon suture is placed in the edge of the tentorium just anterior to the insertion of the fourth nerve. This retraction suture is inserted in the middle fossa dura, with care taken to avoid venous channels, and is tied to provide retraction of the tentorial edge (Fig. 17.4). This maneuver provides further visualization of the area.

With a sharp hook, the arachnoid is opened over the P_1 segment of the posterior cerebral artery and the origin of the superior cerebellar artery (Fig. 17.4). A fine suction (no. 16 gauge) is used at reduced vacuum tension to remove cerebrospinal fluid from the cisterns. Using a fine dissector, the surgeon follows the superior cerebellar artery and P_1 segment to the basilar tip area. The posterior communicating artery is carefully preserved as a source of collateral circulation and because it is the origin of important perforating arteries. The posterior cerebral artery me-

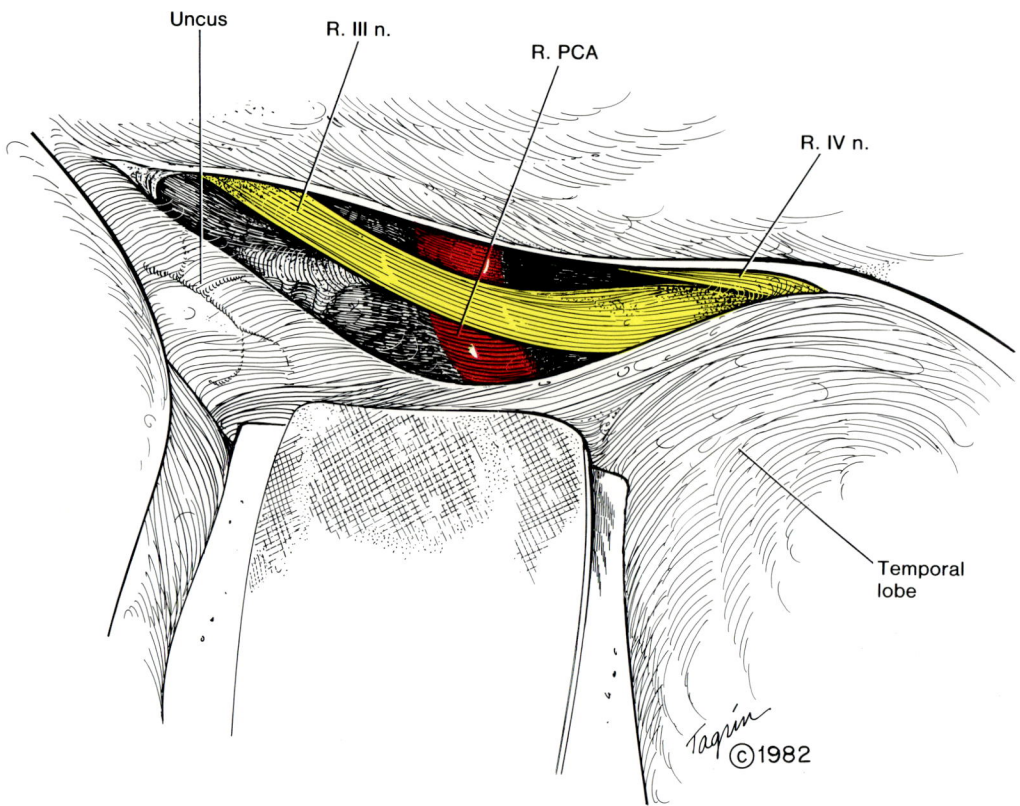

Figure 17.3. Subtemporal approach. Bridging veins are sacrificed and the temporal lobe is gently elevated. The free edge of tentorium comes into view with the third and fourth cranial nerves and the posterior cerebral artery (*PCA*), beneath a sheet of arachnoid.

dial to the third nerve gives off perforating branches to the brain stem. It is absolutely critical to avoid injury or occlusion to these crucial branches; otherwise, devastating brain stem stroke can occur.

Unless the aneurysm points anteriorly, the next maneuver is to dissect anterior to the neck and distal basilar artery to expose the P_1 segment on the opposite side (Fig. 17.5). This critical landmark establishes the relative anatomic positions of the two P_1 segments and the basilar trunk, thus setting up the remainder of the dissection. Reference to the Towne projection of the angiogram will assist in identification of the position of the two P_1 segments. A precise visualization of upward or downward tilting of the left P_1 segment is essential for accurate clipping of the aneurysm without occluding this vessel and its critical perforators. In the case of a large lesion, it is possible to mistake the opposite superior cerebellar artery for the posterior cerebral artery with potentially disastrous consequences. Once the P_1 segment on the left is identified, the proximal neck of the aneurysm may be prepared anteriorly with gentle dissection.

With this anatomy firmly in mind, the most critical dissection may be undertaken along the posterior aspect of the neck (Fig. 17.6). For these maneuvers, the authors use a temporary clip on the basilar artery, or if the wall of the aneurysm appears to be relatively thick, slight hypotension (85–90 torr systolic) may suffice. In most cases, a 16-gauge suction may be used to deflect the neck of the aneurysm forward as a fine microdissector gently sweeps the perforators posteriorly. Gentle but firm dissection must continue until the posterior aspect of the left P_1 segment alongside the origin of the third nerve comes into view. To avoid an unduly narrow pathway with potentially dangerous traction on the aneurysm and perforators, it is useful to dissect a significant length of the perforating arteries away from the aneurysm. Sometimes, a small strip of Gelfoam may be inserted between the aneurysm and the perforators to keep the path open for the posterior blade of the clip. With the perforators slack on either side of the dissection plane, an instrument or clip is less likely to tear them or rupture the aneurysm. Under direct microsurgical vision, it must be precisely ascertained that the perforating arteries have been safely dissected away from the aneurysm. Sacrifice of any of these perforating vessels is likely to result in brain stem infarction and serious neurologic deficit. It is said that one or two tiny perforators may be occluded without deficit, but the authors have noted serious deficit after occlus-

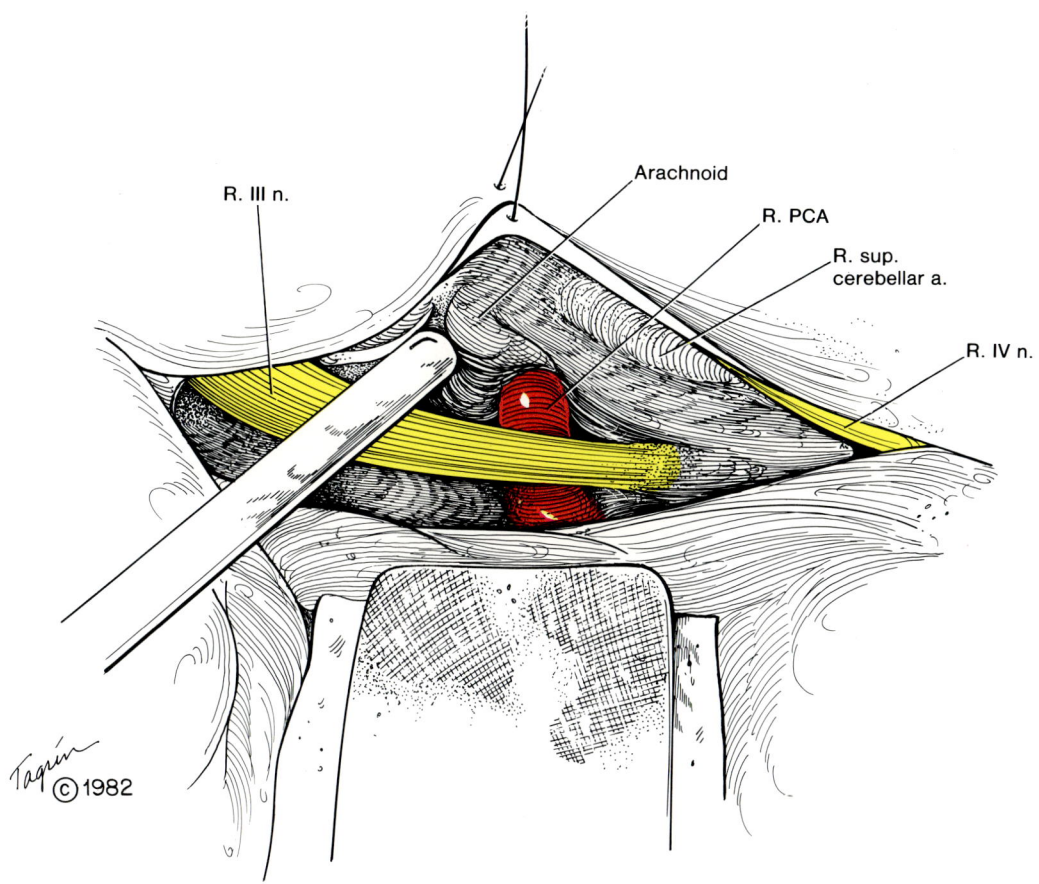

Figure 17.4. Dissecting the right posterior cerebral artery (*PCA*). The edge of the tentorium has been retracted. The arachnoid is opened with a hook, and the right posterior cerebral artery is followed back toward its origin. The third nerve is left attached to the uncus.

sion of a single perforator and thus would now try to avoid such occlusion at all costs (Fig. 17.13).

Obliterating the Aneurysm. Most of these aneurysms can be occluded with a clip, and usually a fenestrated clip is the best choice (Figs. 17.7 and 17.8). For most basilar tip aneurysms, the initial segment of the P_1 segment on the right embraces the neck and lateral dome of the aneurysm. In this situation, much retraction of the lesion and substantial dissection from the P_1 segment can be avoided by the use of a fenestrated clip. Clip selection and application demand precision. The blade length must correspond exactly to the neck width. If it is too long, it overlaps and occludes the left P_1 segment; if it is too short, the lesion is incompletely obliterated. If the aperture is not exactly positioned, the aneurysm may bulge into the fenestration, remaining unclipped, or the blade may occlude the right P_1 segment or the origin of one of its perforators. Measurement on the Towne view from the angiogram and rough measurement of the breadth of the lesion at surgery will be of help in selecting the proper clip (Fig. 17.8). Either a Drake or a Sugita or Yasargil clip with a Drake aperture is satisfactory. The latter have narrower blades, which facilitate introduction into a confined space. Also, the Sugita clips are available in 60° and 90° angulation, which may be useful for certain aneurysms. Note that these clips can be shortened and smoothed with a diamond drill to prevent occlusion of the opposite P_1 segment (see above). For selected cases, some other clip may be preferable. If the P_1 segment is not in the way, a straight clip may be best.

Occasionally, a ligature may be the best answer. In these cramped quarters, the technique of ligature passage without a ligature carrier may offer a satisfactory alternative. In this method, the aneurysmal neck is deflected to one side, and with the bipolar forceps, a waxed, doubled 3-0 silk ligature is passed deep to the lesion. Then the aneurysm is deflected in the opposite direction, and under direct vision the suture is retrieved from its position along the other side of the neck. The extra strand of suture is removed. The ligature may then be tied down for complete obliteration of the lesion or to set the stage for final clipping. Straight slender mosquito hemostats are used

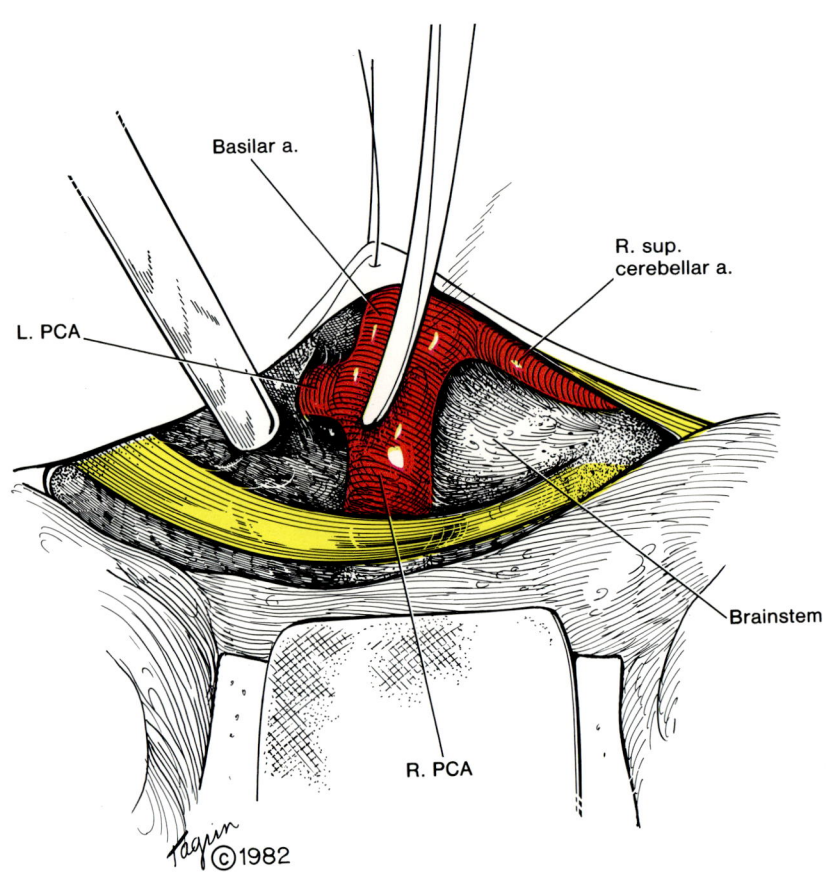

Figure 17.5. Dissecting anteriorly. Unless the aneurysm points forward, one can safely work across the basilar apex and aneurysm neck to define left P_1 segment, thus establishing the key landmarks. *PCA*, Posterior cerebral artery.

to grasp and tighten the suture, which is tied with a surgeon's knot to prevent slippage.

After obliteration, the position of the clip or ligature must be checked carefully. If the position of the clip is not satisfactory, it must be adjusted for precise obliteration of the lesion and preservation of normal arteries. Typically, the authors place and replace the clip once to several times before they are satisfied. In some cases, preliminary clipping may be utilized for further dissection of the aneurysm, followed by repositioning of the clip. The clip is advanced with a gentle wiggling or axial rotation of the blades to decrease frictional drag on the lesion. During clip advancement, the tip of the clip should be inspected under direct vision, if possible, so that it advances just to the point of touching the opposite posterior cerebral artery. After the clip is allowed to close, this tip position is again checked on both sides of the aneurysm. The left P_1 segment and its perforators must be free. The entire neck of the aneurysm must be gathered into the obliterating clip blades. If this objective has been achieved, aspiration of the aneurysm with a 25-gauge spinal needle assures complete obliteration of the lesion. Should there be a tiny dog-ear of unclipped aneurysm that defies clipping, application of muslin may be used to reinforce the lesion. In view of the proximity of the brain stem, cranial nerves, and perforating arteries, the authors have avoided the use of tissue adhesives with their potentially toxic effects.

Special Problems. Although posteriorly pointing basilar tip aneurysms seem most forbidding, good results have been achieved in such cases probably because, in general, these aneurysms have been smaller. After initial dissection across the anterior neck to the posterior cerebral artery, the difficult job is dissecting out the posterior neck from the interpeduncular cistern (Fig. 17.9). The approach is much the same as with the upward-pointing lesions, except that more extensive posterior retraction on the peduncle is required. The pia-arachnoid of the peduncle and all the perforators travel together posteriorly, and care must be taken to avoid tearing of these perforators when retracting posteriorly this arachnoidal layer. Complete dissection to the opposite edge of the neck, with visualization of the P_1 segment, is mandatory to avoid inaccurate clipping. Occasionally, these aneurysms can be clipped with a straight

Posterior Circulation Aneurysms

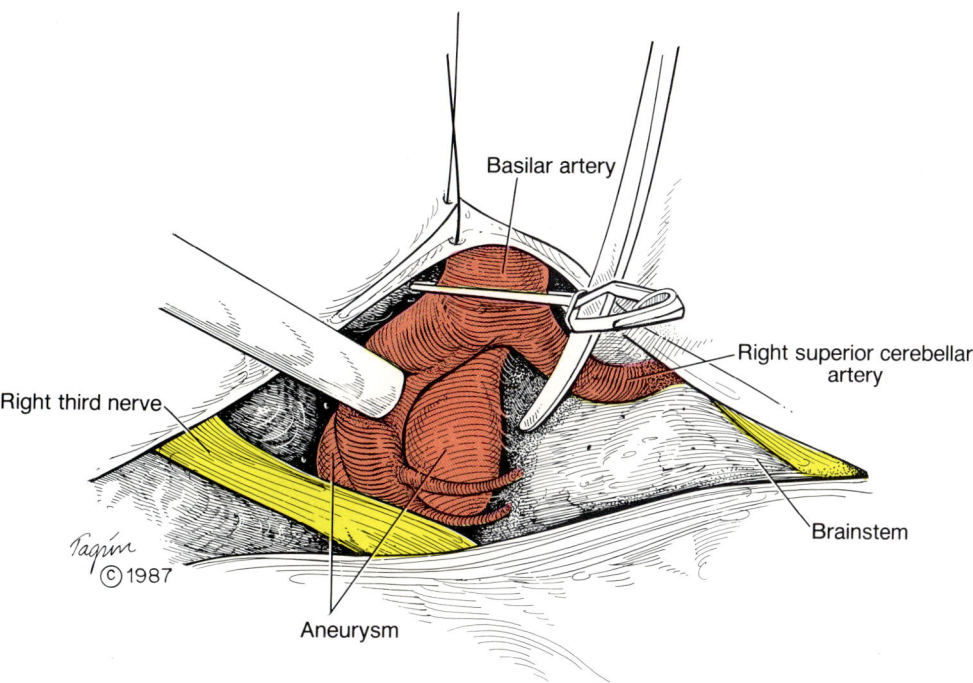

Figure 17.6. Dissecting posteriorly. For most basilar bifurcation aneurysms, this is the most difficult step. A temporary Sugita clip has been placed on the basilar artery trunk. A fine microcurved dissector is convenient to sweep brain stem and perforating arteries away from the neck and proximal dome.

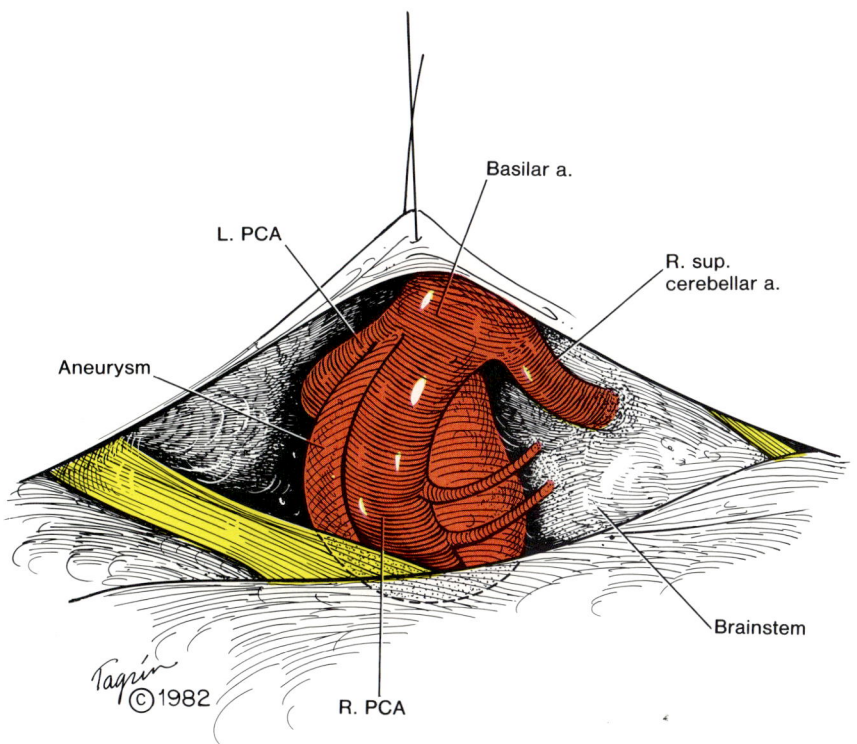

Figure 17.7. Dissection completed. Once the anterior and posterior walls of neck are freed, a clip is selected. In this situation, where the right posterior cerebral artery (PCA) bars the way, a clip with an aperture to go around the artery avoids excess manipulation or kinking of the vessel.

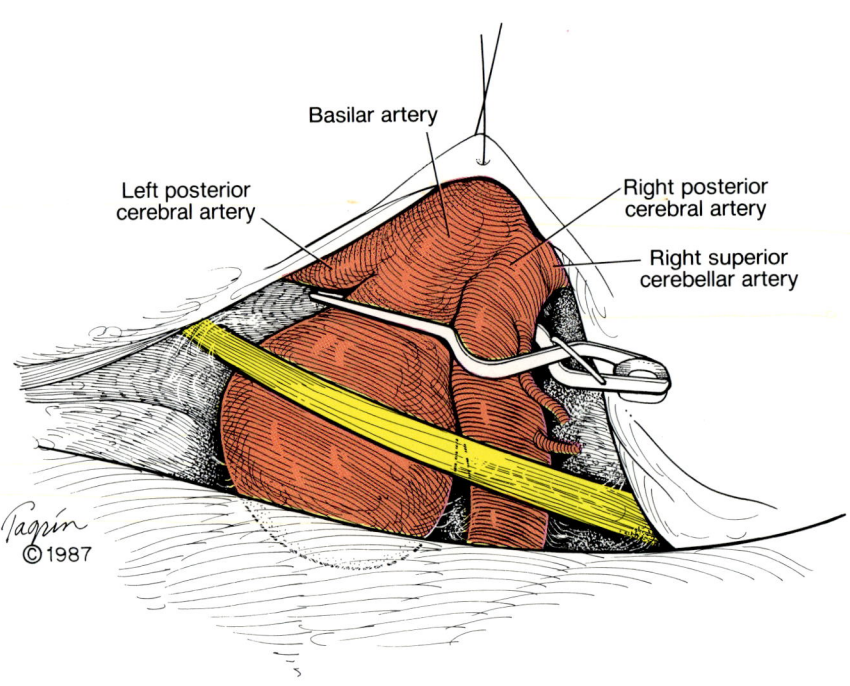

Figure 17.8. Aneurysm clipped. An 8-mm Sugita clip has been applied. The clip just barely crosses the neck, and properly so, for a longer one might occlude the left P_1 segment and a shorter one might inadequately obliterate the lesion. The fenestration encircles the right P_1 segment (but no aneurysm tissue).

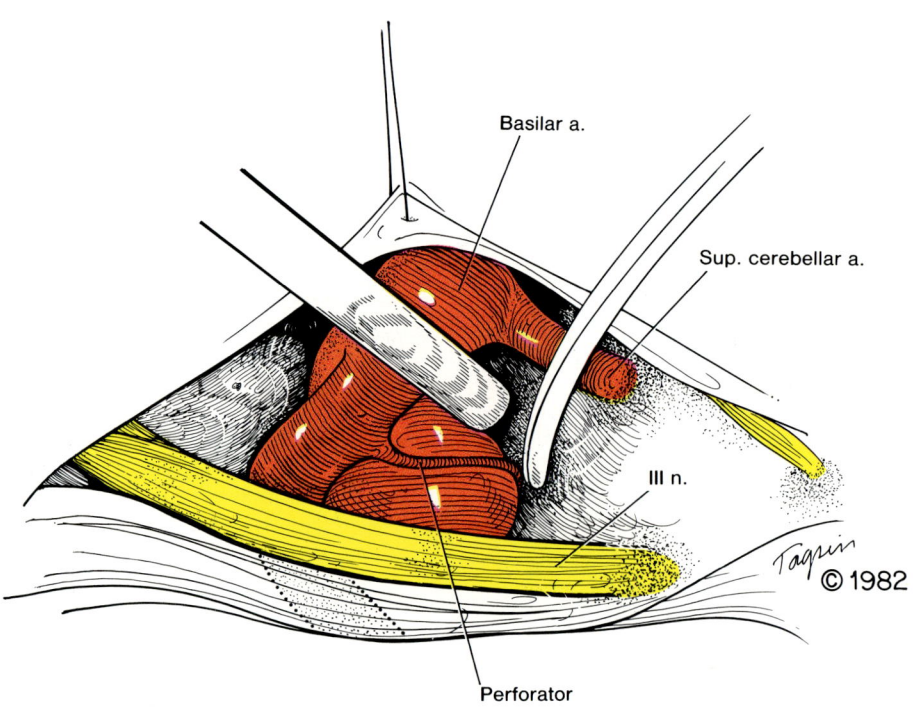

Figure 17.9. Aneurysm pointing back into brain stem. The anterior neck is dissected first. Then brain stem and perforators are swept away from the posterior neck of the aneurysm.

clip applied with both blades behind the right P_1 segment, leaving it outside the clip anterior and superior to it.

The anteriorly pointing lesions, least common of all, present an entirely different problem (Fig. 17.10). Frequently, these aneurysms are adherent to the clivus, and there is great danger of massive hemorrhage from tearing of the aneurysm if one exerts any degree of posterior retraction on the basilar artery. If there is clot present anteriorly, it is wise to proceed outside the clot, providing a bit of extra margin for the dissection. If there is a red "angry" area on the anterior aspect of the lesion, it may be preferable to prepare the posterior aspect of the lesion first. The perforating vessels are usually less adherent in this type of aneurysm, and they tend not to be related to the lesion at all. For large and giant lesions, the bulk interferes with accurate visualization, particularly of the left P_1 segment. Indenting the lesion with a suction under hypotension or temporary clipping may facilitate dissection of the neck and application of the clip. The clip application may be difficult because the bulk of the lesion forces the clip down into the basilar artery itself. To solve this problem, application of the clip well up on the aneurysm may permit sliding of the slip down into perfect position as the blades are closed. When the posterior communicating artery is large, a preliminary ligature around the neck of the lesion or inclusion of the P_1 segment in the blades of the clip may permit obliteration of the neck. With the smaller lesions, a straight clip can usually be applied with both blades anterior to the P_1 segments.

A low-lying basilar bifurcation may require special technique. This situation can be anticipated when the angiogram shows the basilar bifurcation below the posterior clinoid process. Often, adequate exposure can be obtained by section of the tentorium (Fig. 17.11). The incision is placed posterior to the entry of the fourth cranial nerve to avoid injury to this structure. Clips or bipolar cauterization controls bleeding from venous channels in the tentorium. This type of aneurysm almost always should be approached subtemporally because the posterior clinoid will be on the way if one approaches it from the front (pterional approach). There is rarely enough room for application of a temporary clip in these cases, and the surgeon must depend on induced hypotension to soften the aneurysm during dissection and clipping.

Pterional Approach

The pterional approach may sometimes be used for treatment of basilar bifurcation aneurysms (7, 15,

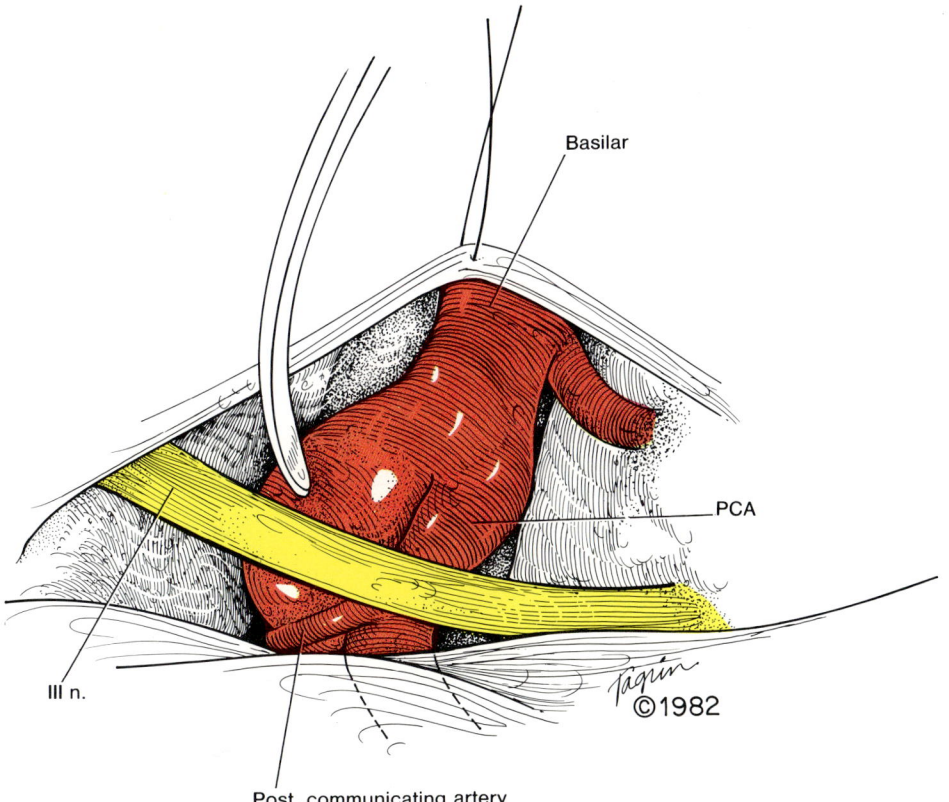

Figure 17.10. Aneurysm adherent to clivus. It may be best to free the posterior aspect first. Then gentle dissection, preferably outside the hematoma, may free the anterior neck. *PCA*, Posterior cerebral artery.

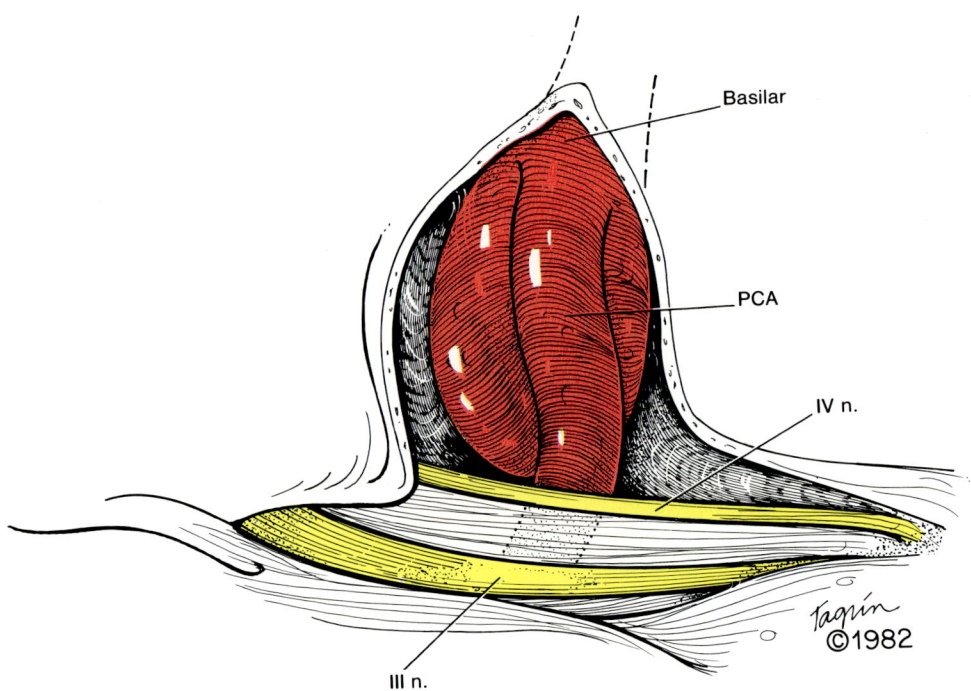

Figure 17.11. Low-lying basilar aneurysm. Section of the tentorium, posterior to incorporation of the fourth nerve, permits access to almost all low-lying basilar apex aneurysms. *PCA*, Posterior cerebral artery.

16, 21) (Fig. 17.12). After a pterional craniotomy is fashioned with removal of the lateral sphenoid ridge, the sylvian fissure is opened widely for visualization of the internal carotid artery. Deeper dissection permits access to the basilar tip, either between the carotid artery and the optic nerve, if that space is very wide, or, most commonly, lateral to the carotid artery. When either space is too narrow, one may work in both spaces, applying the clip in one space (i.e., lateral to the carotid) while viewing the clip application with the line of vision through the other space (between the optic nerve and the carotid). The approach may afford a nice view of a high-lying basilar bifurcation aneurysm that cannot be easily reached even with deep subtemporal retraction. There are several disadvantages that render the approach less useful for most basilar tip lesions: the angle of clip application, oblique rather than direct lateral, is more difficult to visualize anatomically; the space available is less in most cases; in some patients, the aneurysm is obscured by the posterior clinoid process; bilobular basilar tip lesions and those entirely in the interpeduncular fossa cannot be exposed satisfactorily; and, most importantly, the perforators behind the aneurysm may be completely obscured by the lesion itself. However, this approach is particularly advantageous when another aneurysm of the anterior circulation is to be dealt with at the same operation. The exposure through the sylvian fissure has access to the anterior circulation, while the deeper opening then permits dissection of the basilar tip. When the basilar lesion may need a subtemporal approach, it may be wisest to use a combined exposure—a pterional flap extended posteriorly and inferiorly over the temporal lobe.

Results

Over an 8-year period, the authors have operated 50 non-giant basilar bifurcation aneurysms (Table 17.1). There were 41 excellent or good results, 9 poor outcomes, and no deaths. These results are similar to those reported in the literature (5, 6, 10, 15, 16, 18, 21). Poor results were attributable to perforator occlusion (Fig. 17.13), excessive hypotension, or excessive temporal retraction with infarction. Oculomotor palsy has occurred in about 70% with virtual or complete resolution in almost all of these (4).

POSTERIOR CEREBRAL ARTERY ANEURYSMS

Surgical Management

Four sites can be distinguished: (a) P_1 segment at the take-off of a perforator, (b) at the junction of the P_1 segment and the posterior communicating artery, (c) at the first major branching beside the brain stem, and (d) at the separation of calcarine and posterior temporal branches. The second and fourth types are most common.

When the P_1 segment is involved, these lesions are treacherous because the crucial perforator branches are usually immediately adherent to the dome. It may be possible to free the perforators and clip the neck. When this is not safely possible, a P_1 segment occlu-

Posterior Circulation Aneurysms

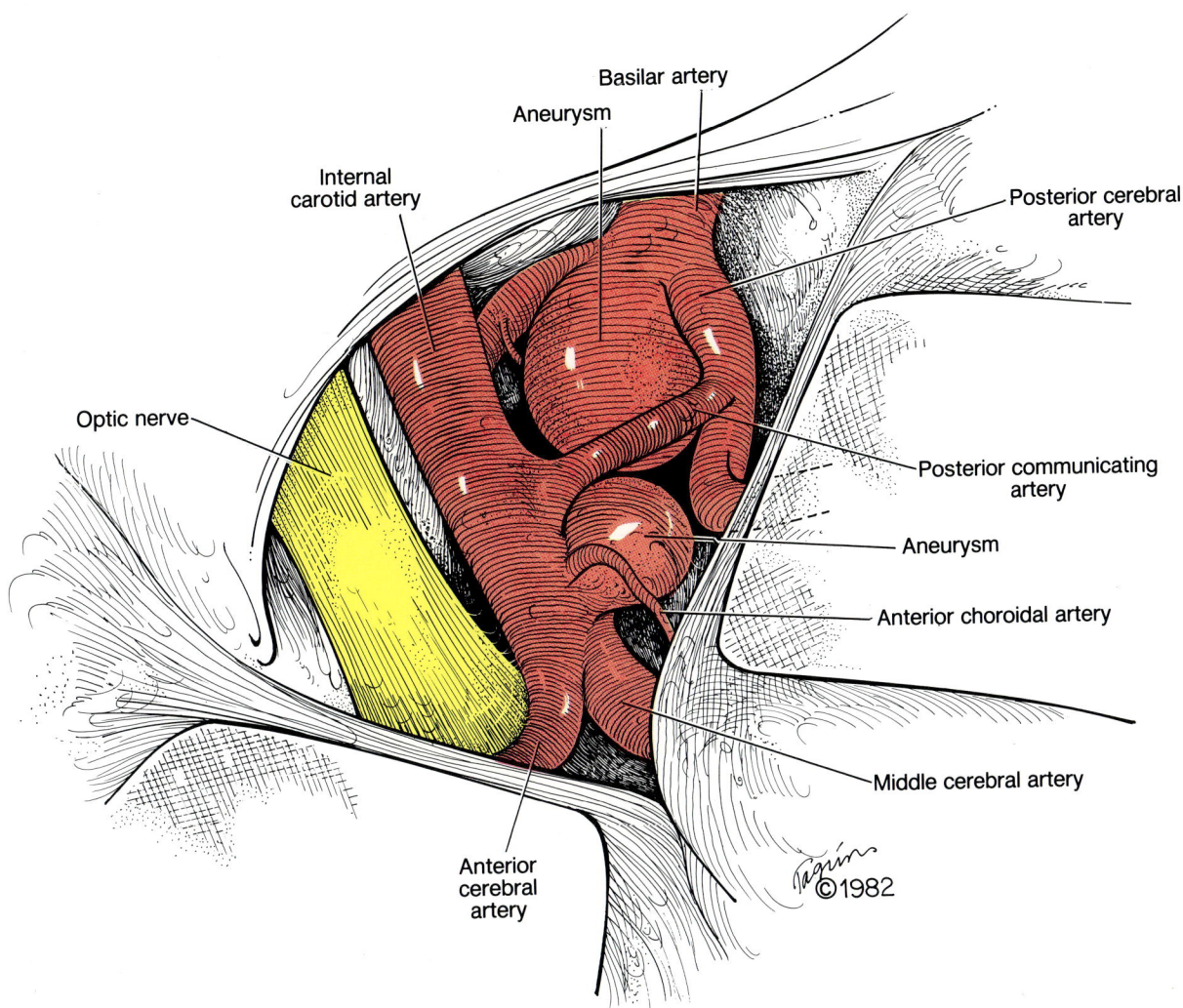

Figure 17.12. Pterional approach. Through a right pterional craniotomy, one can deal with both a basilar apex aneurysm and a right internal carotid–anterior choroidal artery aneurysm. Note the difficulty in visualizing perforating arteries from the P_1 segments.

sion has been suggested (6). However, the authors have seen brain infarction with use of this maneuver and can only recommend it as a last alternative.

When the lesion is distal to the posterior communicating artery, the situation is better because perforators are readily avoided and distal posterior cerebral artery collateral supply is rich, permitting posterior cerebral artery trunk occlusion with less risk of infarction. The latter maneuver is frequently necessary because many of these aneurysms are fusiform. Removal of a bit of hippocampal gyrus may be needed for exposure (Fig. 17.14).

Results

Table 17.1 summarizes the results. Poor results in 2 of 5 patients with P_1 segment aneurysms were related to perforating branch ischemia; the other 3 patients did well. Of the 4 patients with P_2 segment aneurysm, 3 had an excellent outcome. In 2 patients, fusiform nonbacterial postcommunal lesions were trapped with no complications. The third patient underwent an attempt at reconstruction of the artery, and although this was not successful, there was no deficit (Fig. 17.15). The other patient with a large fusiform P_2 segment aneurysm had the posterior cerebral artery occluded accidentally when the aneurysm ruptured. She developed a hemianopia and a thalamic infarct that resulted in a serious chronic pain syndrome; therefore, she is classified as a poor result.

BASILAR TRUNK–SUPERIOR CEREBELLAR ARTERY ANEURYSM

Presentation

Aneurysms of the basilar trunk-superior cerebellar artery arise at the distal crotch of the origin of the superior cerebellar artery and usually project later-

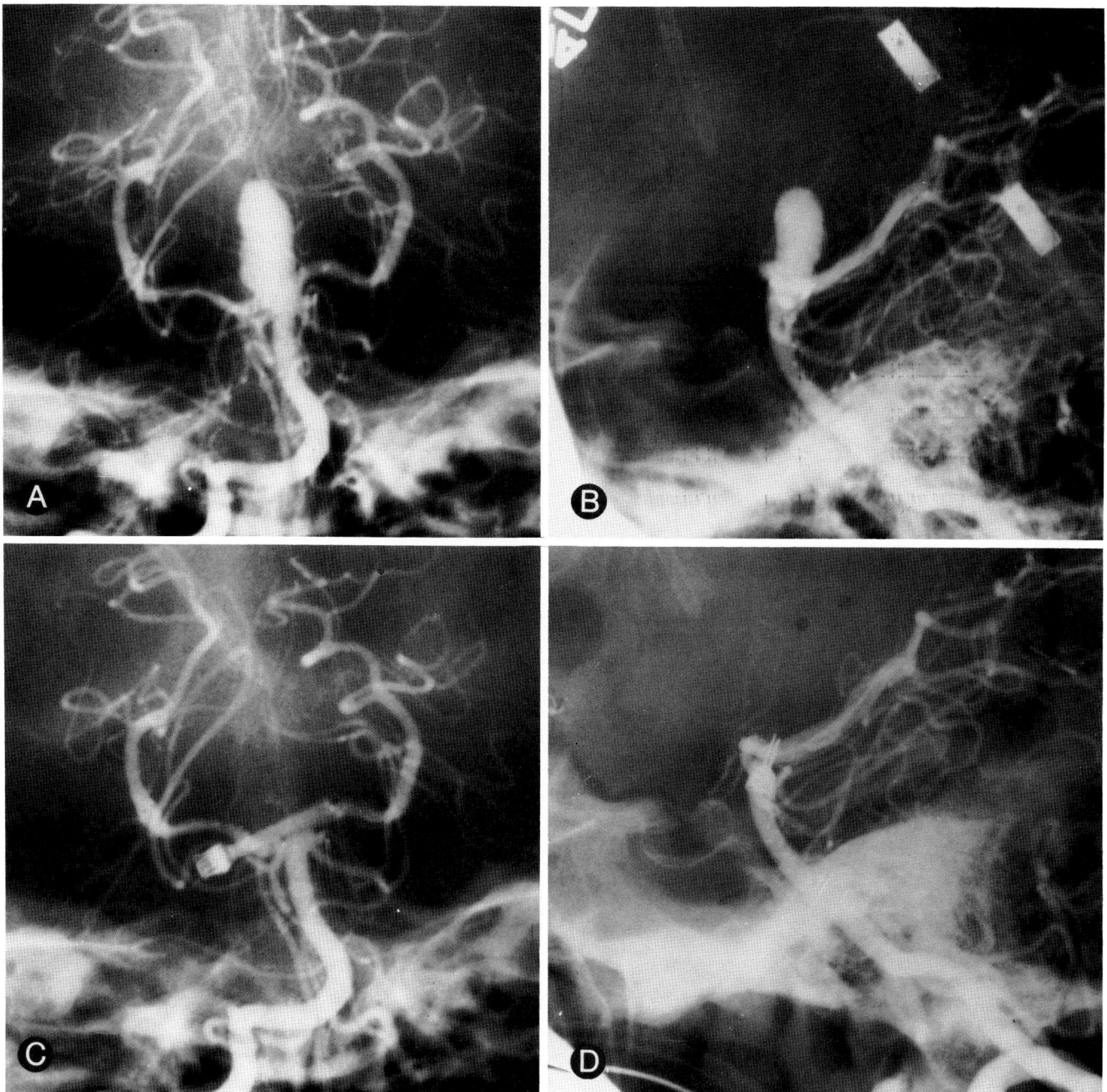

Figure 17.13. Importance of perforating arteries. **A** and **B**, Angiograms show a large aneurysm directed upward. The patient had abulia and hemiparesis. Difficult surgery was performed on day 27; two small perforators from left P_1 could not be excluded from the clip. **C** and **D**, Aneurysm obliterated, P_1 arteries normal. Severe obtundation after operation was probably due to occlusion of two perforant arteries.

ally, occasionally forward (6). Most patients with these aneurysms present with subarachnoid hemorrhage, but signs of brain stem compression may be seen with large and giant aneurysms (Fig. 17.16). There may be a third nerve palsy, since this nerve lies in a close relationship to the aneurysm.

Surgical Management

The subtemporal and pterional approaches described for low-lying basilar bifurcation aneurysms can be used to expose these lesions. Peerless and Drake have described the operative exposure for the

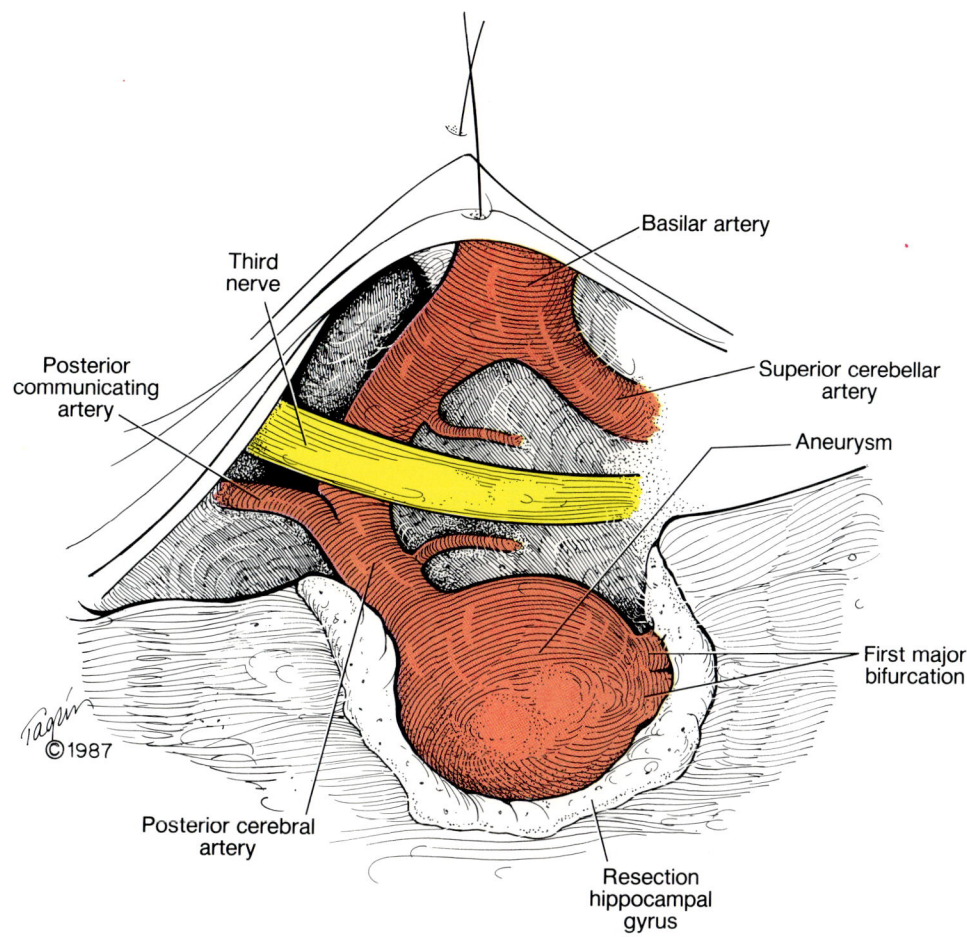

Figure 17.14. Subtemporal approach to fusiform aneurysm of P_2 segment of posterior cerebral artery. Resection of a portion of the hippocampal gyrus uncovers the lesion for obliteration. Distal to the posterior communicating artery junction, trapping is possible with low risk of infarction.

subtemporal approach in detail (9). The approach is from the side of the fundus of the aneurysm. The tentorium is retracted with a suture to aid exposure. In some patients, the tentorium needs to be divided. Care must be taken to prevent injury to the fourth cranial nerve. By first working down the sides of the aneurysm from the front, the surgeon can avoid the dome. Depressing the sac against the peduncle will reveal the neck of the aneurysm emerging from the basilar artery and the superior cerebellar artery below. The P_1 segment may be seen, but if the aneurysm is of significant size, the artery will be hidden above and behind. By working behind the aneurysm, it can be separated from the peduncle by using a microdissector. The waist and neck of the aneurysm are freed from the P_1 segment. With the aneurysm displaced forward, the neck is visualized and any perforating branches are separated. Care must be taken not to injure the third nerve, which frequently winds around the neck. If application of a clip is difficult because of the nerve, a ligature may be used or the neck can be shrunk with coagulation. The superior cerebellar artery may emerge from the side of the neck, and one must be careful not to kink it with the ligature or clip.

The authors prefer the pterional approach (Fig. 17.17)(6, 15, 19, 21) for most basilar-superior cerebellar artery aneurysms because the aneurysmal neck is approached perpendicularly and is not hidden from view by the dome of the aneurysm, which is frequently the case when these aneurysms are approached subtemporally. Fortunately, the relationship of the perforating vessels to the aneurysm is very different from the top of the basilar aneurysms. The

Table 17.1.
Results of Direct Operation in Non-Giant Aneurysms

Location	Results		
	Good	Poor	Dead
Basilar bifurcation	41	9	0
Basilar-superior cerebellar	9	0	1
Posterior cerebral (proximal)	3	2	0
Posterior cerebral (distal)	3	1	0

tors at the origin of the superior cerebellar artery, but these usually run superiorly or directly posteriorly and can be spared after proper development of the neck between the superior cerebellar artery and the posterior cerebral arteries, which is done by applying a clip perpendicularly, leaving the perforators medial to the clip. Another advantage of the pterional approach to these aneurysms is that, at least in the authors' experience, it is easier to preserve third nerve function, since all of the work can be done at the neck usually medial to the nerve (three of the authors' five patients approached in this manner did not experience postoperative third nerve palsy). The main contraindication to the pterional approach is a very low origin of the aneurysm (15, 19). In these cases of low bifurcation, the posterior clinoid obscures the approach from the front. Yasargil has recommended drilling off the posterior clinoid in these cases (20), but, in general, it may be safest to approach these low-lying aneurysms subtemporally.

The pterional approach to the upper basilar artery has been described. It is essential to open the medial aspect of the sylvian fissure widely so that the surgeon has the option of working lateral or medial to the internal carotid artery. Because of the narrow view afforded by either of these spaces, the authors sometimes apply the clip in one direction (i.e., through the space lateral to the internal carotid artery) while directing their line of vision through the other space (between the optic nerve and the internal carotid artery). In some cases, to allow for more working room lateral to the internal carotid artery, they have resected a bit of the uncus on either side without ill effects. This maneuver is particularly helpful with large aneurysms and when the internal carotid artery is atherosclerotic and direct retraction of the artery must be avoided. In these instances, one must be extremely careful with the third nerve, which may be quite adherent to the uncus.

Whether to approach these aneurysms from the ipsilateral or the contralateral side is an unsettled question (20). The contralateral approach allows a more perpendicular approach to the neck in some aneurysms and may be advantageous in cases of large aneurysms, particularly if they project forward, because the dome will not be in the way. The authors believe that in most patients, the critical separation of the origin of the posterior cerebral artery and the superior cerebellar artery from the neck can be done more easily from the ipsilateral side. Also, a rupture at the dome may be more easily controlled from the ipsilateral side.

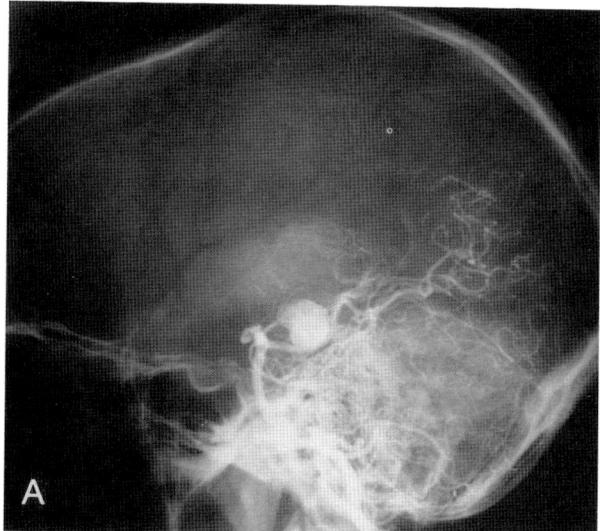
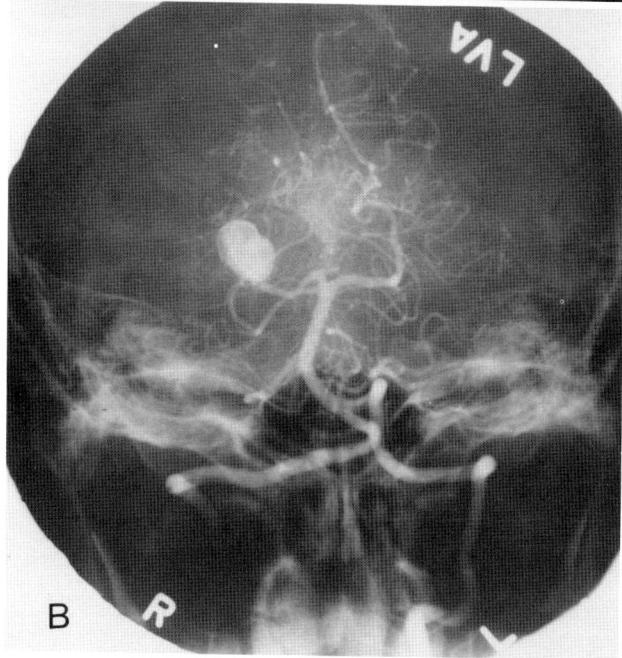

Figure 17.15. **A** and **B**, Posterior cerebral artery aneurysm. At surgery, the aneurysm was found to be giant, fusiform, and partially thrombosed. An attempt to reconstruct the lumen of the posterior cerebral artery was not successful, but there was no neurologic deficit.

perforating arteries from the top of the basilar artery and P_1 segments of the posterior cerebral arteries are not usually a problem in aneurysms at the origin of the superior cerebellar artery. These aneurysms almost always point laterally, and critical perforators are well visualized by depressing the superior aspect of the aneurysm and separating the neck from the posterior cerebral arteries. This can be done optimally via the perpendicular approach afforded by the pterional exposure. Occasionally, there are perfora-

Results

The largest operative experience has been reported by Peerless and Drake (9). They had a high percentage of excellent and good results, as did Yasargil (20) and

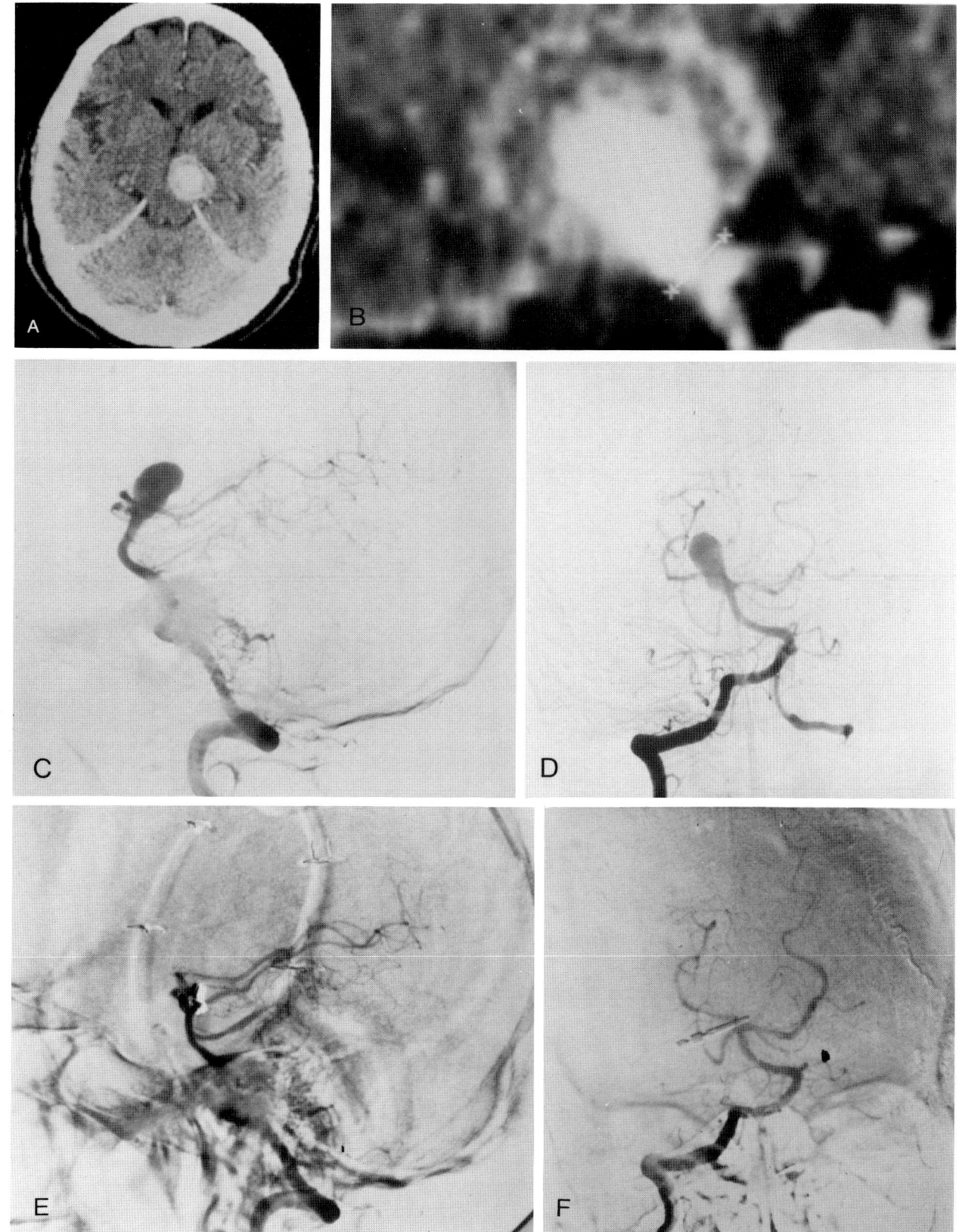

Figure 17.16. Giant superior cerebellar artery aneurysm. Presentation with progressive moderate right hemiparesis in a 62-year-old woman. **A**, Contrast-enhanced CT scan demonstrates residual lumen and mural thrombus in aneurysm. **B**, Reconstructed CT scan shows that the aneurysm neck is free of neural thrombus. **C** and **D**, preoperative vertebral angiograms demonstrate that the origin is from the basilar-superior cerebellar artery junction, not from the basilar artery apex. **E** and **F**, Postoperative angiograms confirm complete obliteration of lesion after subtemporal approach for clipping and evacuation of the aneurysm (hard thrombus was not removed), with resultant gradual and virtually complete recovery of the patient.

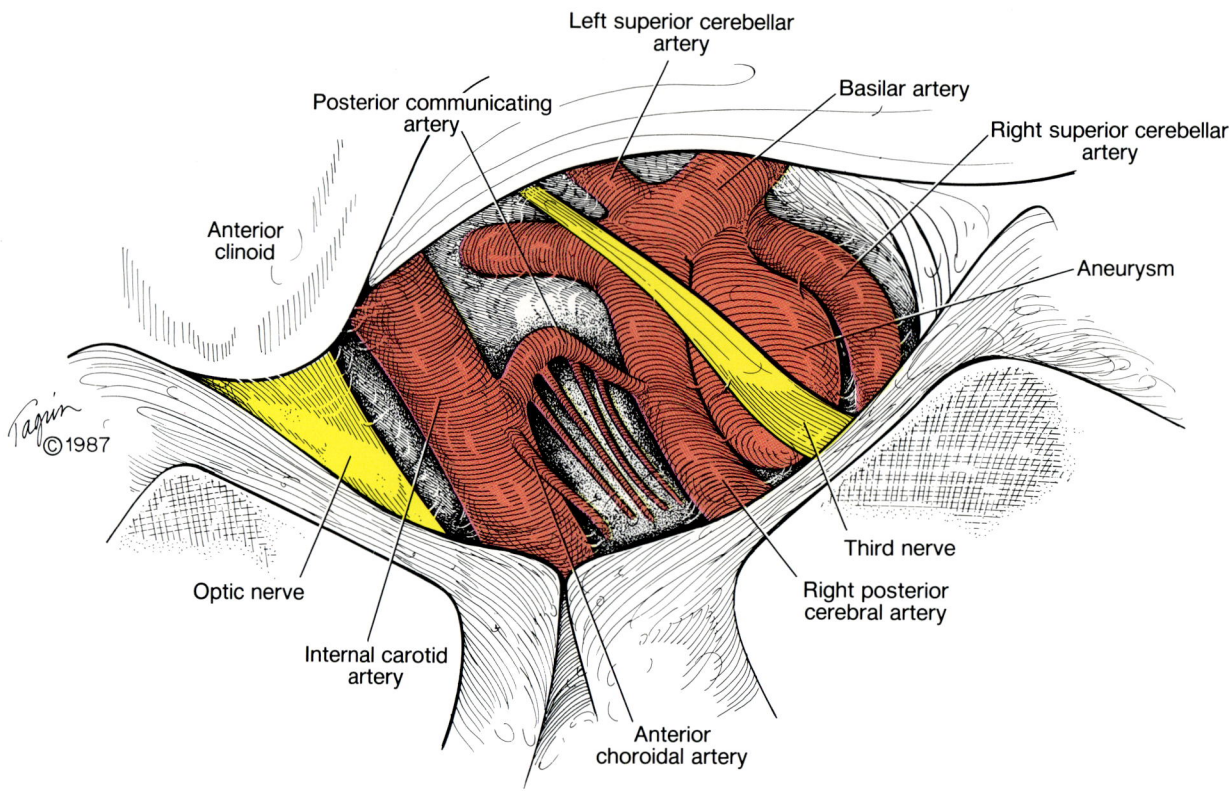

Figure 17.17. Pterional approach to superior cerebellar artery aneurysm. The neck of the aneurysm is well visualized, and the oculomotor nerve need not be disturbed.

Sugita (16). In the present authors' series of 10 patients, nine had excellent results (see Table 17.1). One patient died after intraoperative rupture of a large, partially thrombosed aneurysm. At surgery, the origin of the posterior cerebral artery and probably some vital perforators were occluded, and the patient died some weeks later from a brain stem infarction. Temporary third nerve palsies were noted in some patients.

REFERENCES

1. Andreoli A, Calbucci F, Limoni P, Testa C: Delayed angiographic appearance of a large basilar aneurysm. Surg Neurol 22:377–381, 1984.
2. Andrews BT, Brant-Zawadzki M, Wilson CB: Variant aneurysms of the fenestrated basilar artery. Neurosurgery 18:204–207, 1986.
3. Ausman J, Diaz F, Malik J, Fielding AS, Son CS: Current management of cerebral aneurysms: Is it based on facts or myths? Surg Neurol 24:625–635, 1985.
4. Cruciger MP, Hoyt WF, Wilson CB: Peripheral and midbrain oculomotor palsies from operations for basilar bifurcation aneurysms in a series of 31 cases. Surg Neurol 15:215–216, 1981.
5. Drake CG: The surgical treatment of aneurysms of the basilar artery. J Neurosurg 29:436–446, 1968.
6. Drake CG: The treatment of aneurysms of the posterior circulation. Clin Neurosurg 26:96–144, 1979.
7. Kobayashi S, Sugita K, Nakagawa F: An approach to a basilar aneurysm above the bifurcation of the internal carotid artery. Case report. J Neurosurg 59:1082–1084, 1983.
8. Ljunggren B, Brandt L: Timing of aneurysm surgery. Clin Neurosurg 33:159–175, 1985.
9. Peerless SJ, Drake CG: Management of aneurysm of posterior circulation. In Youmans JR (ed): Neurological Surgery, ed 2. Philadelphia, WB Saunders, 1982, pp 1715–1763.
10. Peerless SJ, Drake CG: Posterior circulation aneurysms. In Wilkins RH, Rengachary S (eds): Neurosurgery. New York, McGraw-Hill, 1986, pp 1422–1437.
11. Pelz DM, Vinuela F, Fox AJ, Drake CG: Vertebrobasilar occlusion therapy of giant aneurysms. J Neurosurg 60:560–565, 1984.
12. Piek J, Lim DP, Bock WJ: Obstructive hydrocephalus caused by a growing, giant aneurysm on the upper basilar artery. Surg Neurol 20:288–290, 1983.
13. Pitelli SD, Almeida GG, Nakagawa EJ, Marchese AJ, Cabral ND: Basilar aneurysm surgery: The subtemporal approach with section of one zygomatic arch. Neurosurgery 18:125–128, 1986.
14. Raudzens PA, Shetter AG: Intraoperative monitoring of brain stem auditory-evoked potentials. J Neurosurg 50:368–373, 1979.
15. Samson DS, Hodosh RM, Clark WK: Microsurgical evaluation of the pterional approach to aneurysms of the distal basilar circulation. Neurosurgery 3:135–141, 1978.
16. Sugita K, Kobayashi S, Shintani A, Mutsuga N: Microneurosurgery for aneurysms of the basilar artery. J Neurosurg 51:615–620, 1979.
17. Tiyaworabun S, Wanis A, Schirmer M, Bock WJ: Aneurysms of the vertebrobasilar system: Clinical analysis and follow-up results. Acta Neurochir (Wien) 63:221–229, 1982.
18. Wilson CB, Hoi Sang U: Surgical treatment for aneurysms of the upper basilar artery. J Neurosurg 44:537–543, 1976.

19. Yamainura A, Ise R, Makino H: Treatment of aneurysms arising from the terminal portion of the basilar artery. *Neurol Med Chir (Tokoyo)* 22:521–532, 1982.
20. Yasargil MG: Vertebrobasilar aneurysms. In Yasargil MG (ed): *Microneurosurgery.* New York, Thieme-Stratton, 1984, vol 2, pp 232–295.
21. Yasargil MG, Antic J, Laciga R, Jain KK, Hodosh RM, Smith RD: Microsurgical pterional approach to aneurysms of the basilar bifurcation. *Surg Neurol* 6:83–91, 1976.
22. Zeumer H, Bruckmann H, Adelt D, Hacke W, Ringelstein EB: Balloon embolization in the treatment of basilar aneurysms. *Acta Neurochir* 78:136–141, 1985.

18

Basilar Trunk and Vertebral Artery Aneurysms

BASILAR TRUNK-ANTERIOR INFERIOR CEREBELLAR ARTERY ANEURYSMS

Presentation

Aneurysms of the basilar trunk-anterior inferior cerebellar artery arise at the carina or origin of the anterior inferior cerebellar artery over the clivus (2, 4, 6, 14) (Fig. 18.1). Patients usually present with subarachnoid hemorrhage. There is a close relationship between the aneurysm and the abducens nerve, so a sixth nerve paresis may be present.

Surgical Management

The surgical approach is either through a subtemporal transtentorial exposure or through a suboccipital craniectomy (3, 5, 7, 14). The origin of the anterior inferior cerebellar artery is usually the border zone for exposure of the basilar trunk from above or below. In general, those lesions over the lower third of the clivus are exposed from the suboccipital opening, while those above are approached through the tentorium. The choice of the approach depends on the location of the aneurysm in relation to the clivus, its size and projection, and a consideration of the disadvantages of each approach (from above, possible injury to the fifth, sixth, seventh, and eighth cranial nerves and dominant temporal lobe; from below, the chance of injury to the ninth, tenth, and eleventh cranial nerves). For example, a high-lying anterior inferior cerebellar artery aneurysm that points laterally is best approached from above.

In some patients, lesions between the anterior inferior cerebellar artery and the vertebrobasilar junction may be hard to expose from below. Here, a combined subtemporal-transtentorial-suboccipital exposure can permit rotation of the brain stem with excellent visualization of the lower basilar trunk (9) (Fig. 18.2A and B). Since section of the transverse sinus is employed, preoperative angiographic visualization of the contralateral sinus is necessary. Because of the deep temporal retraction required, a right-sided approach, whenever possible, is preferred.

For a transtentorial approach, a substantial posterior temporal craniotomy permits subtemporal exposure to the tentorial edge (14). Care must be taken to preserve the vein of Labbé because of the possiblity of venous infarction. The midtemporal lobe is elevated. In cases in which the vein of Labbé is in the way, the authors prefer to suction a bit of the inferior temporal lobe in front of or behind the vein and then approach the tentorial surface through the brain, without stretching the vein of Labbé (Fig. 18.3A–C). If one limits the brain resection to the lateral and inferior portion of the temporal lobe and "re-enters" the pial surface of the inferior temporal lobe lateral to the visual radiation, there should be no ill effect

The tentorium is opened behind the insertion of the fourth nerve and is incised 1 cm posterior to the petrous ridge. This is necessary to avoid injury to the superior petrosal sinus that runs just at the posterior edge of the petrous ridge. The tentorium can be folded forward and sutured to the floor of the middle fossa. This exposes the fourth and fifth cranial nerves and the petrosal vein which is divided. The same retractor may then elevate both the temporal lobe and the edge of the cerebellum just lateral to the fifth nerve, or a separate retractor may be used on the cerebellum posteriorly. This maneuver rotates the brain stem and provides extensive exposure of the basilar trunk. The exposure is through an opening between the fifth nerve medially and the seventh and eighth nerves laterally. The sixth nerve and basilar artery are exposed, and the aneurysm is seen as the basilar artery is followed inferiorly. The aneurysm, which generally points laterally, is carefully dissected near the origin, with care exercised to prevent injury to the sixth nerve which is often adherent to the dome. The anterior inferior cerebellar artery must be freed from the lesion and carefully preserved during final clipping.

Results

Peerless and Drake have reported on 27 patients who were grade 1 or 2 at the time of operation (14). Among this group, there were 18 with excellent results, 3 with good results, 4 with poor results, and 2 deaths. The authors of this text have operated on 5 patients with mid-basilar aneurysms, with good results seen in all, although one patient continues to have a sixth nerve paresis and another has partial sixth and seventh nerve paresis which is improving (Table 18.1).

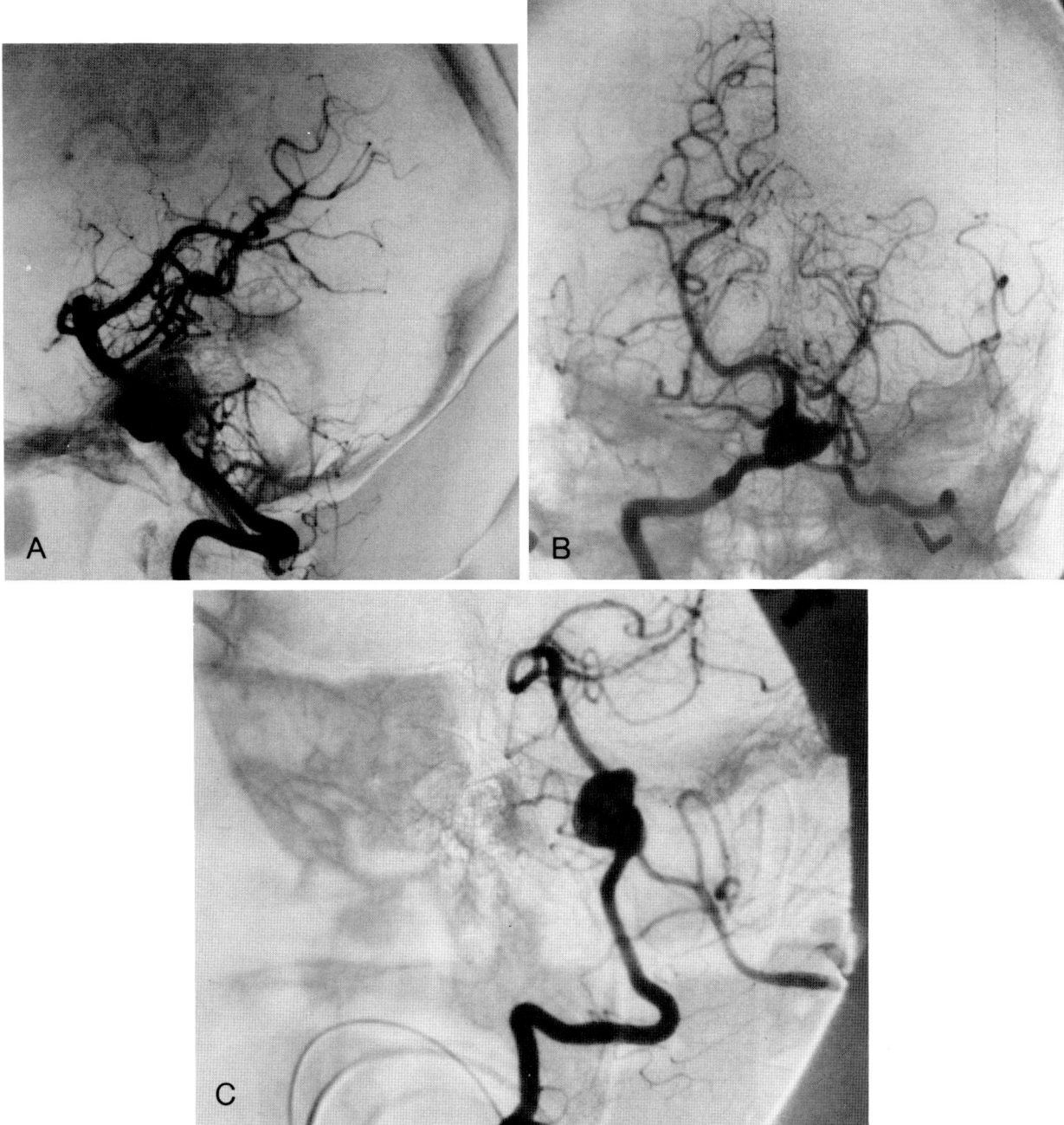

Figure 18.1. Basilar trunk aneurysm at the origin of the anterior inferior cerebellar artery. **A–C**, The aneurysm projected toward the left side. The patient presented with subarachnoid hemorrhage and a left sixth nerve palsy. Because the aneurysm was approximately at the level of the midportion of the clivus, a subtemporal-transtentorial approach in which the tentorium is divided from the transverse sinus to its edge on a line about 1 cm parallel to the posterior ridge of the petrous bone was used. The aneurysm was found to have a complex neck that involved all of the anterior aspect of the basilar artery. The authors worked in the space between the seventh and eighth nerves superiorly and the ninth and tenth nerves inferiorly. The sixth nerve on the right side was stretched by the aneurysm, even though preoperatively the patient had a contralateral sixth nerve palsy, probably because the dome of the aneurysm projected toward the left and it ruptured in that direction. There was not a sufficient amount of space to use a temporary clip on the basilar artery; therefore, the authors had to use deep hypotension in order to be able to clip the aneurysm satisfactorily. The latter was accomplished with a long straight Sugita clip. The aneurysm was opened after clipping. Postoperatively, the patient did well except for partial right sixth and seventh nerve palsies which continue to improve and the contralateral left sixth nerve palsy which remains unchanged.

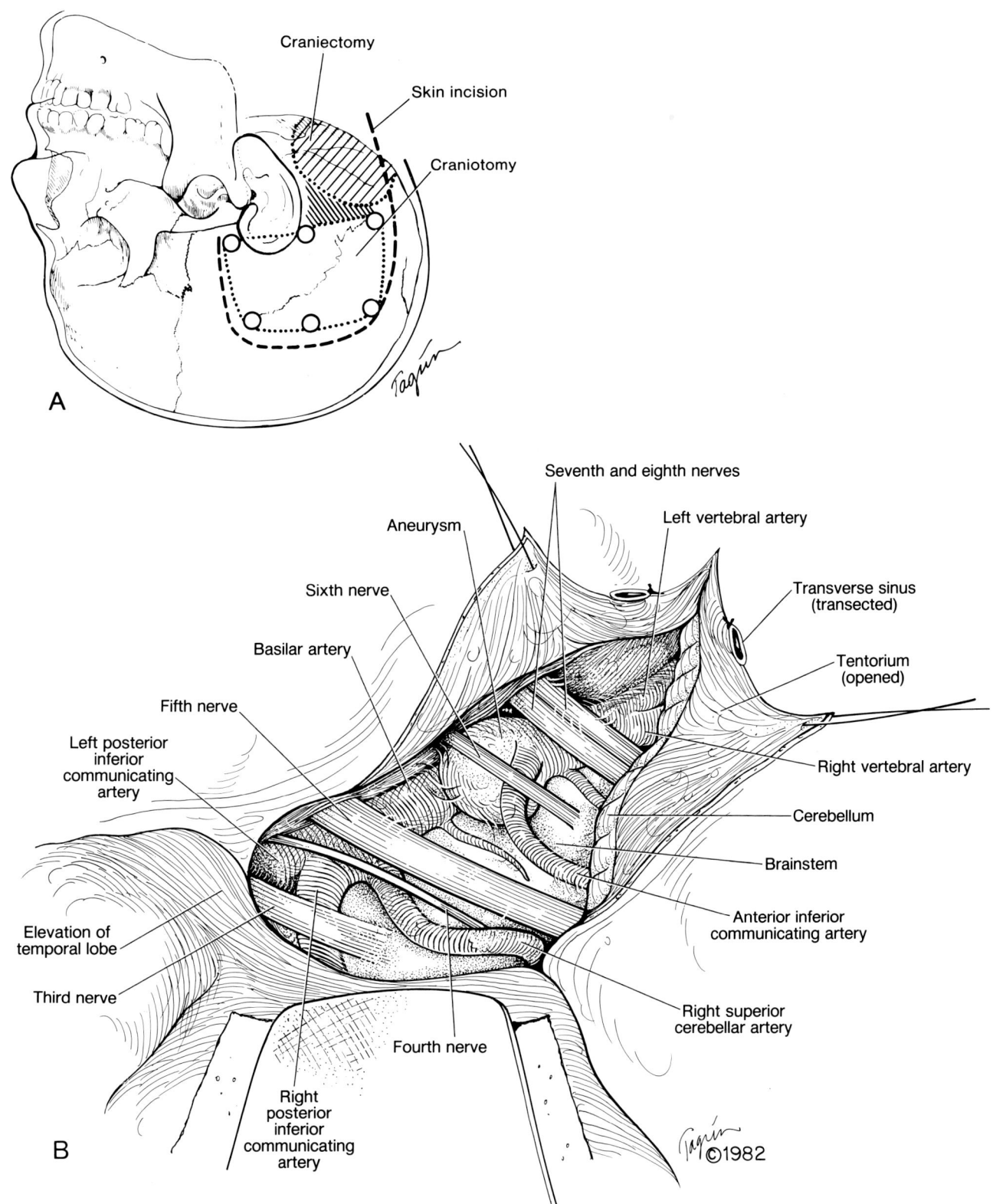

Figure 18.2. Approach to basilar trunk. **A**, Combined subtemporal-suboccipital approach is used. **B**, The tentorium is sectioned widely to expose the length of the basilar artery.

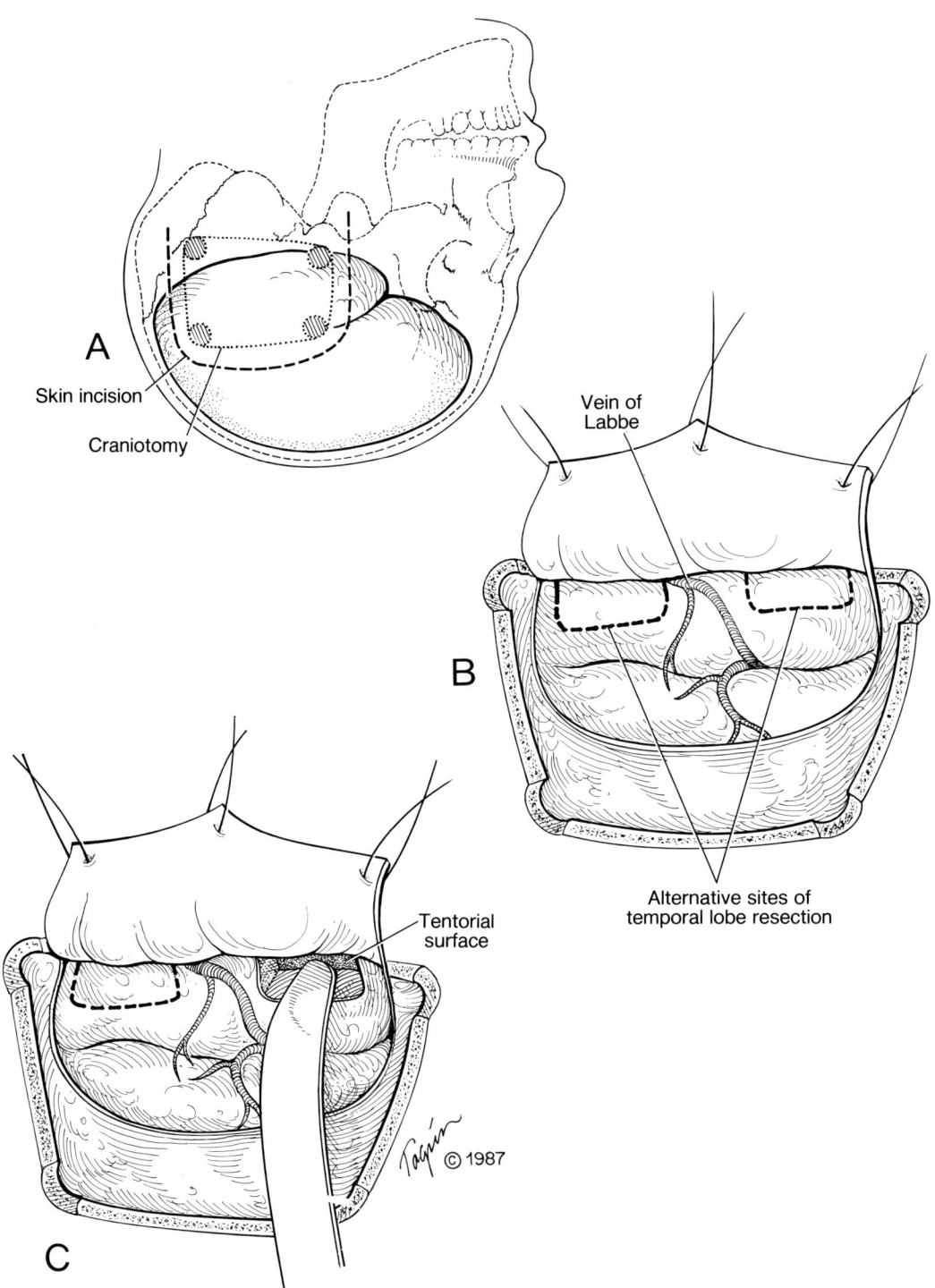

Figure 18.3. Posterior temporal craniotomy for subtemporal-transtentorial approach to the basilar trunk. **A**, The bone edge must be rongeured or drilled down to the temporal floor inferiorly. **B**, Alternative sites of brain retraction or resection, depending on the position of the vein of Labbé. **C**, A small area of brain resection in the inferior temporal gyrus allows the surgeon to place a retractor and expose the deep aspect of the tentorial surface without undue traction and risk of injury to the vein of Labbé.

DISTAL ANTERIOR INFERIOR CEREBELLAR ARTERY ANEURYSMS

Presentation

Aneurysms of the distal anterior inferior cerebellar artery are very rare. Only 14 cases from the literature were collected in a 1983 review (13). Patients with this aneurysm usually present with subarachnoid hemorrhage or a cerebellopontine angle syndrome mimicking an acoustic tumor (13, 18).

Surgical Management

The operative approach is through a suboccipital craniectomy identical to that used for the resection of an acoustic tumor, since these aneurysms are in the cerebellopontine angle. Neck clipping is preferable whenever possible. Sometimes the aneurysm is in close relationship to the internal auditory artery, and care must be exercised to preserve this small artery. Loss of hearing and facial function from probable injury to this artery has been reported in cases in which the nerves themselves were apparently not injured (13). Some of these aneurysms are unclippable, and trapping or excision should be considered, but some patients will have resultant loss of hearing, facial paralysis and, less commonly, brain stem infarction (13). The authors have had no personal experience with aneurysms in this location.

VERTEBROBASILAR JUNCTION ANEURYSMS

Presentation

Aneurysms of the vertebrobasilar junction usually arise from the carina between the basilar artery and the dominant vertebral artery. Occasionally, they occur in relation to a fenestration of the lower basilar artery (8). The patient usually presents with subarachnoid hemorrhage or signs of lower brain stem compression

Surgical Management

The vertebrobasilar junction may be approached in several ways. Most surgeons have abandoned the transoral transclival approach because of very high morbidity, usually associated with meningitis (3, 4, 10). In addition, with this approach one usually encounters the dome of the aneurysm first, and it may be quite adherent to the dura of the clivus. The posterior temporal transtentorial approach can be used to approach these aneurysms, particularly if the basilar origin is relatively high, i.e., above the junction of the lower third and the upper two-thirds of the clivus. If the aneurysm lies over the lower third of the clivus, it may be preferable to combine a subtemporal and a suboccipital approach and divide the transverse sinus to allow the cerebellum to "fall back," thus providing better visualization of the lower basilar artery (9) (Fig. 18.2). A more recent modification, with which the authors have had no experience, is the "transpetrosal" approach (10). This consists of drilling off the anterior portion of the pyramid of the petrosal bone by a subtemporal extradural approach and then opening the dura medially and dividing the tentorium. The main drawback to this approach is the possibility of injuring the cochlea, with resultant deafness. Apparently, however, if one limits the resection to a 1 × 2 cm groove in the anterior pyramid, this can be avoided. All of these subtemporal approaches share the disadvantages of necessitating deep temporal retraction and a substantial risk of injury to the sixth, seventh, or eighth cranial nerves. In addition, the dome of the aneurysm, which will usually point upward and laterally, is encountered first, and it frequently obstructs the view of the aneurysmal neck.

Because of these disadvantages, the authors prefer to approach the vertebrobasilar junction from a suboccipital exposure, except in the rare case of an aneurysm of a very high basilar origin (usually above the lower third of the clivus). This approach, which is a slight modification of the standard lateral suboccipital approach, has been described (7). The patient is placed in the straight lateral position, with a flat folded sheet under the axilla used as padding (Fig 18.4A). The head is maintained in the straight ahead position (nose at 90° angle from the floor), with a 30° angle tilt toward the ipsilateral (upper) shoulder. With the patient in this position, the cerebellum tends to fall away, and therefore, less retraction is necessary. Also, because the head is slightly elevated, cerebrospinal fluid tends to run down and does not need to be suctioned actively. Air embolism is unlikely with the patient in this position, since the head is only slightly higher than the heart. However, placement of a central venous line is still a useful precaution, and the central venous pressure should be kept at a minimum level of 6–8 cm of H_2O.

The skin incision is started at about the level of the top of the ear in a sagittal plane about 3 fingerbreaths medial to the mastoid. The incision first extends straight downward toward the mastoid, then curves sharply medially to the midline, and then proceeds straight downward to the spinous process of C2 (Fig. 18.4B). The incision provides good exposure laterally at the mastoid and also inferiorly over the foramen magnum and arch of C1. The muscle mass is opened with electrocautery along the line of the skin incision down to the suboccipital bone which is then exposed by subperiosteal dissection.

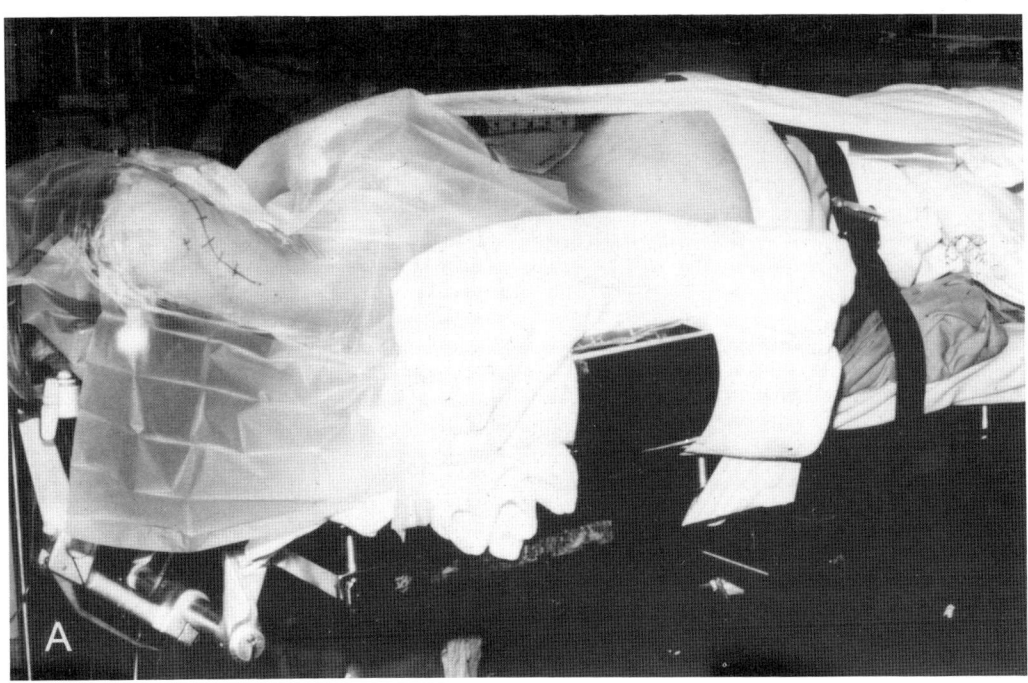
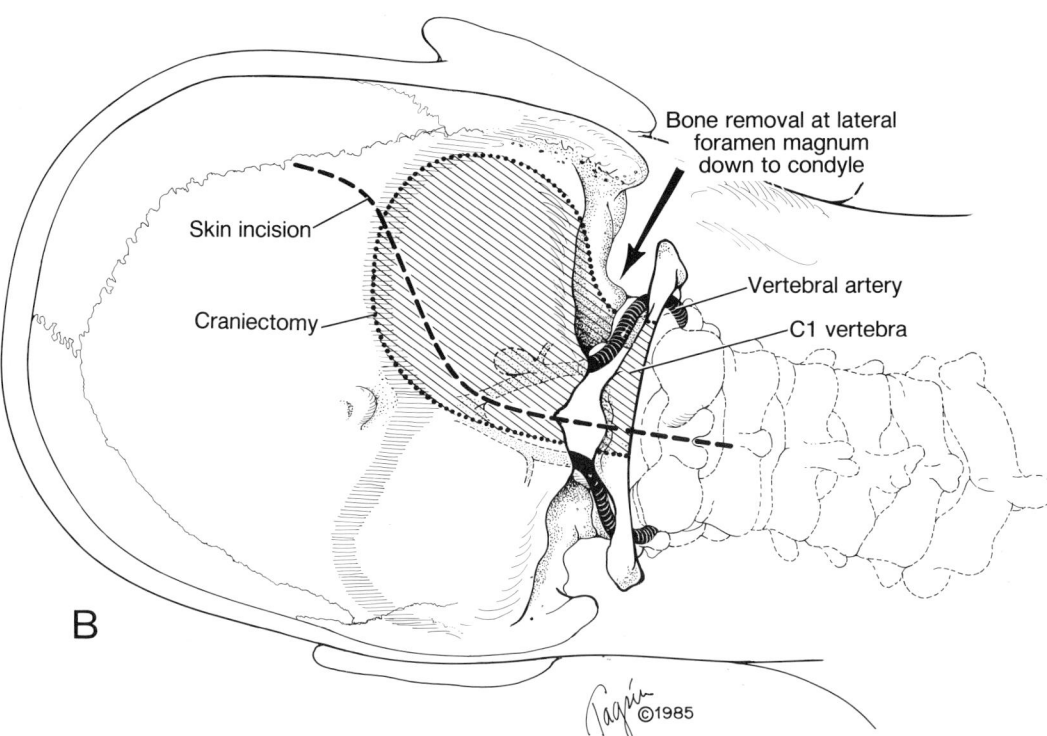

Figure 18.4. Lateral suboccipital approach to the vertebral basilar junction. **A**, Position of the patient. The head is in the straight lateral position, slightly elevated in reference to the heart, and tilted toward the ipsilateral shoulder to allow the cerebrospinal fluid to drain away from the operative field. **B**, Skin incision and craniectomy. Removal of the rim of the foramen magnum is carried laterally to just behind the occipital condyle. The posterior arch of C1 is removed from the arterial sulcus of the vertebral artery laterally to just beyond the midline medially. It is important to expose the vertebral artery so as to avoid injuring it prior to craniectomy and removal of the arch of C1. **C**, After the craniectomy and removal of the posterior arch of C1, the dura is opened in a gentle curve from the junction of the sigmoid and transverse sinus superiorly to the midline just below C1. **D**, After the dura and the arachnoid are opened, the preferred direction of approach is in the space between the eleventh cranial nerve inferiorly and the ninth and tenth cranial nerves superiorly (*arrow*). In this particular sketch, an aneurysm at the origin of the posterior inferior cerebellar artery is illustrated. (**B–D** are from Heros RC: Lateral suboccipital approach for vertebral and vertebrobasilar artery lesions. *J Neurosurg* 64:555–562, 1986.)

Basilar Trunk and Vertebral Artery Aneurysms

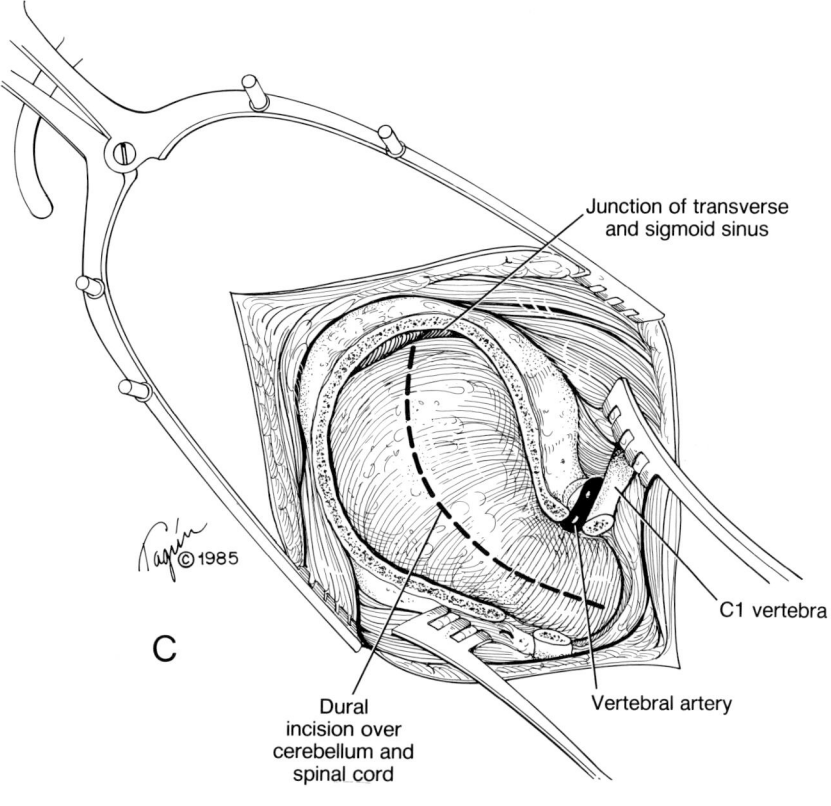

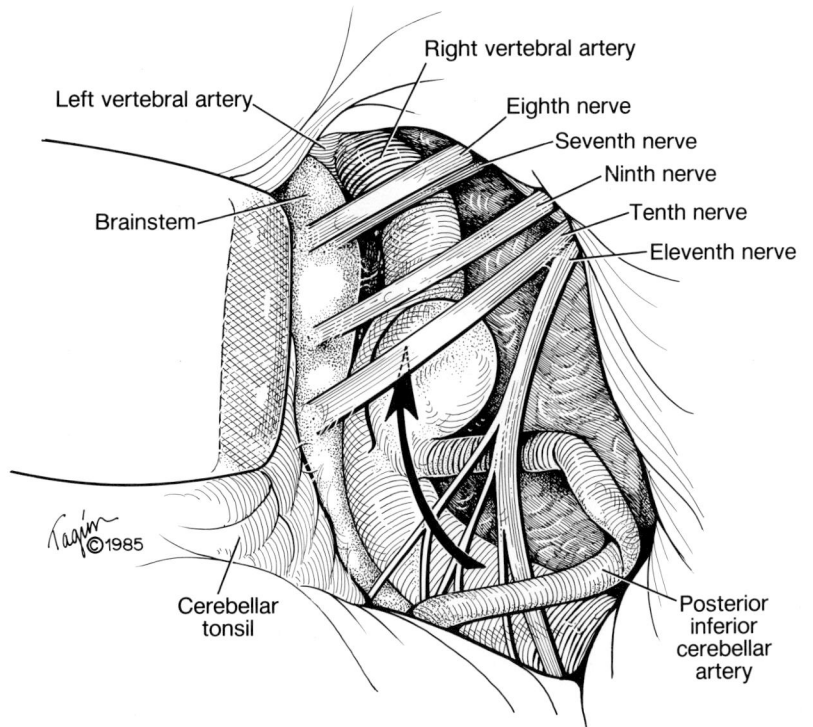

Figure 18.4C and D.

Inferolaterally, sharp dissection is preferred, and the posterior arch of C1 is exposed by subperiosteal dissection, with care exercised especially laterally so as to not injure the vertebral artery. The incision is held open with large (Weitlander) retractors. The craniectomy extends from the junction of the transverse and sigmoid sinuses to just beyond the midline through the foramen magnum in a teardrop fashion (Fig. 18.4C). After the suboccipital craniectomy is accomplished, the arch of C1 is removed from just beyond the midline in the opposite side to the sulcus arteriosus underlying the vertebral artery on the ipsilateral side. Laterally, the perivertebral venous plexus overlying the vertebral artery must be carefully coagulated or packed. It is not uncommon to encounter brisk venous bleeding at this point, but with patience this can usually be controlled. The authors prefer to expose the vertebral artery in order to avoid injuring it. However, with experience this may not be necessary. The removal of the arch of C1 allows an approach from a more inferior direction below the cerebellar tonsil, without the need for retraction of the lateral mass of the cerebellar hemisphere.

The critical aspect of this exposure is extensive removal of bone in the area of the foramen magnum; this removal is carried laterally as far as the condylar fossa just posterior to the occipital condyle and just above and behind the entry of the vertebral artery into the dura (Fig. 18.5). Brisk venous bleeding can also be encountered in this region; it can be controlled with bipolar coagulation and packing with Surgicel. As the bone removal proceeds laterally, the bone edge becomes more vertical, and it becomes impossible to reach under the bone with the footplate of a Kerrison rongeur. A high-speed air drill is very useful for the last 3 or 4 mm of exposure. Not infrequently, a small emissary branch of the vertebral artery is encountered perforating the bone behind the condyle; it is not necessary to carry bone removal beyond this point. This extreme lateral removal of bone in the area of the foramen magnum is the key to the approach to the front of the brain stem from an inferolateral angle with minimal or no brain stem retraction. Each extra millimeter removed from the lateral rim of the foramen magnum gains for the surgeon several extra degrees laterally in the angle of exposure. In this respect, the lateral rim of the foramen magnum represents to the suboccipital exposure what the pterion represents to the frontotemporal exposure.

The dura mater is opened on a gentle curve, starting superoloaterally and coming down toward the midline in the area of the foramen magnum and then continuing straight down to just below the level of the removed arch of C1 (Fig. 18.4C). The lateral aspect of the dura is tented up tightly to the lateral muscle mass to maximize the lateral angle of exposure. After the dura is opened, the microscope is brought into the field, and the arachnoid is opened inferiorly. The vertebral artery is encountered im-

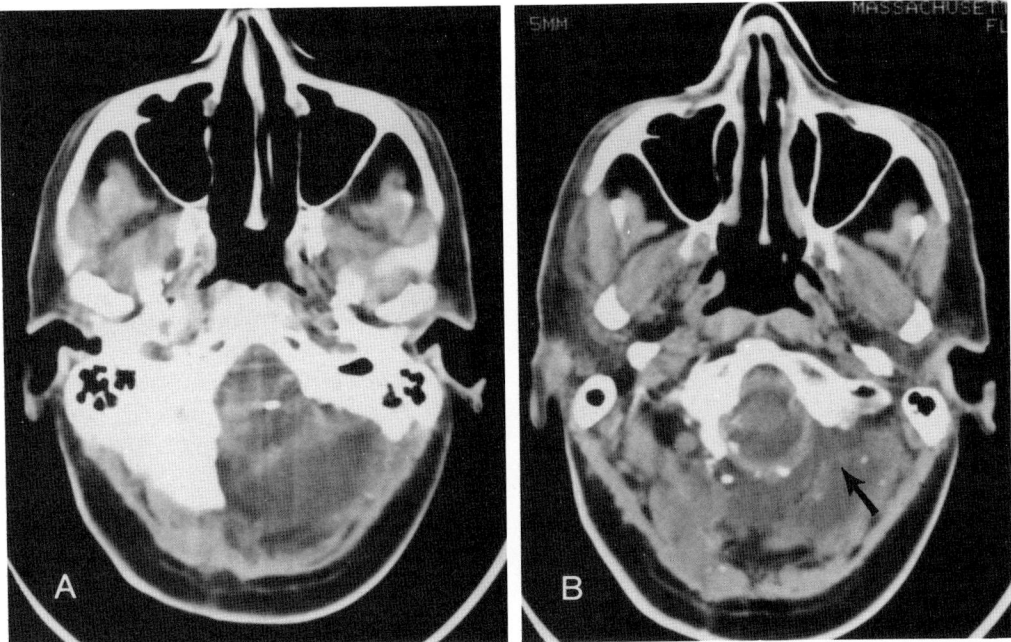

Figure 18.5. Postoperative CT scans of a patient operated via the suboccipital approach. **A,** Scan indicating the amount of bone removal in the suboccipital region. **B,** Scan indicating the amount of bone removal at the level of the foramen magnum and C1. The *arrow* indicates the direction of the operative approach.

mediately (Fig. 18.4D). Sometimes, it is helpful to cut the first dentate ligament to allow the medulla to fall away. The tonsil of the cerebellum is gently lifted upward and medially with a self-retaining retractor. The origin of the posterior inferior cerebellar artery is immediately apparent. The authors then prefer to continue the approach in the direction of the vertebral artery between the eleventh cranial nerve inferiorly and the ninth and tenth cranial nerves superiorly (Fig. 18.4D). The vertebrobasilar junction can be reached through this space in the majority of cases. The authors have found that this space is wider than the space between the ninth and tenth cranial nerves and the seventh and eighth cranial nerves more superiorly. In addition, it is their impression that the seventh and eighth cranial nerves are more sensitive and a complete loss of function of these nerves can develop from even the most gentle manipulation. The ninth and tenth cranial nerves seem to be more resistant to injury, although serious injury to these nerves is more life-threatening than injury to other cranial nerves.

In cases of a relatively high vertebrobasilar junction, the surgeon must move the line of vision upward to the space between the seventh and eighth cranial nerves superiorly and the ninth and tenth nerves inferiorly. Another useful maneuver is to direct the line of vision through the upper space, between the seventh-eighth and ninth-tenth nerve complexes, but apply the clip through the wider space below the ninth and tenth cranial nerves.

With this approach, one can usually see not only the ipsilateral vertebrobasilar junction but also the distalmost portion of the opposite vertebral artery, thus gaining complete control at the origin of the aneurysm. In cases of a large aneurysm, the basilar artery may be obscured by the bulk of the aneurysm, and the aneurysm must be retracted forward or backward to see the basilar artery clearly. It must be emphasized that this exposure is not easy and that the surgeon is working in a very narrow space. When the vertrobasilar junction is very high, a combined approach may be preferable.

Results

During the past 5 years, the authors have operated on 7 patients with aneurysms at the vertebrobasilar junction (see Table 18.1). Five of these patients have done well. Sometimes, it is very difficult to gain complete exposure of the anatomy, and this difficulty resulted in a fatality in one of the patients who had a bilobular aneurysm that ruptured at exposure. The situation was controlled by clipping the aneurysm, but because of the limited exposure, it was not appreciated at the time of surgery that one lobe of the aneurysm projecting behind the basilar to the contralateral side had been left out of the clip. The patient died of a fatal postoperative hemorrhage from

Table 18.1.
Surgical Results in Basilar Trunk and Vertebral Aneurysms

Location	Result		
	Good	Fair	Dead
Basilar trunk	5	0	0
Vertebrobasilar junction	5	0	2
Vertebral-posterior inferior cerebellar artery	11	1	0
Peripheral posterior inferior cerebellar artery	3[a]	0	1[b]

[a]One patient had five different peripheral PICA aneurysms
[b]This patient was operated in extremis (grade 5) after his mycotic aneurysm ruptured into the fourth ventricle.

the unclipped portion of the aneurysm. A second death occurred in a patient with a giant aneurysm of the vertebrobasilar junction that could be exposed but not clipped satisfactorily. The ipsilateral vertebral artery was ligated just proximal to the aneurysm. At surgery, the blood seemed to be "settling" inside of the aneurysm which became much softer. It was intended that an angiogram be performed about a week after surgery and that if the aneurysm remained unthrombosed, contralateral vertebral artery ligation would proceed. The patient died of a massive aneurysmal hemorrhage on the fifth postoperative day. None of these patients had a significant permanent cranial nerve palsy as a result of the surgical approach, although in some there was mild transient difficulty with swallowing and hoarseness.

VERTEBRAL-POSTERIOR INFERIOR CEREBELLAR ARTERY ANEURYSMS

Presentation and Evaluation

Aneurysms of the vertebral-posterior inferior cerebellar artery usually arise at the distal carina at the origin of the posterior inferior cerebellar artery from the vertebral artery (Fig 18.6A). The vertebral artery may have a tortuous course, and the origin of the posterior inferior cerebellar artery may vary. These aneurysms can occur from near the intracranial entry of the vertebral artery to near the vertebrobasilar junction. They tend to point superiorly and slightly posteriorly and lie against the medulla. They usually have an intimate relationship with the vagal and hypoglossal nerves.

Most patients with this aneurysm present with subarachnoid hemorrhage. The headache is more likely to be localized to the neck and occipital region than is the headache from an anterior circulation aneurysm. Subarachnoid hemorrhage with a sixth nerve or lower cranial nerve palsy is often due to this aneurysm. Giant aneurysms may present with symptoms and signs suggesting cerebellopontine angle tumor. The true size may only be seen with the computed tomography (CT) scan. The CT scan alone

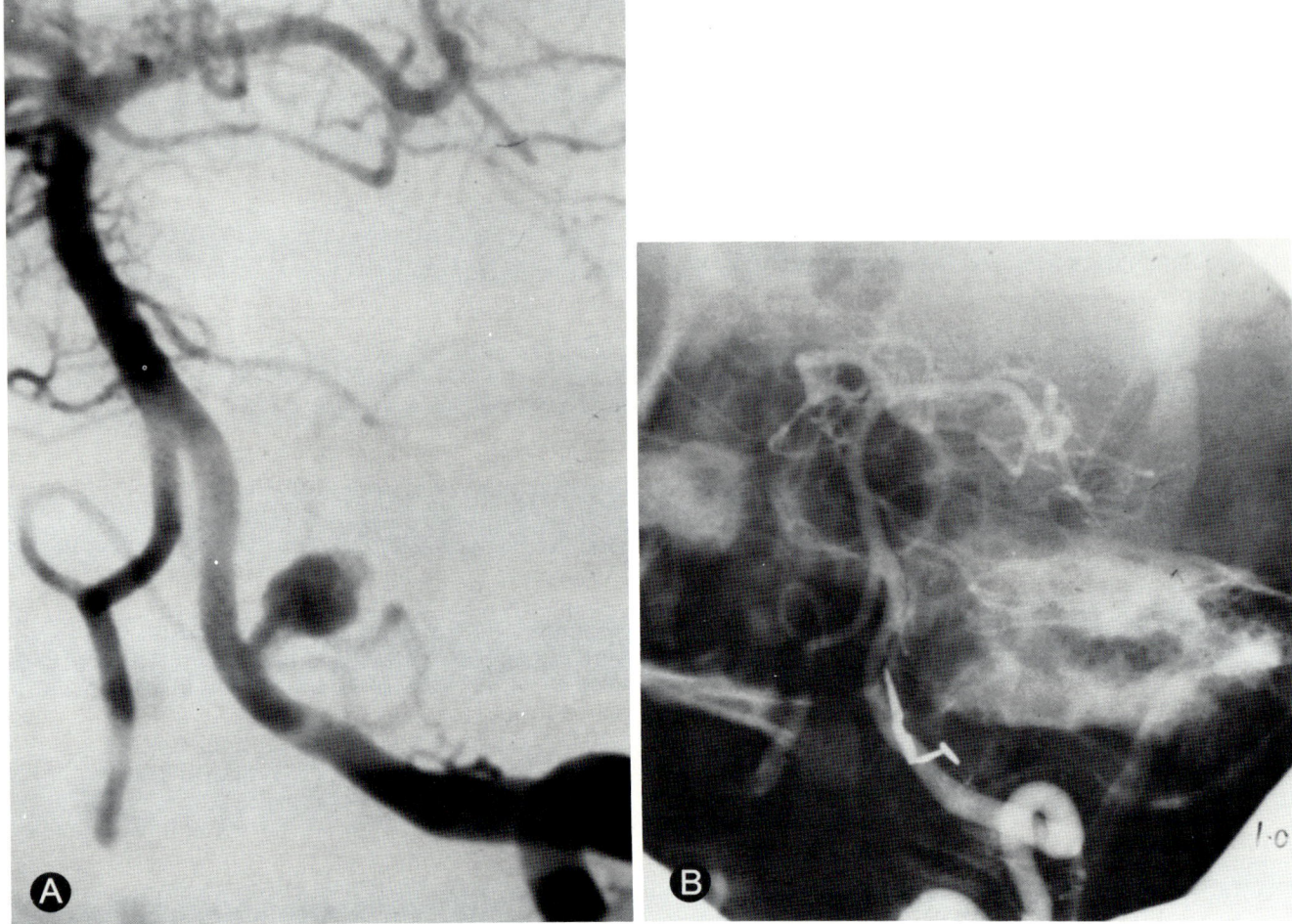

Figure 18.6. Vertebral-posterior inferior cerebellar artery aneurysm. **A**, Preoperative angiogram showing aneurysm arising from distal crotch of origin of the posterior inferior cerebellar artery from the vertebral artery. **B**, Postoperative angiogram demonstrating obliteration of the aneurysm and preservation of the posterior inferior cerebellar artery.

may suggest a posterior interior cerebellar artery aneurysm when there is little blood in the cisterns of the circle of Willis and the blood is concentrated in the cisterna magna, around the lower brain stem, and in the fourth ventricle. When a posterior inferior cerebellar artery aneurysm is suspected or bilateral carotid angiography is negative in subarachnoid hemorrhage, it is important that both vertebral arteries be visualized to include the origin of both posterior inferior cerebellar arteries, even if separate injections of the two vertebral arteries are needed.

Surgical Management

It has been our observation that generalized vasospasm is rare in cases of ruptured posterior inferior cerebellar artery aneurysms, since there is usually little blood around the circle of Willis. This observation coupled with the fact that little retraction is required to clip these aneurysms has led the authors to a policy of considering surgery as early as possible after subarachnoid hemorrhage in these patients, without regard to vasospasm or presumed brain fullness. These aneurysms are approached through a unilateral suboccipital craniectomy (3, 5, 7, 14, 15).

The authors prefer to use the position, skin incision, and craniectomy described in the preceding section (7) (Fig. 18.4). However, posterior inferior cerebellar artery aneurysms usually are more laterally placed, and there is no need to be as aggressive with bone removal in the lateral aspect of the foramen magnum. Likewise, depending on the location of the aneurysm, one may chose not to remove the arch of C1. In general, the more distal and anterior the aneurysm, the more inferolateral the angle of approach should be in order to avoid deep cerebellar and brain stem retraction. Therefore, the authors remove the arch of C1 and in cases of more distal vertebral or vertebrobasilar junction aneurysms, are aggressive in lateral bone removal at the foramen magnum. The more proximal vertebral artery aneurysms are immediately seen after the dura is opened through a simple unilateral suboccipital craniectomy that is carried to the foramen magnum. Other surgeons believe that it is unnecessary in these cases to carry the craniectomy to the foramen magnum (8, 17). However, if one does not do this, more cerebellar retraction is required, since one must work from laterally, around the cerebellum, rather than from inferiorly, under the tonsil of the cerebellum. In the past, the authors used a "hockey stick" skin incision. With use of this incision, muscle mass is in the way, and one loses the advantage of a more lateral angle of vision. Therefore, the authors now use the skin incision shown in Figure 18.4B which allows for the muscle to be divided laterally.

After the dura is opened (Fig.18.4D), the cerebellum is lifted off the medulla with a narrow retractor blade placed on the base of the tonsil (Fig. 18.7A). The eleventh nerve is exposed. The vertebral artery is identified emerging from under the dentate ligament, and the loop of the posterior inferior cerebellar artery is seen. The vertebral artery is traced distally. The origin of the posterior inferior cerebellar artery, almost always just proximal to the lesion, serves as a good landmark. Exposure is gained with patience and gentle dissection (Fig. 18.7B). The access to the lesion and the posterior inferior cerebellar artery is between filaments of the tenth and eleventh nerves which must be protected meticulously against the possibility of injury which can cause disabling hoarseness and dysphagia. In addition, any arterial branches to the medulla should be spared. As the rest of the aneurysm is brought into view, it is best to work on either side of the posterior inferior cer-

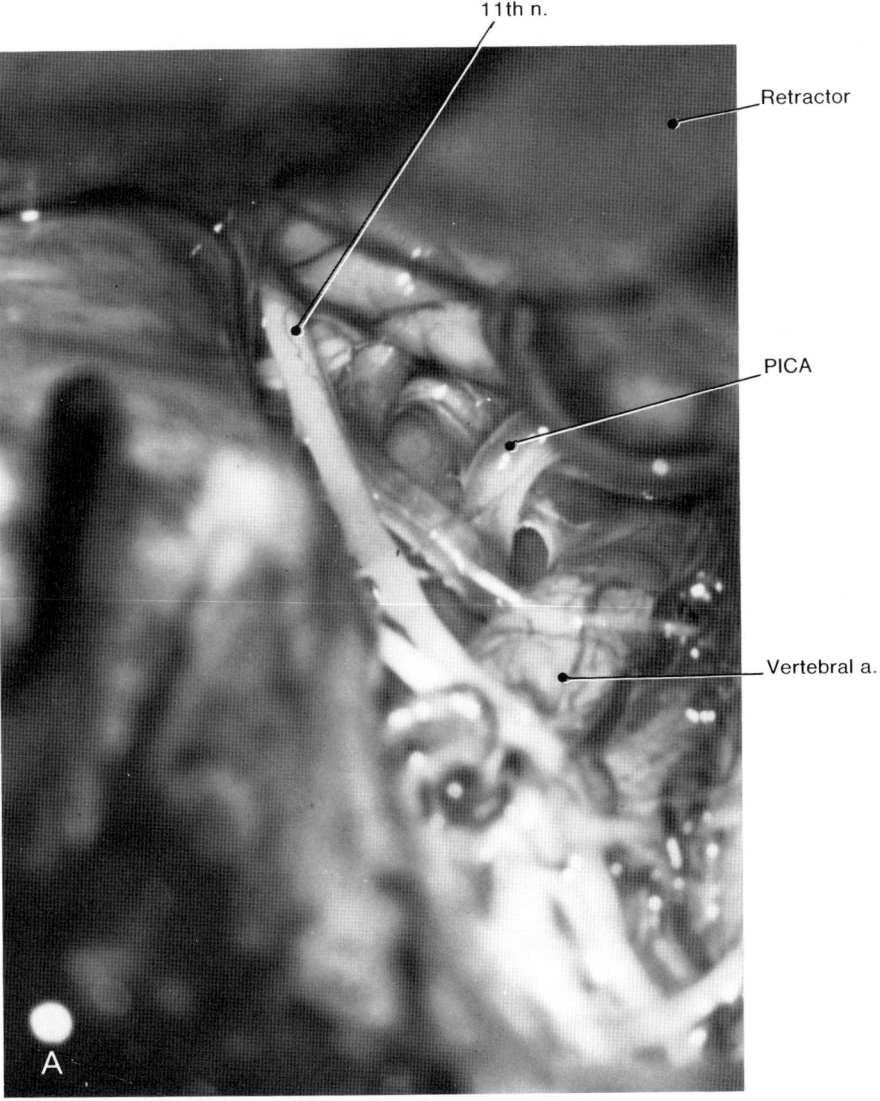

Figure 18.7A. The cerebellum is lifted with a narrow retractor blade placed on the tonsil. The vertebral artery is identified and the loop of the posterior inferior cerebellar artery (*PICA*) is seen.

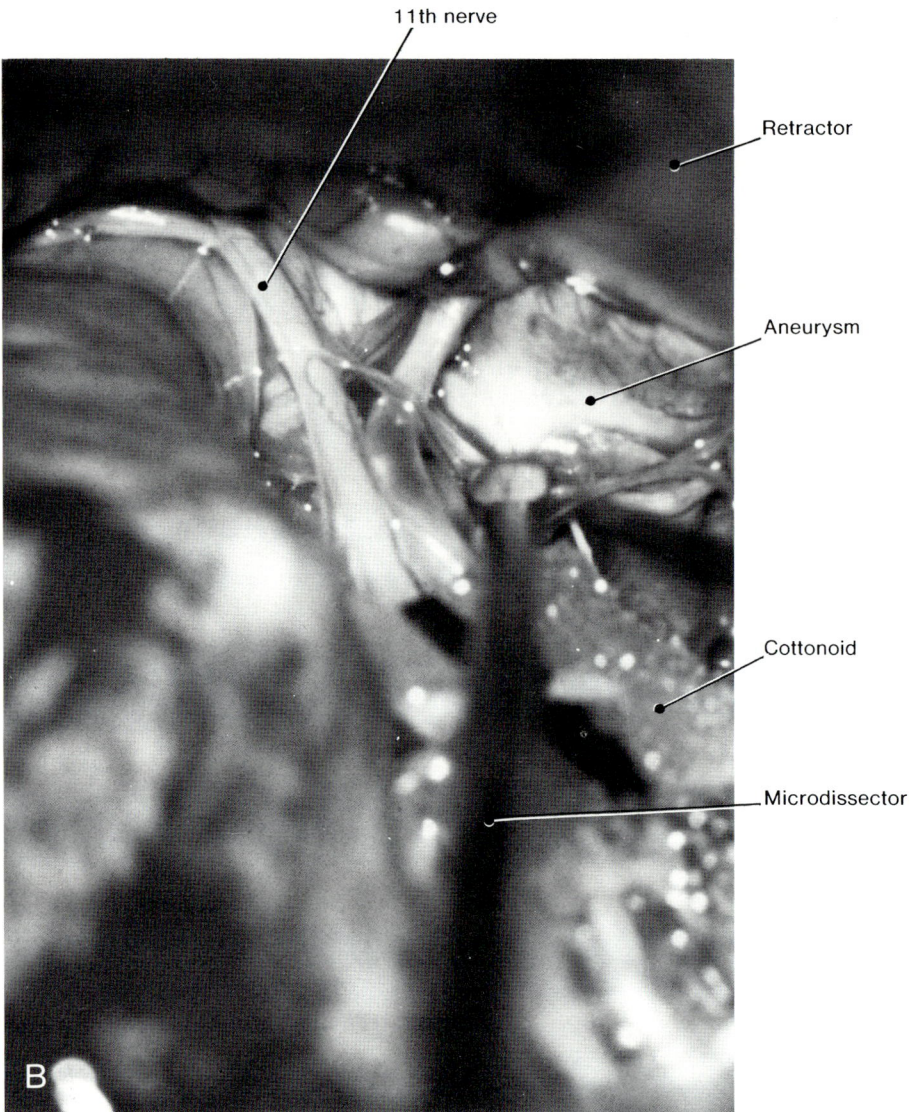

Figure 18.7B. The wall of the aneurysm is visualized. The lateral posterior inferior cerebellar artery loop has been depressed and is covered with a cottonoid. Rootlets of the vagus nerve crossing the posterior surface of the aneurysm are being freed with the straight dissector.

ebellar artery and up the sides of the vertebral artery beyond the neck (Fig. 18.7C). Usually, that portion of the dome of the aneurysm adherent to the medulla can be left undisturbed, and only the neck isolated (Fig. 18.7D). On occasion, depending on the projection of the aneurysm, it may be necessary to dissect it out of a medullary indentation. Bipolar coagulation may be needed to define the neck. Some care will be needed during this maneuver to avoid injury to the twelfth cranial nerve on the far side of the neck. A small straight clip or a clip with a Drake aperture encircling the posterior inferior cerebellar artery may be used after the neck is prepared.

Results

Peerless and Drake have reported on a series of 69 patients who were grade 1 or 2 at the time of operation. There were 59 patients with excellent results, 8 with good results, and 2 who died (14). Yasargil had 9 patients with good results and 1 with a fair result among 10 patients (17). Yamainura et al reported "satisfactory" results in all 17 patients with vertebral-posterior inferior cerebellar artery aneurysm (16). During the past 5 years, the present authors have treated 12 patients with aneurysms in this location with good results, except for 1 patient who

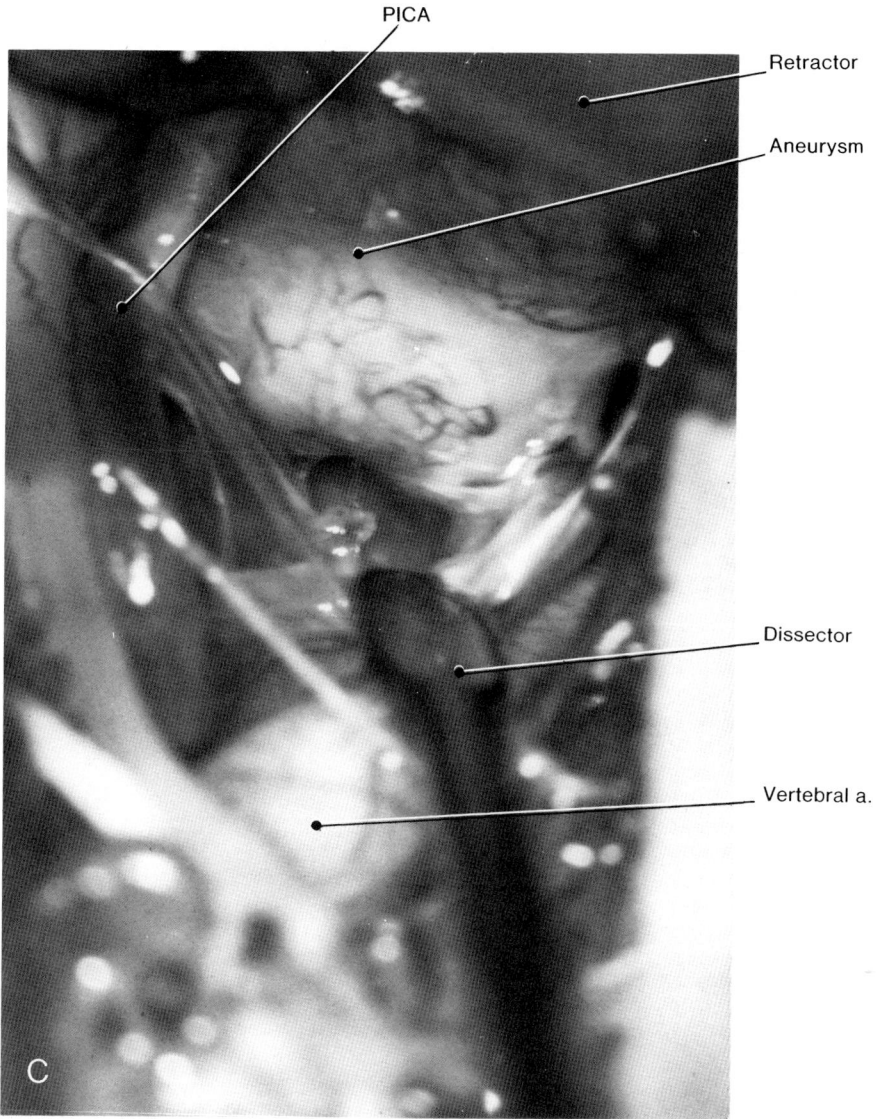

Figure 18.7C. The neck of the aneurysm is exposed. Dissection with a microdissector progresses on each side of the posterior inferior cerebellar artery (*PICA*) and along the vertebral artery.

developed a lateral medullary infarction probably from kinking of the posterior inferior cerebellar artery origin by an improperly placed clip. She had an almost complete recovery within a few months. Some of the patients had mild temporary lower cranial nerve difficulties, but in none was this a serious problem (see Table 18.1).

PERIPHERAL POSTERIOR INFERIOR CEREBELLAR ARTERY ANEURYSMS

Presentation

Aneurysms of the posterior inferior cerebellar artery distal to its origin from the vertebral artery are rare, comprising between 0.5 and 0.7% of all intracranial aneurysms. In a recent review, 61 cases were collated from the literature (1). Whenever these aneurysms are seen, especially if they are multiple or are associated with peripheral aneurysms in other locations, an infectious etiology should be suspected. However, the authors have reported on the remarkable case of a patient with five distinct peripheral posterior inferior cerebellar artery aneurysms without any evidence of an infectious etiology on culture and histology of the excised aneurysmal wall (1).

These aneurysms usually present with subarachnoid hemorrhage with headache localized in the neck and occipital region. There is usually CT scan evidence of clot in the posterior fossa or fourth ventricle with frequent hydrocephalus and little blood in the

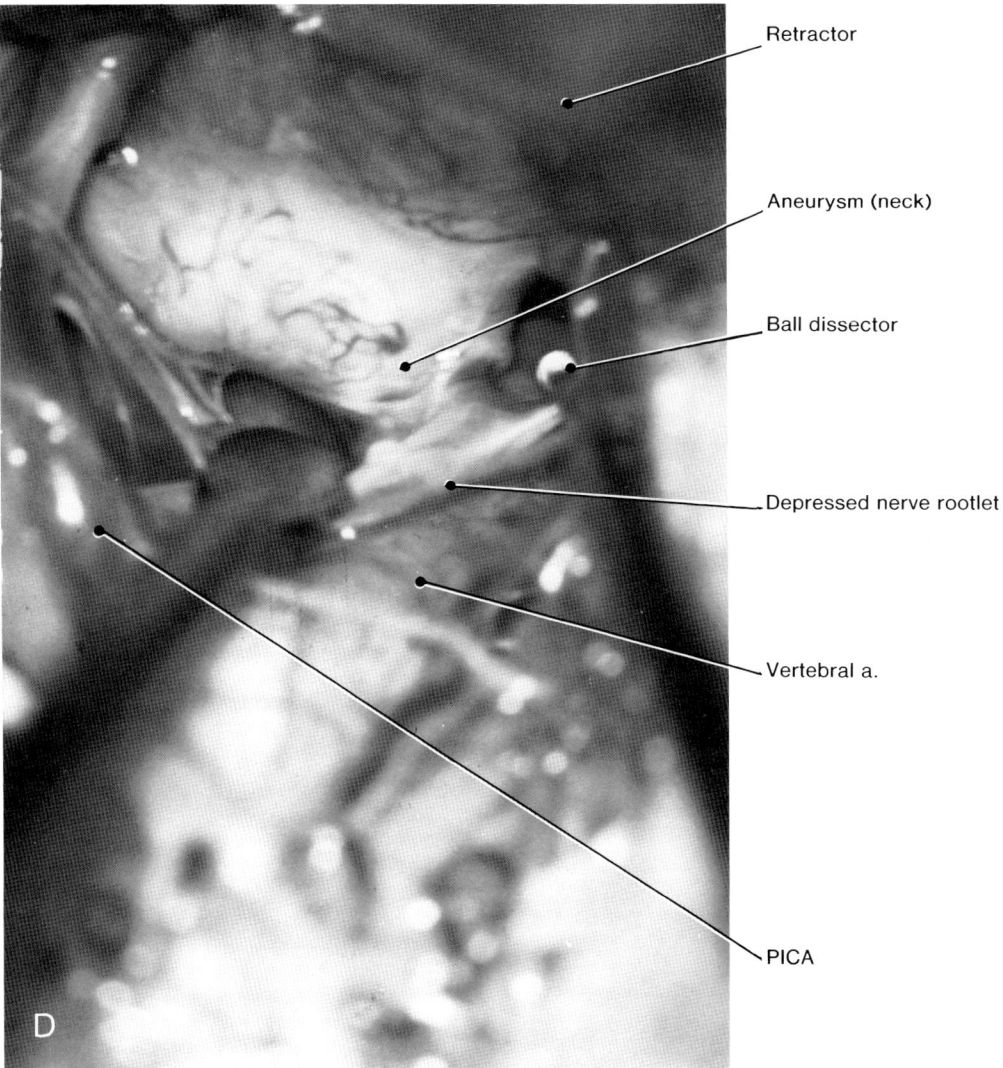

Figure 18.7D. Some of the rootlets of the vagus nerve have been depressed, exposing the lateral side of the neck (straight microdissector) and the medial side of the neck (microball dissector). The aneurysm is ready for clipping. *PICA*, posterior inferior cerebellar artery.

cisterns of the circle of Willis. Whenever an aneurysm in this location is suspected by the CT appearance, full four-vessel angiography is required, since simple reflux into the origin of the contralateral posterior inferior cerebellar artery from a single vertebral injection may fail to opacify a more peripherally located posterior inferior cerebellar artery aneurysm.

Surgical Management

The surgical approach to these aneurysms must be based on a good understanding of the anatomy of the posterior inferior cerebellar artery. This artery can be divided into five segments (12). The first two segments lie anterior and lateral to the medulla. Aneurysms in these locations can be approached inferolaterally by gentle elevation and medial retraction of the tonsil, as described for vertebral-posterior inferior cerebellar artery aneurysms. The next segment, the tonsillomedullary segment, courses behind the medulla in front of the tonsil. For aneurysms in this location, the authors would use a combined lateral and medial suboccipital craniectomy essentially as described for vertebral-posterior inferior cerebellar artery aneurysms but with bone removal extending well past the midline in the inferior aspect of the occipital bone and the foramen magnum as well as the arch of C1. Control of the proximal posterior inferior cerebellar artery is then gained from laterally; this may be useful in case temporary clipping is advisable. Then the surgeon has the option, depending on the location of the aneurysm, of retracting the tonsil upward, medially, or laterally. In most instances, the authors prefer to remove the tonsil by suction and approach the aneurysm by subpial dissection after temporary clipping of the posterior inferior cerebellar artery distal to its medullary branches. In this location, temporary clipping should be safe for a relatively long period, and there is no need to risk a major rupture which could almost certainly be prevented by temporary clipping. The authors prefer to resect rather than retract the tonsil because these aneurysms are adherent to the tonsil and could rupture as the tonsil is retracted.

Aneurysms of the posterior inferior cerebellar artery distal to its cranial loop (televelotonsillar and cortical segments) can be approached by a standard midline suboccipital craniectomy extending through the foramen magnum and with removal of the posterior arch of C1 (11, 16). The aneurysm can be approached between the tonsils by gently retracting them laterally or, if hidden behind one tonsil or adherent to it, by suction of tonsillar tissue and subpial dissection. Aneurysms located more peripherally in a cortical branch of the posterior inferior cerebellar artery are almost always infectious and should be treated by resection of the arterial segment rather than by clipping. It should be safe to resect a branch of the posterior inferior cerebellar artery at this level, since the last important branches to the deep cerebellar nuclei are given at about the choroidal point in the cranial loop (televelotonsillar segment) of the posterior inferior cerebellar artery (12).

Results

Results of operations on peripherally located posterior inferior cerebellar artery aneurysms have almost invariable been excellent (1, 5, 16, 17). In addition to the above-mentioned patient with five posterior inferior cerebellar artery aneurysms successfuly clipped with preservation of the parent vessel, the authors have seen 3 other patients with peripheral posterior inferior cerebellar artery aneurysms (see Table 18.1). In all 3 the aneurysm was in the cranial loop, near the midline, in relation to the floor of the fourth ventricle. One patient had an infectious aneurysm that bled massively, resulting in apnea and decerebration while he was hospitalized, being treated with antibiotics. He died in spite of emergency craniotomy and resection of the aneurysm and blood clot in the cerebellum and fourth ventricle. The other 2 patients did well after uncomplicated clipping of noninfectious aneurysms.

REFERENCES

1. Beyerl BD, Heros RC: Multiple peripheral aneurysms of the posterior inferior cerebellar artery. Neurosurgery 19:285–289, 1986.
2. Chou SN, Oritz-Suarez HJ: Surgical treatment of arterial aneurysms of the vertebrobasilar circulation. J Neurosurg 41:671–680, 1974.
3. Drake CG: The surgical treatment of aneurysms of the basilar artery. J Neurosurg 29:436–446, 1968.
4. Drake CG: The surgical treatment of vertebral basilar aneurysms. Clin Neurosurg 16:114–169, 1969.
5. Drake CG: The treatment of aneurysms of the posterior circulation. Clin Neurosurg 26:96–144, 1979.
6. Hammon WM, Kempe LG: The posterior fossa approach to aneurysms of the vertebral and basilar arteries. J Neurosurg 37:339–347, 1972.
7. Heros RC: Lateral suboccipital approach for vetebral and vertebrobasilar artery lesions. J Neurosurg 64:555–562, 1986.
8. Ito Z: Microsurgery of Cerebral Aneurysms. Amsterdam, Elsevier, 1985, p 227.
9. Kasdon DL, Stein BM: Combined supratentorial and infratentorial exposure for low-lying basilar aneurysms. Neurosurgery 4:422–426,1979.
10. Kawase T, Toya S, Shiobara R, Mine T: Transpetrosal approach for aneurysms of the lower basilar artery. J Neurosurg 63:857–861, 1985.
11. Kempe LG: Operative Neurosurgery. New York, Springer-Verlag, 1970, vol 2, pp 66–71.
12. Lister JR, Rhoton AL, Matsushima T, Peace DA: Microsurgical anatomy of the posterior inferior cerebellar artery. Neurosurgery 10:170–199, 1982.
13. Nishimoto A, Fujimoto S, Tsuchimoto S, et al: Anterior inferior cerebellar artery aneurysm. J Neurosurg 59:697–702, 1983.
14. Peerless SJ, Drake CG: Management of aneurysms of posterior circulation. In Youmans JR (ed): Neurological Surgery, ed 2. Philadelphia, WB Saunders, 1982, pp 1715–1763.
15. Rhoton AL Jr: Anatomy of saccular aneurysms. Surg Neurol 14:59–66, 1980.
16. Yamainura A, Ise H, Makino H: Radiometric study on posterior inferior cerebellar aneurysms with special reference to accessibility by the lateral suboccipital approach. Neurol Med Chir 21:721–733, 1981.
17. Yasargil MG: Vertebrobasilar aneurysms. In Yasargil MG (ed): Microneurosurgery. New York, Thieme-Stratton, 1984, vol 2, pp 232–295.
18. Zlotnik E, Skylut J, Smejanovich A, Stasenko E: Saccular aneurysm of the anterior inferior cerebellar-internal auditory artery. J Neurosurg 57:829–832, 1982.

19

Multiple, Unruptured, and Asymptomatic Aneurysms

MULTIPLE ANEURYSMS

Evaluation and Management

In clinical and angiographic series of intracranial aneurysms, multiple lesions are found in approximately 15% of the patients (20–22). The incidence of multiple aneurysms is a compelling reason to perform four-vessel angiography in all patients known to have one aneurysm.

Multiple aneurysms may be associated with cerebral arterial anomalies (such as a duplicated communicating artery or azygous anterior cerebral artery), moya moya disease (23), polycystic kidney disease, familial incidence (1), and hypertension (26). The existence of multiple aneurysms on a single vessel suggests a developmental defect (13).

When aneurysms are multiple, they often occur in "mirror" locations, e.g., upon both internal carotid or middle cerebral arteries. Multiple lesions can involve anterior and posterior circulations. Sometimes, several aneurysms will be found on a single artery (2, 13).

Although transient ischemic attacks (TIAs) or seizures may occasionally draw attention to multiple aneurysms, the usual presentation is subarachnoid hemorrhage. In this situation, the initial problem facing the clinician is determination of which aneurysm ruptured. On the basis of angiographic criteria, Wood was able to pinpoint the site of bleeding correctly in 90% of the cases, as confirmed at surgery or autopsy (40). In this study, the bleeding lesion was associated with larger size, multiple lobes, local mass effect, or local spasm. Computed tomography (CT) scanning makes the identification of the bleeding source more accurate. Demonstration of local subarachnoid hematoma in relation to an aneurysm is strong evidence of its rupture. On the other hand, subarachnoid clot demonstrated by CT scanning may be misleading. A hematoma in the interpeduncular cistern may come from an internal carotid-posterior communicating artery aneurysm instead of from a basilar artery aneurysm. Clinical, CT, and angiographic data should be weighed carefully in the determination of the site of bleeding. In one study with surgical or pathologic confirmation, the overall accuracy of determining the site of bleeding was 97.5% (24). Irregular shape was the most significant indicator of site of rupture. Focal spasm, focal mass effect, and serial change were highly reliable but infrequent signs.

Once the source of the subarachnoid hemorrhage has been ascertained, therapy for this lesion proceeds according to the plan described in Chapters 10 and 11. If, during the procedure to obliterate the bleeding aneurysm, one or more asymptomatic lesions are easily exposed and can be clipped with little or no increased risk to the patient, this is done (30). This approach also provides the surgeon with the opportunity to examine several aneurysms, particularly if at surgery the presumed bleeding aneurysm shows no local signs of hemorrhage. If none of the lesions examined at surgery seems to have bled, then one must conclude that the source is elsewhere, and if another aneurysm is known to exist, this lesion should be treated during the same anesthesia if the patient's condition is satisfactory; if this is not practical, it must be treated at the earliest opportunity.

If the bleeding lesion has been clipped and one or more aneurysms exist outside the operative field, therapy for these lesions is guided by the criteria outlined for asymptomatic aneurysms because the likelihood of bleeding from the unruptured aneurysm is low. If the patient has no significant neurologic deficit after surgery, the authors usually wait about 6 weeks between operations to allow sufficient recovery from the first procedure. If, however, the patient has a neurologic deficit after the initial surgery, a greater period of time between procedures should be considered.

Operative Technique

For multiple aneurysms, the scalp and bone flap may be modified to provide access to as many lesions as possible (29). A frontotemporal bone flap may be carried posteriorly into the temporal region to provide both a subfrontal access to the internal carotid circulation and a subtemporal approach to the basilar artery bifurcation. In some cases, a standard pterional approach may provide satisfactory exposure to the internal carotid artery and basilar artery bifurcation. A coronal incision with the bone flap extending across the midline and low into the pterional area can provide access to both internal carotid and middle cerebral artery lesions, as well as to a distal anterior cerebral artery aneurysm (Fig. 19.1). A generous frontotemporal flap may provide access to both internal carotid arteries and even both middle cerebral arteries if cerebrospinal fluid is drained extensively. An S-shaped suboccipital incision with a lateral bone exposure to the foramen magnum (Chapter 18) may be used to clip multiple aneurysms in the posterior fossa (Fig. 19.2A and B). It should be emphasized, however, that inadequate exposure should not be accepted (Fig. 19.3). When an asymptomatic aneurysm cannot be dealt with safely through the exposure being used for a symptomatic aneurysm, it is better practice to defer its therapy for another day when optimum surgical exposure can be obtained.

When multiple lesions are exposed in an operative field, a major decision is to determine which lesion to clip first. In principle, one prefers to eliminate the ruptured aneurysm. It is important to maintain exposure to the other lesions in question. If a ruptured superficial lesion is clipped, the clip may obstruct the path to a more deeply placed aneurysm. In this situation, it may be wiser to deal with the more deeply placed lesion first, even if it is unruptured.

UNRUPTURED SYMPTOMATIC ANEURYSMS

Occasionally, an unruptured aneurysm presents with focal neurologic deficit, headache, TIAs, or seizure. When compressive or embolic symptoms develop, the risk of hemorrhage appears to be great. In the Cooperative Study, 28% of such cases managed medically went on to fatal hemorrhage, and another 16% were functionally disabled (17). In the study from the Mayo Clinic, 11 of the 15 unruptured aneurysms that bled had nonhemorrhagic symptoms prior to rupture (37). All symptomatic lesions in this study were 10 mm in diameter or larger.

Among patients with compressive symptoms from aneurysm, the most common presentation is partial or complete third nerve palsy, usually but not always with periorbital pain and a fixed, dilated pupil. This syndrome is usually caused by enlargement of an internal carotid-posterior communicating artery aneurysm, but occasionally a superior cerebellar-basilar artery aneurysm is the culprit. Compression of the optic nerves or chiasm may be caused by an enlarging carotid-ophthalmic or anterior communicating artery aneurysm. Other cranial nerves, including the abducens nerve, can be involved (5, 18). Of course, a giant aneurysm can compress local structures to cause focal signs (see Chapter 20).

Headaches may indicate the presence of a cerebral aneurysm. The precise mechanism for the headaches is obscure. In some patients, pain probably comes from aneurysmal involvement with the dura. In others, it has been suggested that enlargement of the aneurysm may be the cause of headaches.

Intracranial aneurysms may present as TIAs or cerebral infarction (8–10, 28, 33). Proving a causal relationship is difficult and will depend on demonstration of emboli in the distal territory of the parent artery. The mechanism in these cases appears to be dislodgement of mural thrombus within the aneurysm and subsequent distal embolization. CT demonstration of mural thrombus in such a case is strong presumptive evidence for an embolic mechanism. The exact risk of stroke after TIA by such mechanism is unknown but must increase the overall threat from such a lesion.

Seizure may be the first warning of an intracranial aneurysm (16) (Fig. 19.4). Such lesions are generally large with protrusion into frontal or temporal lobes. Gliotic reaction to the mass lesion produces an epileptogenic focus. The appearance of seizures may be related to the increasing size of the lesion.

Evaluation (often detection) of such lesions depends on CT, with and without contrast, and angiography. When the patient is medically stable and the aneurysm accessible, surgical therapy is usually indicated to prevent further neurologic deterioration and to guard against the risk of subarachnoid hemorrhage. Surgery is particularly warranted, on an urgent basis, when there is evidence of aneurysmal enlargement as in the painful third nerve palsy from aneurysmal compression. In some older patients, medical instability and a difficult lesion could favor a conservative approach, with follow-up angiography after 1 year. Interval CT scanning can also detect aneurysmal enlargement, which would favor surgical correction.

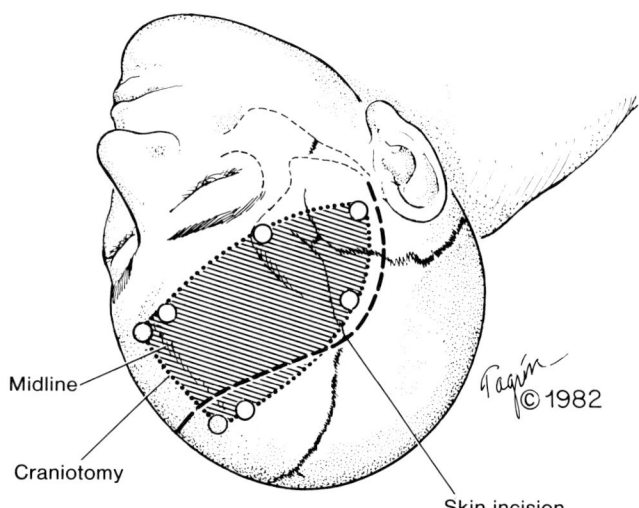

Figure 19.1. Exposure for multiple aneurysms. Coronal skin incision and large bone flap extending across midline provide access to circle of Willis and distal anterior cerebral artery.

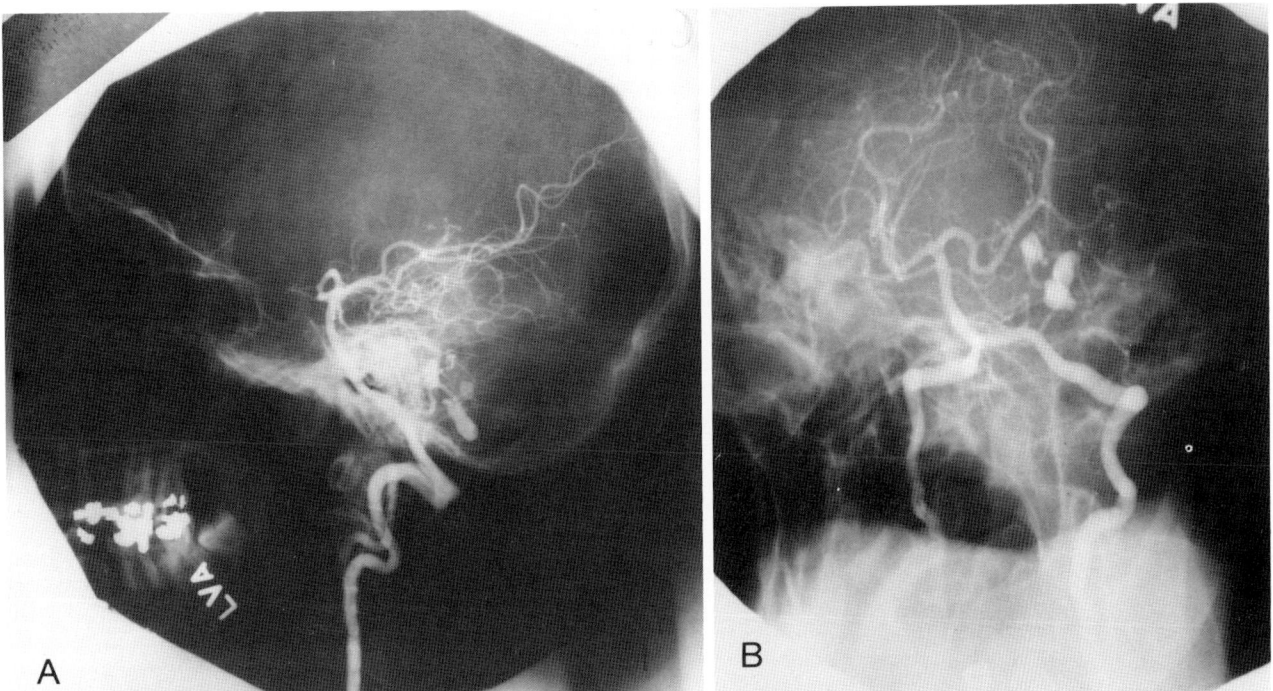

Figure 19.2. **A** and **B**, Preoperative lateral and oblique vertebral angiograms of patient presenting with subarachnoid hemorrhage. The angiograms were interpreted as showing four different aneurysms of the left posterior cerebellar artery. At surgery, five different aneurysms were found at different locations from near the origin to the peripheral tonsillar branches. None of the aneurysms was mycotic in origin. Postoperative angiograms showed obliteration of all the aneurysms with preservation of the posterior inferior cerebellar artery.

ASYMPTOMATIC ANEURYSMS

Not uncommonly, an intracranial aneurysm may be discovered as an incidental finding on CT scanning, magnetic resonance imaging, or cerebral angiography. The combination of carotid stenosis and intracranial aneurysm is discussed in Chapter 1. Unruptured multiple aneurysms, discovered during identification of a separate ruptured lesion, likewise are regarded as asymptomatic aneurysms. CT with contrast and thin sections may be performed, with reformatting in various projections, to delineate unruptured asymptomatic aneurysms (41). Virtually all lesions 10 mm in diameter or larger can be detected with CT.

What is the threat from such asymptomatic aneurysms? Every bleeding aneurysm was once an asymptomatic aneurysm. Growth and rupture of asymptomatic lesions have been documented (12, 21). In this sense, the asymptomatic aneurysm is the precursor of a major threat to life. However, autopsy studies have demonstrated that many intracranial aneurysms, particularly the very small ones, never cause a bleeding episode during life (4, 6, 15).

The frequency of aneurysms in the general population is about 5%, but the average annual incidence of aneurysmal subarachnoid hemorrhage is only 10/100,000 population (27). These data indicate that the vast majority of intracranial aneurysms never rupture nor cause other symptoms.

The selection of patients for surgical treatment depends on the ability to predict which aneurysms pose a substantial threat of rupture. The Cooperative Study suggested that lesions 7 mm in diameter or larger may be regarded as high risk (17). Zacks et al (42) noted no hemorrhages in 7 weeks to 7½ years in a study of aneurysms less than 10 mm in diameter. In the follow-up of multiple intracranial aneurysms, Winn et al (38) noted subarachnoid hemorrhage in 10 of 50 patients (20%) with surgical treatment of a previously ruptured aneurysm; three hemorrhages were believed to emanate from a previously intact aneurysm. Jane and colleagues suggest a bleeding rate of 1%/year for unruptured aneurysm (14). Heiskanan presented data on 61 patients in whom 7 unruptured aneurysms bled over 10 years for a bleeding rate of 1.1%/year (11).

The Mayo Clinic group has presented the largest well-studied series of unruptured aneurysms (161 aneurysms in 130 patients followed 7 years) (34, 36, 37). Of 102 aneurysms smaller than 10 mm, none ruptured, whereas 15 of the 51 aneurysms 10 mm in diameter or greater eventually ruptured. Older patients were more likely to sustain aneurysmal bleeding: for those younger than the median age (59 years) the risk was 3.4%/year, and for those older than the

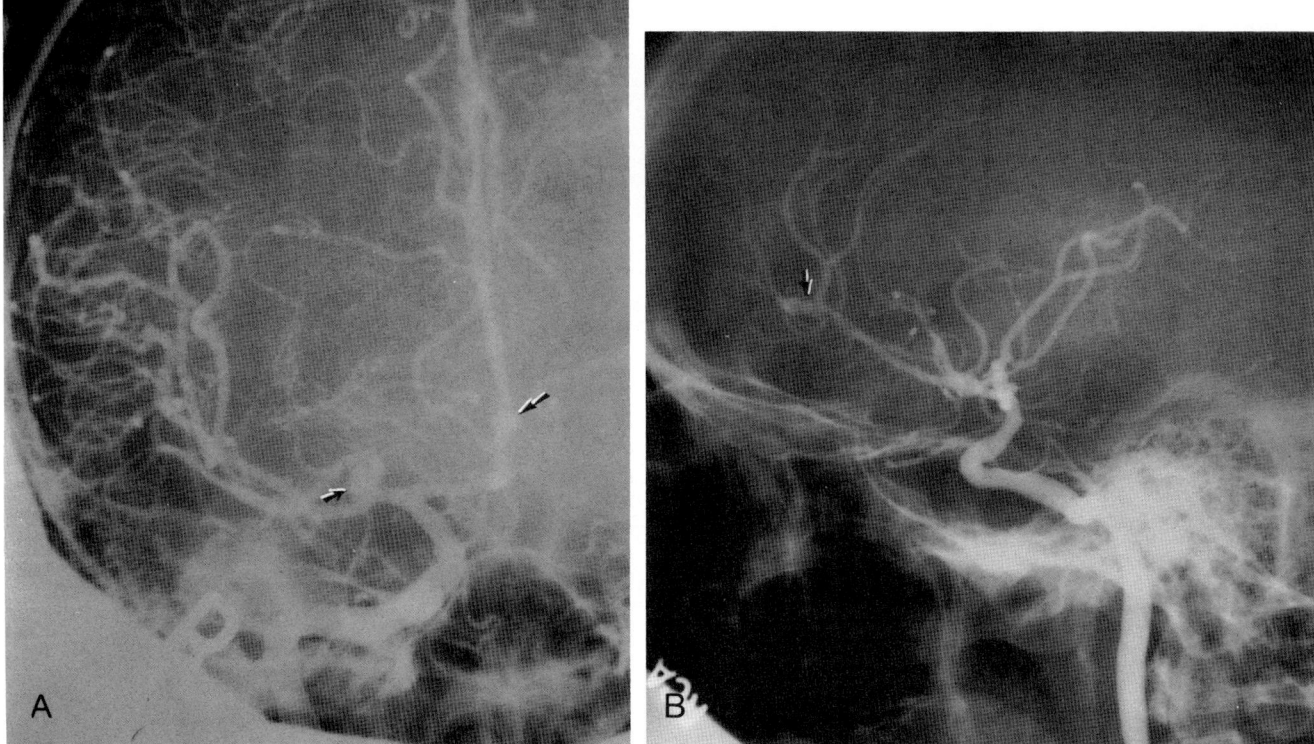

Figure 19.3. Operative approach to multiple aneurysms. **A–E,** Right anteroposterior (AP) and left AP, lateral, and oblique angiograms show four aneurysms (*arrows*): bilateral middle cerebral artery bifurcations, anterior communicating artery, and pericallosal artery. There is also evidence of hydrocephalus. There is no indication as to which aneurysm bled. Comment: This 46-year-old man had subarachnoid hemorrhage with drowsiness but no focal signs. Angiography was done on the ninth day after subarachnoid hemorrhage. The CT scan did not localize the site of the hemorrhage. To approach these lesions, a large left frontal temporal flap that crossed the midline was used. First, the left middle cerebral aneurysm was exposed and clipped via a sylvian fissure approach. This was not the site of hemorrhage. The right middle cerebral aneurysm was seen by going over the optic chiasm and under the frontal lobe to the opposite carotid bifurcation and then exposing the middle cerebral bifurcation. This exposure was not easy, and the aneurysm was clipped with difficulty. Next, the anterior communicating aneurysm was exposed and clipped. This was the lesion that had bled. The dura was opened to the right of midline, the right frontal lobe was retracted laterally, and microdissection was done to expose the aneurysm at the junction of the pericallosal and callosomarginal arteries. **F–I,** Right AP and oblique, left AP, and lateral carotid angiograms show obliteration of all aneurysms except the one on the right middle cerebral artery where the clip either had slipped or had not been satisfactorily placed. Reoperation was done through a right frontal temporal approach. **J,** Postoperative right carotid angiogram shows obliteration of the remaining aneurysm. The patient made a good recovery, with the only deficit being a loss of smell.

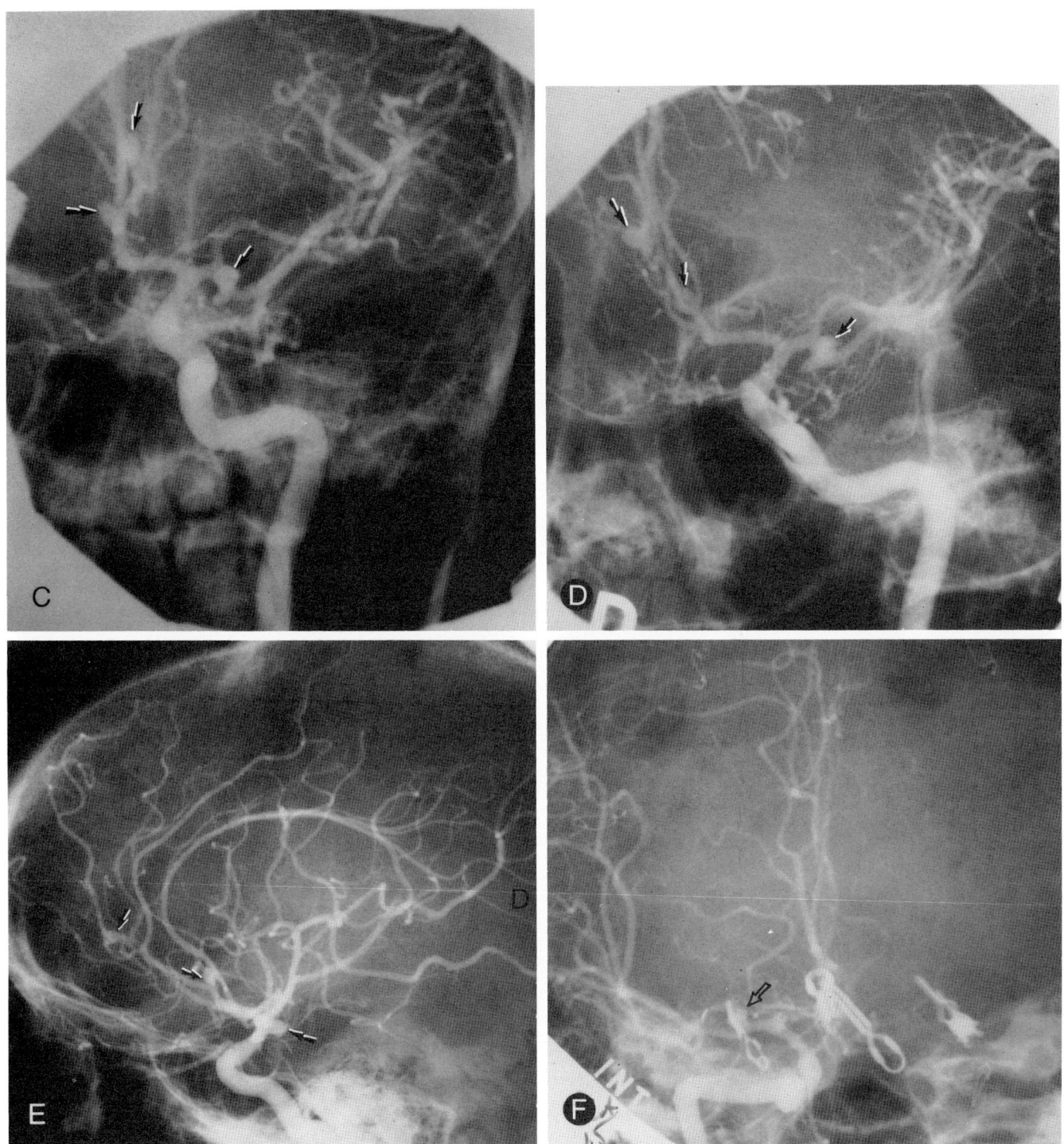

Figure 19.3C–F.

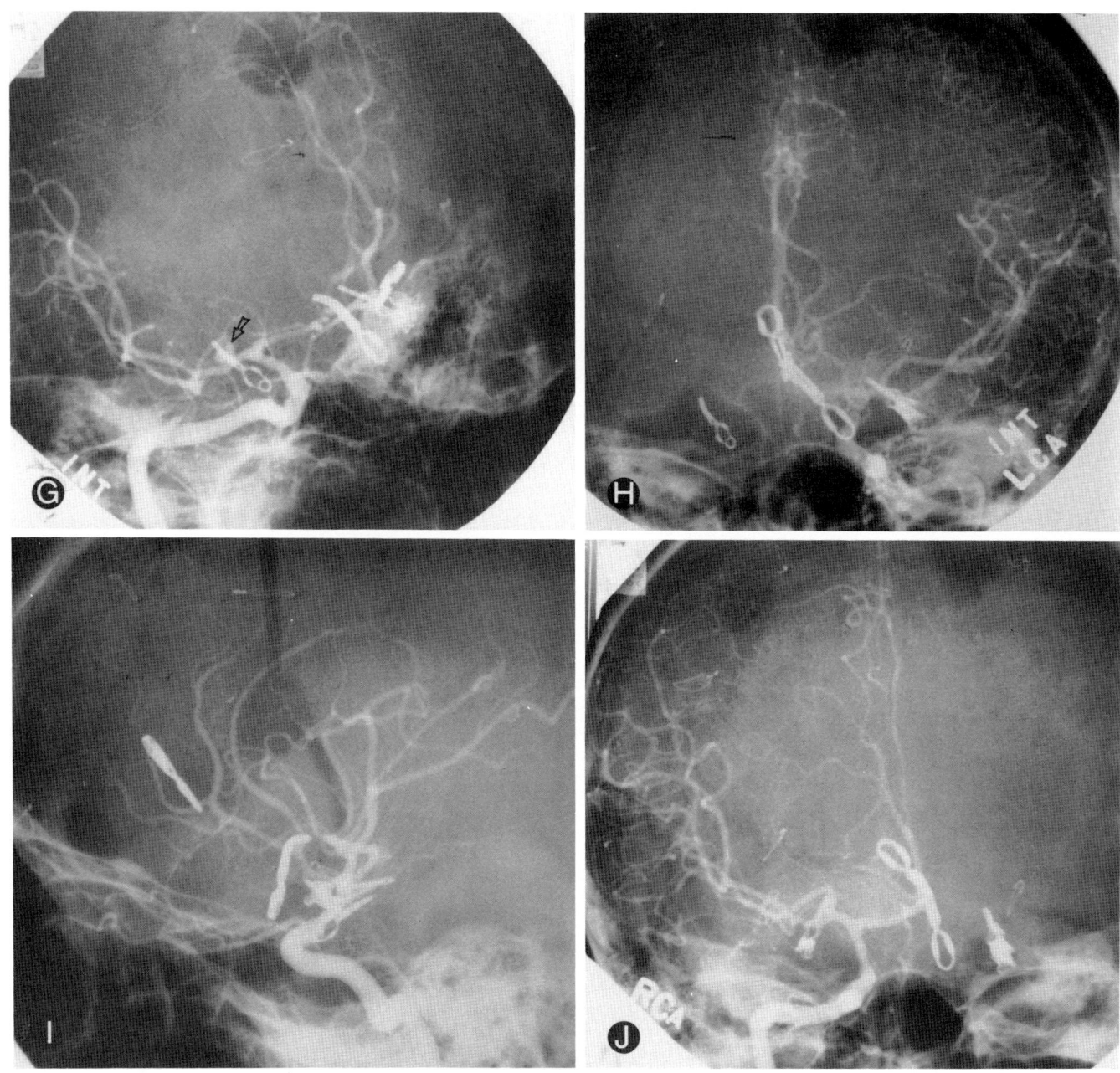

Figure 19.3G–J.

median age the risk was 6.9%/year. Aneurysms that bled were in the range of 10–40 mm in diameter (mean, 21.3 mm), which differs from the size of all ruptured aneurysms seen at Mayo Clinic (mean, 7.5 mm in diameter). This discrepancy is probably due to a decrease in the filling compartment of the aneurysm after rupture and stabilization of aneurysmal size at less than 10 mm in the absence of rupture shortly after formation. They noted a high frequency of eventual rupture in aneurysms causing compressive or embolic symptoms.

Unruptured aneurysms may occur in association with polycystic kidney disease (19). Some have recommended cerebral angiography for all patients with polycystic kidney disease and surgery for identified aneurysms (35). Inasmuch as aneurysms smaller than 10 mm are unlikely to bleed and because CT recognizes almost all lesions of 10 mm or more, the authors recommend CT without and with contrast for such patients.

The results of surgical treatment of intracranial aneurysm have improved markedly, with mortalilty

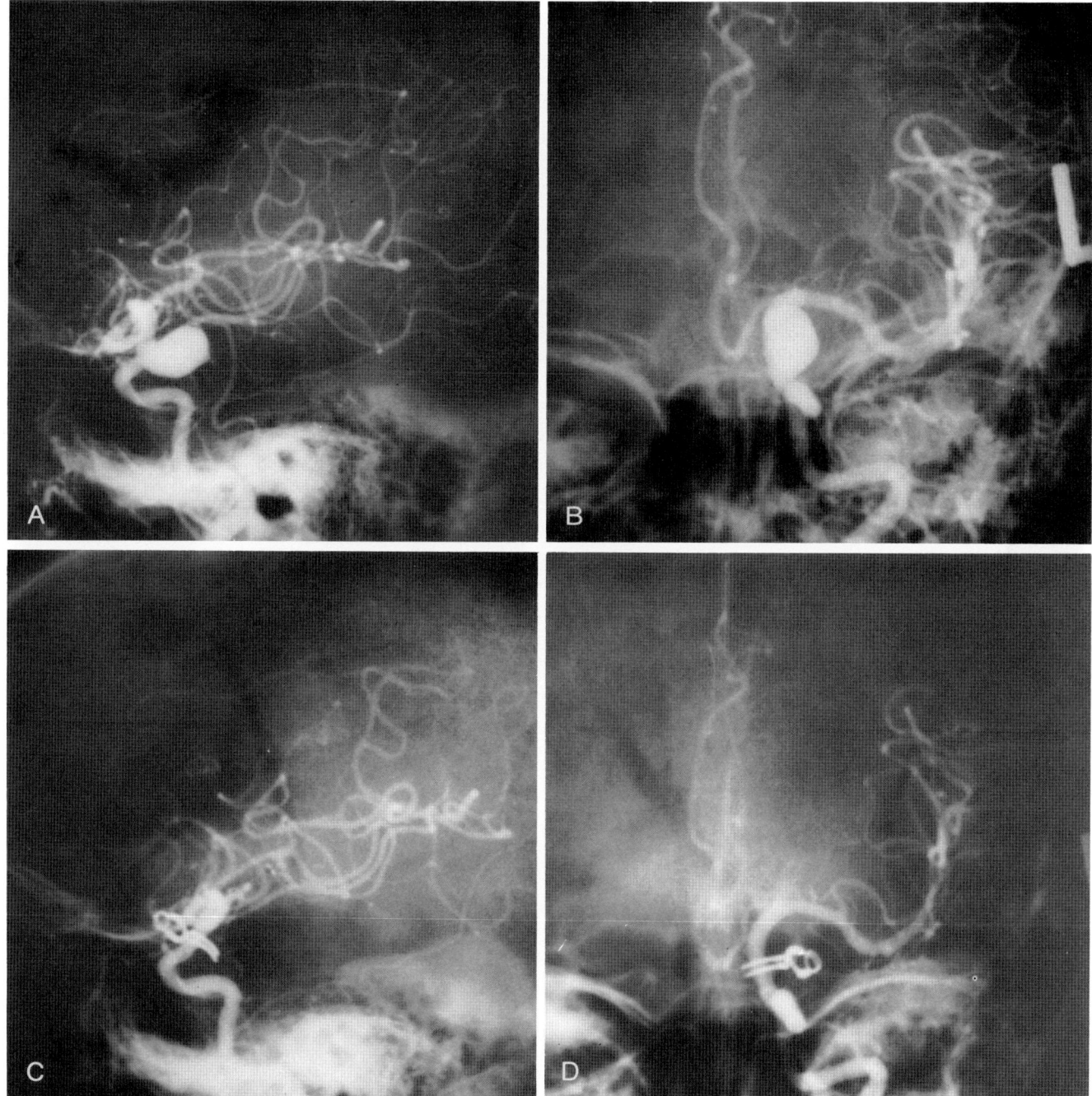

Figure 19.4. Internal carotid artery aneurysm presenting with seizures. **A** and **B**, Left carotid angiograms show large internal carotid-posterior communicating artery aneurysm. Comment: At surgery, patient's lesion was adherent to medial temporal lobe. Aneurysm was obliterated by ligation and clipping. **C** and **D**, Postoperative angiograms confirm clipping. The patient experienced severe dysphasia beginning 4 days after operation, which gradually cleared.

figures of 5% or less in most centers (31, 34). Surgery on unruptured aneurysms is usually thought less risky than that for ruptured lesions, but even unruptured aneurysms may be associated with postoperative vasospasm (3). In a study of surgery for unruptured intracranial aneurysms, 107 patients in 12 centers were reported with 7% operative morbidity and no mortality (39).

Particular features of each individual case modify risk. Location of the aneurysm is important; internal carotid artery lesions are of lesser risk, and vertebrobasilar artery lesions are of higher risk. Obviously,

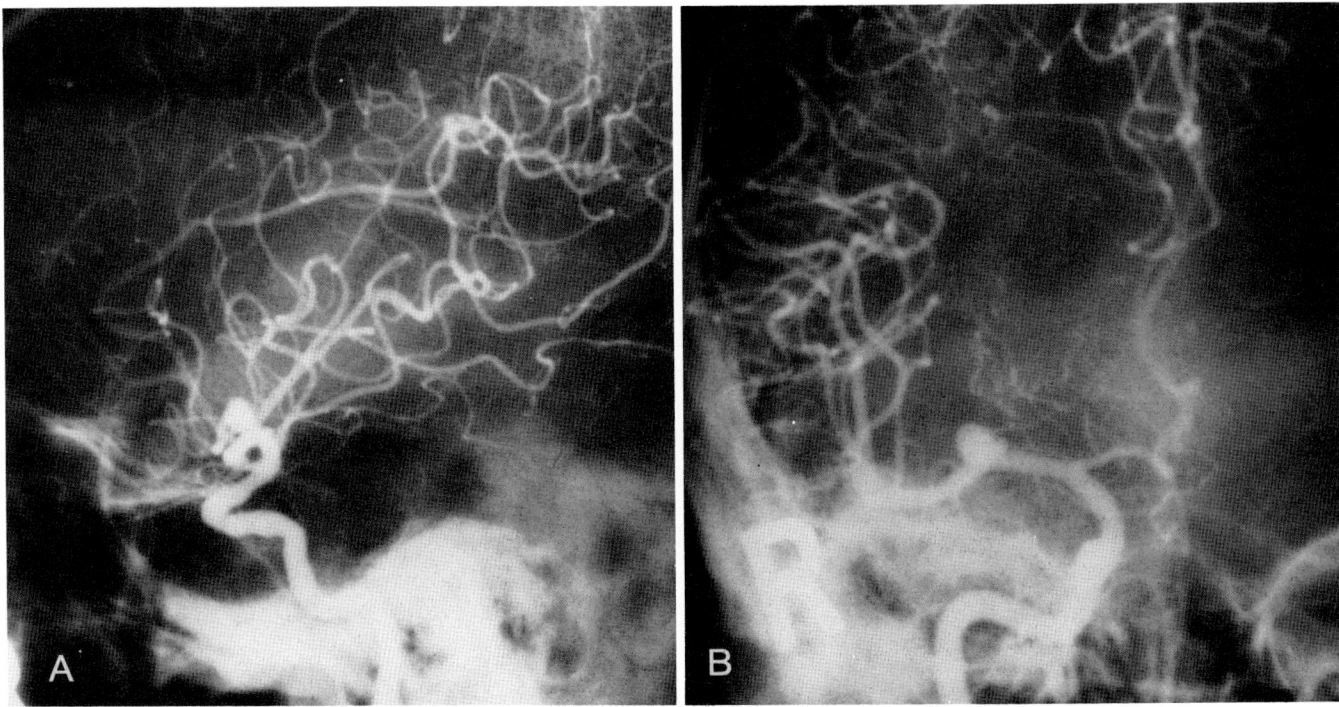

Figure 19.5. Asymptomatic aneurysm. **A** and **B**, Right carotid angiogram demonstrates 7-mm aneurysm of the middle cerebral artery. Comment: The angiogram was done because the patient had nonspecific headaches, her mother had had an aneurysm, and the patient was very anxious regarding subarachnoid hemorrhage. The aneurysm was clipped. Postoperative angiography confirmed obliteration of the lesion. Neurologic examination was normal.

giant aneurysms are more risky. The patients's age and general medical status must be taken in account, with younger patients in sound condition being more suitable for surgery. In addition, the surgeon must gauge surgical risk in light of personal experience rather than reports in the literature.

In general, the authors suggest surgical therapy for most asymptomatic aneurysms 10 mm or greater in medically fit patients under 60 years of age (7, 21, 22, 25, 31, 32, 37). In older patients who are in very good health or in younger patients with aneurysms 7–10 mm in diameter (Fig. 19.5), individual judgment on a case by case basis, considering factors such as location of the aneurysm and experience of the surgeon, are in order. Note that CT or magnetic resonance screening could in almost all cases detect asymptomatic aneurysms appropriate for surgery.

REFERENCES

1. Ambrosetto P, Gulassi E: Familial occurrence of multiple intracranial aneurysms. Case reports and review of the literature. *Acta Neuryochir (Wien)* 56:233–238, 1981.
2. Beyerl BD, Heros RC: Multiple aneurysms of the posterior inferior cerebellar artery. *Neurosurgery* 19:285–289, 1986.
3. Bloomfield SM, Sonntag VK: Delayed cerebral vasospasm after uncomplicated operation on an unruptured aneurysm: Case report. *Neurosurgery* 17:792–796, 1985.
4. Chasen JL, Hindman WM: Berry aneurysms of the circle of Willis: Results of a planned autopsy study. *Neurology* 8:41–44, 1958.
5. Coppeto JR, Chan YS: Abducens nerve paresis caused by unruptured vertebral artery aneurysm. *Surg Neurol* 18:385–387, 1982.
6. Dell S: Asymptomatic cerebral aneurysm: Assessment of its risk of rupture. *Neurosurgery* 10:162–166, 1982.
7. Drake CG, Girvin JP: The surgical treatment of subarachnoid hemorrhage with multiple aneurysms. In Morley TP (ed): *Current Controversies in Neurosurgery*. Philadelphia, WB Saunders, 1976, pp 274–278.
8. Fisher M, Davidson RI, Marchs EM: Transient focal cerebral ischemia as a presenting manifestation of unruptured cerebral aneurysms. *Ann Neurol* 8:367–372, 1980.
9. Fukuoka S, Suematsu K, Nakamura J, Matsuzaki T, Satoh S, Hashimoto I: Transient ischemic attacks caused by unruptured intracranial aneurysm. *Surg Neurol* 17:464–467, 1982.
10. Graff-Redford NR, Adams HP Jr, Smoker WR, Biller J, Boarini DJ: Unruptured fusiform aneurysms of the posterior circulation with thalamic infarction. *Neurosurgery* 17:495–499, 1985.
11. Heiskanan O: Risk of bleeding from unruptured aneurysms in cases with multiple intracranial aneurysms. *J Neurosurg* 55:524–526, 1981.
12. Heiskanan O, Martilla I: Risk of rupture of a second aneurysm in patients with multiple aneurysms. *J Neurosurg* 32:295–299, 1970.
13. Hiscott P, Crockard A: Multiple aneurysms of the distal posterior inferior cerebellar artery. *Neurosurgery* 10:101–102, 1982.
14. Jane JA, Kassell NF, Torner JC, Winn HR: The natural history of aneurysms and arteriovenous malformations. *J Neurosurg* 62:321–323, 1985.
15. Jellinger K: Patholody of intracerebral hemorrhages. *Zentralb Neurochir* 38:29–42, 1977.
16. Leibrock LG, Bennett DR, Block S: Complex partial seizures associated with unruptured thrombosed basilar artery apex aneurysm. *Surg Neurol* 19:17–20, 1983.

17. Locksley HB: Report on the Cooperative Study of Intracranial Aneurysms and Subarachnoid Hemorrhage. Section V, Part II. Natural history of subarachnoid hemorrhage, intracranial aneurysms and arteriovenous malformations. J Neurosurg 25:321–368, 1966.
18. Markwalder TM, Meienberg O: Acute painful carernous sinus syndrome in unruptured intracavernous aneurysms of the interal carotid artery. Possible pathogenetic mechanisms. J Clin Neuro Ophthalmol 3:31–35, 1983.
19. Matsumura M, Wada H, Nojiri K, Ohwada A, Shinoda T: Unruptured intracranial aneurysms in polycystic kidney disease. Acta Neurochir (Wien) 79:94–99, 1986.
20. McKissock W, Richardson A, Walsh L, Owen E: Multiple intracranial aneurysms. Lancet 1:623–626, 1964.
21. Mount LA, Brisman R: Treatment of multiple aneurysms—symptomatic and asymptomatic. Clin Neurosurg 21:166–170, 1974.
22. Moyes PD: Surgical treatment of multiple aneurysms and of incidentally discovered unruptured aneurysms. J Neurosurg 35:291–295. 1971.
23. Nagamine Y, Takahashi S, Sonobe M: Multiple intracranial aneurysms associated with moya moya disease. Case report. J Neurosurg 54:673–676, 1981.
24. Nehls DG, Flom RA, Carter LP, Spetzler RF: Multiple intracranial aneurysms: Determining the site of rupture. J Neurosurg 63:342–348, 1985.
25. Ojemann RG: Management of the unruptured intracranial aneurysm. N Engl J Med 304:725–726, 1981.
26. Osterfgaard JR, Heg E: Incidence of multiple intracranial aneurysms. Influence of arterial hypertension and gender. J Neurosurg 63:49–55, 1985.
27. Phillips LH II, Whisnant JP, O'Fallon WM, Sundt TM Jr: The unchanging pattern of subarachnoid hemorrhage in a community. Neurology 30:1034–1040, 1980.
28. Przelomski MM, Fisher M, Davidson RI, Jones HR, Marcus EM: Unruptured intracranial aneurysm and transient focal cerebral ischemia: A follow-up study. Neurology 36:584–587, 1986.
29. Rodriguez y Baena R, Rainoldi F, Sulvani V, Gaetani P, Bonezzi C: Surgical treatment of multiple supratentorial aneurysms. Neurochirurgia 29:20–24, 1986.
30. Salazar JL: Surgical treatment of asymptomatic and incidental intracranial aneurysms. J Neurosurg 53:20–21, 1981.
31. Samson D: Surgery for unruptured intracranial aneurysms. In Wilkins RH, Rengachary SS (eds): Neurosurgery. Philadelphia, WB Saunders, 1986, pp 1437–1439.
32. Samson DS, Hodosh RM, Clark WK: Surgical management of unruptured asymptomatic aneurysms. J Neurosurg 46:731–734, 1977.
33. Stewart RM, Samson D, Diehl J, Hinton R, Ditmore QM:Unruptured cerebral aneurysms presenting as recurrent transient neurologic deficits. Neurology 30:47–51, 1980.
34. Sundt TM Jr, Kobayashi S, Fode NC, Whisnant JP: Results and complications of surgical management of 809 intracranial aneurysms in 722 cases: Related and unrelated to grade of patient, type of aneurysm, and timing of surgery. J Neurosurg 56:753–765, 1982.
35. Wakabayashi T, Fujita S, Ohbora Y, Suyama T, Tamaki N, Matsumoto S: Polycystic kidney disease and intracranial aneurysms. Early angiographic diagnosis and early operation for the unruptured aneurysm. J Neurosurg 58:488–491, 1983.
36. Wiebers DO, Whisnant JP, O'Fallon WM: The natural history of unruptured intracranial aneurysms. N Engl J Med 304:696–698, 1981.
37. Wiebers DO, Whisnant JP, Sundt TM Jr: The significance of unruptured intracranial aneurysms. J Neurosurg in press.
38. Winn HR, Almaani WS, Berga SL, Jane JA, Richardson AE: The long-term outcome in patients with multiple aneurysms: Incidence of late hemorrhage and implications for treatment of incidental aneurysms. J Neurosurg 59:642–651, 1983.
39. Wirth FP, Laws ER Jr, Piepgras D, Scott RM: Surgical treatment of incidental intracranial aneurysms. Neurosurgery 12:507–511, 1983.
40. Wood EH: Angiographic identification of the ruptured lesion in patients with multiple cerebral aneurysms. J Neurosurg 21:182–198, 1964.
41. Yamamoto Y, Asari S, Sunami N, Kunishio K, Fukui K, Sadamoto K: Computed angiotomography of unruptured cerebral aneurysms. J Comput Assist Tomogr 10:21–27, 1986.
42. Zacks DJ, Russell DB, Miller JDR: Fortuitously discovered intracranial aneurysms. Arch Neurol 37:39–41, 1980.

20
Giant Aneurysms

Intracranial aneurysms larger than 25 mm in diameter are considered giant aneurysms and these comprise about 5% of all intracranial aneurysms (22, 48, 59, 77, 143). The age at which giant intracranial aneurysms become symptomatic seems to be about the same as for intracranial aneurysms in general with the peak during the fourth and fifth decades (48). Although intracranial aneurysms are rare in children, there seems to be a slightly higher proportion of large and giant aneurysms in this age group (48). Aneurysms in general are more common in females, but this is not true for giant aneurysms except in the ophthalmic and paraclinoid region where they are far more common in females (25, 29, 52, 105).

PATHOLOGY

It is not clear what factors cause some aneurysms to rutpure and others to grow to reach giant proportions (4, 6, 98, 101). In giant aneurysms there is broadening of the parent artery and splaying of branch vessels at the neck of the aneurysm. This is what creates many of the difficulties encountered in trying to clip these aneurysms. Atherosclerosis and calcification within the neck and the fundus of the lesion are common. Mural thrombus frequently develops and may protect some portions of the aneurysmal wall from rupture but other areas remain paper-thin and this may account for the fact that subarachnoid hemorrhage appears to be as common with giant aneurysms as with aneurysms of smaller size. (22, 48, 59).

Giant aneurysms can also be fusiform (69). These aneurysms are frequently associated with atherosclerosis and some may be related to arterial dolichoectasia (Fig. 20.1). They are common in the basilar artery but can occur in the supraclinoid segment of the internal carotid artery, the main trunk of the middle cerebral artery, the vertebral artery and the P_1 and P_2 segments of the posterior cerebral artery. Most of these aneurysms present with symptoms due to compression of adjacent intracranial structures or with ischemia. The frequency of subarachnoid hemorrhage from these aneurysms is unknown. Another unusual type of giant intracranial aneurysm is the serpentine aneurysm. These aneurysms occur almost exclusively in the middle cerebral artery. The characteristic feature is a long, tortuous lumen ending in normal branches associated with a large mass effect from the mostly thrombosed aneurysmal mass. These aneurysms may be special types of fusiform giant aneurysms where a portion of the wall enlarges in a globular form and thromboses (139).

The mechanism of thrombosis in giant intracranial aneurysms is poorly understood (16, 94, 101). The high incidence of thrombus formation within giant intracranial aneurysms is probably related to a critical ratio between aneurysmal volume and aneurysmal neck size above which intraaneurysmal thrombosis occurs (7, 139). Partial thrombosis does not protect the patient from the risk of subarachnoid hemorrhage. The incidence of subarachnoid hemorrhage in partially thrombosed giant aneurysms is between 30 and 40% which is the same incidence as in nonthrombosed giant aneurysms (22, 59, 129, 139). Even almost complete thrombosis of a giant aneurysm does not protect against the risk of a future hemorrhage (Fig. 20.2) (129). Sudden clinical deterioration may be associated with acute intraaneurysmal thrombosis (48, 99, 129, 139). Occasionally, massive cerebral edema has been observed on computed tomography (CT) scanning in these cases (51). Deterioration may be a result of acute aneurysmal enlargement, by intramural bleeding and thrombosis, or occlusion of the parent vessel or one of its branches by extension of the intramural thrombus (99).

CLINICAL PRESENTATION

About one-third of giant intracranial aneurysms present with subarachnoid hemorrhage indistinguishable from rupture of smaller intracranial aneurysms (22, 48, 140). Nonspecific presenting symptoms include headaches in the absence of subarachnoid hemorrhage, signs of increased intracranial pressure such as papilledema and epilepsy (10, 45, 48, 97). If the seizures are of the "partial complex type" the aneurysm is likely to be on the middle cerebral artery compressing the medial temporal lobe. Ischemic symptoms due to intracranial aneurysms are rare but

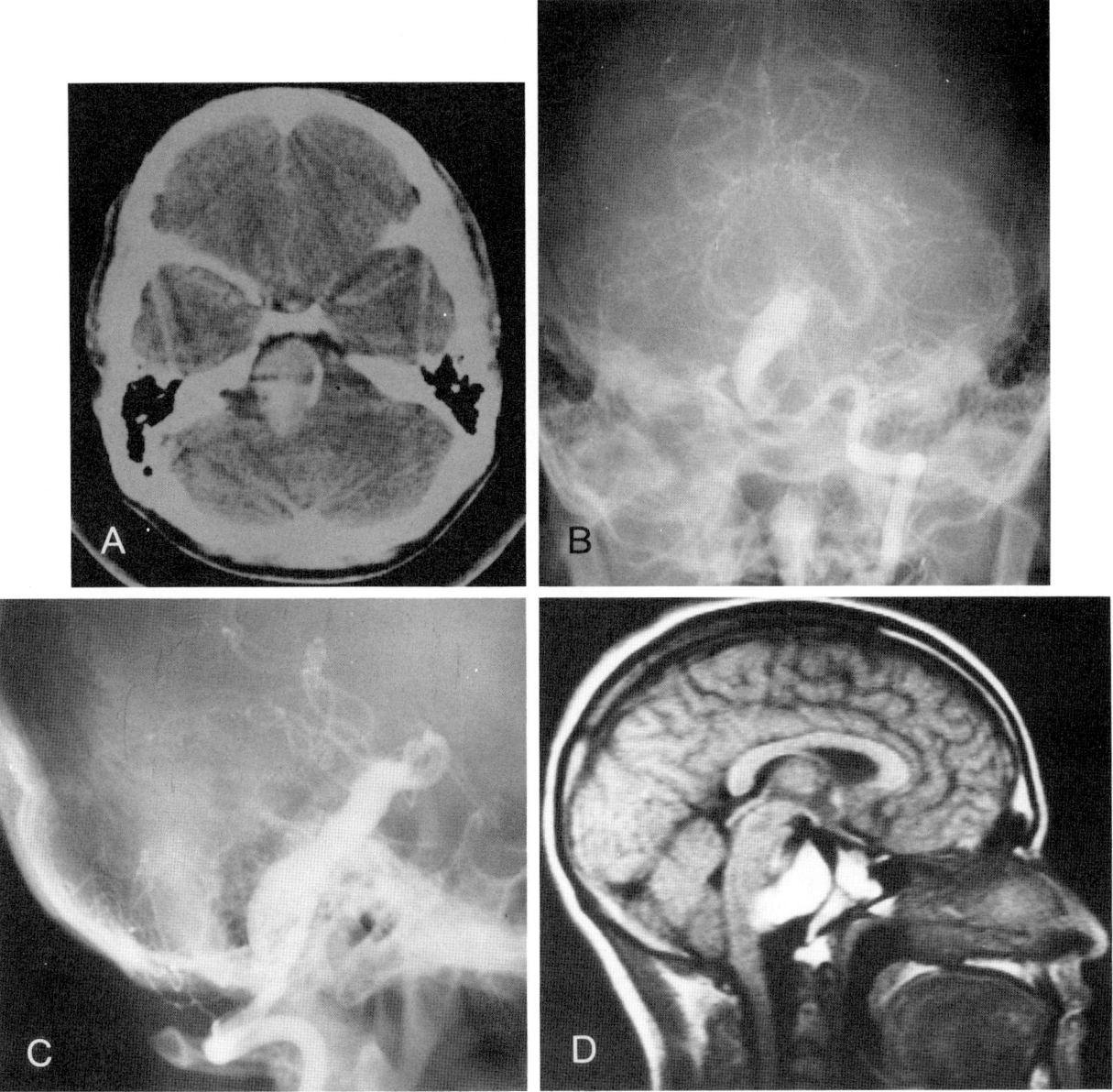

Figure 20.1. Partially thrombosed fusiform aneurysm of the basilar trunk as seen on: **A**, CT scan; **B** and **C**, vertebral angiogram; and **D**, MRI. Note the excellent anatomic definition of the clot within the aneurysm by MRI (**D**). The authors were unable to offer any treatment to this patient who presented with progressive deterioration from brain stem compression and/or ischemia.

when they occur, the aneurysm is more likely to be giant (94, 115).

Giant aneurysms occasionally present with massive cerebral edema simulating a brain tumor. This phenomenon has been seen mostly in cases of middle cerebral artery giant aneurysms and in each case the aneurysm has been massive and partially thrombosed (51) (Fig. 20.3). The mechanism whereby these aneurysms produce massive hemispheric edema is unclear. Apparently a critical size is exceeded leading to a breakdown of autoregulation and swelling, possibly the result of thrombosis or local ischemia (22, 51).

RADIOLOGIC DIAGNOSIS

Plain skull films may show "ring calcification" which is essentially pathognomic for these lesions, and bony erosion from chronic pressure. Aneurysms of the internal carotid artery in its petrous segment can produce erosion of the petrous pyramid and in the distal portion of the cavernous segment can result

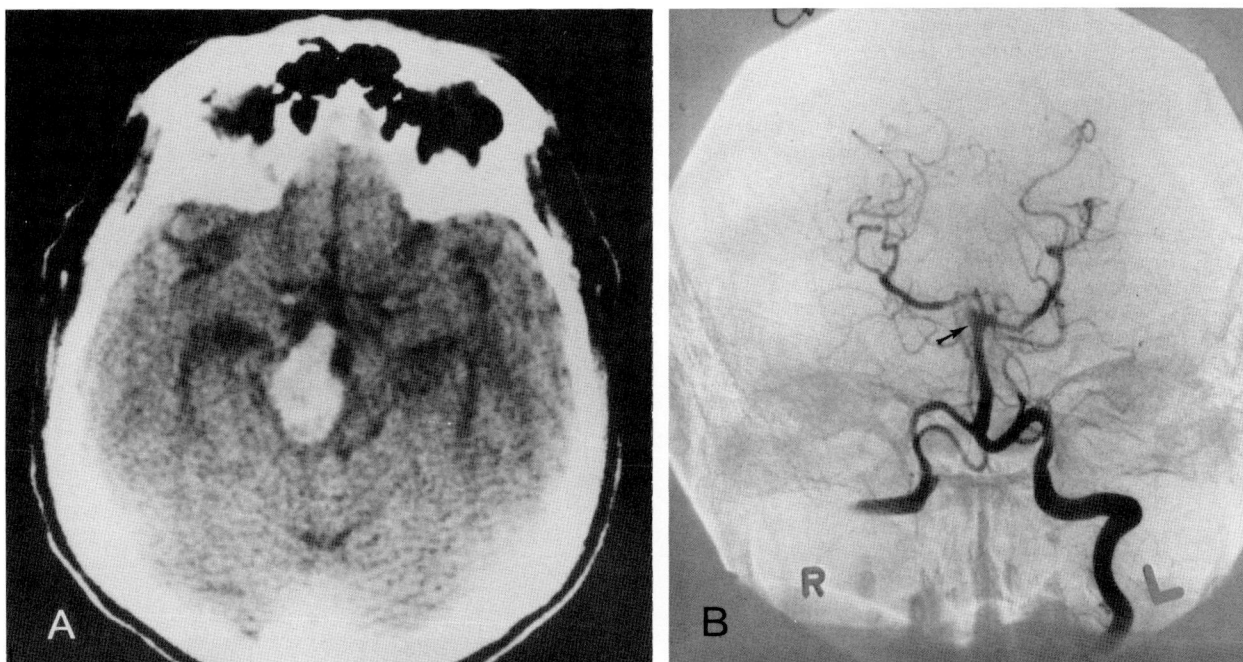

Figure 20.2. Recently thrombosed giant aneurysm of basilar artery. **A**, The CT scan shows a homogeneous hyperdense lesion on the plain scan that did not change significantly with contrast enhancement. **B**, Towne's view of left vertebral angiogram shows an area of irregularity between the right superior cerebellar and posterior cerebral arteries (*arrow*). There is also displacement of these vessels. The studies were interpreted as showing an almost completely thrombosed aneurysm with only a tiny residual area of patency in the neck (*arrow*). This patient presented with a 6-month history of weakness of his left arm and leg that became suddenly much worse 3 weeks before admission. There was a right partial third nerve palsy. He was treated conservatively and reassured that his aneurysm had "thrombosed" and would never bleed. He improved significantly with physical therapy, but 4 months later he died of a massive rupture of his aneurysm.

in erosion of the optic strut (48). Paraclinoid aneurysms may erode the anterior and posterior clinoid processes or extend into the sella and produce sellar enlargement (92, 138).

The CT scan is almost invariably positive (12, 15, 34, 40, 44, 68, 83, 88, 89). CT scan demonstrates recent subarachnoid hemorrhage and secondary effects such as intracerebral hemorrhage, hydrocephalus and surrounding edema. Three general patterns of CT scan visualization of giant intracranial aneurysms have been seen: (a) nonthrombosed aneurysms usually produce a slightly hyperdense image on the plain CT scan and "enhance" with a dense, round uniform stain after contrast injection; (b) partially thrombosed aneurysms produce an inhomogeneous pattern of variable density on the plain scans which may be associated with ring calcifications or intraaneurysmal calcification. Usually there is no significant perianeurysmal low density or edema but, as stated above, some of the massive lesions may be associated with significant edema. With contrast injection, these partially thrombosed aneurysms can present a pathognomonic target sign with a central or eccentric dense staining area surrounded by an area of no uptake and enclosed within a densely staining rim (Fig. 20.4); (c) completely thrombosed aneurysms present with a variable picture, depending on the "age" of the thrombus. Recent thrombus is hyperdense on the plain scan (Fig. 20.2). An older clot may be hypodense. No significant central uptake is seen after contrast enhancement, but rim enhancement continues to be visible for variable periods of time and occasionally indefinitely. Absence of surrounding brain edema usually differentiates these lesions from brain tumors.

Venous digital subtraction angiography has been used with some success, particularly when combined with dynamic CT scan, to study giant aneurysms (65). Selective arterial angiography with or without digital subtraction technique, remains the definitive test. Angiography may be negative in cases of completely or almost completely thrombosed aneurysms (Fig. 20.2). Only the portion of the lumen that remains patent is visible angiographically. Mass effect resulting in splaying and stretching of surrounding branches is almost always apparent. Special projections may be required to demonstrate the neck of the aneurysm.

Cross-compression studies to assess collateral circulation are important for planning therapy. For ca-

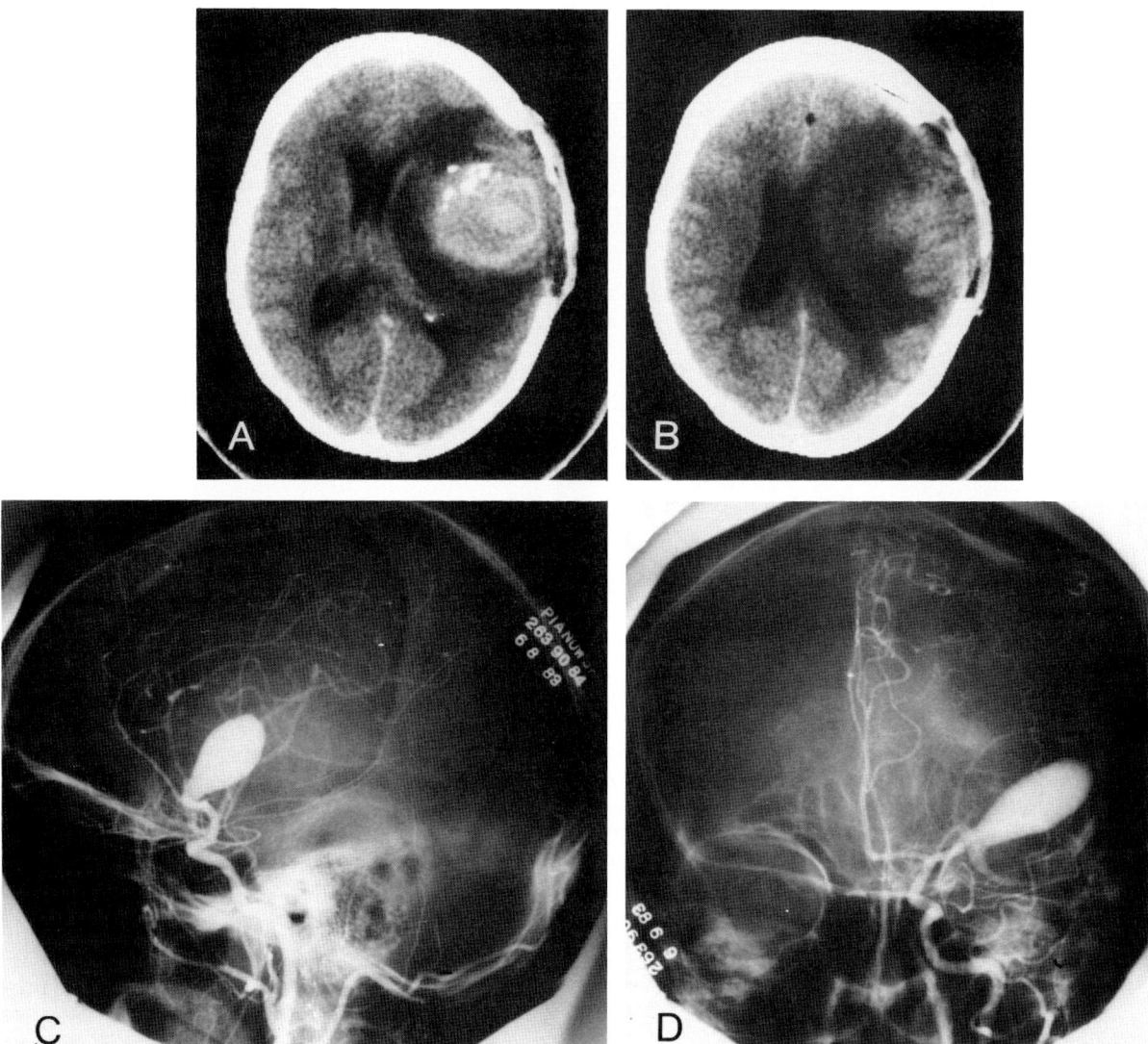

Figure 20.3. Partially thrombosed aneurysm of middle cerebral artery with massive cerebral edema. **A** and **B**, CT scan shows a partially thrombosed aneurysm with massive surrounding hemispheric edema and shift. **C** and **D**, Left carotid angiogram shows that the central aspect of the aneurysm is still patent. This middle-aged lady presented with progressive hemiparesis and aphasia. She was operated at another hospital after a CT scan (not shown) had suggested a brain tumor. At surgery, the diagnosis of a partially thrombosed aneurysm was made. At the time of transfer, she had a severe hemiparesis and aphasia. At reoperation a preliminary bypass graft was attempted but no satisfactory cortical vessel was found on the markedly edematous cortical surface of the hemisphere. Aneurysmorrhaphy was then attempted under cardiopulmonary bypass. A tear was produced at the base of the aneurysm, and the middle cerebral artery complex was reconstructed only with considerable difficulty. Postoperatively, she was hemiplegic and aphasic and showed little sign of recovery over the subsequent several months.

rotid aneurysms the contralateral carotid artery and a vertebral artery are sequentially injected while the involved carotid artery is compressed. For vertebrobasilar aneurysms, Allcock has introduced the procedure of injecting a vertebral artery while each carotid artery is sequentially compressed. In this manner, the size of each posterior communicating artery may be ascertained (22). Intraarterial balloons may be inflated temporarily to determine tolerance of the patient to arterial occlusion.

Magnetic resonance imaging (MRI) is helpful in the diagnosis of thrombosed, angiographically "silent" lesions and in the estimation of the age of the mural thrombus in partially thrombosed lesions (Fig. 20.5). However, it is still too early to know whether MRI is superior to CT scanning in this respect.

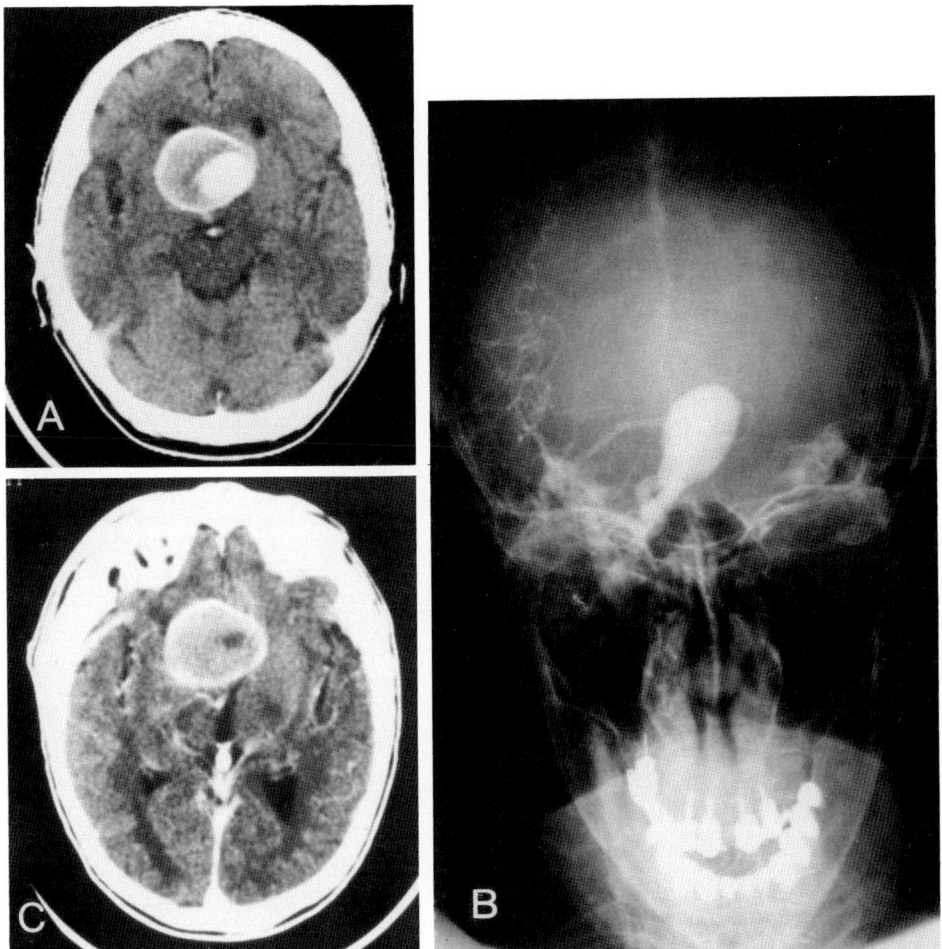

Figure 20.4. Partially thrombosed giant paraclinoid aneurysm. **A**, CT scan shows the typical appearance of a partially thrombosed aneurysm. **B**, Angiogram shows that the aneurysm arises from the paraclinoid region. This patient presented with headaches and visual loss in the right eye. She tolerated temporary occlusion of the right internal carotid artery for 15 minutes during angiography. At intracranial exploration, the aneurysm was found to be unclippable. Therefore, the authors proceeded to close the craniotomy site and awaken the patient (the carotid bifurcation had already been exposed). During a 15-minute period of temporary carotid occlusion, the patient's neurologic examination remained normal and the stump pressure fell by about 60% to a mean pressure of 45 torr. The distal common carotid artery was ligated acutely. **C**, Postoperative CT scan 1 week after surgery shows complete thrombosis of the aneurysm.

NATURAL HISTORY AND INDICATIONS FOR TREATMENT

Indications for treatment must be based on an understanding of natural history. The natural history of asymptomatic giant aneurysms is not well known (48). Many of these lesions are currently being diagnosed when CT scans are obtained for unrelated symptoms. Not enough of these patients have been followed over the years to provide a clear understanding of their natural history. There is no reason to suspect that the natural history of these aneurysms is any more benign than that of nongiant aneurysms. Whether or not treatment should be offered to these patients depends on a variety of factors such as the age and general health of the patient, the size and location of the aneurysm and anticipated safety of surgical treatment. Treatment of these lesions is more hazardous than treatment of ordinary aneurysms (see Results). However, giant aneurysms appear more likely to grow than ordinary aneurysms (4, 96, 101); and since the treatment is likely to be more hazardous as the aneurysm grows, consideration must be given to treating these aneurysms, even though asymptomatic, in selected cases.

The prognosis of syptomatic giant intracranial aneurysms is better known and it appears to be very grave. A review of several series indicates that approximately 80% of symptomatic patients (subarachnoid hemorrhage or mass effect) who remain untreated

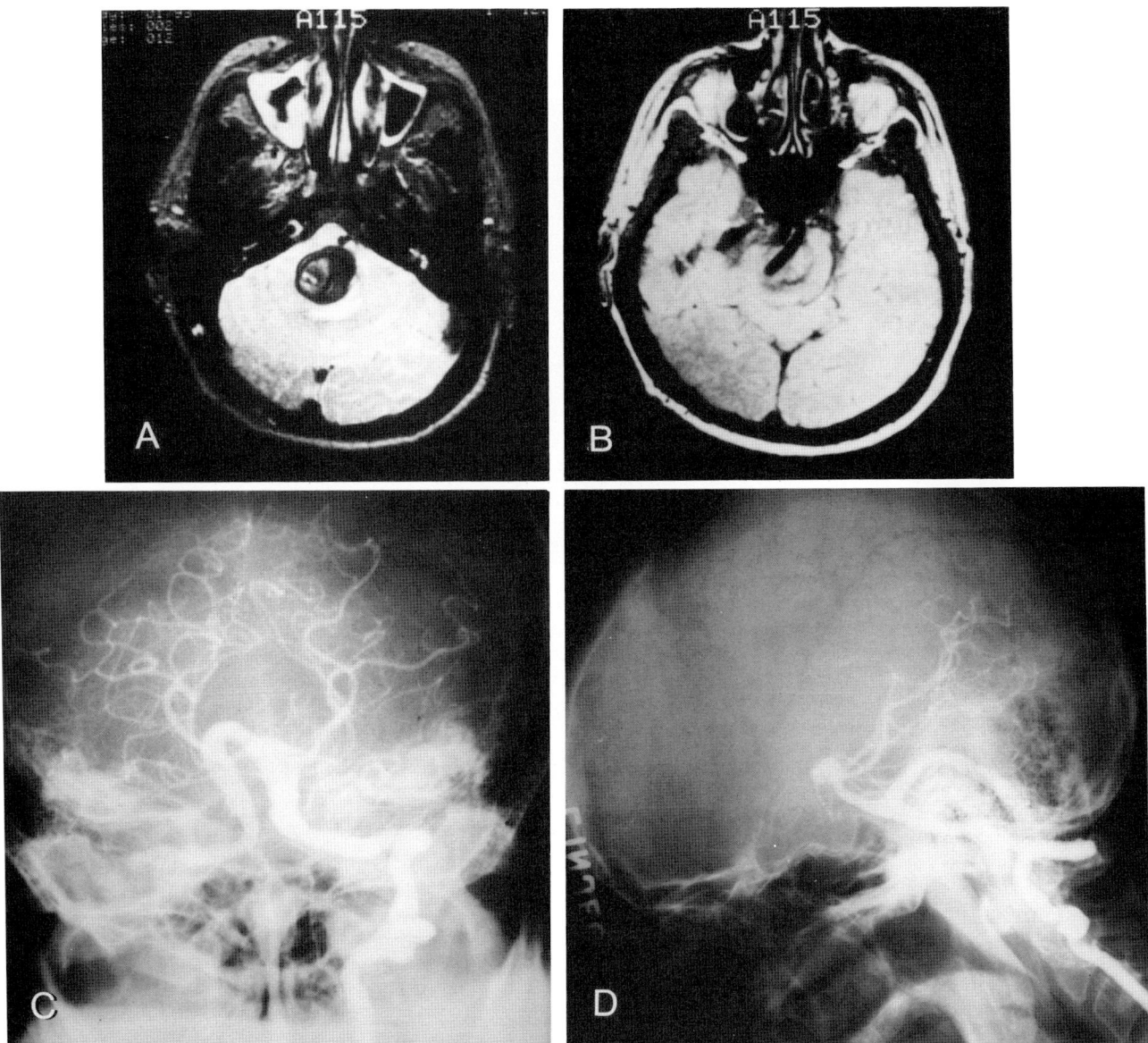

Figure 20.5. Giant fusiform vertebral aneurysm. **A** and **B**, MRI shows a prepontine mass with void signal in the shape of a channel suggestive of a residual lumen. **C** and **D**, Left vertebral angiogram shows some beaded irregularity, suggestive of fibromuscular dysplasia, of the left vertebral artery. There is reflux into a residual lumen of the right vertebral artery which is displaced posteriorly by the mass of intraaneurysmal thrombus. This 57-year-old man presented with ataxia, diplopia, and facial numbness. He was treated with balloon occlusion of the right vertebral artery. **E** and **F**, Left vertebral angiogram after right vertebral artery occlusion by balloon. There is no filling of the aneurysm in this study or in the right vertebral angiogram. The patient improved gradually.

are dead or totally incapacitated within 5 years of diagnosis (10, 22, 59, 77). Patients who present with visual deterioration as a result of compression of the optic apparatus by a giant aneurysm usually continue to deteriorate steadily and, without treatment, become blind within a few years, (25, 29, 52). Patients presenting with brain stem compression progress to total disability and death usually within a few months (22). A more benign natural history is that of giant aneurysms in the cavernous portion of the internal carotid artery. These aneurysms are relatively protected against subarachnoid hemorrhage but the cavernous syndrome that they produce usually progresses to complete ophthalmoplegia and blindness if the aneurysm is left untreated. Once a giant aneurysm results in subarachnoid hemorrhage, the frequency

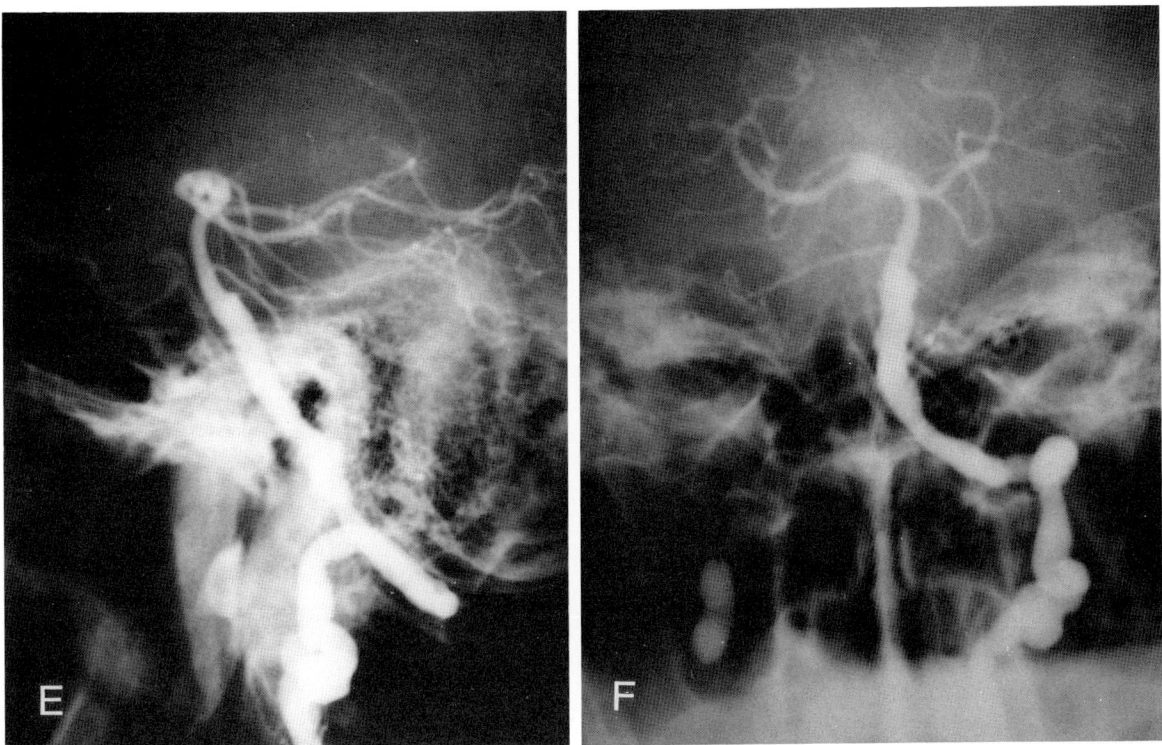

Figure 20.5E and F.

of rebleeding is at least as high as in ordinary aneurysms (22, 48, 59).

In view of the above, every effort should be made to treat symtomatic giant aneurysms whatever their presentations. An exception is the patient with limited life expectancy from advanced age or poor medical condition. In addition, large fusiform aneurysms of the basilar artery (see Fig. 20.1) and some giant aneurysms with limited potential for collateral circulation, are simply untreatable by presently available techniques. Furthermore, in some aneurysms the treatment is probably more dangerous than the expected natural history. As always, individual judgment must be exercised in each case.

If direct obliteration appears impossible or too risky, the surgeon may choose indirect treatment by proximal arterial occlusion, either by open operation or by detachable balloon. This may be preceded by a bypass graft if collateral circulation is inadequate. Since the issues are different for aneurysms in various locations, indirect techniques will be discussed according to specific aneurysm sites. Either preoperatively or intraoperatively after direct inspection, delicate surgical judgment permits the surgeon to weigh comparative risks to select the safest procedure for the patient. During surgery there is a point of no return; once the aneurysm is opened or ruptured, one cannot go back. Mature judgment needs the restraint to stop short of catastrophic rupture for truly unclippable aneurysms along with the perseverance to obliterate clippable lesions.

SURGICAL MANAGEMENT

Intracranial Procedure

The preoperative preparation of patients with giant aneurysms is not significantly different than in patients with smaller aneurysms (see Chapter 11). Patients with significant mass effect on CT scan will probably benefit from corticosteroid administration for several days before surgery. In these patients, a balanced anesthetic technique to avoid an exacerbation of intracranial hypertension is preferable. Whenever there is anticipation of need for temporary arterial occlusion or trapping, it is a useful precaution to have the patient well-hydrated which usually can be ensured by intravenous administration of colloid starting the night before surgery.

The position for surgery depends on the site of the aneurysm. It is important to have the neck prepared and draped in the operative field whenever one is dealing with giant aneurysms of the paraclinoid region. The postoperative care of these patients does not differ significantly from the care of other aneurysm patients.

The decision of whether an aneurysm may be amenable to intracranial obliteration either by clipping or aneurysmorrhaphy is a difficult one that needs to be made from correlating the angiogram and the CT scans. If there is doubt intracranial exploration is recommended since the ideal treatment for a giant aneurysm is direct obliteration if it can be done safely (22). At intracranial exploration, many of these aneurysms initially appear to be unclippable either because of location, calcification or atherosclerosis of the base, partial thrombosis, branches coming from the neck, or massive size. There are several options that may make it possible to deal with such aneurysms.

Deep Hypotension

Not infrequently an aneurysm that appears impossible to clip upon first inspection may become soft and pliable enough to accept a clip under deep hypotension (i.e., mean systemic pressure of 35–45 torr for several minutes and mean pressures of 45 torr if a more prolonged period of hypotension is necessary). Relative contraindications are poor cardiovascular condition, advanced age, preoperative vasospasm, and poor preoperative neurologic condition. It is essential to have an experienced anesthesiologist whenever deep hypotension is to be used. Moderate hypotension can usually be achieved by increasing the inhaled concentration of anesthesic agents. When deep levels of hypotension are required, nitroprusside is preferred because it is fast, predictable in its action and its effect, and it is rapidly reversible. Cyanide toxicity is not a problem when the agent is used for a short period of time (1). In some patients nitroglycerin is just as effective but it has been found that approximately half the patients do not respond well to nitroglycerin. Ganglionic blockers are also effective but they can result in some postoperative drowsiness and pupillary irregularity. After prolonged hypotension, dysautoregulation may develop, rendering the brain intolerant to subsequent hypertension which has been seen to cause parenchymal hemorrhage. Significant postoperative hypertension is avoided in these cases.

Temporary Proximal Arterial Occlusion or Trapping

For many years, neurosurgeons have used proximal arterial occlusion or trapping in emergency situations such as a major rupture of the aneurysm during dissection. This maneuver has saved many lives but also has caused much neurologic morbidity. In many instances, the surgeon was not prepared for temporary occlusion and the patient may have been hypotensive or dehydrated and there was no time for cerebral "protective" measures to be undertaken under such circumstances. Also temporary proximal arterial occlusion is particularly dangerous at a time when the aneurysm is bleeding massively since the blood loss compounds the problem by causing hypotension and reducing further the availability of collateral circulation.

It is far better to perform temporary proximal occlusion or trapping under controlled circumstances. This has been recommended by Suzuki for many years (84, 127) but it has only recently been adopted widely in aneurysm surgery. The authors have found this technique extremely useful and have become increasingly dependent on it for large and giant aneurysms or for any other complicated aneurysm that appears difficult to clip. It is important to avoid the use of concomitant hypotension with temporary vessel occlusion; the patient is usually kept normotensive or the pressure is raised to slightly higher than normal levels. Only low pressure clips should be used for temporary occlusion. It has been shown that normal and high pressure clips used for permanent aneurysmal occlusion can cause significant arterial damage even when used for a short period of time on normal arteries (26). Several types of aneurysm clips offer special low force temporary clips which are adequate for this purpose (the temporary Yasargil and Sugita clips which have been found to be very useful are marked by gold head or shanks on the clip).

Several operative approaches permit use of temporary arterial occlusion if needed. For paraclinoid aneurysm the carotid bifurcation is exposed in the neck for proximal control (52). Digital carotid compression by an anesthesiologist is not reliable enough to be recommended for general use. In cases of basilar tip aneurysms where the basilar bifurcation is relatively low, it may be necessary to cut the tentorium for some distance in order to get a more proximal basilar exposure (see Chapter 17). For middle cerebral artery aneurysms approached laterally through the sylvian fissure or superior temporal gyrus, the surgeon can usually work around the base of the aneurysm to prepare a small space on the distal M_1 segment for temporary clipping (53). In anterior communicating artery aneurysms, the authors routinely approach the aneurysm from the side of the dominant A_1 segment to achieve early proximal control of at least the major afferent vessel. Usually the contralateral A_1 segment can also be controlled before dealing with the aneurysm (see Chapter 14). Suzuki routinely uses a bifrontal approach in order to achieve easy control of both A_1 segments and both A_2 segments before aneurysmal dissection (125).

Duration of temporary arterial occlusion is critical. Suzuki has routinely used periods of 20–30 minutes and he advocates occlusion as long as 40 minutes with cerebral protection (mannitol, fluorocarbons, vitamin C) (126, 127). Such long periods are required to do the entire dissection of the aneurysm but this is only exceptionally necessary. For these unusual situations we have used successfully the following regimen: (a) 50 gm mannitol is given intravenously 15 minutes before cross-clamping; (b) albumin is administered to raise central venous pressure to 8–10 cm; (c) during cross-clamping the systolic blood pressure is elevated to 140–160 torr; and (d) temporary clips are opened for 1 minute for every 5 minutes of occlusion. The authors prefer this approach, which improves cerebral blood flow, over the use of barbiturates (103), which may cause hypotension and postoperative drowsiness.

For most aneurysms, much of the dissection can be done safely without temporary occlusion. The authors recommend reserving temporary clips for these cases for the final critical dissection and clipping. These maneuvers require 3–5 minutes, during which moderate hypertension (140–150 torr systolic) suffices for protection.

Wrapping

The technique of aneurysmal wrapping has been reviewed by Selverstone (104). In general this approach is effective only in middle cerebral artery aneurysms that can be dissected completely. It is almost impossible to expose completely the more centrally located aneurysms that are too large to be clipped and unless the aneurysm can be wrapped completely, wrapping is ineffective (22). With microsurgery, it has become increasingly clear that most aneurysms that were previously "wrapped" can usually be clipped and that what appeared to be vessels that were coming off the dome of the aneurysm are actually vessels that come off the neck and are simply adherent to the dome and can be dissected away from it with care under high magnification (53). Therefore, the recent experience of the authors with aneurysmal wrapping is confined to partial reinforcement of small segments of the aneurysm left out of the clip to avoid arterial compromise. For this purpose muslin gauze, which causes intense local reaction and helps prevent hemorrhage, can be used (27, 79). Muslin must not be placed on cranial nerves in order to avoid deficit from arachnoiditis (13). Cyanoacrylate adhesives are not recommended for they are neither effective nor safe (27, 56, 109).

Suction Aspiration

Flamm uses a 21 butterfly-needle for suction aspiration of the aneurysm (31). This procedure has been found to be helpful in some cases; however, the needle may become dislodged just at the time when the clip is being applied, and if the aneurysm cannot be clipped, bleeding from the needle hole is bothersome.

Special Clipping Methods

A variety of clipping techniques permit obliteration of many aneurysms hitherto considered unclippable. The aneurysm surgeon should be familiar with these methods, have the requisite armamentarium of clips at hand, and be ready to improvise creative solutions for the aneurysm he exposes. Drake has long advocated such methods (22), and Sugita has beautifully illustrated a range of complex obliteration techniques in his recently published atlas (117) (Fig. 20.6).

Tandem Clips. Clips may be applied side-by-side when a single clip is insufficient. Use of one big bayonet clip helps in placement by avoiding interference of the hubs. Alternatively, a second Sugita clip can be placed over the first, either parallel or oblique or a Sundt booster clip may be applied over the initial clip to close its tips (122) (Fig. 20.6D).

Preliminary Clipping. A permanent clip is placed on the aneurysm neck so as to occlude inflow and permit complete dissection without need for cerebral protection. Then the initial clip is repositioned or replaced for final precise obliteration.

Multiple Clips. This is commonly the key to obliteration of a giant aneurysm. Extraordinarily useful are the fenestrated clips, both straight and angled, introduced by Drake and ingeniously modified by Sugita (117). The possibilities with these newly developed clips are too numerous to present but a few are illustrated in Figure 20.6. As suggested by Sugita, we have found it easy to shorten his clip with a diamond drill to the precise length needed.

Ultralong Clips. At times these clips are needed to deal with the very wide necks of some giant aneurysms (22, 119). Since such necks broaden as they are occluded, the clip should be placed at some distance from the parent artery to avoid arterial compromise. Such clips have also been found useful for obliteration of aneurysms deep in a crevice too narrow to admit the jaws of a clip applier (Chapter 17).

Aneurysmorrhaphy

With hard atherosclerotic plaque and/or thrombus at the neck of the aneurysm, a clip may dislodge emboli or slip back onto the parent vessel. Also the major divisions of the parent vessel may come off the neck of the aneurysm. The only way to handle these situations is with aneurysmorrhaphy. Complete trapping of the aneurysm is necessary for aneurysmorrhaphy (102). The period of trapping is usually prolonged and cerebral protection is necessary, as described. Others have suggested performing a bypass graft in preparation for a prolonged period of trapping for aneurysmorrhaphy even though it is anticipated that the parent vessel will be spared (121). The technique of aneurysmorrhaphy is difficult and dangerous and should be used only by experienced surgeons. Often an indirect treatment is safer. When aneurysmorrhaphy is done removing too much of the atheroma in the area of the neck is avoided because it is easy to make a hole right through the neck which

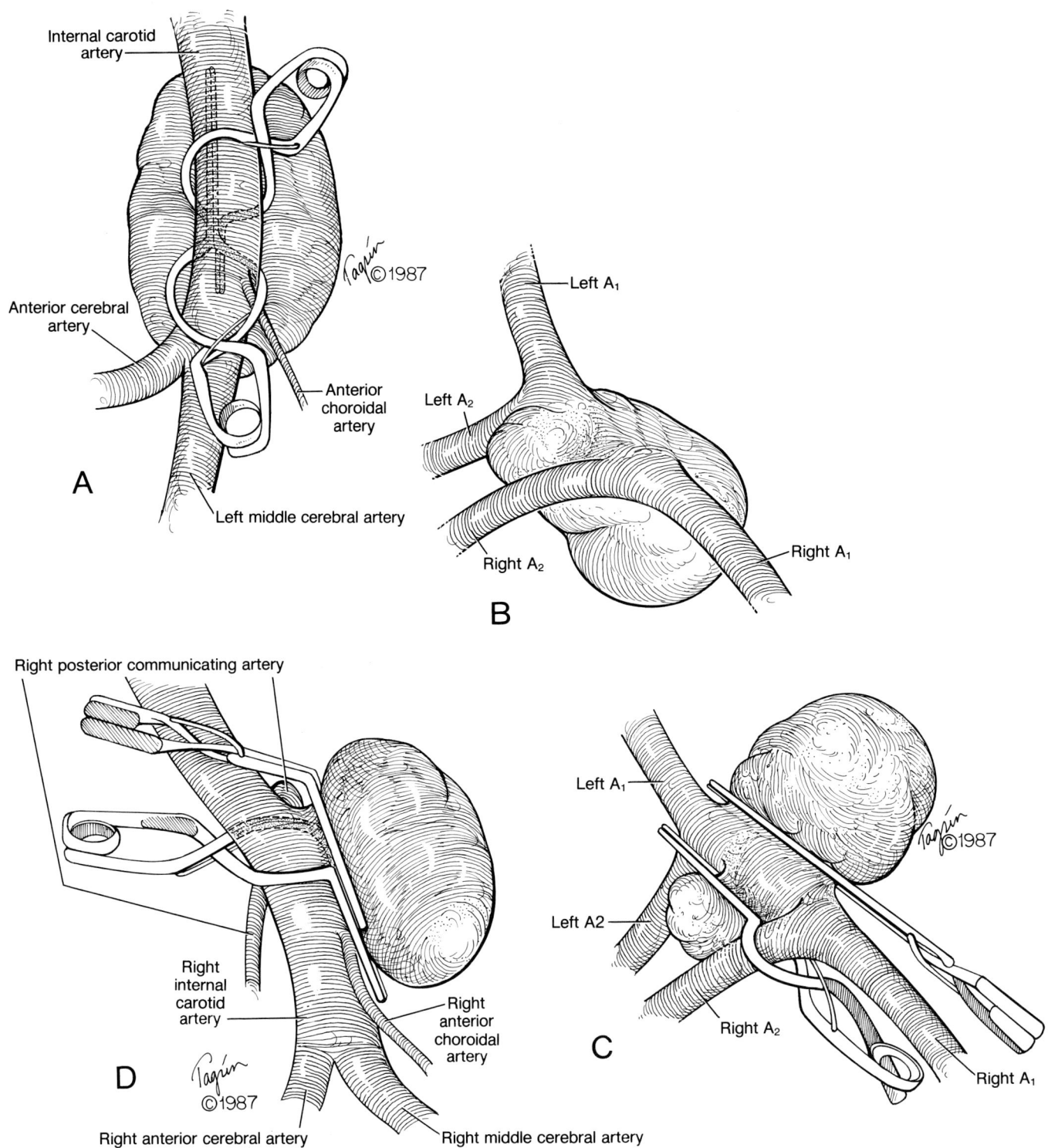

Figure 20.6. Clipping techniques for giant aneurysms. **A**, Globular aneurysm of the supraclinoid portion of the internal carotid artery has been clipped with "reconstruction" of the lumen of the carotid artery with two angled Sugita clips with Drake apertures placed in opposition with the aperture of the shorter clip going over the blades of the longer clip. **B** and **C**, A large bilobular aneurysm of the anterior communicating artery is clipped with a long straight Sugita clip obliterating the larger lobule which projects anteriorly and a straight Sugita clip with a Drake aperture used to obliterate the smaller lobule that projects superiorly. The right A_2 is encircled by the Drake aperture of the second clip. This technique preserves the perforators which arise from the posterior aspect of the anterior communicating artery (not shown). **D**, A large aneurysm of the dorsal wall of the supraclinoid internal carotid artery is clipped in "tandem" by using first a right-angle Sugita clip encircling the carotid artery but leaving some of the neck which is then obliterated with an oblique unfenestrated Sugita clip. (Modified after Sugita K: *Microsurgical Atlas*. Tokyo, Springer-Verlag, 1985.)

will make it impossible to reconstruct the normal anatomy. The ultrasonic aspirator (CUSA) is useful in removing the hard organized thrombus from the inside of the aneurysm. It is not necessary to remove all the thrombus or dissect all the dome to achieve a satisfactory aneurysmorrhaphy. It is best to leave a generous cuff to close with continuous suture (7-0 or 8-0 nylon is usually satisfactory) or with a clip (Fig. 20.7).

Some form of monitoring could be useful. A variety of methods have included EEG, cortical excitability (28) and cortical blood flow by thermal dilution (14).

Cerebral protection by any of the methods previously discussed is recommended in all these cases.

Cardiopulmonary Bypass

Prolonged cardiocirculatory arrest can be tolerated under deep hypothermia and artificial extracorporeal circulation (24, 38, 41, 60, 74, 107, 108, 123, 137, 142). Initially this technique carried very significant morbidity related mostly to systemic problems after extracorporeal circulation (22). For this reason this procedure has been abandoned by most surgeons. However, there are some centers in which the tech-

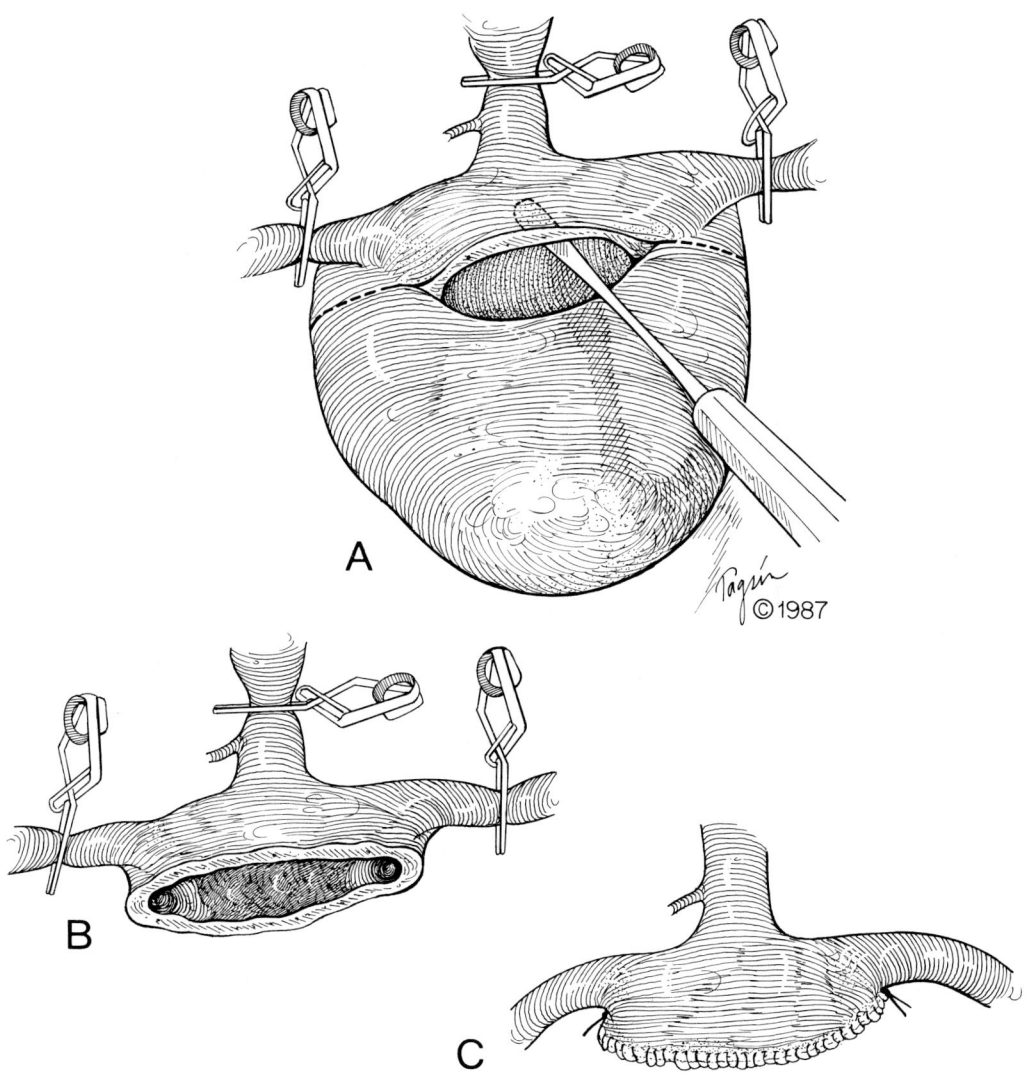

Figure 20.7. Technique of aneurysmorrhaphy. **A**, After placement of temporary clips in the afferent and efferent arteries, an incision is made in the front wall of the base of the aneurysm and then the organized clot and/or atheroma is carefuly separated from the wall of the aneurysm with a dissector. Sometimes this material is so tenacious and gritty that the use of the ultrasonic cavitron may be required to facilitate its removal. **B**, After removal of the organized clot, a circumferential excision of the aneurysm is acomplished. In doing this it is extremely important to leave a wide enough "cuff" so that it can be closed without encroaching on the origins of the main efferent vessels. **C**, The cuff has been closed with a running suture. Alternatively, sometimes it is possible to close the cuff with an aneurysm clip.

nique, particularly by the closed chest method of transfemoral cannulation, continues to be used with a considerable measure of success. The techniques involved are very complicated and the authors' personal experience with this method has been very limited and generally unsuccessful; therefore it will not be described in further detail.

Carotid Occlusion

When carotid ligation is considered, there are a number of choices to be made. The internal or the common carotid artery may be occluded. The occlusion may be abrupt or gradual. The aneurysm may be trapped by occluding the carotid artery distal to the aneurysm. A preliminary bypass graft may or may not be done. The artery may be occluded by ligature, clamp, or balloon. To make these choices intelligently, the surgeon must have as much information as possible about the potential for collateral circulation. Our approach is to perform three-vessel angiography with detailed cross-compression studies (the contralateral carotid and a vertebral artery are sequentially injected while the ipsilateral carotid artery is temporarily occluded). Prompt filling of the ipsilateral middle cerebral artery territory either through the anterior circle of Willis by contralateral carotid injection or through the posterior communicating artery by vertebral injection while the ipsilateral carotid is occluded is usually a good indication that the patient will tolerate carotid occlusion. Since angiography is usually performed with the patient awake, the patient can also be tested clinically while the internal or the common carotid artery is occluded temporarily by balloon for 15 minutes (17). The authors prefer to have the patient heparinized for this procedure. If heparin cannot be used either because there has been a recent subarachnoid hemorrhage or craniotomy, test occlusion is limited to 5 minutes.

The controversies surrounding the use of carotid ligation have been extensively discussed in the literature which has been reviewed by the authors in several recent publications (47, 49, 52, 130). The authors' interpretation of the data leads to the conclusion that, in general, common carotid artery occlusion is associated with less morbidity than internal carotid artery occlusion. This may be due to the fact that the internal carotid artery usually stays open with flow either from the external carotid artery to the internal carotid or vice versa reducing the risk of thromboembolic complications from distal clot in the internal carotid artery. In the cooperative study, Nishioka (81) reported that the rate of ischemic complications was 49% with internal carotid artery litigation and 28% with common carotid artery ligation. Other authors have reported similar figures (64, 78). The literature also reflects very little difference in effectiveness (i.e., rate of rebleeding and incidence of thrombosis or size reduction in the aneurysm) between internal carotid and common carotid artery ligation (36, 37, 64, 78, 81, 82, 90, 133). These data refer to internal carotid artery occlusion at its origin by ligature or clamp. There are no data comparing common carotid artery occlusion with occlusion of the internal carotid artery just below the aneurysm by balloon.

There does not seem to be significant difference in the rate of ischemic complications after gradual or abrupt carotid occlusion (67, 81). Even though the rate of ischemic complications in the cooperative study was slightly higher for patients with abrupt occlusion, Nishioka points out that in these instances the occlusion occurred earlier after subarachnoid hemorrhage and that the ischemic problems that these patients suffered in many instancs were undoubtedly related to vasospasm rather than directly related to the carotid occlusion itself (81). About 20% of the patients will not tolerate abrupt occlusion (75). Of these a few will tolerate gradual occlusion over a period of several days.

Proximal carotid artery occlusion alone is not adequate treatment for patients who present with rapidly progressing visual loss or neurologic deterioration from compression of the brain by the aneurysm. These patients should have their aneurysms trapped and decompressed directly by aneurysmorrhaphy. This is also necessary in those patients who develop significant visual loss or brain compression from aneurysmal enlargement related to thrombosis after carotid ligation (22). The authors have not felt compelled to decompress the aneurysm in those patients who develop only pain or oculomotor palsies after carotid ligation, since these problems usually resolve with time.

It should also be noted that Jane, Winn and colleagues have reported that carotid ligation reduces the early frequency of recurrent subarachnoid hemorrhage but the long-term rate of recurrent hemorrhage is not significantly altered (63, 141). Therefore, patients must continue to be followed indefinitely after carotid ligation unless the aneurysm has been trapped or has thrombosed completely.

A situation where carotid occlusion is contraindicated is illustrated in Figure 20.8. This patient had bilateral internal carotid artery aneurysms. The smaller aneurysm on the left side had its origin in the cavernous sinus and could not be clipped. The larger aneurysm on the right side arose from the paraclinoid region. When there is an intact aneurysm that cannot be clipped on the contralateral carotid artery, it is recommended that every effort be made to clip the giant aneurysm directly. If this is not possible it may be best to perform an extracranial-intracranial (EC-IC) bypass graft if carotid occlusion is to be done.

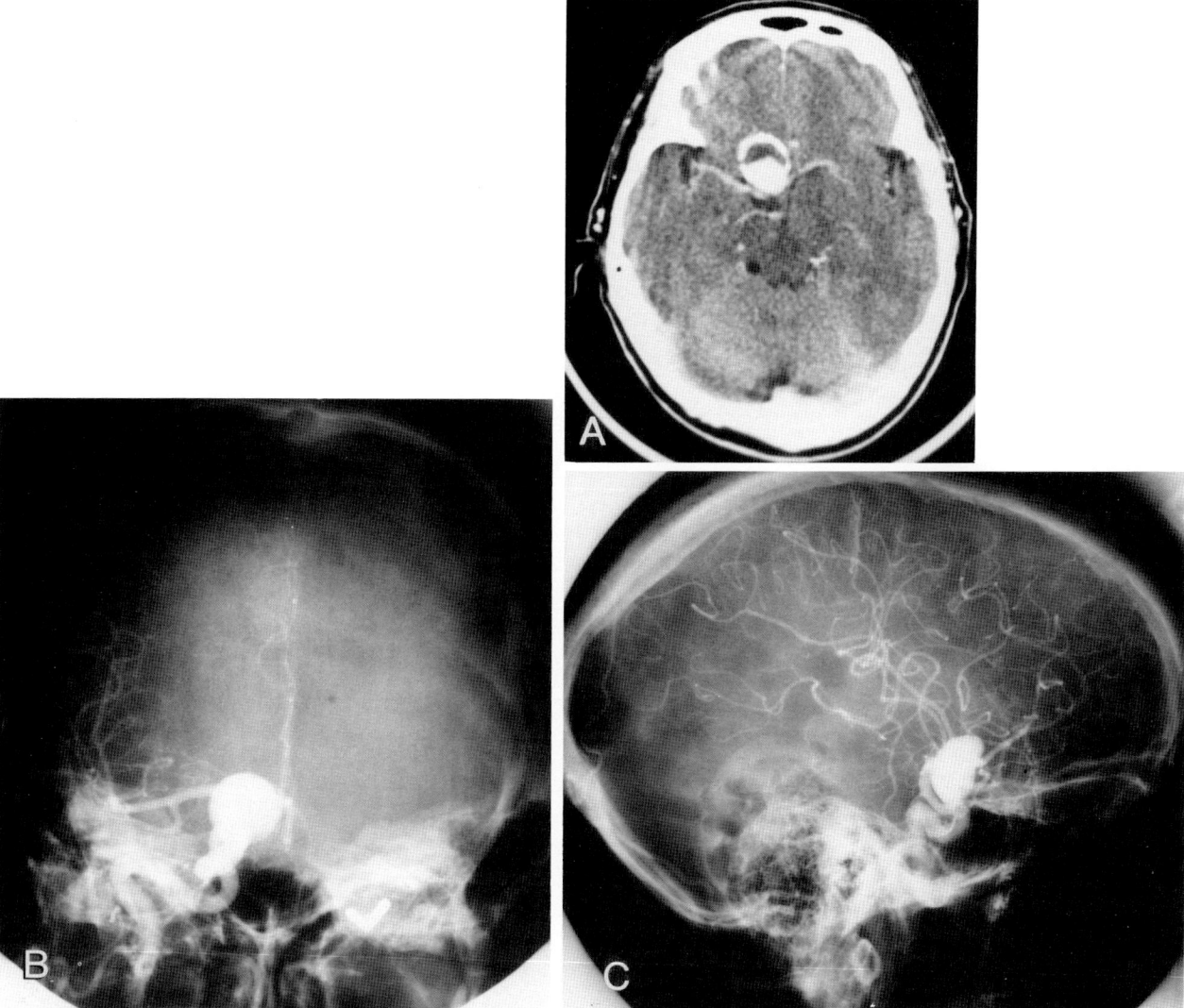

Figure 20.8. Bilateral carotid aneurysms. A relative contraindication to carotid occlusion. **A–C**, CT scan and right carotid angiogram, respectively, show a partially thrombosed giant paraclinoid aneurysm. **D** and **E**, Left carotid angiogram shows a smaller paraclinoid aneurysm on the left side. The authors could not be sure whether the aneurysm took origin from the paraclinoid region, and therefore could be clipped, or whether, as it appeared more likely from studying the angiograms, the origin was from the infraclinoid region in the cavernous sinus which would make it unclippable. This middle-aged lady presented with visual loss in the right eye. Because of the high likelihood of not being able to clip the aneurysm on the left side, the authors decided to make every effort to clip the aneurysm on the rigt side. Indeed the authors were able to do so with temporary occlusion of the exposed cervical portion of the internal carotid artery. **F** and **G**, Postoperative right carotid angiogram shows that the aneurysm has been completely occluded and the carotid artery has been preserved. Tandem clips were necessary using first a straight Sugita clip with an angled handle. A straight Sugita clip with a Drake fenestration was then placed distal to the initial clip. The handle of the initial clip was left under fenestration of the second clip. Unfortunately the patient's vision in the right eye was much worse postoperatively but she has regained some vision as the months have gone by. Several weeks after the first operation, the second aneurysm was explored and indeed it was found that the origin was in the cavernous sinus and therefore it could not be clipped. Since the right internal carotid artery was preserved, there is the option of treating the second aneurysm by left carotid occlusion in the future should symptoms develop or the aneurysm show any enlargement.

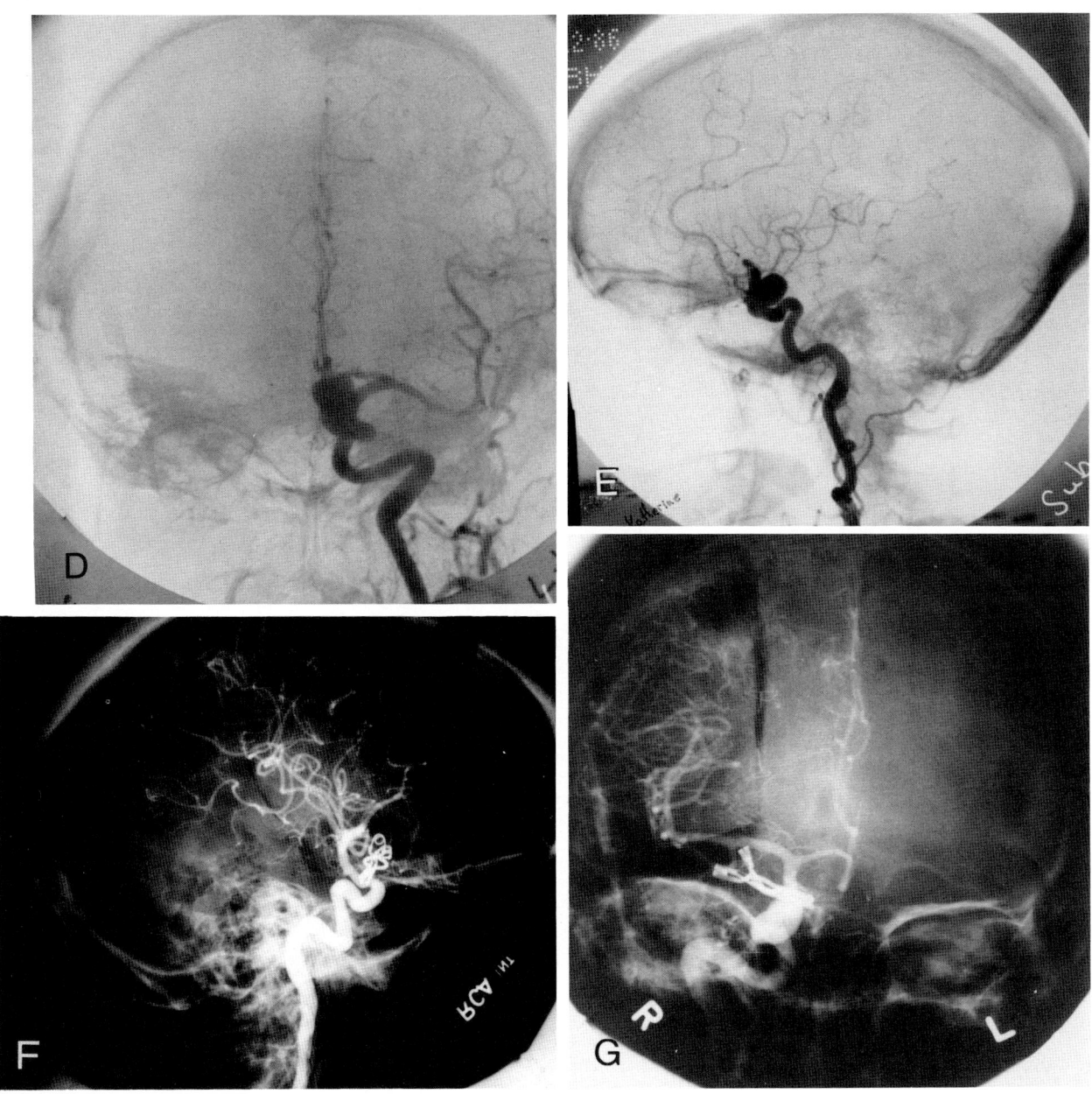

Figure 20.8D–G.

Common Carotid Occlusion

With the above considerations in mind, the authors have developed an approach that is outlined in Figure 20.9. If collateral circulation is estimated to be inadequate by either angiographic cross-compression studies or because the patient did not tolerate temporary occlusion during angiography, an EC-IC bypass procedure is performed first. This is followed 2–5 days later by an attempt to occlude the internal carotid artery with a balloon with the patient awake in the angiographic suite. An angiogram is performed initially to ensure that the bypass is open. Sometimes all that can be seen is filling of a few intracranial branches but this is sufficient. Next the patient is tested with the balloon inflated but not detached. This period of test occlusion lasts 15 minutes if the patient can be heparinized but it should be restricted to 5 minutes if the use of heparin is contraindicated because of recent subarachnoid hemorrhage. If the patient tolerates this temporary occlusion, the procedure is continued by detaching the balloon as close as possible to the neck of the aneurysm but without

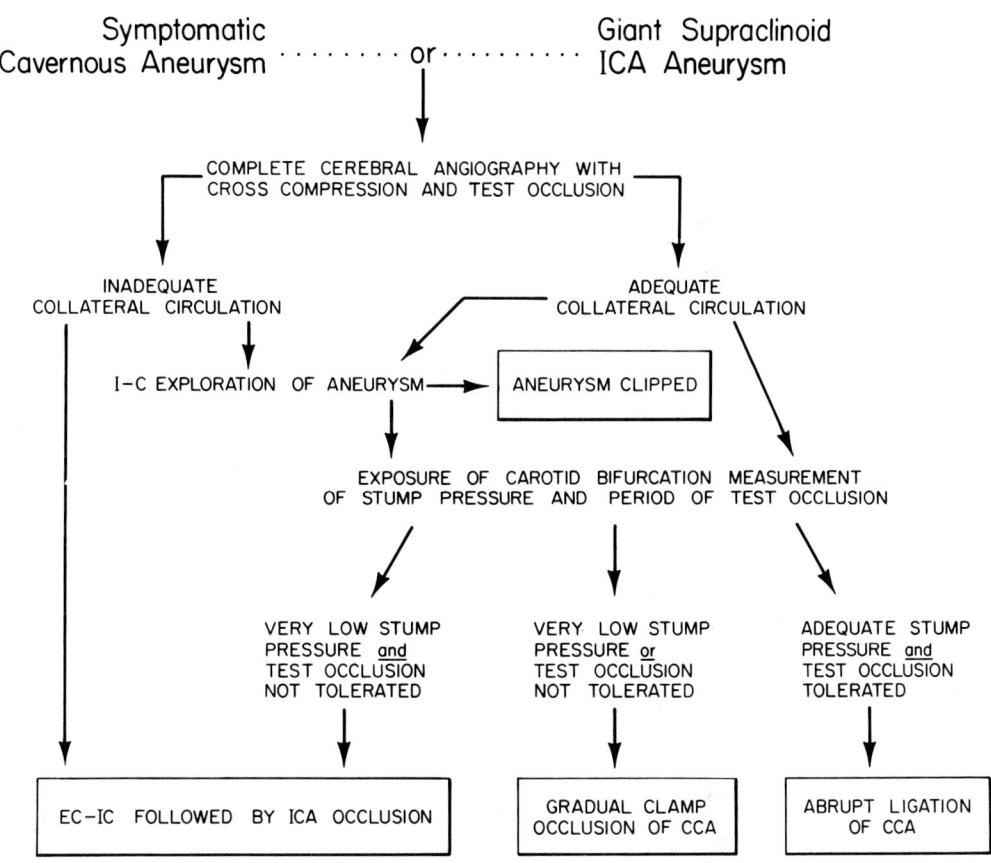

Figure 20.9. Schematic representation of the decision making process presently used with giant aneurysms of the internal carotid artery at the MGH. (From Swearingen B, Heros RC: Common carotid occlusion for unclippable carotid aneurysms. *Neurosurgery*, in press.)

making an attempt to detach it directly in the neck of the aneurysm. When the latter is attempted problems can develop from the balloon protruding partially into the aneurysm or occluding the origin of the ophthalmic artery or other important vessels (17). An angiogram is obtained to study the degree of filling through the bypass graft after the carotid is occluded. The degree of dilatation of the superficial temporal artery from the preocclusion to the immediate postocclusion angiogram can sometimes be quite impressive (Fig. 20.10).

If collateral circulation was estimated to be adequate by cross-compression studies and the patient tolerated temporary occlusion during the angiogram, the authors prefer to occlude the common carotid artery in view of the greater safety and equal effectiveness of this procedure when compared with internal carotid artery occlusion. In cases where intracranial exploration was carried out first, the neck will already be prepared and if the carotid bifurcation is not exposed this can be done quickly while the patient is still asleep and then the patient can be awakened to be tested clinically during the period of test occlusion to be described. The authors prefer to use EEG monitoring for all these cases but are aware of the limitations imposed on its interpretation by the fewer number of scalp leads that can be placed around a craniotomy field. Still, in several instances the EEG information has been found to be useful although the authors cannot vouch for its reliability in all cases.

If intracranial exploration is not done, the carotid bifurcation in the neck is exposed with the patient awake under local anesthesia or, preferably, under regional anesthesia. If the patient is asleep, EEG monitoring is important and the authors prefer to use it even when the patient is awake. Once the bifurcation is exposed, the common carotid, internal carotid, and external carotid arteries are isolated with tapes. While the patient is monitored by EEG, and if awake by clinical examination, the distal common carotid artery is occluded for a period of 15 minutes. When there has not been a recent subarachnoid hemorrhage and the patient has not had a simultaneous craniotomy, the patient is heparinized during this period (5,000 units of heparin as a bolus) and reversed with Protamine after ligature. If there has been a recent subarachnoid hemorrhage or a concurrent crani-

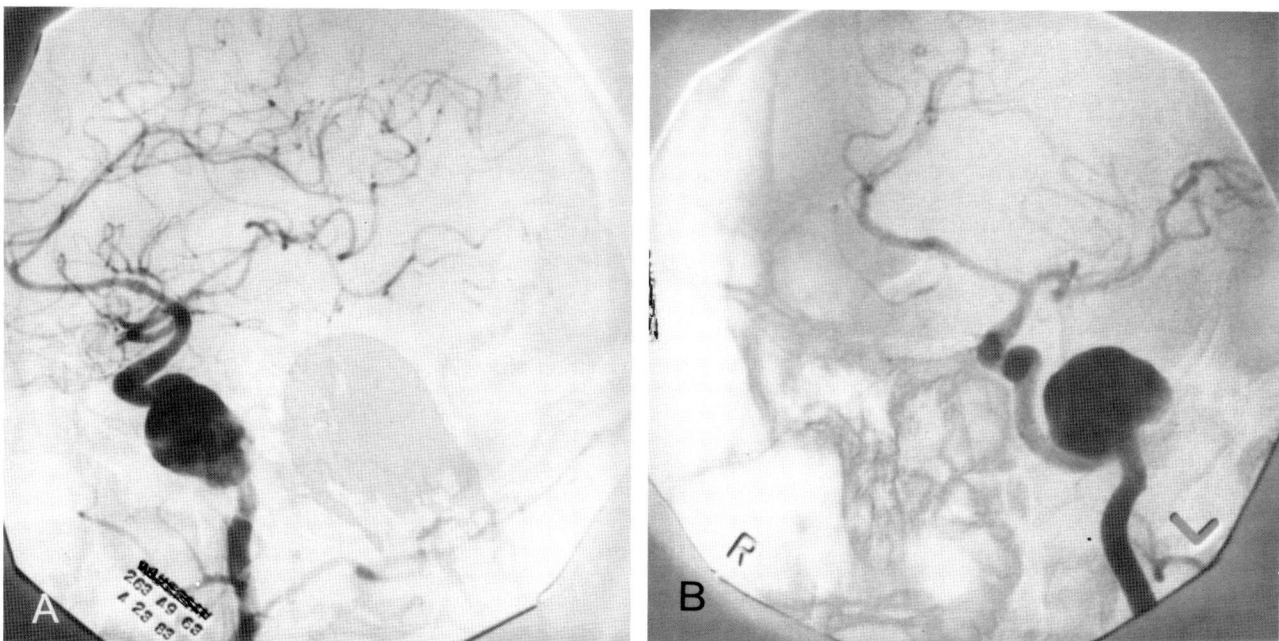

Figure 20.10. Giant petrous aneurysm treated by internal carotid artery balloon occlusion after EC-IC bypass. **A** and **B**, Angiography revealed a giant aneurysm of the petrous portion of the left internal carotid artery. The patient presented with pain in the left side of the face and a sixth nerve palsy. A right hemiparesis developed during temporary occlusion of the left internal carotid artery with a balloon. The deficit resolved promptly with deflation of the balloon. Because of this demonstrated intolerance to carotid occlusion, the authors proceeded with a superficial temporal to middle cerebral artery bypass graft. Two days later the patient was rearteriographed. **C**, Selective left external carotid angiogram shows that the bypass graft is patent but it only supplied a few branches of the middle cerebral artery. Test occlusion of the left internal carotid artery by balloon was well tolerated for 15 minutes; therefore, the authors proceeded with balloon occlusion of the internal carotid artery. Initially, a balloon was detached distal to the aneurysm to prevent distal thromboembolic problems. Two more balloons were then detached in the internal carotid artery proximal to the origin of the aneurysm. **D** and **E**, Immediate postocclusion angiography shows significant dilation of the superficial temporal artery (*double arrow*) and the position of the balloons (*single arrow*). Note that the superficial temporal artery is now able to supply not only the entire middle cerebral artery but also, by retrograde flow, the anterior cerebral territory on the left side (**E**).

otomy, the authors do not hesitate to proceed with temporary common carotid occlusion without heparinization since blood flow usually continues in the internal carotid and external carotid arteries. However, the period of test occlusion is limited to 5 minutes under these circumstances. If flow needs to be reestablished, it is important to direct flow first into the external carotid artery by brief temporary clamping of the internal carotid artery to avoid embolic problems.

During the period of temporary occlusion, the stump pressure is measured in the internal carotid artery. An alternative would be to use intraoperative blood flow measurements where such are available (121). A very marked fall in pressure (more than 70% fall in the mean pressure or a mean pressure below 30 torr), together with a change in the clinical examination or EEG during temporary occlusion, makes the authors abandon the attempt at carotid occlusion and proceed to an EC-IC bypass procedure followed by an attempt at internal carotid artery occlusion by balloon (35, 112, 114). The bypass may be performed under the same anesthetic if the patient has been so advised. If either the stump pressure falls markedly but the neurologic examination and the EEG remain normal or if the examination or EEG change but the stump pressure does not fall markedly, the authors prefer to apply a clamp and proceed with gradual occlusion over the next several days. The use of the Crutchfield clamp for this procedure is illustrated in Figure 20.11. When gradual occlusion is used, the patient is heparinized for the last critical 2 or 3 days of clamp closure if there has been no recent subarachnoid hemorrhage.

When the clinical examination and/or the EEG remain normal during the period of temporary occlusion and the stump pressure falls less than 70% and is greater than 30 torr, the authors proceed with abrupt ligation of the common carotid artery with three ligatures applied just below the bifurcation. A useful

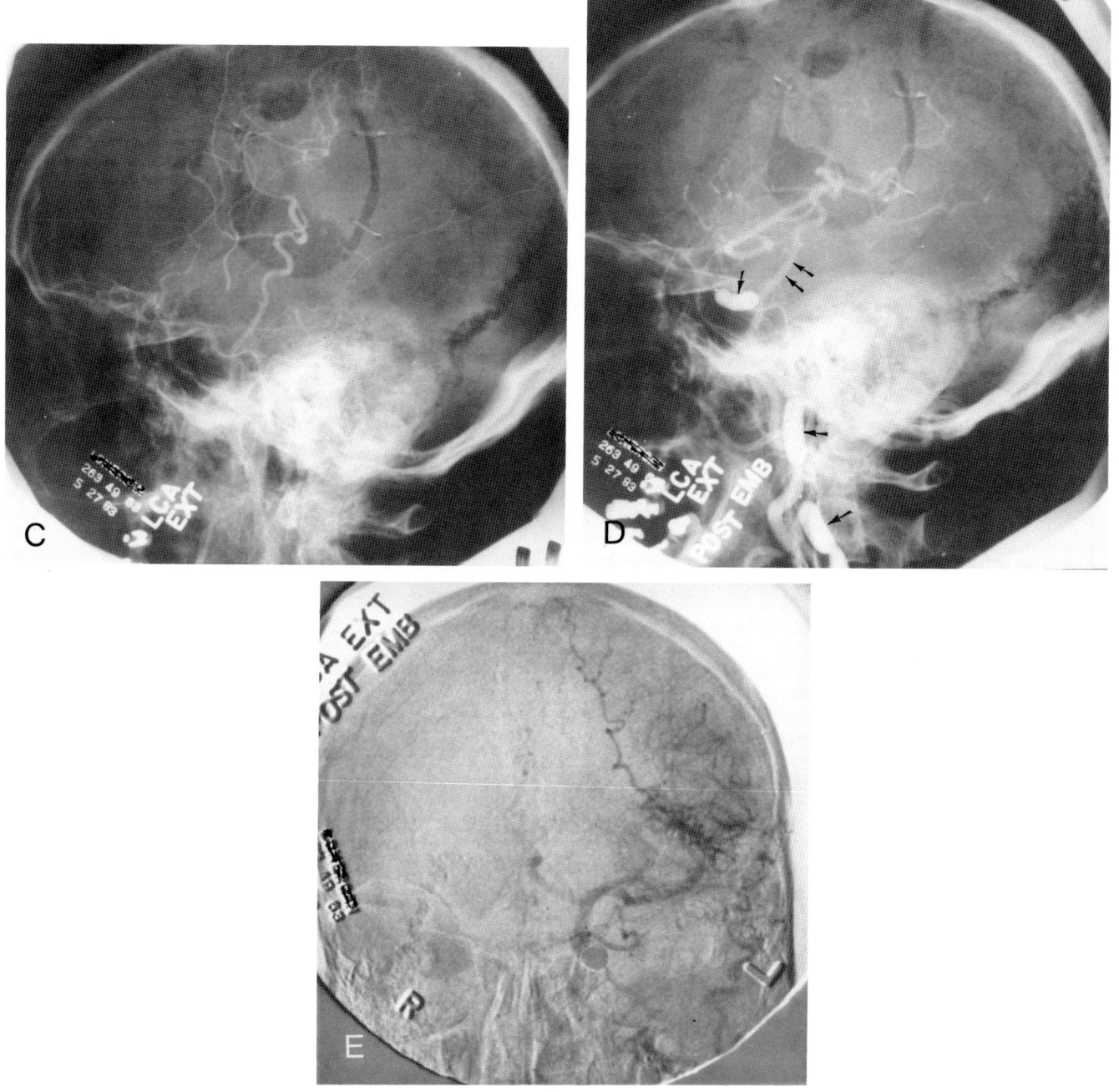

Figure 20.10C–E.

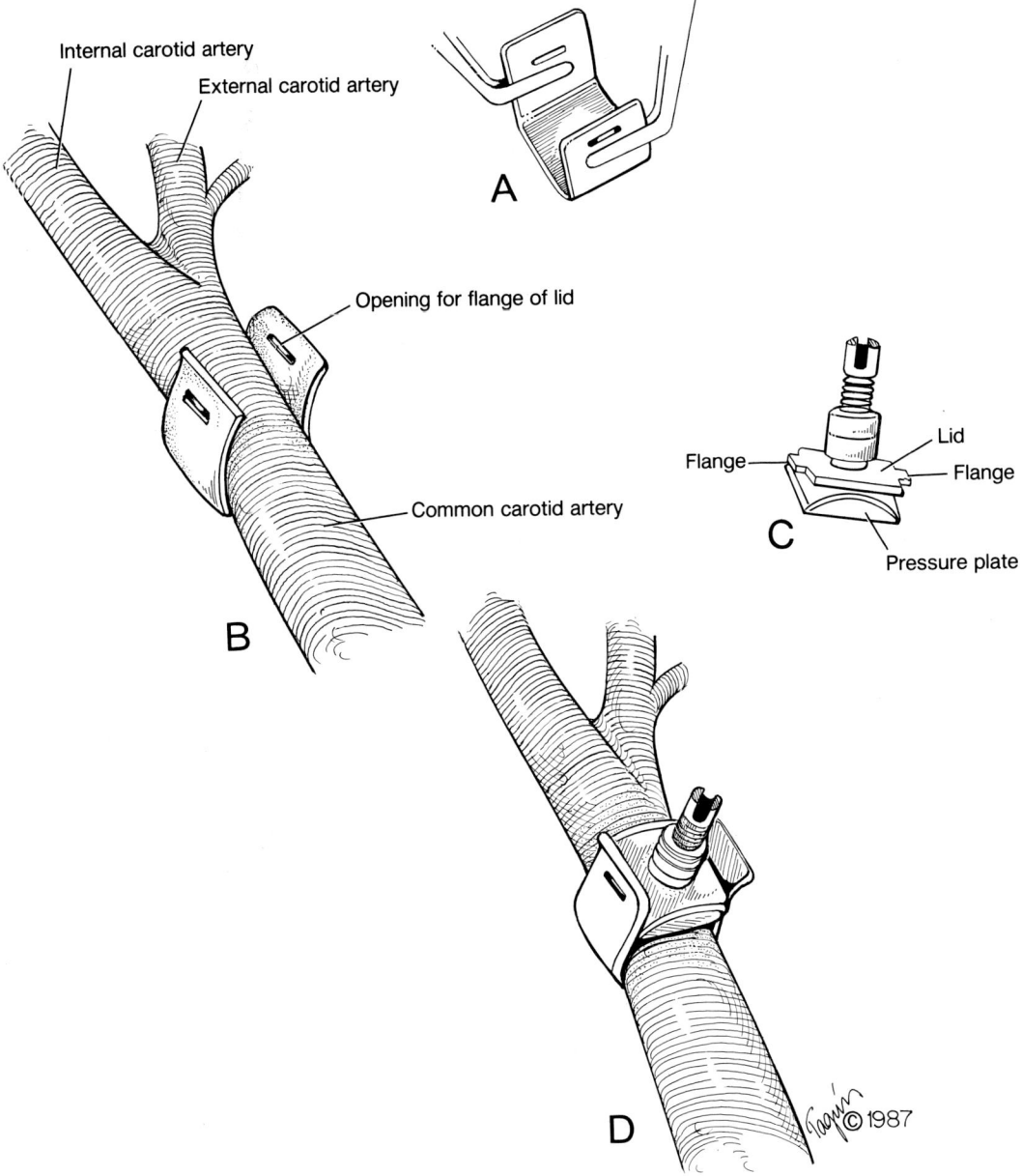

Figure 20.11. Placement of Crutchfield clamp. **A**, The U-shaped portion of the clamp may be held open with right-angle clamps to permit removal or replacement of the lid assembly (see **C**). **B**, With the lid assembly removed, the U-shaped portion of the clamp is gently positioned at the distal portion of the common carotid artery. **C**, The lid assembly consists of a screw through the lid to a pressure plate. Flanges on the lid fit into slots in the U-shaped portion. **D**, The lid assembly is fitted into place with flanges engaging slots as shown. Right-angle clamps open the U-shaped portion as shown in **A**. **E**, The control assembly consists of a screwdriver, handle, and locks. This assembly is pushed through a lateral stab wound with the cap in place to protect the tip of the screwdriver. **F**, The U-shaped portion is rotated to receive the control assembly. Turning the screw occludes the artery. **G**, Recording of intraarterial pressure when clamp must be left partially opened. Note that pressure in this patient starts to drop between four and five turns. The pressure with complete occlusion is about 40 mm. The clamp is left at a point where a slight reduction in pressure has occurred.

Giant Aneurysms

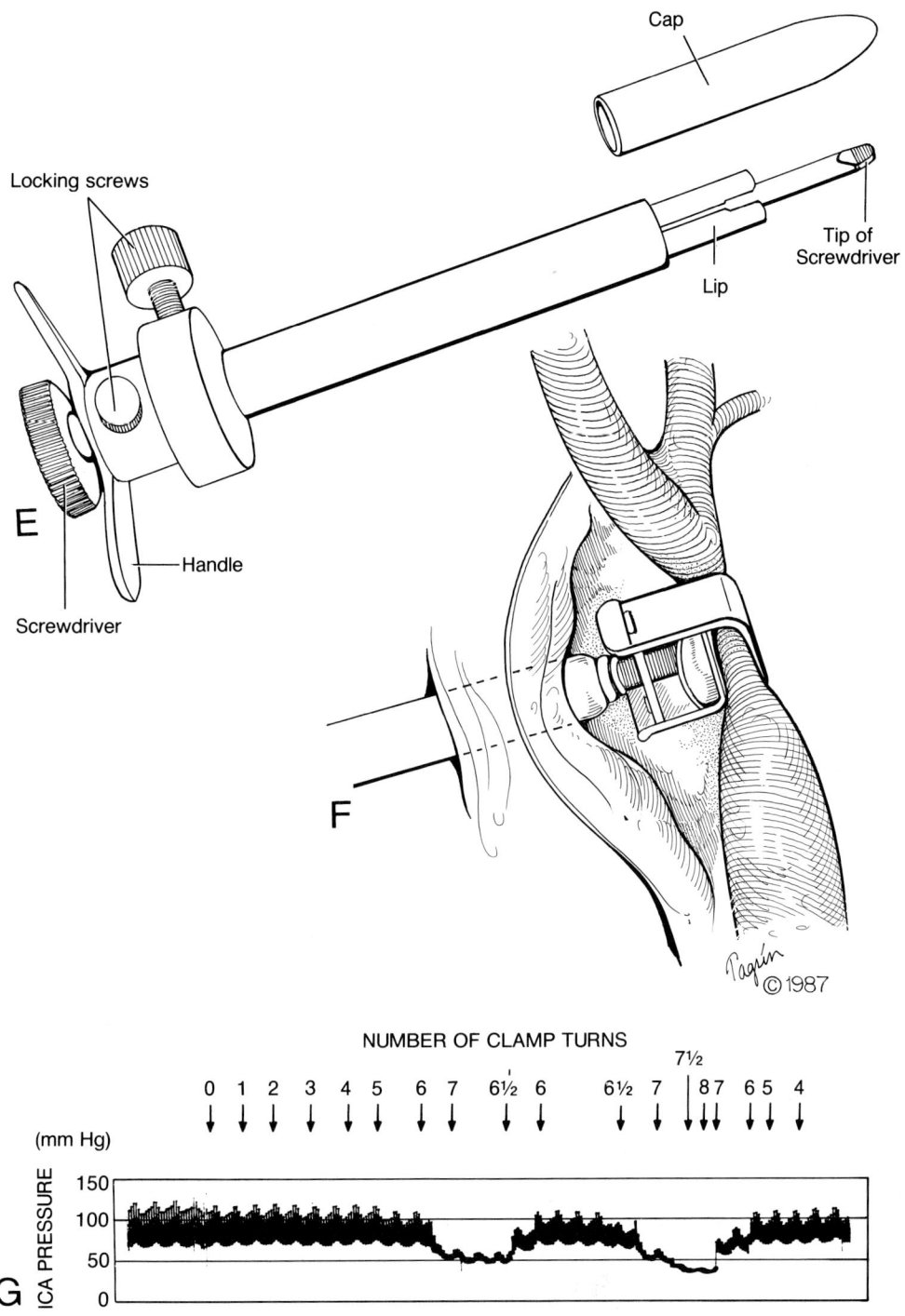

Figure 20.11E–G.

precaution, particularly if the systemic pressure during test occlusion is abnormally high, is to "stress" the patient by artificially lowering the blood pressure by 20 or 30 torr during the time of test occlusion.

In cases where there is very little drop in stump pressure (i.e., less then 30%), there is little hope of aneurysmal thrombosis with common carotid artery ligation alone. One may temporarily occlude the origin of the internal carotid artery and see if the pressure then falls significantly. This would be unusual but if it occurs, internal carotid artery occlusion would be indicated. Occlusion of the internal carotid artery with a balloon is preferred so as to avoid a long distal stump with its inherent risk of thromboembolism. For the same reasons, anticoagulants are used whenever possible if the internal carotid artery is to be occluded. If the internal carotid artery stump pressure still does not fall significantly after proximal occlusion, the only useful alternative left is to trap the aneurysm with proximal internal carotid artery ligation in the neck and distal ligation intracranially. With trapping there is some risk of ophthalmic ischemia and blindness but since the external carotid artery is left open, retrograde ophthalmic flow should be adequate and the risk of blindness very small.

Postoperatively, continuous monitoring of blood pressure allows prompt treatment of hypotension. Patients are mobilized slowly to prevent orthostatic hypotension. CT scans are obtained before discharge from the hospital and then at regular intervals (i.e., 3 months) until aneurysmal thrombosis is confirmed. Sometimes, particularly with large intracavernous aneurysms, thrombosis is heralded by the development of a cranial nerve palsy or severe retro-orbital pain. The deficit or pain has resolved completely in our cases. If the aneurysm remains unthrombosed by CT scan after a period of 3-6 months, it is probably reasonable to assume that it will not thrombose. Repeat angiography is done to determine how the aneurysm is being supplied. If the aneurysm is below the posterior communicating artery and the flow is retrograde from the other carotid artery or from the vertebral circulation, a simple trapping procedure ligating the internal carotid artery intracranially below the posterior communicating artery will usually deal with the problem. If the flow is from the external to the internal carotid artery, ligation of the external carotid artery in the neck usually suffices. Table 20.1 summarizes nine patients with unclippable carotid aneurysms treated in this manner at the Massachusetts General Hospital (MGH) over the past 5 years.

Internal Carotid Occlusion by Balloon

With the development of balloon catheter methods the risk of internal carotid occlusion can be assessed at the time of angiography by evaluation of collateral circulation, neurologic status and, when available, blood flow studies during temporary carotid occlusion (17, 18, 32, 33, 62). From this information the need for a preliminary EC-IC bypass is determined. This procedure is done only when collateral circulation appears to be insufficient. If a bypass appears to be unnecessary, balloon occlusion can be attempted during the initial angiographic session. Before balloon detachment a 15-minute period of test occlusion with the patient heparinized is undertaken. If the patient tolerates test occlusion the balloon can be detached just proximal to the neck of the aneurysm. It is best to detach a second balloon proximally to avoid deflation and distal embolization of the first balloon; a complication that has been reported by the authors (128). Another complication of balloon occlusion that has been observed is distal thromboembolism after balloon detachment. This complication may be prevented by pretreatment with antiplatelet drugs, full heparinization during the procedure and antiplatelet drugs and/or at least partial heparinization for 2 or 3 days after balloon detachment (86). If delayed ischemic events develop they can be treated vigorously with volume expansion and elevation of the systemic pressure if necessary. The authors make sure, whenever carotid occlusion by any method is contemplated that the patient is hypervolemic at the time of carotid occlusion and for several days thereafter; this is accomplished by regular infusions of colloid solutions such as albumin or dextran.

When a bypass is done, internal carotid occlusion by intraluminal balloon is attempted 2–5 days after the bypass procedure. If the patient has a functional bypass and still does not tolerate test occlusion, the choices are between no treatment and an attempt at gradual occlusion of the internal carotid artery by clamp.

SPECIFIC SITES

Internal Carotid Artery Aneurysms

Petrous Aneurysms

Several recent publications have described in detail the symptomatology and treatment of these relatively rare aneurysms (9, 39, 55, 71, 73, 76, 96, 131). These aneurysms may be mycotic, posttraumatic, or congenital in origin. Patients may have a history of chronic otitis media often with purulent otorrhea. A traumatic etiology can be suspected if there has been antecedent serious head injury with or without a documented basilar skull fracture. Petrous aneurysms become symptomatic as a result of hemorrhage into or mass effect on structures adjacent to the carotid canal. Spontaneous hemorrhage into the eustachian tube or middle ear cavity has resulted in dramatic episodes of epistaxis and otorrhagia. Frequently patients complain only of decreased hearing, pain, or pulsatile tinnitus in the affected ear. Ill-ad-

Table 20.1.
Summary of Nine Consecutive Patients with Unclippable Carotid Aneurysms[a]

CASE NO.	AGE & SEX	CLINICAL PRESENTATION	RADIOLOGIC FINDINGS	OPERATIVE PROCEDURE	STUMP PRESSURE	EEG	RESULT
1	56 F	HEADACHE	GIANT CAVERNOUS	CCA CLAMP CLOSED 1 DAY P-OP	90 → 65 MEAN	nl	DEVELOPED PARTIAL III 2 DAY P-OP CLEARED CT: THROMBOSED
2	38 M	VISUAL LOSS O.D.	GIANT R PARACLINOID, L OPHTHALMIC L CAROTID BIFURCATION	1. L OPHTHALMIC BIFURCATION CLIPPED 2. R CCA LIGATED, WITH WAKE-UP	100 → 30 MEAN	–	VISION NORMAL CT: THROMBOSED
3	58 F	RIGHT VI PALSY	GIANT, CAVERNOUS	TEST OCCLUSION ONLY	90 → 15	FLAT	EC-IC RECOMMENDED
4	38 F	HEADACHE	GIANT, CAVERNOUS	CCA LIGATION, REGIONAL ANESTH.	120 → 80	–	R RETRO-ORBITAL PAIN CT: THROMBOSED
5	59 F	COMPLEX PARTIAL SEIZURES	GIANT BIFURCATION	CCA LIGATION WITH WAKE-UP	110 → 40	nl	PARTIAL R III 4 DAY P-OP CLEARED CT: THROMBOSED
6	38 F	HEADACHE	FUSIFORM, GIANT	1. I-C EXPLORATION 2. CCA LIGATION WITH WAKE-UP	100 → 65	nl	CT: NO THROMBOSIS NO CHANGE IN SIZE
7	67 F	PARTIAL VI PALSY	GIANT CAVERNOUS	CCA LIGATION, REGIONAL ANESTH.	200 → 90 SYSTOLIC OCCLUSION TOLERATED TO 100 SYSTOLIC	nl	CT: THROMBOSED
8	68 F	VISUAL LOSS OD	GIANT PARACLINOID	1. I-C EXPLORATION 2. CCA LIGATION WAKE-UP	110 → 37 MEAN	nl	CT: THROMBOSED
9	61 F	VISUAL LOSS OU	GIANT PARACLINOID	1. I-C EXPLORATION 2. CCC LIGATION WITH WAKE-UP	95 → 35 MEAN	Min. chg.	CT: THROMBOSED

[a]The protocol outlined in Figure 20.9 was followed for these patients. (From Swearingen B, Heros RC: Common carotid occlusion for unclippable carotid aneurysms. *Neurosurgery*, in press.

vised transtympanic biopsy of these lesions has often resulted in massive hemorrhage which can usually be controlled with packing of the external auditory canal. These aneurysms may also present with symptoms of compression of adjacent cranial nerves, most frequently V, VI, and VII.

Direct surgical approach to these deep lesions is very difficult although feasible (39). The most frequent treatment for these aneurysms has been proximal ligation of the ipsilateral internal or common carotid artery. The patient illustrated in Figure 20.10 was treated with balloon occlusion of the internal carotid artery after a bypass graft because the patient did not tolerate temporary occlusion of the carotid artery during preoperative angiography.

Intracavernous Aneurysms

Aneurysms in this location present most commonly with a cavernous sinus syndrome. The third nerve is most frequently involved but the fourth and sixth nerves can also be affected. The patient usually has mild proptosis and slight conjunctival injection without the pulsating exophthalmus, chemosis, and bruit that are characteristic of carotid cavernous fistulae. When the aneurysm is large the optic nerve may be involved. Severe retro-orbital pain may be the first complaint. Sympathetic fibers may become involved as they course through the cavernous sinus resulting in oculosympathetic paralysis. The fifth nerve is variably affected with the first and second divisions being most frequently involved. Both massive epistaxis from erosion into the ethmoid or sphenoid sinuses and subarachnoid hemorrhage from transdural rupture can result but such events have been very rare.

Smaller asymptomatic aneurysms of this area may be treated conservatively but giant aneurysms, in the authors' opinion, should always be considered for treatment provided the patient can tolerate it. Direct approaches to aneurysms of the cavernous sinus have been reported (20), but these techniques are dangerous. Carotid occlusion is the preferred method of treatment.

Paraclinoid Aneurysms

These aneurysms arise at the origin of the ophthalmic artery or from the posterior or lateral wall of the carotid artery. Aneurysms of this general region are reviewed in detail in Chapter 13. They usually present either with subarachnoid hemorrhage or with signs of compression of the visual apparatus.

An attempt should be made to treat all giant aneurysms of this region whether symptomatic or not unless the patient's condition will not allow any form of treatment. A direct approach is recommended whenever there is any reasonable hope of clipping the aneurysm. The techniques involved, which include removal of the anterior clinoid process intracranially and exposure of the carotid artery extracranially have been reviewed and are presented in detail in Chapter 13 (21, 25, 29, 30, 32, 42, 43, 46, 52, 105, 120, 144). With persistence, many of these aneurysms that initially appear unclippable can be clipped satisfactorily (Figs. 20.8 and 20.12). When safe direct obliteration is not possible, one must proceed with proximal ligation or a trapping procedure.

Supraclinoid Aneurysms

Under this designation all aneurysms are included between the paraclinoid region and the internal carotid artery bifurcation. Smaller aneurysms of this area usually arise either at the origin of the posterior communicating artery or at the origin of the anterior choroidal artery. With giant aneurysms it is usually impossible to tell the precise site of origin since these aneurysms involve most of the supraclinoid segment of the internal carotid artery. They are frequently globular involving all of the posterior wall of the carotid artery and they can also be fusiform in shape involving all of the supraclinoid segment. These aneurysms present with subarachnoid hemorrhage or with optic compression. Occasionally they grow backward and compress the brain stem (Fig. 20.13).

The treatment should be direct clipping whenever possible. From the preoperative angiogram it is frequently possible to predict which aneurysms will not be amenable to clipping (i.e., massive globular or fusiform aneurysms). If there is any suggestion of a neck on the preoperative angiogram, the aneurysm should be explored (Fig. 20.13).

When the aneurysm is unclippable, carotid ligation is the treatment of choice. This tends to be less effective as the origin of the aneurysm becomes more distal on the internal carotid artery and there is greater

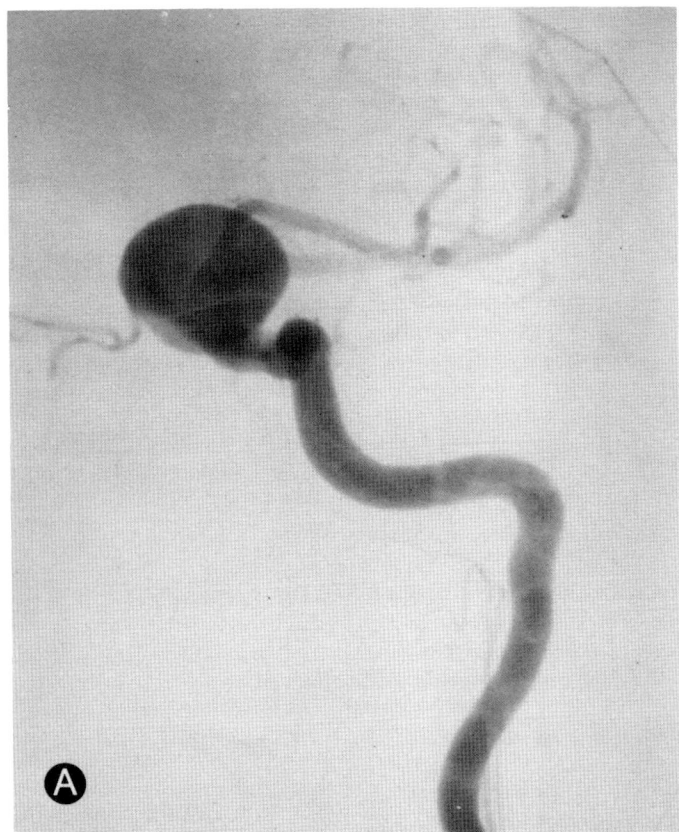
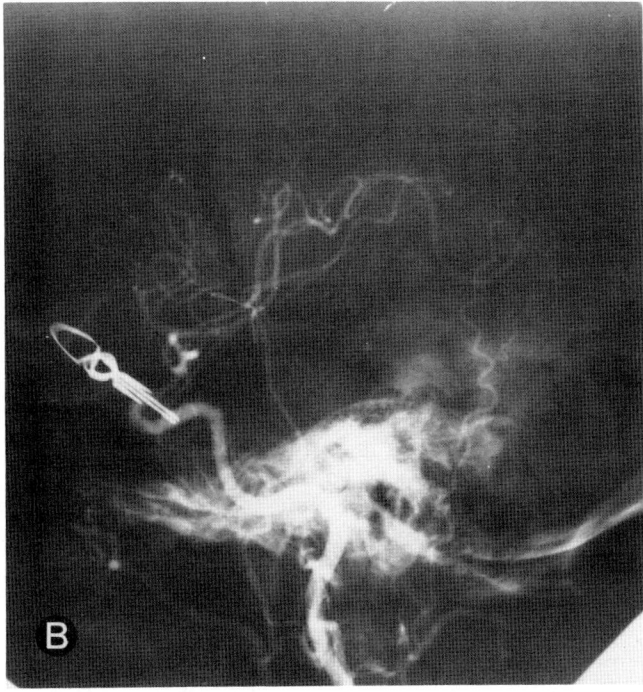

Figure 20.12. Giant ophthalmic artery aneurysm. **A,** The aneurysm projects superiorly compressing the optic nerve. **B,** Postoperative angiogram shows one of the tricks to use in occluding the aneurysm. A long clip has been placed across the neck of the aneurysm preserving internal carotid circulation. A second clip holds the blades of the first clip closed. Before placing the second clip, the blades of the long clip would open with each pulsation of systolic blood pressure.

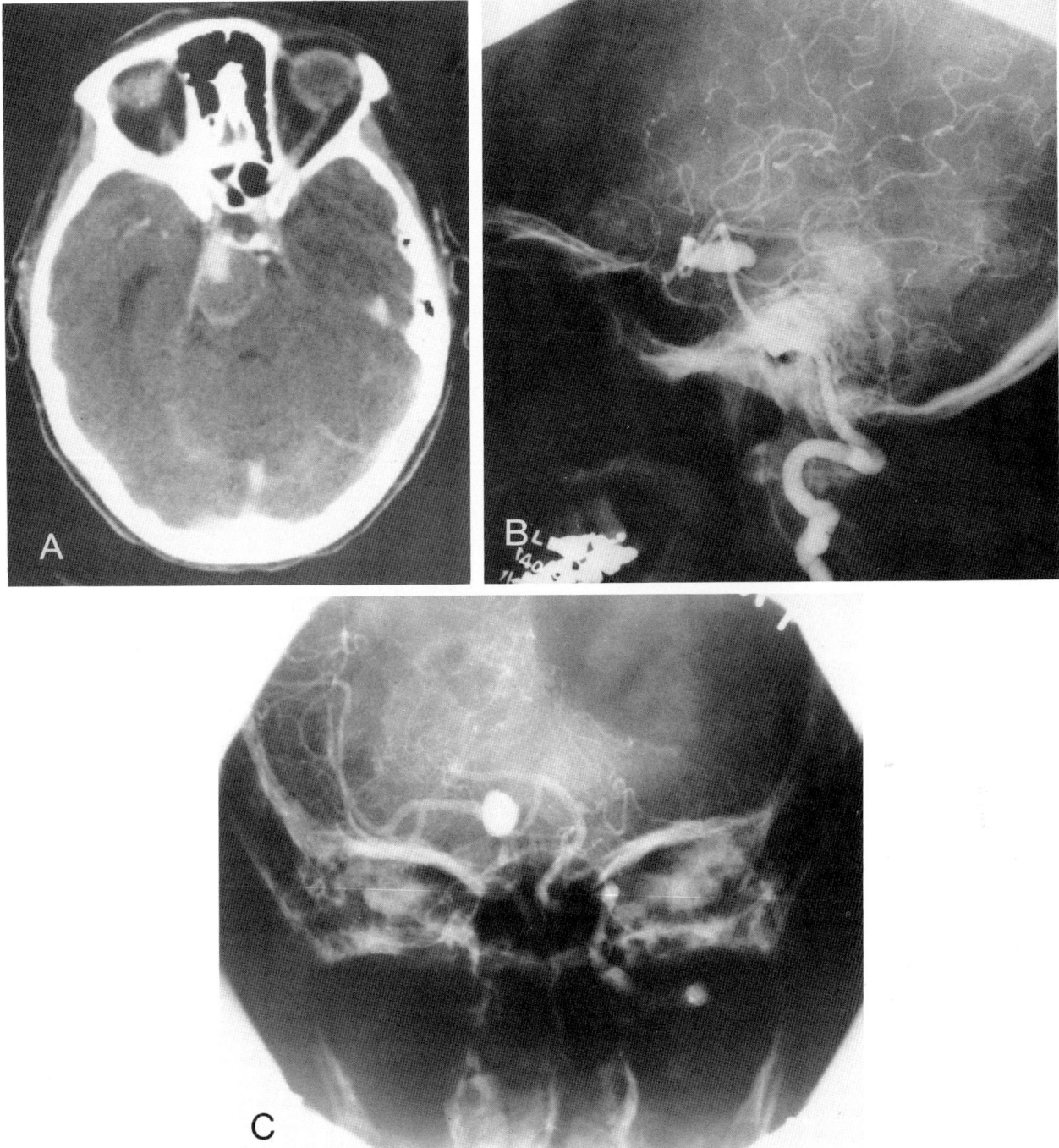

Figure 20.13. Partially thrombosed giant supraclinoid aneurysm treated by direct clipping. **A**, CT scan shows a typical "eccentric target sign" of a partially thrombosed aneurysm. **B** and **C**, Vertebral angiogram shows that the aneurysm continues to fill via the right posterior communicating artery. This lady presented initially with a right third nerve palsy and a subarachnoid hemorrhage. She was treated with common carotid ligation for a giant right internal carotid aneurysm that was thought to be unclippable. Several years later, she presented with progressive deterioration from brain stem compression. At operation the aneurysm was found to have a clippable neck. After clipping, the partially thrombosed aneurysmal mass was excised in order to relieve the brain stem compression. The patient improved markedly over the next several weeks.

availability of collateral circulation first through the ophthalmic artery, then through the posterior communicating artery and choroidal arteries and finally through the anterior cerebral artery in the case of carotid bifurcation aneurysms. It is not known whether globular and fusiform aneurysms should be treated by carotid ligation. Proximal ligation might induce aneurysmal thrombosis which could be catastrophic if embolization occurred or there was occlusion of the origin of the posterior communicating or choroidal arteries as well as other important perforators.

Carotid Artery Bifurcation Aneurysms

These aneurysms usually project upward and can grow deeply into the basal ganglia frequently simulating a tumor on CT scan. They can present with subarachnoid hemorrhage or focal signs from pressure on the basal ganglia and internal capsule. Treatment is most difficult. Several of these aneurysms have been explored but the authors have never been able to clip one successfully because the origin of the middle and anterior cerebral arteries is usually at some distance from the entrance of the carotid artery into the aneurysm. In addition, the vital perforators along the posterior wall of the aneurysm are extremely difficult to handle. Carotid ligation also tends to be less successful with these aneurysms because of the increased potential for antegrade flow across the anterior circle of Willis. Nevertheless, in some cases carotid ligation can result in complete thrombosis of these aneurysms (Fig. 20.14).

Anterior Cerebral Artery Aneurysms

Giant aneurysms of the anterior communicating region are much less frequent than one would expect from the frequency of smaller aneurysms in this location (22, 48, 59, 121). They present either with subarachnoid hemorrhage or as basifrontal tumors with signs of compression of the visual apparatus, frontal lobes, and hypothalamus (10, 22, 72, 77, 97).

Direct clipping should be attempted in almost every case since carotid ligation is not generally effective. Many of these lesions can be clipped successfully particularly with temporary clipping of the A_1 segments (Fig. 20.15).

Proximal ligation has been used for these aneurysms. Logue suggested clipping of the dominant anterior cerebral artery; i.e., the artery that fills the aneurysm primarily (70). This operation is often effective but has an ischemic complication rate of 10–20%. The clip must be carefully placed so as not to injure the perforating vessels from the anterior cerebral artery or the recurrent artery of Heubner. Tindall, Odom, and associates reported a modification of this procedure which consists of clipping of the dominant anterior cerebral artery at its origin and contralateral common carotid ligation (134, 135). Proximal arterial occlusion is recommended only when aneurysmal anatomy or patient condition contraindicate direct attack.

Giant aneurysms of the anterior cerebral artery distal to the anterior communicating artery complex are very rare (91), and the present authors have not had experience with them.

Middle Cerebral Artery Aneurysms

Patients with giant aneurysms of the middle cerebral artery present with subarachnoid hemorrhage or mass effect (lateralizing hemispheric signs, temporal lobe epilepsy, or headache and papilledema). The headache is commonly on the side of the aneurysm. Occasionally patients present with either ischemic symptoms from embolism from intraaneurysmal clot or from vascular compression.

Indirect forms of treatment for middle cerebral artery aneurysms are either dangerous (middle cerebral artery occlusion) or not effective (carotid occlusion); therefore direct exploration is strongly recommended for most of these aneurysms. The exception may be in large fusiform or "serpentine" type of aneurysms where there appear to be important branches coming off the dome of the aneurysm. Ordinarily saccular giant aneurysms do not give off branches although branches can be adherent to the wall and may appear to arise from the dome (Fig. 20.16).

To explore these aneurysms, a modified frontotemporal craniotomy is usually performed, extending the bone removal more posteriorly in the temporal region to have exposure of the anterior portion of the temporal lobe and the anterior aspect of the sylvian fissure (see Chapter 16) (53). This exposure is important because it is often helpful to resect the thin mantle of the anterior temporal lobe overlying these aneurysms. The head is turned about 60° to deal with the anterior temporal lobe. The pterion is removed as deeply as possible to gain access to the M_1 trunk. Complete circumferential exposure of the aneurysm can usually be achieved since brain can be suctioned with impunity in the anterior temporal region. Because of this feature, this is the one type of giant aneurysm that occasionally can be encased completely when it appears impossible to preserve all major divisions even after aneurysmorrhaphy (22). Aneurysmorrhaphy is frequently necessary since the origin of the divisions usually is separated from the point at which the middle cerebral artery enters the aneurysm by as much as 1 cm. An alternative is to sacrifice one of the divisions and reimplant it with an end-to-side anastomosis into the second division that is left intact after careful clip application (61).

When the surgeon decides direct obliteration is too dangerous, the alternative procedure is occlusion of the middle cerebral artery. Drake suggested using an

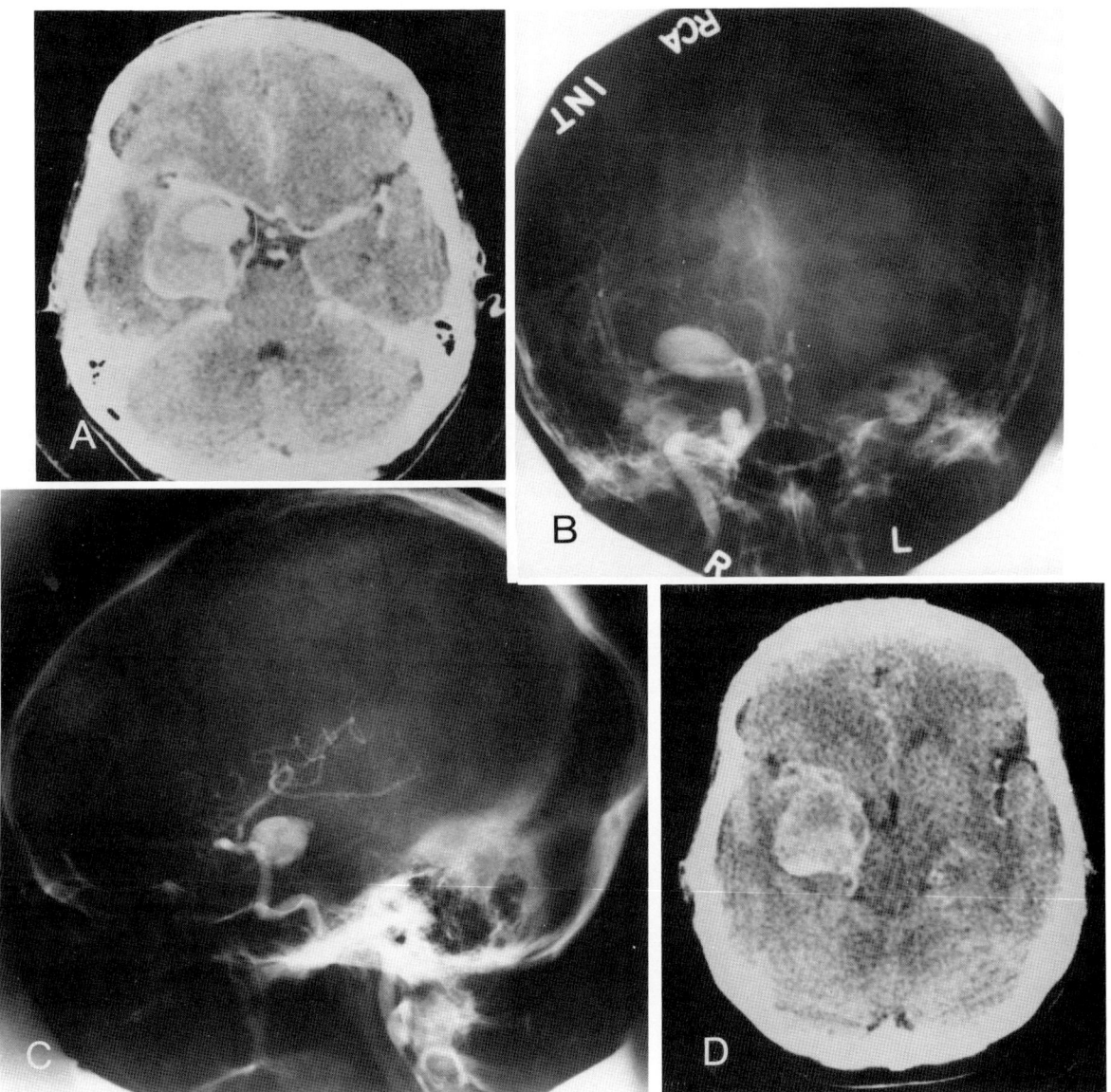

Figure 20.14. Partially thrombosed giant carotid bifurcation aneurysm treated by carotid ligation. **A**, Contrast CT scan shows a typical "eccentric target sign" of a partially thrombosed aneurysm. **B** and **C**, Right carotid arteriogram shows that the aneurysm is located in the right carotid bifurcation. This patient presented with headaches and temporal lobe epilepsy. She tolerated the period of test occlusion of the right carotid artery and was treated with common carotid ligation. **D**, The postoperative CT scan done 7 days after common carotid ligation shows that the aneurysm has thrombosed completely.

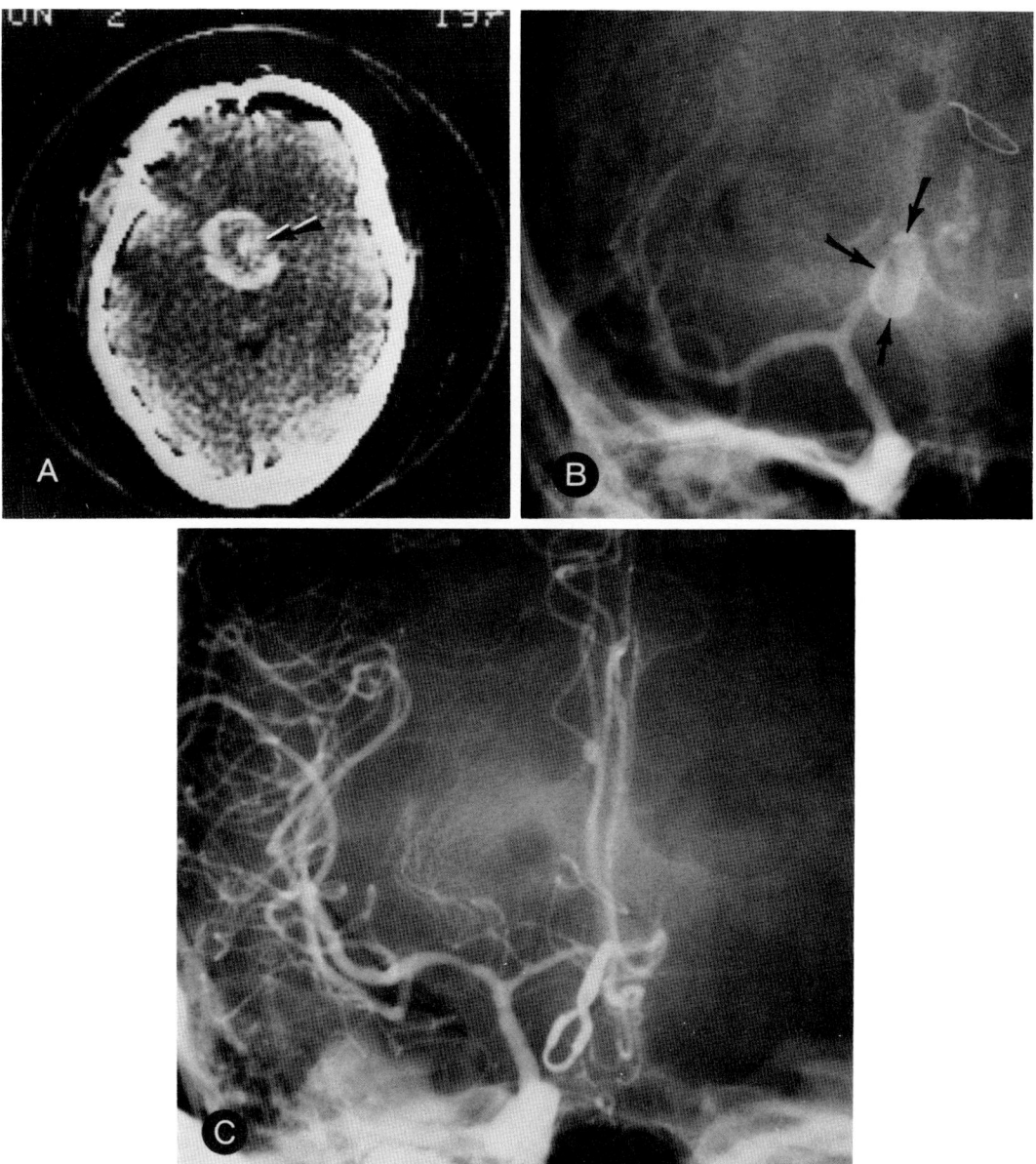

Figure 20.15. Giant anterior communicating aneurysm. **A**, CT scan shows area of enhancement (*arrow*) within a ring lesion. This is characteristic for a giant, partially thrombosed aneurysm. **B**, Right carotid angiogram demonstrates the aneurysm (*arrows*). Note the discrepancy in the size of the lesion seen on the CT scan and angiogram. **C**, Postoperative angiogram showing the aneurysm to be occluded and the mass effectively reduced. Comment: Patient seen at another hospital with evidence of optic chiasm compression. Exploration was done based on the CT scan and without angiography. At reoperation, the aneurysm was clipped and debulked. This was followed by relief of symptoms.

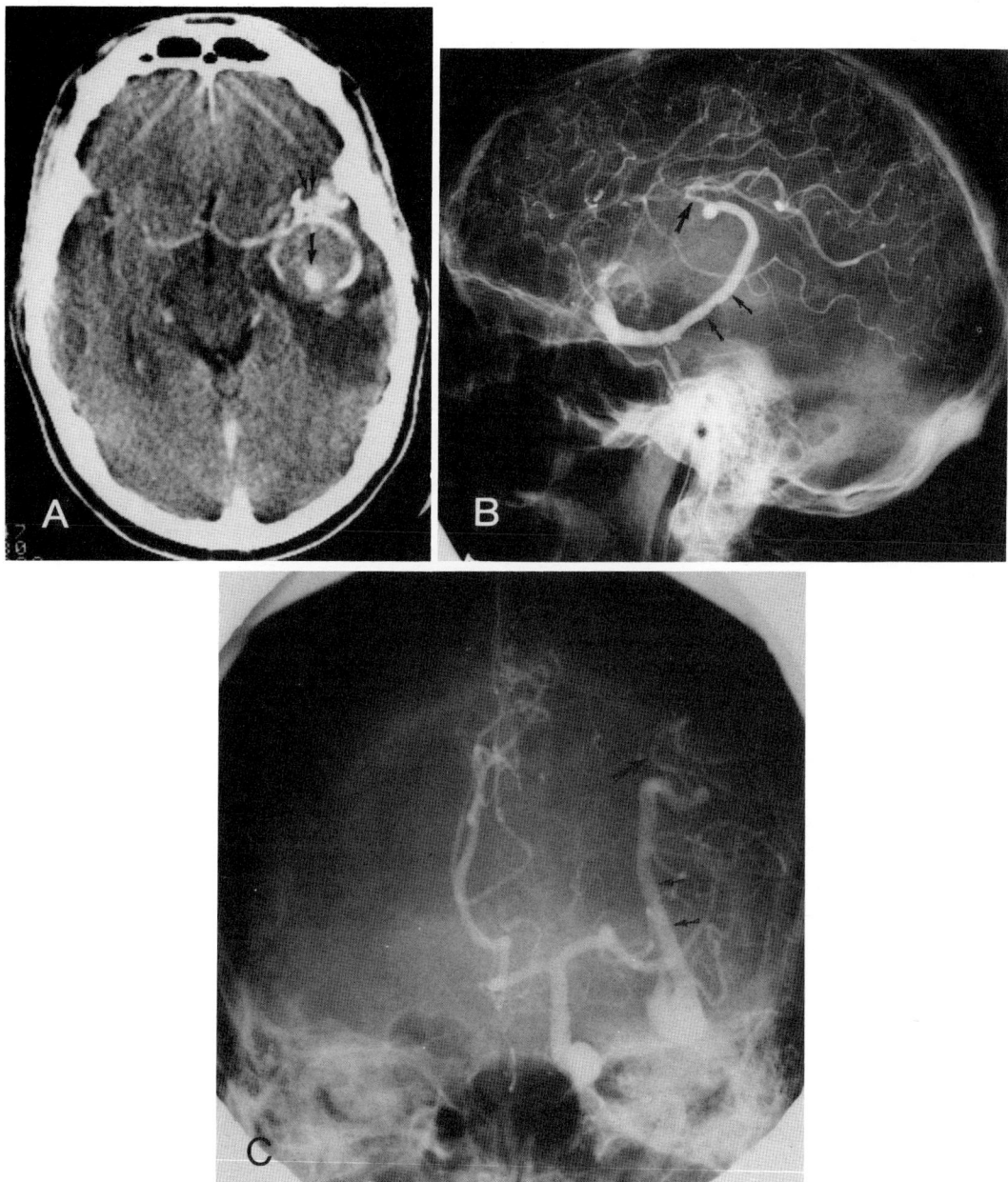

Figure 20.16. Giant partially thrombosed middle cerebral artery aneurysm simulating a "serpentine" aneurysm. **A**, CT scan shows that the aneurysm was almost completely thrombosed except for a small eccentrically located lumen (*single arrow*). It was also noted that there was an area of calcification that appeared to be outside but immediately adjacent to the aneurysm (*double arrow*). In addition, there was an extensive area of either edema or infarction throughout the temporal lobe. **B** and **C**, Left carotid angiogram was interpreted as showing a typical "serpentine" aneurysm with a residual lumen (*double arrow*) leading to a major division of the middle cerebral artery (*single arrow*). This 59-year-old physician had a history of speech difficulty which developed abruptly about 8 months before admission. He was diagnosed as having an untreatable giant aneurysm. He was referred because of progression in this speech difficulty. In retrospect it appears that he had had a remote subarachnoid hemorrhage from which he made a good recovery. The aneurysm was explored with the intention of performing a saphenous vein bypass graft, sacrificing the middle cerebral artery and excising the aneurysm. Surprisingly, the aneurysm could be dissected completely and no branch was found coming from its dome. There was one major division of the middle cerebral artery that was closely adherent to the back wall of the aneurysm but it could be dissected off the aneurysm and preserved. After aneurysmorrhaphy, the aneurysmal mass could be excised completely leaving a long cuff which could be simply ligated with silk sutures since the neck was relatively narrow. **D** and **E**, Postoperative plain and contrast CT scans, respectively, show the same area of calcification which at surgery was found to be anterior and outside the aneurysm, and the same preoperatively existing area of either edema or infarction in the temporal lobe. The aneurysmal mass has been excised completely. The patient was unchanged by the operation but gradually improved markedly in the ensuing few months.

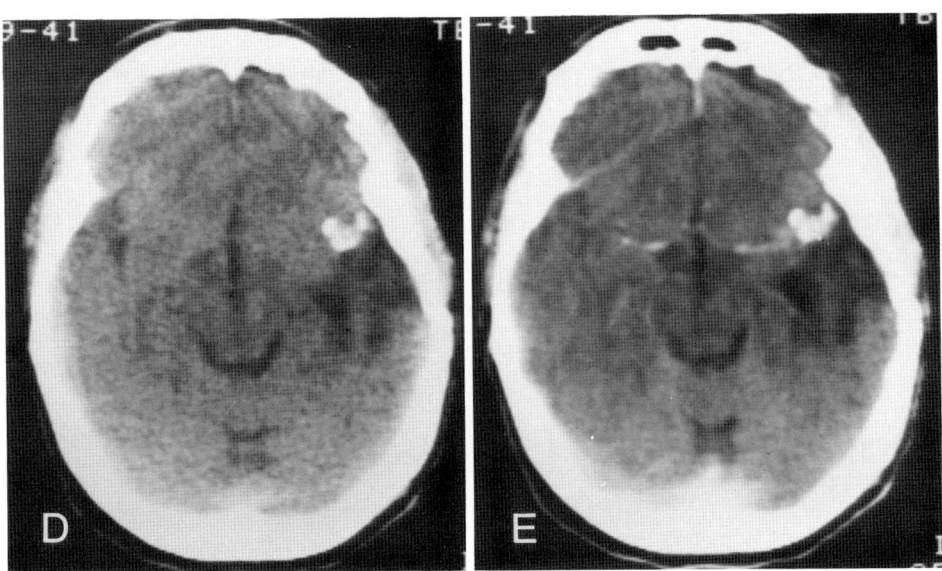

Figure 20.16D and E.

implanted tourniquet around the distal middle cerebral artery just proximal to the origin of the aneurysm. The tourniquet is brought out through the skin for subsequent occlusion with the patient awake under angiographic control (22). As Drake pointed out, this procedure should always be preceded by an EC-IC bypass. However, even after successful anastomosis of the superficial temporal artery to a middle cerebral branch some patients will not tolerate middle cerebral artery occlusion and develop infarction (19, 22, 57, 95). Hemorrhage from the aneurysm has been reported after bypass (100). Still, a number of patients have been successfully treated by EC-IC bypass and subsequent occlusion of the middle cerebral artery either directly or by tourniquet (3, 11, 22, 35, 57, 111, 112, 124, 136).

Because of the uncertainty about the ability of the superficial temporal artery to middle cerebral artery bypass to support the entire middle cerebral circulation, a "high flow" bypass with a vein graft followed by direct middle cerebral artery clipping is preferred (85, 112, 113, 116, 121) (Fig. 20.17). The technique for saphenous vein bypass grafts has been given in detail in Chapter 4.

When the aneurysm can be clipped by sacrificing only one division and leaving the other intact it is preferable to do so. However, in these cases one must be very careful to perform the bypass graft to a branch in the area of supply of the division to be sacrificed. In general, those branches above the sylvian fissure will belong to the superior division and those below the fissure to the inferior division but this is not always the case and one must review carefully the preoperative angiogram. If the middle cerebral artery trunk itself is to be sacrificed, then one can perform a single anastomosis to one division and by retrograde flow usually the other division is irrigated. Alternatively, the vein can be anastomosed to both divisions using a side-to-side anastomosis to one division and an end to side anastomosis to the second (85). The authors prefer to perform the anastomosis to either a division (M_2 segment) or a major secondary branch (M_3 segment). The divisions can usually be identified along the walls of the aneurysm if the aneurysm is exposed circumferentially. The authors proceed immediately after bypass with occlusion of the middle cerebral artery by clipping it as distally as possible, preserving all the perforators (Fig. 20.17). The vein should provide enough blood to support the middle cerebral artery circulation. Immediate clipping is preferable to delayed occlusion because the aneurysm can rupture during the period between completion of anastomosis and subsequent occlusion of the artery (50, 100).

After the saphenous vein bypass, excision of the aneurysm may be indicated. If the aneurysm is not excised and the vein graft is quite large, the aneurysm may not thrombose (50). A moderate caliber vein (4 mm distended) is probably ideal; big enough to avoid ischemia, small enough to permit aneurysm thrombosis.

Vertebrobasilar Aneurysms

Posterior Cerebral Artery Aneurysms

Giant aneurysms of the proximal portion of the posterior cerebral artery are most commonly fusiform (22). Therefore, they can generally not be clipped and proximal ligation of the posterior cerebral artery or

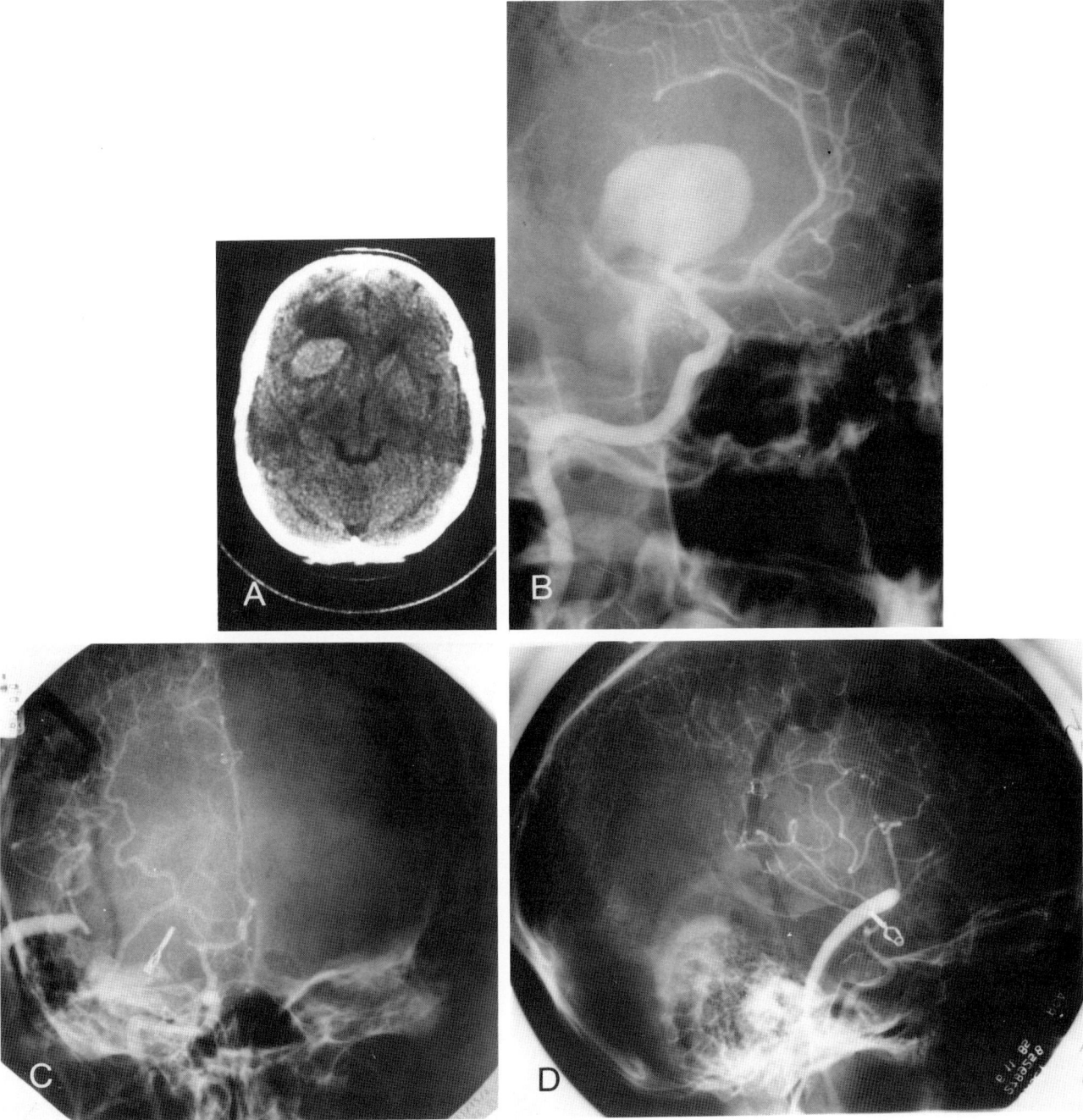

Figure 20.17. Giant middle cerebral artery aneurysm treated by occlusion after saphenous vein bypass graft. **A** and **B**, CT scan and right carotid angiogram, respectively, show a giant middle cerebral artery aneurysm without any evidence of thrombosis. This 32-year-old lady presented with temporal lobe epilepsy and had a normal neurologic examination. At surgery the aneurysm was found to be unclippable because each division arose at some distance from the point of entrance of the middle cerebral artery into the aneurysm. The authors elected to treat the patient with a saphenous vein bypass graft to a major division within the sylvian fissure. The middle cerebral artery was clipped just proximal to the aneurysm and distal to the lenticulostriate arteries. **C** and **D**, Postoperative angiogram shows that the middle cerebral artery is occluded proximal to the clip, there is no filling of the aneurysm and the vein graft fills the distal middle cerebral territory. The patient had no deficit from the operation.

trapping are the only available treatment. It is remarkable that, in Drake's experience, this procedure was often tolerated without a neurologic deficit. However, serious deficits can result from this procedure. Drake suggests that puncturing the aneurysm after proximal ligation may give a clue as to the degree of collateral circulation. If this appears to be poor he prefers to use a tourniquet on P_1 distal to the perforators for subsequent occlusion with the patient awake. His results with these aneurysms were generally good (22).

Distal posterior cerebral artery aneurysms can be either fusiform or saccular. They have occasionally resulted in hemianopsia either from embolic phenomena or from direct occlusion of the posterior cerebral artery. Some of the fusiform aneurysms in this area can be "reconstructed" using right-angle fenestrated clips (117). Plenty of wall must be left within the fenestrations of the clips; the tendency is to make the reconstruction too narrow. What appears to be intraoperatively a successful "reconstruction" of a fusiform aneurysm may thrombose postoperatively (Fig. 20.18).

Basilar Artery Bifurcation Aneurysm

Giant aneurysms at the top of the basilar artery can present either with subarachnoid hemorrhage or can act as a tumor with brain or cranial nerve compression (8, 132). These aneurysms usually project superiorly into the diencephalon and sometimes produce obstructive hydrocephalus (66, 87). They may also grow posteriorly into the interpeduncular fossa resulting in pseudobulbar palsy, ataxia, and quadriparesis. This latter syndrome is more common with aneurysms of the basilar trunk. Basilar tip aneurysms occasionally can grow asymmetrically and compress the cerebral peduncle and the third nerve resulting in a Weber's syndrome with contralateral hemiparesis and ipsilateral oculomotor paralysis. Isolated third nerve compression, however, is more common with aneurysms originating from the basilar-superior cerebellar junction.

These aneurysms present one of the most difficult neurosurgical challenges. The authors have never been able to clip basilar tip aneurysms without morbidity (Fig. 20.19). Drake, however, has had success with direct occlusion of the neck of many of these aneurysms (22). He has also introduced basilar ligation and unilateral or bilateral vertebral ligation for the treatment of these aneurysms (23). Basilar ligation can be accomplished by tourniquet with the patient awake (22) or directly by clip when one is sure of adequate collateral circulation. It would be ideal to ligate the basilar artery between the superior cerebellar and the posterior cerebral arteries but this is rarely possible because with these aneurysms the entire top of the basilar, including the origin of the superior cerebellar arteries, is dilated. A prerequisite to distal basilar occlusion is the demonstration of at least one normal sized posterior communicating artery by the Allcock maneuver (injection of the vertebral artery while each internal carotid artery is sequentially occluded) (22). Drake has used prophylactic bypass only occasionally in a large series of ligations (22, 23). In an early report of his experience with 42 giant basilar bifurcation aneurysms, Drake treated 14 patients with seven good results by basilar artery occlusion without bypass (22). Others have preferred to use a bypass graft, usually a saphenous vein graft to the proximal posterior cerebral artery, when basilar occlusion is planned (121). The planned arterial occlusion should be done soon after establishment of the bypass graft, particularly if this is a high flow type of graft, to avoid rupture of the aneurysm in the interval of time between establishment of the bypass and basilar occlusion. The latter is a complication that the authors have reported (129).

Basilar-superior cerebellar artery giant aneurysms are more amenable to clipping, and the authors have been able to clip two of these lesions successfully. The surgical approach is the same as for basilar tip aneurysms.

Aneurysms of the Basilar Trunk, Vertebrobasilar Junction, and Vertebral Artery

Aneurysms of the basilar trunk simulate extrinsic tumors such as clival meningiomas or cerebellopontine angle tumors with involvement of cranial nerves as well as symptoms from compression of the brain stem. They also frequently result in ischemic symptoms simulating occlusive vertebrobasilar disease (Fig. 20.1).

Aneurysms of the vertebrobasilar junction and the vertebral artery can compress the lower cranial nerves and the medulla, resulting in difficulties with swallowing, ataxia and hemiparesis or quadriparesis (5, 110) (Fig. 20.20). Giant aneurysms of the intracranial portion of the vertebral artery are frequently fusiform and can produce a cerebellopontine angle syndrome or simulate a meningioma of the foramen magnum or clivus. Giant aneurysms of the distal posterior inferior cerebellar artery are extremely rare but the authors recently had such a case treated sucessfully by excision and end-to-end anastomosis of the posterior inferior cerebellar artery (Fig. 20.21).

These aneurysms can sometimes be clipped successfully using a subtemporal transtentorial approach for basilar trunk aneurysms (Chapter 18 and Fig. 20.22) and either a subtemporal transtentorial approach or a lateral suboccipital approach for vertebrobasilar junction aneurysms (Chapter 18). When unclippable, these aneurysms can be treated by unilateral or bilateral vertebral ligation. Whether fusiform and dolichoectatic lesions can be so treated is not known since this treatment may result in basilar thrombosis and neurologic catastrophe (Chapter 18). Unilateral vertebral ligation is usually well tolerated, provided there is a patent contralateral vertebral ar-

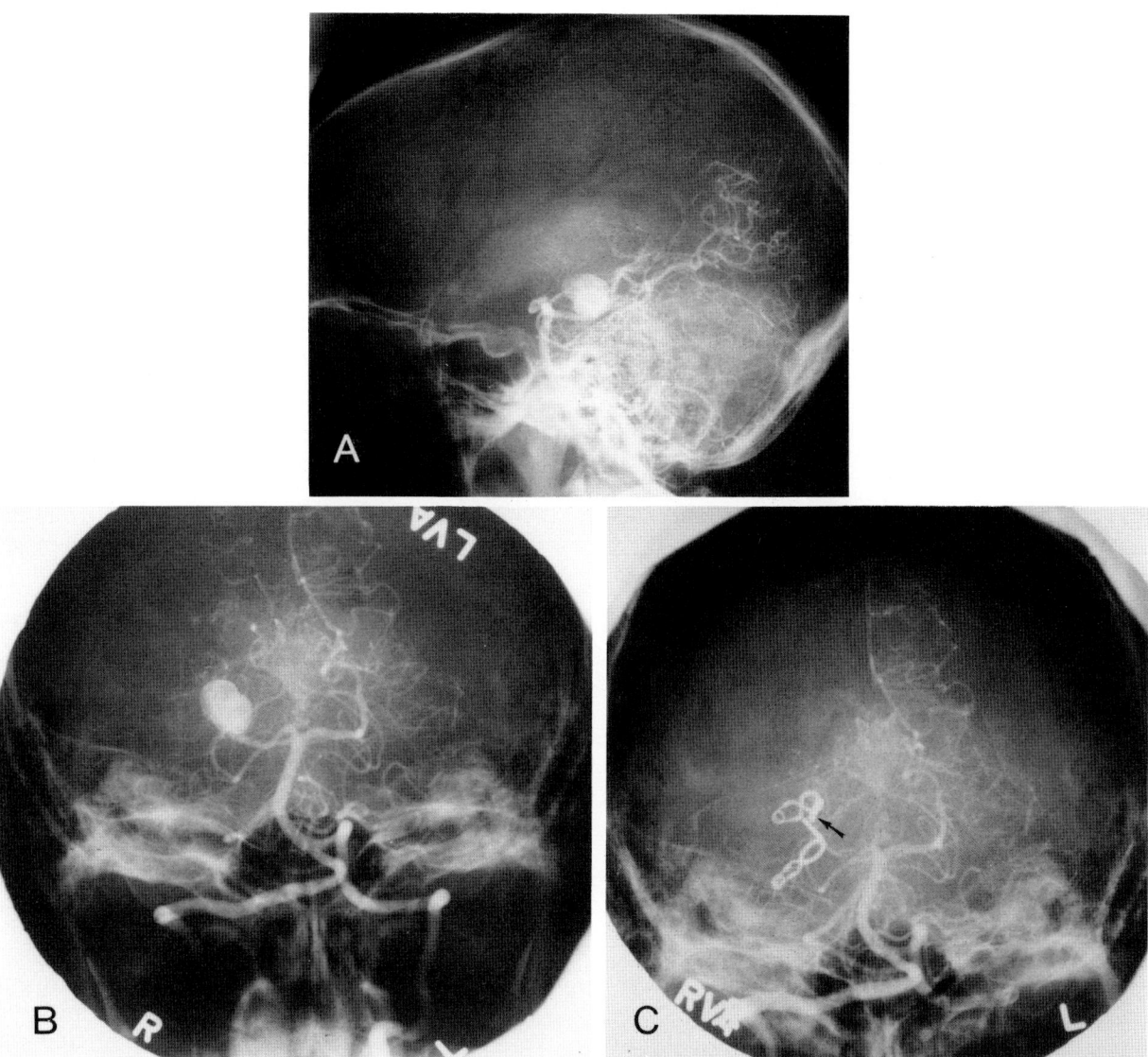

Figure 20.18. Giant partially thrombosed fusiform posterior cerebral artery aneurysm. **A** and **B**, Vertebral angiogram showed an aneurysm of the P_2 segment of the right posterior cerebral artery. By CT scan (not shown) the aneurysm was seen to be larger and partially thrombosed. This patient presented with headaches and hallucinations in his left visual field suggestive of migraine. He also had one episode of transient left hemiparesis. At surgery the aneurysm was found to be fusiform involving a long segment (about 1½ cm) of the posterior cerebral artery. After aneurysmorrhaphy to remove some of the blood clot, the authors were able to "reconstruct" the lumen of the posterior cerebral artery with two right-angle Sugita clips with Drake fenestrations leaving the lumen of the posterior cerebral artery within the fenestrations of the clips. The clips were placed in opposing directions meeting at their tip. It took the length of these two long clips to occlude the long base of the aneurysm. The authors were very satisfied at surgery since the posterior cerebral artery appeared to be patent and it pulsated very vigorously within the fenestrations of the clips and also distal to the clips. The patient had no neurologic deficit from the surgery. **C**, Postoperative angiogram shows that the posterior cerebral artery is occluded. It is of note that the clips now appear to be at a relatively acute angle to each other whereas, when placed at surgery, they appeared to be essentially in a straight line following the normal direction of the posterior cerebral artery. It is possible that the occlusion was related to "kinking" of the clips (*arrow*) that developed postoperatively. Remarkably, the patient has remained free of any neurologic difficulty.

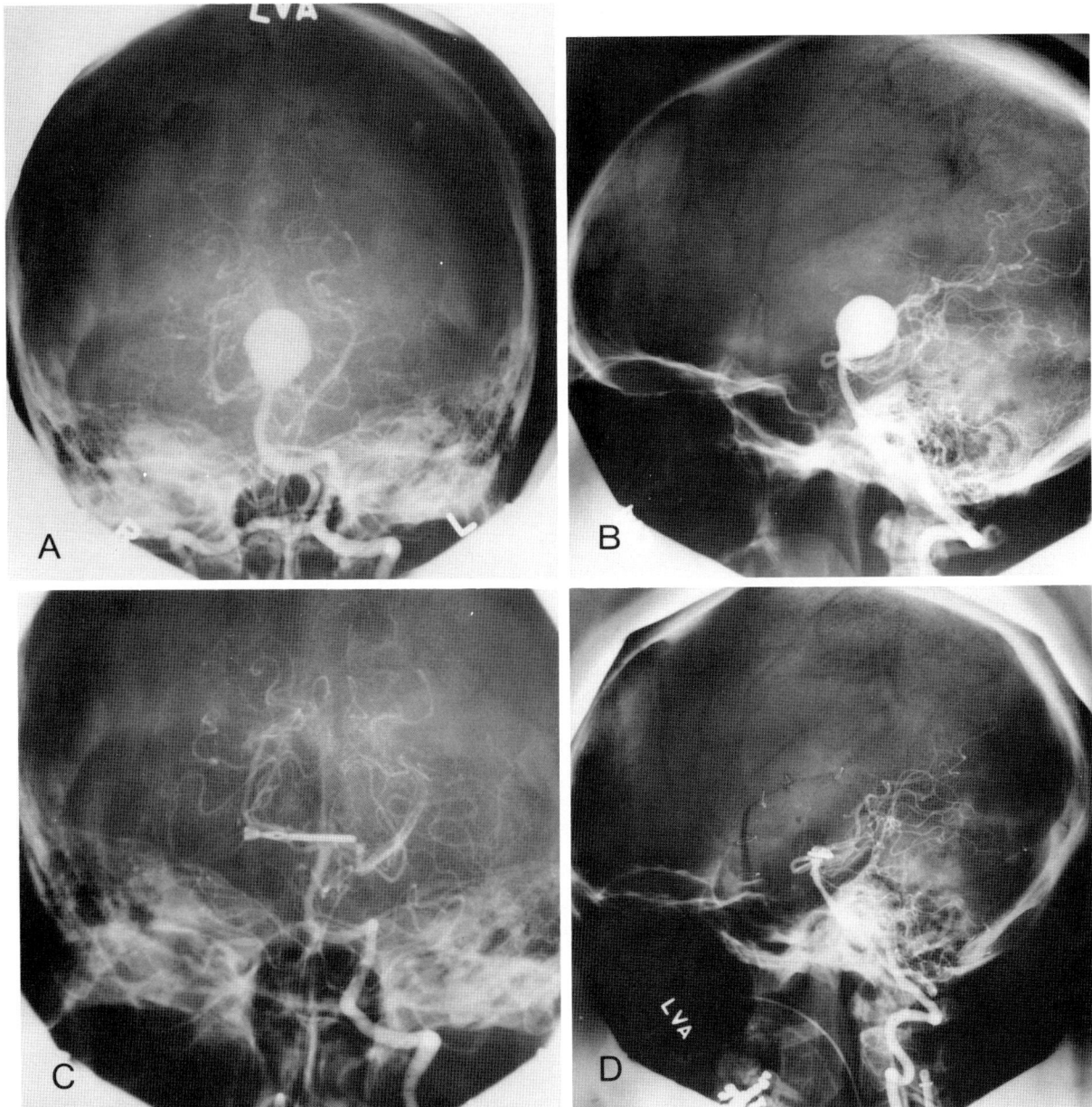

Figure 20.19. Giant basilar tip aneurysm. **A** and **B**, Angiography showed a giant basilar tip aneurysm. This 32-year-old lady presented with progressively more severe headaches. At surgery an attempt was made several times to clip the aneurysm with a straight Sugita clip with a Drake fenestration leaving the right P_1 on the fenestration of the clip. Each time the clip slipped down into the top of the basilar artery occluding the origin of the right P_1 and some of the perforators. Finally the authors were able to clip the aneurysm preserving the origin of both P_1s and all the perforators by using a straight Sugita clip inserted from behind the right P_1 and ending slightly behind the left P_1. This was done under temporary basilar occlusion by tilting the aneurysm backwards as we applied the clip. Since the clip was against the crotch of both P_1s it could not slip down. The authors were pleased with the clipping; however, the patient failed to awaken satisfactorily. **C** and **D**, Emergency angiography was performed and shows preservation of both P_1s and complete obliteration of the aneurysm. She has remained in poor neurologic condition with a severe right hemiparesis and bilateral third nerve palsies. Multiple CT scans have shown neither hydrocephalus nor any visible brain stem or thalamic infarction. Undoubtedly, she has suffered brain stem damage, possibly from damage to some of the perforators that had been occluded temporarily during the several attempts at clipping.

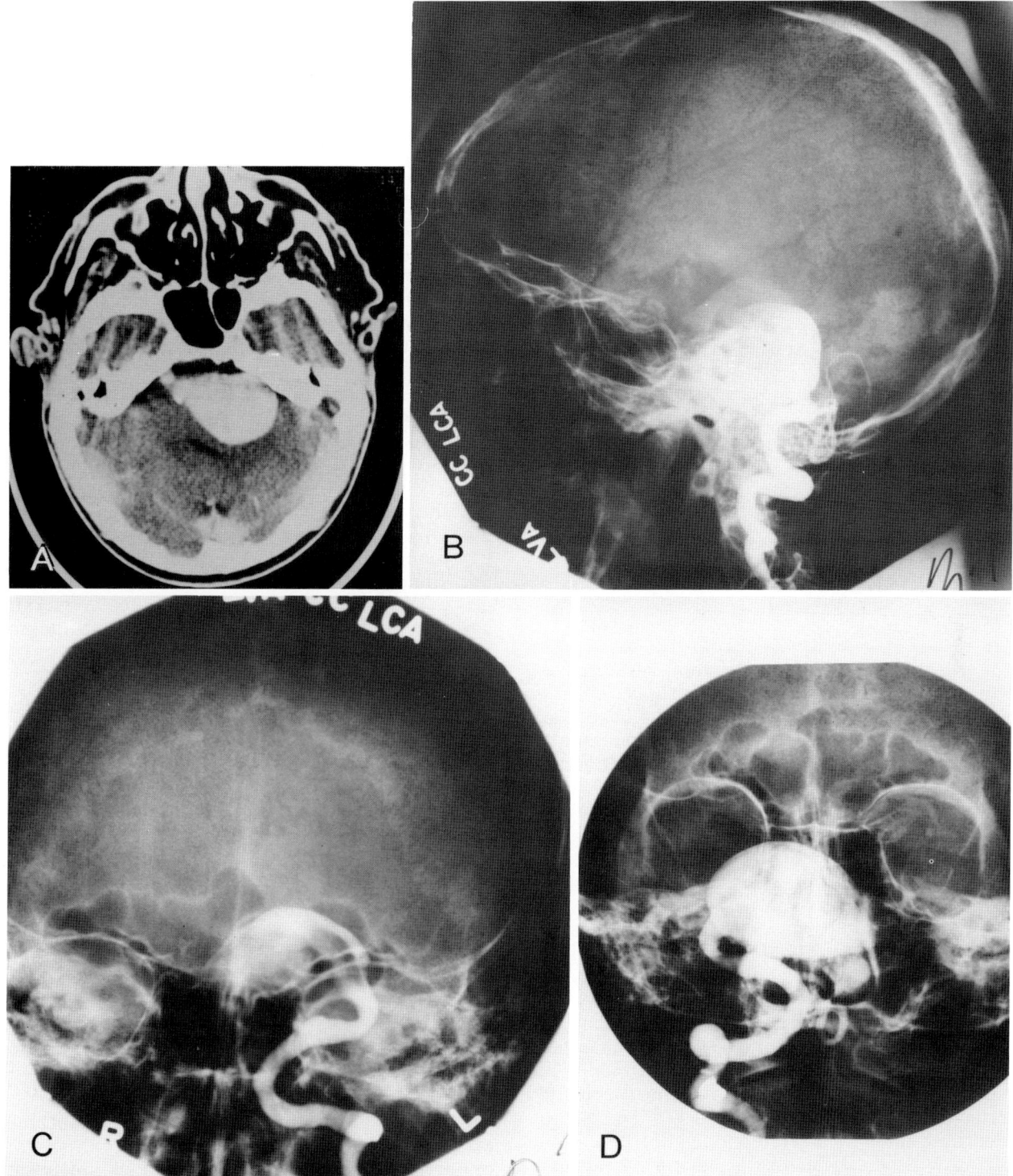

Figure 20.20. Giant vertebral-basilar aneurysms. **A**, CT scan shows a very large prepontine mass extending into the left cerebellar pontine angle. **B–D**, Left (**B**, **C**) and right (**D**) vertebral angiography, respectively, shows a massive aneurysm of the vertebrosbasilar junction that filled equally well from both vertebral arteries. This 63-year-old man presented with progressive ataxia, left-sided hearing loss, facial numbness and facial weakness on the left side, dysarthria, and difficulty swallowing. In addition, he had several spells of profound left hemiparesis which resolved over a period of hours. After angiography he had a severe subarachnoid hemorrhage from which he made a fairly good recovery. **E**, He was treated with balloon occlusion of the left vertebral artery just distal to the origin of the posterior inferior cerebellar artery. This was done in hope of reducing the total blood flow to the aneurysm and inducing aneurysmal thrombosis. The contralateral vertebral artery could not be ligated because the Allcock's maneuver had demonstrated essentially no collateral circulation to the vertebrobasilar system from the carotid arteries. Subsequent to vertebral ligation, he had another episode of profound left hemiparesis which this time did not resolve. He continued to deteriorate progressively and died of aspiration pneumonitis.

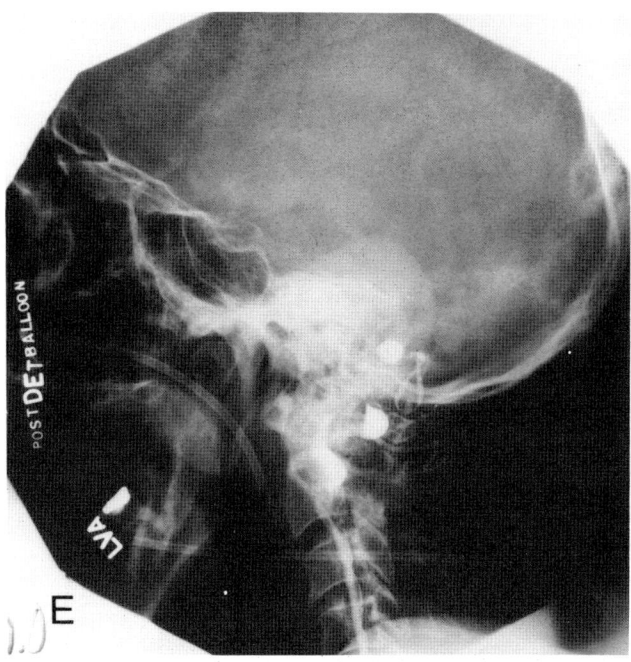

tery of at least moderate size. Bilateral vertebral occlusion is extremely dangerous unless there is extraordinarily good collateral flow to the basilar artery from the carotid circulation (22, 23). Usually vertebral artery occlusion should be done intracranially or just before the artery enters the skull upon the sulcus arteriosus of the atlas. If the vertebral occlusion is carried out more proximally, the usually abundant collateral circulation from muscular branches in the neck will maintain the patency of the distal vertebral artery and possibly the aneurysm. The occlusion can be performed openly at surgery or intravascularly by detachable balloon; the authors have had some success with the latter technique.

Giant aneurysms of the vertebral artery are usually fusiform although some of the aneurysms arising at the origin of the posterior inferior cerebellar artery can be saccular. Some of the fusiform aneurysms can be reconstructed successfully using the special fenestrated clips designed by Sugita (117, 118). For most of these aneurysms, vertebral ligation or balloon occlusion will be satisfactory provided there is evidence of adequate perfusion of the basilar artery by the opposite vertebral artery. A lateral medullary syndrome from ischemia in the distribution of the posterior inferior cerebellar artery may result from this form of treatment, but the prognosis in these cases is relatively good and seven out of eight cases reported by Drake did well (22).

RESULTS

The surgical results of the authors with giant aneurysms are summarized in Table 20.2. These results include some previously reported giant paraclinoid aneurysms operated by one of the authors at the University of Pittsburgh (52). Otherwise, the results are from patients operated at the MGH during the past 6 years. The results are generally satisfactory for internal carotid aneurysms (this series contains a disproportionately large number of paraclinoid aneurysms) and for middle cerebral aneurysms. The experience of the authors with aneurysms of the anterior communicating complex is very limited. The results with vertebrobasilar aneurysms leave much to be desired.

In the group of internal carotid aneurysms, one patient died from a massive hemorrhage when a piggybacked clip slipped in the recovery room. Another patient died of recurrent aneurysmal hemorrhage 1 year after common carotid occlusion. This patient, operated about 8 years ago, had refused angiography after follow-up CT scan demonstrated that her aneurysm remained patent. The two poor results and the death after internal carotid occlusion were due to thromboembolic complications. In the middle cerebral artery group one patient had a poor result from occlusion of a major branch. The second poor result and the death were in patients with massive aneurysms who were in poor preoperative condition with large mass effect from cerebral edema surrounding the aneurysm (51). The poor result in a patient with a giant anterior cerebral artery aneurysm was probably due to perforator injury since the patient developed marked difficulty with memory and personality which has not recovered and from which he remains totally incapacitated. The bad results with giant basilar tip aneurysms were also due to perforator injury and the death was due to a massive intraoperative rupture from avulsion of the neck which required sacrifice of the origin of the posterior cerebral artery with subsequent brain stem infarction. The patient who died after basilar ligation had a fatal rupture the night after a tourniquet was placed around the upper basilar artery after a saphenous vein bypass to the posterior cerebral artery (50). One patient who died after vertebral ligation had a giant aneurysm at the vertebrobasilar junction that was treated by ligation of one vertebral artery just proximal to the aneurysm and distal to the origin of the posterior inferior cerebellar artery. The contralateral vertebral artery was smaller and the authors thought that unilateral vertebral ligation would deal with the problem. She suffered a fatal rupture of her aneurysm on the fifth postoperative day. The second death in this group occurred in a patient with a massive vertebrobasilar aneurysm. He presented in poor condition from brain stem compression and/or ischemia and continued to deteriorate and die in spite of balloon occlusion of the dominant vertebral artery (Fig. 20.20). The aneurysm never thrombosed.

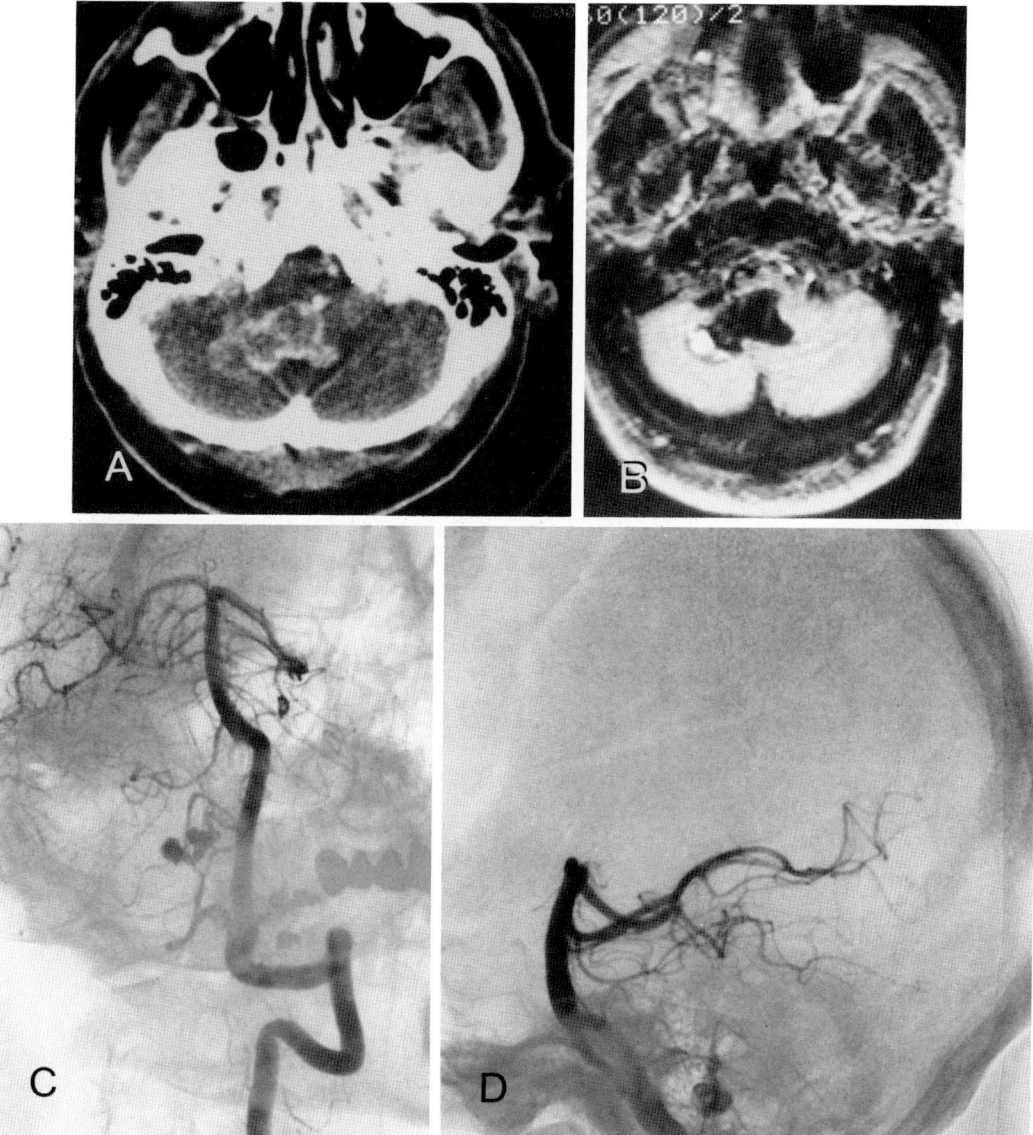

Figure 20.21. Giant aneurysm of the posterior inferior cerebellar artery mimicking a cerebellar hemorrhage. **A** and **B**, CT scan and MRI, respectively, are suggestive of a partially resolved cerebellar hemorrhage. There is substantial heterogenicity in the MRI appearance and therefore either a tumor which had bled or an arteriovenous malformation could not be ruled out and an angiogram was performed. **C** and **D**, Vertebral angiogram showed what appeared to be either two small aneurysms or a bilobular aneurysm arising from the peripheral portion of the posterior inferior cerebellar artery. This middle-aged man presented with sudden development of headache, ataxia, and dizziness. The initial diagnosis at another institution was a probable cerebellar tumor with hemorrhage. The symptoms remained stable and he was referred for evaluation. A suboccipital craniectomy was performed and a giant aneurysm of the retromedullary portion of the posterior inferior cerebellar artery was found. The aneurysm was completely excised, and the vessel was mobilized and anastomosed on an end-to-end fashion. It was felt that it was necessary to preserve flow through the posterior inferior cerebellar artery because there were branches to the brain stem and to the deep cerebellar nuclei arising distally from the origin of the aneurysm. There was an excellent pulse in the vessel after the anastomosis and the patient awoke from the surgery unchanged and gradually has improved neurologially over the ensuing few weeks. In view of his substantial improvement, no postoperative angiography has been performed.

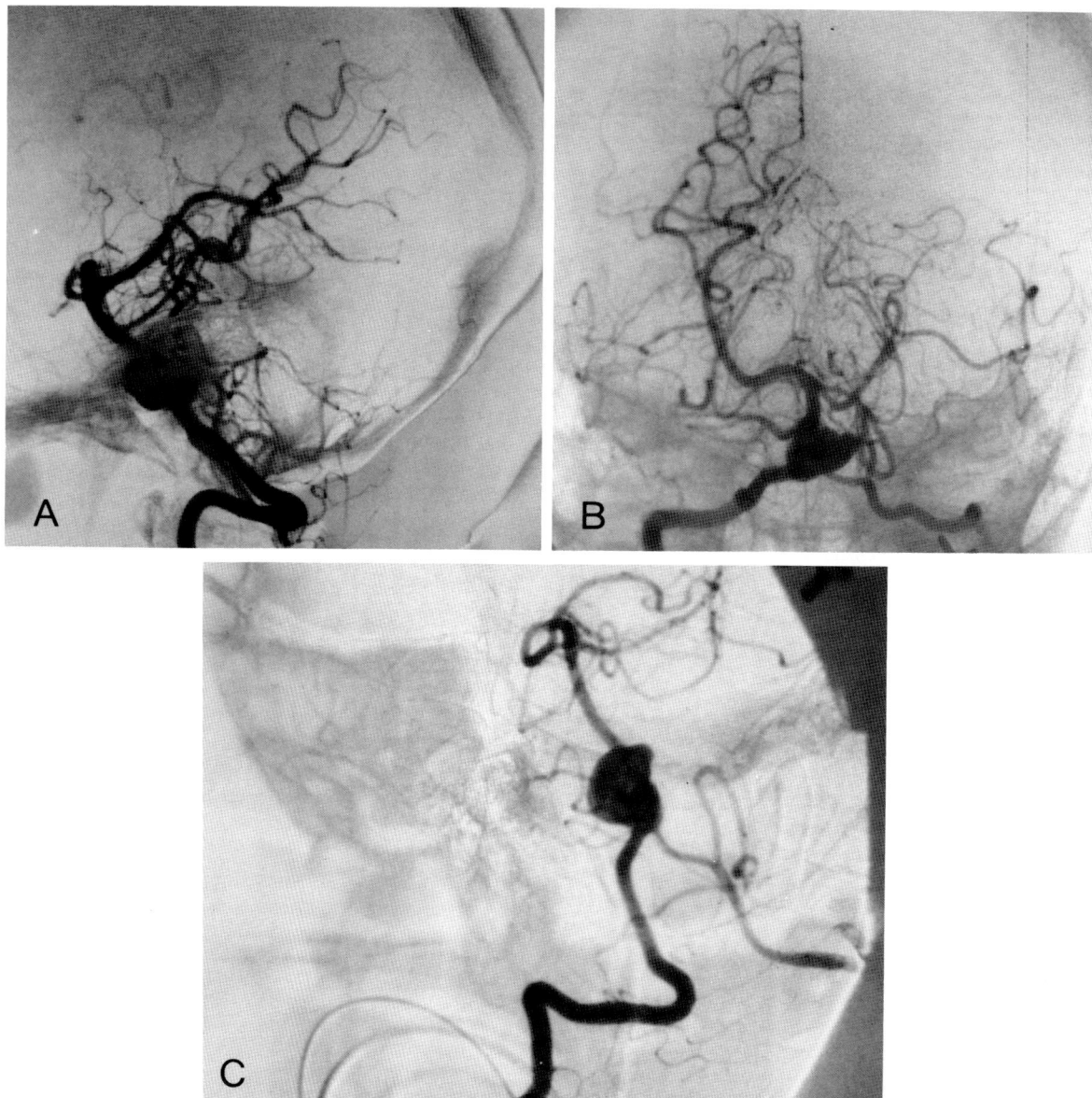

Figure 20.22. Partially thrombosed giant aneurysm of the basilar trunk successfully clipped by a subtemporal transtentorial approach. **A–C**, Lateral, anteroposterior, and oblique views, respectively, from a left vertebral angiogram show an irregular large aneurysm of the basilar trunk in the general region of the anterior inferior cerebellar artery. This lady presented with a subarachnoid hemorrhage and a left sixth nerve palsy. The aneurysm was located approximately at the midclival level and therefore it was approached by a right subtemporal transtentorial exposure. The aneurysm which was found to be much larger and partially thrombosed, could be clipped successfully with a large bayonet Sugita clip working in the plane between the fifth cranial nerve superiorly and the seventh and eighth cranial nerves inferiorly. Postoperatively, she had a partial sixth nerve palsy on the right side in addition to her already existing complete sixth nerve palsy on the left side. Fortunately both of these deficits resolved within a 3-month period and she has had no other neurologic deficit.

Table 20.2.
Surgical Results in Giant Aneurysms

	Good	Poor	Dead
Internal carotid Aneurysms[a,b]			
Intracranial occlusion	25		1
CCA ligation[c]	13		1[d]
ICA ligation (usually with EC-IC bypass)	5	2	1
Middle cerebral aneurysms[b]			
Intracranial occlusion	12	2	1
Encasement	3		
MCA ligation (with EC-IC bypass)	2		
Anterior cerebral aneurysms[b]	2	1	
Posterior cerebral aneurysms			
Intracranial occlusion	2	1	
Upper basilar aneurysms			
Intracranial occlusion	2[e]	2	1
Basilar ligation (with EC-IC bypass)	1		1
Basilar trunk aneurysms			
Intracranial occlusion	2		
Vertebral and vertebrobasilar aneurysms			
Intracranial occlusion	3		
Vertebral ligation (with balloon in some cases)	3		2
Posterior inferior cerebellar artery aneurysms			
Excision and end-to-end anastomosis	1		
Total (92)	76 (83%)	8	8

[a] Results ignore visual problems and refer only to neurologic outcome; CCA = common carotid artery, ICA = internal carotid artery.
[b] Many of these patients had aneurysmorrhaphy.
[c] Two of these patients had a trapping procedure.
[d] Patient died of hemorrhage 1 year after CCA ligation.
[e] The two successfully clipped giant upper basilar aneurysms were basilar-superior cerebellar aneurysms.

Drake reported overall good or excellent results in 71.5% of his giant aneurysms (22). Over half the giant aneurysms in that series were in the vertebrobasilar circulation and, remarkably, 71% of these patients had a good or excellent result. Yasargil reported good results in 66.7% of 30 patients with giant aneurysms; of these 12 were in the vertebrobasilar circulation (143). Sundt and Piepgras obtained good or excellent results in 77.5% of patients with giant aneurysms (121). Hosobuchi had good results in 80% of his 40 patients using in several the technique of intramural thrombosis by wire injection into the aneurysm (58, 59). Mullan has also used this technique to treat some patients with giant aneurysms (80).

In summary, when compared with the grim natural history of these lesions, the surgical results in patients with giant aneurysms of the anterior circulation appear to be satisfactory. However, there still remains the problem of how to deal with patients with massive aneurysms that result in significant cerebral edema and hemispheric shift. Except for one center that has accumulated an extraordinary experience with vertebrobasilar aneurysms (22) the results with these cases in general are poor. It may be that new techniques such as aneurysmal obliteration by intraluminal detachable balloon (17, 54, 93, 106, 145), intraluminal thrombosis (2, 58, 80), or cardiopulmonary bypass (107, 108) will improve these results in the future.

REFERENCES

1. Albin MS: Neuroanesthesia and aneurysmal surgery. In Hopkins LM and Long DM (eds): *Clinical Management of Intracranial Aneurysms*. New York, Raven Press; 1982, pp 163–272.
2. Alksne JF, Smith RW: Iron-acrylic compound for stereotaxic aneurysm thrombosis. *J Neurosurg* 47:137–141, 1977.
3. Ammerman BJ, Smith DR: Giant fusiform middle cerebral artery aneurysm: Successful treatment utilizing microvascular bypass. *Surg Neurol* 7:255–257, 1977.
4. Artmann H, Vonofakos D, Muller H, Grau H: Neuro-radiologic and neuropathologic findings with growing giant intracranial aneurysm. *Surg Neurol* 21:381–401, 1984.
5. Beck DW, Boarini DJ, Kassell NF: Surgical treatment of giant aneurysm of vertebral-basilar junction. *Surg Neurol* 12:283–285, 1979.
6. Bjorkesten G, Troupp H: Changes in the size of intracranial arterial aneurysms. *J Neurosurg* 19:583–588, 1962.
7. Black SPW, German WJ: Observations on the relationship between volume and size of the orifice of experimental aneurysms. *J Neurosurg* 17:948–990, 1960.
8. Bose B, Northrup B, Osterholm J: Giant basilar artery aneurysm presenting as a third ventricular tumor. *Neurosurgery* 13:699–702, 1983.
9. Brihaye J: Internal carotid aneurysms arising in the carotid canal. In Pia HW, Langmaid C, Zierski J (eds): *Cerebral Aneurysms: Advances in Diagnosis and Therapy*. New York, Springer-Verlag, 1977, pp 48–57.
10. Bull J: Massive aneurysms at the base of the brain. *Brain* 92:535–570, 1969.
11. Bushe KA, Bockhorn J: Extracranial-intracranial arterial bypass for giant aneurysms. *Acta Neurochir (Wien)* 54:107–115, 1980.
12. Byrd SE, Bentson JR, Winter J, Wilson GH, Joyce PW, O'Connor L: Giant intracranial aneurysms simulating brain neoplasms on computed tomography. *J Comput Assist Tomogr* 2:303–307, 1978.
13. Carney PG, Oatey PE: Muslin wrapping of aneurysm and delayed visual failure; a report of three cases. *J Clin Neurol Ophthalmol* 3:91–96, 1983.
14. Carter LP, Erspamer R, White WL, Yamagata S: Cortical blood flow during craniotomy for aneurysm. *Surg Neurol* 17:203–208, 1982.
15. Davis KR, Kistler JP, Heros RC, Davis JM: A neuroradiologic approach to the patient with a diagnosis of subarachnoid hemorrhage. *Radiol Clin North Am* 20:87–93, 1982.
16. Davila S, Oliver B, Molet J, Bartumeus F: Spontaneous thrombosis of an intracranial aneurysm. *Surg Neurol* 22:29–32, 1984.
17. Debrun G, Fox A, Drake C, Peerless S, Girvin J, Ferguson G: Giant unclippable aneurysms: Treatment with detachable balloons. *AJNR* 2:167–173, 1981.
18. Debrun G, Lacour P, Caron JP: Detachable balloon and calibrated leak balloon techniques in the treatment of cerebral vascular lesions. *J Neurosurg* 49:635–649, 1978.

19. Diaz FG, Ausman JI, Pearce JE: Ischemic complications after combined internal carotid artery occlusion and extracranial-intracranial anastomosis. Neurosurgery 10:563–570, 1982.
20. Dolenc VV: Direct microsurgical repair of intracavernous vascular lesions. J Neurosurg 58:824–831, 1983.
21. Dolenc VV: A combined epi- and subdural direct approach to carotid ophthalmic artery aneurysms. J Neurosurg 62:667–672, 1985.
22. Drake C: Giant intracranial aneurysms: Experience with surgical treatment in 174 patients. Clin Neurosurg 26:12–95, 1979.
23. Drake CG: Ligation of the vertebral (unilateral or bilateral) or basilar artery in the treatment of large intra-cranial aneurysms. J Neurosurg 43:255–274, 1975.
24. Drake CG, Barr HWK, Coles JC, Gergely NF: The use of extracorporeal circulation and profound hyothermia in the treatment of ruptured intracranial aneurysm. J Neurosurg 21:575–581, 1964.
25. Drake CG, Vanderlinden RG, Amacher AL: Carotid ophthalmic aneurysms. J Neurosurg 29:24–31, 1968.
26. Dujovny M, Wakehut N, Kossovsky N, Gomes CW, Laha RK, Leff L, Nelson D: Minimum vascular occlusive force. J Neurosurg 51:662–668, 1979.
27. Ebina K, Iwabuchi T, Suzuki S: A clinico experimental study on various wrapping material of cerebral aneurysms. Acta Neurochirurg 72:61–71, 1984.
28. Eisenberg HM, Turner JW, Teasdale G, Rowan J, Feinstein R, Grossman RG: Monitoring of cortical excitability during induced hypotension in aneurysm operations. J Neurosurg 50:595–602, 1979.
29. Ferguson GG, Drake CG: Carotid-ophthalmic aneurysms: The surgical management of those cases presenting with compression of the optic nerves and chiasm alone. Clin Neurosurg 27:263–308, 1980.
30. Ferguson GG, Drake CG: Carotid-ophthalmic aneurysms: Visual abnormalities in 32 patients and the results of treatment. Surg Neurol 16:1–8, 1981.
31. Flamm ES: Suction decompression of aneurysms. Technical note. J Neurosurg 54:275–276, 1981.
32. Fox JL: Techniques of aneurysm surgery. III. Internal carotid artery aneurysms: In Fox JL (ed): Intracranial Aneurysms. Berlin, Springer-Verlag, 1983, vol II, pp 949–1011.
33. Fox AJ, Vinuela F. Pelz DM, Peerless SJ, Ferguson GC, Drake CJ, Debrun G: Use of detachable balloons for proximal artery occlusion in the treatment of unclippable cerebral aneurysms. J Neurosurg 66:40–46, 1987.
34. Ganti SR Steinberger A, McMrutry JG, Hilal SK: Computed tomographic demonstration of giant aneurysms of the vertebrobasilar system: Report of eight cases. Neurosurgery 9:261–267, 1981.
35. Gelber BR, Sundt TM: Treatment of intracavernous and giant carotid aneurysms by combined internal carotid ligation and extracranial-intracranial bypass. J Neurosurg 52:1–10, 1980.
36. German WJ, Black SPW: Cervical ligation for internal carotid aneurysms. J Neurosurg 23:572–577, 1965.
37. Giannotta SL, McGillicuddy JE, Kindt GW: Gradual carotid artery occlusion in the treatment of inaccessible carotid artery aneurysms. Neurosurgery 5:417–421, 1979.
38. Gissen AJ, Matteo RS, Housepian EM, Bowman O Jr: Elective circulatory arrest during neurosurgery for basilar artery aneurysms. JAMA 207:1315–1318, 1969.
39. Glassock ME, Smith PG, Whitaker SR, et al: Management of aneurysms of the petrous portion of the internal carotid artery by resection and primary anastomsis. Laryngoscope 93:1445–1453, 1983.
40. Golding R, Peatfield RC, Shawdon HH, Edwards JMR: Computer tomographic features of giant intracranial aneurysms. Clin Radiol 31:41–48, 1980.
41. Guegan JM, Scarabin JM, LeGuilcher C, Gillou L, Logeais Y, Pecker J: Extracorporal circulation with deep hypothermia and circulatory arrest in the treatment of intracranial arterial aneurysms. Surg Neurol 24:441–448, 1985.
42. Guidetti B, LaTorre E: Management of carotid-ophthalmic aneurysms. J Neurosurg 42:438–442, 1975.
43. Guidetti B, Nicole S: Carotid-ophthalmic aneurysm. In Fein JM, Flamm ES (eds): Cerebrovascular Surgery. Berlin, Springer-Verlag, 1985, vol III, pp 805–839.
44. Handa J, Nakano Y, Aii H, Handa H: Computed tomography with giant intracranial aneurysms. Surg Neurol 9:257–263, 1978.
45. Heiskanen O, Nikki P: Large intracranial aneurysms. Acta Neurol Scand 38:195–208, 1962.
46. Heros RC: Surgical management of large paraclinoid aneurysms. Contemp Neurosurg 12:1–6, 1983.
47. Heros RC: Thromboembolic complications after combined internal carotid ligation and extracranial to intracranial bypass. Surg Neurol 21:75–79, 1984.
48. Heros RC: Giant intracranial aneurysms. In Long DM (ed): Current Therapy in Neurological Surgery. Philadelphia, BC Decker, 1985, pp 80–84.
49. Heros RC: Management of non-clippable aneurysms. In Schmidek HH, Sweet WH (eds): Operative Neurosurgical Techniques. New York, Grune & Stratton, 1987.
50. Heros RC, Ameri AM: Rutpure of a giant basilar aneurysm after saphenous vein interposition graft to the posterior cerebral artery. Case report. J Neurosurg 61:387–390, 1984.
51. Heros, RC, Kolluri S: Giant intracranial aneurysms presenting with massive cerebral edema. Neurosurgery 15:572–577, 1984.
52. Heros RC, Nelson PB, Ojemann RG, Crowell RM, Debrun G: Large and giant paraclinoid aneurysms: Surgical techniques, complications and results. Neurosurgery 13:153–163, 1983.
53. Heros RC, Ojemann RG, Crowell RM: Superior temporal gyrus approach to middle cerebral artery aneurysms. Technique and Results. Neurosurgery 10:308–313, 1982.
54. Hieshima GB, Higashida RT, Wapenski J, Halbach VV, Cahan L, Bentson JR: Balloon embolization of a large distal basilar artery aneurysm. J Neurosurg 65:413–416, 1986.
55. Holtzman RNN, Parisier SC: Acute spontaneous otorrhagia resulting from a ruptured petrous carotid aneurysm. J Neurosurg 51:258–261, 1979.
56. Hood TW, Mastri AR, Chou SN: Neural and vascular tissue reaction to cyanoacrylate and adhesives: A further report. Neurosurgery 11: 363–366, 1982.
57. Hopkins LN, Grand W: Extracranial-intracranial arterial bypass in the treatment of aneurysms of the carotid and middle cerebral arteries. Neurosurgery 5:21–31, 1979.
58. Hosobuchi Y: Electrothrombosis of carotid-cavernous fistula. J Neurosurg 42:76–85, 1975.
59. Hosobushi Y: Direct surgical treatment of giant intracranial aneurysms. J Neurosurg 51:743–756, 1979.
60. Housepian EM, Bowman FO Jr, Gissen AJ: Elective circulatory arrest in intracranial surgery. J Neurosurg 26:594–597, 1967.
61. Ito Z: Microsurgery of Cerebral Aneurysms. New York, Elsevier, 1982.
62. Jafar JJ, Tan WS, Abejo R: Balloon occlusion of giant intracranial aneurysms under cerebral blood flow control. Neurosurgery, in press.
63. Jane N, Butler P, Lye RH, Fawcitt RA: Carotid ligation: What happens in the long term? J Neurol Neurosurg Psychiatry 49:893–898, 1983.
64. Kak VK, Taylor AR, Gordon DS: Proximal carotid ligation for internal carotid aneurysms. A long term follow-up study. J Neurosurg 39:503–513, 1973.
65. Kataoka K, Yamada K, Nakao K, Hayakawa T, Ikeda T, Kawai R, Miura T: Digital subtraction angiography and dynamic computed tomography for evaluating the hemodynamics in cases of giant intracranial aneurysm. Surg Neurol 20:355–360, 1983.

66. Koga H, Mori K, Kawano T, Tsutsumi K, Jinnouchi T: Parinaud's syndrome in hydrocephalus due to a basilar artery aneurysm. *Surg Neurol* 19:548–553, 1983.
67. Landolt AM, Millikan CHL: Pathogenesis of cerebral infarction secondary to mechanical carotid artery occlusion. *Stroke* 1:52–62, 1970.
68. Lavyne MH, Kleefield J, Davis KR, Ojemann RG, Crowell RM: Giant intracranial aneurysms of the anterior circulation: Clinical characteristics and diagnosis by computed tomography. *Neurosurgery* 3:356–363, 1978.
69. Little JR, St. Louis P, Weinstein M, Dohn DF: Giant fusiform aneurysm of the cerebral arteries. *Stroke* 12:183–188, 1981.
70. Logue V: Surgery in spontaneous subarachnoid hemorrhage. Operative treatment of aneurysm of the anterior cerebral and anterior communicating artery. *Br Med J* 1:473, 1956.
71. Lynch JC, Amaral MA, Pareira A: Giant aneurysm of the petrous portion of the carotid artery. *J Neurol Neurosurg Psychiatry* 46:685–687, 1983.
72. Maxwell RE, Chou SN: Aneurysm tumors of the basifrontal region. *J Neurosurg* 46:438–455, 1977.
73. McGrail KM, Heros RC, Debrun G, Beyerl BD: Aneurysm of the petrous segment of the internal carotid artery. *J Neurosurg* 65:249–252, 1986.
74. Michenfelder JD, Kirklin JW, Uihlein A, Svien HJ: Clinical experience with a closed-chest method of producing profound hypothermia and total circulatory arrest in neurosurgery. *Ann Surg* 199:125–158, 1984.
75. Miller JD, Jawak K, Jennet B: Safety of carotid ligation and its role in the management of intracranial aneurysms. *J Neurol Neurosurg Psychiatry* 40:64–72, 1977.
76. Morantz RA, Kirchner FR, Kishore P: Aneurysms of the petrous portion of the internal carotid artery. *Surg Neurol* 6:313–318, 1976.
77. Morley TP, Barr HWK: Giant intracranial aneurysms: Diagnosis, course and management. *Clin Neurosurg* 16:73–94, 1969.
78. Mount LA: Results of treatment of intracranial aneurysms using the Selverstone clamp. *J Neurosurg* 16:611–618, 1959.
79. Mount L, Antunes JL: Results of treatment of intracranial aneurysm by wrapping and coating. *J Neurosurg* 42:189–193, 1975.
80. Mullan S: Experiences with surgical thrombosis of intracranial berry aneurysms and carotid cavernous fistulas. *J Neurosurg* 41:657–670, 1974.
81. Nishioka H: Report on the cooperative study of intracranial aneurysms and subarachnoid hemorrhage. Section VIII. Part I. Results of the treatment of intracranial aneurysms by occlusion of the carotid artery in the neck. *J Neurosurg* 25:660–682, 1966.
82. Odom GL, Tindall GT: Carotid ligation in the treatment of certain intracranial aneurysms. *Clin Neurosurg* 15:101–116, 1968.
83. O'Neill M, Hope T, Thomson G: Giant intracranial aneurysms: Diagnosis with special reference to computerized tomography. *Clin Radiol* 31:27–39, 1980.
84. Onuma T, Suzuki JL: Surgical treatment of giant intracranial aneurysms. *J Neurosurg* 51:33–36, 1979.
85. Peerless SJ, Hampf CR: Extracranial to intracranial bypass in the treatment of aneurysms. *Clin Neurosurg* 32:114–154, 1985.
86. Pelz DM, Buchan A, Fox AJ, Barnett JH, Vinuela F: Intraluminal thrombus of the internal carotid arteries: Angiographic demonstration of resolution with anticoagulant therapy alone. *Radiology* 160:369–373, 1986.
87. Piek J, Lim DP, Bock WJ: Obstructive hydrocephalus caused by a growing, giant aneurysm on the upper basilar artery. *Surg Neurol* 20:288–290, 1983.
88. Pinto, RS, Cohen WA, Kricheff II, Redington RW, Berninger WH: Giant intracranial aneurysms: Rapid sequential computed tomography. *AJNR* 3:495–499, 1982.
89. Pinto RS, Kricheff II, Butler AR, Murali R: Correlation of computed tomographic, angiographic, and neuropathological changes in giant cerebral aneurysms. *Neuroradiology* 132:85–92, 1979.
90. Pozzati E, Fagioli L, Servadei F, Gaist G: Effect of common carotid ligation on giant aneurysms of the internal carotid artery. *J Neurosurg* 55:527–531, 1981.
91. Pozzati E, Nuzzo G, Gaist G: Giant aneurysms of the pericallosal artery. Case report. *J Neurosurg* 57:566–569, 1982.
92. Raymond LA, Tew J: Large suprasellar aneurysms imitating pituitary tumour. *J Neurol Neurosurg Psychiatry* 41:83–87, 1978.
93. Romodanov PA, Sheheglov VI: Intravascular occlusion of saccular aneurysm of the cerebral arteries by means of a detachable balloon catheter. In Krayenbuhl H (ed): *Advances and Technical Standards in Neurosurgery*. New York, Springer-Verlag, 1982, vol 9, pp 25–49.
94. Sakaki T, Kinugawa K, Tanigake T, Miyamoto S: Embolism from intracranial aneurysms. *J Neurosurg* 53:300–304, 1980.
95. Samson DS, Neuwelt EA, Beyer CW, Ditmore QM: Failure of extracranial-intracranial arterial bypass in acute middle cerebral artery occlusion: Case report. *Neurosurgery* 6:185–188, 1980.
96. Sarwar M: Abducens nerve paralysis due to giant aneurysms in the medial carotid canal. *J Neurosurg* 46:121–123, 1977.
97. Sarwar M. Batnizky S, Schechter MM: Tumorous aneurysms. *Neuroradiology* 12:79–97, 1976.
98. Sarwar M, Batnitzky S, Schechter MM, Liebeskind A, Zimmer AE: Growing intracranial aneurysms. *Radiology* 120:603–607, 1976.
99. Scott RM, Ballantine HT Jr: Spontaneous thrombosis in a giant middle cerebral artery aneurysm: Case report. *J Neurosurg* 37:361–363, 1972.
100. Scott RM, Liu HC, Yuan R, Adelman L: Rupture of a previously unruptured giant middle cerebral artery aneurysm after extracranial-intracranial bypass surgery. *Neurosurgery* 10:600–603, 1982.
101. Sekhar LN, Heros RC: Origin, growth and rupture of saccular aneurysms; A review. *Neurosurgery* 8:248–260, 1981.
102. Sekhar LN, Nelson PB: A technique of clipping giant intracranial aneurysms with the preservation of the parent artery. *Surg Neurol* 20:361–368, 1983.
103. Selman WR, Spetzler RF, Roessman UR, Rosenblatt JI, Crumrine RC: Barbiturate-induced coma therapy for focal cerebral ischemia: Effect after temporary and permanent MCA occlusion. *J Neurosurg* 55:220–226, 1981.
104. Selverstone B: Coating of intracranial aneurysms with nontoxic adherent plastics. In HH Schmidek, WH Sweet (eds): *Operative Neurosurgical Techniques*. New York, Grune & Stratton, 1982, vol 2, pp 949–955.
105. Sengupta RP, Gryspeerdt GL, Hankinson J: Carotid-ophthalmic aneurysms. *J Neurol Neurosurg Psychiatry* 39:387–853, 1976.
106. Serbinenko FA: Balloon catheterization and occlusion of major cerebral vessels. *J Neurosurg* 41:125–145, 1974.
107. Silverberg GD, Reitz BA, Ream AK: Hypothermia and cardiac arrest in the treatment of giant aneurysms of the cerebral circulation and hemangioblastoma of the medulla. *J Neurosurg* 55:337–346, 1981.
108. Silverberg GD, Reitz BA, Ream AK, Taylor G, Enzmann DR: Operative treatment of a giant cerebral artery aneurysm with hypothermia and circulatory arrest: Report of a case. *Neurosurgery* 3:301–305, 1980.
109. Smith TW, DeGirolami V, Crowell RM: Neuropathological changes associated with the transorbital application of ethyl 2-cyanoacrylate adhesive to the basal cerebral arteries of cats. *J Neurosurg* 62:108–114, 1985.
110. Spallone A: Giant, completely thrombosed intracranial aneurysm simulating tumor of the foramen magnum. *Surg Neurol* 18:372–376, 1982.
111. Spetzler RF: Extracranial-intracranial arterial anastomosis for cerebrovascular disease. *Surg Neurol* 11:157–161, 1979.

112. Spetzler RF, Roski RA: The role of EC-IC in the treatment of giant intracranial aneurysms. Neurol Res 2:345–359, 1980.
113. Spetzler RF, Rhodes RS, Roski RA, Kikavel MJ: Subclavian to middle cerebral artery saphenous vein bypass graft. J Neurosurg 53:465–469, 1980.
114. Spetzler RF, Schuster H, Roski RA: Elective extracranial-intracranial arterial bypass in the treatment of inoperable giant aneurysms of the internal carotid artery. J Neurosurg 53:22–27, 1980.
115. Stewart RM, Samson D, Diehl J, Hinton R, Ditmore QM: Unruptured cerebral aneurysm presenting as recurrent transient neurologic deficits. Neurology 30:47–51, 1980.
116. Story JL, Brown WE Jr, Eidelberg E: Cerebral revascularization: Common carotid to distal middle cerebral artery bypass. Neurosurgery 2:131–134, 1978.
117. Sugita K: *Microsurgical Atlas*. Tokyo, Springer-Verlag, 1985.
118. Sugita K, Kobayashi S, Inoue T, Banno T: New angled fenestrated clips for fusiform vertebral artery aneurysms. J Neurosurg 54:346–350, 1981.
119. Sugita K, Kobayashi S, Inoue T, Takemae T: Characteristics and use of ultralong aneurysm clips. J Neurosurg 60:145–150, 1984.
120. Sugita K, Kobayashi S, Kyoshima K, Nakagawa F: Fenestrated clips for unusual aneurysms of the carotid artery. J Neurosurg 57:240–246, 1982.
121. Sundt TM Jr, Piepgras DG: Surgical approach to giant intracranial aneurysms. Operative experience with 80 cases. J Neurosurg 51:731–742, 1979.
122. Sundt TM Jr, Piepgras DG, Marsh WR: Booster clips for giant and thickened aneurysms. J Neurosurg 60:761–762, 1984.
123. Sundt TM, Pluth JR, Gronert GA: Excision of giant basilar aneurysm under profound hypothermia. Mayo Clin Proc 47:631–634, 1972.
124. Sundt TM Jr, Siekert RG, Piepgras DG, Sharbrough FW, Houser OW: Bypass surgery for vascular disease of the carotid system. Mayo Clin Proc 51:677–692, 1976.
125. Suzuki J, Kodama N, Ebina T, Keiji K: Surgical treatment of anterior communicating artery aneurysms: From the experiences of 346 cases. In Suzuki J (ed): *Cerebral Aneurysms*. Tokyo, Neuron, 1979, pp 238–243.
126. Suzuki J, Tanaka S, Yoshimoto T: Suppression of brain swelling with mannitol and perfluorochemicals—an experimental study. Acta Neurochir (Wien) 58:149–160, 1981.
127. Suzuki J, Yoshimoto T: The effect of mannitol in prolongation of permissible occlusion time of cerebral arteries: Clinical data of aneurysm surgery. In Suzuki, J (ed): *Cerebral Aneurysms*. Tokyo, Neuron, 1979, pp 330–337.
128. Swann K, Heros RC, Debrun G, Nelson C: Inadvertent middle cerebral artery embolism by a detachable balloon: Management by embolectomy. J Neurosurg 64:309–312, 1986.
129. Swearingen B, Heros RC: Fatal rupture of a thrombosed giant basilar artery aneurysm. Surg Neurol 23:299–302, 1985.
130. Swearingen B, Heros RC: Common carotid occlusion for unclippable carotid aneurysms: An old but still effective operation. Neurosurgery, in press.
131. Teal JS, Bergeron RT, Rumbaugh CL, Segall HD: Aneurysms of the petrous or cavernous portions of the internal carotid artery associated with non-penetrating head trauma. J Neurosurg 38:568–574, 1973.
132. Thron A, Bockenheimer S: Giant aneurysms of the posterior fossa suspected as neoplasms on computed tomography. Neuroradiology 18:93–97, 1979.
133. Tindall GT, Goree JA, Lee JF, Odom GL: Effect of common carotid ligation on size of internal carotid aneurysms and distal intracarotid and retinal artery pressures. J Neurosurg 25:503–511, 1966.
134. Tindall GT, Kapp J, Odom LG, Robinson SC: A combined technique for treating certain aneurysms of the anterior communicating artery. J Neurosurg 33:41–47, 1970.
135. Tindall GT, Odom GL: Treatment of intracranial aneurysm by proximal carotid ligation. Prog Neurol Surg 3:66–114, 1969.
136. Tognetti F, Andreoli A, Testa C: Giant fusiform aneurysm of the middle cerebral artery treated with extracranial-intracranial arterial bypass and Drake tourniquet. Surg Neurol 22:33–35, 1984.
137. Uihlein A, MacCarty CS, Michenfelder JD, Terry HR, Daw EF: Deep hypothermia and surgical treatment of intracranial aneurysms. JAMA 195:127–129, 1966.
138. White JC, Ballantine HT Jr: Intrasellar aneurysms simulating hypophyseal tumors. J Neurosurg 18:34–50, 1961.
139. Whittle IR, Dorsch NW, Besser M: Spontaneous thrombosis in giant intracranial aneurysms. J Neurol Neurosurg Psychiatry 45:1040–1047, 1982.
140. Whittle KR, Dorsch N, Besser M: Giant intracranial aneurysms: Diagnosis, management and outcome. Surg Neurol 21:218–230, 1984.
141. Winn HR, Richardson AE, Jane JA: Late mortality and morbidity of common carotid ligation for posterior communicating aneurysms. J Neurosurg 47:727–736, 1977.
142. Woodhall B, Sealy WC, Hall KD, Floyd WL: Craniotomy under conditions of quinidine-protected cardioplegia and profound hypothermia. Ann Surg 152:37–44, 1959.
143. Yasargil MG: Giant intracranial aneurysms. In: *Microsurgery*. New York, Thieme-Stratton, 1984.
144. Yasargil MG, Gasser JC, Hodosh RM, Rankin TV: Carotid-ophthalmic aneurysms: Direct microsurgical approach. Surg Neurol 8:155–165, 1977.
145. Zeumer H, Bruckmann H, Adelt D, Hacke W, Ringelstein EG: Balloon embolization in the treatment of basilar aneurysms. Acta Neurochir (Wien) 78:136–141, 1985.

21
Infectious Aneurysms

INTRODUCTION

Since 1885, when William Osler described an aortic aneurysm associated with bacterial endocarditis, the term "mycotic" aneurysm has been used to designate any aneurysm that develops following infection in the wall of an artery (48). Until a few years ago, almost every publication concerning intracranial "mycotic" aneurysms reported a bacterial cause for the aneurysm, usually in association with endocarditis. Reports of aneurysms associated with meningitis and cavernous sinus thrombophlebitis, as well as true mycotic (fungal) aneurysms, have subsequently appeared (45,46). The designation, bacterial intracranial aneurysm, should be used for those aneurysms that result from bacterial infection (8). It is suggested that all types of aneurysms due to infection be grouped under the heading of infectious aneurysms (45).

Several publications have reviewed the subject of bacterial intracranial aneurysms (8, 10, 15, 20, 45). In one, 85 cases found at angiography, operation, or autopsy between 1954 and 1978 were summarized (8). In another, the authors analyzed infectious intracranial aneurysms documented by angiography and reported in the 20 years from 1959 through 1978 (45). This included 53 patients with bacterial intracranial aneurysm associated with definite or probable endocarditis (1, 3, 5–8, 10, 16, 18, 20, 21, 24–28, 35, 36, 39, 40, 42–45, 49, 52, 54, 61, 64, 65), 5 with aneurysms due to meningitis (18, 47, 59, 60), 7 with aneurysms associated with cavernous sinus thrombophlebitis (30, 55, 59, 61), and 5 with fungal aneurysms (2, 13, 19, 33, 63). Subsequently, further reports of patients with bacterial aneurysms documented by angiography have appeared, bringing to 81 the total number of cases through 1980 (4, 15, 17, 23, 34, 41, 53, 56, 57, 62).

BACTERIAL INTRACRANIAL ANEURYSMS

Clinical Manifestations

The majority of bacterial intracranial aneurysms occur in patients with subacute bacterial endocarditis, some of whom have associated congenital or rheumatic heart disease. In a few patients with bacterial intracranial aneurysms, a diagnosis of endocarditis is not established. Usually, there has been a history of infection such as pharyngitis, infected laceration, or drug addiction.

Bacterial aneurysms are due to infected emboli reaching the cerebral circulation and are most often located on a distal branch of an intracranial artery, usually a middle cerebral artery branch. This location tends to differentiate bacterial aneurysm from the more common developmental aneurysm usually found on the circle of Willis or proximal cerebral arteries.

Neurologic problems are frequent in patients with bacterial endocarditis and may be the presenting symptoms (24, 32, 51). Neurologic symptoms were found by Jones et al in 29% (110 of 385) and by Pruitt et al in 39% (84 of 218) of patients with bacterial endocarditis (24, 51). The majority of patients have evidence of cerebral embolism with infarction, but hemorrhage (subarachnoid or intracerebral) and infarction followed by hemorrhage may occur. A few patients have had brain abscess or meningitis. Occasionally, headache has been noted without evidence of hemorrhage (26).

Intracranial bacterial aneurysms occur in 4–10% of patients with bacterial endocarditis (8). The incidence may be even higher, since some aneurysms are asymptomatic. Multiple aneurysms occur in about 20% of patients with an aneurysm, but the true figure is unknown, since very few patients have had full angiography. The lesions may occur at any age.

When a patient with endocarditis develops a bacterial aneurysm, the most common presentation is subarachnoid or intracerebral hemorrhage. Patients without a previous diagnosis of bacterial endocarditis may have onset of hemorrhage from a bacterial aneurysm as the first manifestation of the disease. Another clinical group first presents with symptoms and signs of cerebral ischemia, but an aneurysm is discovered with angiography. A few patients with cerebral infarction later develop a subarachnoid or intracerebral hemorrhage from an aneurysm (51). Recurrent hemorrhage occurs but the incidence is unknown.

In our review of 81 patients with documented bacterial aneurysms due to endocarditis, there was enough clinical information on 65 to determine the probable initial neurologic event that led to the angiogram (Table 21.1). This was definite or probable hemorrhage in 42, infarction in 16, infarction followed by hemorrhage in 5, and headache without hemorrhage in 2. In 16 patients with a ruptured bacterial aneurysm reported by Pruitt et al, 8 had a history suggesting embolization and infarction prior to the hemorrhage (51). At angiography, an occluded vessel was often found in association with the aneurysm.

The most frequent organism cultured in patients with bacterial aneurysms due to endocarditis has been Streptococcus (Table 21.2). However, Staphylococcus has become a common organism in the reports during the past few years. In some cases, no organisms can be isolated from the blood culture due to prior antibiotics. In spite of the improvement in the recovery rate from infectious endocarditis with antibiotic treatment, the incidence of neurologic complications of the disease has not been significantly reduced (26, 30). It is important to note that aneurysms can develop and hemorrhage can occur in a patient who is receiving adequate antibiotic treatment.

Diagnostic Studies

When there is evidence to suggest subarachnoid hemorrhage in a patient with bacterial endocarditis, a computed tomography (CT) scan followed by a cerebral angiogram should be obtained. It has been suggested that the presence of cerebral embolization during the course of bacterial endocarditis is a strong indication for cerebral angiography (40).

CT scanning should be carried out with and without contrast enhancement. It may localize the aneurysm either directly or by demonstrating adjacent hematoma. The extent of intracerebral or intraventricular hemorrhage is determined. The CT scan may also show edema, infarction, abscess, and/or hydrocephalus.

Angiography is the definitive study to outline the location of the aneurysm and its relationship to the parent vessels (Figs. 21.1–21.4). If the diagnosis of associated subarachnoid hemorrhage is in doubt or if meningitis is suspected, a lumbar puncture is indicated after the CT scan has been obtained.

There is a striking predilection for involvement of the middle cerebral artery. No less dramatic is the tendency for involvement of a distal intracranial branch, regardless of which artery is involved (Table 21.3). In the 71 patients in whom the site of the angiographically proven bacterial aneurysm was definitely established on the initial angiogram, 64 had at least one aneurysm on a distal branch of an intracranial artery, and 55 had involvement of a middle cerebral artery branch. Very few patients have had complete angiography, so the true incidence of multiple aneurysms is unknown.

Follow-up angiography was reported in 27 patients, who had not had surgery, within a few days to 8 months after the first study but usually within 2–8 weeks. A few patients had more than one follow-up study. A new aneurysm was found in 8 patients, with 3 having had a normal initial angiogram. At the time of the last angiographic study, the aneurysm was no longer visualized in 8, was smaller in 5, unchanged in 4, and larger in 6; and in 4 patients, a new aneurysm was found but no further study was reported. Seven other patients had postoperative angiography. The original aneurysm was gone in all cases, but one patient had a new distal middle cerebral aneurysm that had ruptured.

Decisions regarding Management

A program of treatment for patients with bacterial intracranial aneurysm can be outlined based on a review of the literature (7, 8, 15, 38, 45, 51, 52). Medical treatment should include the appropriate intravenous antibiotics and, if indicated, the correction of the responsible cardiac lesion. It has been recommended that the cardiac operation be performed before repair of the intracranial aneurysm, unless the patient is threatened by mass effect from a hematoma, to remove the source for further emboli and correct

Table 21.1.
Clinical Presentation in Patients Found to Have Bacterial Intracranial Aneurysms (Summary of Reported Cases through 1980)

Hemorrhage	42
Infarction	16
Infarction followed by hemorrhage	5
Headache without hemorrhage	2
No data	16

Table 21.2.
Bacteriology in Patients Found to Have Bacterial Intracranial Aneurysms (Summary of Reported Cases through 1980)

Streptococcus	36
Staphylococcus	15
Pseudomonas	2
Enterococcus	1
Corynebacterium	1
Cardiobacterium	1
Multiple organisms	4
No growth	10
No data	11

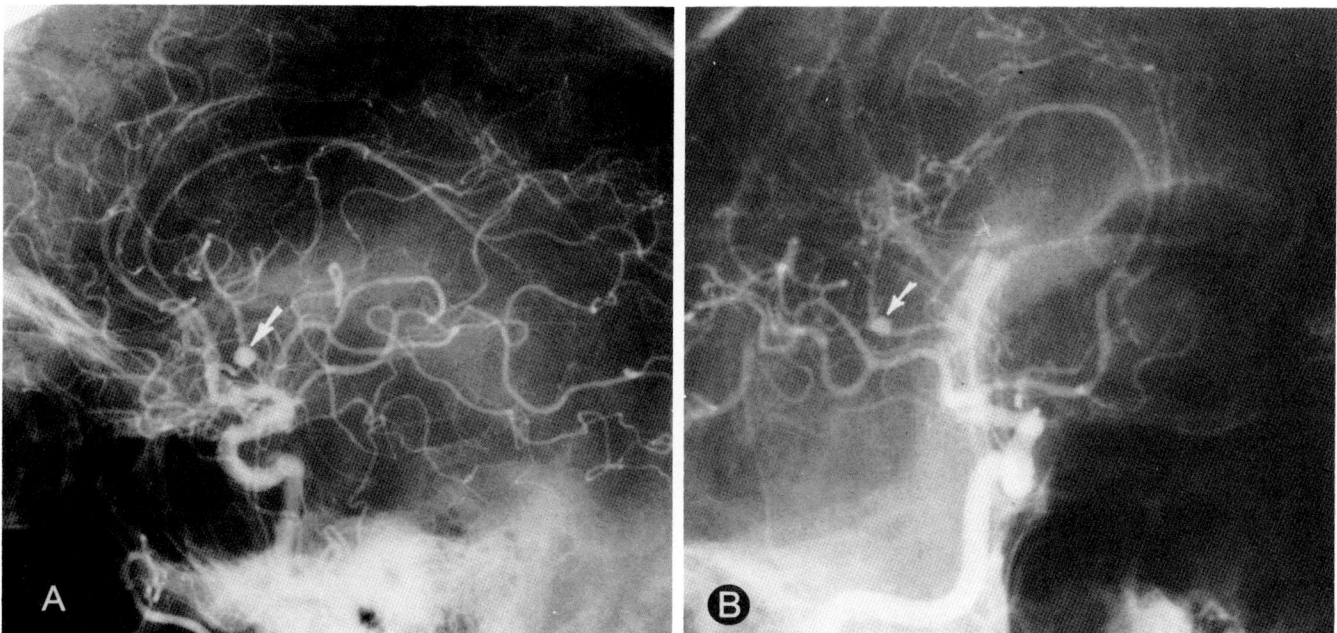

Figure 21.1. Bacterial intracranial aneurysm in distal middle cerebral artery branch. **A**, Lateral angiogram shows the aneurysm *(arrow)* on the ascending frontal parietal branch of the middle cerebral artery. **B**, Oblique angiogram defines the relationship of the aneurysm *(arrow)* to the parent artery. Comment: The patient presented with an intracerebral hemorrhage and was found to have subacute bacterial endocarditis.

any hemodynamic problem (38). There has been no increased morbidity with the cardiopulmonary bypass and associated heparinization. The use of antifibrinolytic agents has not been studied in this illness.

The place of surgical treatment has been discussed in several reports. Bingham reviewed 45 cases of bacterial intracrancial aneurysms of all types where it was thought that adequate antibiotic treatment had been given and where angiography had been performed (7). He concluded that there did not appear to be a clear-cut advantage to the use of surgery plus antibiotics over the use of antibiotics alone. Twenty patients received only antibiotic treatment, but 3 died from hemorrhage while under treatment. In the 25 patients who had combined antibiotic and surgical treatment, 6 died, but most of these were poor risk patients. He noted that the mortality associated with a definitive surgical procedure for bacterial intracranial aneurysm on distal arterial branches appeared to be quite low if one eliminated the poor-risk surgical candidates from death due to cardiac or other medical problems and from fatal hemorrhage due to a second previously undiagnosed aneurysm. He recommended an operation only if the aneurysm enlarged or did not change in size after 6 weeks of antibiotic therapy. Bohmfalk et al reviewed reports on 17 patients who had surgical removal of bacterial aneurysms of distal arterial branches (8). There was no mortality. These authors also noted 6 patients in the literature who did not develop hemorrhage until after completion of their antibiotic treatment for endocarditis. Cantu et al reported on 5 patients brought to autopsy who died due to rupture of a bacterial aneurysm; all 5 were receiving intensive antibiotic therapy at the time of the hemorrhage (10). Pruitt et al reported 9 patients who were adequately treated with antibiotics prior to aneurysmal ruptures (51). Frazee et al concluded that patients with a diagnosis of bacterial endocarditis who develop sudden severe headache, focal neurologic signs, or symptoms of seizures should undergo serial angiography every 7–10 days throughout their hospitalization (15). Morawetz and Karp noted that new aneurysms may appear and existing ones may enlarge during the first 4–6 weeks of antibiotic therapy and these changes do not mandate surgery but that surgical intervention is indicated following intracerebral or subarachnoid hemorrhage or when an aneurysm enlarges after the completion of a full course of antibiotic therapy (38). If an aneurysm is identified, it should be excised whenever possible.

The results from a review of the literature of 81 patients who had angiography because of neurologic symptom and were found to have a bacterial aneurysm are outlined in Table 21.4. Of 30 patients treated with antibiotics in whom the outcome was known, 13 died. Elective surgery was performed in 29 patients: 2 patients died, but both had recovered from

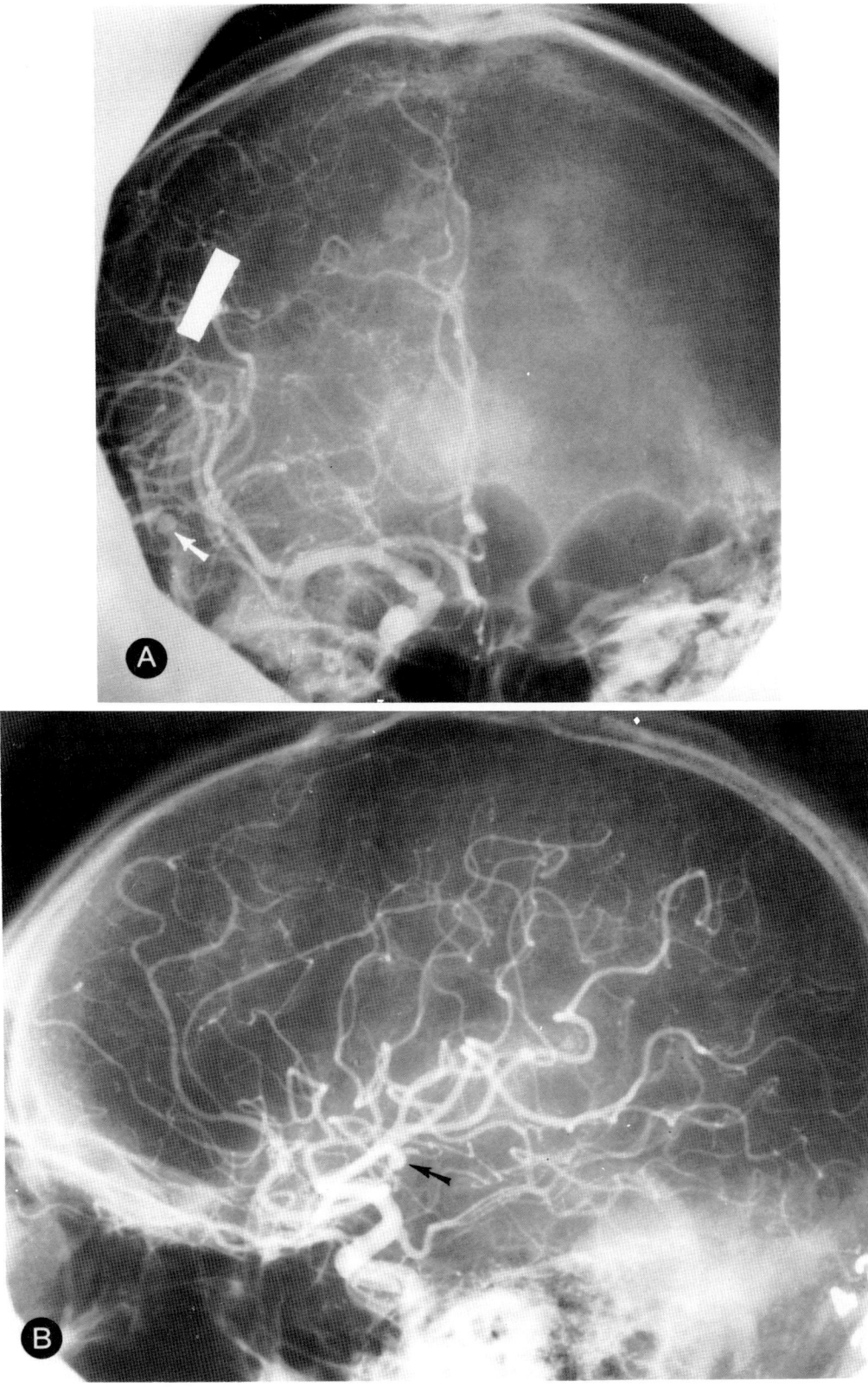

Figure 21.2. Bacterial intracranial aneurysm in distal middle cerebral artery branch. **A** and **B,** Anteroposterior and lateral angiograms show aneurysm on a superior temporal branch of the middle cerebral artery. Comment: The patient presented with a history of pharyngitis and then subarachnoid hemorrhage. There was no evidence of subacute bacterial endocarditis. The aneurysm was excised at operation. Pathologic findings were consistent with an infectious lesion.

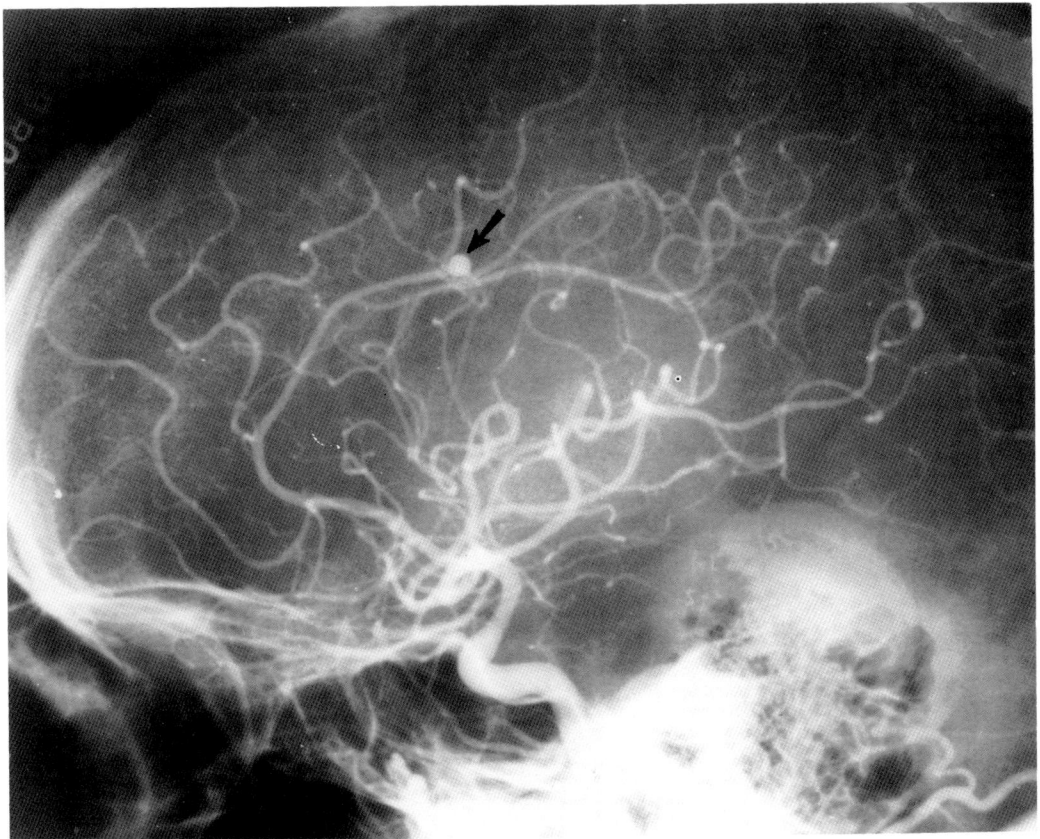

Figure 21.3. Bacterial intracranial aneurysm in distal anterior cerebral artery branch. This lateral angiogram shows the aneurysm *(arrow)* several centimeters distal to the site of the usual developmental pericallosal aneurysm. Comment: The patient had subacute bacterial endocarditis. The lesion healed with antibiotic therapy.

surgery only to die from rupture of a second unrecognized aneurysm. As would be expected, the results were worse when emergency surgery was required, usually because an intracranial hematoma had caused a serious neurologic deficit.

The authors' recommendations are: (a) a single bacterial aneurysm on a distal middle cerebral artery branch associated with subarachnoid or intracerebral hemorrhage should be excised if the patient's medical condition is stable; and (b) for bacterial aneurysm on the proximal arterial trunks, unruptured aneurysms, or aneurysms involving arteries whose excision is very likely to cause a serious neurologic deficit, a program of antibiotics and serial angiography is indicated. How often the angiogram should be obtained has not been established, and recommendations have ranged from one to several weeks (15, 31, 38, 45, 46, 50). The authors of this text suggest 10–14 days. If the aneurysm is larger at follow-up angiography, surgery is considered. If it is the same size or smaller, antibiotic treatment is continued. Angiography is repeated at an appropriate interval and again when antibiotic treatment is completed. If the aneurysm does not disappear after treatment, surgery is usually indicated.

The literature does not give a definitive answer as to what to do with the patient when multiple bacterial aneurysms are found. A review of 15 reported cases of multiple bacterial aneurysms, due to all causes including meningitis, revealed that 11 were treated nonsurgically and none died as a direct result of this treatment (15). Analysis of reports of 10 patients with multiple bacterial aneurysms seen on angiography and related to established or probable endocarditis revealed that 7 were treated with antibiotics alone, with only one death occurring (45). This was in a patient who also was a heroin addict and had brain abscess and infarction. There is no explanation for these findings of a low mortality rate with antibiotic therapy alone compared with the higher mortality rate for nonsurgically treated patients with a single aneurysm. However, the authors have already noted that 2 patients who had recovered from elective surgery for removal of a single aneurysm subsequently died because of hemorrhage from a second unrecognized aneurysm. Frazee et al proposed that if mul-

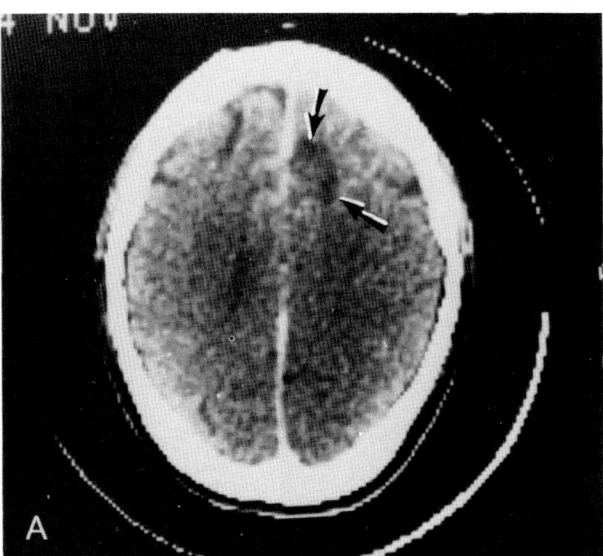
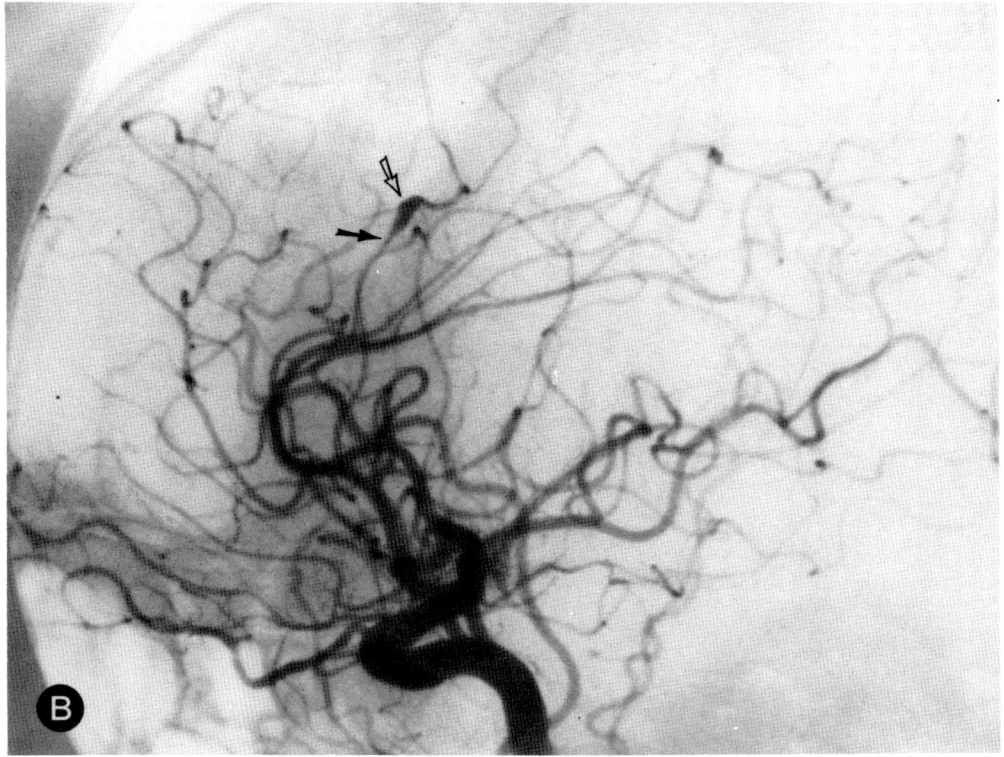

Figure 21.4. Bacterial intracranial aneurysm and associated brain abscess **A,** Initial CT scan of a patient who presented with a febrile episode (upper respiratory infection) and a rapidly progressive disturbance in mental function shows a low-density area with minimal adjacent enhancement *(arrows)*. **B,** Angiogram of the same patient shows a fusiform lesion *(open arrow)* on a distal branch of the anterior cerebral artery *(closed arrow)*, consistent with a bacterial aneurysm. The low-density area seen on CT scan was aspirated and an abscess was confirmed. The patient was treated with antibiotic therapy. There was no evidence of subacute bacterial endocarditis. **C,** CT scan 2 weeks later shows a smaller abscess with a well-defined capsule which enhances. **D,** Angiogram of the same patient at this time shows the aneurysm to be smaller *(open arrow)* and marked narrowing of the parent vessel *(closed arrow)*. Complete recovery followed a full course of antibiotic treatment.

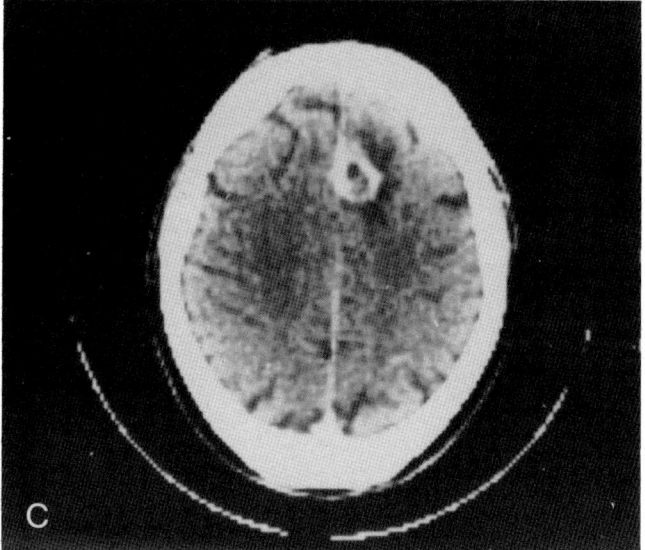
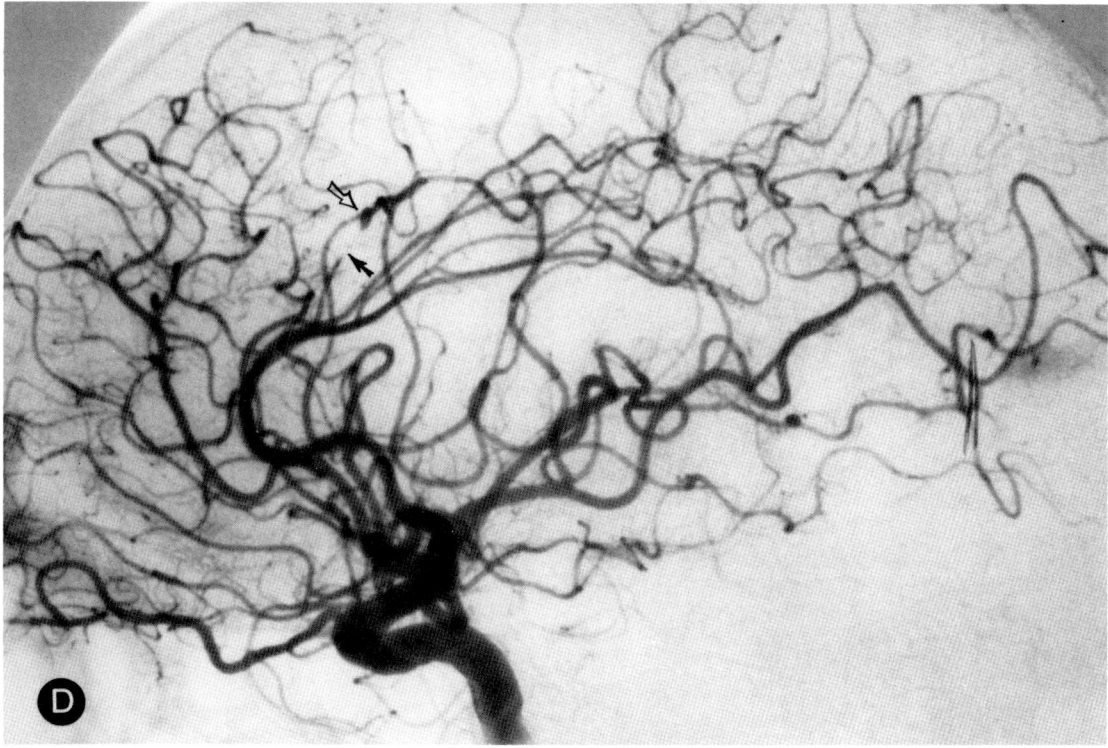

Figure 21.4C and D.

Table 21.3.
Findings on Initial Angiogram in Patients Found to Have Bacterial Intracranial Aneurysms (Summary of Reported Cases through 1980)

Aneurysm location	
Single	61
Distal middle cerebral artery	44
Distal anterior cerebral artery	3
Distal posterior cerebral artery	4
Proximal intracranial artery	7
Not specified: middle cerebral artery	3
Multiple	15
Distal middle cerebral artery only	4
Distal middle cerebral artery and other vessels	7
Combinations not including distal middle cerebral artery	2
Not specified	2
No aneurysm seen	5
Occluded artery in addition to aneurysm	13

tiple aneurysms are unilateral, they should be excised at one operation wherever possible, and if they are bilateral, the largest or the one presumed to have bled should be excised and then the patient should be followed by angiography (15). Another suggestion is to treat the patient with antibiotics and to repeat the angiogram at 2-week intervals and when therapy is completed. If the lesions become larger or do not disappear after treatment, surgery may be indicated.

In planning the surgical treatment, it is important to remember that these aneurysms have an inflamed, friable wall that may easily fragment. For peripheral lesions, the aneurysm can be excised with the small vessel from which it arises, usually with little or no neurologic deficit. The less common proximal or less accessible lesions may present a more serious technical problem. Treatment with antibiotics may allow the arteritis to resolve with fibrosis in the wall of the aneurysm and parent artery. The lesion can then be handled more safely at surgery (52). If surgery is needed for a proximal lesion or aneurysm involving a critical artery, a bypass graft may be required as the initial procedure, since in these cases, the parent artery frequently needs to be sacrificed. This has been reported in 2 patients (12).

At the time of surgery, the neurosurgeon may encounter not only an intracerebral hematoma or an area of infarction but also a brain abscess (Fig. 21.4). In the series of cases reported through 1980, 5 patients had associated brain abscesses.

BACTERIAL INTRACRANIAL ANEURYSMS ASSOCIATED WITH MENINGITIS

Arterial lesions have been described in patients with meningitis caused by a variety of organisms. Extensive arterial changes can occur with a panarteritis that may result in thrombosis, but on occasion the wall is weakened and an aneurysm forms (18, 45, 46, 59, 60). Patients may present with hemorrhage or seizures and neurologic deficit. These aneurysms are more likely to involve the distal anterior cerebral artery branches. Treatment considerations are the same as those outlined for bacterial aneurysm associated with endocarditis.

BACTERIAL ANEURYSMS OF THE INTERNAL CAROTID ARTERY ASSOCIATED WITH CAVERNOUS SINUS THROMBOPHLEBITIS

Cavernous sinus thrombophlebitis can be associated with development of an aneurysm of the internal carotid artery (30, 45, 55, 59, 61). Bilateral aneurysms have been reported (14). The thrombophlebitis may be associated with an infection near the eye or on the face or with a remote abscess or infection causing septicemia. Where a culture is available, *Staphylococcus* is usually reported. Persistent evidence of exophthalmus and ophthalmoplegia should lead to use of angiography. These symptoms or enlargement of the aneurysm on repeat angiography has led to treatment, and these patients have been treated by carotid ligation and by a trapping operation. An extracranial-intracranial arterial bypass has been used (14).

BACTERIAL ANEURYSMS OF THE EXTRACRANIAL AND PETROUS PORTION OF THE INTERNAL CAROTID ARTERY

Patients with aneurysms of infectious origin involving the petrous portion of the internal carotid artery have presented with epistasis and otorrhagia (11). Patients with infectious aneurysms of the extracranial internal carotid artery have presented with (a) painful pulsatile mass in the neck which may be associated with tenth or twelfth cranial nerve palsy (29, 58), (b) bleeding into the pharynx (9), and (c) intracranial abscesses, presumably from a septic embolus from the aneurysm (22). Treatment has been

Table 21.4.
Treatment of and Results in Patients Found to Have Bacterial Intracranial Aneurysms (Summary of Reported Cases through 1980)

	Recovered[a]	Died	No information	Total
Antibiotics	17	13	1	31
Elective surgery[b]	27	2	0	29
Emergency surgery[b]	8	6	0	14
No treatment	1	1	1	3
No data	0	0	4	4

[a]Some patients who recovered from their neurologic illness subsequently died from a cardiac cause and some were left with a neurologic disability.
[b]Patients who had surgery also received antibiotics.

some form of carotid occlusion which may have needed to be performed as an emergency procedure.

FUNGAL INTRACRANIAL ANEURYSMS

The reports of 13 patients with fungal or "true" mycotic aneurysms have been reviewed (37). The most common causative organisms are: *Asperigillus*, which spreads from sinuses or follows cranial surgery; *Phycomycetes*, found in patients with diabetes mellitis or systemic illness; and *Candida*, found in patients with endocarditis and systemic infections.

The fungal aneurysm is usually located on a proximal major intracranial artery. However, in one case in which the aneurysm was due to emboli from endocarditis, involvement was in the distal middle and anterior cerebral arteries. Associated thrombosis in contiguous or remote basal arteries is common.

Treatment of the local sinus condition or systemic illness with antifungal medication and an attempt at direct surgical therapy have been tried. There is no reported case with survival.

REFERENCES

1. Agnoli A, Bettag W: Endokarditis und Subarachnoidalblutung. *Z Neurol* 199:295–305, 1971.
2. Ahuja GK, Jain N, Vijayaraghavan M, Roy S: Cerebral mycotic aneurysm of fungal origin. *J Neurosurg* 49:107–110, 1978.
3. Alajouanine T, Castaigne P, Lhermitte F, Cambier J: The cerebral arteritis of bacterial endocarditis: Its late complications. *JAMA*, 170:1858, 1959.
4. Almazan V, Pulpon A. DeTeresa L, Catalan E, Burgui L, Artaza-Andrade M: Mycotic aneurysm secondary to bacterial endocarditis. *Arch Inst Cardiol Mex* 48:1224–1232, 1978.
5. Amine AR: Neurosurgical complications of heroin addiction: Brain abscess and mycotic aneurysm. *Surg Neurol* 7:385–386, 1977.
6. Bell WE, Butler C II: Cerebral mycotic aneurysms in children. Two case reports. *Neurology* 18:81–86, 1968.
7. Bingham WF: Treatment of mycotic intracranial aneurysms. *J Neurosurg* 46:428–437, 1977.
8. Bohmfalk GL, Story JL, Wissinger JP, Brown WE Jr: Bacterial intracranial aneurysm. *J Neurosurg* 48:369–382, 1978.
9. Bolender NF, Bassett MR, Loeser JD, Patterson HC: Mycotic aneurysm of the internal carotid artery. A surgical emergency. *Ann Otol Rhinol Laryngol* 93:273–276, 1984.
10. Cantu RC, LeMay M, Wilkinson HA: The importance of repeated angiography in the treatment of mycotic-embolic intracranial aneurysms. *J Neurosurg* 25:189–193, 1966.
11. Chiappetta F, Vasnselista J, Pirrone R: Recurrent massive otorrhagia caused by a petrous carotid aneurysm. *J Neurosurg Sci* 26:205–207, 1982.
12. Day AL: Extracranial-intracranial bypass grafting in the surgical treatment of bacterial aneurysm. Report of two cases. *Neurosurgery* 9:583–588, 1981..
13. Davidson P, Robertson DM: A true mycotic (*Aspergillus*) aneurysm leading to fatal subarachnoid hemorrhage in a patient with hereditary hemorrhagic telangiectasia. Case report. *J Neurosurg* 35:71–76, 1971.
14. Esuchi T, Nakasomi T, Teraoka A: Treatment of bilateral mycotic intracavernous carotid aneurysms. Case report. *J Neurosurg* 56: 443–447, 1982.
15. Frazee JG, Cahan LD, Winter J: Bacterial intracranial aneurysms. *J Neurosurg* 53:633–641, 1980.
16. Gilroy J, Andaya L, Thomas VJ: Intracranial mycotic aneurysms and subacute bacterial endocarditis in herion addiction. *Neurology* 23:1193–1198, 1973.
17. Grinberg M, Lage SH, de Almeida GG, Stolf N, DeCourt LV: Infectious endocarditis, cerebral mycotic aneurysm and meningeal hemorrhage. *Arq Bras Cardiol* 32:257–261, 1979.
18. Harrison MJG, Hampton JR: Neurological presentation of bacterial endocarditis. *Br Med J* 2:148–151, 1967.
19. Horten BC, Abbott GF, Porro RS: Fungal aneurysms of intracranial vessels. *Arch Neurol* 33:577–579, 1976.
20. Hourihane JB: Ruptured mycotic intracranial aneurysm. A report of three cases. *Vasc Surg* 4:21–29, 1970.
21. Ishikawa M, Waga S, Moritake K, Handa H: Cerebral bacterial aneurysms: Report of three cases. *Surg Neurol* 2:257–261, 1974.
22. Imamura J, Watanabe Y: Multiple brain abscesses associated with a mycotic aneurysm of the left common carotid artery. *J Neurosurg* 64:325–327, 1986.
23. Jara FM, Lewis JF Jr, Magilligan DJ Jr: Operative experience with infective endocarditis and intracerebral mycotic aneurysm. *J Thorac Cardiovasc Surg* 80:28–30, 1980.
24. Jones HR Jr, Siekert RG, Geraci JE: Neurologic manifestations of bacterial endocarditis. *Ann Intern Med* 71:21–28, 1969.
25. Katz RI, Goldberg HI, Selzer ME: Mycotic aneurysm.. Case report with novel sequential angiographic findings. *Arch Intern Med* 134:939–942, 1974.
26. Kaufman SL, White RI Jr, Harrington DP, Barth KH, Siegelman SS: Protean manifestations of mycotic aneurysm. *Am J Roentgenol* 131:1019–1025, 1978.
27. King AB: Successful surgical treatment of an intracranial mycotic aneurysm complicated by a subdural hematoma. *J Neurosurg* 17:788–791, 1960.
28. Laguna J, Derby BM, Chase R: *Cardiobacterium hominis* endocarditis with cerebral mycotic aneurysm. *Arch Neurol* 32:438–439, 1975.
29. Lambert MJ III, Johns ME, Mentzer R, Fitz-Hugh GS: Mycotic carotid artery aneurysm. *Otolaryngol Head Neck Surg* 87:624–627, 1979.
30. Lansky LL, Maxwel JA: Mycotic aneurysm of the internal carotid artery in an unusual intracranial location. *Dev Med Child Neurol* 17:79–88, 1975.
31. Leipzig TJ, Brown FD: Treatment of mycotic aneurysms. *Surg Neurol* 23: 403–407, 1985.
32. Lerner PI: Neurologic complications of infective endocarditis. *Med Clin North Am* 69:385–398, 1985.
33. Mahaley MS, Spock A: An unusual case of intracranial aneurysm. In Smith JL (ed): *Neuro-ophthalmology*. St Louis, CV Mosby, 1968, vol 4, pp 148–166.
34. Maly Z: Paraventicular hemorrhage from a mycotic aneurysm. *Cesk Neurol Neurochir* 41:394–396, 1978.
35. Matson DD: Intracranial arterial aneurysms in childhood. *J Neurosurg* 23:578–583, 1965.
36. McNeel D, Evans RA, Ory EM: Angiography of cerebral mycotic aneurysms. *Acta Radiol Diagn* 9:407–412, 1969.
37. Mielke B, Weir B, Oldring D, von Westarp C: Fungal aneurysm: Case report and review of the literature. *Neurosurgery* 9:578–582, 1981.
38. Morawetz RB, Karp RB: Evolution and resolution of intracranial bacterial (mycotic) aneurysms. *Neurosurgery* 15:43–49, 1984.
39. Morin MA, Talalla A: Angiography for mycotic aneurysm. *N Engl J Med* 281:1249–1250, 1969 (letter).
40. Moskowitz MA, Rosenbaum AE, Tyler HR: Angiographically monitored resolution of cerebral mycotic aneurysms. *Neurology* 24:1103–1108, 1974.
41. Nishmura T, Aoki N, Aruga T, Hashimoto I, Imanaga H, Kuboto M, Mizutani H, Tanishima K: A case of mycotic aneurysm after open heart surgery. *No Shinkei Geka* 7:371–375, 1979.
42. Ng KK, Wong WK, Skene-Smith H: Ruptured mycotic intracranial aneurysm. *Australas Radiol* 19:255–257, 1975.
43. Noonan JA, Wilson CB, Spencer FC, Talbert WM Jr: Cerebral

44. North-Coombes D, Schonland MM: Cerebral mycotic aneurysm. A case report. S Afr Med J 48:1808–1810, 1974.
45. Ojemann RG: Infectious intracranial aneurysms. In Fein JM, Flamm ES (eds): Cerebrovascular Disease. New York, Springer-Verlag, 1985, vol 3, pp 1047–1060.
46. Ojemann RG: Surgical management of bacterial intracranial aneurysms. In Schmidek HK, Sweet WH (eds): Operative Neurosurgical Techniques. New York, Grune & Stratton, 1982, pp 933–940.
47. Ojemann RG, New PFJ, Fleming TC: Intracranial aneurysms associated with bacterial meningitis. Neurology 16:1222–1226, 1966.
48. Osler W: Gulstonian lectures on malignant endocarditis. Lancet 1:415–418, 459–464, 505–508, 1885.
49. Pool JL, Potts DG: Aneurysms and Arteriovenous Anomalies of the Brain. New York, Harper & Row, 1965, pp 60–62.
50. Pootrakul A, Canter LP: Bacterial intracranial aneurysms: Importance of sequential angiography. Surg Neurol 17:429–431, 1982.
51. Pruitt AA, Rubin RH, Karchmer AW, Duncan GW: Neurologic complications of bacterial endocarditis. Medicine 57:329–343, 1978.
52. Roach MR, Drake CG: Ruptured cerebral aneurysms caused by micro-organisms. N Engl J Med 273:240–244, 1965.
53. Sato T, Sakuta Y, Suzuki J, Takaku A: Successful surgical treatment of intracranial mycotic aneurysm with brain abscess. Acta Neurochir 47:53–61, 1979.
54. Schold C, Earnest MP: Cerebral hemorrhage from a mycotic aneurysm developing during appropriate antibiotic therapy. Stroke 9:267–268, 1978.
55. Shibuya S, Igarashi S, Amo T, Sato H, Fukumitsu T: Mycotic aneurysms of the internal carotid artery. Case report. J Neurosurg 44:105–108, 1976.
56. Shillito J Jr: Strokes in children. Clin Neurosurg 23:185–219, 1976.
57. Simmons KC, Sage MR, Reilly PL: CT of intracerebral hemorrhage due to mycotic aneurysm. Case report. Neuroradiology 19:215–217, 1980.
58. Slade-Howell H, Baburao T, Graziano J: Mycotic cervical carotid aneurysm. Surgery 81:357–359, 1977.
59. Suwanwela C, Suwanwela N, Charuchinda S, Hongsaprabhas C: Intracranial mycotic aneurysms of extravascular origin J Neurosurg 36:552–559, 1972.
60. Sypert GW, Young HF: Ruptured mycotic pericallosal aneurysm with meningitis due to Neisseria meningitidis infection. Case report. J Neurosurg 37:467–469, 1972.
61. Tanemura H, Sakai N, Yamamori T, Yamada H: Intracranial mycotic aneurysm. Report of a case. Neurol Surg (Tokyo) 5:871–875, 1977.
62. Valadares JB, deSouza MT, Hankinson J, Hall K, Sengupta R: Multiple intracranial mycotic aneurysms. Case report. Arq Neuropsiquiatr 37:311–318, 1979.
63. Visudhiphan P, Bunyaratavej S, Khantanaphar S: Cerebral aspergilllosis. Report of 3 cases. J Neurosurg 38:472–476, 1973.
64. Yarnell PR, Stears J: Intracerebral hemorrhage and occult sepsis. Neurology 24:870–873, 1974
65. Ziment I, Johnson BL Jr: Angiography in the management of intracranial mycotic aneurysms. Arch Intern Med 122:349–352, 1968.

22

Arteriovenous Malformations of the Brain

Vascular malformations are developmental anomalies that result from a failure of normal involution of embryonic vascular networks (104, 105). These lesions are non-neoplastic although some exhibit a tendency to grow during childhood and early adulthood (78, 94, 192). Even though they are thought to be congenital, they are generally not familial, there being only seven reported cases of familial arteriovenous malformations in the English literature in a review in 1985 (13).

The prevalence of vascular malformations of the brain is not well known. The best available prevalence study indicated a 4.05% prevalence in a series of 4069 consecutive autopsies (152). This study revealed 165 vascular malformations of which only 24 were true arteriovenous malformations (AVMs), a prevalence of 0.6%, and the rest were mostly venous malformations and a smaller number of cavernous angiomas and telangiectasias.

There are more data on the incidence of AVMs. In the cooperative study, AVMs accounted for 8.6% of the cases of subarachnoid hemorrhage (133). Since subarachnoid hemorrhage accounts for roughly 10% of all strokes this means that subarachnoid hemorrhage from AVMs accounts for about 1% of all strokes. Similar figures have been reported in other studies (114, 115). The prevalence and incidence of AVMs are about one-tenth that of intracranial aneurysms. Males seem to be affected slightly more often than females (46, 56, 105, 133, 136).

PATHOLOGY

McCormick has classified vascular malformations of the brain into four major types (104, 105). *Telangiectases* are typically small (0.3–1.0 cm) lesions composed of capillary-type vessels separated from each other by more or less normal-appearing neural parenchyma. These lesions are most common in the brain stem, rarely bleed, and usually are found incidentally at autopsy. *Cavernous angiomas* are well-defined, grossly visible lesions that may reach a significant size and can easily be confused with a brain tumor. They are composed of a compact mass of sinusoidal-type vessels immediately in apposition to each other without any recognizable intervening neural parenchyma. The lesion appears grossly as a purplish mass which may resemble a blood clot from a recent hemorrhage. There is frequently microscopic evidence of small hemorrhages with numerous hemosiderin-laden macrophages in the adjacent, often gliotic neural parencyma. Calcification and even ossification is very common. There is no recognizable direct arterial input, which makes them "silent" angiographically. *Venous angiomas* are composed of anomalous veins with no recognizable direct arterial input. The veins within the malformation are separated by normal neural parenchyma. Calcification of these lesions is rare. An unusual type of venous abnormality is a venous varyx which sometimes has been classified as a separate type of vascular malformation (104, 105) but which should probably be considered as a variant of a venous angioma where the draining vein has become very dilated. *Arteriovenous malformations* are the most significant lesions from the clinical point of view. They are composed of masses of arteries and arterialized veins. The vessels vary greatly in diameter but in general the veins are larger than the arteries. The parenchyma between the vessels is usually abnormal and gliotic. There is frequently evidence of old hemorrhage and hemosiderosis.

CLINICAL PRESENTATION

The clinical manifestations of AVMs of the brain are well known (20, 114, 122, 153, 175). These lesions frequently become symptomatic during childhood or early adulthood. Hemorrhage is the most common presenting symptom in childhood and seizures appear to be the most common presenting symptom in adulthood. However, seizures can occur early in childhood and hemorrhages can occur at any age. Approximately 50% of AVMs present clinically as an intracranial hemorrhage (117, 127, 128, 133, 136, 179). The hemorrhage is most frequently intraparenchymal, but in about half of the cases there is subarachnoid extension with clinical signs and symptoms of a subarachnoid hemorrhage. The symptomatology related to the parenchymal hemorrhage is determined by the site of the hemorrhage. In 5–10% of the cases, the hemorrhage is primarily intraventricular (133, 136). AVMs with no history of previous hemorrhage show evidence, at surgery or autopsy, of previous bleeding in 15–30% of the cases indicating that many hemorrhages escape clinical detection (95, 104, 187). It has been suggested that the smaller AVMs are more frequently associated with hemorrhage than the larger ones. However, the data in this respect are uncertain since the relative incidence of large versus small AVMs is not clearly indicated in most of the series (56, 77, 105, 116, 117). Whether hemorrhage from an AVM is related to strenous activity is not clear. Perret found that hemorrhage from an AVM occurs during sleep in 36% of the patients, but activities such as heavy lifting, defecation, coitus, and emotional stress are associated with almost 25% of the hemorrhages (132).

The second most important clinical manisfestation of AVMs is epilepsy. Seizures are the presenting symptom in 28–67% of reported cases (116, 117, 127, 128, 133, 136, 166, 176). Seizures can be generalized or focal. Lesions involving the motor-sensory cortex frequently result in typical Jacksonian attacks whereas lesions involving the deep structures of the temporal lobe frequently result in partial complex seizures. It is clear that seizures are a frequent manifestation of hemorrhage from the AVM (116, 117, 132, 136, 166, 192). However, it is less clear whether AVMs that present with a seizure, without associated hemorrhage, have a greater chance of bleeding in the future than AVMs that do not result in seizures (62).

Recurrent headaches are probably the next most common symptom of AVM. The relationship of headaches to AVM is difficult to define precisely because many patients with recurrent headaches are subjected to CT scanning and a few are found to have an AVM. Still, there is no doubt that some types of headaches are related to AVMs. Large lesions with prominent meningeal vascular supply frequently produce unilateral headaches that can be relieved by embolization of the meningeal supply or by complete removal of the lesion (62). The relationship of AVMs, particularly in the occipital lobe, and the migraine-like headaches is also well known. One study concluded that AVMs do not produce a typical aura of scintillating scotomata (178). However, the experience of the authors as well as that of others indicates that patients with occipital lobe AVMs can have symptoms that are indistinguishable from classic migraine (38, 62, 88). In some patients with recurrent classic migrainous symptoms, the headaches have been totally relieved by removing the occipital AVM (62). More common but less well-defined is the relationship between generalized severe recurring headaches and AVMs. Not infrequently these patients undergo a CT scan after an episode of severe headache and the CT scan demonstrates the AVM but no evidence of hemorrhage. Sometimes the AVM in these patients is not particularly large and it is difficult to understand how it could result in headaches. In these patients the headaches may not be cured by removal of the AVM.

Less common but more dramatic is the syndrome of progressive neurologic deterioration related to an AVM. The etiology of this syndrome is not well understood although it is usually associated with large AVMs (Fig. 22.1). The most commonly invoked mechanism is that of a "steal phenomenon" whereby blood is shunted preferentially through the low resistance channels of the AVM with consequent ischemia in the surrounding brain (44, 81, 92, 166, 167). This old theory has received some modern support from the fact that occluding some of the major feeders to the malformation can result in amelioration of the symptoms (62, 81, 92). There are, however, other mechanisms that may be playing a role in some of these progressive deficits. Obstructive hydrocephalus from ventricular compression by dilated deep veins is one such mechanism (141). Venous hypertension from arterialization of the deep or superficial venous drainage system may also account for symptomatology (188). Mass effect has also been demonstrated by CT scanning in some of the larger AVMs that have no history of previous hemorrhage but show areas of hypodensity (edema) around the lesion (79). Occlusive vascular disease of the proximal feeding vessels to the AVM with a moya moya pattern of deep collateral circulation has been described in a report of 13 patients; these patients were generally young (103).

There has been considerable literature concerning the clinical association of intracranial aneurysms with AVMs (41, 58, 73, 113, 120, 133, 196, 204). This literature can be summarized by saying that the incidence of AVMs in patients with aneurysms appears to be only about twice as high as would be expected and a patient with an AVM appears to have about a 10% chance of having an associated intracranial aneurysm. These aneurysms often are located in one of the feeding vessels to the lesion. When these two lesions coexist and there is a hemorrhage a CT scan will frequently suggest whether the hemorrhage occurred from the aneurysm or from the AVM. If there is diffuse subarachnoid hemorrhage and it is not clear whether the patient bled from the AVM or from the aneurysm, it appears that the aneurysm is slightly more likely to have been the source of bleeding than the AVM. If it is clear which lesion bled, that lesion should be treated first if possible. The associated lesion can be treated at the same operation if that is convenient. When the AVM is removed and the aneurysm is in the arterial distribution of the AVM but not immediately accessible at surgery, it may be wiser to follow the patient with periodic angiography since these aneurysms may involute in time (58). However, contrasting advice has been given based on the presumption that early postoperative hemorrhage may

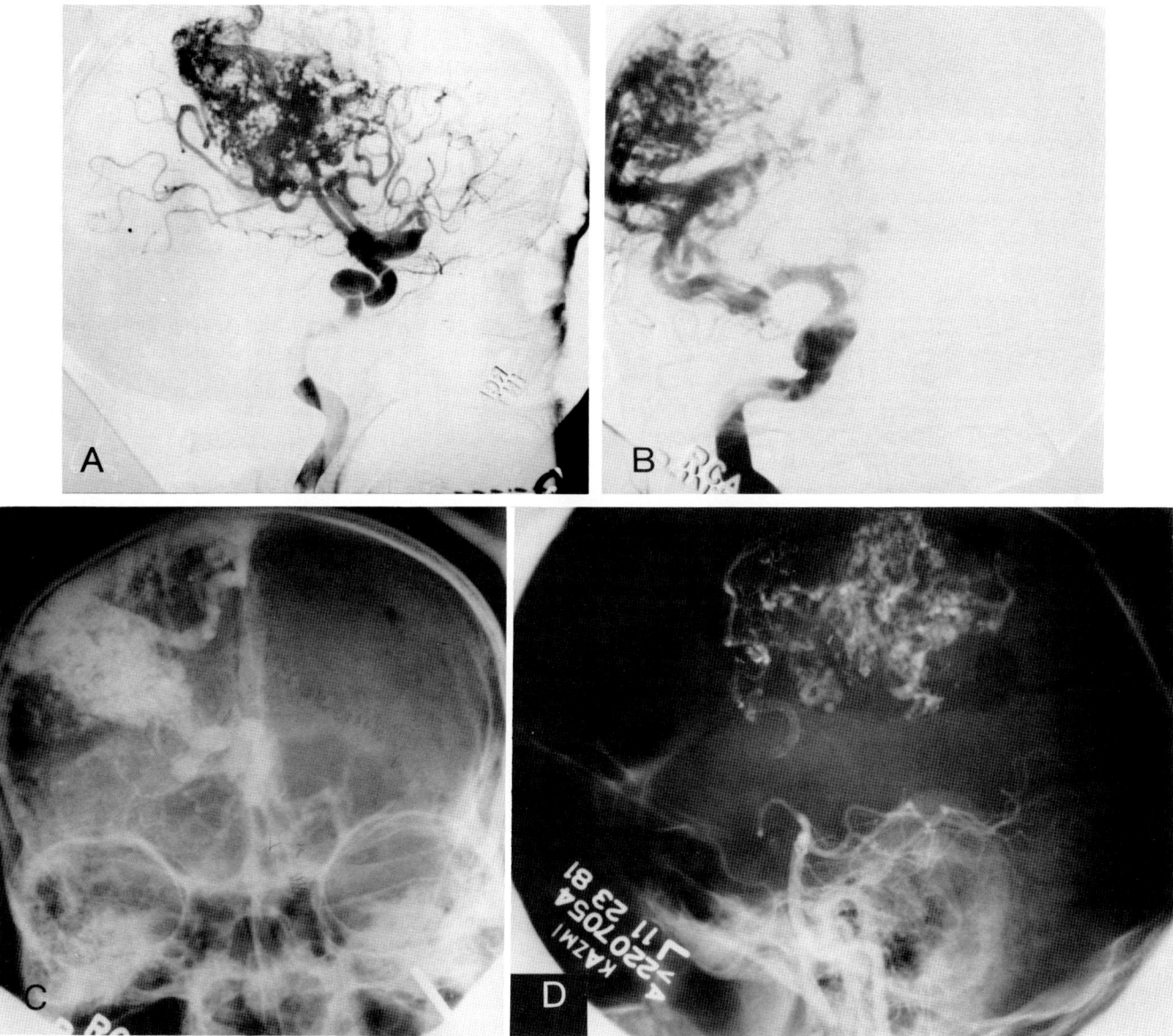

Figure 22.1. Cerebral convexity AVM with progressive neurologic deficit. This dentist presented with a progressive left hemiparesis which started to develop slowly about 5 years before admission. Over the last year his deficit had progressed more rapidly and he became unable to work because his left hand was essentially useless. It was decided to handle the lesion in three stages. The first stage was embolization of the pericallosal blood supply which was primarily from the left internal carotid artery and which supplied the medial (parasagittal) segment of the malformation. **A–C**, right carotid angiogram after embolization of the pericallosal supply. The second stage was direct operative embolization of the right middle cerebral artery feeders to the malformation. **D**, The bucrylate cast left after this procedure. The final stage was a complete excision of the malformation. **E**, Postexcision right carotid angiogram. The lesion has been excised completely. Note that the pericallosal arteries now fill well from the right side whereas they did not fill at all from the right-sided injection before excision of the lesion. Immediately postoperatively, the patient had a very dense left hemiparesis but with time he has improved to the point that he ambulates with only a minimal limp and can use his left upper extremity although his hand remains very clumsy. He is working effectively as an executive hospital administrator.

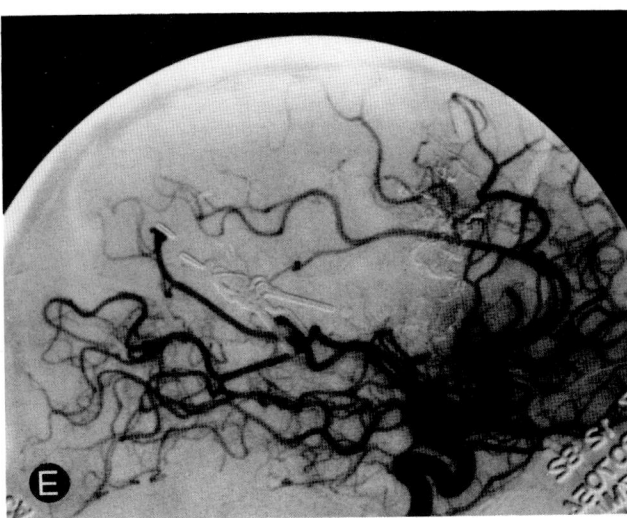

Figure 22.1E.

be related to increased blood flow in the proximal vasculature (73, 113). If it is not clear whether the aneurysm or the AVM has bled, the aneurysm should be treated first since the incidence of rebleeding is higher and the hemorrhages are more dangerous with intracranial aneurysm.

NATURAL HISTORY AND INDICATIONS FOR TREATMENT

An understanding of the natural history of AVMs is essential prior to any discussion of the indications for treatment (62, 63, 90, 131). AVMs that have bled ("ruptured" AVMs) have approximately a 6% chance of rebleeding during the first year (55, 177). This risk is evenly distributed throughout the first year without the early peak of rebleeding associated with ruptured intracranial aneurysms. After the first year, the incidence of recurrent hemorrhage seems to be about 3% per year which is very similar to the incidence of rehemorrhage for a patient with a ruptured intracranial aneurysm (55, 146, 177). Using a different type of analysis, another report observed a 25% risk of rehemorrhage within the 4 years after the first hemorrhage from an AVM (46). These authors also found that after the second hemorrhage, there was a 25% chance of rehemorrhage within a year.

Hemorrhage from an AVM in general is not as devastating as hemorrhage from an intracranial aneurysm, possibly because of the low incidence of vasospasm. However, mortality rates of 6–30% with an average of about 15% after a first hemorrhage and serious morbidity in 15–80% with an average of about 30% have been reported (46, 48, 55, 67, 74, 94, 132, 133, 171). Therefore, it appears that the combined morbidity and mortality of a hemorrhage from an AVM may be as high as 40–45%.

The natural history of a patient with an AVM presenting with epilepsy is less well known but it has been estimated that there is a 25% chance of hemorrhage within 15 years (46). Long-term follow-up from the cooperative study of subarachnoid hemorrhage shows an incidence of hemorrhage of approximately 3% per year (177). Less is known about the prognosis of epilepsy in these patients. Seizures tend to be sporadic and infrequent and medical control is usually successful (171). The prognosis for seizures after surgery is also uncertain, but in the occasional patient who is incapacitated because of poorly controlled epilepsy, operation may reduce the frequency of seizures.

The natural history of the totally asymptomatic patient has taken on an increasing clinical significance since many asymptomatic AVMs are being detected in patients who have a CT scan for a variety of reasons. The risk of hemorrhage in such patients is not very different from the risk of hemorrhage in patients who have epilepsy or who have had a hemorrhage more than a year previously (55, 62, 63, 177). This risk appears to be about 2–3% per year. Table 22.1 gives a summary of the natural history of AVMs that have never bled. A bleeding rate of 25–39% with a combined morbidity and mortality rate of from 30–46% over an average follow-up from 12.5 to more than 20 years can be gleaned from this table.

With an understanding of the natural history of AVMs, indications for surgery can be discussed more intelligently. With the exception of patients who have life-threatening intracerebral hematoma, AVM surgery should be elective. Even in patients with such hematomas, the approach has been to evacuate enough of the hematoma to achieve adequate decompression, trying not to provoke bleeding from the AVM, and to defer excision of the lesion for a later date unless the lesion is small and easily excised with the hematoma.

The indications for treatment of patients with unruptured AVMs are not substantially different from those in patients with AVMs that have previously bled. The risk of hemorrhage is similar in these two groups of patients, although if a patient has had multiple hemorrhages the risk of another hemorrhage is higher (46). One must also remember that it is not always clear whether or not the patient has bled in the past. There have been patients who have presented with a history suggestive of hemorrhage but no evidence of hemorrhage was seen either by CT scan or at surgery (62). Conversely, patients with no history of hemorrhage have frequently been found to have evidence of hemorrhage by CT scan or at surgery (62, 95, 98, 164). Pathologically as many as 25–33% of all AVMs without a previous clinical history of hemorrhage show evidence of previous bleeding (98, 104).

It is frequently said that surgery is easier and safer in patients who have bled but the authors have not found this to be the case. In three different surgical

Table 22.1.
Conservative Treatment of Unruptured AVMs[a]

Author (Reference)	No. of Cases	Bleeding (%)	Morbidity (%)	Mortality (%)	Average Years of Follow-up
Kelly et al (71)	26	—	34.5	11.5	12.5
Moody and Poppen (116)	6	—	—	17	3–10
Graf et al (55)	71	39	—	—	20
Fults and Kelly (48)	26	26.9	19.2	11.6	8.7
Forster et al (46)	46	25	20	17	15
Henderson and Gomez (59)	11	36.4	—	18.2	5–20
Perret and Nishioka (133)	77	30	—	—	>20

[a]Modified from Heros R, Tu YK: Unruptured arteriovenous malformations. A dilemma in surgical decision making. *Clin Neurosurg* 33:187–236, 1986.

series where the results of ruptured and unruptured AVMs were separated, the morbidity and mortality were almost identical in both groups (62, 116, 133).

Patients with unruptured AVMs are frequently devastated psychologically by the knowledge that they have an AVM particularly when inadvisable terms such as "a time bomb in the head" or "sitting on a powder keg" have been used to describe their condition. Some patients can live with the knowledge that they have an AVM without being substantially bothered by it whereas others are overwhelmed by this thought. Sometimes this problem becomes an indication for surgery.

Another important factor in deciding about treatment is the safety and effectiveness of the operation or other treatment modality on that particular patient with that particular AVM. Overall surgical results have little relation to the probable morbidity and mortality of surgery for an individual patient with an AVM. The morbidity and mortality that can be expected with a particular AVM depend on the size, location, and configuration of the AVM as well as the age and general medical and neurologic condition of the patient. The surgeon's personal experience with similar lesions is also a very important factor.

Once the patient with an AVM reaches middle age without a hemorrhage, it is much less likely he will bleed in the future (94, 133). At younger ages AVMs tend to enlarge (34, 78, 94, 192) and they seem to reach a stable size and occasionally decrease in size after middle age (94). Another important aspect of age is the well-known capacity of younger patients for neurologic recovery. The patient's neurologic condition is also clearly important in that a pre-existing neurologic deficit makes additional surgical morbidity less likely; on the other hand if the neurologic deficit is devastating, little is to be gained by operation. The patient's hobbies and occupation are also important in evaluating what effect the neurologic deficit that may possibly result from surgery would have on this particular patient's life.

The recommendation of treatment for a patient with an AVM is a highly individual decision made only after careful consideration of all the factors discussed. Since AVMs can be the most difficult of neurosurgical cases, the surgeon must bear in mind personal operative experience and results as well as the natural history when considering operative intervention.

SURGICAL TREATMENT

Timing of Operation

Unless there is an intracerebral or subdural hematoma that demands early intervention, the operation on an AVM can wait until there is recovery from the diffuse effects of subarachnoid hemorrhage and stabilization from any neurologic deficit resulting from a parenchymal hemorrhage. This can be expected to take between 3 and 4 weeks. Since the risk of rehemorrhage is not high, epsilon aminocaproic acid is not used in patients with ruptured AVMs during the waiting period. There is little point in waiting beyond 3–4 weeks since existing intracerebral hematoma is usually at a stage of becoming liquified at this time which facilitates operative dissection.

Preoperative Preparation and Anesthesia

Steroids and anticonvulsants are used routinely in preparation for surgery and prophylactic antibiotics are used just before surgery and continued for 1 day.

The general aspects of the anesthesia and the measures to reduce brain tension are the same as descibed for aneurysms in Chapter 11. Hypotension has not been used routinely but occasionally it has been helpful in controlling bleeding from the small fragile vessels encountered at the depth of the exposure in some cases of large AVMs.

Positioning

Positioning for surgery is critical in the management of these patients. The position varies with the approach to each lesion but in general it is important that no compression of the veins in the neck be present since this can exacerbate intraoperative problems with bleeding and swelling. One may wish to have the flexibility of changing the position of the head during surgery for different stages of the operation. It is important to remember that the surgeon's comfort is of significance in these operations which can be relatively long. The authors prefer to position the patient in such a way that the surgeon can sit and rest the arms comfortably.

General Aspects of Technique

Credit is generally given to Olivecrona for having developed the modern art of surgical excision of AVMs (41, 126). Most of the convexity lesions are roughly conical in shape wtih the apex pointing toward the ventricle. The operation must be planned to pursue the apex of the cone right down to the ventricle if necessary. Small AVMs may not reach the ventricular surface, but in any AVM of significant size, extension to the ventricle must be suspected. Some small convexity lesions are not visible on the surface, and in these sometimes a red draining vein may guide the surgeon to the lesion. Ultrasound may prove helpful in finding these smaller AVMs that are not evident on the surface.

The operating microscope is invaluable in defining the plane around the AVM, particularly in eloquent areas of the brain, where one must stay right on the edge of the AVM in order to avoid damage to the surrounding tissue. It is critical in AVM surgery in general to try to eliminate the large arterial feeders, or as many of them as possible, in the early stages of the operation. Sometimes there is some doubt as to which vessels are feeding arteries and which are arterialized draining veins of the AVM. However, by opening the arachnoid around those vessels close to the lesion and under high magnification, the experienced surgeon will have little difficulty in differentiating arteries from veins. When in doubt a temporary clip can be applied to the vessel to confirm distal (toward the AVM) damping of pulsations of feeding arteries. The vessel is coagulated with the bipolar coagulator and then a permanent hemoclip is applied before dividing any vessel larger than about 1.5 mm in diameter. The larger feeding arteries sometimes will not shrink with bipolar coagulation and the use of a temporary aneurysm clip may aid in making the vessel amenable to coagulation. The aneurysm clip is then removed (because of the cost), and it is replaced with a permanent hemoclip. The arterial supply must be taken only when the surgeon is convinced that the vessel goes exclusively to the AVM rather than being a vessel of passage which gives some branches to the AVM but goes on to supply distal brain. When in doubt, it is preferable not to divide the vessel and place a temporary aneurysm clip to facilitate dissection; the vessel can be permanently cauterized and divided later if it is confirmed that it supplies only AVM. This precaution is particularly important when one is working in the sylvian fissure where not infrequently a branch of the middle cerebral artery mingles with the coils of a parasylvian AVM only to continue later on as a branch supplying normal brain.

In general, veins should be preserved until the end of the operation. Occasionally, however, if the angiogram demonstrates the presence of a large deep draining vein, one can divide the superficial venous drainage if such a maneuver would be of significant help in dissecting the AVM. When there are several superficial draining veins, one can usually leave the larger vein and divide the others so as to be able to complete the plane around the surface of the AVM. This helps the operation since frequently there are small arterial branches that hide on the undersurface of draining veins. Even after the dissection has been completed around the AVM down to the ventricle, the lesion may still appear "alive" with arterial blood and it is not until one divides the final venous pedicle that a small arterial feeder is recognized on the undersurface (or sometimes even in the adventitia) of the large draining vein.

In convexity lesions, after securing as much arterial supply as possible, the next step should be to develop a corticectomy to a depth of about 2–3 cm all around the AVM. This depth is chosen because some of the superficial arterial supply to the lesion may come along the depth of a sulcus and may not be visible on the surface. By carrying a circumferential corticectomy of such depth all around the lesion, one is sure to eliminate all of the major superficial arterial supply. There should be no other large arterial branches encountered until one reaches the depth of the malformation when deep branches from other arterial territories may reach the lesion.

In most convexity lesions, once the superficial arterial supply has been secured, the AVM should be relatively "soft" and compressible. Bleeding from the AVM should be relatively easy to control by packing the area of hemorrhage with cottonoids and returning to the same area at a later time. There is usually a gliotic plane around the AVM but, in the authors' experience, this plane may not be present around the entire circumference of the AVM and it is an easy matter to enter the AVM as one proceeds with the dissection. With lesions in critical brain one tries to stay right at the edge of the lesion which means that there will be frequent bleeding as the surgeon gets into the lesion. If no bleeding is encountered this usually means the surgeon is too far into normal brain and the plane of resection must be brought closer to the AVM.

In noneloquent brain the surgeon has the luxury of working in a plane a few millimeters away from the AVM leaving some intervening brain which simplifies the surgery. In cases of temporal tip or frontal tip AVMs, a modified lobectomy staying behind and outside the lesion is done. Most other lesions reach the ventricle and it is here when problems with bleeding become more serious. Small vessels in the wall of the ventricle or from adjacent arterial territories ("transitional vessels") are extraordinarily fragile and sometimes burst when the bipolar coagulator is applied to them and then keep retracting into the brain tissue as one tries to stop the bleeding. This is usually brain that must be spared to avoid neurologic damage. There is no "trick" to recommend for dealing with this problem. Hemoclips are generally ineffective. The surgeon must persist with bipolar coagulation to control the bleeding. Occasionally aneurysm clips are necessary although they are not always effective and some of these fine vessels have been seen continuing to bleed through the clip. One must resist the temptation to "pack" the bleeding since the bleeding in these cases is not from the AVM but from vessels coming to the AVM from normal brain or the ventricle and a significant intracerebral or intraventricular hematoma can develop with devasting consequences. This is very different than packing bleeding from the AVM. Usually there are one or more small transventricular vessels keeping the AVM alive and once these are secured, the AVM will collapse and become "blue" unless there are some unsecured superficial feeders hiding under the draining veins.

Finally, the remaining venous pedicle is divided and the malformation removed. The surgeon may be quite tired at this stage but patience is required to inspect the area of resection carefully and ensure absolute hemostasis. Whenever one has carried the resection of the AVM right to its margin, there is the risk of having divided a portion of the malformation which may still bleed. The walls of the resection are systematically inspected by "rubbing" them with a cottonoid to stimulate bleeding from any remnants of AVM. Then the bed of the malformation is lined with a single layer of Surgicel and the blood pressure elevated gently to the level expected postoperatively. If there is no bleeding after 10 minutes, one can proceed to close.

The authors have had no experience with the laser in AVM surgery. Published reports indicate that the neodynium-YAG laser may be of help in defining the plane between AVM and the brain, in coagulating dural components of the AVM and in achieving hemostasis of the AVM bed after resection of the lesion (43, 194). The laser does not seem to be of help in dealing with the small fragile vessels at the depth of the malformation that is the major remaining surgical problem with these lesions.

Perfusion Breakthrough

This problem has been described and reviewed by several surgeons (41, 119, 124, 161, 198). Though the etiology is not completely understood, it is clear that after resection of some of these large lesions, one can encounter severe, protracted, and unexplained brain swelling accompanied by diffuse hemorrhage or focal deep hemorrhages in the parenchyma immediately adjacent to the area of resection. This can occur even when the resection appears to have gone very smoothly without significant retraction on the surrounding brain.

Anatomic and physiologic criteria help predict when this problem is likely to occur (41, 124, 134, 161, 198). The most important criteria are the size of the lesion (it is rare to encounter this phenemenon when the nidus is less than 4–5 cm) and the caliber of the feeding vessels which are almost always large in cases where this problem develops. However, these factors are certainly not the entire answer. AVMs have been treated that are almost identical in size and in the caliber of their feeding vessels as well as in the smoothness with which the surgery proceeded, and yet protracted serious postoperative swelling occurred in one case but not in another (Figs. 22.2 and 22.3). Another angiographic clue in predicting the development of this syndrome is preferential shunting into the lesion with lack of opacification of normal vessels to surrounding brain. There may be a "shift" of the watershed area from adjacent arterial territories attempting to supply the ischemic regions around the lesion (Figs. 22.3 and 22.4). There is often very rapid filling of the nidus with complete opacification within the first second after arterial injection. A progressive neurologic deficit due to "steal" phenomenon from surrounding brain is a good predictor of danger for the development of this syndrome. Measurement of blood flow over the carotid arteries may also predict trouble when there is a markedly increased flow velocity as does loss of autoregulation in the brain surrounding some of the large malformations that presumably are at risk for this phenomenon (134). Measurement of the pressure in the feeder arteries just before they entered the malformation before and after temporary distal occlusion revealed that if proximal pressure increases markedly as the feeder is being occluded, there may be increased risk of postoperative difficulty with swelling and hemorrhage (124). These criteria were used to help decide when to stage operations and even to decide how many "stages" were needed. It was also found that not only the caliber of the feeding vessels but also their length was important in the development of perfusion breakthrough. The authors have not seen this syndrome develop after one-stage resection of relatively large malformations where the feeding vessels were large but very short.

When the phenomenon of "perfusion breakthrough" is predicted, the key maneuver to prevention is to reduce the blood supply to the malformation by stages ("staging"). This can be accomplished by

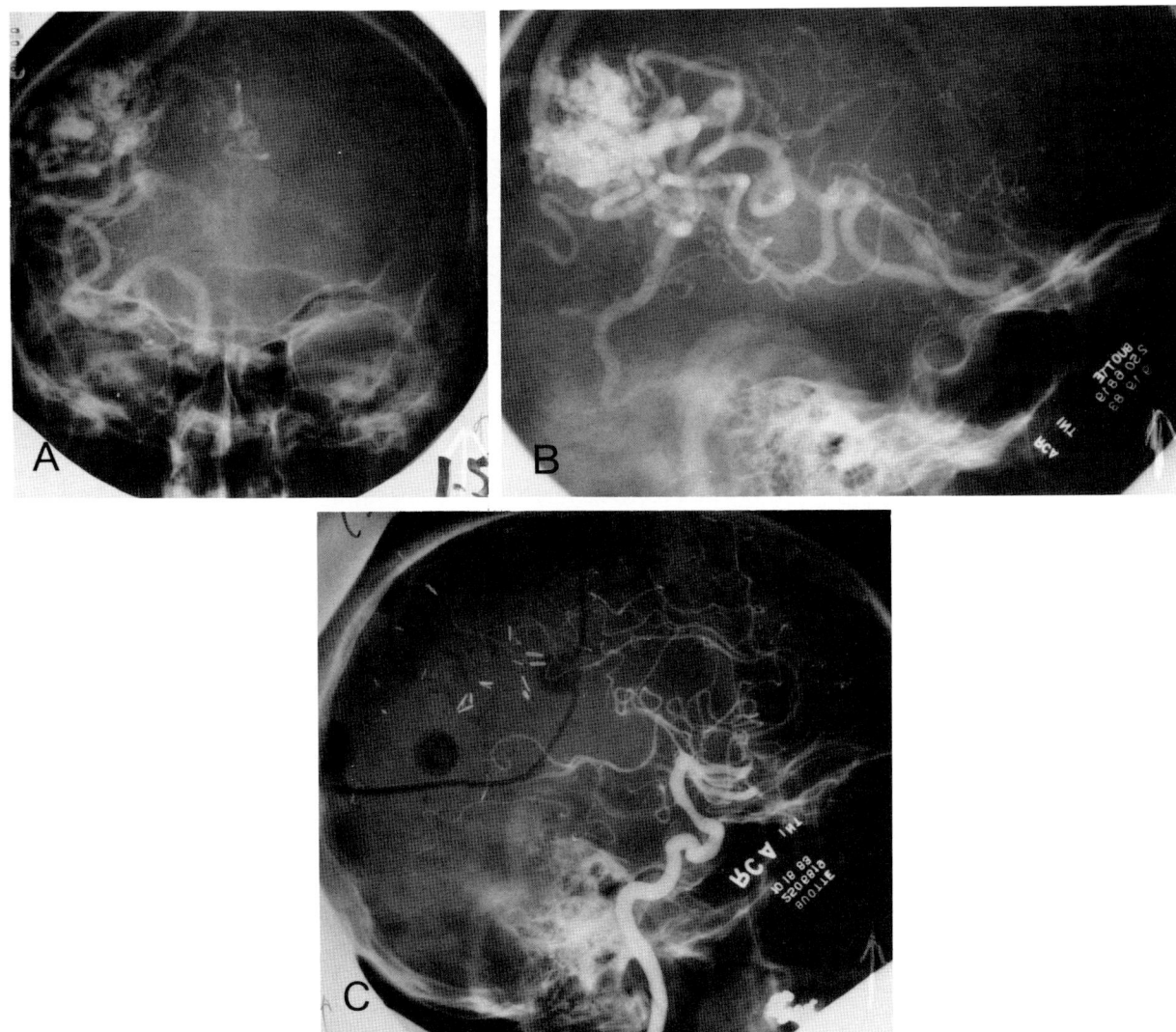

Figure 22.2. Right parietal AVM with intractable seizure disorder. **A** and **B**, Preoperative angiogram. The lesion was resected in one stage. **C**, Postoperative angiogram showed no residual malformation. Even though this lesion was very similar in location and size to the lesion shown in Figure 22.3, the patient did well without major postoperative difficulties. One cannot always predict when the "perfusion breakthrough phenomenon" will develop. This patient has been seizure-free since this operation.

surgical ligation of feeders (6, 41, 119, 124, 134, 180, 198) or by embolization which can be percutaneous (endovascular) (32, 87, 94, 165, 186, 198) or by direct catheterization of the feeding vessels at open craniotomy (25, 36, 37, 41, 149) (Fig. 22.1). Simple feeder ligation at craniotomy has been condemned by many because of the presumption that blood supply would simply be recruited from adjacent arterial territories and no doubt if enough time is allowed this will happen. However, it has been demonstrated that the sector of the AVM corresponding to a certain feeding artery does not fill angiographically after ligation of that artery (134). Therefore, it is likely that if the subsequent stages are not delayed for more than a few days, simple feeder ligation is effective.

Feeder occlusion can be accomplished percutaneously by injection of spheres that are large enough to lodge in the feeder rather than go into the nidus of the malformation (94). Most surgeons have been using embolization into the nidus of the malformation to occlude the feeder and reduce significantly the amount of residual patent nidus. Such embolization can be accomplished with liquid polymers such as Isobutyl-2-cyanoacrylate (bucrylate) or with solid particles such as small spheres or emulsions of Gelfoam or polyvinyl alcohol. With modern neuro-

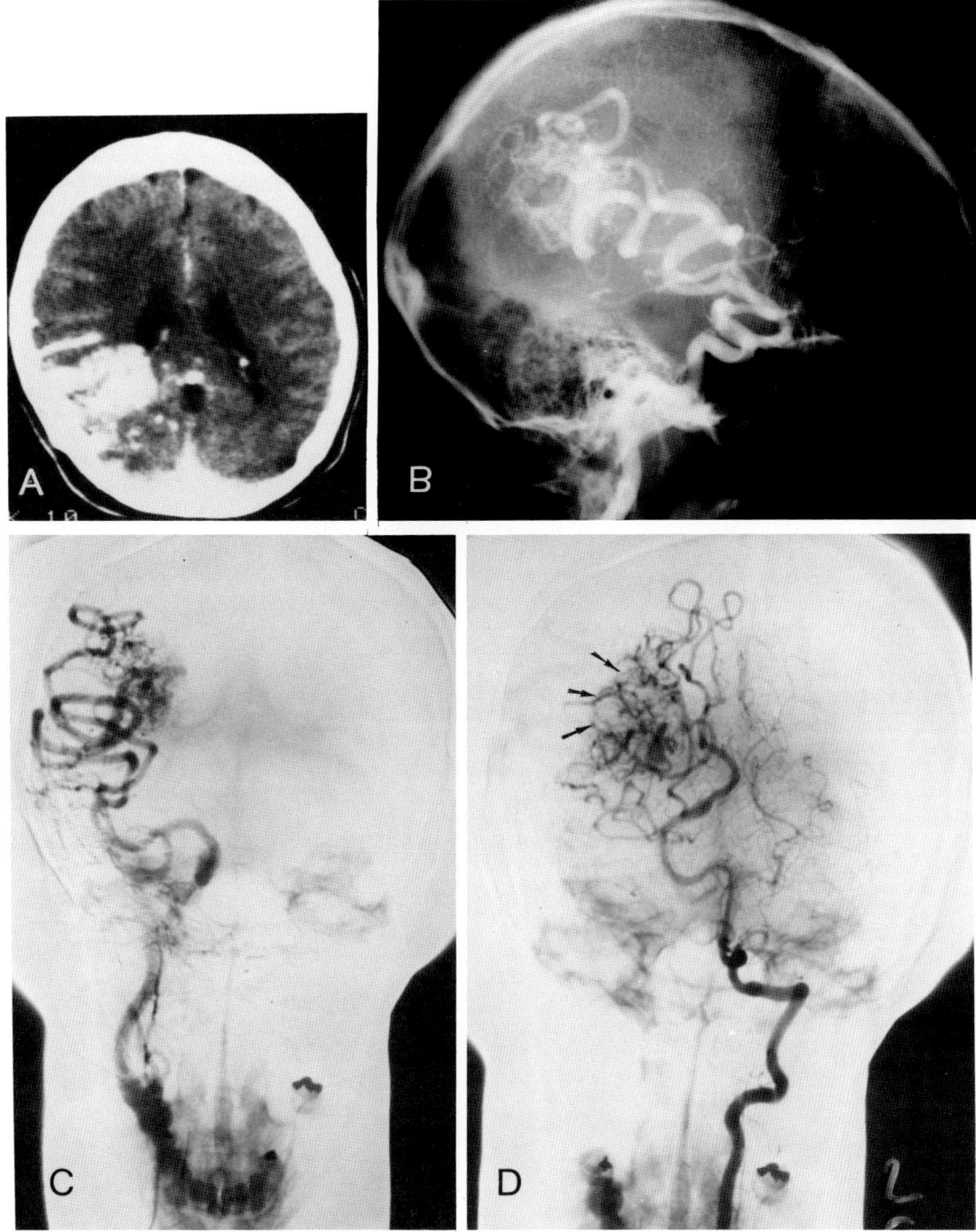

Figure 22.3. Right parietal AVM with seizures and deterioration in ability to concentrate and memory. **A**, Preoperative CT scan. **B–D**, Angiogram. Note the long, tortuous large caliber feeders (**B** and **C**), the relative lack of filling of the rest of the middle cerebral artery territory (**B**) and the ill-defined margin and presence of transitional vessels from the posterior circulation (*arrows* in **D**). The lesion was resected completely in one stage. **E–G**, Postoperative angiography showing no residual malformation. Note better filling of the rest of the hemisphere with the right carotid injection. Also note residual dilatation and either slow filling or retrograde thrombosis of some of the major feeders that fail to opacify for a considerable distance proximal to the clips with which they were occluded (*arrows* in **F**). This patient had a stormy postoperative course with significant brain edema, left hemiparesis, and stupor. With vigorous medical treatment, she gradually recovered but she does have a complete hemianopsia as a residual deficit. Retrospectively, this patient may have done better with embolization before definitive resection.

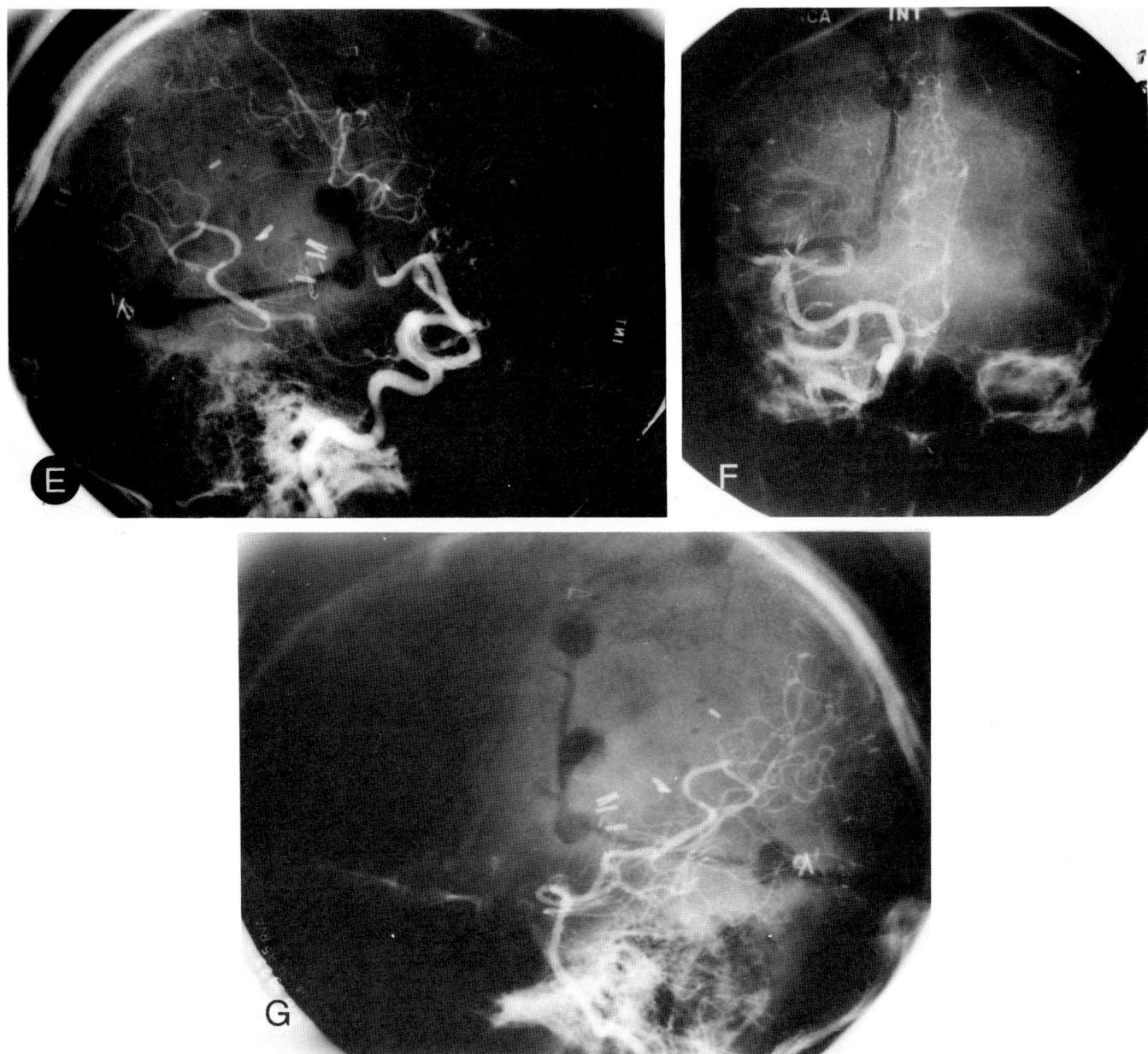

Figure 22.3E–G.

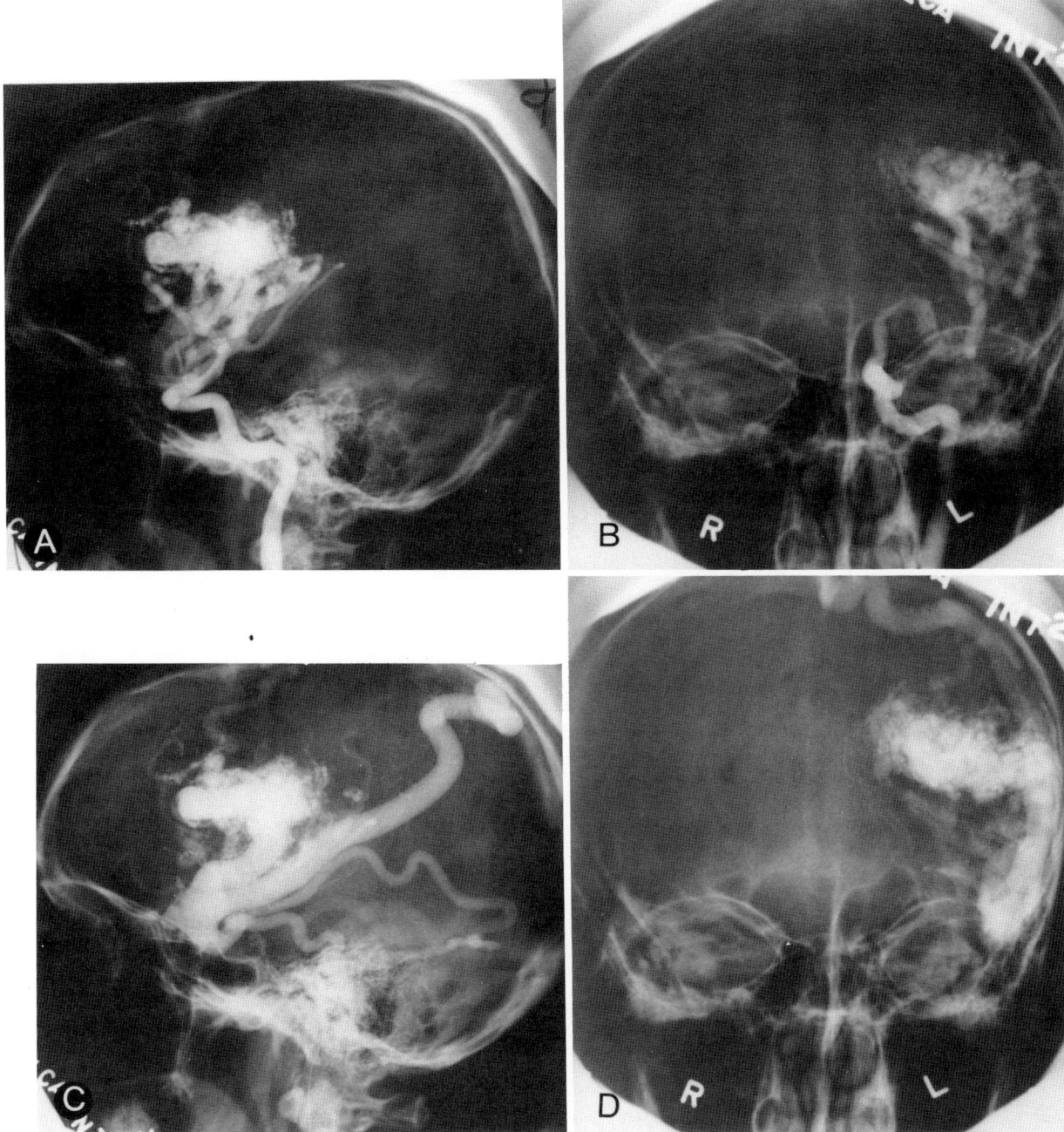

Figure 22.4. Left cerebral convexity AVM with seizures. This semiprofessional weightlifter wanted to continue to lift weights competitively. He felt that he could tolerate a speech impediment. **A** and **B**, Very early arterial phase of the left carotid angiogram showing the "true" nidus of the malformation. **C** and **D**, Later films from the same sequence showing the venous drainage. **F**, The right carotid injection shows large feeders to the malformation (*solid arrows*). Also note the "transitional" vessels that are in the area of the brain above the malformation and do not belong to the malformation proper (*open arrows*). Because of the fear of "perfusion breakthrough" with this high volume rapid flow malformation, endovascular preoperative embolization was performed about 1 week before complete resection. **G** and **H**, Postoperative left carotid angiogram shows no residual AVM. Note some residual bucrylate in vessels proximal to the malformation (*arrows*) and that there is good filling of the pericallosal system as well as the rest of the middle cerebral artery territory. In the preoperative studies (**A** and **B**), essentially only the malformation filled. As expected, the patient had significant expressive aphasia and moderate left hand clumsiness after surgery. Over several months his left-sided strength and coordination returned to normal and he resumed his weightlifting activities. His speech improved significantly but he has lost some fluency.

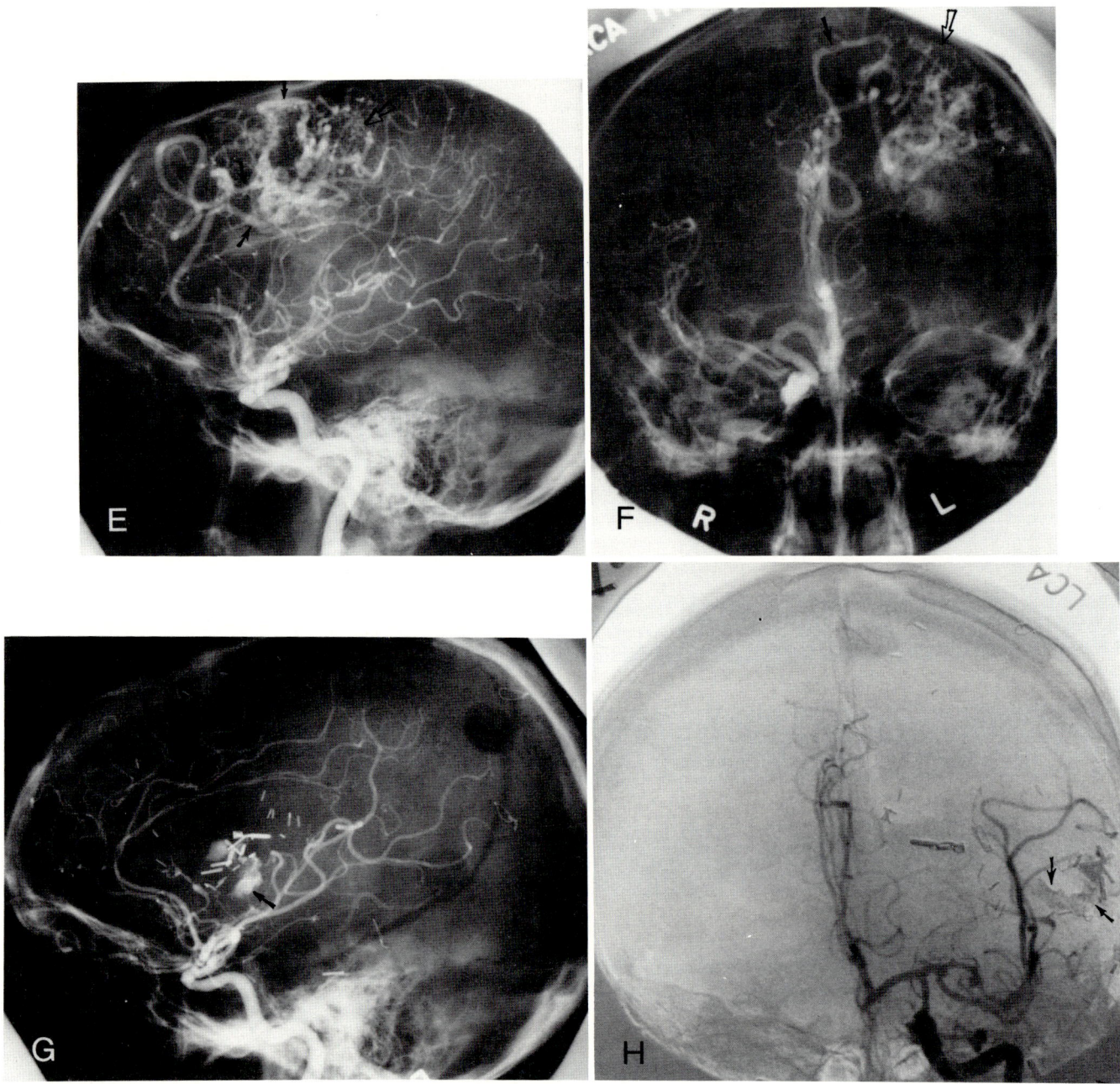

Figure 22.4E–H.

radiologic techniques, it is very frequently possible to reach the feeder to the AVM percutaneously by endovascular navigation. However, when the technique is not well-developed or in cases of tortuous feeders that cannot be reached by endovascular navigation, the problem can be solved by intraoperative catheterization. For this technique it is best to proceed with the craniotomy flap which will eventually be used for complete excision. The AVM can then be directly exposed and the surrounding feeders can be catheterized as they enter the AVM, as in the case of middle cerebral feeders to a convexity AVM. Alternatively, deep feeders may be reached and catheterized through an approach remote from the eventual approach for the AVM excision such as in the case of large branches of the posterior cerebral artery than can be catheterized by a subtemporal approach in cases of AVMs of the parietal-occipital area which eventually will have to be excised through a convexity approach. Both endovascular as well as direct intraoperative embolization are difficult techniques which require considerable experience and will be described in further detail later.

The decision to use one, two, or more stages prior to final definitive resection is difficult and is usually made empirically depending on the experience of the surgeon. The authors have never used more than two stages before the definitive resection. The authors have never electively planned to remove part of the malformation leaving segments for a later date. This has been accomplished with success by others but the risk of postoperative hemorrhage appears high. It has been recommended that a circumscribing incision around the lesion be carried to a depth of about 3 cm to eliminate all of the superficial supply to the lesion and then return a few days later to finalize the resection (134). This appears to be reasonable since this is a form of "feeder ligation." Not all surgeons agree that it is necessary to stage these operations. Some have reported good results by removing the lesion in one stage under hypotensive anesthesia or by placing a temporary clamp on the carotid artery and reducing flow by about 50% if the primary supply is in carotid territory (12, 97).

Whether one stage or a multiple stage resection is accomplished, the postoperative care of these patients after the final excision of the malformation is critical. Hypertension must be avoided in order to prevent hyperemia of dysautoregulated chronically ischemic brain surrounding the malformation (21, 89, 149, 180).

One must be sure that the blood pressure does not exceed the level at which hemostasis was ensured. The authors prefer to use a rapidly acting intravenous medication such as nitroprusside if the blood pressure reaches a certain prestated level. One sensible recommendation has been to keep the patient anesthetized for 2–3 hours after a long operation in an effort to avoid early rebleeding. In this manner one can delay the hypertension sometimes associated with extubation and allow time for the small coagulated vessels to become more solidly sealed (134). It has also been recommended, in cases where some brain swelling is already evident at the time of closure, to keep the patient under barbiturate anesthesia for hours or sometimes days (28, 180). Even patients who have developed frank postoperative hemorrhage have been treated successfully with high dose barbiturate anesthesia and hypotension for several days with eventual evacuation of the blood clot once the brain swelling starts to subside (28). Not infrequently these patients make a dramatic recovery even after a prolonged period of postoperative disability (Figs. 22.3 and 22.4).

Routine postoperative angiography has not been used during the immediate postoperative period as has been suggested by others (150). Rather, the authors depend on the intraoperative check as described, and so far there has only been one patient who has bled during the immediate postoperative period. This hemorrhage occurred in the operating room at the time when the patient was being awakened (residual AVM was found in this particular patient as the wound was promptly reopened). Postoperative angiography is usually done after 1 week or later if there have been complications.

Steroids are continued for at least 5 days or longer if brain swelling is suspected. Prophylactic antibiotics are used for 24 hours after surgery. Anticonvulsants are continued.

Management of AVMs in Specific Locations

Large AVMs of the Cerebral Convexity

Since many of these lesions involve critical areas of the brain, careful surgical judgment must be exercised before surgery is recommended to these patients. All the factors previously discussed under surgical decison-making should be kept in mind. Often lesions that appear to involve critical areas of the convexity can be removed with little or no permanent residual neurologic deficit (12, 35, 41, 80, 198). Patients, particularly when they are young, show a remarkable capacity to recover from what immediately postoperatively appears to be a very severe neurologic deficit. This may be related to the congenital nature of AVMs with critical areas being displaced by the lesion. Adjacent areas of the brain or corresponding areas in the contralateral hemisphere may compensate for some of the lost function. This is particularly true in cases where a large hemorrhage has occurred early in life. However, one must be very cautious not to assume that large AVMs involving the primary motor, sensory, visual, or speech areas can be removed without neurologic deficit. In general the experience of the authors has been that the patient will awaken from the operation with the kind of neurologic deficit that one would predict from the location of the AVM. Many patients improve very significantly after weeks and months go by but still the surgeon must be sure that the patient is prepared to accept a substantial neurologic deficit after excision. Treatment must be individualized. Hemiparesis of any degree may not be acceptable to a pianist or to a surgeon and a speech impediment may not be acceptable to a professor.

Large lesions of the cerebral convexity present special problems. They are very likely to involve eloquent cortex. They can be associated with "perfusion breakthrough phenomenon." These lesions almost always reach the wall of the ventricle and have deep venous drainage which implies deep arterial supply. They commonly involve at least two and frequently all three main arterial territories which means that some of the main arterial supply reaches the lesion deeply. These large lesions of the convexity frequently recruit sizable dural and transcranial supply from the meningeal and external carotid circulations (26, 42).

The margins of these lesions tend to be less well-defined and frequently one encounters abnormally dilated vessels in the periphery of the lesion. It is difficult at times to know whether these vessels belong to the malformation proper or may be dilated "watershed" vessels supplying the ischemic brain around the lesion (Figs. 22.3D and 22.4E and F). The safest assumption is to think of the malformation as being defined only by the compact arterial nidus seen in the very earliest arterial phase of the angiogram (Fig 22.4). The surrounding dilated transitional vessels must be assumed not to belong to the malformation and must be left in place.

Because of the size of these lesions and the different arterial territories involved, the surgeon may wish to perform different aspects of the operation with the patient in different positions (ie., with the head in the lateral position and tilted toward the floor for subtemporal control of the posterior cerebral artery supply and then a second stage with the head straight up for parasaggital control of the pericallosal artery supply in some large parieto-occipital lesions).

Dealing with the meningeal and external carotid supply can sometimes be quite difficult. With the help of preoperative embolization much of the meningeal blood supply to the malformation can be dealt with. If embolization is not available or not feasible, the surgeon should plan the bone flap considering the meningeal supply to the AVM. Burr holes are made which can be enlarged with a rongeur over the area where the meningeal arteries cross the edge of the planned bone flap. The meningeal arteries are ligated at this point to reduce blood loss as the bone flap is removed. To avoid bleeding from dural attachments of the AVM the dura is opened away from the malformation and then cut perpendicularly to where the malformation seems to be attached. The dura is then cut in a circle around the malformation, leaving it attached to the malformation much as in surgery for a convexity meningioma. The dural defect can be closed with a dural graft; the authors usually use pericranial tissue. Transcranial blood supply in the authors' experience is more of a problem. Planning the skin incision in such a way as to interrupt the external supply (usually from the superficial temporal artery, the occipital artery and the supraorbital arteries), is usually preferable to preoperative embolization. Necrosis of the scalp has been seen after preoperative embolization of scalp arteries. Even after the major external arterial supply is proximally interrupted, there remains the fact that the bone flap is attached to the dura which in turn is attached to the AVM and torrential blood loss can occur during removal of the bone flap. To try to avoid this problem a number of burr holes are made close to the area of presumed attachment and then gradually the bone is rongeured toward the area of attachment, individually coagulating and separating the dural attachments from the bone before removing the rest of the bone plate.

Sylvian AVMs

This particular group of lesions is considered separately because of the problems related to their intimate relationship with normal branches of the middle cerebral artery within the sylvian fissure (Figs. 22.5 and 22.6). For the most anterior of these lesions (Fig. 22.5), a pterional approach is used, except that the bone flap is made slightly larger inferiorly, to visualize the anterior temporal pole and posterosuperiorly to have access to the anterior sylvian fissure. The head is turned slightly more than for the standard pterional approach (about 60°). The pterion and the lesser wing of the sphenoid are removed. The carotid artery is exposed and the sylvian fissure opened medially. Arterialized veins draining the tip of the temporal lobe must be protected. There will usually be other anteriorly draining veins which may be coagulated to allow for better exposure. If there are adequate veins draining posteriorly, the arterialized venous drainage that crosses the sylvian fissure may be divided to mobilize the lesion (Fig. 22.5). The middle cerebral artery is followed from medial to lateral and this artery and all its branches are dissected within the sylvian fissure by separating the malformation to one side or the other without taking any feeders until the anatomy is well understood.

The key to the operation is to coagulate, clip, and divide the branches to the malformation only after the surgeon is convinced that the branch goes to the malformation and nowhere else. This requires tedious dissection of each of the suspected feeders until it definitely enters the mass of the malformation.

Arteriovenous Malformations of the Brain

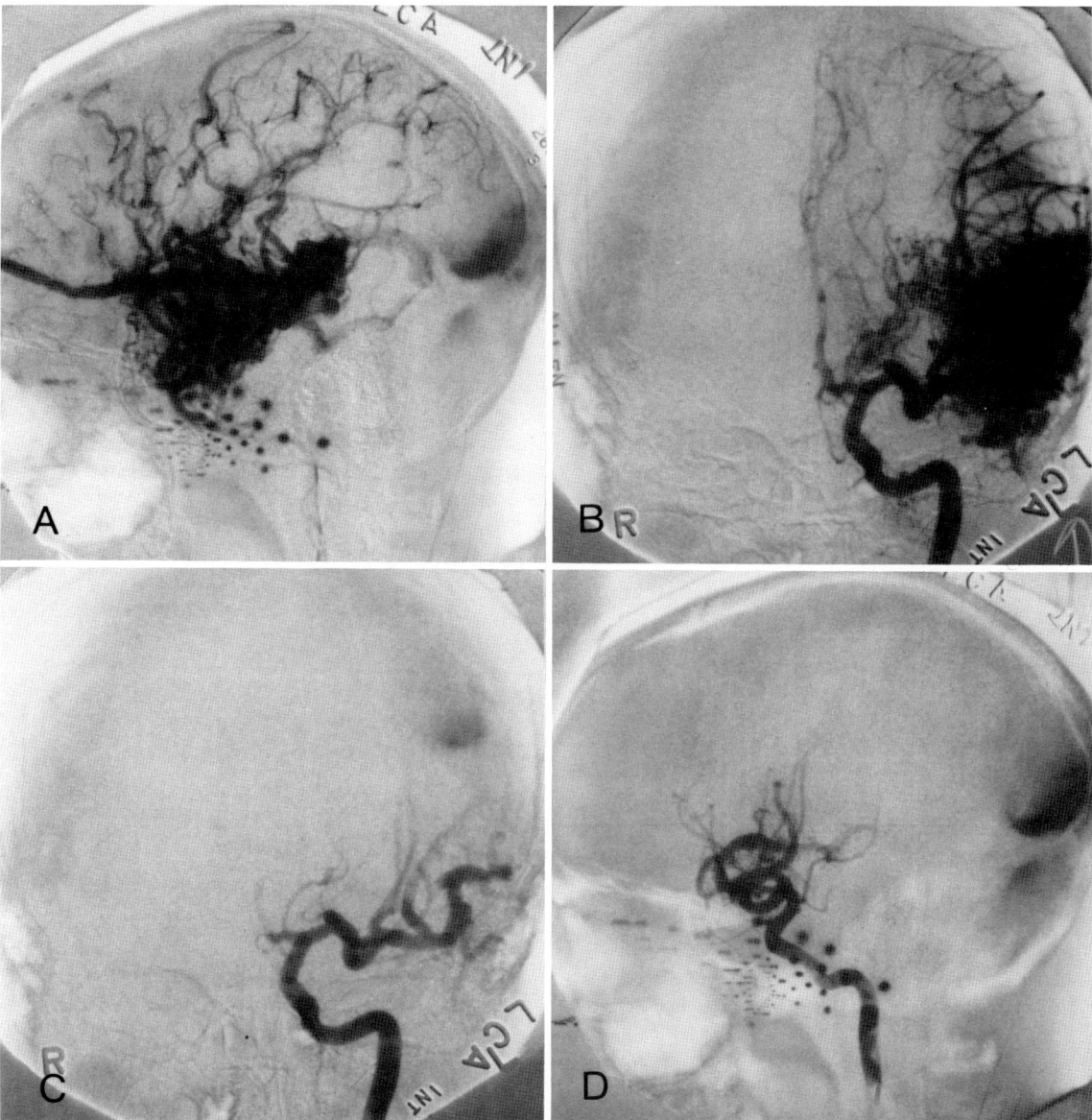

Figure 22.5. Sylvian AVM in a teenager with an intracerebral temporal hemorrhage. Over a period of 6 weeks, his initial neurologic deficit recovered completely. **A** and **B**, Preoperative angiogram. Note significant lateral lenticulostriate supply across the insula (**B**). **C** and **D**, Earliest films of the arterial phase of the left carotid angiogram showing the complexity of the feeders within the sylvian fissure. These were helpful in planning resection. The lesion was resected completely in one stage. **E**, Postoperative angiogram. The patient had a mild hemiparesis and speech difficulty which cleared completely over the ensuing 2 weeks. There was no problem with "perfusion breakthrough" with this rather large lesion. Perhaps this is attributable to the fact that the feeders, though of relatively large caliber, were relatively short. The age of the patient is also important. An older patient with a similar lesion would have probably had a more prolonged period of disability and may not have recovered completely.

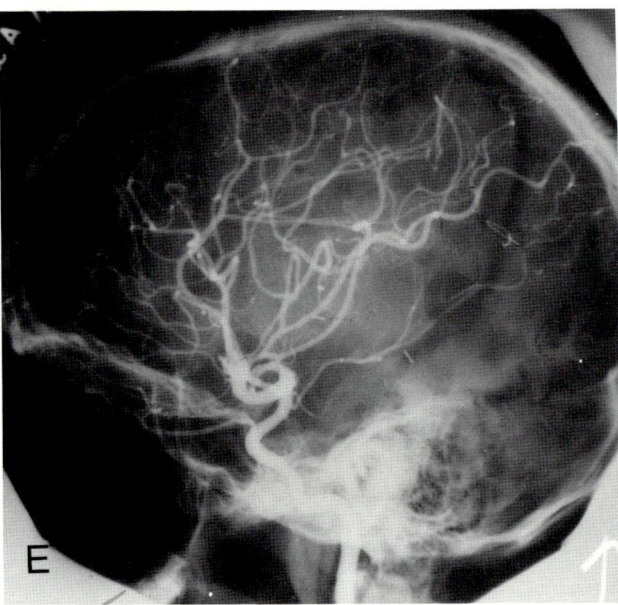

Figure 22.5E.

When in doubt, the surgeon can use a temporary aneurysm clip on the branch and follow it along taking the small branches that go to the malformation and preserving the major trunk unless one is sure that it eventually enters the malformation. Not infrequently, it has been found that a branch that initially appears to go to the malformation eventually goes on to supply distal brain. To take such a branch is the danger with these lesions. Another problem with these AVMs is that they may obtain deep blood supply from the insula via lateral lenticulostriate vessels (Fig. 22.5B). This deep supply to the lesion can be very fragile and difficult to coagulate and one must be extremely careful to avoid a deep hemorrhage by "packing" bleeding in this area. However, these lesions can be removed with no resulting neurologic deficit (Fig. 22.5).

More posteriorly located lesions can be approached by opening the fissure more posteriorly (Fig. 22.6). In these cases, the head is held in the straight lateral position and the bone flap is more posterior using a standard temporal horseshoe type of incision centered above the ear. It is not necessary to remove the pterion in these cases nor is it necessary to open the medial aspect of the sylvian fissure. The exact location of the sylvian fissure in this more posterior location may be obscure but one can usually find an arterialized vein on the surface that can be followed to the lesion. A minimal amount of subpial dissection may be necessary superficially when the fissure is not well defined, but as one proceeds more deeply usually the fissure becomes better defined. Temporary clips may help identify feeders. If the lesion does not change in turgency or color, the clips are removed and a search is made for deeper branches. After clipping the deep feeders, coagulation of the partially collapsed coils causes them to shrink away from the critical surrounding brain. In this manner the AVM may be gradually "pulled" away from the brain to avoid significant postoperative deficit (Fig. 22.6).

Deep Temporal AVMs.

Under this subheading deep AVMs of the anterior and middle portions of the temporal lobe will be considered. Trigonal AVMs present a slightly different problem and will be considered separately. It is frequently difficult to decide when these lesions are operable. If a substantial amount of the basal ganglia or thalamus is involved, the lesion should be left alone. The following neuroradiologic criteria have been used to suggest that the lesion is probably operable: (a) primary supply by the anterior choroidal artery and laterally directed branches of the posterior cerebral artery (as opposed to medially directed branches); (b) primary drainage into the vein of Rosenthal and medial sylvian vein (as opposed to directly into the internal cerebral vein or the vein of Galen); (c) projection beneath the plane of the middle cerebral artery on the lateral view of the carotid injection (if the lesion projects superior to this plane, it is likely to involve the internal capsule or thalamus); (d) projection lateral to the sweep of the posterior cerebral artery on the anteroposterior or Towne's view of the vertebral arteriogram (if the lesion is medial to this sweep, it will involve the midbrain) (61).

Anterior medial temporal lobe AVMs involve the uncus, the hippocampus and parahippocampal gyrus, the amygdala, and frequently extend into the inferolateral aspect of the basal ganglia (Fig. 22.7). Though these lesions may be approached through an incision in the inferior temporal gyrus (61), the pterional approach is now preferred (163). These lesions are fed by early branches of the middle cerebral artery (usually anterior temporal branches), by branches of the anterior choroidal artery, and by perforating branches of the posterior communicating artery and the posterior cerebral artery. One has ready access to all these branches by opening widely the medial aspect of the sylvian fissure (Fig. 22.8E and F). The position and craniotomy are as for the standard pterional approach except for the more generous inferior and posterior temporal bone removal and the slightly more lateral turning of the head (about 60°). With careful dissection, the sylvian fissure can be opened widely retracting the AVM with the temporal lobe. The branches going to the AVM are then on tension and can be readily identified (Fig. 22.8E). Great care must be taken to preserve the branches of the anterior choroidal artery continuing on to supply the cerebral peduncle. Branches from the posterior communicating artery and from the P_2 segment of the posterior cerebral artery are also clearly seen and placed on

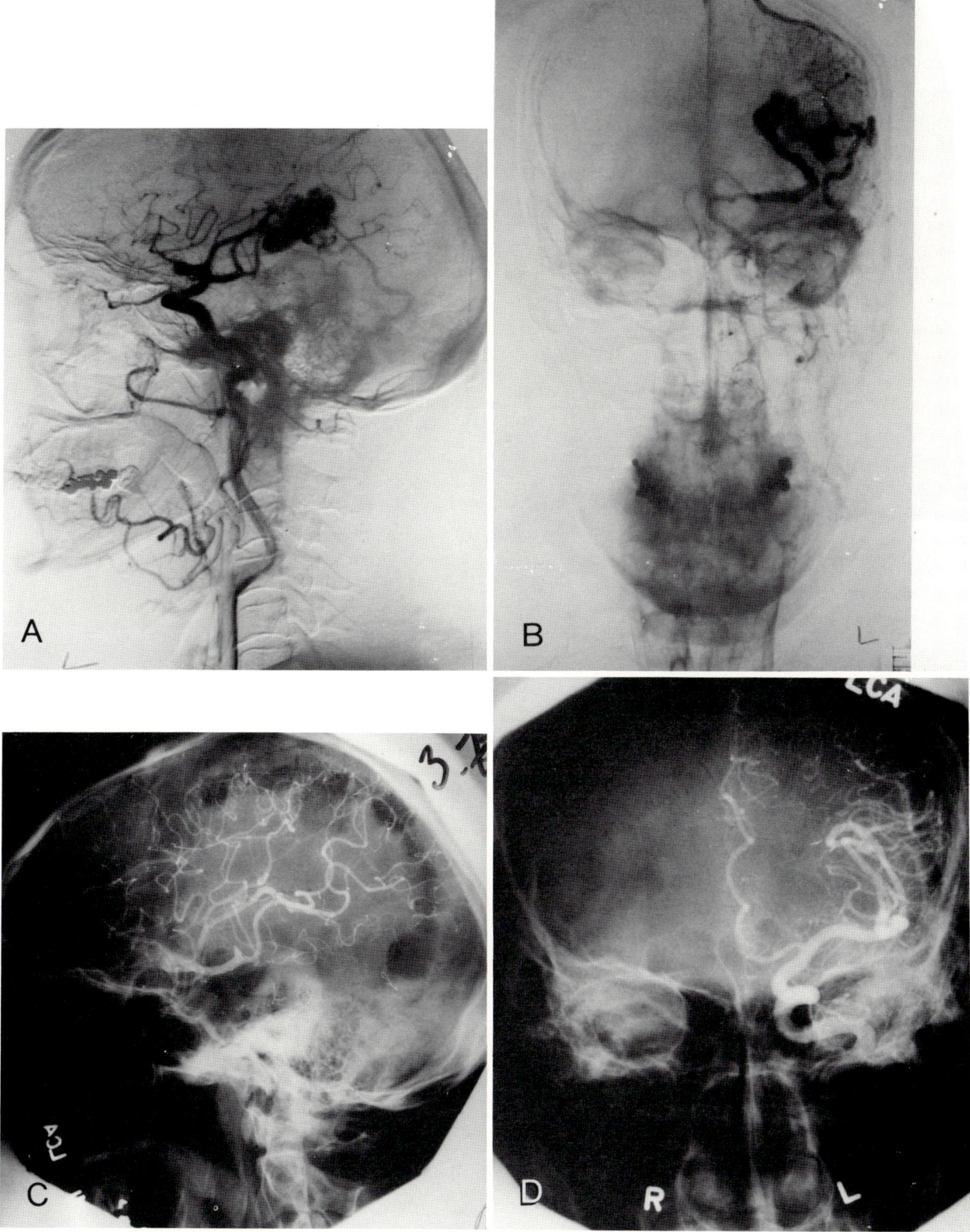

Figure 22.6. Posterior sylvian AVM. This middle-aged man had a hemorrhage from which he had recovered completely. **A** and **B**, Preoperative angiogram. The lesion was excised by opening the posterior aspect of the sylvian fissure and following the feeders to the lesion. There was no postoperative speech difficulty or hemiparesis. **C** and **D**, Postoperative angiography showed complete removal of the lesion.

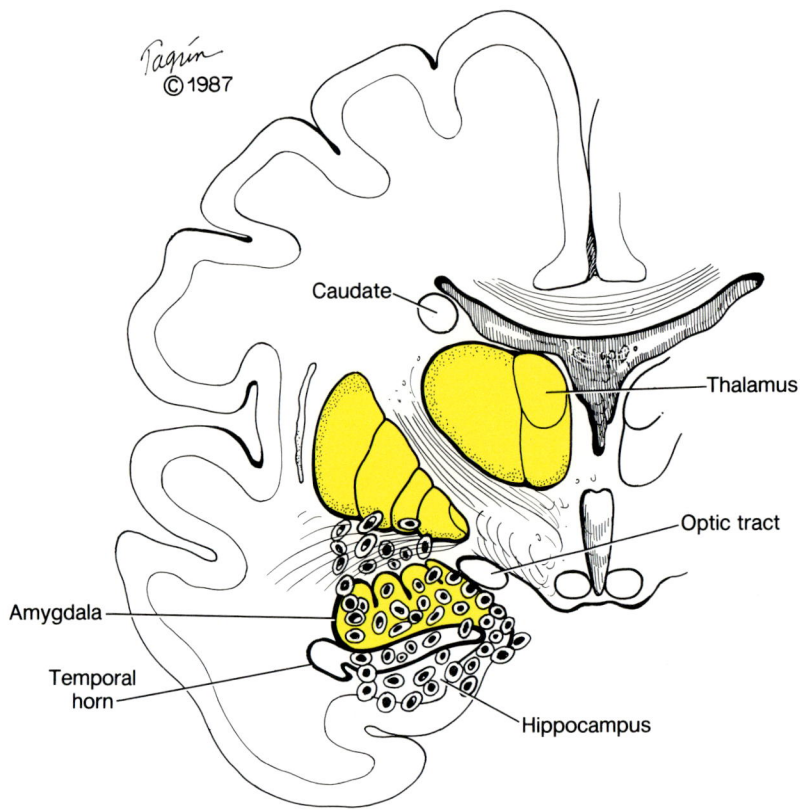

Figure 22.7. Deep anterior temporal AVM. Coronal section at the level of the amygdala showing typical anatomical relationships.

stretch with retraction of the malformation laterally. With this approach one can see all the way to the first anterior temporal branch of the posterior cerebral artery. Finally an anterior temporal lobectomy is performed staying on a plane just behind the malformation and working right down to the medial plane along the sylvian fissure.

Posteriorly located lesions involve the walls of the temporal horn, the hippocampus and parahippocampal region, and sometimes the posteroinferior aspect of the thalamus including the lateral geniculate body (Fig. 22.9). These lesions are approached through an incision (or sometimes a small amount of resection) in the inferior temporal gyrus (Fig. 22.10) (61). This incision can be on either side of the vein of Labbé but if the vein is in the usual position, the incision is usually anterior to it. A subtemporal approach has been used by other surgeons (41, 163) but this carries some danger of injury to the vein of Labbé and for this reason a small amount of resection of the inferior temporal gyrus is preferred. An incision in the superior or middle temporal gyrus may offer a more direct approach but results in injury to the optic radiations and, in the dominant hemisphere, it will incur some danger of speech deficit (130). The approach is through a standard temporal craniotomy using a horseshoe incision with the head in the straight lateral position and tilted back to allow the temporal lobe to fall away. Spinal drainage allows maximal relaxation of the temporal lobe.

The initial approach is to the anterior portion of the temporal horn where the anterior choroidal artery can be identified in the arachnoid of the choroidal fissure (Fig. 22.9). In the temporal horn anatomic orientation becomes easier and the anterior choroidal artery, which invariably feeds these lesions, can be followed to the malformation. It is important to interrupt only actual feeders to the malformation and to preserve the medially directed branches of the anterior choroidal artery to the brain stem and the basal ganglia. Then one must deal with the branches from the posterior cerebral artery by either continuing to work through the same incision and identifying the posterior cerebral branches as they come to the lesion transcortically along the inferior aspect of the malformation or, if too much bleeding is encountered in this plane of dissection, by a subtemporal approach identifying the posterior cerebral artery in the ambient cistern, and then following the branches that come to the temporal lobe until it is clear that they go to the malformation. One then returns to the previous plane of dissection and proceeds with ex-

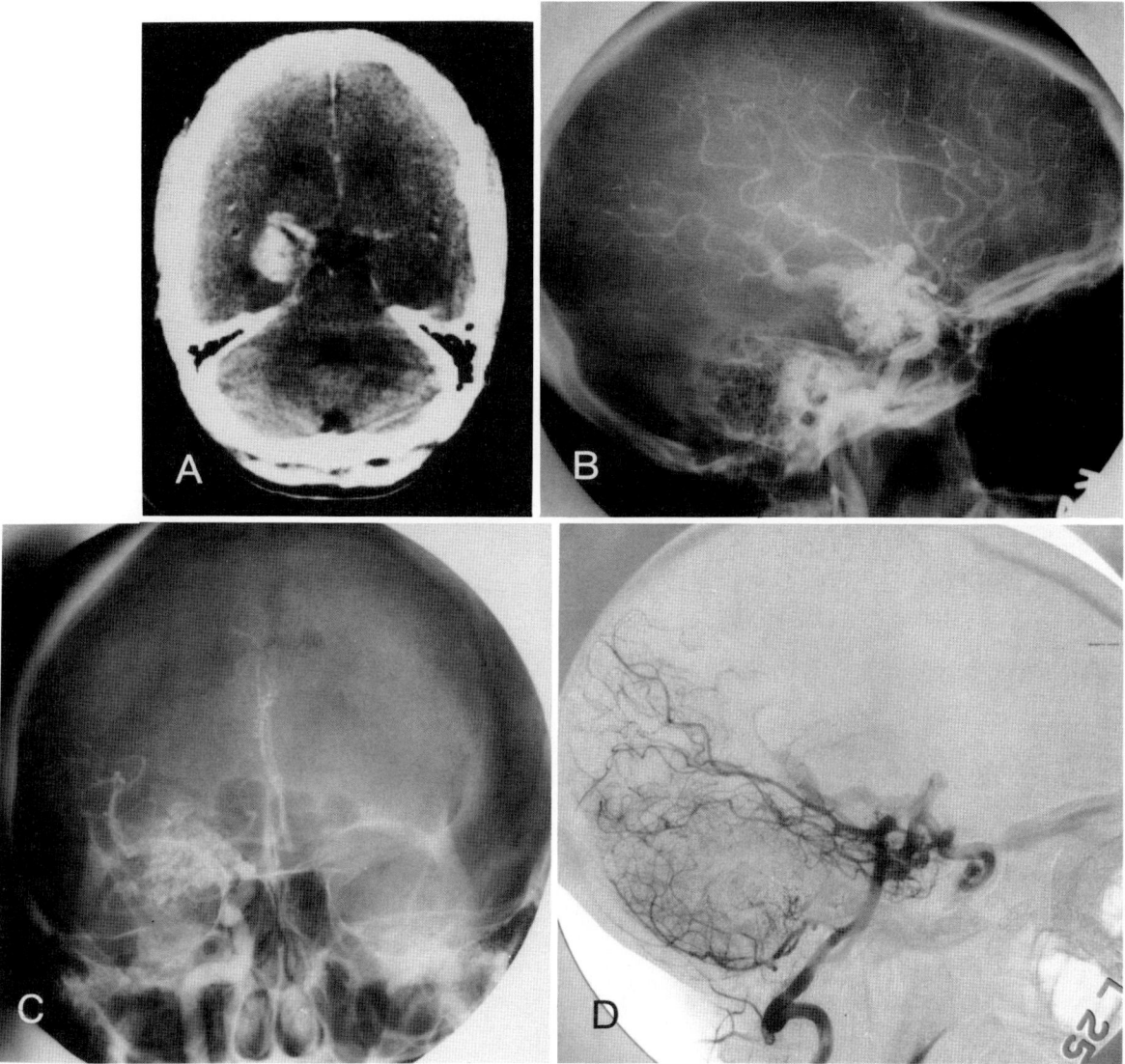

Figure 22.8. Deep anterior temporal AVM. This young lady presented with temporal lobe epilepsy. **A**, Initial CT scan. **B** and **C**, The lesion was fed by branches of the middle cerebral artery and by small branches from the posterior cerebral artery (**D**). **E** and **F**, Operative photographs. The approach was to open the sylvian fissure and first identify and clip a large anterior temporal branch (*arrow* in **E**). After division of this large branch, the sylvian fissure could be opened further by retracting the AVM (*open arrows* in **F**). In this manner, the posterior cerebral artery (*large solid arrow* in **F**) and the anterior choroidal artery (*small solid arrows* in **F**) could be seen with their small branches being taken close to the AVM as the lesion was being retracted away from these vessels. After all these feeders were eliminated, the lesion was essentially collapsed and could be removed without difficulty through a small anterior temporal lobectomy. **G** and **H**, Postoperative angiogram shows complete removal of the lesion with preservation of the anterior choroidal artery (*arrow* in **G**). The patient has no postoperative neurologic deficit.

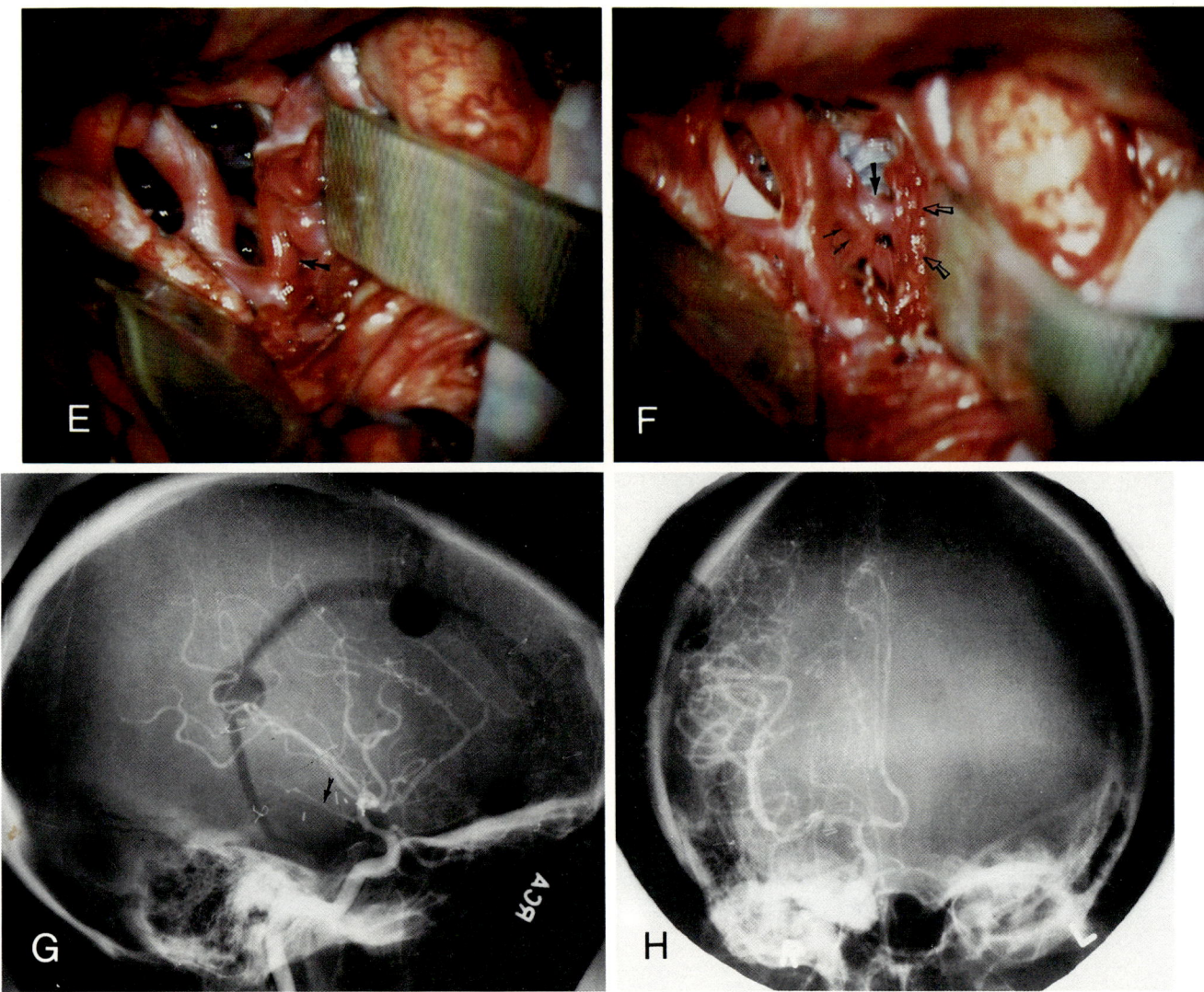

Figure 22.8E–H.

cision of the malformation working anteriorly to posteriorly since the drainage almost invariably is from the posteromedial aspect of the lesion into the basal vein of Rosenthal. At this point the lesion is usually soft and pliable and the loops of the malformation abutting the inferior aspect of the thalamus can be gradually coagulated and shrunken away. If the lesion is imbedded in the lateral geniculate body, there will be a postoperative hemianopsia and this must be taken into consideration before surgery is recommended. If there has been preoperative hemorrhage, many of these patients already will have significant field deficits and the surgery can be accomplished without additional resulting disability (Fig. 22.11). Even if the lesion does not involve the lateral geniculate body, it is very likely the resection will result in at least a superior quadrantic field defect from interruption of the inferior aspect of the visual radiations. This is quite tolerable to most patients and is a small price to pay for elimination of the threat of hemorrhage.

An alternative approach to the posteromedial temporal AVMs is through a limited anteromedial lobectomy as used in epilepsy surgery (159). This route provides good access to the lesion with only modest retraction, provided the AVM does not extend behind the brain stem on axial CT. Thus, posteromedial temporal lesions have been removed without postoperative field defects.

Trigonal and Deep Temporal-Occipital AVMs

These lesions are difficult. They involve the superior, medial, and inferior walls of the trigone and are adjacent to the thalamus (Figs. 22.12 and 22.13). The arterial supply is from the posterior cerebral artery and its posterolateral choroidal branches. The

Arteriovenous Malformations of the Brain

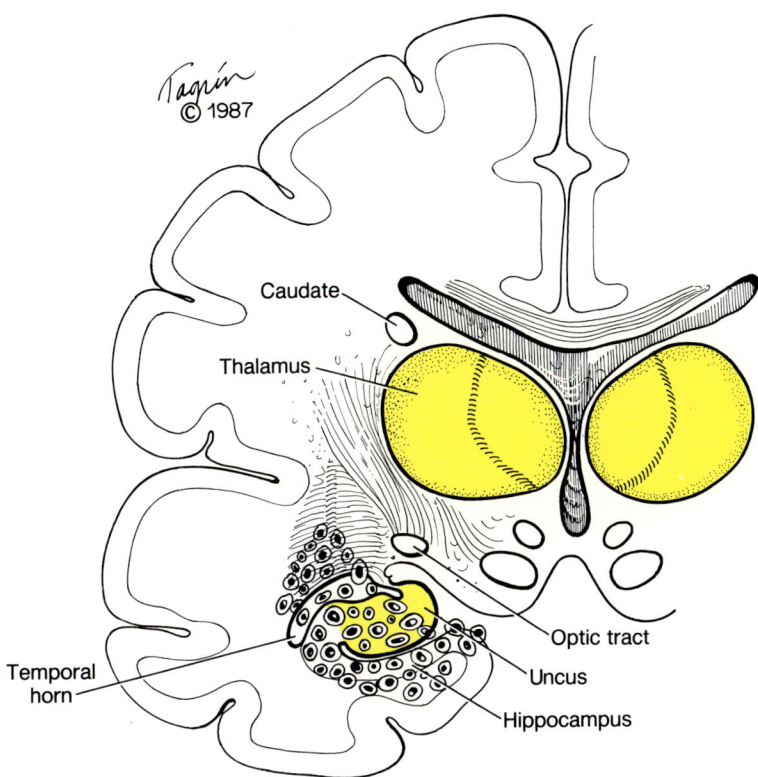

Figure 22.9. Deep medial midtemporal AVM. Coronal cross-section at the midthalamic level showing the important anatomic relationships.

venous drainage is usually into the vein of Rosenthal. If the lesion is on the right side, it can be approached directly through an incision in the superior temporal gyrus. In the dominant hemisphere, however, such an approach will often result in postoperative speech difficulty. One alternative is to approach the atrium superiorly using a cortical incision in the parasagittal region at a point about 9 cm above the inion and 2 cm from the midline which will usually be above the visual radiations and below (or posterior to) the primary sensory radiations (Fig. 22.14). The disadvantage of this superior approach to the atrium is that one encounters the malformation before its blood supply which usually comes from inferiorly. This approach, however, is very good when the lesion is located entirely posterior to the atrium (Fig. 22.13). In these cases, one enters the atrium for orientation and then works in the plane anterior to the malformation to interrupt the blood supply from the posterior cerebral arteries which comes transcerebrally from anterior and inferior to the lesion.

In the more complex type of lesion involving the inferior as well as the medial wall of the atrium (Fig. 22.12), an incision in the inferior temporal gyrus (Fig. 22.10) provides early access to feeders. If the vein of Labbé is relatively anterior, one may make the incision just posterior to that vein. One has to work in an upward direction toward the atrium which is relatively clumsy (163). Nevertheless, it is possible in this manner to stay below the bulk of the optic radiations, although it is quite likely that at least a superior quadrantic defect will result from such an approach. If the inferior temporal access to feeders is limited, one can go subtemporally to control the posterior cerebral artery feeders prior to excision through the atrial exposure.

Splenial AVMs

These difficult lesions are supplied by the pericallosal branch of the anterior cerebral artery, the posteromedial and posterolateral choroidal arteries and, if the lesion extends much below the splenium, by direct branches of the posterior cerebral artery (Fig. 22.15) (201). The lesions drain directly into the internal cerebral vein and the vein of Galen. The only logical surgical approach is the interhemispheric approach, working from the side with the bulk of the AVM (even though these AVMs involve the midline, they usually extend preferentially to one side or the other and, in fact, may reach the atrium laterally in one side) (Fig. 22.15). The patient is placed in a semi-sitting position. This position carries the well-known risk of air embolism and requires the use of a central venous catheter, a doppler monitor and end-tidal CO_2

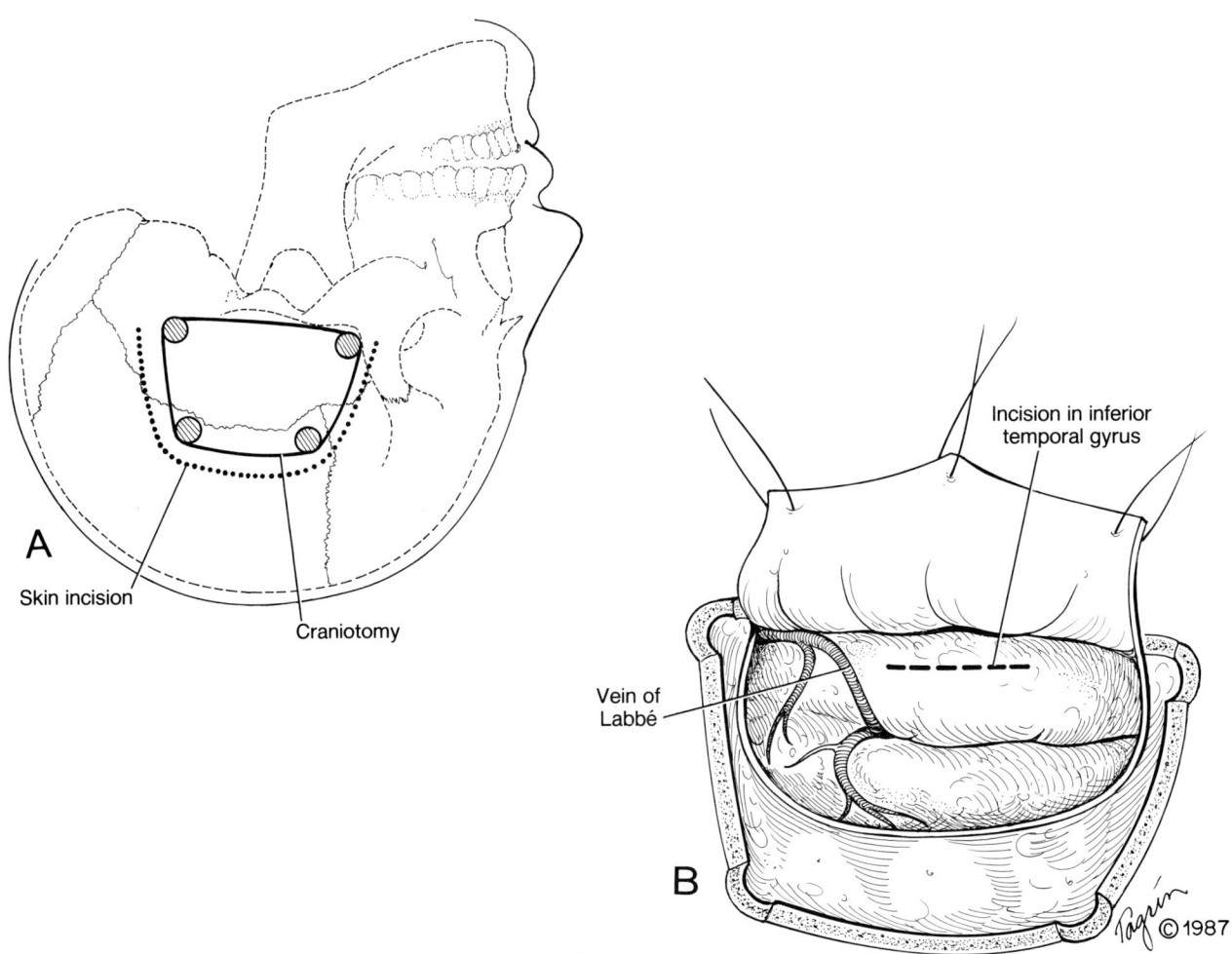

Figure 22.10. Deep medial midtemporal AVM. **A**, The skin incision and craniotomy are outlined. The craniotomy should be low with bone rongeured inferiorly if necessary right down to the temporal floor. **B**, An incision (or small amount of brain resection) in the inferior temporal gyrus is preferable to elevation of the temporal lobe which incurs the risk of injury to the vein of Labbé. If the vein of Labbé drains more anteriorly the incision or brain resection can be immediately behind the vein (see Fig. 22.18).

monitor. Yasargil has found the prone and supine positions unsatisfactory and, therefore, also recommends the semi-sitting position (201).

The bone flap is a parietal-occipital flap extending to the opposite side of the midline (Fig. 22.14A). The usual precautions must be taken in separating the sinus from the bone before removing the bone flap. A relatively large flap in the anteroposterior direction (approximately 6 or 7 cm) permits inspection of the venous anatomy to choose a site of approach between two draining veins. A small draining vein can frequently be sacrificed. Retractors are then placed on the medial aspect of the hemisphere and on the falx and the sinus. One must be careful not to obstruct the sinus mechanically with the retractor. Retraction of the brain must be kept to a minimum. The pericallosal branches to the malformation can then usually be seen and controlled as they come from anteriorly over the corpus callosum. Dissection of the malformation usually begins with an incision in the cingulate gyrus defining the superior and anterior planes of the malformation. The medial plane of the malformation is defined by sectioning the splenium. This may well be on the other side of the midline and the falx may be divided to aid exposure. The malformation is retracted toward the side of its greater bulk. Small vessels from the posteromedial choroidal system, which come posteroinferiorly, can be placed on a stretch, coagulated, and divided. The splenium is then split along the radiation of its fibers laterally toward the atrium of the ventricle. This may require significant retraction of the hemisphere. On the lateral aspect of the malformation the feeders from the posterolateral choroidal arteries are coagulated and

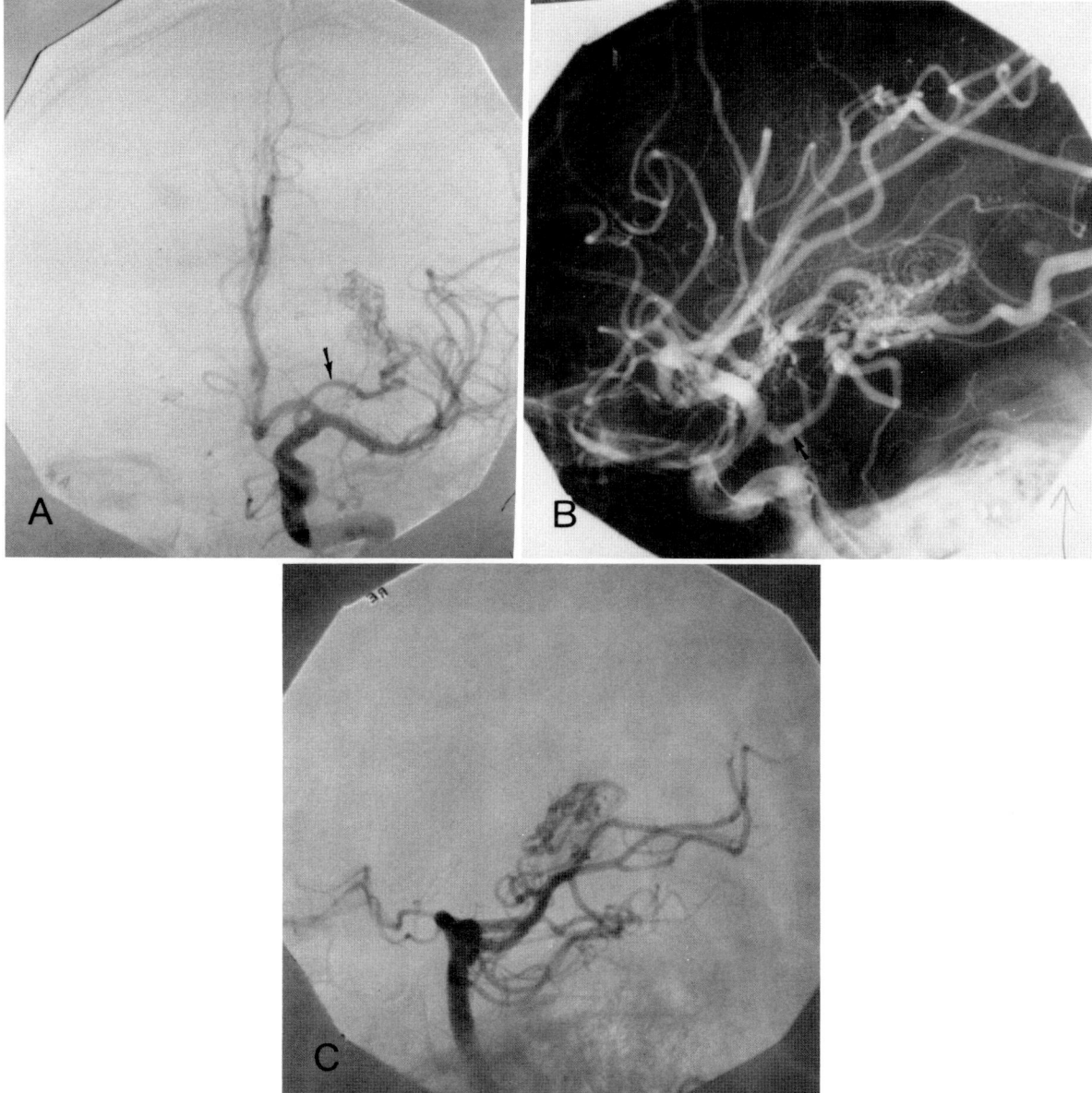

Figure 22.11. Deep temporal AVM with multiple hemorrhages. **A–C**, Preoperative angiogram. The lesion was fed by an enlarged anterior choroidal artery (*arrow* in **C**). The patient had a hemianopsia preoperatively. **D** and **E**, The lesion was completely excised without additional neurologic deficit through an incision in the inferior temporal gyrus on the left side. Note decrease in caliber of the preserved anterior choroidal artery (*arrow* in **D**).

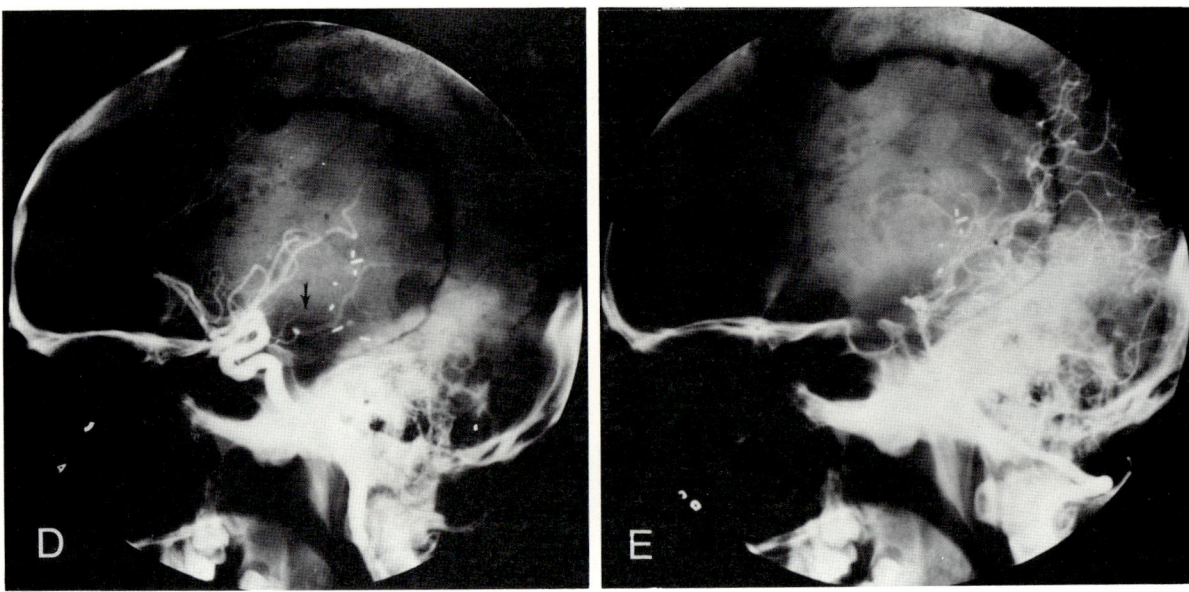

Figure 22.11D and E.

divided. Sometimes the choroid plexus has to be divided because it is continuous with the malformation. The malformation must be separated very carefully from the internal cerebral vein to which it can be quite adherent. Sometimes there are also small direct drainers into the vein of Galen that must be handled with care. A small portion of the cingulate gyrus may be resected for exposure if neeed. Preoperative embolization carries a risk of visual field defect and is probably of little help (Fig. 22.16).

Some surgeons have recommended the contralateral parafalcine approach to these malformations suggesting that one has better vision toward the contralateral side with less need for retraction (29) but this is contrary to the authors' experience. Contralateral exposure has been found to be limited even when the falx and inferior sagittal sinus are sectioned.

Parasagittal AVMs

The anterior frontal parasagittal AVMs are approached through a unilateral frontal craniotomy extending to the midline with the patient in the neutral supine position. The occipital parasagittal AVMs also present no great technical difficulty unless they extend anteriorly to the atrium of the ventricle in which case they are treated essentially as described for AVMs of the region of the atrium. Medial occipital AVMs frequently involve the visual cortex or associated areas and, therefore, careful judgment must be exercised before recommending surgery particularly if the patient has no preoperative field defect. It has been shown that many of these lesions can be removed with considerable preservation of vision and overall excellent results (197), and the authors' experience has been similar.

Posterior frontal and parietal parasagittal AVMs are much more of a problem because they involve the primary or association motor-sensory regions. The lesions are fed almost invariably by pericallosal branches of the anterior cerebral artery and by convexity branches of the middle cerebral artery. The more posteriorly located lesions may also have some posterior cerebral artery supply coming from around the splenium. In staging the operation, which is frequently desirable when these lesions are large, the semi-sitting or "lounging" position with the patient's head flexed and in a neutral (looking straight ahead) position may be used for the limited parasagittal approach to ligate the pericallosal arterial supply. Medially draining veins must be carefully spared. To do this the surgeon frequently must come from some distance in front of the lesion. It is generally fairly safe to ligate large branches of the pericallosal artery that are obviously going to go to the malformation even 2 or 3 cm in front of the lesion. This is not ideal but it is sometimes a necessary compromise. An alternative is to embolize the pericallosal supply endovascularly.

For the definitive resection, it is preferable to have the patient in the full lateral position or, if the neck is quite supple, in the supine position with a role under the ipsilateral shoulder (Fig. 22.17). The head is then turned completely laterally and elevated only slightly. Since the parasagittal feeders are difficult to reach in this position, they are usually eliminated by a prior operation or by percutaneous embolization, as described above. On occasion, the authors have

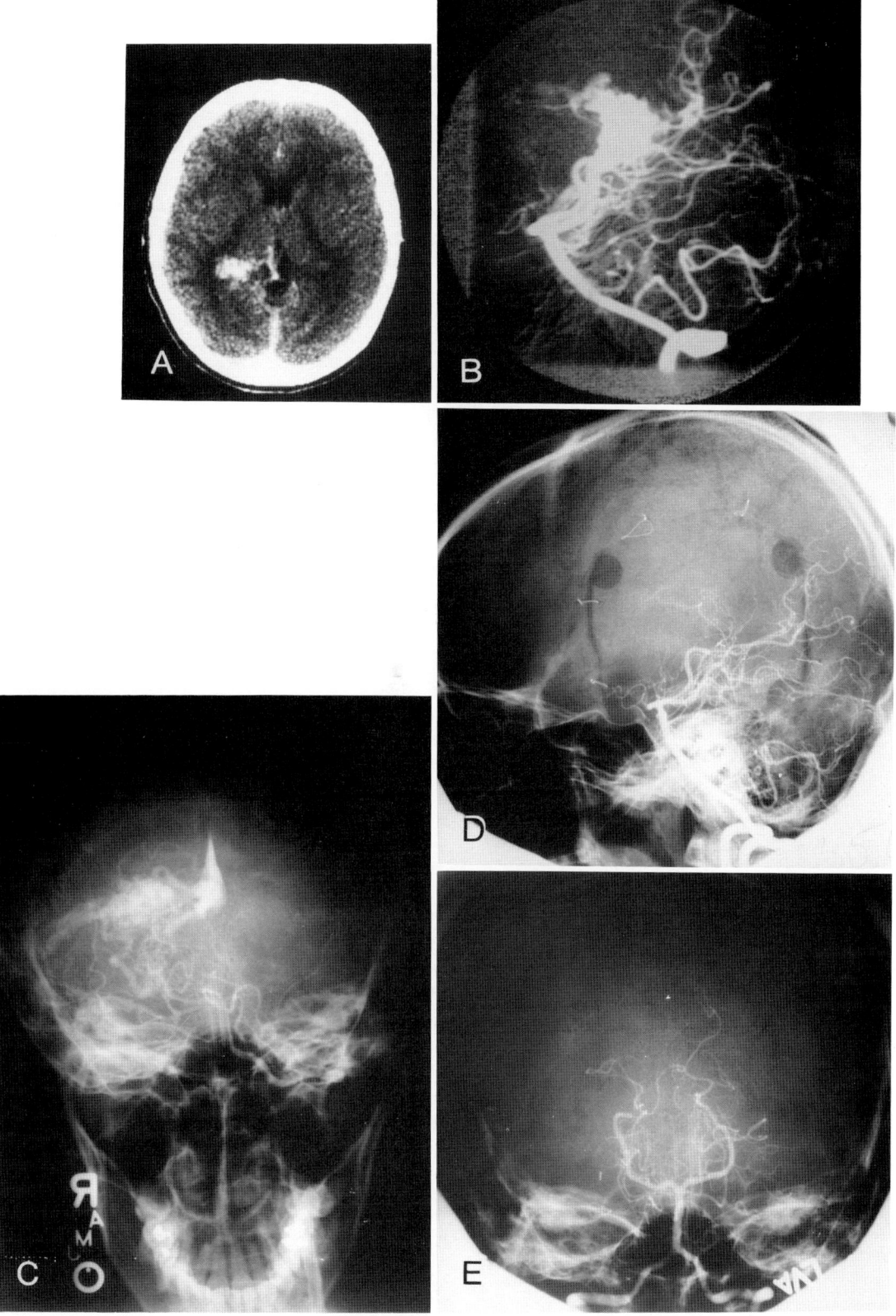

Figure 22.12. Deep temporal AVM in a 21-year-old woman. **A**, She presented with a small hemorrhage. **B**, and **C**, The lesion was fed by direct branches from the posterior cerebral artery. It drained medially into the vein of Galen (**C**). The lesion was removed through an approach to the atrium through the inferior temporal gyrus. **D** and **E**, Postoperatively she initially had a complete hemianopsia but over the ensuing few months, the vision returned in the left inferior field.

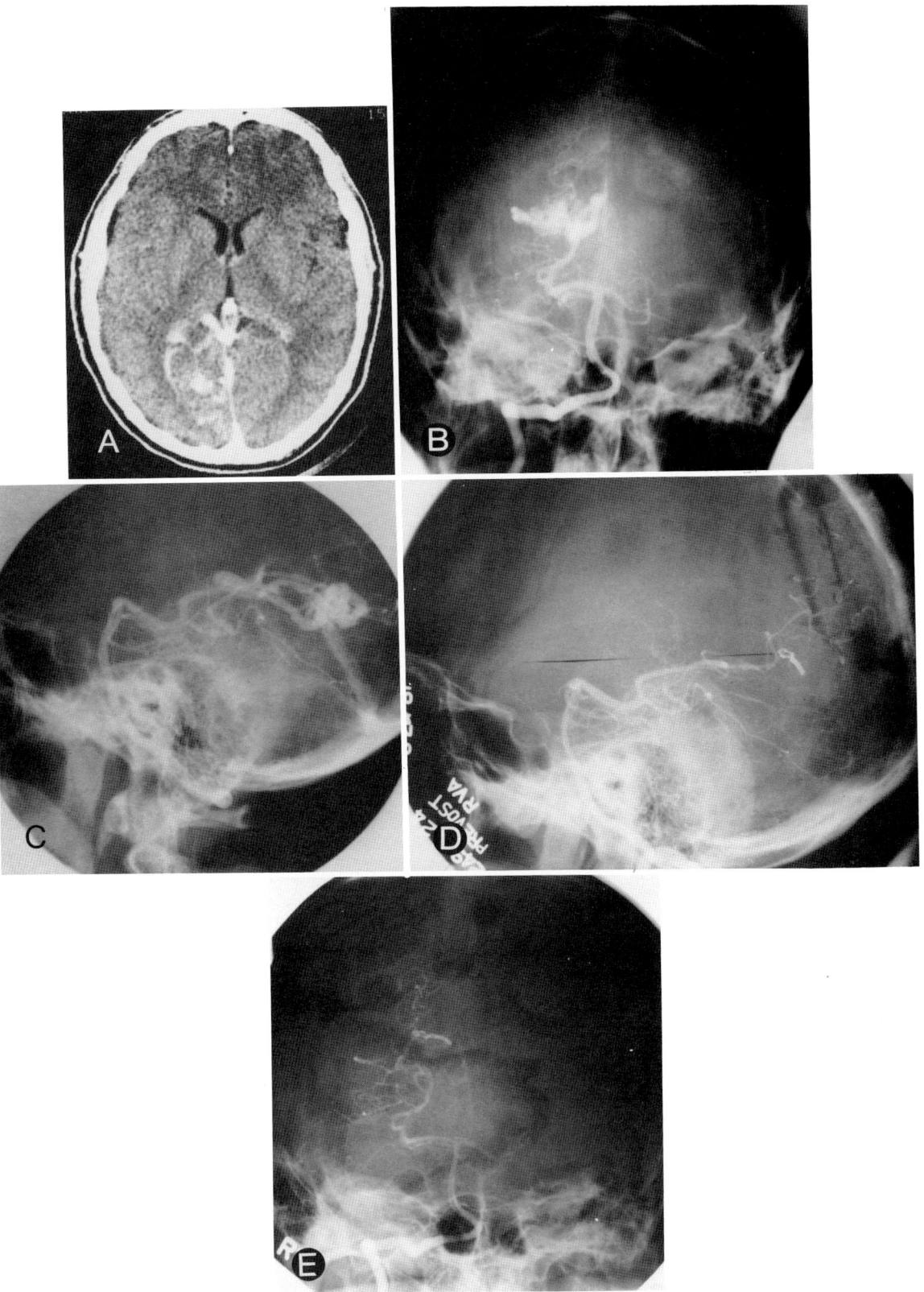

Figure 22.13. Retroatrial AVM. **A–C**, The patient presented with a hemorrhage. **D** and **E**, the lesion was removed through a small parasagittal incision in the posterior parietal lobule (at the parietal-occipital junction) with a direct approach to the atrium of the ventricle. The small transverse incision in the brain was located 9 cm above the inion. The patient had no postoperative neurologic deficit.

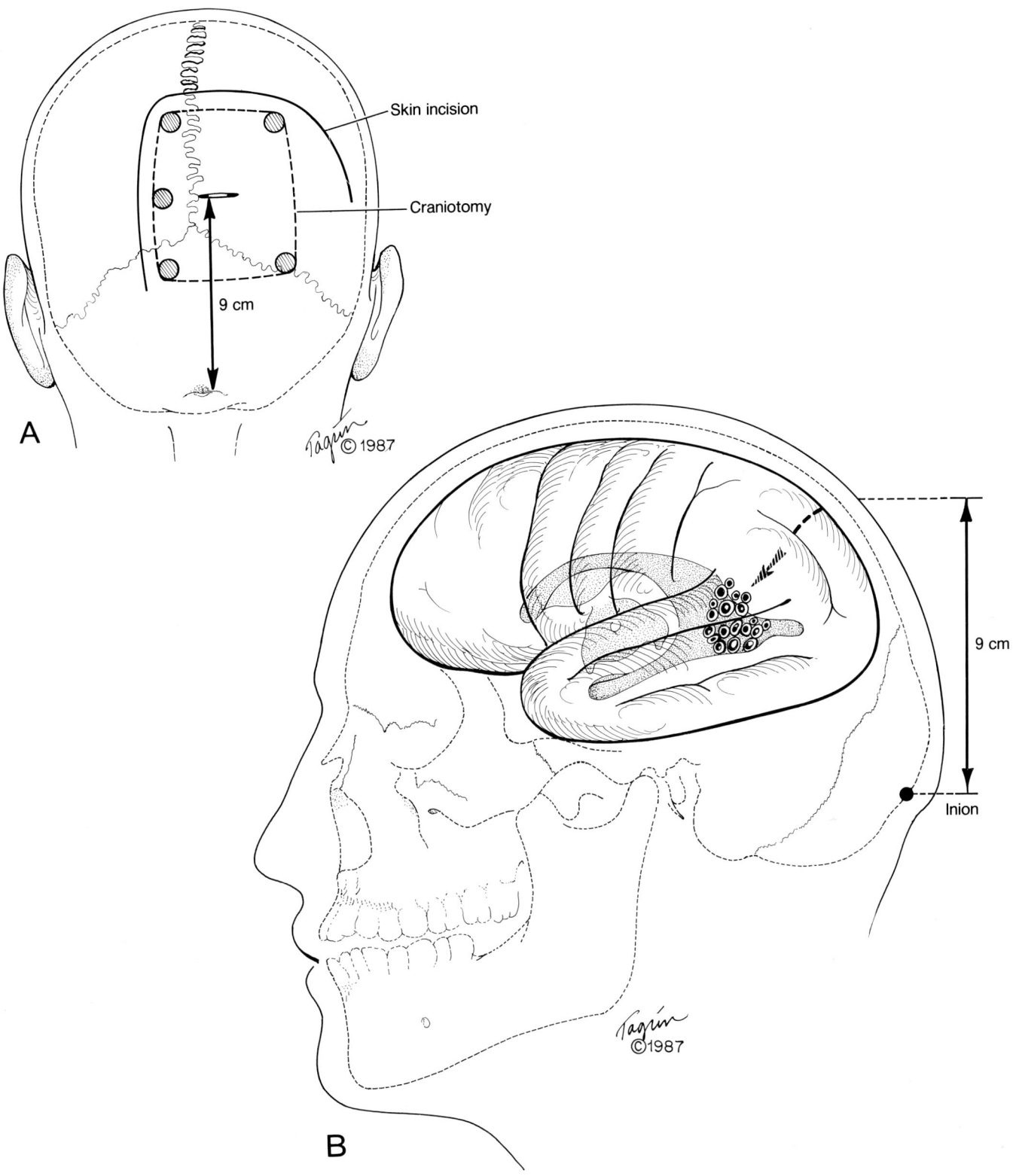

Figure 22.14. AVM of atrium of lateral ventricle. **A**, Craniotomy and skin incision for a parasagittal approach to the splenium or for a transcortical approach to the atrium of the right lateral ventricle through the posterior parietal lobule. The craniotomy can be centered approximately 9 cm above the inion. This point will usually be approximately 7 cm above the tip of the occipital lobe which can be confirmed once the dura is open. An incision in the parasagittal region in this area of the brain should result in no major sensory or visual deficit. The craniotomy is carried to the left of the midline to have ready parasagittal access which is useful both for splenial lesions (where it is the approach of choice) or for the transcortical approach to the ventricle when one may wish to identify the splenium by gently separating the brain from the falx in order to guide the direction of the transcortical approach to the atrium (the atrium is at the same level as the splenium but it is located 2.5–3.0 cm lateral to this structure). **B**, The transcortical approach to the atrium is through a parasagittal incision in the brain centered approximately 9 cm above the inion (about 7 cm above the tip of the occipital lobe as determined intradurally).

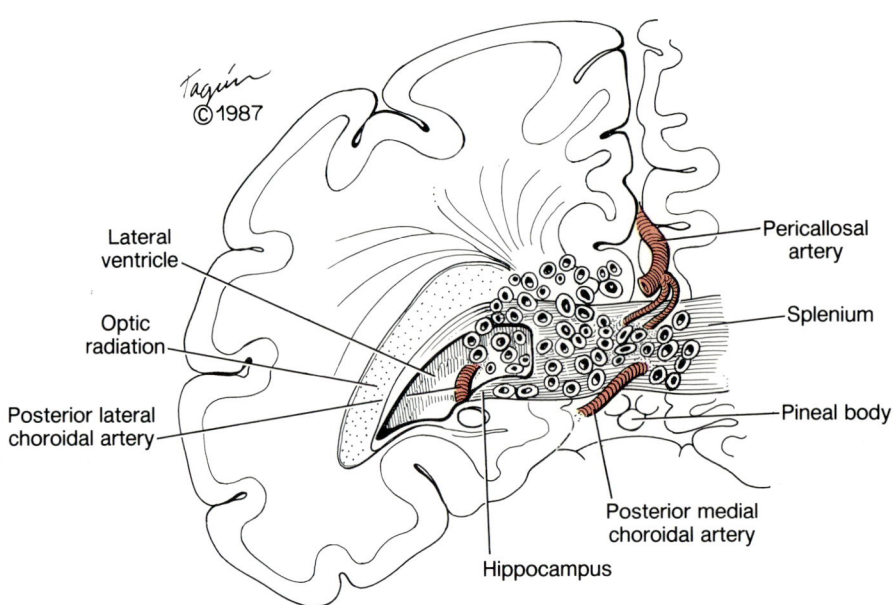

Figure 22.15. Splenial AVM. The anatomical relationships of a typical splenial AVM extending laterally to the atrium of the ventricle are illustrated. These lesions are usually fed by pericallosal branches and by posterior medial and posterior lateral choroidal branches of the posterior cerebral artery which reach the lesion posteriorly and laterally, respectively, as indicated in the sketch.

proceeded with a one-stage operation with the patient's head in the lateral position. The first step is to eliminate the middle cerebral feeders on the surface as they enter the malformation. Then, a circumscribing incision is made around the malformation to the falx anteriorly and posteriorly. In doing this, some of the venous drainage is interrupted, but this should not be a problem, since there are usually major draining veins directly attached to the sagittal sinus. If the latter is not the case, which can be ascertained by studying the preoperative angiogram, then one must preserve at least one large draining vein on the surface. The circumscribing incision around the lesion is taken to a depth of at least 2 cm, which interrupts most of the middle cerebral supply. At this stage, the remaining pericallosal arterial supply is dealt with. Even if the major pericallosal branches have been occluded by prior operation or embolization, there are almost always other smaller branches left to be secured. This can be done by extending the anterior incision through the pia of the parasagittal region against the falx and down toward the corpus callosum. Branches of the posterior cerebral artery coming around the callosum can be taken by extending the posterior plane of dissection against the falx to the inferior aspect of the AVM. Although major arterial supply is now interrupted, the lesion will remain relatively turgid from deep arterial branches that are usually located in relation to the deep (subependymal) venous drainage. Completing the lateral and then inferior plane of the malformation is a tedious process, in that one must stay at the edge of the lesion to avoid unnecessary damage to the brain. The advantage of the lateral position in these cases is that the malformation can be retracted against the falx maintaining orientation by working in reference to the falx. It is important to have the patient's head somewhat flexed (elevated) (Fig. 22.17), which permits the brain to fall away from the AVM with little retraction. Figures 22.18 and 22.19 are representative of these lesions; both patients had their AVM resected in a two-stage procedure.

Anterior Callosal and Deep Frontal AVMs

Lesions of the anterior part of the corpus callosum usually involve the cingulate gyrus on one side and frequently extend to the deep basal medial portion of the frontal lobe. These lesions can involve the head of the caudate nucleus and extend deep into the basal ganglia (Fig. 22.20). The arterial supply is primarily by anterior cerebral artery branches, usually from both sides. They may also be supplied by medial lenticulostriate branches and by the recurrent artery of Heubner from one side. If the lesions are supplied by lateral lenticulostriate arteries, they usually involve the internal capsule, and therefore, operation is contraindicated. If they extend to the basal medial aspect of both frontal lobes, they are inoperable because injury to this region bilaterally will result in severe memory, personality, and intellectual diffi-

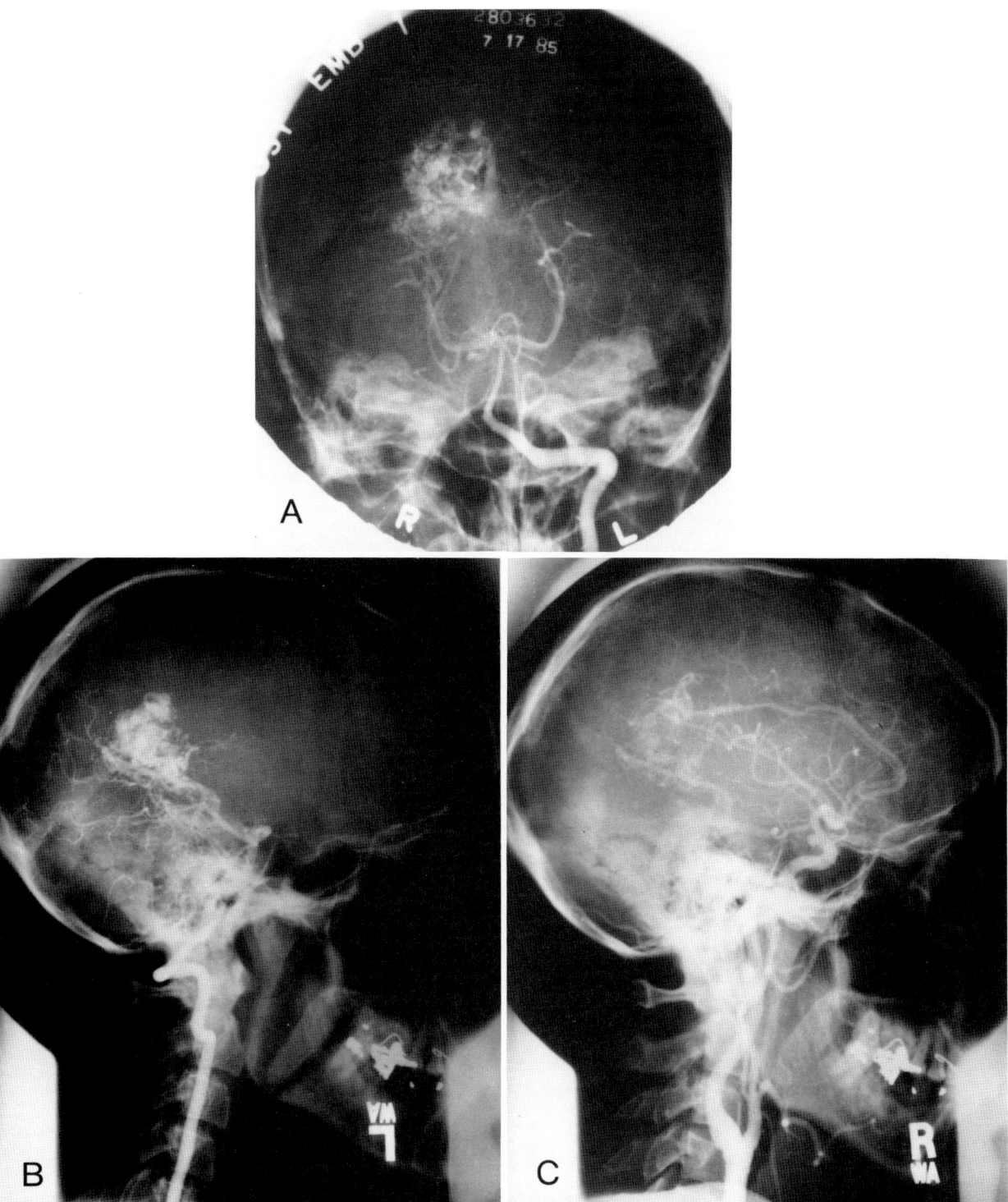

Figure 22.16. Splenial AVM with hemorrhage. **A–C,** The AVM extended on the right side to the atrium. In order to facilitate excision, the posterior cerebral artery was embolized preoperatively. Unfortunately, this resulted in a complete hemianopsia which has never recovered. The lesion was then excised through a parasagittal approach with early control of the pericallosal supply. **D** and **E,** Postoperative angiogram showed complete resection of the lesion. The patient had no neurologic deficit other than the preexisting hemianopsia. Retrospectively, it was believed that this lesion could have been resected without preoperative embolization with little, if any, additional difficulty.

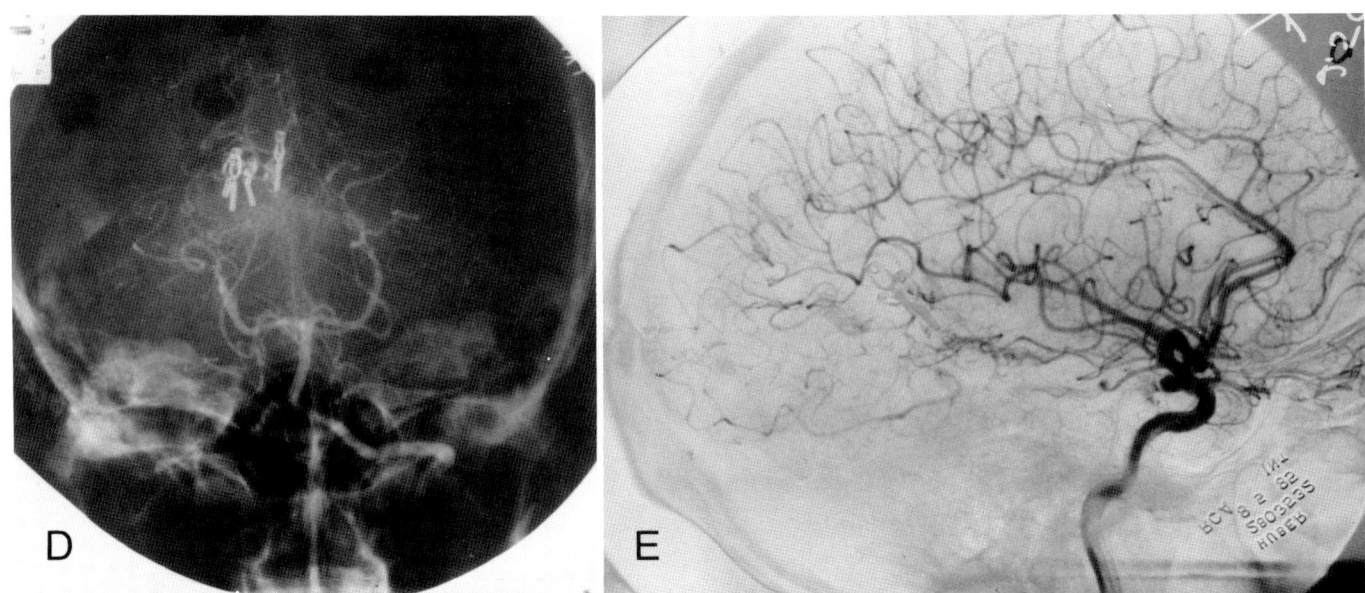

Figure 22.16D and E.

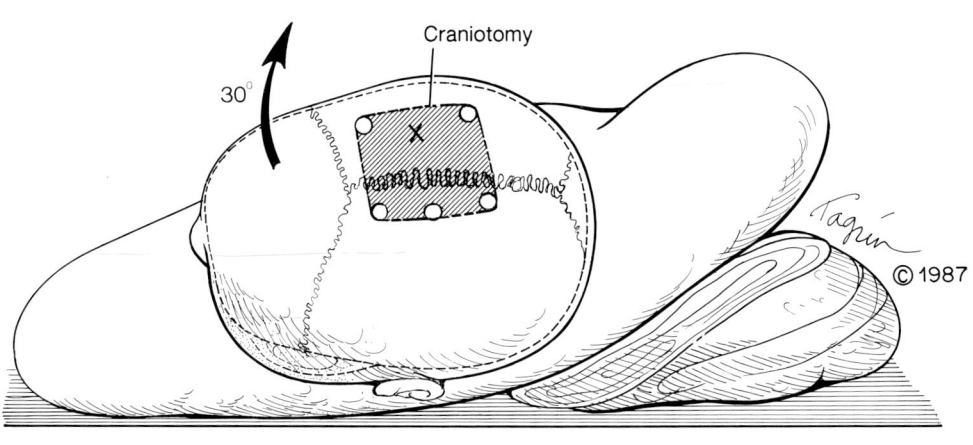

Figure 22.17. Parasagittal AVM. The craniotomy extends to the opposite side of the midline which allows for an initial approach to the parasagittal region for control of the pericallosal blood supply (usually on a separate operation with the patient semi-sitting and the head looking straight ahead.) The same craniotomy allows for the definite resection of the lesion once the pericallosal supply is controlled. It is preferable to perform this stage with the head in the lateral position and slightly elevated. This allows for the AVM to fall against the falx as it is being resected. It also allows for better access to the deeper portions of the AVM which usually reach the ventricular surface.

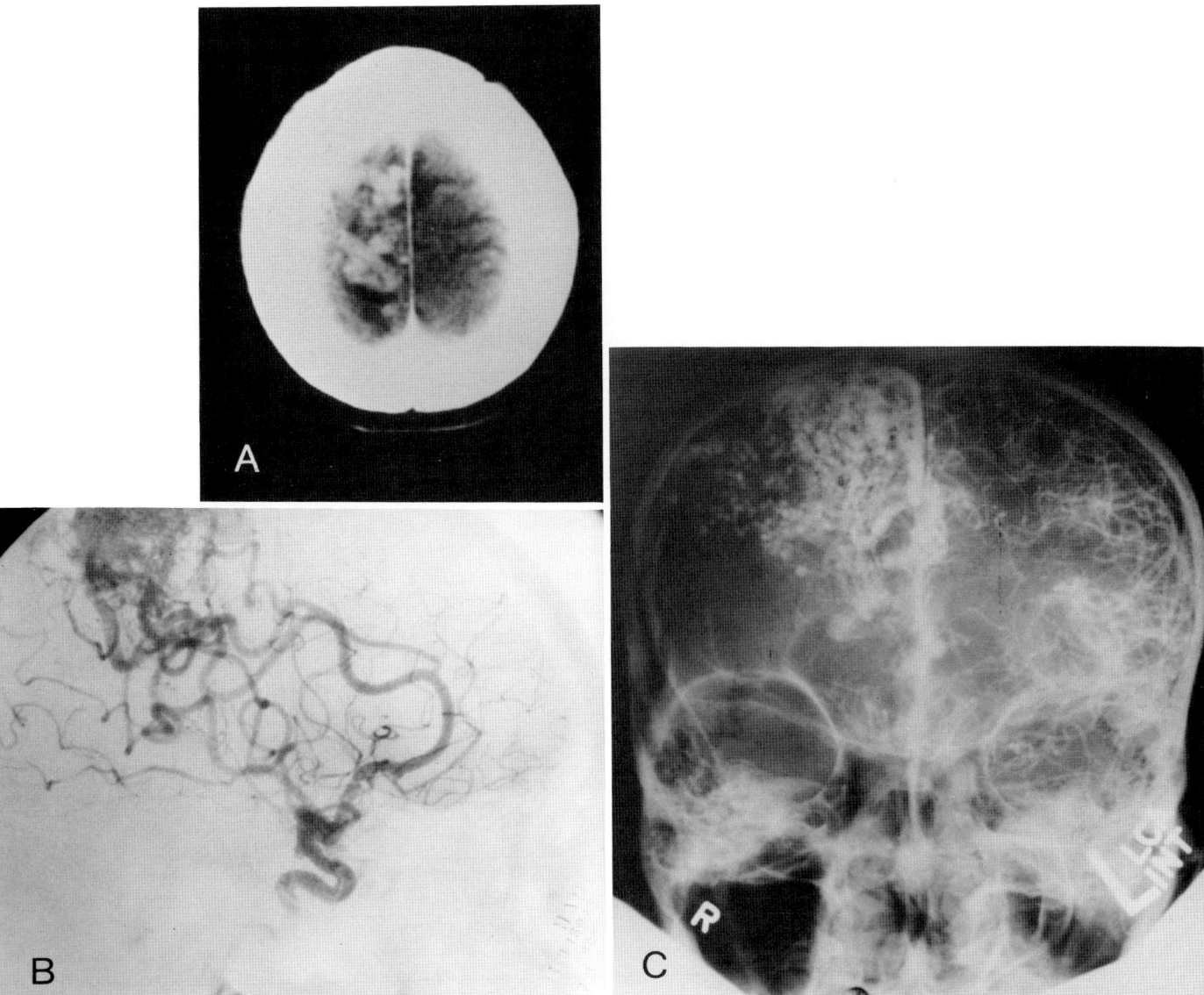

Figure 22.18. Large right parietal AVM. This 38-year-old lady had progressive weakness of the left leg and shoulder as well as clumsiness of the left hand. **A–C,** The CT scan and preoperative angiogram. The lesion was removed in a two-stage surgical procedure. The first stage was in the semi-sitting postition for a parasagittal approach to the pericallosal artery feeders which were clipped and divided. At the same operation, some of the readily visible middle cerebral artery feeders were divided as they approached the lesion in the convexity. The second stage was for complete resection with the head moderately elevated in the lateral postition. **D** and **E,** Postoperative angiogram shows complete excision of the lesion. There was considerable operative difficulty with the deep arterial supply which had to be controlled with large aneurysm clips. The patient awoke with a moderate left hemiparesis but she improved remarkably over the next several months to the point that she walks only with a slight limp and has essentially normal function of the left upper extremity.

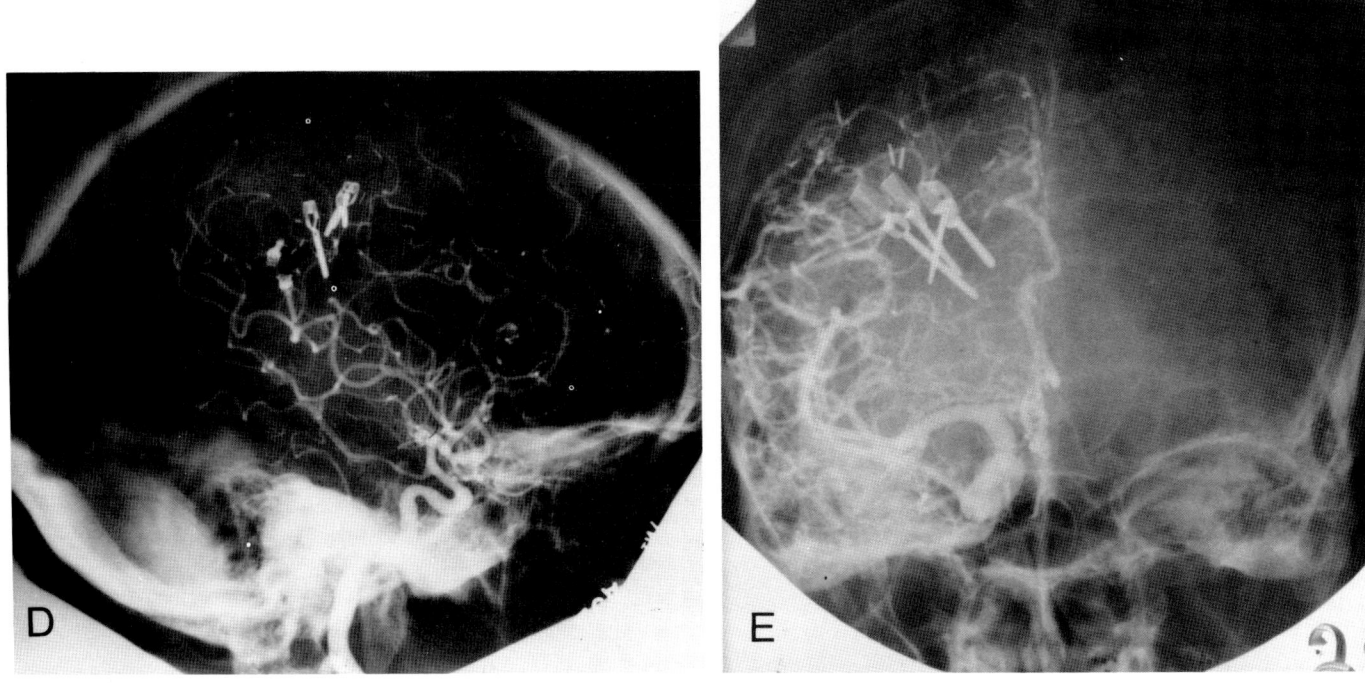

Figure 22.18D and E.

culties. This is unusual in that AVMs usually do not cross pial planes and respect the interhemispheric fissure, although at times the lesion can appear to be bilateral because the loops of the AVM protrude into the opposite side of the midline (62, 63) (Fig. 22.21B and C). One-stage removal of even large and deep lesions can be accomplished in this area without significant deficit (Fig. 22.21).

The choice of approach in these cases depends on whether or not the lesion extends into the basal frontal region. If it does not, the AVM can be approached with the patient in the supine position, the head essentially neutral, and a bone flap that crosses the midline utilized (Fig. 22.22A). If the lesion extends to the subfrontal region (Fig. 22.21), there are two choices. One can perform the operation in two stages by using a pterional craniotomy to take feeders from the anterior communicating artery complex and develop the posterior and inferior planes of the AVM. The final stage can be accomplished with the patient supine, with the patient's head straight ahead, and with a frontal bone flap placed slightly more anteriorly to allow access to the AVM inferior to the genu. The alternative is to perform the entire operation in one stage through a large bone flap extending from across the midline to the pterion. The flap must be both low, to allow for a subfrontal exposure, and high, to allow dissection of the superior and posterior portion of the AVM in the cingulate gyrus and the genu of the corpus callosum (Fig. 22.22B). On the genu and the cingulum, pericallosal arteries are "skeletonized," taking all the branches to the AVM that is retracted with the hemisphere. The medial plane of the AVM is developed by sectioning the genu. To approach the anterior cerebral complex, the patient's head is then turned about 30°. The posterior plane of the AVM is developed by taking the feeders from the anterior communicating artery complex to the base of the AVM and gradually retracting the AVM anteriorly. One A_1 segment may be sacrificed to facilitate dissection if the other is substantial and irrigates both A_2 segments (Fig. 22.21). The lamina terminalis may be opened into the third ventricle. With the patient's head back in the neutral position, the medial plane of the AVM is developed. Finally, the lateral plane of the AVM in the ventricle is completed. Most AVMs of the genu of the corpus callosum are not this large and do not involve the subfrontal region and can be excised through a small frontal craniotomy (202).

Hypothalamic-Basal Frontal AVMs

These AVMs are usually small and involve the general area of the anterior communicating artery complex, the chiasm, and the anterior hypothalamic and septal regions. When the lesions are restricted to the subfrontal region, they can be approached through a pterional exposure (Fig. 22.23). The problem with these lesions is to separate the branches that go to the AVM from those branches going to

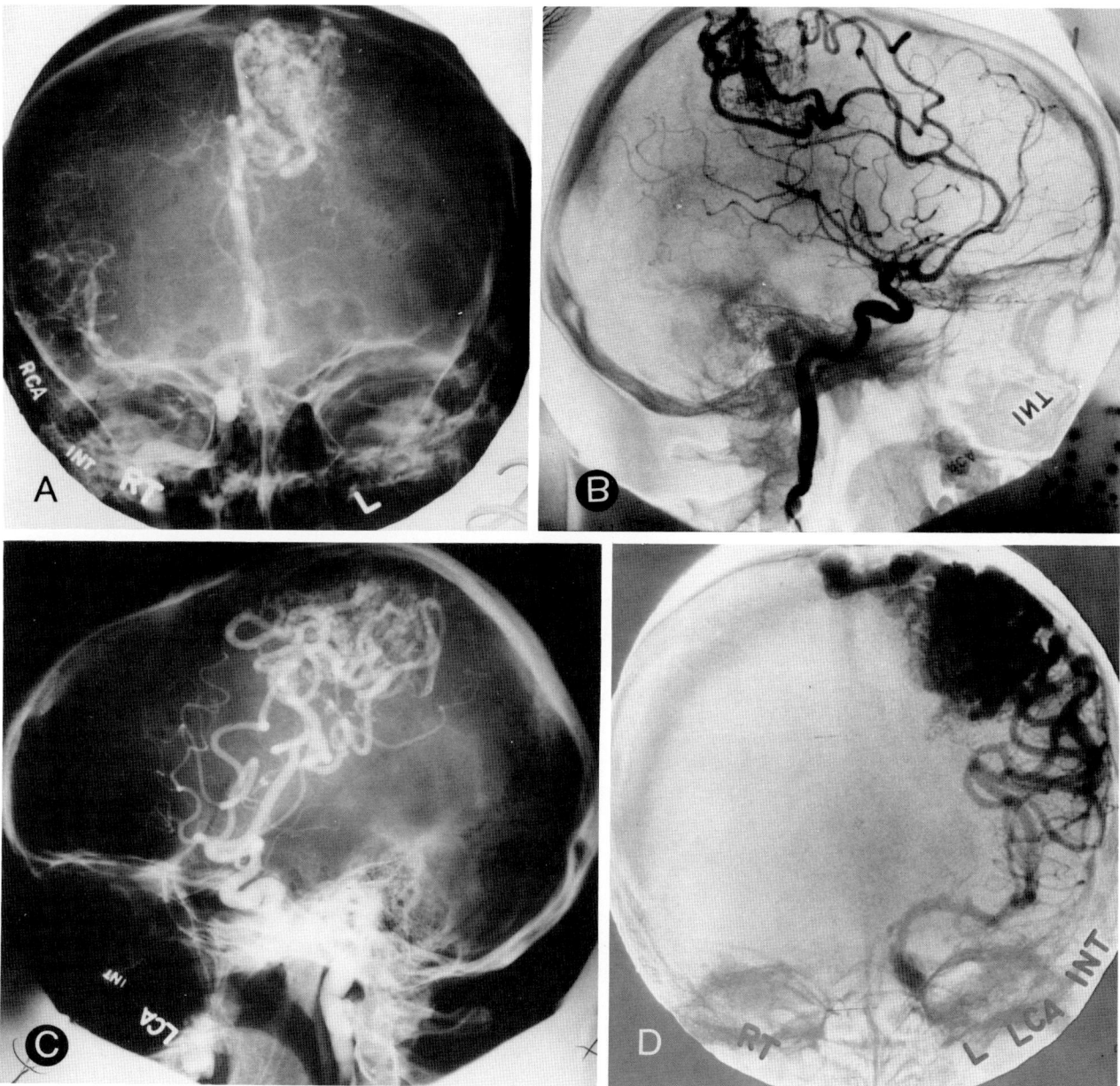

Figure 22.19. Large left parietal AVM which presented as seizures in a 20-year-old woman. **A–C**, Preoperative angiograms. The lesion was fed by the pericallosal branches opacified on the right cartoid injection (**A** and **B**), by left middle cerebral artery branches (**C** and **D**), and by posterior cerebral artery branches (**E**). The lesion was resected in two stages exactly as described for the previous patient (Fig. 22.18). Significant difficulty was encountered with deep bleeding during the second stage. After the lesion was completely removed, there was very severe brain swelling. Shortly after the patient began to wake up, the left pupil dilated and she started to decerebrate. The wound was reopened promptly and a large intracerebral hemorrhage was found and was evacuated. Again there was diffuse bleeding which could be controlled only with difficulty. She has remained with a severe right hemiparesis and aphasia and is incapacitated because of this deficit. Postoperative angiography has not yet been performed. Retrospectively, this patient with only seizures should have been treated conservatively.

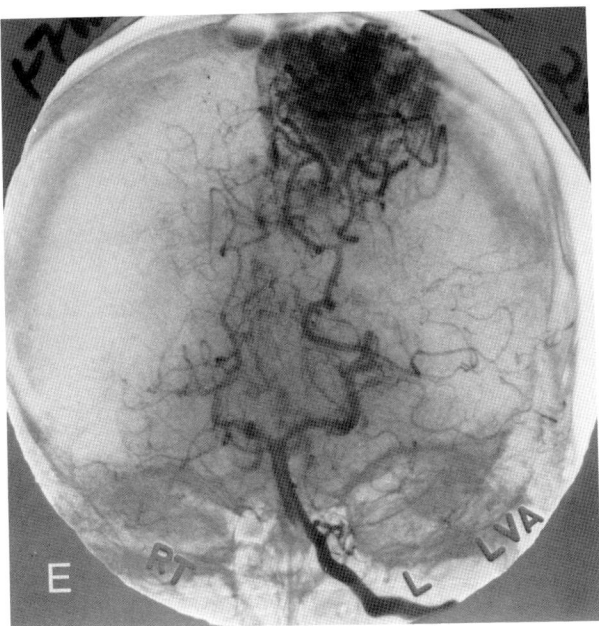

Figure 22.19E.

normal brain. A very early arterial phase on the angiogram may be helpful in understanding the sometimes complex anatomy of these lesions (Fig. 22.23E).

Intraventricular, Thalamic, and Basal Ganglia AVMs

These have been included together because, in general, the only AVMs of the thalamus and basal ganglia that are operable are those small lesions that present in the ventricle. Therefore, the surgical approach is the same as for purely intraventricular AVMs. Deep AVMs of the temporal lobe or trigone involving the basal ganglia or thalamus have been described in detail and are documented in preceding sections (8, 14, 41, 61, 70, 83, 135, 144, 163, 180, 182, 190, 197).

There have been some reports of removal of malformations located primarily within the substance of the basal ganglia or the thalamus (14, 17, 50, 144, 180, 190, 198). However, some degree of neurologic disability, which can be quite severe, must be expected from this type of surgery. The only exception is a lesion of the ventricular surface of the thalamus or caudate nucleus. The distinguishing angiographic clue in the case of thalamic malformations is that, in the lesions that are operable, the blood supply is from choroidal vessels (47, 49, 60, 142). The posteromedial choroidal arteries, which come through the quadrigeminal cistern and around the posterior aspect of the pulvinar to the choroid plexus of the roof of the third ventricle, supply the more medially located lesions. These lesions can be reached either in the transverse cerebral fissure by a midline parasagittal transplenial approach (Fig. 22.24) or, if more laterally located, by the transcortical approach to the atrium through a small incision in the parietal-occipital junction in the parasagittal region described before for atrial AVMs (Fig. 22.14). The more lateral lesions are supplied by posterolateral choroidal branches from the posterior cerebral artery as it courses through the ambient cistern. These branches pass superiorly around the lateral aspect of the thalamus. In the area of the atrium they can anastomose with branches of the anterior choroidal artery so there is a possibility of arterial supply to lateral thalamic AVMs by the anterior choroidal artery but this is unusual. Choroidal branches can be controlled on the surface as they go into the AVM and this is why these lesions are amenable to resection. Conversely, if the lesions are supplied mostly by deep thalamic perforating branches then the operation will be very dangerous because one must approach the lesion on the surface before the arterial supply is controlled. As one dissects along the deep aspect of the lesion, within the parenchyma of the thalamus, the small perforating vessels of supply can hemorrhage and shrink away creating the possibility of major neurologic deficits.

Small AVMs of the head of the caudate nucleus can be operated successfully as long as they do not extend laterally as far as the internal capsule. These lesions are supplied by medial branches of the lenticulostriate group of arteries and at times by branches from the recurrent artery of Heubner. The arterial supply enters the lesion from its depth and the same potential problem as described with thalamic lesions supplied by perforating vessels applies. The authors prefer a transventricular approach over the interhemispheric transcallosal route but the latter is also adequate and may be preferable when the ventricles are small. With the head in the neutral position, a small unilateral frontal exposure centering the small bone flap at about the coronal suture is made for a transfrontal approach to the ventricle (Fig. 22.25).

Purely intraventricular lesions involving the choroid plexus have also been reported (15, 18, 39, 64, 138, 172, 183). These lesions are generally small and can be handled by resecting a large segment of the choroid plexus in continuity with the AVM. The anterior lesions are approached transfrontally or transcallosally and the posterior lesions through the atrium (18, 64, 106, 183).

Brain Stem AVMs

AVMs of the brain stem usually present with hemorrhage. Some of these AVMs, even though they may be occult angiographically, can present with a progressive course mimicking either an intrinsic brain stem tumor or demyelinating disease (145, 162). Drake (40), Chou and collaborators (22), and Lapras (84) were the first to report the possibility, difficulty, and risk of resecting intrinsic brain stem AVMs. Subsequently, others have reported removal of brain stem

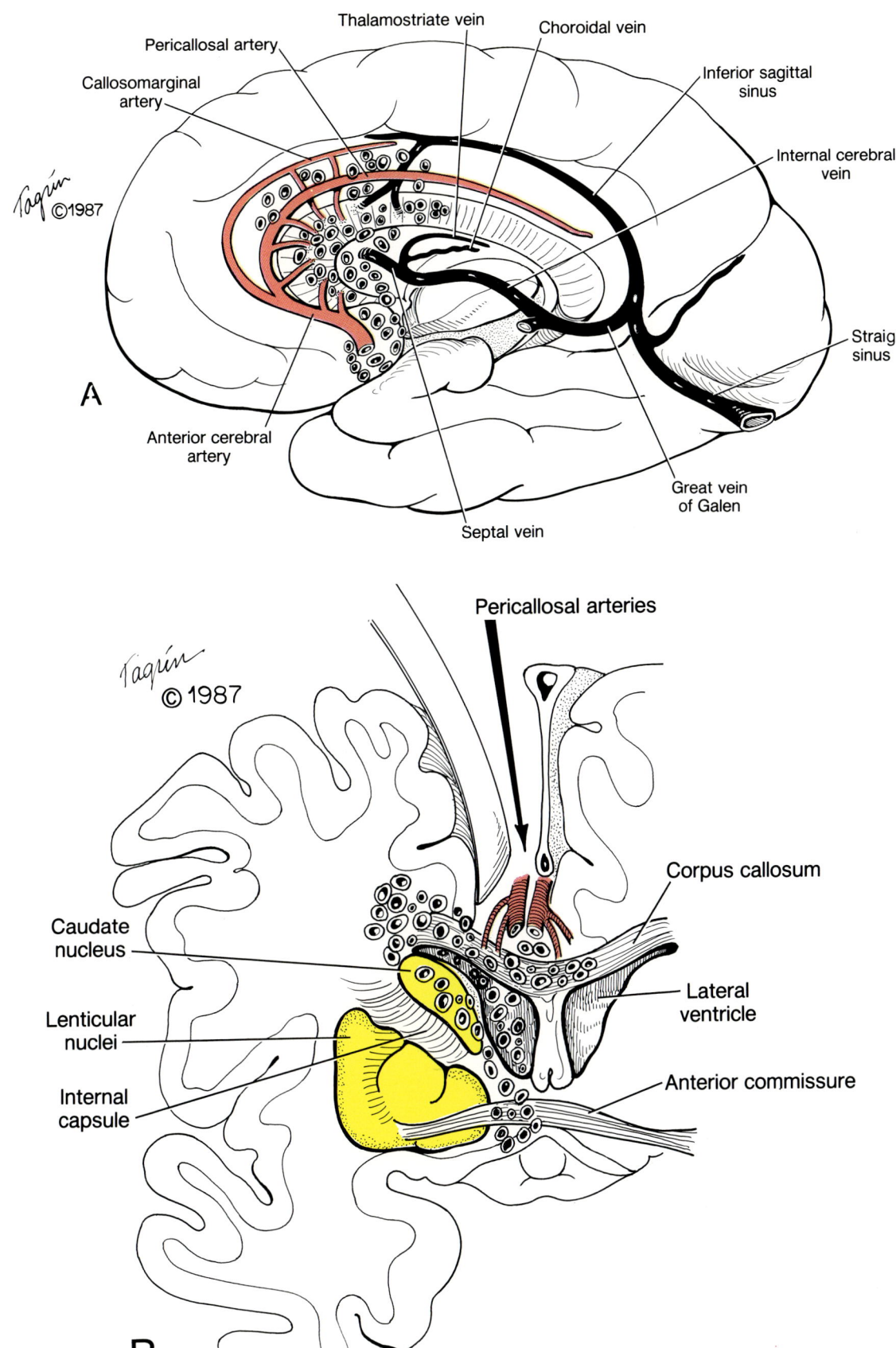

Figure 22.20. AVM of the anterior aspect of the corpus callosum extending into the deep subfrontal region and involving the caudate nucleus. **A** and **B**, Parasagittal and coronal anatomical relationships, respectively, are shown.

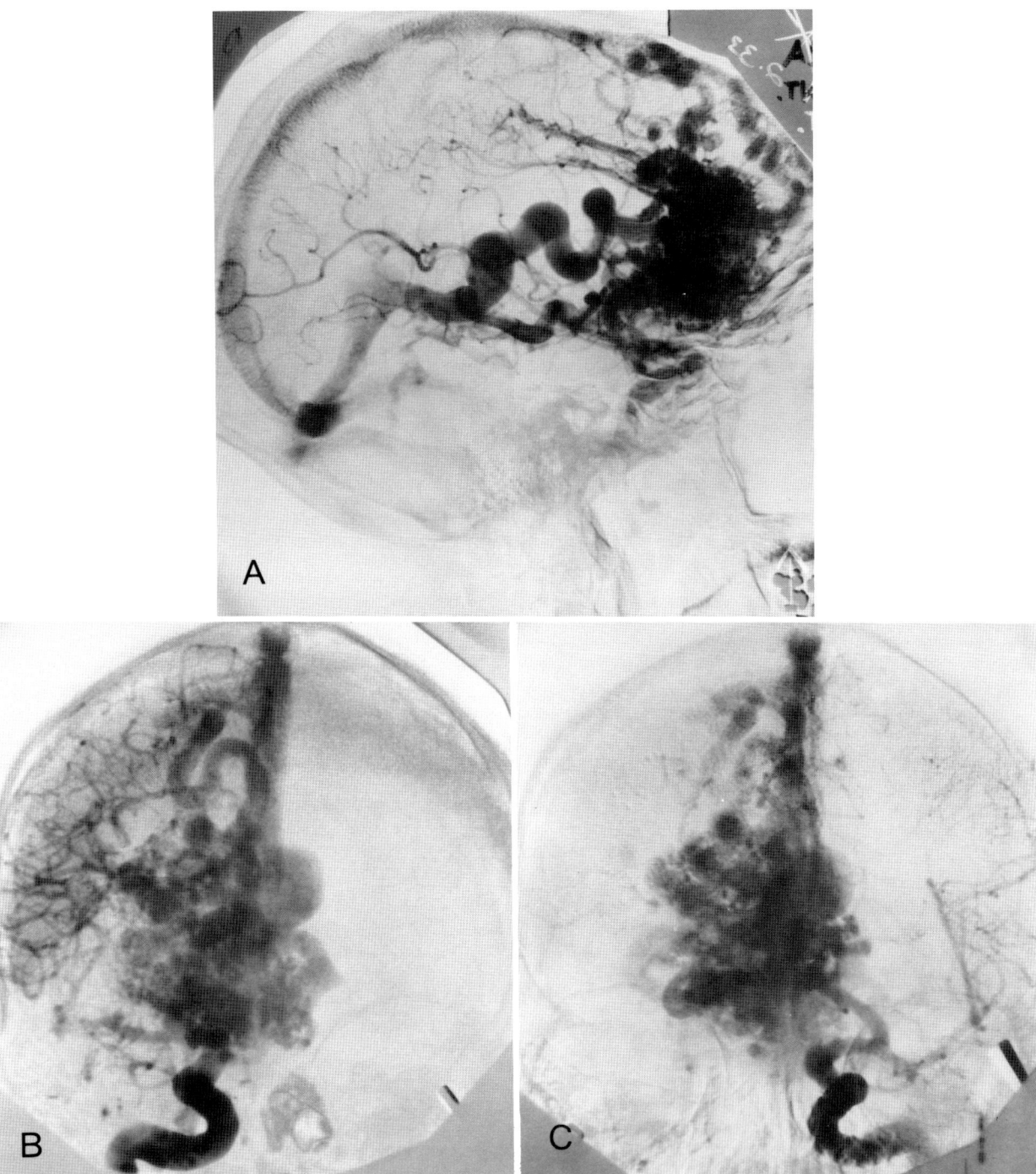

Figure 22.21. Anterior callosal and frontal AVM. This young man had an intractable seizure disorder. **A–C,** Preoperative angiogram. Even though the lesion appears to involve the left frontal lobe (**B** and **C**), the lesion is actually restricted to the right frontal lobe even though loops of the AVM protrude into the left. The lesion was resected in a single stage but the operation lasted approximately 24 hours. A combined bifrontal and right pterional bone flap was used to allow parasagittal control of the pericallosal vessels and intraventricular dissection of the portion of the AVM on the caudate nucleus. The pterional exposure was used for control of the branches from the anterior communicating complex and for dissection of the subfrontal portion of the AVM. **D** and **E,** The postoperative angiogram shows complete resection of the lesion. The right A_1 segment was sacrificed after confirmation of a patent anterior communicating complex supplied from the left A_1 segment. There is good filling of both pericallosal arteries from the left (**E**). The patient initially had some problems with electrolyte balance due to hypothalamic damage but this cleared within 2 weeks. He was intact neurologically otherwise, and he has only had two seizures during the ensuing 4 years.

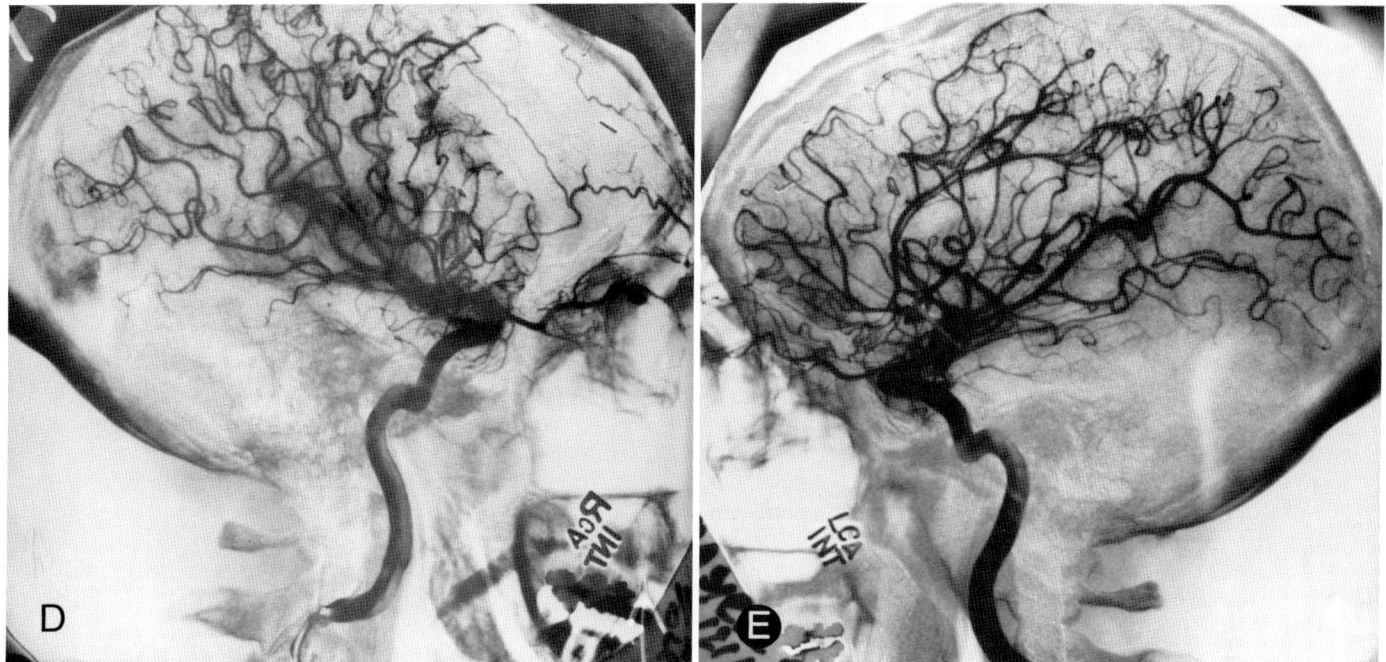

Figure 22.21D and E.

AVMs (9, 86, 100, 102, 129, 158). The lesions that have been removed successfully have been small AVMs located either on the surface of the brain stem, in the cerebellopontine angle, in the floor of the fourth ventricle, or in the region of the quadrigeminal plate.

Lesions of the lateral surface of the brain stem located at the cerebellopontine angle can be approached with the same lateral suboccipital exposure used for acoustic neuromas. More superior lesions of the mesencephalum can be approached subtemporally.

Lesions of the floor of the fourth ventricle can be approached by a standard midline suboccipital exposure with the patient either prone or semi-sitting. The lesion is readily visualized upon spreading the cerebellar tonsils. The problem is that most of these lesions are intimately related to the sixth nerve nucleus, the lateral gaze center, and the genu of the seventh nerve. Therefore, unless the patient has already had a hemorrhage producing the expected deficits in this region, it is very likely that a new neurologic deficit will be present after surgery (Fig. 22.26).

AVMs of the area of the tectum can be operated by the supracerebellar subtentorial approach that is used for pineal region tumors (Fig. 22.27A and B) or through a paraoccipital transtentorial approach (7, 148). The supracerebellar subtentorial approach is preferred because there is better access to circum-mesencephalic branches and because these lesions are usually located below rather than anterior to the vein of Galen. Sometimes the lesion is not obvious in the surface but an arterialized vein may lead directly to it (Fig. 22.28).

Cerebellar AVMs

AVMs of the cerebellum usually present with hemorrhage but at times progressive ataxia develops either from a "steal" phenomenon or from venous hypertension in the posterior fossa. Hydrocephalus is another presentation and is usually caused by mechanical distortion of the aqueduct by dilated arterialized veins.

When the AVM is restricted to one cerebellar hemisphere, a unilateral suboccipital approach is sufficient. The deeper midline lesions involving the vermis and deep nuclei medially and/or the cerebellar peduncle and lateral brain stem more laterally are difficult (Figs. 22.29 and 22.30). The preferred exposure for these lesions is a large bilateral suboccipital craniectomy with the patient in the sitting position (9, 158) (Fig. 22.27). With the patient in this position, the cerebellum falls away by its own weight after dividing the draining veins that hold it superiorly to the tentorium (Fig. 22.27B) (158). These veins can usually be taken because there is almost always prominent venous drainage from the AVM anteriorly by the precentral cerebellar vein and related tributaries to the vein of Galen. Lesions of the vermis are almost invariably supplied by superior cerebellar artery branches that can be identified as they turn around the mesencephalon to pass from the ambient cistern to the cistern of the quadrigeminal plate (150). When one sees over the surface of the cerebellum abnormally enlarged branches that penetrate the anterior cerebellar parenychma in the region of the AVM, one can take these branches with safety since by this time the important mesencephalic branches have already been given. The authors prefer to do this part of the operation first by just opening the superior dural flap to keep the cerebellum from "falling out" as one depresses the cerebellum to look in front.

Once the superior aspect of the lesion has been devascularized, attention is turned to the posterior inferior cerebellar arteries. After opening the dura inferiorly with a vertical incision along the midline, the posterior inferior cerebellar arteries can be identified medially between the tonsils of the cerebellum by gently spreading the tonsils with self-retaining retractors. They are followed upward to the choroidal loop and possible branches to the AVM can be identified at that point. Any significant branches beyond the choroidal loop can be taken if they are presumed to go to the AVM because the important branches of the posterior inferior cerebellar arteries to the brain stem and to the deep cerebellar nuclei have been given off. The floor of the ventricle must then be exposed to define the medial plane of the malformation if it is predominantly located to one side.

Once the malformation is isolated medially from the posterior inferior cerebellar arteries, the authors like to come laterally to the cerebellopontine angle and look for branches of the anterior inferior cerebellar artery coming to the lateral recess of the fourth ventricle. One then returns to the midline and develops the posterior plane of the AVM, the lateral plane, and finally the anterior plane. In the anterolateral aspect of the AVM, small fragile vessels coming across the cerebellar peduncle can be quite troublesome.

Deep cerebellar lesions confined mostly to one cerebellar hemisphere can be removed without a resulting major neurologic deficit (Fig. 22.29). When the lesion is bilateral, however, there is no way to avoid some degree of permanent ataxia from damage to the cerebellar nuclear complex bilaterally (Fig. 22.30). Therefore, one must be very conservative in advising surgery for these large bilateral lesions un-

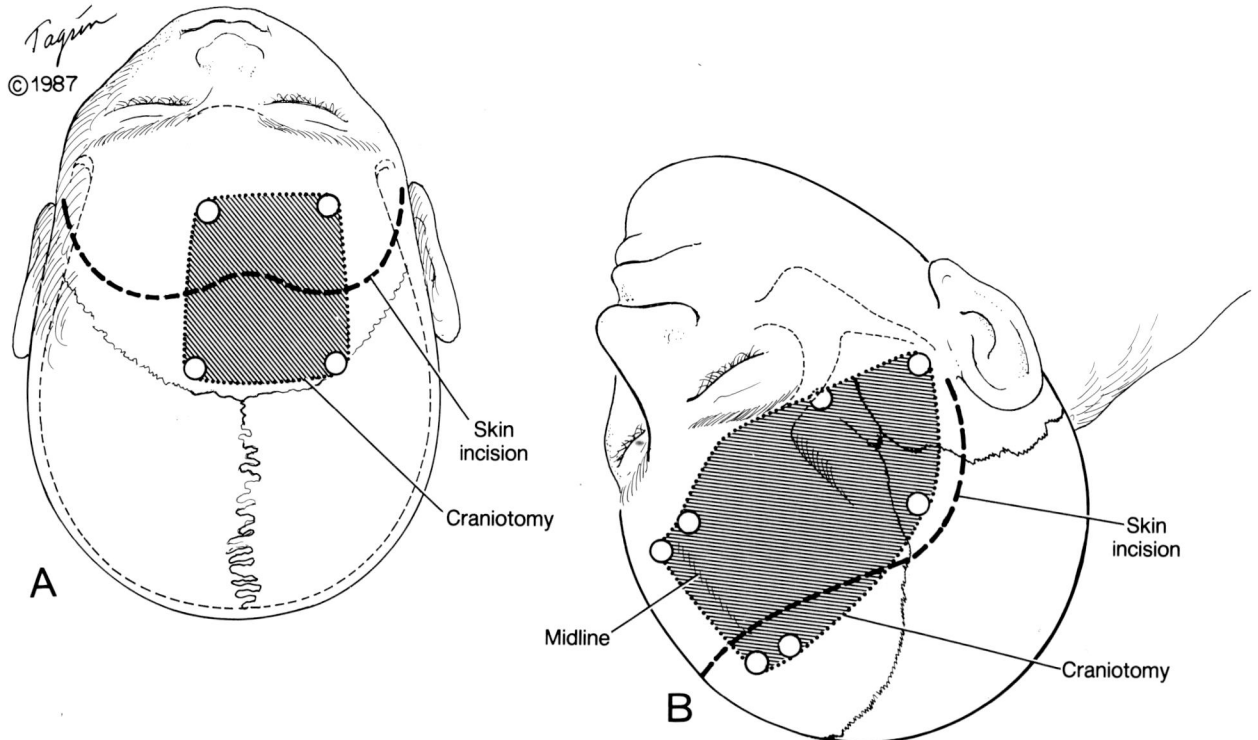

Figure 22.22. Anterior callosal AVMs. **A**, Bicoronal skin incision and right frontal bone flap extending to the left of the midline. This flap can be used for anterior callosal AVMs that do not extend into the deep subfrontal region. **B**, Combined right pterional and frontal bone flap extending to the left of the midline. This flap is useful for anterior callosal AVMs that extend into the deep subfrontal region and have significant blood supply from the anterior communicating artery complex and proximal A_2 segments of the anterior cerebral arteries.

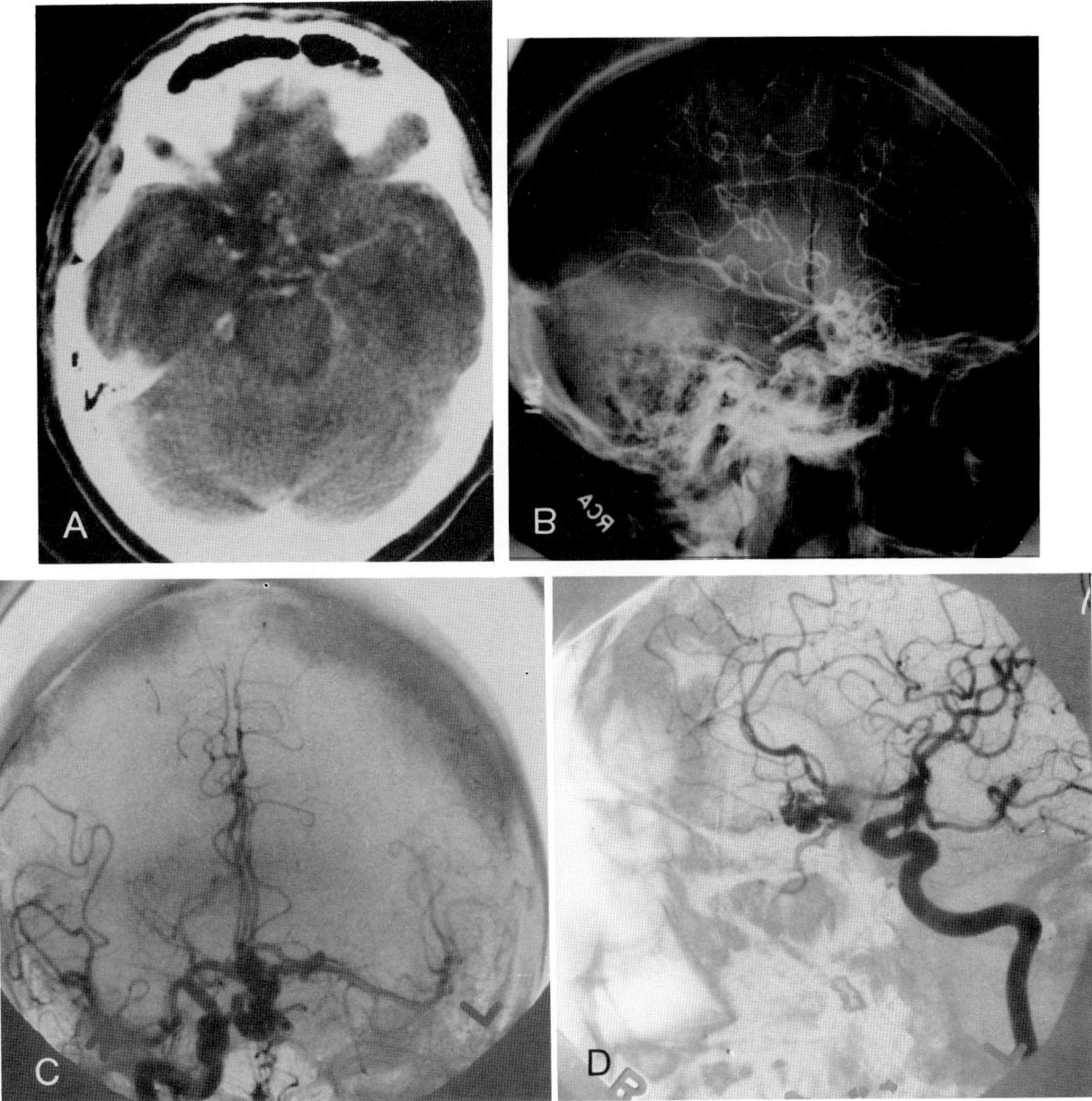

Figure 22.23. Subfrontal AVM. This middle-aged man had significant difficulties with personality and judgment secondary to a large frontal hemorrhage several months prior to admission. **A,** Initial CT scan. **B–D,** On the angiogram the lesion was best seen with the left oblique cartoid injection (**D**). **E,** A very early film of the arterial phase showed clearly the two large feeders from the malformation (*solid arrows*) and their relation to the two A_2 segments (*open arrows*). Such an early arterial film is invaluable in planning operative resection. The lesion was removed without difficulty by a right pterional approach with complete dissection of the anterior communicating artery complex and early division of the two large branches to the AVM. **F** and **G,** Postoperative angiogram confirms complete resection.

less the patient has a neurologic deficit or has bled repeatedly. The exception to this may be in younger patients who have a very substantial capacity to compensate for their ataxia. Sometimes it is very difficult to be sure that some of these deeper lesions do not involve the brain stem. When they do disabling neurologic deficits may result from resection (Fig. 22.31). For such lesions conservative treatment or proton beam therapy may be preferable. In the future the MRI scan may be helpful in demonstrating better the degree of brain stem extension.

An interesting adjunct to surgery of large posterior fossa lesions has been suggested by Suzuki and collaborators (170). They used temporary balloon occlusion of the basilar artery and its branches combined with mannitol, perfluorochemicals and vitamin E, a free radical "scavenger," to achieve some degree of brain protection, in order to facilitate removal of a large cerebellar AVM. The authors have had no experience with this method and would not recommend it for general use.

SURGICAL RESULTS

Surgical results will be discussed only briefly since statistics have restricted meaning for a surgeon faced

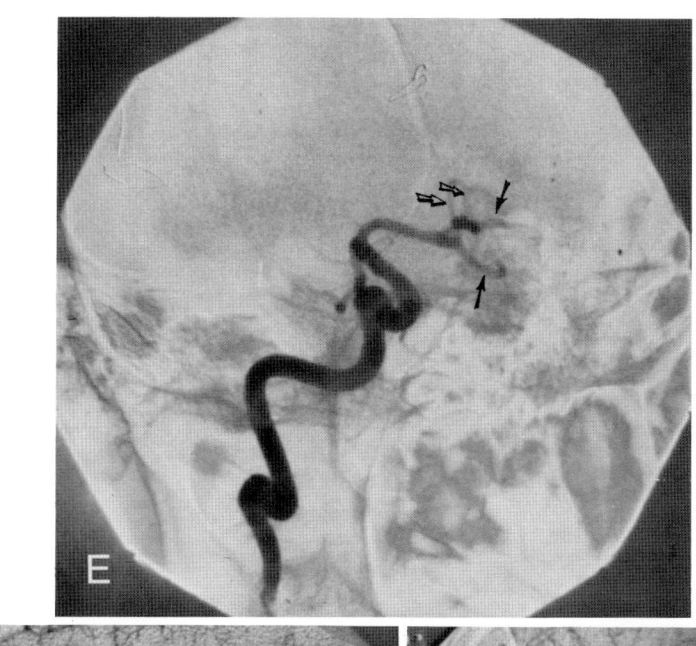

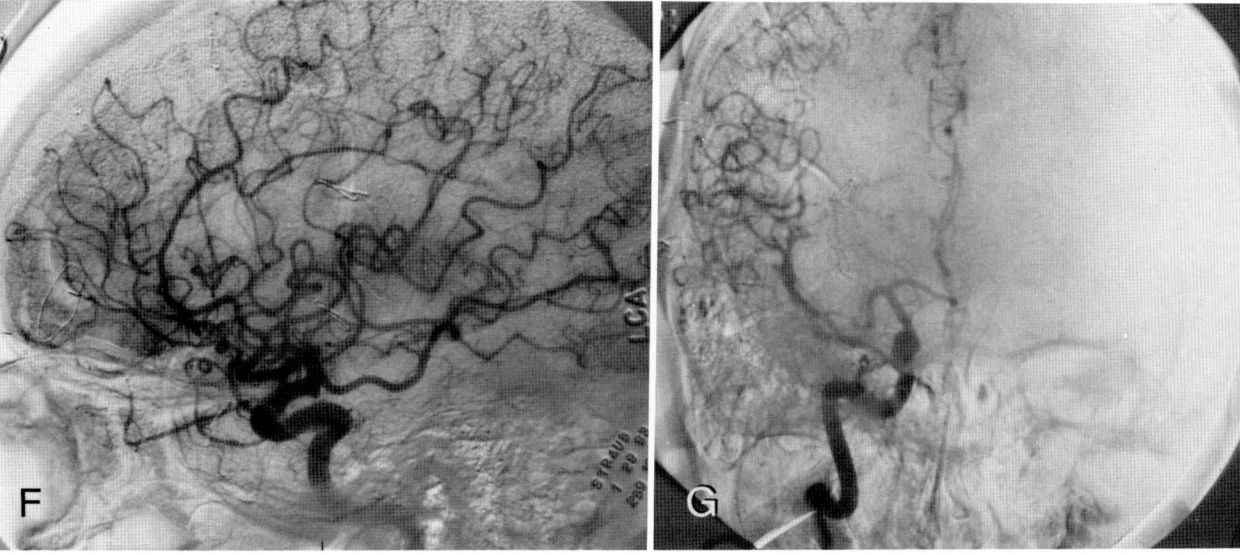

Figure 22.23E–G.

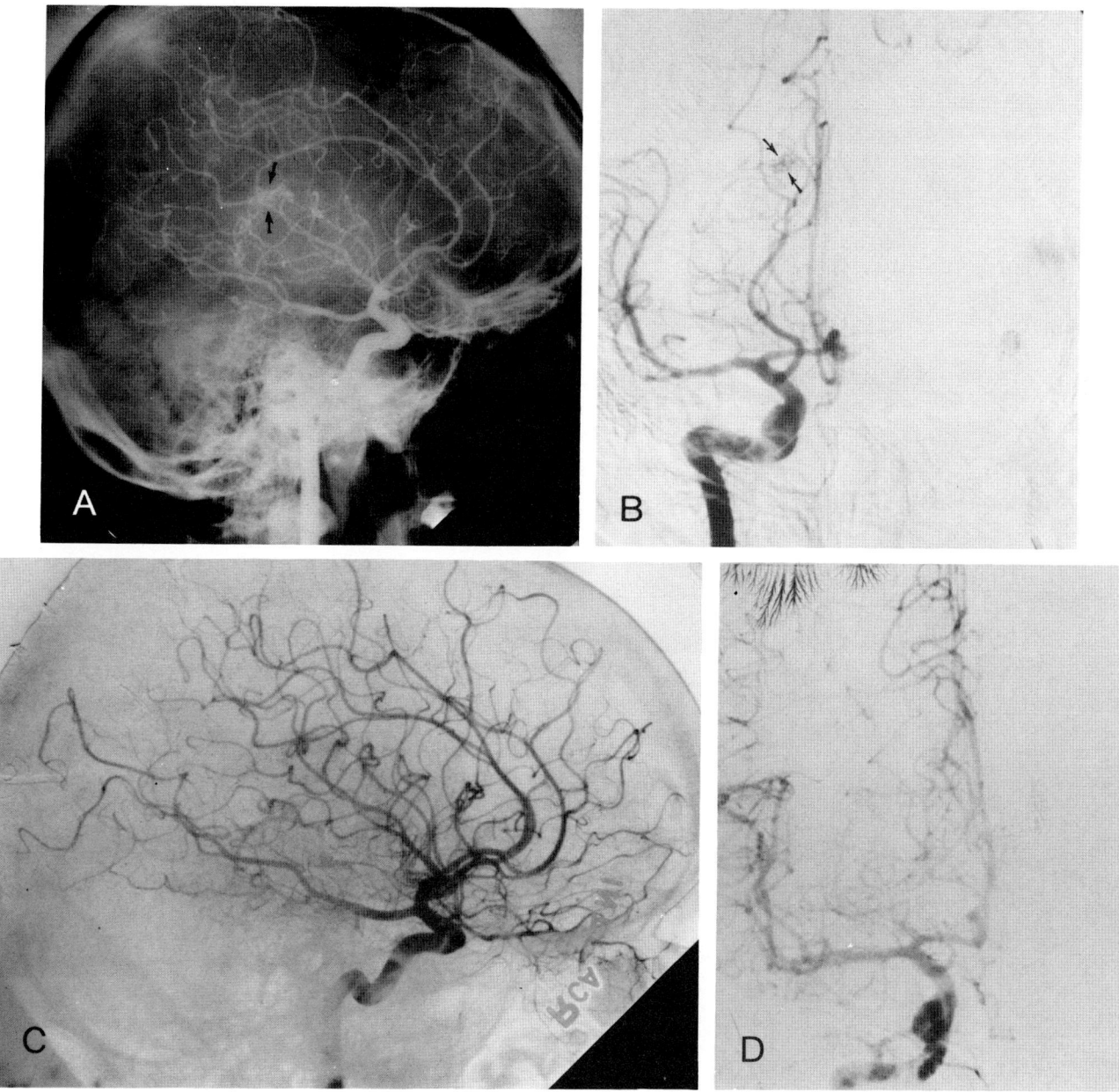

Figure 22.24. Subsplenial AVM in a young man who had suffered three intraventricular hemorrhages. **A** and **B**, The AVM is seen (*arrows*). Initially the location of the lesion was misinterpreted and it was approached through the atrium of the lateral ventricle. No evidence of the lesion in this location was found. From a parasagittal direction the splenum was divided over a length of about 1 cm. The lesion was located to the right of midline in the subsplenial region in the area of the tela choroidea of the roof of the third ventricle. The lesion was then cauterized and excised without difficulty. **C** and **D**, Postoperative angiogram showed no residual AVM. The patient had no deficit from the operation.

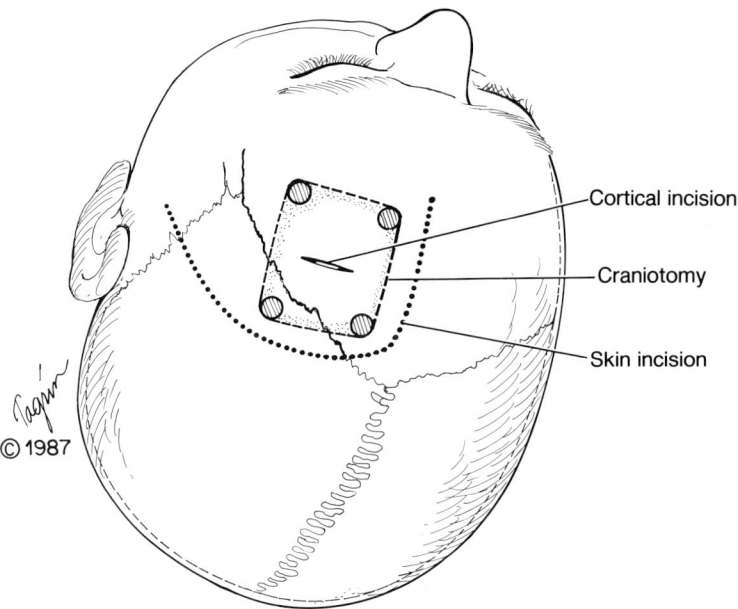

Figure 22.25. Intraventricular AVM. Left frontal craniotomy for transcortical approach to the anterior aspect of the left lateral ventricle.

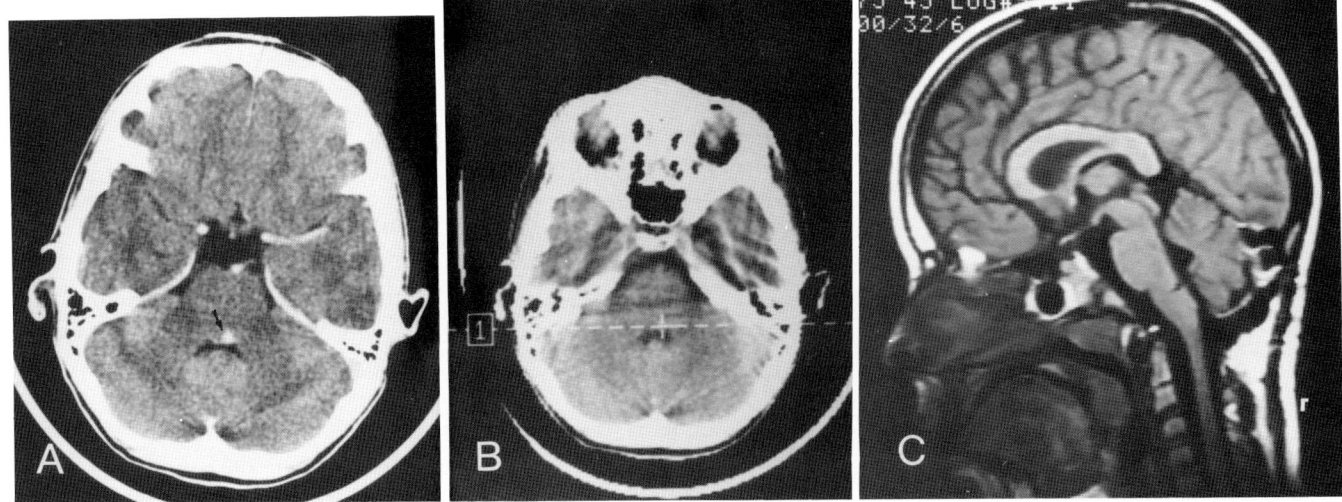

Figure 22.26. Brain stem AVM. This 13-year-old boy presented with a partial left abducens palsy and a moderately severe left facial paralysis of abrupt onset. The angiogram was normal. **A**, The CT scan shows a small parenchymal hemorrhage in the floor of the fourth ventricle (*arrow*). MRI was not available at the time. The patient was explored and abnormal blood vessels were seen to go into the substance of the pons. The authors chose not to pursue these abnormal vessels for fear of producing a serious neurologic deficit (by the time of the operation the patient had recovered almost completely). Subsequently, the patient was given proton beam therapy. Six months thereafter he started to deteriorate again in a progressive fashion without a history to suggest recurrent hemorrhage. Radiation necrosis was suspected; however, neither **B**, the CT scan, nor **C**, the MRI scan, show definite evidence of radiation necrosis.

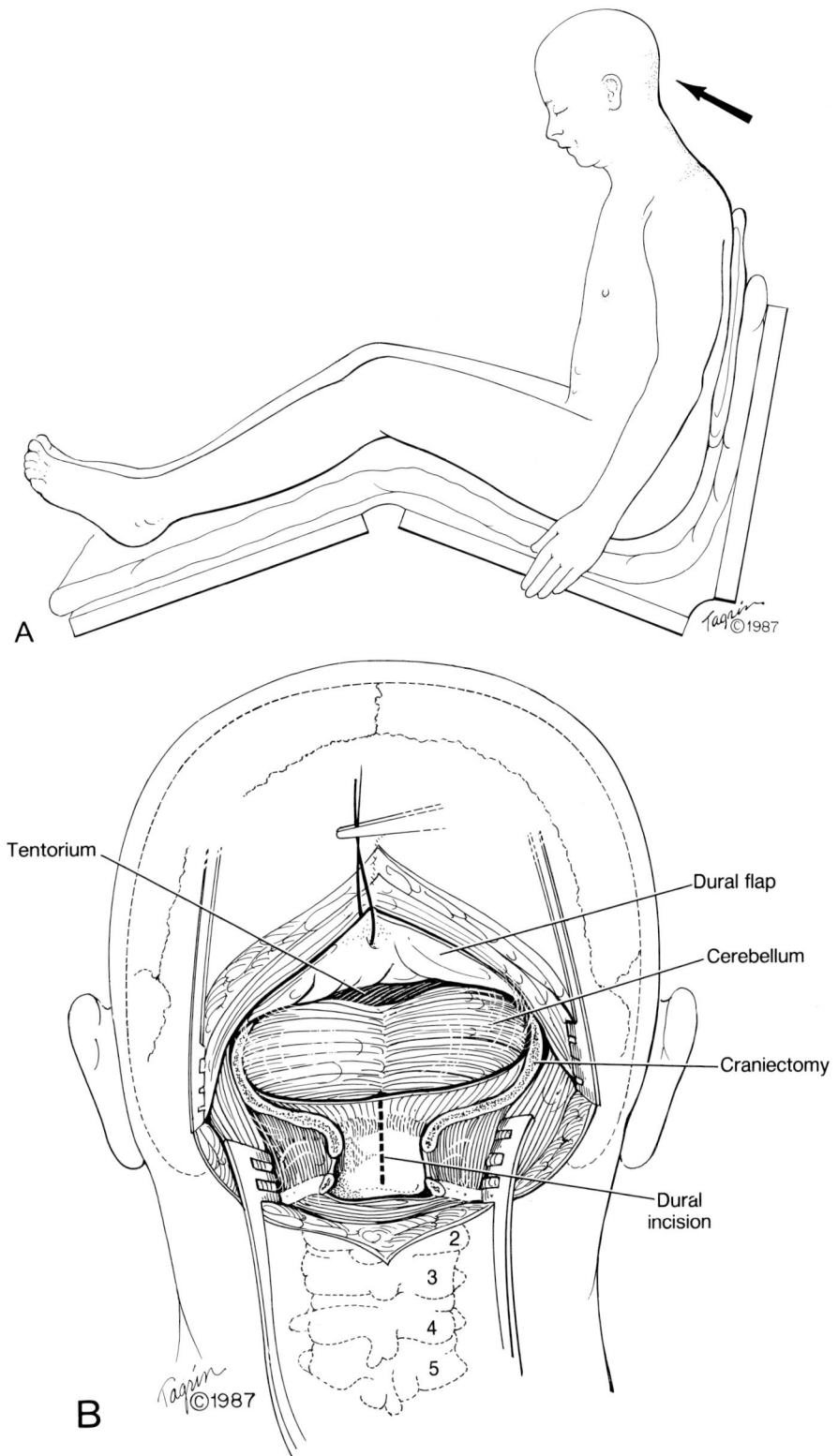

Figure 22.27. Cerebellar AVMs. **A**, Position used for most cerebellar AVMs and **B**, Craniotomy used for cerebellar AVMs that have blood supply from the three major arterial territories of the posterior circulation. With this exposure the surgeon has ready access to the superior cerebellar artery supply (supracerebellar, infratentorial approach), to the anterior inferior cerebellar artery supply (at the cerebellopontine angle), and to the posterior inferior cerebellar artery supply (by working inferiorly between the tonsils of the cerebellum). It is useful to remove the arch of the C_1 for the later aspect of the operation but it is preferable to approach the superior cerebellar artery supply initially over the cerebullum without opening the dura inferiorly in the midline. Otherwise the cerebellum tends to herniate through the dural opening. The same position can be used for access to the tectum and pineal region but in these cases it is not necessary to carry the craniotomy as far laterally or inferiorly and it is not necessary to remove C_1 or open the dura inferiorly.

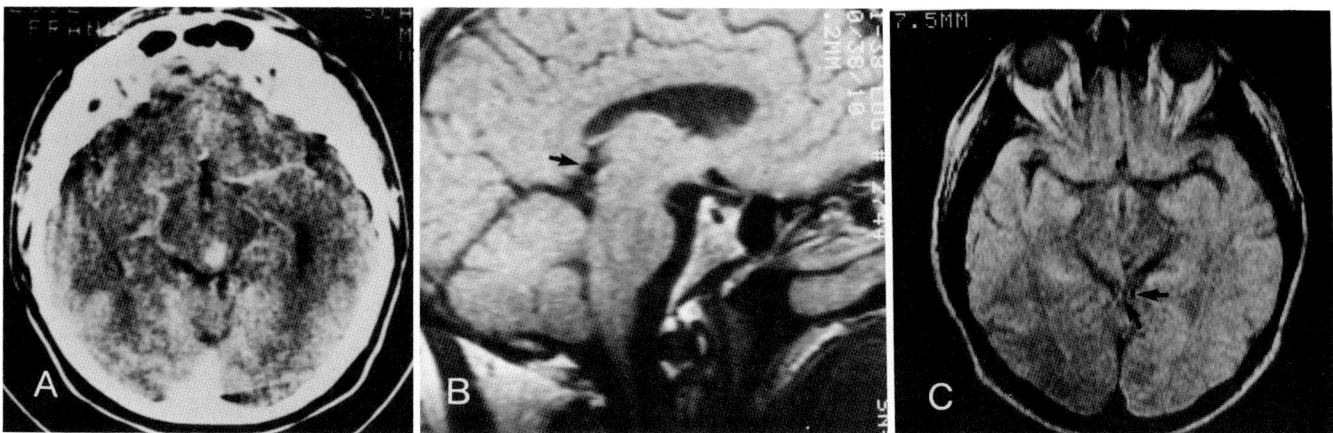

Figure 22.28. Brain stem AVM. This patient had two previous hemorrhages. **A**, CT scans showing a small lesion in the left side of the tectum of the mesencephalon. The angiogram was negative except for a questionable early draining vein. **B** and **C**, The MRI showed small areas of signal void compatible with blood flow in an AVM (*arrow*). The lesion was approached by a supracerebellar infratentorial exposure. The AVM was not obvious on the surface but an arterialized vein could be followed right to the lesion which was only about 0.5 cm from the surface. After coagulation of the AVM, the arterialized vein became blue. No postoperative angiography has been obtained since the preoperative angiogram did not show the lesion. The patient's pre-existing partial Parinaud's syndrome improved slightly over the ensuing several weeks. He had no other neurologic deficit from the surgery.

with a particular patient with an AVM. In one series, for example, combined morbidity and mortality of lesions of less than 4 cm was 4% and for lesions larger than 4 cm, it was 66.5% (94). In another series combined morbidity and mortality rate of "good risk" patients was 10.5% and in "poor risk" patients, the rate was 62% (41). Overall results give only an indication of the seriousness of this kind of surgery. Table 22.2 gives the overall morbidity and mortality figures for most of the large series reported since 1978. Pooled average morbidity is about 9% and the average mortality about 6%. Each surgeon must carefully evaluate all factors including personal operative experience, when recommending treatment for an individual patient with an AVM.

In order to make comparison more meaningful and to help surgeons predict morbidity, Luessenhop and Gennarelli have suggestd a grading scheme of I–IV

Table 22.2.
AVMs—Modern Surgical Results[a]

Year	Author (Reference)	No. of Cases	Morbidity	Mortality
1978	Cophignon et al (24)	45	?	4 (8.5%)
1978	Mingrino (111)	98	2 (2%)	4 (4.1%)
1979	Drake[b] (41)	106	5 (4.8%)	6 (5.7%)
1979	Nornes et al (125)	63	2 (3.2%)	3 (4.7%)
1979	Wilson et al (198)	83	21 (25.3%)	4 (4.8%)
1980	Pellettieri et al (130)	116	18 (15.5%)	6 (5.2%)
1980	Stein and Wolpert (167)	55	3 (10%)	1 (2%)
1980	Guidetti and Delitala[b] (56)	92	6 (6.3%)	3 (3.2%)
1980	Parkinson and Bachers (127)	90	18 (20%)	10 (11%)
1982	Albert[b] (2)	140	?	10 (7%)
1982	Suzuki et al (169)	173	8 (4.6%)	8 (4.6%)
1984	Luessenhop and Rasa (94)	90	10 (11%)	2 (2.2%)
1984	Fults and Kelly (48)	48	3 (6.2)	9 (18.8%)
1985	Adelt et al (1)	43	3 (7%)	3 (7%)
1985	Davis and Symon (27)	69	6 (8.7%)	1 (1.5%)
1985	Jomin et al (69)	128	6 (8.5%)	16 (12.5%)
1986	Heros and Tu (63)	103	16 (15.5%)[b]	1 (0.9%)

[a] Modified from Heros RC, Tu YK: Unruptured arteriovenous malformations. A dilemma in surgical decision making. *Clin Neurosurg* 33:187–236, 1986; and Is surgical therapy needed for unruptured arteriovenous malformations? *Neurology* 37:279–286, 1987.
[b] Includes all new permanent postoperative neurologic deficits, many of which were visual field deficits. Disabling morbidity was only 2.9%.

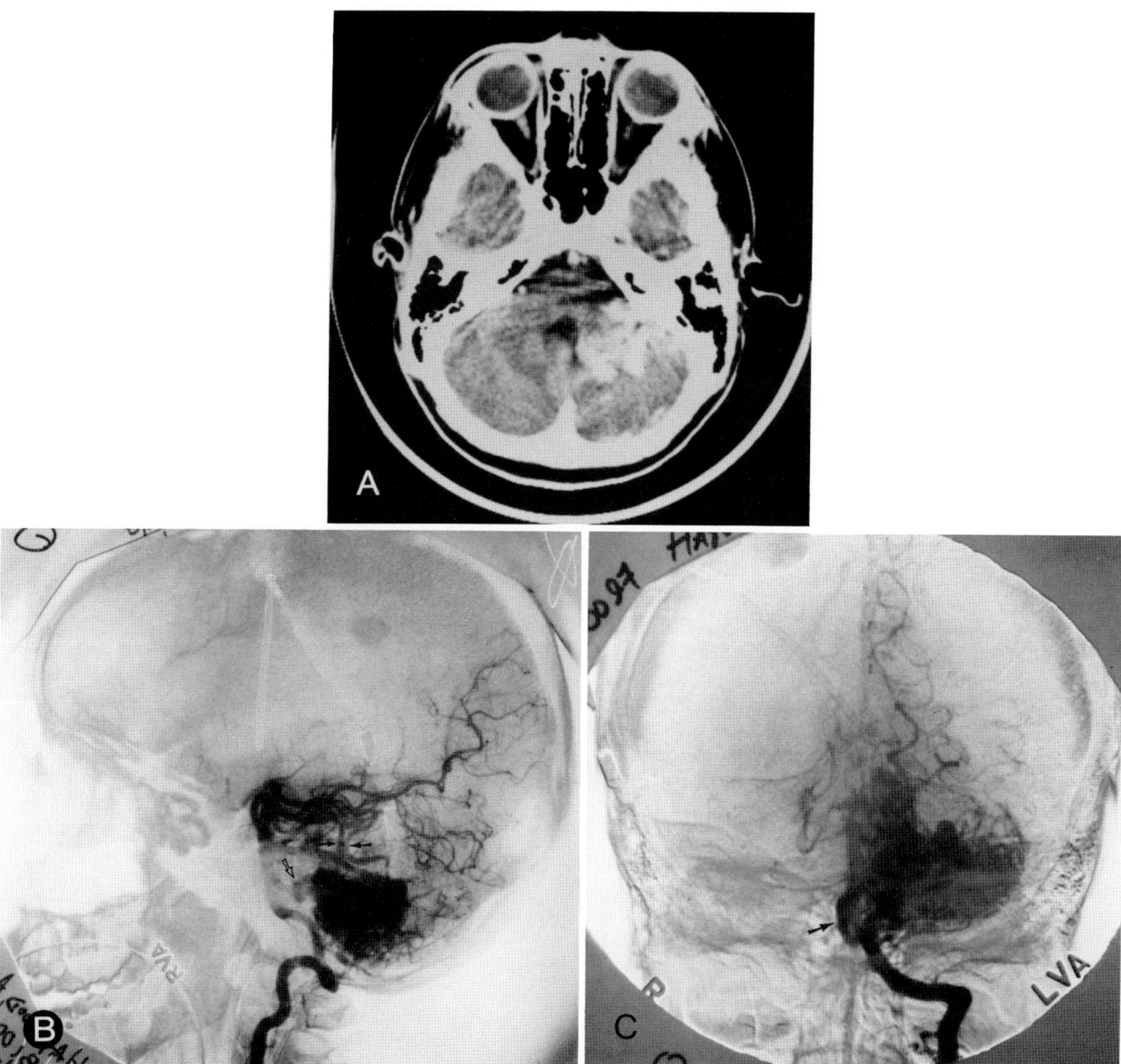

Figure 22.29. Cerebellar AVM. **A**, This 35-year-old man presented with a posterior fossa hemorrhage. **B** and **C**, The lesion was fed by superior cerebellar artery branches (*solid arrows* on **B**), anterior inferior cerebellar artery branches (*open arrow* on **B**), and posterior inferior cerebellar artery branches (*arrow* on **C**). The lesion was removed through a bilateral occipital craniotomy as described in the text. **D** and **E**, Postoperative angiogram confirmed complete resection of the lesion. The patient was unchanged neurologically by the procedure.

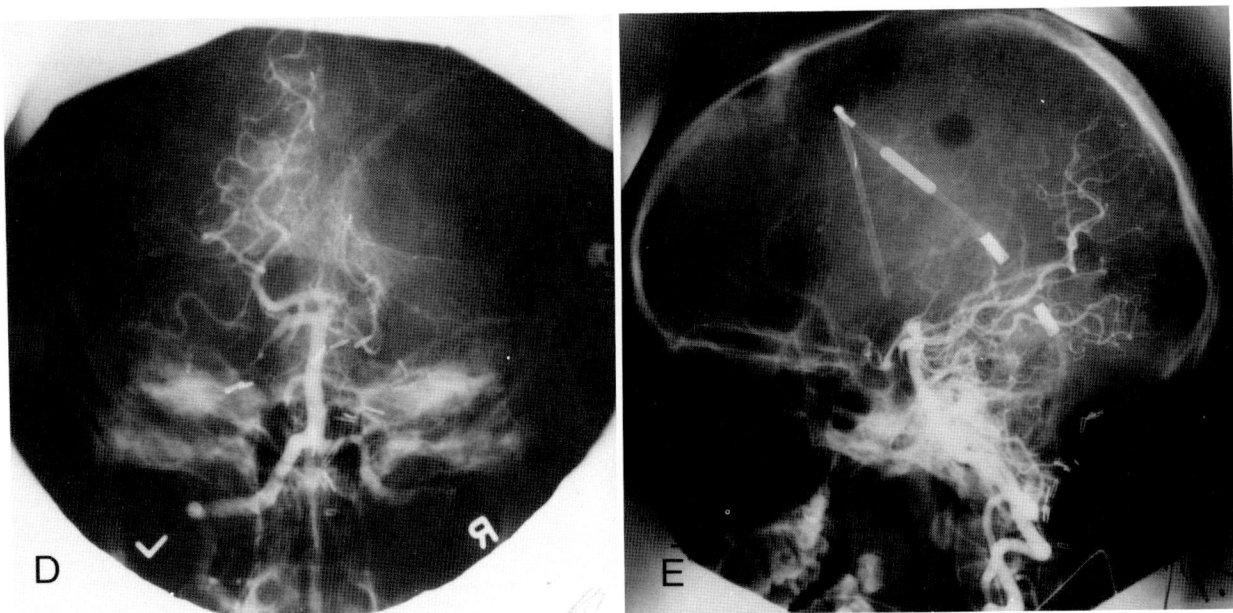

Figure 22.29D and E.

to predict surgical difficulty for total obliteration of an AVM (91). The grading system is based on the number of "named" arteries feeding the AVM. This grading system correlates with the size of the AVM, since the larger the AVM, the more branches will feed it. More recently Spetzler and Martin have suggested another grading system which depends on size, location, and deep drainage to predict risk (160). The reported correlation with surgical outcome coincides with the authors' experience.

The authors have reported a series of 103 patients operated within the past 5 years with a morbidity of 15.5% and a mortality of 0.9% (one patient) (63). The major (disabling) morbidity rate was 2.9% (three patients). The patient who died was a middle-aged gentleman with a history of heavy drinking who developed hepatic failure postoperatively. The 16 cases with morbidity include seven patients who had varying degrees of hemiparesis and/or dysphasia. Two of these patients remain incapacitated but the rest have been able to resume a useful occupation. Another patient remains incapacitated because of a severe lateral medullary syndrome as a result of resection of his deep cerebellar AVM which extended into the lateral medulla. Another patient with a giant AVM treated with multiple embolizations and surgical procedures remains relatively incapacitated because of persistent headaches and seizures (Fig. 22.32). The rest of the patients with morbidity had only visual field defects and all are back to their previous occupation. In reporting these results the condition of the patient at last follow-up was considered, usually four or more months after surgery. Temporary postoperative morbidity which resolved in time was not counted as permanent morbidity. The appearance of postoperative epilepsy in a few patients is not reported as permanent morbidity since the problem has been well-controlled without significant disability. Many patients who presented with preoperative epilepsy were improved in their seizure control. All patients in this series except one were treated with complete excision of the malformation. The one exception is the patient who was treated with multiple embolization procedures, some of them at open craniotomy (Fig. 22.32). She still has a small amount of malformation left in the thalamus. All but five patients have had postoperative angiography and in every instance, the angiogram has confirmed complete excision of the malformation. In addition to the one patient who died, two patients have not had postoperative angiography because of poor neurologic condition. The other two patients who did not have postoperative angiography had small AVMs of the brain stem that were not well visualized before surgery.

Since the above series was reported, the authors have operated on an additional 21 patients with cerebral AVMs. One patient with a large parasagittal lesion remains incapacitated with a severe hemiparesis and moderate aphasia (Fig. 22.19). Another patient suffered an incomplete hemianopsia after the removal of a lesion of the region of the right atrium (Fig. 22.12). The rest of the patients have done well.

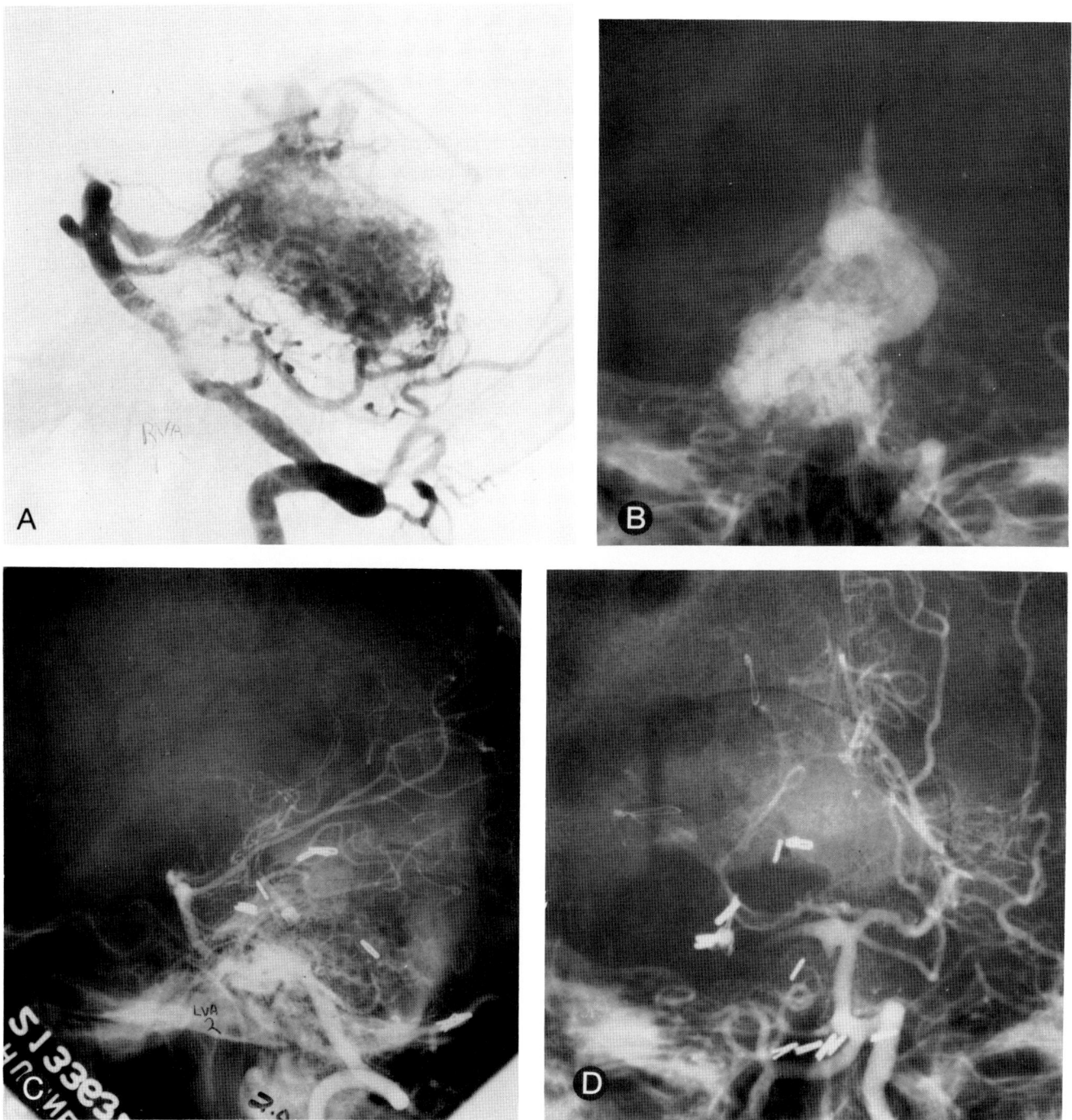

Figure 22.30. Cerebellar AVM. **A** and **B**, A large midline and right cerebellar hemisphere AVM is demonstrated. **C** and **D**, Postoperative angiogram shows no evidence of the AVM. This patient had a history of seven subarachnoid hemorrhages which had left a significant neurologic deficit, but he was still able to make decisions about his business. After operation he resumed his previous level of activity. The only new difficulty was an increase in difficulty with swallowing due to incoordination.

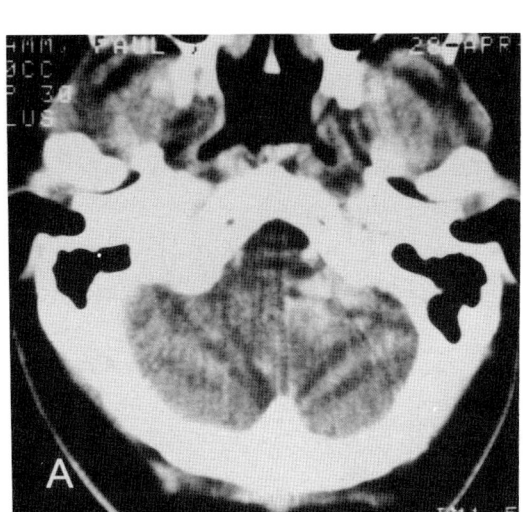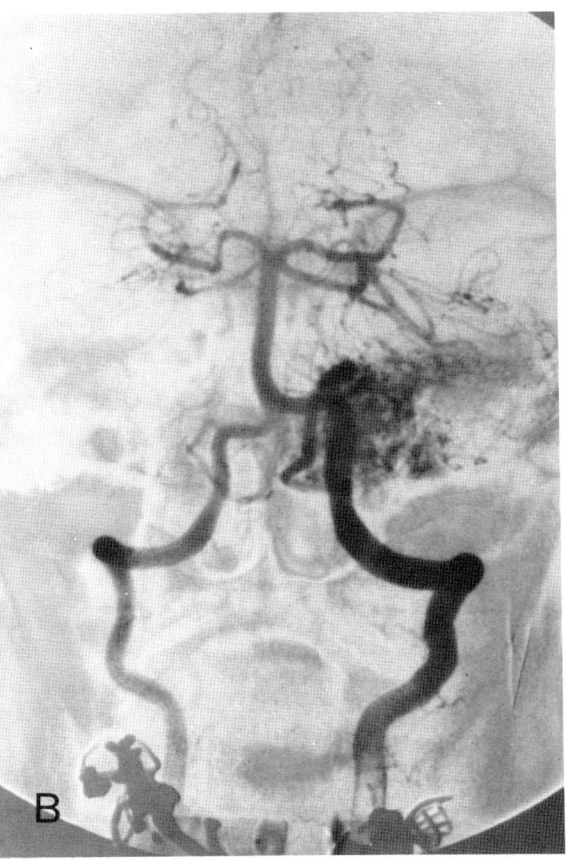

Figure 22.31. Cerebellar AVM. **A** and **B**, This 52-year-old man presented with a hemorrhage that resembled very much the lesion shown in Figure 22.29. At surgery, however, the lesion extended through the cerebellar peduncle into the lateral aspect of the medulla which had not been predicted from the preoperative studies. In that area considerable bleeding was encountered from small fragile parenchymal vessels that retracted upon attempted coagulation. As a result of the resection, the patient has very serious neurologic disabilities including difficulty with swallowing, hoarseness, severe ataxia, numbness of the face, and constant dizziness. An MRI, which was not available at the time, might have been helpful in predicting the extension of the lesion into the brain stem which would have dissuaded recommending excision.

OTHER TREATMENT MODALITIES

Embolization

Embolization of intracranial AVMs was introduced by Luessenhop (89). Since then this technique has been used widely both as primary treatment and more frequently as a preparatory treatment to facilitate surgical excision. Initially embolization was done by introducing Silastic spheres of different size into the carotid and vertebral arteries in the neck ("flow guided" embolization) (32 89, 92, 93). This technique depends on the fact that blood flows primarily to the malformation if the sphere is injected in the corresponding arterial territory. The choice of size of spheres is critical and it depends on the size of the feeding vessels. In general it is difficult for the spheres to negotiate sharp curves, such as those encountered at the take off of the anterior cerebral artery, and spheres usually will not take a right-angle turn as required for embolization of lenticulostriate or perforating vessels. The spheres usually lodge in the feeding vessel and do not occlude the nidus of the malformation. Smaller particles can be injected using the flow guidance technique and some obliteration of the nidus of the malformation can be achieved with this technique (109, 165, 199).

Embolization with polymers that can be injected in liquid form and solidify upon contact with blood has been developed (32, 82, 85, 149, 151, 187). These polymers can only be used if a catheter can be navigated into the feeders of the malformation (or alternatively, by direct surgical catheterization). Sophisticated intravascular navigation to place small catheters right into the feeders has been developed (31–33, 72, 137, 156). Occasionally, an AVM may be completely obliterated by this method. As an adjunct to surgery, embolization may reduce the risk of perfusion breakthrough after resection of very large lesions.

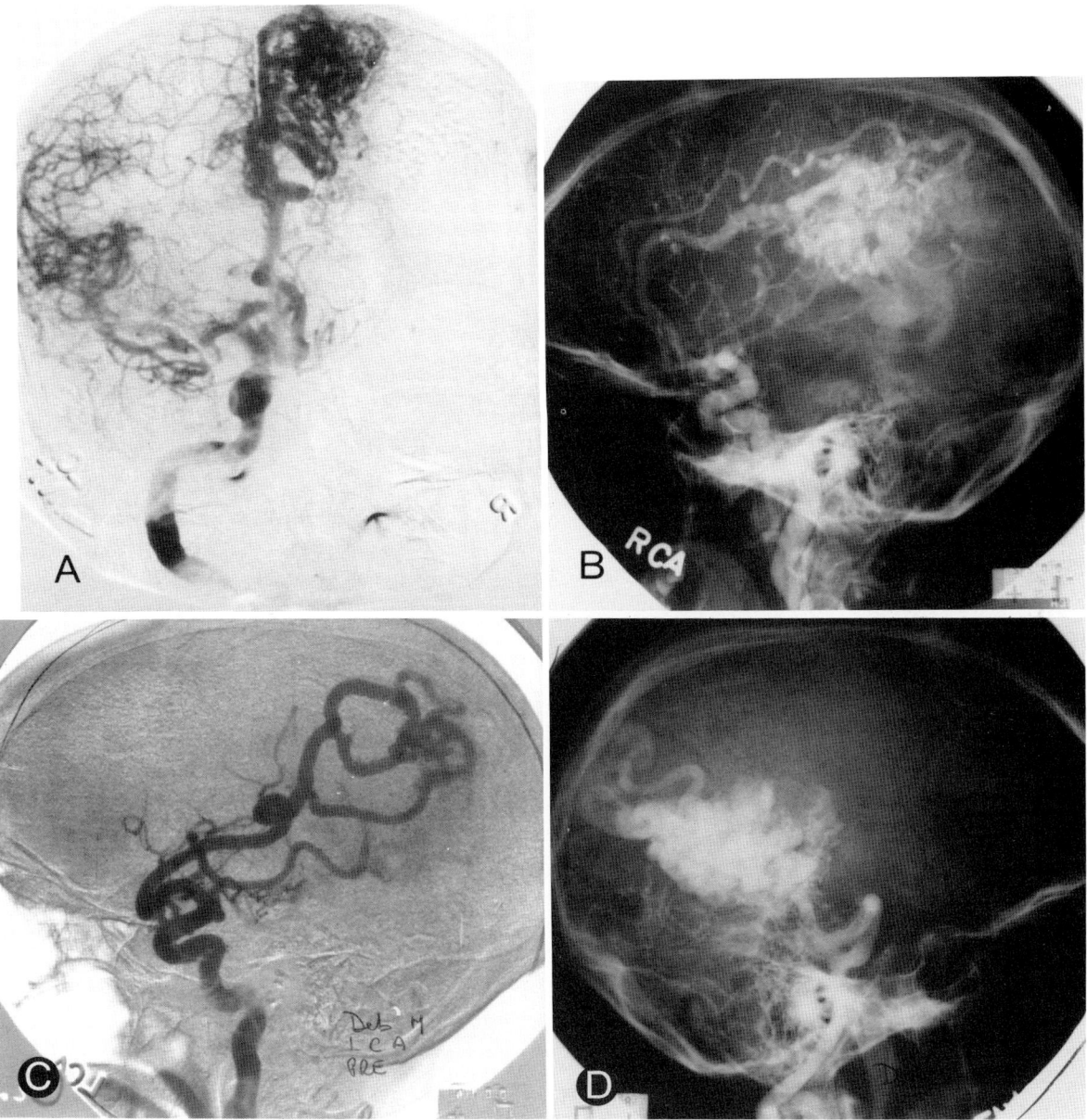

Figure 22.32. Large cerebral convexity AVM. This teenager presented with progressive, incapacitating headaches and seizures. She had never had a known intracranial hemorrhage. **A–D,** The left sided AVM is fed by pericallosal branches (**A** and **B**), middle cerebral artery branches (**C**), and posterior cerebral artery branches (**D**). The lesion was initially treated with embolization in three stages. The pericallosal supply was embolized percutaneously and then several middle cerebral branches were catheterized and embolized directly at open craniotomy. Finally, the posterior cerebral artery, distal to the posterolateral choroidal arteries, was catheterized and embolized. **E–G,** The result of these multiple embolizations shows that most of the AVM is occluded except for a deep thalamic portion fed by posterolateral choroidal branches as well as thalamoperforating branches. In spite of this apparently successful subtotal embolization, the patient's headaches have continued and her seizure disorder is worse than pre-embolization. She also has had at least one subarachnoid hemorrhage since embolization. She has a complete hemianopsia as a result of embolization of the posterior cerebral artery. A partial explanation for her continuing severe headaches may be the development of prominent external carotid supply to the lesion (**H** and **I**). Subsequently, some of this supply has been embolized percutaneously and surgically with some improvement in her headaches. Retrospectively, one must wonder whether this patient might not have been better treated conservatively.

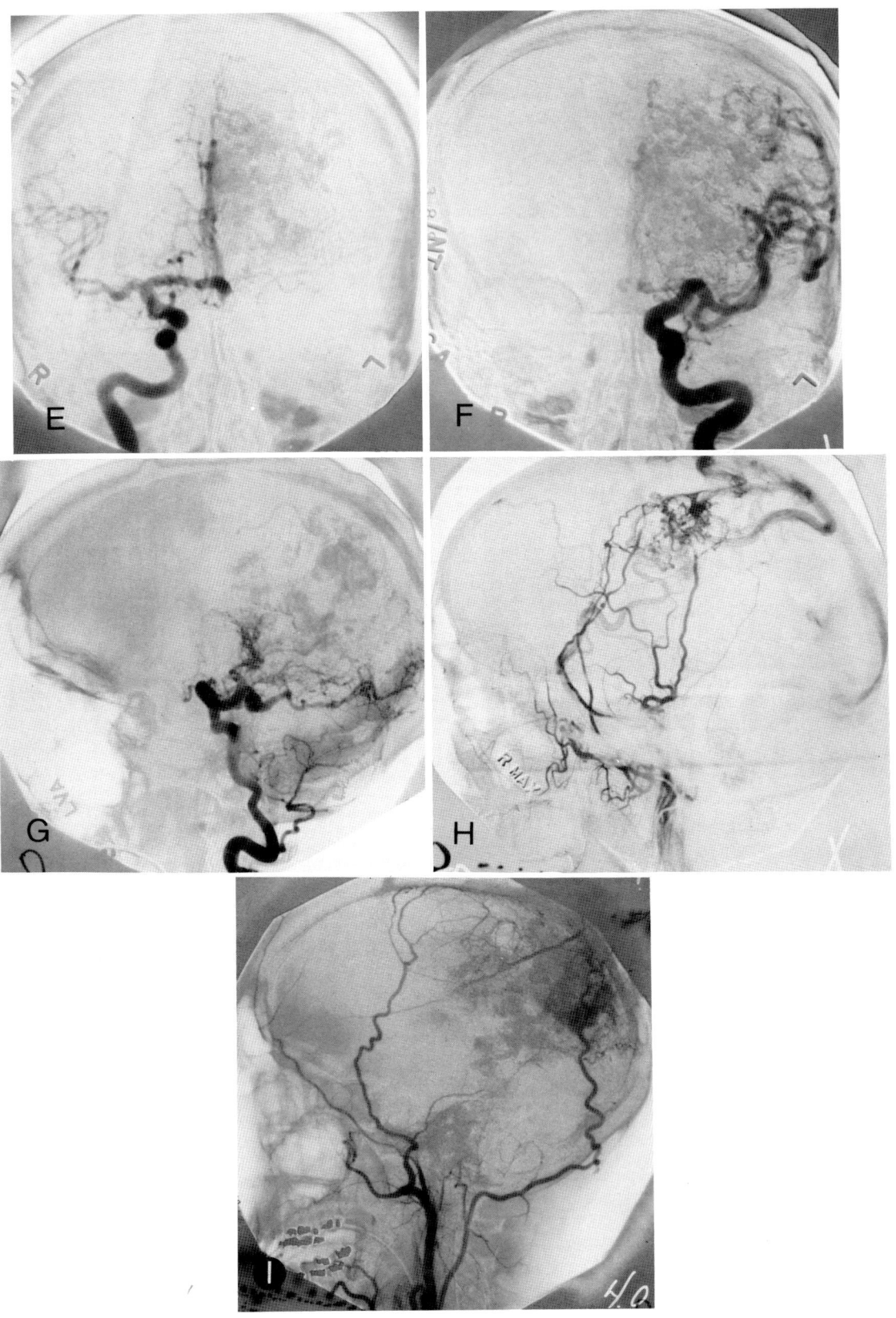

Figure 22.32E–I.

Cyanoacrylate embolization can also be achieved by direct surgical cannulation of feeder arteries. This approach seems attractive for large central lesions with tortuous feeders which cannot be easily entered by endovascular navigation. Particularly suitable are patients with progressive neurologic deficit suggesting a "steal" mechanism. Encouraging results have been reported utilizing local anesthesia, as used in epilepsy surgery (53), and with patients anesthetized (25). Under the operative microscope, a feeder is cannulated with a 22-gauge catheter and angiography is performed to determine if the feeder goes to brain as well as the AVM. If the feeder serves only the AVM, the cyanoacrylate is injected, the volume being determined by the extent of angiographic filling (usually 1 ml or less). After allowing 5 minutes for the adhesive to harden, the catheter is cut off flush with the feeder artery. The brain and AVM are inspected and palpated regarding effects of embolization, which may include white discoloration, palpable cyanoacrylate mass, or newly blue coloration of draining veins suggesting at least partial obliteration of the AVM. If there are no adverse changes, further feeders may be embolized. The authors have been encouraged by a limited experience with this approach.

Despite these advances, problems remain. The balloon and the catheter can become glued in place if the catheter is not withdrawn quickly (32). The polymer may pass through the malformation and into the venous system thus creating a situation of relative hypertension within the malformation which can lead to hemorrhage. The injected substance may reflux into the normal cortical arteries with a consequent neurologic deficit. The long-term histologic effects of these polymers is not known although some early reports suggest considerable tissue reaction (76, 184, 185). It is also not clear whether embolization with polymers facilitates surgery or makes it more difficult because of the solid mass that cannot be easily retracted. It is also difficult to cut across some of the vessels that have been injected with bucrylate because there may be continuing bleeding around the bucrylate when one cuts across these partially occluded vessels that cannot be coagulated. In the authors' experience embolization has been helpful in some cases but an impediment in others and it is difficult to predict these effects.

A difficult question to answer is whether there is any role for embolization as a primary treatment for cerebral AVMs. It is clear that some of these lesions can be eliminated completely with embolization (32). Review of the angiograms of the lesions that have been obliterated completely, indicates that most of them would have been amenable to surgery since they were small and accessible. Most larger lesions that cannot be eliminated completely surgically, are not amenable to complete embolic obliteration (Fig. 22.32). Is there a role for "partial" reduction in flow by repeated embolization with these lesions? Some patients presenting with a progressive neurologic deficit due to "steal" have been improved with this technique and this situation seems a reasonable indication for partial embolization as primary treatment when the lesion is inoperable (32). Whether embolization with polymers that penetrate the nidus will prevent future hemorrhage by decreasing the total blood supply remains to be seen. More patients and longer follow-up are needed for evaluation of embolization as primary therapy.

Electrothrombosis

Handa has introduced the technique of wire-induced electrothrombosis for deep seated or large AVMs (57). It is still too early to see if this complicated technique will be of value.

Radiation Therapy

Radiation causes more injury to endothelium than to normal brain. This differential effect provides a rationale for conventional radiation therapy for AVMs. Sporadic reports have been enthusiastic (68, 174), but in general conventional radiation has not been useful.

More encouraging are the results of proton beam therapy, developed by Kjellberg at the Massachusetts General Hospital (MGH) (74, 75). The Bragg peak of proton energy delivers highly focused heavy particle radiation to a deeply placed target. The proton beam is generated by a cyclotron (160 MeV) and administered via stereotactic technique under local anesthesia. Radiation effects develop gradually, requiring 12–24 months to reach maturity and confer protection. Since the treatment confers little or no protection during this time, hemorrhage at the usual rate is encountered during this interval. Pathologic studies suggest a thickening of vessel walls which may lessen the possibility of hemorrhage. Angiographic follow-up studies have shown obliteration of some of the lesions (Fig. 22.33). Many other lesions show a reduction in size but whether this means a decreased chance of hemorrhage remains to be seen. Early reports have suggested a reduction in the frequency of hemorrhage after the initial 2 years (74, 75).

Complications from proton therapy appear to be uncommon but cases of serious disability from radiation necrosis, particularly when brain stem lesions have been radiated, have been observed at our institution. Hosobuchi, using the heavy particle beam at Berkeley, California, noted serious neurologic deterioration possibly due to sudden thrombosis of the lesion or to direct parenchymal necrosis, in three of 70 cases; all were deep lesions (66).

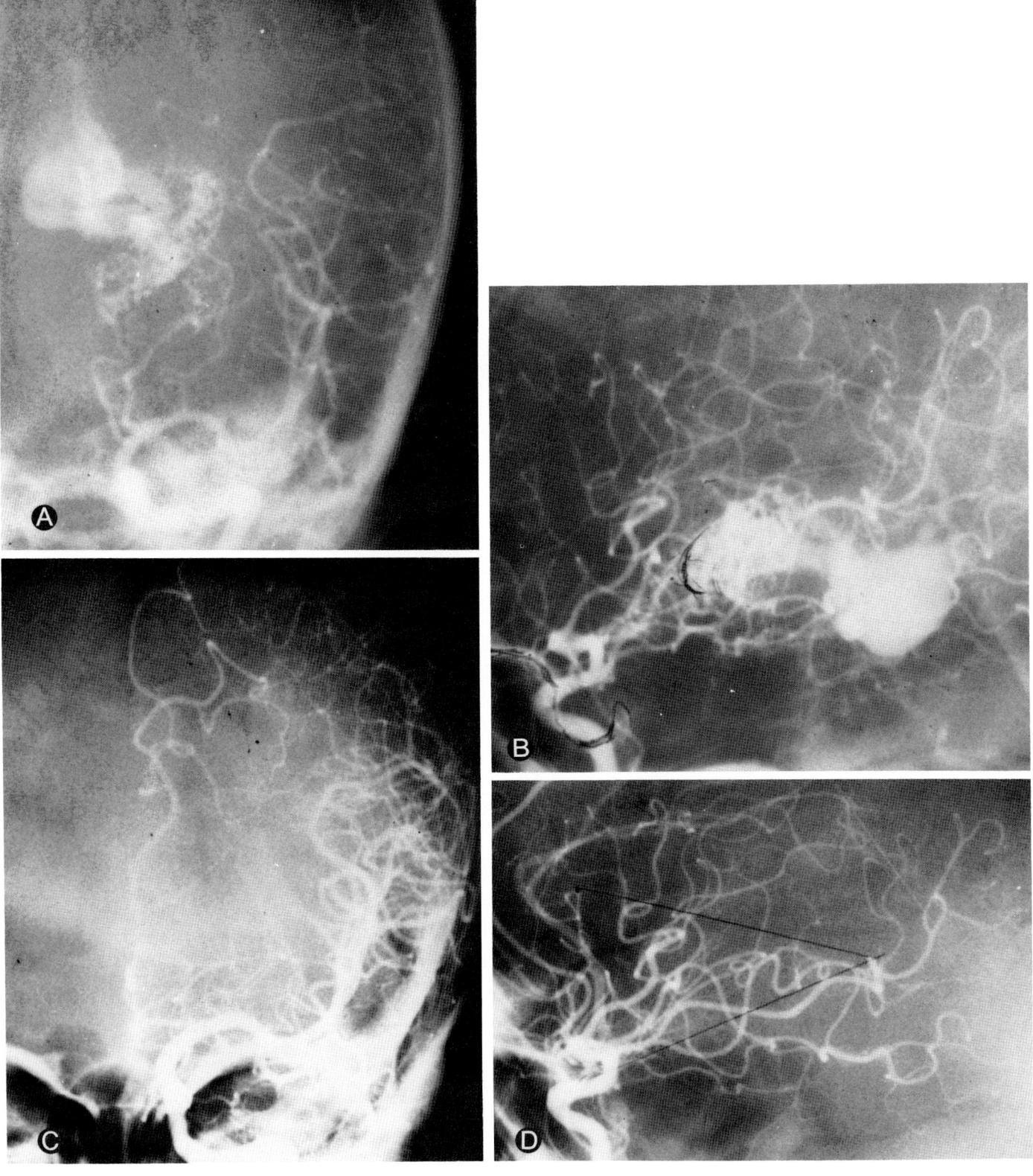

Figure 22.33. Treatment of AVM with proton beam. **A** and **B**, Left carotid angiogram shows AVM involving the basal ganglia. **C** and **D**, Repeat angiogram done 1 year after proton beam treatment showing obliteration of the AVM. This 39-year-old woman had two hemorrhages with a residual right hemiparesis. Proton beam treatment was given 4 months after the last hemorrhage. The patient remains well with a stable neurologic deficit. (These pictures are reproduced through the courtesy of Dr. R. N. Kjellberg.)

Good results have also been reported by Steiner et al using highly collimated gamma irradiation delivered via Leksell's stereotactic method (168). This technique is confined to lesions 3 cm or smaller and so far has not been utilized significantly outside Sweden.

Long-term analysis of the sizable MGH, Berkeley, and Sweden series will be needed to indicate precisely the benefits and risks of focused irradiation of AVMs. The size limits need to be established. Caution is in order when recommending radiation therapy for AVMs. The ideal lesion appeared to be a small inoperable lesion of the basal ganglia or brain stem; however, the recently encountered cases of progressive deterioration from radiation necrosis of the brain stem has given cause for concern. The oncogenic potential of radiation should always be kept in mind when advising radiotherapy for lesions that are compatible with a very long survival. In general, radiotherapy is considered only for AVMs in patients that otherwise meet surgical indications but, because of the location of the lesion, present an unacceptable surgical risk.

CONSERVATIVE THERAPY

Finally, it is well to remember that AVMs are not malignant lesions that progress inexorably to disability or death. Many of these patients live a long and normal life without any disability from these lesions. Therefore, conservative treatment must be an alternative considered in every case and in some patients it will be the alternative of choice (5, 62, 63, 67).

When conservative therapy is elected, the surgeon should not overemphasize the danger of the lesion to the patient. Realistic estimates of probability of hemorrhage are in order but the use of such phrases as "a bomb in your head," is to be condemned. Except for activities such as weight lifting and contact sports, it is recommended that conservatively treated patients resume their normal life activities. There is usually no point in recommending periodic follow-ups with CT scans which can aggravate anxiety. The lesion may be seen to enlarge on that study but it is unlikely that it would become more "operable." Seizures can be treated medically, usually with good control. Future hemorrhages or a progressive neurologic deficit are indications for reassessment of more vigorous treatment, including radiotherapy or embolization if surgical excision is not feasible.

OTHER TYPES OF VASCULAR MALFORMATIONS

Vein of Galen Aneurysms

Primary aneurysms of the vein of Galen are due to multiple arterial vessels emptying directly into the vein of Galen. Secondary aneurysms occur when a separate AVM drains to the vein of Galen and causes it to enlarge. The five clinical syndromes caused by primary aneurysms of the vein of Galen are summarized in Table 22.3. The poor prognosis of the untreated malformation and the poor surgical outcome in the neonate and older child has been emphasized (65).

In infancy, the malformation is associated with uncontrollable cardiac failure. Even with careful stepwise obliteration of the feeding arteries and intensive medical therapy, the prognosis in this age group is poor with very few survivors being reported (3, 4, 107). When the symptoms develop after the first year, the cardiac failure will respond to surgical treatment of the malformation. In older children and adults, symptoms associated with hydrocephalus are more common. Thrombosed aneurysms of the vein of Galen usually present with hydrocephalus (30, 157). Subarachnoid hemorrhage has been reported in the older age group (200).

The diagnosis is suggested by the CT scan and confirmed by angiography. The arterial supply is usually bilateral and comes from the posterior cerebral arteries as well as the anterior pericallosal, superior cerebellar, and thalamic perforating arteries and occasionally from middle cerebral arteries (4, 200) (Fig. 22.34). A thrombosed aneurysm may show a blood-fluid level within the aneurysm and marked enhancement of the periphery of the mass on the CT scan (157).

The lesion is exposed through a parietooccipital craniotomy and is approached along the falx. The technique has been described (4, 200) and a similar

Table 22.3.
Presenting Clinical Syndromes in Patients with Vein of Galen Aneurysms

Group[a]	No. of Patients	Age	Presenting Syndrome
1	11	Neonatal	Severe cardiac failure, cranial bruit
2	3	Neonatal or infancy	Mild heart failure (neonatal), then craniomegaly within 1–6 months; cranial bruit
3	22	1–12 months	Craniomegaly, cranial bruit
4	6	3.5–27 years	Headache, exercise syncope
5	9	6 months–45 years	Drowsy, irritable, hydrocephalus, spasticity

[a]Groups 1–4 are modified from Amacher AL, Shillito J Jr: The syndromes and surgical treatment of aneurysms of the great vein of Galen. J Neurosurg 39:89–98, 1973. Group 5 cases with thrombosed aneurysms are modified from Dean DF: Management of clotted aneurysm of the vein of Galen. Neurosurgery 8:589–592, 1981; and from Six et al: Thrombosed aneurysm of the vein of Galen. Neurosurgery 7:274–278, 1980.

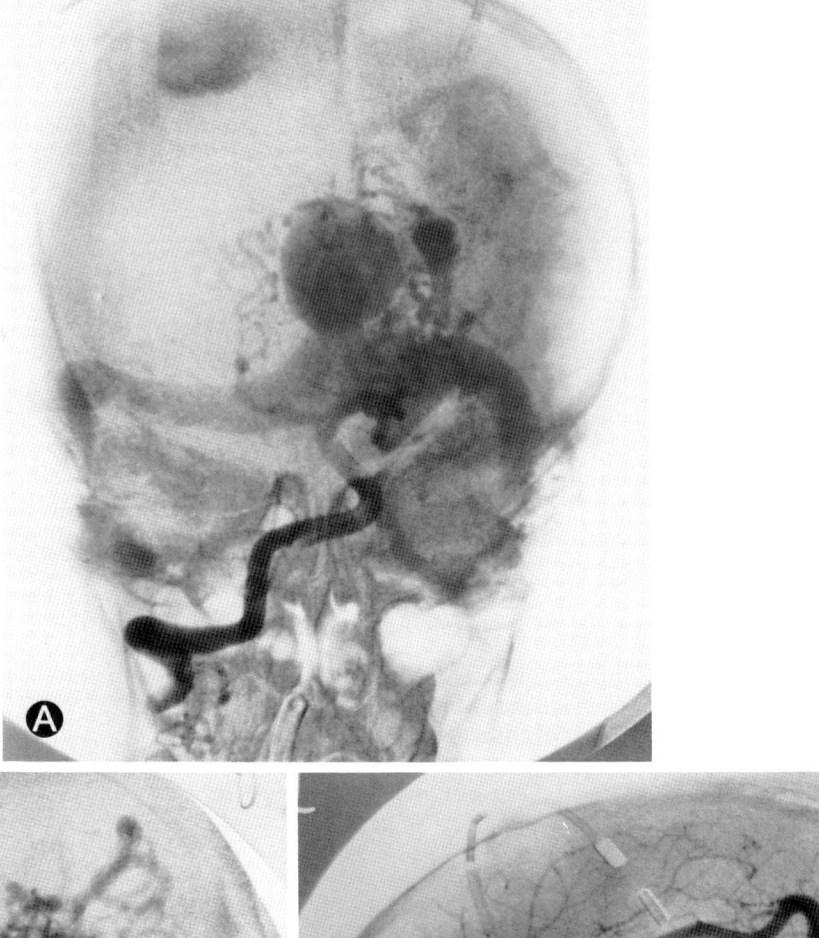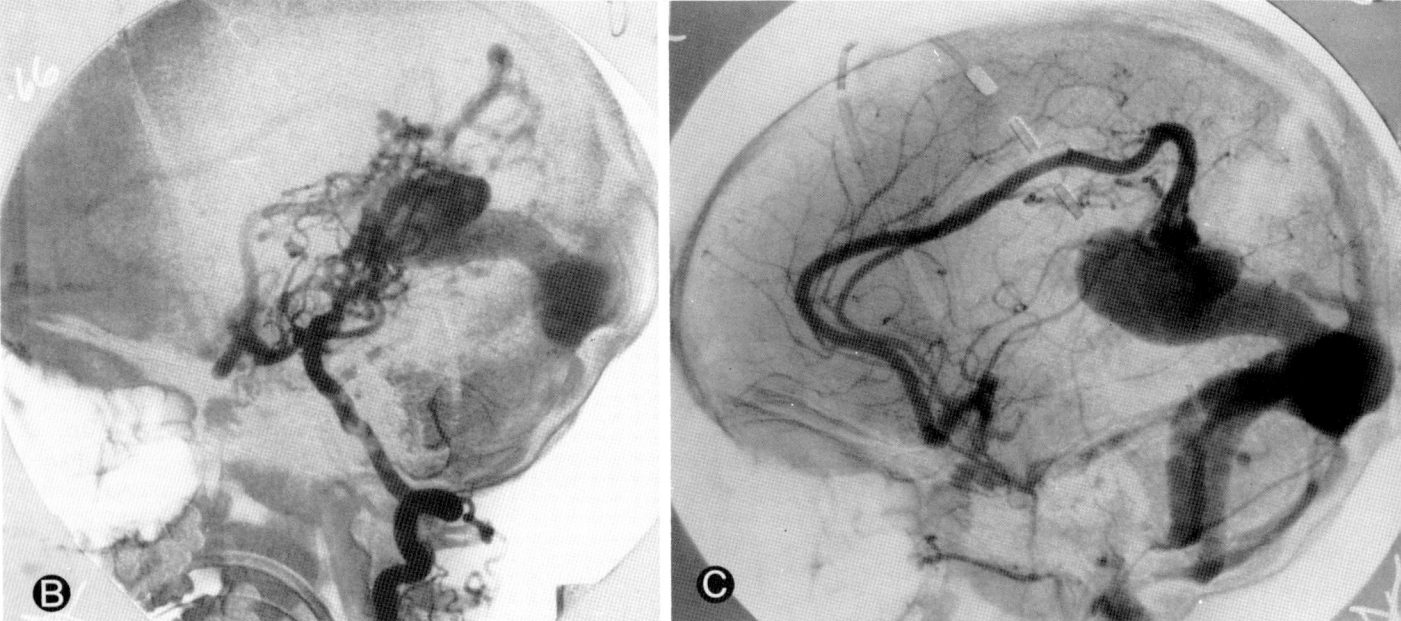

Figure 22.34. Vein of Galen malformation. **A** and **B**, AP and lateral vertebral angiogram shows arterial supply from both posterior cerebral arteries with filling of the vein of Galen aneurysm and transverse sinuses in the arterial phase of the study. Lateral vertebral angiogram better outlines the filling from the posterior branches of the left middle cerebral artery. **C**, Branches from the pericallosal artery enter the top of the aneurysm. The ventricular portion of the shunt system is also seen.

operative approach with good results has been used by others (19, 30, 107, 157). The sac of the aneurysm is identified in the region formed by the falx and tentorium posteriorly and under the splenium of the corpus callosum anteriorly. To expose the aneurysm, it may be necessary to split the splenium and divide the falx or tentorium. Yasargil first occludes the anterior paricallosal arteries by going over the splenium to the dome of the malformation (200). Then the right posterior cerebral artery is identified in the ambient cistern and followed to the malformation where feeders are divided. Next, the right superior cerebellar artery is identified behind the posterior cerebral artery in the ambient and quadrigeminal cisterns and is also followed to the malformation. After a flap is made in the falx, attention is turned to the left side of the aneurysm and the feeders from the left posterior cerebral and superior cerebellar arteries are occluded. In some cases, this will completely take care of the problem, but more often there will still be inflow through the large perforating posterior thalamic vessels from the peduncular segment of the posterior cerebral artery. The aneurysm is reflected inferiorly to expose these arteries as they enter at the anterior base. At times the aneurysm must be elevated to expose the posterior inferior surface to reach all the feeding arteries. The vein of Galen should now be blue. To further check on the completeness of the occlusion, the skull can be auscultated and a blood sample drawn from the vein of Galen and sent for blood gas analysis. Because the sac is usually tough, it can be manipulated with relative safety. The sac is usually not excised. It has been recommended that thrombosed aneurysms of the vein of Galen be decompressed but not removed (30, 157). A much smoother postoperative course was noted when no attempt was made to excise the lesion.

Postoperative complications include heart failure, subdural hematoma, hemiparesis, seizure, and hydrocephalus. In view of the generally poor surgical results (65), methods of embolization by polymer of the feeders to the malformation, either as primary treatment or combined with surgery, have been introduced with moderate success (10). Mickle and Quisling have treated three children with a method involving introduction of wire coils directly into the vein of Galen through the torcula in an effort to induce thrombosis (110). In two of the children they achieved essentially complete thrombosis and they have done well. The third child was in poor cardiac condition and died after surgery.

Cavernous Angiomas

Cavernous angiomas are circumscribed lesions that are best considered as hamartomas. They are composed of dilated collagenized vascular channels lined with a single layer of endothelial cells and without any intervening normal neural parenchyma (104, 105). Their clinical spectrum, prognosis, and recommended form of treatment have been reviewed in several publications (21, 101, 138, 139, 181, 189, 203). These malformations are encountered most commonly in adults in the third through the fifth decades. They are most frequently located in the white matter of the cerebral hemispheres but they can be paraventricular in location and are also found in the posterior fossa particularly in the brain stem. They are rare in childhood but some cases have been reported (139, 203). The presenting symptom has been seizures in about half of the cases, a tumor-like syndrome with moderate mass effect and signs of increased intracranial pressure as well as focal neurologic deficits in one-third, and hemorrhage in about 10–15%, although in one series the incidence of hemorrhage was higher (52). There is often evidence of previous hemorrhage either grossly at surgery or later upon pathologic examination. It is not clear whether these lesions grow in time, but progression of neurologic deficits without new hemorrhage or evidence of thrombosis at surgery in some of the patients suggest expansion (101). With increased use of CT scanning for a number of vague neurologic complaints, most of these lesions are now diagnosed in patients who have no symptoms referable to the lesion.

On plain CT scan the lesions are almost invariably hyperdense and are usually nodular and well-circumscribed. With administration of contrast, there is only slight or no enhancement (Fig. 22.35). Commonly there is a small hypodense zone surrounding the lesion. Calcifications within the nodule are very common. Major mass effect is rare but occasionally local mass effect makes differentiation from tumor much more difficult. MRI done in a few cases has had the characteristic appearance to be described later under occult AVMs. Angiographically most of these lesions are silent but may show an avascular mass effect. Sometimes there is a faint capillary blush and in some of the larger lesions abnormally enlarged draining veins can be noted. There is almost never visible arterial supply.

Since the natural history of cavernous angiomas is not well known, it is difficult to make any definite recommendations as to treatment. They can bleed and some have bled several times. Therefore, if there has been a hemorrhage and the lesion is accessible, surgical excision is recommended. This is particularly true when one cannot be sure that the lesion is not a neoplasm. In patients who present with seizures, surgery is recommended when the lesion is accessible. Lesions located in critical areas should be followed with periodic CT scan since most of these patients run a fairly benign course.

The operation for cavernous angiomas in accessible areas is usually relatively straightforward since they tend not to bleed much during surgery and there

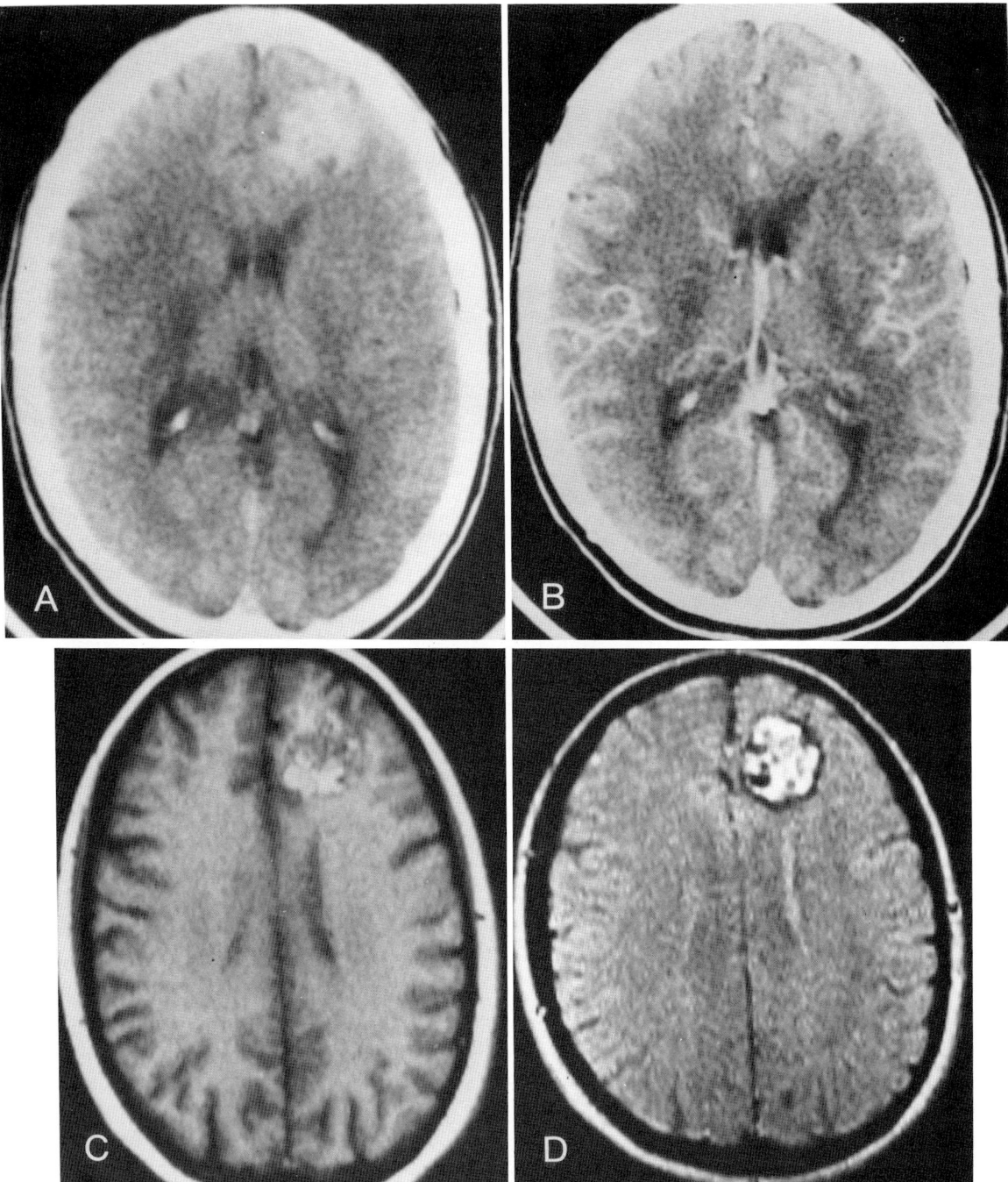

Figure 22.35. Cavernous angioma. This patient presented with a seizure disorder. **A**, Plain CT scan showed a left frontal hyperdense lesion which **B**, did not change significantly with contrast administration. **C**, MRI showed a typical inhomogeneous pattern of increased signal on the T_1 weighted image. **D**, The T_2 weighted image shows again an inhomogeneous pattern of increased signal intermixed with areas of signal void which probably indicates either hemosiderin deposition or active blood flow. The lesion was avascular on angiography. It had a well-defined surrounding plane and could be removed completely without producing any neurologic deficit. The main indication for surgery in this case was the fact that, because this was early in the authors' experience with MRI, it was not certain whether or not the lesion was a tumor. A similar lesion with the same pattern on MRI in a less accessible location probably should be treated conservatively with periodic follow-up by CT scan and MRI.

is most frequently, although by no means always, a well-defined plane around the lesion. At surgery the lesions look reddish or purple and they are frequently multilobulated. They are usually small and are best removed in toto unless they are large in which case they can be decompressed and removed piecemeal. The surgical prognosis for accessible lesions is generally excellent.

Venous Angiomas

Venous angiomas are probably the most common type of vascular malformation (105, 152, 167). Much has been written about these lesions, particularly from the radiologic point of view (16, 23, 45, 96, 101, 108, 118, 140, 143, 147, 152, 154, 155, 193). These malformations consist of a radial array of small veins that converge into a dilated, much larger vein which then drains into a normal sinus. The vascular channels appear histologically like normal veins although they may be hyalinized. There may be some gliosis and, rarely, evidence of previous hemorrhage.

In the past the majority of these lesions were diagnosed at autopsy and had never produced symptoms during life. Lately, many are being diagnosed because of CT scans obtained for a variety of reasons. The immense majority of these lesions are totally asymptomatic. Only 11 patients who had presented with a hemorrhage clearly related to the venous angioma were collected in a review (101). Whether or not these lesions can produce seizures is controversial. Patients with seizures who undergo a CT scan may be found to have a venous angioma, but in several patients an abnormal EEG focus was in a site remote from the venous angioma and, therefore, the lesion probably had nothing to do with the seizures (101).

About half the venous angiomas appear in the plain CT scan as nodular or linear high density lesions (Fig. 22.36A). With injection of contrast their appearance is characteristically an irregular, sometimes nodular or linear area of enhancement deep within the white matter of the cerebrum or the cerebellum (Fig. 22.37A). Sometimes all that can be seen on the CT scan is the linear density which represents the draining transcerebral vein. The appearance is so characteristic that it is usually unnecessary to proceed with angiography. When the angiogram is done, it is usually diagnostic (Figs. 22.36E and 22.37B). The lesion is typically described as having the appearance of a "caput-medusa" with small radial vessels converging centrally into a dilated venous channel which drains to the cortical surface. The lesions are seen during the venous phase although some have been reported to show early filling during the capillary phase (118).

The natural history of these lesions is clearly very benign. Almost invariably, they should be left alone. Even when the lesions are thought to be producing epilepsy, surgery is dangerous since the lesions are deep in the white matter and usually form part of the normal venous drainage. It is particularly dangerous to operate on those in the cerebellum and cases have resulted in death because of venous infarction of the cerebellum after excision (11). The rare case that presents with a hemorrhage may need operation if the hematoma is causing pressure symptoms but again one must be conservative and not remove extensively the venous plexus so as to not interfere with the normal venous drainage (Fig. 22.36).

Occult Vascular Malformations

Separate from cavernous angiomas are two groups of vascular malformations of the brain that are "occult" angiographically and are diagnosed by CT scan, MRI, or pathologically after removal of an intracerebral clot. One group includes patients with the usual AVM that may have bled but are not seen on angiography. These are dangerous lesions. In the other group are patients with a thrombosed lesion that often presents with seizures or focal symptoms and shows specific CT scan findings and an avascular mass on angiogram. The MRI may be of considerable diagnostic help (121).

Typical AVMs Not Seen on Angiography

There are three main reasons why typical AVMs fail to visualize angiographically: pressure from the hematoma, thrombosis, and small size. In some patients a hematoma compresses the AVM (usually small lesions) and, therefore, it fails to appear during an angiogram obtained early after the hemorrhage. When the angiogram is repeated several weeks after the hemorrhage and once the mass effect subsides, some of these lesions can be seen (Fig. 22.38). At surgery one usually finds a typical, small AVM. Wakai et al reviewed the literature and found that up to 50% of the patients with lobar hemorrhage of unknown cause and normal early angiograhpy will be found to have an AVM at surgery or on subsequent angiography (191). In this same review, the authors found a very high incidence of a history of previous hemorrhage. The hemorrhages were frequently large and devastating. For these reasons, they recommended removal of the hematoma in the majority of these patients. They have described in detail an elegant microsurgical technique whereby a small corticotomy is made over the thinnest portion of the cortex over the hematoma. The brain is then gently retracted and only a small portion of the hematoma is aspirated at a time, progressively separating the hematoma from the wall of the cavity and systematically inspecting the walls under the microscope all around the hematoma as it is gradually evacuated. The presence of the malformation is usually heralded by more solid clot which is firmly adherent to the wall. One can then usually see under the microscope abnormal ves-

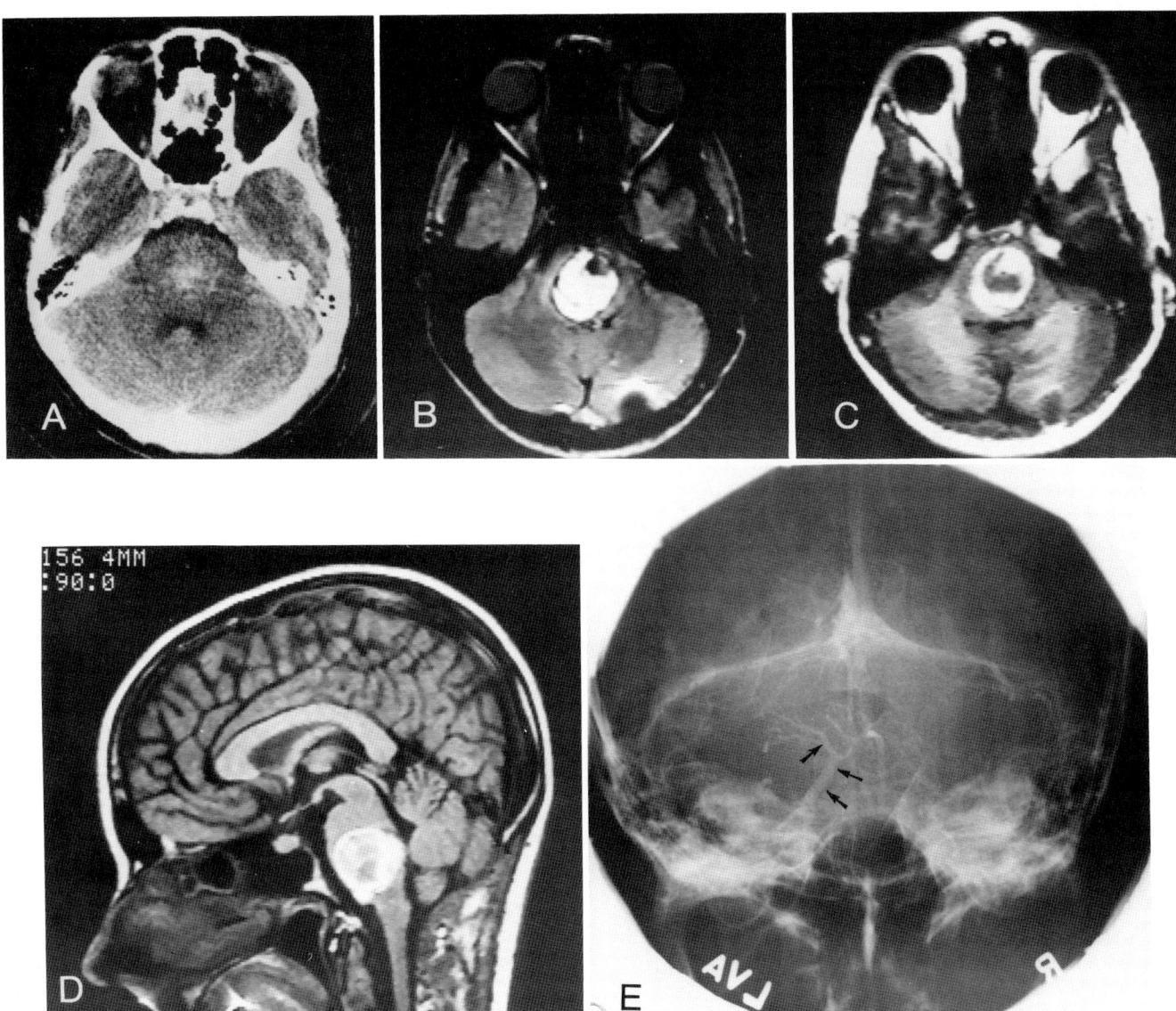

Figure 22.36. Venous angioma. This 21-year-old lady presented with a progressive history of long tract and cranial nerve deficits. **A**, CT scan showed a high-density lesion of the brain stem which did not enhance significantly with contrast. **B–D**, MRI showed an inhomogeneous round lesion of the brain stem that was interpreted as being consistent with hemorrhages of different ages; however, a hemorrhagic tumor could not be ruled out. Angiogram done preoperatively was normal. Because of the progressive sympomatology and the possibility that the lesion represented a "chronic expanding hematoma", the patient was explored through a lateral suboccipital craniectomy since the area of abnormality seemed to "point" in the left anterolateral region of the pons. An incision was made anterior to and between the root entry zones of the 11th and the 9th and 10th cranial nerves. A chronic encapsulated hematoma was found which was easily drained. Biopsies of the capsule of the hematoma as well as the surrounding brain stem showed no evidence of tumor. The patient had no additional neurologic deficit from surgery. **E**, Postoperative angiogram showed a classic venous angioma of the brain stem (*arrows*) seen only in the very late venous phase. Comparing this angiogram with the preoperative angiogram, it was realized that the initial (preoperative) study did not include late venous filming and this is probably the reason the venous angioma was missed. The plan is to observe the patient clinically since, in the authors' opinion, it would be impossible to remove the venous angioma without resulting major neurologic deficit.

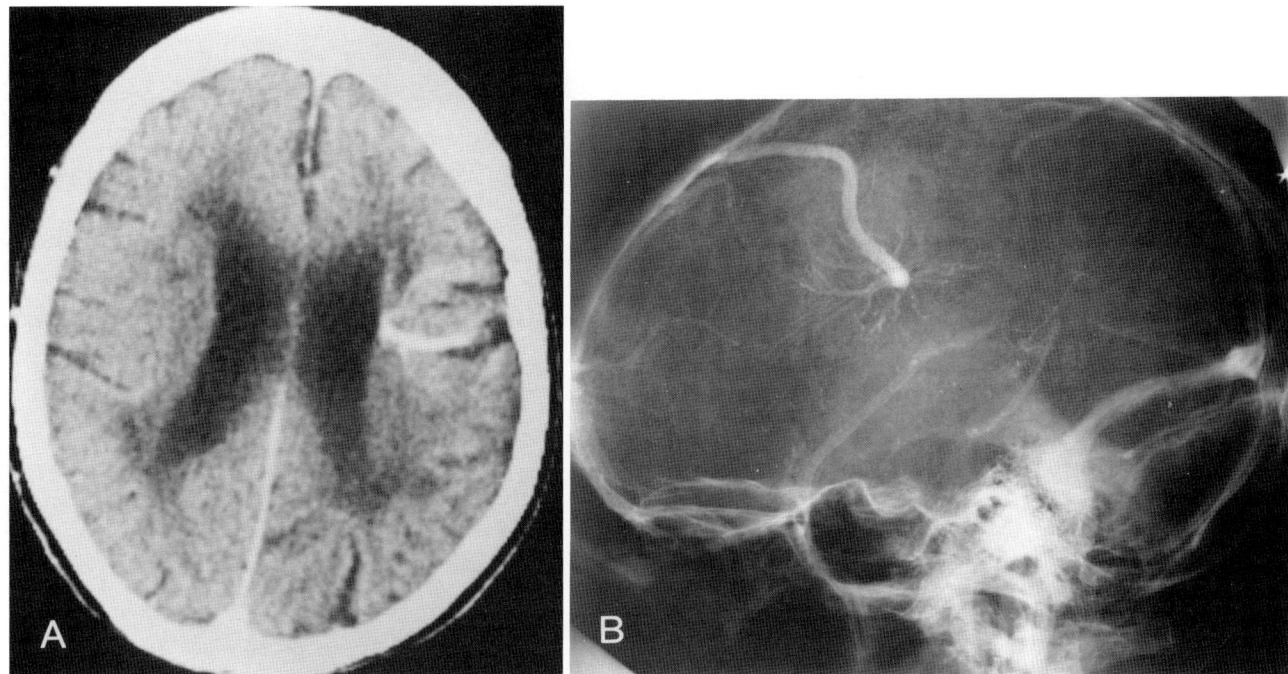

Figure 22.37. Venous angioma. This patient had migraine. **A**, CT scan shows the typical linear density seen on the contrast scan in patients with venous angiomas. **B**, Angiogram shows the typical "spoke-wheel" appearance of a venous angioma in the late venous phase. The lesion was almost certainly unrelated to the patient's symptoms and, therefore, she was treated conservatively.

sels in the region which can be coagulated and excised.

In patients with an intracerebral hemorrhage of unknown etiology and negative initial angiography the angiogram is repeated in 6–12 weeks after the initial hemorrhage depending on the neurologic condition of the patient. The authors wait longer with patients in poor neurologic condition to allow for maximal recovery. When the angiogram is negative many of these patients will show a nodular, irregular area of enhancement on the wall of the hematoma cavity on CT scanning (112, 121, 173, 191). The MRI in these patients may show circumscribed regions of low intensity, most prominent on T_2-weighted images, interspersed with areas of mixed signal intensity patterns which correspond to different stages of evolution within the hematoma. Whether the circumscribed areas of low intensity (or signal void) indicate blood flow within a malformation or a draining vein or whether they are related to hemosiderin deposits is not clear but the latter appears to be the most likely case (54, 121). This pattern is thought to be diagnostic of an AVM; however, exceptions have been seen particularly in patients with gliomas and metastatic tumors in whom the MRI characteristics have led to the incorrect preoperative diagnosis of occult AVM. Also, an identical appearance on MRI has been seen in patients with pathologically proven cavernous angiomas. When a CT scan shows nodular enhancement in the wall of the hematoma or when the MRI shows the typical picture described, exploration is indicated and an AVM will usually be found. The authors have not had a case where the CT scan was completely normal and the MRI was diagnostic of AVM. Whether cases with only abnormal CT should be explored is not clear but this would be justified if the patient were young and the hematoma in an accessible location. Cases in which neither the CT scan nor the MRI suggest an abnormality probably should be observed with periodic repetition of these tests since it is unlikely that an AVM would be found. These cases probably represent either small cryptic AVMs that destroy themselves with hemorrhage or small AVMs that have completely thrombosed.

Another reason for AVMs not being visualized angiographically is thrombosis. Thrombosis of an AVM is usually associated with hemorrhage and compression of the lesion by the blood clot but it also may occur spontaneously.

Some AVMs fail to be visualized angiographically or on CT scan because they are very small, true "cryptic" AVMs. The association of these small lesions with intracerebral hemorrhage was first described by Margolis et al (99). The subject was later reviewed by Gerlack who proposd the term "microangiomas" (51). These lesions are suspected as the cause of many,

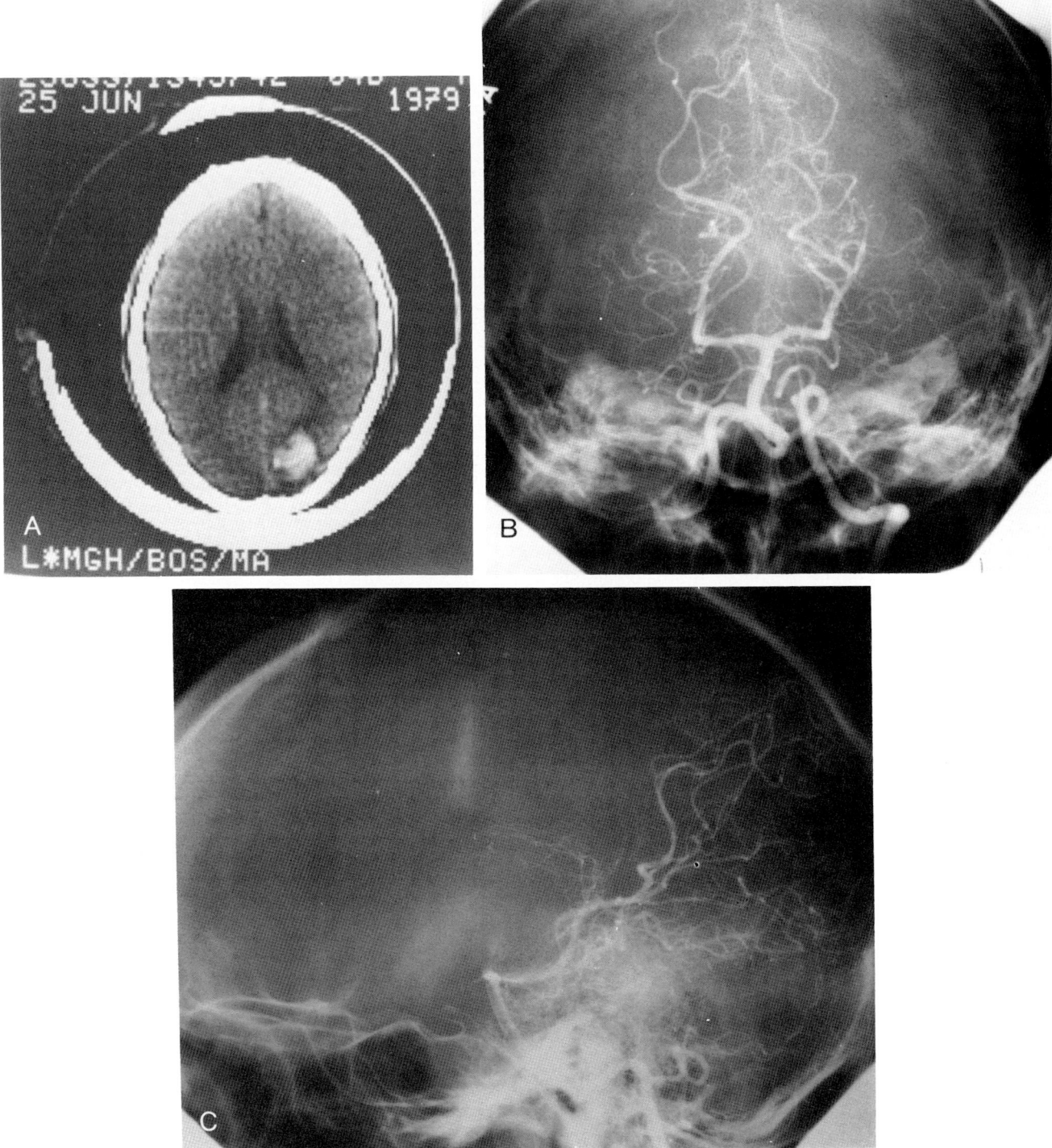

Figure 22.38. Demonstration of AVM on delayed angiogram. **A,** CT scan shows a right occipital lobe hematoma. **B** and **C,** AP and lateral vertebral angiogram reveals no abnormality. The carotid studies were also normal. **D** and **E,** AP and lateral vertebral angiogram 3 weeks later show filling of a small AVM and an early draining vein (*arrows*). This 19-year-old boy had the sudden onset of a headache. The second angiogram was done at a planned interval of time.

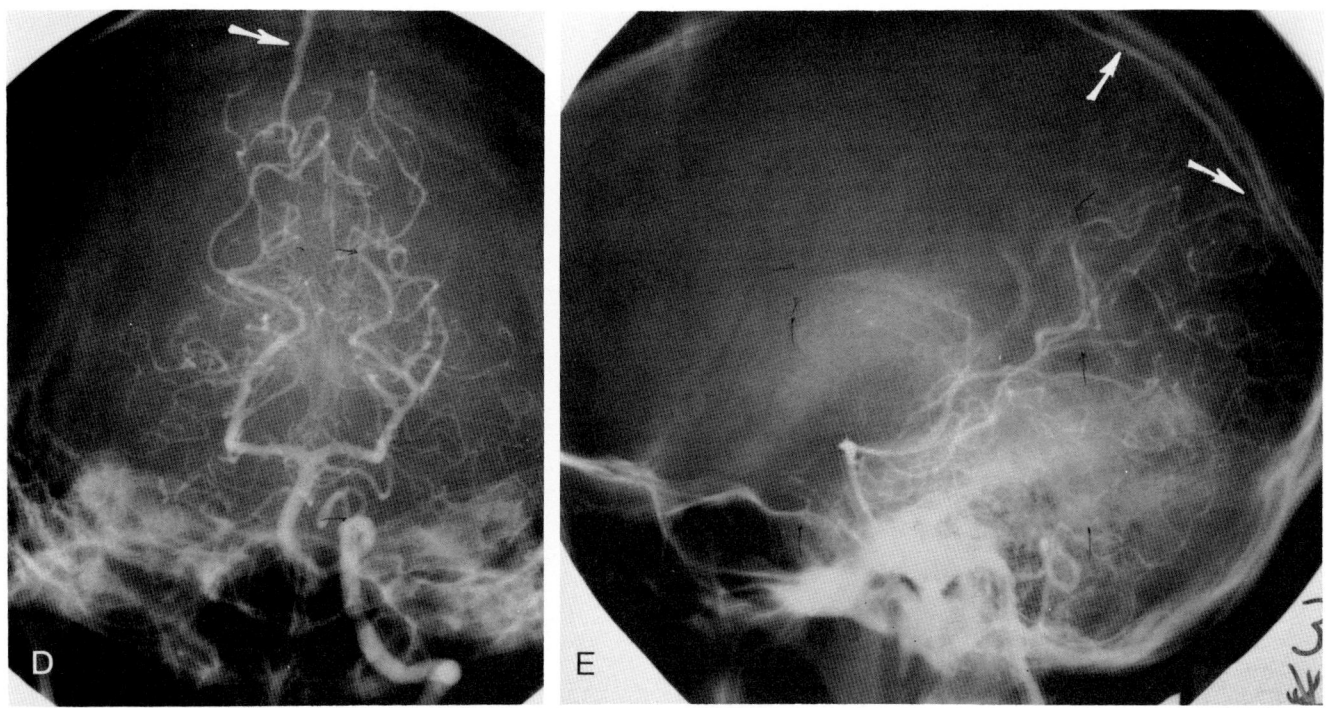

Figure 22.38D and E.

if not most, intracerebral hemorrhages occurring in young adults in whom angiograms and CT scans fail to demonstrate an etiologic cause. The diagnosis is usually made when the patient is operated for a large intracerebral hemorrhage and a small abnormal tuft of blood vessels is found in the wall of the cavity at surgery or, more commonly, in the pathologic specimen. Primary intraventricular hemorrhage has also occasionally been caused by these small malformations (15, 39). The presumption is that most of these small malformations "destroy" themselves with the hemorrhage. It is not clear whether surgical extirpation should be recommended for a patient who recovers from an intracerebral hemorrhage and subsequently has not only a negative angiogram but also a negative CT scan and MRI. For now it appears safe to recommend that nothing be done in these patients if delayed (at least 2 months) CT scan and MRI show nothing but evidence of an old hematoma cavity.

Thrombosed Vascular Malformations Presenting as a Mass Lesion

A separate category of patients with occult AVMs are those with thrombosed vascular malformations that become manifested either because they result in seizures or less commonly, because of a focal or progressive neurologic syndrome (Figs. 22.39 and 22.40) (195). On CT scan these lesions are usually round or lobulated and are hyperdense on the plain scan and become either minimally enhanced or do not change with contrast administration. There is usually little or no associated surrounding edema (112, 121, 195). A neoplasm is usually the primary consideration when the patient presents with seizures or with a focal or progressive neurologic syndrome. Some lesions in deep critical areas of the brain have been radiated blindly under the assumption that they were gliomas. At autopsy thrombosed vascular malformations have then been found (123). These thrombosed lesions can also cause intracerebral hemorrhage. Some of the authors' cases had a history of multiple hemorrhages and in a few patients with a negative angiogram, subsequent hemorrhage occurred (121). The most probable explanation for their continuing potential for clnical manifestation is incomplete thrombosis. In the majority of the cases that the authors have explored, pathologic examination showed that while most of the malformation was thrombosed other parts had open vascular channels.

The MRI may make the specific diagnosis in these patients (54, 121) but it is doubtful that in the near future it will replace the operation which is needed both to establish the diagnosis and to eliminate the risk of future hemorrhage and continuing neurologic deterioration. Whenever this diagnosis is suspected, operative excision is recommended to avoid the risk of hemorrhage associated with stereotactic biopsy. Even in the ventricular surface of the thalamus or caudate nucleus, these lesions can be excised with

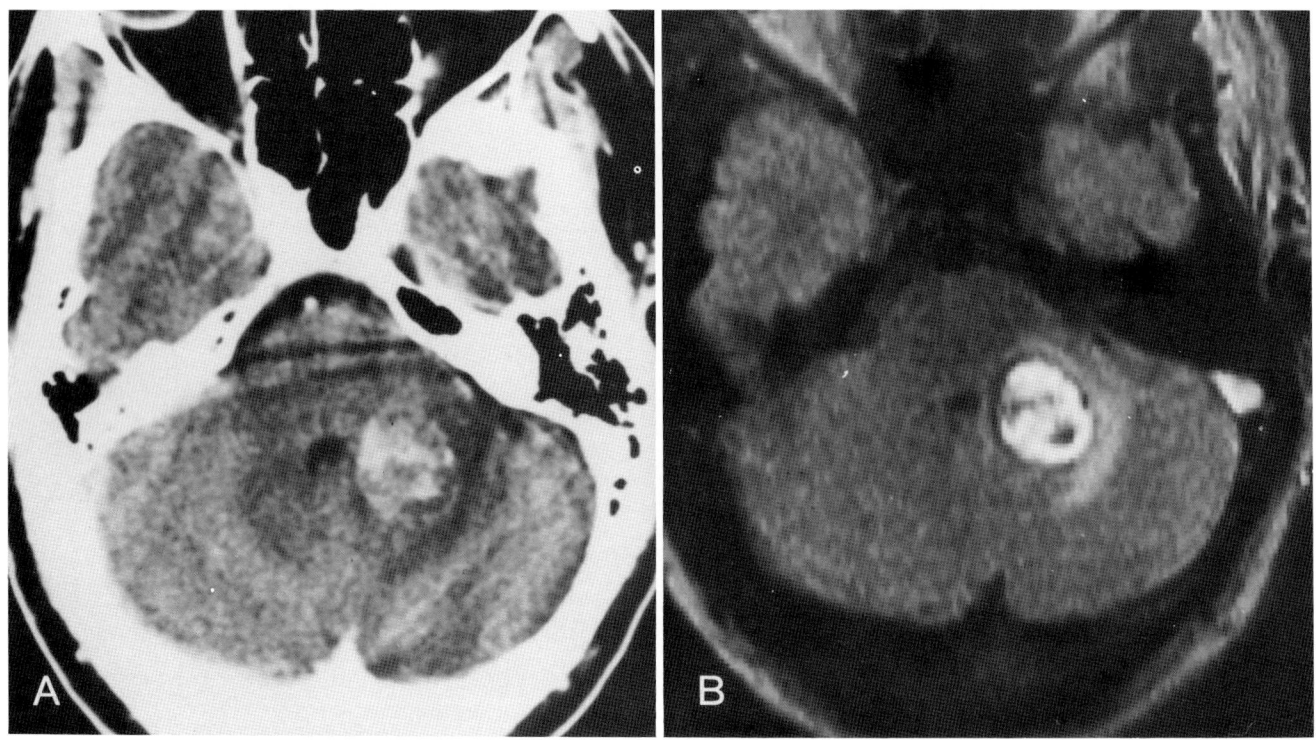

Figure 22.39. Occult thrombosed AVM. This 37-year-old man presented with progressive left-sided appendicular ataxia and gait difficulty. **A**, CT scan shows a hyperdense lesion which enhanced moderately in an inhomogeneous pattern. **B**, MRI shows an inhomogeneous pattern of high signal with a few areas of signal void surrounded by a thin rim of signal void which probably represented hemosiderin in the periphery of the lesion. The angiogram was normal. The lesion was approached over the cerebellum and coagulation and excision were possible through an incision in the anterior paravermian surface of the cerebellum. The AVM was partially thrombosed but some of the vessels were patent; however, they were under very low pressure and could be coagulated readily without significant bleeding. The patient was unchanged neurologically after surgery.

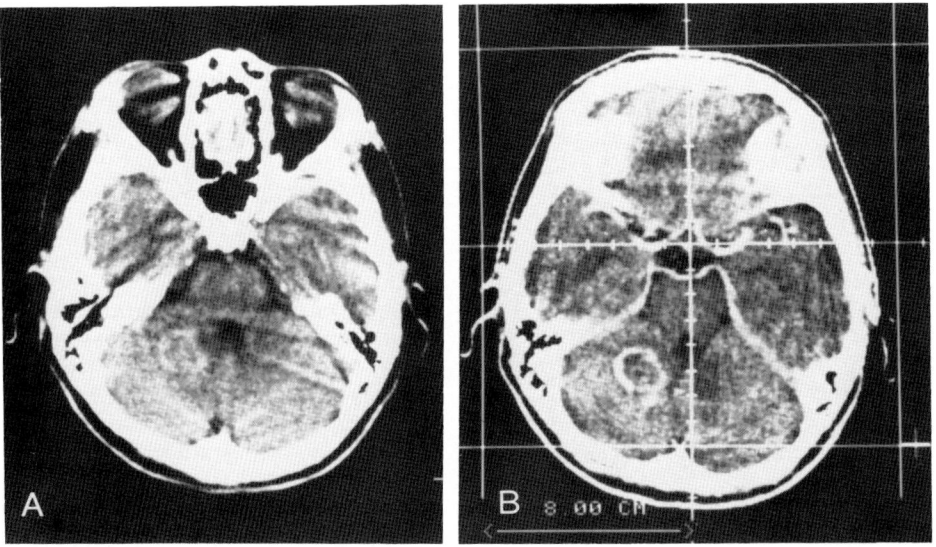

Figure 22.40. Occult (thrombosed) AVM. **A**, CT scan done without contrast. Note hyperdense paraventricular lesion in the right cerebellar hemisphere. **B**, CT done after intravenous contrast injection shows enhancement in the periphery of the lesion. Patient presented with onset of difficulty using her right hand and slight unsteadiness of gait and had right cerebellar signs on examination. The cerebellar dysfunction persisted and she developed nausea. Angiogram was normal. At operation, a localized lesion was found and excised. There had been a small old hemorrhage. Pathologic examination revealed a thrombosed AVM.

relatively low risk because they are low pressure lesions which can be readily coagulated and excised. Ultrasound may prove of help in guiding the surgeon to the deeper lesions of the hemisphere. Lesions deep within the thalamus or the brain stem should not be operated unless they are associated with major neurologic deficits not likely to be worsened by operation. In most thalamic and brain stem lesions, where MRI and CT scan suggest a thrombosed AVM, it will probably be best to observe the patient and repeat these studies periodically. If there are progressive symptoms, proton beam radiation can be considered.

REFERENCES

1. Adelt D, Zeumer H, Walters J: Surgical treatment of cerebral arteriovenous malformations. Follow-up study of 43 cases. *Acta Neurochir (Wien)* 76:45–49, 1985.
2. Albert P: Personal experience in the treatment of 178 cases of arteriovenous malformations of the brain. *Acta Neurochir (Wien)* 61:207–226, 1982.
3. Alvarez-Garijo JA, Mangual MV, Gomila DT, Martin AA: Giant arteriovenous fistula of the vein of Galen in early infancy treated successfully with surgery. *J Neurosurg* 53:703–706, 1980.
4. Amacher AL, Shillito J Jr: The syndromes and surgical treatment of aneurysms of the great vein of Galen. *J Neurosurg* 39:89–98, 1973.
5. Aminoff MJ: Management of unruptured cerebral arteriovenous malformations. *Clin Neurosurg* 33:177–185, 1986.
6. Andrews BT, Wilson CB: Staged treatment of arteriovenous malformations of the brain. *J Neurosurg*, in press.
7. Aoki N: Combined occipital transtentorial and infratentorial supracerebellar approach in the concorde position for the treatment of an arteriovenous malformation in the upper vermis: Case report. *Neurosurgery* 17:815–817, 1985.
8. Batjer H, Samson D: Surgical approaches to trigonal arteriovenous malformations. Paper presented at the American Association of Neurological Surgeons meeting, Denver, CO, 1985.
9. Batjer H, Samson D: Arterioveneous malformations of the posterior fossa. Clinical presentation, diagnostic evaluation, and surgical treatment. *J Neurosurg* 64:849–856, 1986.
10. Berenstein A, Epstein F: Vein of Galen malformations: combined neurosurgical and neuroradiologic intervention. In: *Surgery of the Developing Nervous System*. New York, Grune & Stratton, 1982, pp 637–647.
11. Biller J, Toffol J, Shea FJ, Fine M, Azar-Kia B: Cerebellar venous angiomas. A continuing controversy. *Arch Neurol* 42:367–370, 1985.
12. Bonnal J, Born JD, Hans P. One-stage excision of high-flow arteriovenous malformations. *J Neurosurg* 62:128–131, 1985.
13. Boyd MC, Steinbok P, Paty DW: Familial arteriovenous malformations. *J Neurosurg* 62:597–599, 1985.
14. Bushe K-A, Bockhorn J, Schafer ER: Macro- and microsurgery of central angiomas. In Pia HW, Gleave JR, Grote E, Zierski J (eds): *Cerebral Angiomas. Advances in Diagnosis and Therapy*. Berlin, Springer-Verlag, 1975, pp 123–128.
15. Butler AB, Partain RA, Netsky MG: Primary intraventricular hemorrhage. A mild and remediable form. *Neurology* 22:475–687, 1972.
16. Cabanes J, Blasco R, Garcia M, Tamarit L: Cerebral venous angiomas. *Surg Neurol* 11:385, 1979.
17. Caram PC, Sharkey PC, Alvord EC Jr: Thalamic angioma and aneurysm of the anterior choroidal artery with intraventricular hematoma. *J Neurosurg* 17:347–352, 1960.
18. Carleton CC, Cauthen JC: Vascular ("arteriovenous") malformations of the choroid plexus. *Arch Pathol* 99:286–288, 1975.
19. Carson LV, Brooks BS, Gammal TE, Massey CE, Beveridge WE, Allen MB: Adult arteriovenous malformation of the vein of Galen: A case report with pre- and postoperative computed tomographic findings. *Neurosurgery* 7:495–498, 1980.
20. Celli P, Ferrante L, Palma L, Cavedon G: Cerebral arteriovenous malformations in children. *Surg Neurol* 22:43–49, 1984.
21. Chadduck WM, Binet EF, Farrell FW Jr, Araoz CA, Reding DL: Intraventricular cavernous hemangioma: Report of three cases and review of the literature. *Neurosurgery* 16:189–197, 1985.
22. Chou SN, Erickson DL, Ortiz-Suarez HJ: Surgical treatment of vascular lesions in the brain stem. *J Neurosurg* 42:23–31, 1975.
23. Constans JP, Dilenge D, Vendrenne C: Angiomes neineux cerebraux. *Neurochirurgie* 14:641, 1968.
24. Cophignon J, Thurel C, Djindjian R, Rey A, Visot A, LeBesneraie Y, Houdart R: Cerebral arteriovenous malformations. Modern aspects of investigations and treatment. *Prog Neurol Surg* 9:195–237, 1978.
25. Cromwell LD, Harris B: Treatment of cerebral arteriovenous malformations. A combined neurosurgical and neuroradiologic approach. *J Neurosurg* 52:705–708, 1980.
26. Dahl RE, Kline DG: Intraparenchymal arteriovenous malformations with predominant external cartoid artery contribution. *J Neurosurg* 41:681–687, 1974.
27. Davis C, Symon L: The management of cerebral arteriovenous malformations. *Acta Neurochir (Wien)* 74:4–11, 1985.
28. Day AL, Friedman WA, Sypert GW, Mickle JP: Successful treatment of the normal perfusion pressure breakthrough syndrome. *Neurosurgery* 11:625–630, 1982.
29. deAlmedia GM, Shibata MK, Nakagawa EJ: Contralateral parafalcine approach for parasagittal and callosal arteriovenous malformations. *Neurosurgery* 14:744–746, 1984.
30. Dean DF: Management of clotted aneurysm of the vein of Galen. *Neurosurgery* 8:589–592, 1981.
31. Debrun G, Lacour P, Caron J: Detachable balloons and calibrated-leak ballon techniques in the treatment of cerebral vascular lesions. *J Neurosurg* 49:635–649, 1978.
32. Debrun G, Vinuela F, Fox A, Drake CG: Embolization of cerebral arteriovenous malformations with bucrylate. Experience in 46 cases. *J Neurosurg* 56:615–627, 1982.
33. Debrun G, Vinuela D, Fox AJ, Kan S: Two different calibrated-leak balloons: Experimental work and application in humans. *AJNR* 3:407–414, 1982.
34. Delitala A, Delfini R, Vagnozzi R, Esposito S; Increase in size of cerebral angiomas. Case report. *J Neurosurg* 57:556–558, 1982.
35. DePian R, Pasqualin A, Schienza R, Vivenza C: Microsurgical treatment of ten arteriovenous malformations in critical areas of the cerebrum. *J Microsurg* 1:305–320, 1980.
36. Deruty R, Lapras C, Bret P, Taboada F, et al: Embolisation per-operatoire des malformations arterior-veinueses cerebrales inextirpables: Tentative d'obliteration par un melange a polymerisation retardee A propos de deux cas. *Neurochirurgie* 27:5–14, 1981.
37. Deruty R, Lapras C, Pierluca P, Patet JD, et al: Embolisation peroperatoire des malformations arterio-veineuses cerebrales par le butyl-cyanoacrylate (18 cas). *Neurochirurgie* 31:21–29, 1985.
38. Dimsdale H: Discussion of the neuro-ophthalmological aspects of the cerebral angioma. *Proc R Soc Med* 50:85, 1957.
39. Doe FD, Shuangshoti S, Netsky MG: Cryptic hemangioma of the choroid plexus. *Neurology* 22:1232–1293, 1972.
40. Drake CG: Surgical removal of arteriovenous malformations from the brain stem and cerebellopontine angle. *J Neurosurg* 43:661–670, 1975.
41. Drake CG: Cerebral arteriovenous malformations: considerations for and experience with surgical treatment in 166 cases. *Clin Neurosurg* 26:145–208, 1979.
42. Faria MA, Fleischer AS: Dual cerebral and meningeal supply

to giant arteriovenous malformations of the posterior cerebral hemisphere. *J Neurosurg* 52:153–161, 1980.
43. Fasano VA, Urchioli R, Lombard GF, Benech F, Ponzio RM: Treatment of cerebral arterio-venous malformations with laser. *Neurol Res* 6:127–132, 1984.
44. Feindel W, Yamamoto YL, Hodge CP: Cerebral microcirculation: red cerebral veins and the cerebral steal syndrome: evidence for fluorescein angiography and microregional blood flow by radioisotopes during excision of an angioma. *J Neurosurg* 35:167, 1971.
45. Fierstein T, Pribram HW, Hieshima A: Angiography and computed tomography in the evaluation of cerebral venous malformations. *Neuroradiology* 17:137–142, 1979.
46. Forster DMC, Steiner L, Hakanson S: Arteriovenous malformations of the brain. A long-term clinical study. *J Neurosurg* 37:562–570, 1972.
47. Fujii K, Lenkey C, Rhoton AL Jr: Microsurgical anatomy of the choroidal arteries: Lateral and third ventricles. *J Neurosurg* 52:165–188, 1980.
48. Fults D, Kelly DL: Natural history of arteriovenous malformations of the brain. A clinical study. *Neurosurgery* 15:658–662, 1984.
49. Galatius-Jensen F, Ringberg V: Anastomosis between the anterior choroidal artery and the posterior cerebal artery demonstrated by arteriography. *Radiology* 81:942–944, 1963.
50. Garrido E, Stein B: Removal of an arteriovenous malformation from the basal ganglion. *J Neuro Neurosurg Psychiatry* 41:992–995, 1978.
51. Gerlach J: Intracerebral hemorrage caused by microangiomas. *Prog Neurol Surg* 3:363–396, 1969.
52. Giombini S, Morello G: Cavernous angiomas of the brain (account of 14 personal cases and review of the literature). *Acta Neurochir (Wien)* 40:61–82, 1978.
53. Girvin JP, Fox AJ, Vinuela F, Drake CG: Intraoperative embolization of cerebral arteriovenous malformations in the awake patient. *Clin Neurosurg* 31:188–247, 1983.
54. Gomori JM, Grossman RI, Goldbert HI, Hackney DB, Zimmerman RA, Bilanuik LT: Occult cerebral vascular malformations: High-field MR imaging. *Radiology* 158:707–713, 1986.
55. Graf CJ, Perret GE, Torner JC: Bleeding from cerebral arteriovenous malformations as part of their natural history. *J Neurosurg* 58:331–337, 1983.
56. Guidetti B, Delitala A: Intracranial arteriovenous malformations. Conservative and surgical treatment. *J Neurosurg* 53:149, 1980.
57. Handa H, Yoneda S, Matuda M, Shimizu Y, Goto H: The surgical treatment of deep-seated or large arteriovenous malformations of the brain by means of electrically induced thrombosis. In Carrea R (ed): *Neurological Surgery (with Emphasis on Non-Invasive Methods of Diagnosis and Treatment)*. Amsterdam, Excerpta Medica, 1978, pp 143–148.
58. Hayashi S, Arimoto T, Itakura T, Fujii T, Nishiguchi T, Komai N: The association of intracranial aneurysms and arteriovenous malformation of the brain. *J Neurosurg* 55:971–975, 1981.
59. Henderson WR, Gomez R: Natural History of cerebral angiomas. *Br Med J* 4:571–577, 1967.
60. Herman LH, Fernando OU, Gurdjian ES: The anterior chorodial artery: An anatomical study of its area of distribution. *Anat Rec* 154:95–102, 1966.
61. Heros RC: Arteriovenous malformations of the medial temporal lobe. *J Neurosurg* 56:44–52, 1982.
62. Heros RC, Tu YK: Unruptured arteriovenous malformations. A dilemma in surgical decision making. *Clin Neurosurg* 33:187–236, 1986.
63. Heros RC, Tu YK: Is surgical therapy needed for unruptured arteriovenous malformations? *Neurology* 37:279–286, 1987.
64. Hodge CJ, King BB: Arteriovenous malformation of choroid plexus. Case report. *J Neurosurg* 42:457–461, 1975.
65. Hoffman HJ, Chuang S, Hendrick EB, Humphreys RP: Aneurysms of the vein of Galen. Experience at the Hospital for Sick Children, Toronto. *J Neurosurg* 57:316–322, 1982.
66. Hosobuchi Y, Fabricant J, Lyman J: Stereotaxis heavy-particle irradiation of intracerebral arteriovenous malformation. Paper presented at the American Association of Neurological Surgeons meeting in Denver, CO, 1986.
67. Iansek R, Elstein AS, Balla JI: Application of decision analysis to management of cerebral arteriovenous malformations. *Lancet* 1:1132–1136, 1983.
68. Johnson RT: Radiotherapy of cerebral angiomas, with a note on some problems in diagnosis. In Pia HW, Gleave JRW, Grote E, Zierski J (eds): *Cerebral Angiomas. Advances in Diagnosis and Therapy*. Berlin, Springer-Verlag, 1975, pp 256–266.
69. Jomin M, Lesom F, Lozes G: Prognosis for arteriovenous malformations of the brain in adults based on 150 cases. *Surg Neurol* 23:362–366, 1985.
70. Juhasz J: Surgical treatment of arteriovenous angiomas localised in the corpus callosum, basal ganglia and near the brain stem. *Acta Neurochirurg* 40:83–191, 1978.
71. Kelly DL Jr, Alexander E Jr, Davis CH Jr, Maynard DC: Intracranial arteriovenous malformations: Clinical review and evaluation of brain scans. *J Neurosurg* 31:422–428, 1969.
72. Kerber CW: Balloon catheter with a calibrated leak. *Radiology* 120:547–550, 1976.
73. Kikuchi K, Kowada M, Yoneya M: Association of arteriovenous malformation and intracranial aneurysms in the posterior fossa. *Surg Neurol* 22:499–502, 1984.
74. Kjellberg RN, Hanamura T, Davis KR, Lyons SL, Adams RD: Bragg-peak proton-beam therapy for arteriovenous malformations of the brain. *N Engl J Med* 309:269–274, 1983.
75. Kjellberg RN, Poletti CE, Robertson GH, Adams RD: Bragg peak proton-beam treatment of arteriovenous malformations of the brain. In Carrea R (ed): *Neurological Surgery (with Emphasis on Non-Invasive Methods of Diagnosis and Treatment)*. Amsterdam, Excerpta Medica, 1978, pp 181–187.
76. Klara PM, George ED, McDonnell DE, Pevsner PH: Morphological studies of human arteriovenous malformations. *J Neurosurg* 63:421–425, 1985.
77. Krayenbuhl H, Siebenmann R: Small vascular malformations as a cause of primary intracerebral hemorrhage. *J Neurosurg* 22:7–20, 1965.
78. Krayenbuhl HA: Angiographic contribution to the problem of enlargement of cerebral arteriovenous malformations. *Acta Neurochir* 36:215–242, 1977.
79. Kumar AJ, Fox AJ, Vinuela F, Rosenbaum AE: Revisited old and new CT findings in unruptured large arteriovenous malformations of the brain. *J Comput Assist Tomogr* 8:648–655, 1984.
80. Kunc Z: Surgery of arteriovenous malformations in the speech and motor-sensory regions. *J Neurosurg* 40:293–303, 1974.
81. Kusske JA, Kelly WA: Embolization and reduction of the "steal" syndrome in cerebral arteriovenous malformations. *J Neurosurg* 40:313–321, 1974.
82. Kvam DA, Michelsen WJ, Quest DO: Intracerebral hemorrhage as a complication of artificial embolization. *Neurosurgery* 7:491–494, 1980.
83. Laine E, Delandsheer JM, Pruvot P, Jomin M: Les anevrysmes cirsoides choroidiens anterieurs et les anevrysmes chirsoides stries. *Neurochirurgie* 16:383–396, 1970.
84. Lapras C: Angiomas of cerebellum and brainstem. In Pia HW, Gleave JRW, Grote E, Zierski J (eds): *Cerebral Angiomas. Advances in Diagnosis and Therapy*. Berlin, Springer-Verlag, 1975, pp 136–141.
85. Lasjaunias P, Halimi PH, Lopez-Ibor, Sichez JP, Hurth M, DeTribolet N: Traitement endovasculaire des malformations vasculaires durales (MVD) pures spontanees. Revue de 23 cas explores et traites entre mai 1980 et octobre 1983. *Neurochirurgie* 30:207–223, 1983.

86. LaTorre E, Delitala A, Sorano V: Hematoma of the quadrigeminal plate. J Neurosurg 49:610–613, 1978.
87. Lazar L, Pasztor E, Czirjak S, Lanyi F, Deak G: Experiences in the endovascular treatment of cerebral arteriovenous angiomas. Neurol Res 4:242–252, 1982.
88. Lees F: The migrainous symptoms of cerebral angiomata. J Neurol Neurosurg Psychiatry 25:45–50, 1962.
89. Luessenhop AJ: Artificial embolization for cerebral arteriovenous malformations. Prog Neurol Surg 3:320–362, 1969.
90. Luessenhop AJ: Natural histroy of cerebral arteriovenous malformations. In Wilson CB, Stein BM (eds): Intracranial Ateriovenous Malformations. Baltimore, Williams & Wilkins, 1984, pp 12–33.
91. Luessenhop AJ, Gennarelli TA: Anatomical grading of supratentorial arteriovenous malformations for determining operability. Neurosurgery 1:30–35, 1977.
92. Luessenhop AJ, Mujica PH: Embolization of segments of the circle of Willis and adjacent branches for management of certain inoperable cerebral arteriovenous malformations. J Neurosurg 54:573–582, 1981.
93. Luessenhop AJ, Presper JH: Surgical embolization of cerebral arteriovenous malformations through the intracranial carotid and vertebral arteries. Long-term results. J Neurosurg 42:443–451, 1975.
94. Luessenhop AJ, Rosa L: Cerebral arteriovenous malformations. Indications for and results of surgery, and the role of intravascular techniques. J Neurosurg 60:14–22, 1984.
95. MacKenzie I: The clinical presentation of the cerebral angioma: A review of 50 cases. Brain 76:184–214, 1953.
96. Maehara T, Tasaka A: Cerebral venous angioma: computerized tomography and angiographic diagnosis. Neuroradiology 16:296, 1978.
97. Malik GM: Surgical treatment of large cerebral arteriovenous malformations. In Smith RR, Haerer AF, Russell WF (eds): Vascular Malformations and Fistulas of the Brain. New York, Raven Press, 1982, pp 77–99.
98. Malis LI: Arteriovenous malformations of the brain. In Youmans JR (ed): Neurological Surgery, ed 2. Philadelphia, WB Saunders, 1982, pp 1786–1806.
99. Margolis G, Odom GL, Woodhall B, Bloor BM: The role of small angiomatous malformations in the production of intracerebral hematomas. J Neurosurg 8:564–575, 1951.
100. Martin NA, Stein BM, Wilson CB: Arteriovenous malformations of the posterior fossa. In Wilson CB, Stein BM (eds): Intracranial Arteriovenous Malformations. Baltimore, Williams & Wilkins, 1984, pp 209–221.
101. Martin NA, Wilson CB, Stein BM: Venous and Cavernous malformations. In Wilson CB, Stein BM (eds): Intracranial Arteriovenous Malformations. Baltimore, Williams & Wilkins, 1984, pp 234–245.
102. Matsumura H, Makita Y, Someda K, Kondo A: Arteriovenous malformations in the posterior fossa. J Neurosurg 47:50–56, 1977.
103. Mawad ME, Hilal SK, Michelsen WJ, Stein B, Ganti SR: Occlusive vascular disease associated with cerebral arteriovenous malformations. Radiology 153:401–408, 1984.
104. McCormick WF: The pathology of vascular ("arteriovenous") malformations. J Neurosurg 24:807–812, 1966.
105. McCormick WF: Classification, pathology, and natural history of angiomas of the central nervous system. Neurol Neurosurg Wkly Update 1:3–7, 1978.
106. McGuire TH, Greenwood J Jr, Newton BL: Bilateral angioma of the choroid plexus. Case report. J Neurosurg 11:428–430, 1954.
107. Menezes AH, Graf CJ, Jacoby CC, Cornell SH: Management of vein of Galen aneurysms. Report of two cases. J Neurosurg 55:457–462, 1981.
108. Michels LG, Bentson JR, Winter J: Computed tomography of cerebral venous angiomas. J Comput Assist Tomogr 1:149–154, 1977.
109. Michelsen WJ: Natural history and pathophysiology of arteriovenous malformations. Clin Neurosurg 26:307–313, 1979.
110. Mickle JP, Quisling RG: The transtorcular embolization of vein of Galen aneurysms. J Neurosurg 64:731–735, 1986.
111. Mingrino S: Supratentorial arteriovenous malformations of the brain. In Krayenbuhl H (ed): Advances and Technical Standards in Neurosurgery. New York, Springer-Verlag, 1978, vol 5, pp 93–123.
112. Mitnick JS, Pinto RS, Lin JP, Rose H, Lieberman A: CT of thrombosed arteriovenous malformations in children. Radiology 150:385–389, 1984.
113. Miyasaka K, Wolpert SM, Prager RJ: The association of cerebral aneurysms, infundibula, and intracranial arteriovenous malformations. Stroke 13:196–203, 1982.
114. Mohr J: Neurological manifestations and factors related to therapeutic decisions. In Wilson CB, Stein BM (eds): Intracranial Arteriovenous Malformations. Baltimore, Williams & Wilkins, 1984, pp 1–11.
115. Mohr JP, Caplan LR, Melski JW, Goldstein RJ, Duncan GW, Kistler JP, Pessin MS, Bleich H: The Harvard Cooperative Stroke Registry: A prospective registry. Neurology 28:754–762, 1978.
116. Moody RA, Poppen JL: Arteriovenous malformations. J Neurosurg 32:503–511, 1970.
117. Morello G, Broghi GP: Cerebral angiomas. A report of 154 personal cases and a comparison between the results of surgical excision and conservative management. Acta Neurochir (Wien) 28:135–155, 1973.
118. Moritake K, Handa H, Mori K, Ishikawa M, Morimoto M, Takebi Y: Venous angiomas of the brain. Surg Neurol 14:95–105, 1980.
119. Mullan S, Brown FD, Patronas NJ: Hypermic and ischemic problems of surgical treatment of arteriovenous malformations. J Neurosurg 51:757–764, 1979.
120. Nehls, DG, Carter LP: Multiple unusual aneurysms and arteriovenous malformations in a single patient: A case report. Neurosurgery 17:97–100, 1985.
121. New PFJ, Ojemann RG, Davis KR, Rosen BR, Heros RC, Kjellberg RN, Adams RD, Richardson EP: Magnetic resonance imaging and CT of occult vascular malformations of the brain. AJNR 7:771–779, 1986.
122. Newton TH, Trost BT: Arteriovenous malformations and fistulae. In Newton TH (ed): Radiology of the Skull and Brain. St Louis, CV Mosby, 1974, vol II, book 4, pp 2490–2565.
123. Norcross K, Ciric IS, Mikhael MA, Vick NA: Vascular malformation of the thalamus with normal angiograms. J Neuro-Oncol 3:69–76, 1985.
124 Nornes H, Grip A: Hemodynamic aspects of cerebral arteriovenous malformations. J Neurosurg 53:456–464, 1980.
125. Nornes H, Lundar T, Wikeby P: Cerebral arteriovenous malformations: Results of microsurgical management. Acta Neurochir (Wien) 50:243–257, 1979.
126. Olivecrona H, Riives J: Arteriovenous aneurysms of the brain: their diagnosis and treatment. Arch Neurol Psychiatry 59:567–602, 1948.
127. Parkinson D, Bachers G: Arteriovenous malformations. Summary of 100 consecutive supratentorial cases. J Neurosurg 53:285–299, 1980.
128. Paterson JH, McKissok W: A clinical survey of intracranial aneurysms with special reference to their mode of progression and surgical treatment: A report of 110 cases. Brain 79:223–226, 1956.
129. Patil AA: Surgical excision of arteriovenous malformation of the cerebellum and brainstem: A case presentation. Acta Neurochir (Wien) 54:117–125, 1980.
130. Pellettieri L, Carlsson AA, Grevsten S, Norlen G, Uhlemann C: Surgical vs conservative treatment of intracranial arteriovenous malformations: A Study in surgical decision making. Acta Neuochir (Wien) (Suppl)29:1–86, 1980.
131. Perret G: Conservative management of inoperable arterio-

venous malformations. In Pia HW, Gleave JRW, Grote E, Zierski J (eds): *Cerebral Angiomas. Advances in Diagnosis and Therapy*. New York, Springer-Verlag, 1975, pp 268–270.
132. Perret G: The epidemiology and clinical course of arteriovenous malformations. In Pia HW, Gleave JRW, Grote E, Zierski J (eds): *Cerebral Angiomas. Advances in Diagnosis and Therapy*. New York, Springer-Verlag, 1975, pp 21–26.
133. Perret G, Nishioka H: Report on cooperative study on intracranial aneurysms and subarachnoid hemorrhage. Section VI: Arteriovenous malformations. Analysis of 545 cases of cranio-cerebral arteriovenous malformations and fistulae reported to cooperative study. *J Neurosurg* 25:467–490, 1966.
134. Pertuiset B, Ancri D, Sichez JP, Chauvin M: Radical surgery in cerebral AVM. Tactical procedures based upon hemodynamic factors. In Krayenbuhl H (ed): *Advances and Technical Standards in Neurosurgery*. New York, Springer-Verlag, 1983, vol 10, pp 81–144.
135. Pertuiset B, Sachs M, Guyot J-F: Les anevrysmes arterioveineux des parois juxta-pedonculaires de la fente de bichat. *La Presse Med* 71:2341–2342, 1963.
136. Pertuiset B, Sichez JP, Philippon J: Mortalite et morbidite apres exerese chirurgicale totale de 162 malformations arterioveineuses intracraniennes (1958–1978). *Rev Neurol (Paris)* 35:319, 1979.
137. Pevsner PH: Microballoon catheter for superselective angiography and therapeutic occlusion. *AJR* 128:225–230, 1977.
138. Pozzati E, Gaist G, Poppi M, Morrone B: Microsurgical removal of paraventricular cavernous angiomas. Report of two cases. *J Neurosurg* 55:308–311, 1981.
139. Pozzati E, Padovani R, Morrone B, Finizio F, Gaist G: Cerebral cavernous angiomas in children. *J Neurosurg* 53:826–832, 1980.
140. Preissig RS, Preissig SH, Goree SA: Angiographic demonstration of a cerebral venous angioma. Case Report. *J Neurosurg* 44:628–631, 1976
141. Pribil S, Boone SC, Waley R: Obstructive hydrocephalus at the anterior third ventricle caused by dilated veins from an arteriovenous malformation. *Surg Neurol* 20:487–492, 1983.
142. Rhoton AL Jr, Fujii K, Fradd B: Microsurgical anatomy of the anterior choroidal artery. *Surg Neurol* 12:171–187, 1979.
143. Rothfus WE, Albright AL, Casey KF, Latchaw RE, Roppolo HM: Cerebellar venous angioma: "Benign" entity? *AJNR* 5:61–66, 1984.
144. Rutka JT, Tucker WS: Successful removal of an arteriovenous malformation in the basal ganglia. *Neurosurgery* 14:472–474, 1984.
145. Sadeh M, Shacked I, Rappaport ZH, Tadmor R: Surgical extirpation of a venous angioma of the medulla oblongata simulating multiple sclerosis. *Surg Neurol* 17:334–337, 1982.
146. Sahs, AL, Perrett GE, Locksley HB, Niskioka H (eds): *Intracranial Aneurysms and Subarachnoid Hemorrhage: A Cooperative Study*. Philadelphia, JB Lippincott, 1969.
147. Saito Y, Kobayashi N: Cerebral venous aniomas. Clinical evaluation and possible etiology. *Radiology* 139:87–94, 1981.
148. Salcman M, Nudelman RW, Bellis EH: Arteriovenous malformations of the superior cerebellar artery: Excision via an occipital transtentorial approach. *Neurosurgery* 17:749–756.
149. Samson D, Ditmore QM, Beyer CW Jr: Intravascular use of isobutyl 2-cyanoacrylate: Part I. Treatment of intracranial arteriovenous malformations. *Neurosurgery* 8:43–51, 1981.
150. Samson D, Hatjer H: Arteriovenous malformations of the cerebellar vermis. *Neurosurgery* 16:341–349, 1985.
151. Sano K, Jimbo M, Saito I, Baseiji N: Artificial embolization of inoperable angioma with polymerizing substance. In Pia HW, Gleave JRW, Grote E, Zierski J (eds): *Cerebral Angiomas. Advances in Diagnosis and Therapy*. Berlin, Springer-Verlag, 1975, pp 222–229.
152. Sarwar M, McCormick WF: Intracerebral venous angioma. *Arch Neurol* 35: 323–328, 1978.
153. Scott WG, Simril WA, Seaman WB: Intracerebral arteriovenous malformations. *Am J Roentgenol Radium Ther Nucl Med* 71:762–776, 1954.
154. Scotti LN, Goldman RL, Rao GR: Cerebral venous angioma. *Neuroradiology* 9:125–128, 1975.
155. Senegar M, Dohrmann GJ, Wollman RL: Venous angiomas of the posterior fossa should be considered as anomalous venous drainage. *Surg Neurol* 19:26–32, 1983.
156. Serbinenko FA: Balloon catheterization of occlusion of major cerebral vessels. *J Neurosurg* 41:125–145, 1974.
157. Six EG, Cowley AR, Kelly DL Jr, Laster DW: Thrombosed aneurysm of the vein of Galen. *Neurosurgery* 7:274–278, 1980.
158. Solomon RA, Stein BM: Management of arteriovenous malformations of the brain stem. *J Neurosurg* 64:857–864, 1986.
159. Spencer DD, Spencer S, Mattson RH, Williamson PD, Novelly RA: Access to posterior medial temporal lobe structures in the surgical treatment of temporal lobe epilepsy. *Neurosurgery* 15:667–671, 1984.
160. Spetzler RF, Martin NA: A proposed grading system for arteriovenous malformations. *J Neurosurg* 65:476–483, 1986.
161. Spetzler RF, Wilson CB, Weinstein PR: Normal perfusion pressure breakthrough theory. *Clin Neurosurg* 25:651–672, 1978.
162. Stah SM, Johnson KP, Malamud N: The clinical and pathological spectrums of brain-stem vascular malformations. Long-term course simulates multiple sclerosis. *Arch Neurol* 37:25–30, 1980.
163. Stein BM: Arteriovenous malformations of the medial cerebral hemisphere and the limbic system. *J Neurosurg* 60:23–31, 1984.
164. Stein BM: General techniques for the surgical removal of arteriovenous malformations. In Wilson CB, Stein BM (eds): *Intracranial Arteriovenous Malformations*. Baltimore, Williams & Wilkins, 1984, pp 143–155.
165. Stein BM, Wolpert SM: Surgical and embolic treatment of cerebral arteriovenous malformations. *Surg Neurol* 7:359–369, 1977.
166. Stein BM, Wolpert SM: Arteriovenous malformations of the brain. I: Current concepts and treatment. *Arch Neurol* 37:1–5, 1980.
167. Stein BM, Wolpert SM: Arteriovenous malformations of the brain. II: Current concepts and treatment. *Arch Neurol* 37:69–75, 1980.
168. Steiner L, Leskell L, Forster DMC, Greitz T, Backlund E-O: Stereotactic radiosurgery in intracranial arteriovenous malformations. *Acta Neurochir* 21:195–209, 1974.
169. Suzuki J, Onuma T, Kayama T: Surgical treatment of intracranial arteriovenous malformations. *Neurol Res* 4:191–207, 1982.
170. Suzuki J, Takahashi A, Yoshimoto T, Seki Hirobumi: Use of balloon occlusion and substances to protect ischemic brain during resection of posterior fossa AVM: Case report. *J Neurosurg* 63:626–629, 1985.
171. Svien HJ, McRae JA: Arteriovenous anomalies of the brain. Fate of patients not having definitive surgery. *J Neurosurg* 23:23–28, 1965.
172. Tahmouresie A, Quest, DO: Vascular malformation of the medial posterior choroidal artery. *Surg Neurol* 12:235–237, 1979.
173. Terao H, Hori T, Matsutani M, Okeda R: Detection of cryptic vascular malformations by computerized tomography. Report of two cases. *J Neurosurg* 51:546–551, 1979.
174. Tognetti F, Andreaoli A, Cuscina A, Testa C: Successful management of an intracranial arteriovenous malformation by conventional irradiation. *J Neurosurg* 63:193–195, 1985.
175. Tonnis W, Schieffer W, Walter W: Signs and symptoms of supratentorial arteriovenous aneurysms. *J Neurosurg* 15:471–480, 1958.
176. Tonnis W, Walter W: Differential diagnose, Klinik und Behandlung der cerebralen Gefassmissbildungen. In *Biologie*

und Klinik des Zentralnervensystems. Basel, Sandoz, 1967.
177. Torner JC: Natural history of arteriovenous malformations. Paper presented at the American Association of Neurological Surgeons meeting, San Francisco, CA, April 12, 1984.
178. Troost BT, Newton TH: Occipital lobe arteriovenous malformations. Arch Ophthalmol 93:250–256, 1975.
179. Troupp H: Arteriovenous malformations of the brain: What are the indications for operation? In Morley TP (ed): Current Controversies in Neurosurgery. Philadelphia, WB Saunders, 1976, pp 210–216.
180. U HS: Microsurgical excision of the paraventricular arteriovenous malformations. Neurosurgery 16:293–303, 1985.
181. Vaquero J, Leunda G, Martinez R, Bravo, G: Cavernomas of the brain. Neurosurgery 12:208–210, 1983.
182. Viale GL, Turtas S, Pau A: Surgical removal of striate arteriovenous malformations. Surg Neurol 14:321–324, 1980.
183. Vianello A: Angiome arterio-veineux (A.A.V.) due glomus choroidien gauch. Neuro-chirurgie 4:327–332, 1969.
184. Vinter HV, Debrun G: Pathology of arteriovenous malformation embolized with isobutyl-2-cynoacrylate (bucrylate). Report of two cases. J Neurosurg 55:819–825, 1981.
185. Vinter HV, Lundi MJ, Kaufmann CE: Long-term pathological follow-up of cerebral arteriovenous malformations treated by embolizations with bucrylate. New Engl J Med 314:477–483, 1986.
186. Vinuela F, Debrun GM, Fox AJ, Girvin JP, Peerless SJ: Dominant hemisphere arteriovenous malformations; therapeutic embolization with isobutyl-2 cyanoacrylate. AJNR 4:959–966, 1983.
187. Vineula F, Fox AJ, Debrun G, Pelz D: Preembolization superselective angiography: Role in the treatment in brain arteriovenous malformations with isobutyl-2-cyanoacrylate. AJNR 5:765–769, 1984.
188. Vineula F, Nombela L, Roach MR, Fox AJ, Pelz DM: Stenotic and occlusive disease of the venous drainage system of deep brain AVM's. J Neurosurg 63:180–184, 1985.
189. Vorght K, Yasargil MG: Cerebral cavernous hemangiomas or cavernomas. Neurochirugia (Stuttg) 19:59–68, 1976.
190. Waga S, Shimosaka S, Kojima T: Arteriovenous malformations of the lateral ventricle. J Neurosurg 63:185–192, 1985.
191. Wakai S, Ueda Y, Inoh S, Nagai M: Angiographically occult angiomas: A report of thirteen cases with analysis of the cases documented in the literature. Neurosurgery 17:549–556, 1985.
192. Walter W: Conservative treatment of cerebral arteriovenous angiomas. In Pia HW, Gleave JRW, Grote E, Zierski J (eds): Cerebral Angiomas. Advances in Diagnosis and Therapy. New York, Springer-Verlag, 1975, pp 271–278.
193. Wendling LR, Morre JS, Kieffer SA, Goldberg HI, Latchaw RE: Intracerebral venous angioma. Radiology 119:141–147, 1976.
194. Wharen RD, Anderson RE, Sundt TM: The Nd:YAG laser in neurosurgery. J Neurosurg 60:540–547, 1984.
195. Wharen RE Jr, Scheithauer BW, Laws ER Jr: Thrombosed arteriovenous malformations of the brain. J Neurosurg 57:520–526, 1982.
196. Wilkins RH: Multiple aneurysms and associated arteriovenous malformations: Operative considerations. In Hopkins LN (ed): Clinical Management of Intracranial Aneurysms. New York, Raven Press, 1982, pp 193–200.
197. Wilson CB, Martin NA: Deep supratentorial arteriovenous malformations. In Wilson CB, Stein BM (eds): Intracranial Arteriovenous Malformations. Baltimore, Williams & Wilkins, 1984, pp 184–208.
198. Wilson CB, U HS, Domingue J: Microsurgical treatment of intracranial vascular malformations. J Neurosurg 51:446–454, 1979.
199. Wolpert SM, Stein BM: Catheter embolization of intracranial arteriovenous malformations as an aid to surgical excision. Neuroradiology 10:73–85, 1975.
200. Yasargil MG, Antic J, Laciga R, Jain K, Boone SC, Arteriovenous malformations of vein of Galen: Microsurgical treatment. Surg Neurol 6:195–200, 1976.
201. Yasargil MG, Jain KK, Antic J, Laciga R: Arteriovenous malformations of the splenium of the corpus callosum: Microsurgical treatment. Surg Neurol 5:5–14, 1976.
202. Yasargil MG, Jain KK, Antic J, Laciga R, Kletter C: Arteriovenous malformations of the anterior and middle portions of the corpus callosum: Microsurgical treatment. Surg Neurol 5:67–80, 1976.
203. Yamasaki T, Handa H, Yamashita J, Moritake K, Nagasawa S: Intracranial cavernous angioma angiographically mimicking venous angioma in an infant. Surg Neurol 22:461–466, 1984.
204. Zellem RT, Buchheit WA: Multiple intracranial arteriovenous malformations: Case report. Neurosurgery 17:88–93, 1985.

23

Dural Arteriovenous Malformations

PATHOLOGY

Arteriovenous malformations (AVMs) involving the dura consist of abnormal communications between branches of the external carotid, internal carotid, and vertebral arteries and the venous sinuses within the dura, tentorium, or falx. Most dural AVMs involve the transverse and sigmoid sinuses (17). The next most common site is the cavernous sinus, and these malformations are discussed in Chapter 24. A few cases of dural AVMs involving the anterior fossa and the sphenoparietal sinus have been reported (4, 38). The present authors have experience with one case involving the region of the torcula (Fig. 23.1) and another in the area of the tentorial incisura and petrosal sinus (Fig. 23.2). About 200 cases of dural AVMs have been reported in the literature.

Rarely is there a history of trauma (30) or surgery (39). Some dural AVMs are probably developmental in origin (2, 30). Most lesions, however, appear to be acquired (2, 17). Several lines of evidence support this concept. Clinical presentation is usually in midlife, and lesions are rarely identified in children (1). Spontaneous resolution is common, particularly for cavernous sinus lesions (11, 19, 25, 31). Angiography often shows sinus occlusion or irregularities suggesting recanalization (13, 17). Finally, fistulas have been demonstrated in patients known previously to have normal angiography or sinus occlusion without arteriovenous fistula (7, 17).

On the basis of these observations, it is believed that inflammation and/or thrombosis results in partial or total sinus occlusion (5). Preexisting minute arteriovenous channels in the sinus wall then open and enlarge to form an AVM. The initial sinus occlusion may recanalize. Spontaneous resolution may result from sinus thrombosis (7, 17). This general mechanism could explain childhood cases that might be due to perinatal sinus injury.

CLINICAL PRESENTATION

Dural AVMs of the transverse and sigmoid sinuses can occur at any age and affect both sexes but are more common in women older than 40 years of age. Pulsatile tinnitus is the most common presenting symptom. Headaches are the next most common complaint and may be due to raised intracranial pressure. Other manifestations of intracranial hypertension are visual obscurations and visual dimming or blindness, sometimes in relation to papilledema or proptosis (6, 16, 17, 20, 22, 30, 34).

Occasionally, patients present with hemiparesis, speech disturbance, tic douloureux, gait ataxia, seizures, brain stem signs, hydrocephalus, or hemorrhage, which may be subarachnoid or intracerebral (14, 19, 24, 29, 30, 37). These symptoms may be due to arterialized cortical venous drainage. "Steal" phenomena may rarely explain focal symptoms (37).

On examination, a bruit is usually heard over the mastoid region. Papilledema may be associated with decreased visual acuity. Unusual cases may show signs of local neural compression. A few patients exhibit meningismus and other signs typical of subarachnoid hemorrhage.

These lesions can be asymptomatic, being an incidental finding at the time of angiography (2). Spontaneous thrombosis and disappearance of symptomatology have been reported (3, 11, 21, 25, 33).

RADIOGRAPHIC EVALUATION

Computed tomography outlines ventricular size and may show abnormal decreased density in the white matter, patchy enhancement, and hemorrhage when this has occurred (8, 9, 28). The malformation itself is usually not seen, but dilated veins may be outlined. In one case, it was observed that after obliteration of the shunt the decreased density in the white matter disappeared, suggesting that it was due to the edema from the raised venous sinus pressure (28).

Adequate angiography requires selective studies of the external and internal carotid and vertebral arteries (18, 21, 23). Subtraction angiography and special oblique views may be needed to characterize the fistulous communications. The center of the malformation is usually at the junction of the transverse and sigmoid sinuses (17) (Figs. 23.3 and 23.4).

Kühner et al have classified the possible sources of blood supply into three groups (21). In the external group, arteries from the scalp and neck reach the dura through perforations in the skull. This includes perforating branches from the occipital, superficial temporal, and posterior auricular arteries and muscular branches from the ascending cervical and vertebral arteries. In the intermediate group, meningeal branches from both the middle meningeal and vertebral arteries supply the malformation. The internal group inclues the tentorial branches from the internal carotid artery and, less commonly, leptomeningeal branches from the posterior and middle cerebral arteries.

Retrograde filling of the venous system may be striking (Fig. 23.4A and B). In some cases, thrombosis of a sinus may be seen (13). In the 14 patients reported by Houser et al, 10 had occlusion or narrowing of the transverse or sigmoid sinus (17). Particular attention should be paid to cortical venous engorgement because of the poor prognosis associated with this feature (37).

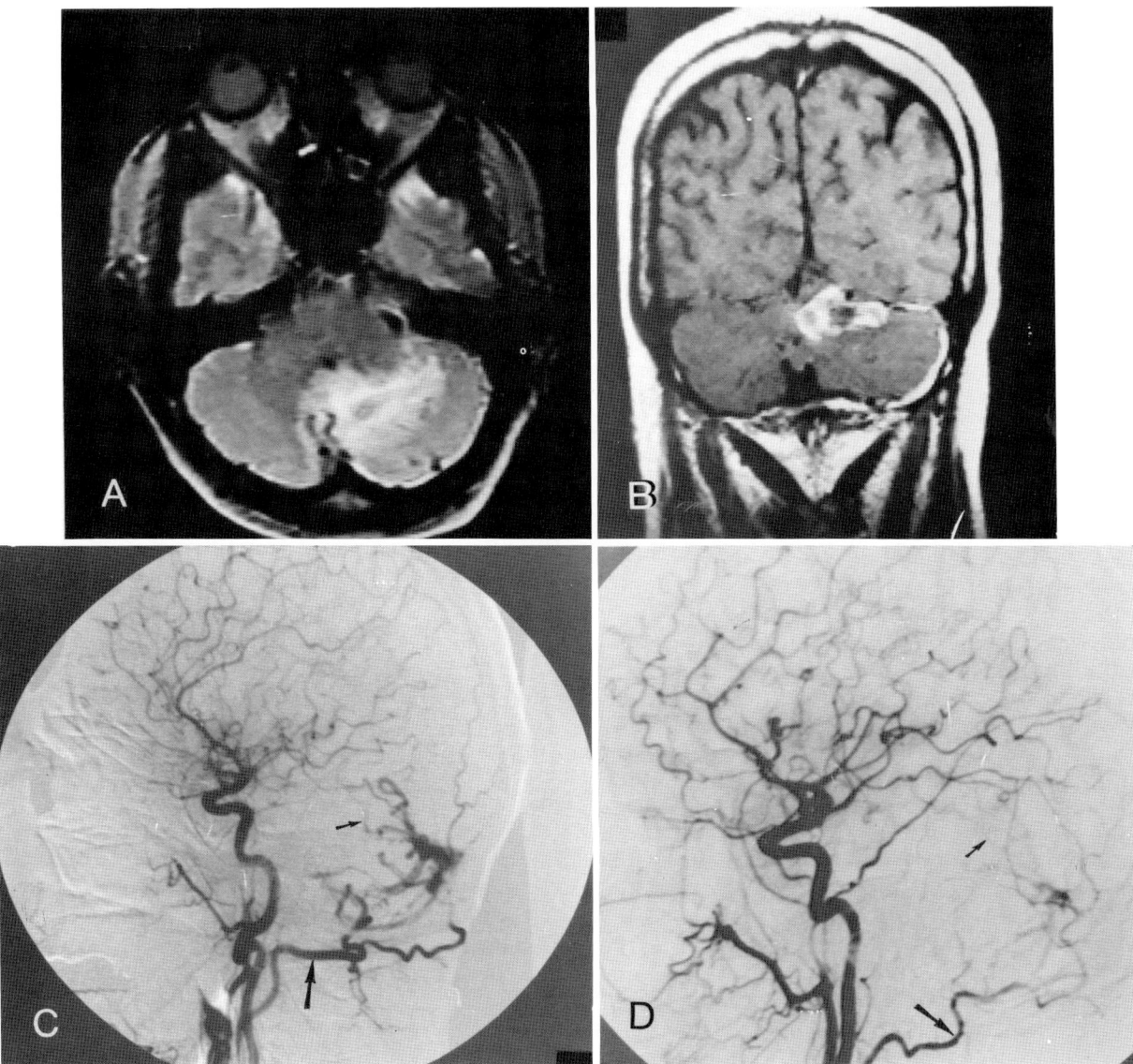

Figure 23.1. Dural AVM of the torcular region in a patient who presented with a cerebellar hemorrage. **A** and **B**, Magnetic resonance imaging of cerebellar region in transverse and coronal planes shows cerebellar hemorrhage and large vessels (signal void). Note the relatively high position of the hemorrhage. **C** and **D**, Right and left common carotid injections, respectively, show the fistula in the region of the torcula fed mostly by the occipital (*large arrows*) and tentorial (*small arrows*) arteries. **E**, Vertebral injection. The fistula does not fill, emphasizing the importance of performing common carotid angiography in cases of suspected cerebellar AVM when vertebral angiography is negative. The fistula was obliterated successfully by skeletonization of the inferior sagittal sinus and the medial aspect of both the transverse sinuses and the torcula (by bilateral division of the tentorium). The operation was performed via a bilateral occipital and suboccipital craniotomy through a long linear skin incision.

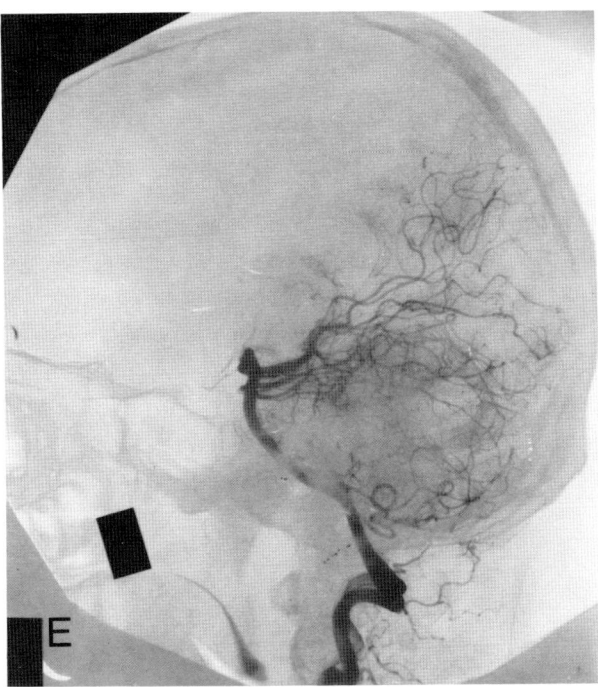

Figure 23.1E.

SURGICAL MANAGEMENT

Indications

When patients present with minor complaints of noise in the head or headaches, often no treatment need be offered. However, in patients with progressive disabling symptoms or in those in whom an intracranial hemorrhage has occurred, surgical treatment of the dural AVM is indicated unless the general medical condition offers a contraindication. Surgery may also be indicated for removal of intracranial hematomas from dural AVMs. The presence of arterialized cortical drainage on angiography is a feature favoring aggressive treatment.

Several reports have concluded that surgical resection of the transverse and proximal sigmoid sinuses is the preferred treatment for fistulas of this region (17, 20, 30, 33, 34). The difficulty of treating recurrent, incompletely treated lesions has been emphasized (34). Hugosson and Bergstrom have described the exposure and dural incisions, although they ligated the sinus, they did not resect it (18). The present authors have experience with both approaches with good results so far but without a long enough follow-up period to recommend either the more aggressive approach (sinus excision) or the more conservative approach (skeletonization of the sinus). When there is no occlusion of the sinus and no reversal of venous drainage from normal cortex, they prefer to skeletonize the sinus and leave it patent to avoid the risk of venous infarction. Occasionally, a shunt will be required for relief of hydrocephalus.

Technique

During the exposure, Lasix and mannitol may be given to facilitate brain retraction, particularly if tentorial section is planned. For the common unilateral transverse-sigmoid fistula, the supine position is used, with the patient's ipsilateral shoulder elevated on a roll and the head slightly elevated and rotated laterally (Fig. 23.5A). The incision is marked in front of the ear and extends back a variable degree, depending on the medial extent of the fistula along the transverse sinus, and then obliquely downward to cross over the anterior border of the sternocleidomastoid muscle (Fig. 23.5B). This lower extension of the incision is opened first to provide access to the carotid artery bifurcation for ligation of the occipital artery and for temporary occlusion of the external carotid artery, as necessary, to help reduce bleeding during the rest of the exposure. As the scalp flap is turned back, individual perforating arteries entering the bone are coagulated and the bone is waxed. In some patients, the bone may look like a sieve with blood pouring out of each small hole. Hemostasis at this stage can sometimes be quite difficult but can usually be achieved with bone wax.

The bone removal must extend above and below the transverse sinus. Usually, a suboccipital craniectomy is performed and a bone flap is turned over the sinus. Torrential, fatal hemorrhage after removing the bone flap has been described (34). In some patients, the present authors use the technique of raising a single bone flap over the temporal, occipital, and suboccipital regions. This is done by placing multiple burr holes and then carefully separating the dura from the bone. Separation of the area of the sinuses and the fistula is deferred until after the rest of the bone flap has been cut and separated from the dura. Just before the bone flap is ready to be raised, the last bone cuts are made across the sinus. Two maneuvers have been found to be extremely helpful in preventing excessive blood loss at this stage. The first is to place the burr holes and enlarge them as necessary with a craniectomy so that the meningeal vessels can be occluded prior to raising the bone flap. There is usually at least a large posterior branch of the middle meningeal artery (Figs. 23.3A and 23.4B). The second helpful maneuver is to expose the carotid bifurcation region as the first step and temporarily occlude the external carotid artery as needed. The occipital artery, which is almost always a major external feeder, can be permanently occluded before the craniotomy is even started. To control the dural bleeding, packing and pressure may be required. The packs are gradually removed with stepwise electrocoagulation of the dural bleeders, which can be a very tedious process.

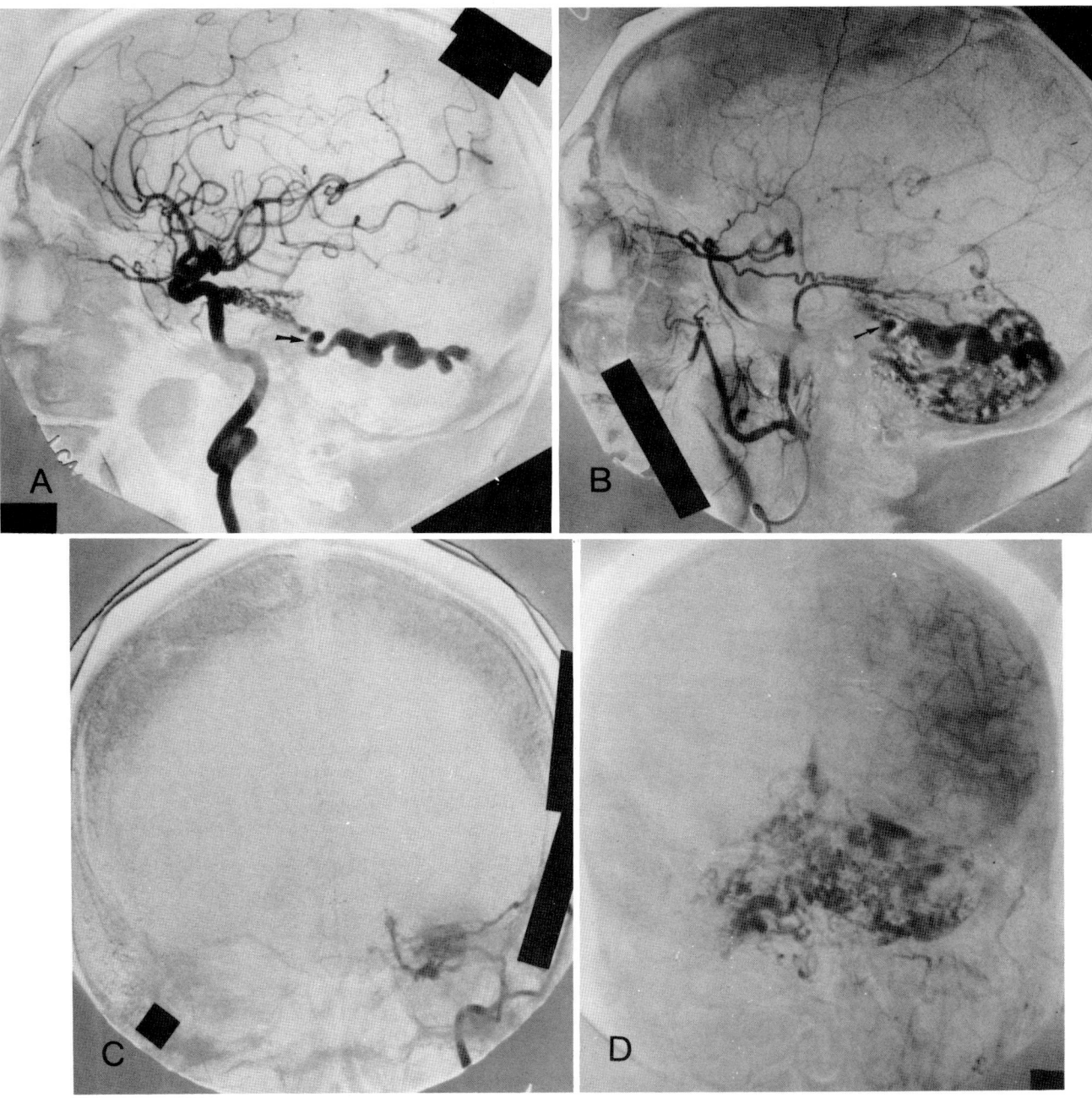

Figure 23.2. Dural fistula of the region of the left tentorial incisura in a patient who presented with papilledema and mild but progressive brain stem and cerebellar dysfunction. **A,** Left internal carotid injection shows multiple tortuous tentorial arterial branches draining into a large single vein in the area of the superior petrosal vein (*arrow*). **B** and **C,** Left external carotid injection shows filling of the fistula (*arrow*) by meningeal and tentorial branches. **D,** Late arterial phase shows extensive early filling of a complex of tortuous, dilated veins throughout the posterior fossa. The fistula was occluded through a left subtemporal craniotomy with extensive cauterization and division of the tentorial edge behind the insertion of the fourth nerve and over the petrous pyramid. The connection of the fistula to the venous system of the posterior fossa was through a single, dilated superior petrosal vein which was divided after it had become blue and collapsed after obliteration of the fistula. **E** and **F,** Postoperative internal and external carotid angiograms show no residual fistula.

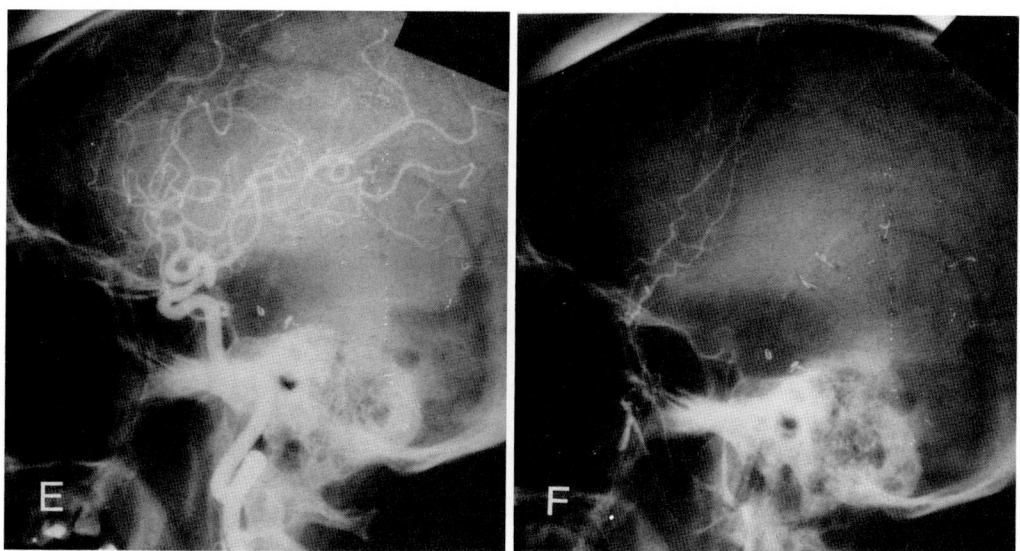

Figure 23.2E and F.

The sigmoid sinus is uncovered by using the high-speed air drill (Fig. 23.5). The only area that cannot be exposed is the outer wall of the basal portion of the sigmoid sinus. In the authors' experience, failure to take the exposure far enough laterally can result in failure to obliterate the lesion, thus special effort is warranted here.

There are numerous small feeders coming to the area of the fistula directly through the mastoid and petrous bones across the dura lateral to the sigmoid sinus. These feeders can only be obliterated by thorough drilling through the mastoid bone and into the posterior aspect of the petrous bone so that the dura lateral to the sigmoid sinus can be cut or at least thoroughly coagulated. Familiarity with the anatomy of this region or the assistance of an otolaryngologist is important to avoid damage to hearing or to the facial nerve during this stage of the operation. This is usually the most difficult part of the operation because of the problems controlling bleeding from the petrous bone (Fig. 23.5C).

The dura is opened above, below, and parallel to the sinus, with the feeding arteries occluded as they are encountered (Fig. 23.5B and C). The incision above the transverse sinus ends at the superior petrosal sinus. The dura lateral to the sigmoid sinus but below the superior petrosal sinus should ideally be coagulated and divided, but if this is too difficult, at least thorough coagulation should be carried out. The incision in the cerebellar dura is carried below the transverse and sigmoid sinuses as close to the jugular foramen as possible (38). Great care must be taken to prevent injury to the congested brain, since uncontrollable edema and bleeding may result even from minor injury to the hyperemic cortex. An incision is made in the tentorium anterior to the transverse sinus from just lateral to the torcula to the superior petrosal sinus. This step may be omitted when there is lack of angiographic evidence of tentorial feeders and one can confirm at surgery, by looking above and below the tentorium, that the tentorium contains no arterialized feeders to the fistula. The transverse sinus is then clamped, ligated, and oversewn lateral to the torcula. A second ligation, as far lateral as possible, is performed and the sinus is excised (Fig. 23.2D). To occlude feeders from the petrous bone that cannot be reached laterally by excision, the sinus is plugged with muscle or plastic (Fig. 23.5D). The dural defect is closed with a graft of pericranial tissue (Fig. 23.5E).

An alternative is to skeletonize the sinus and leave it in place, particularly when there is normal venous cortical drainage (e.g., the vein of Labbé) into a patent transverse sinus. If the opposite transverse sinus is open on preoperative angiography, the sigmoid sinus can be divided, packed, and occluded below the superior petrosal sinus. It is easier to leave the sigmoid sinus patent, but then one must ensure, by very thorough bone removal lateral to the sigmoid sinus, that no arterial feeders are left from the petrous bone.

Closure after dural grafting involves replacement of the bone flap and obliteration of the mastoid air cells and any defect in the petrous bone to avoid postoperative cerebrospinal fluid leakage. The authors routinely prepare the abdomen in order to obtain some fat, if necessary, for this maneuver. Gelfoam and bone wax may suffice in cases in which pneumatization is not extensive and one is sure that the dural closure is watertight.

For certain paraclinoid lesions, a frontotemporal craniotomy will be needed for excision (37). For the

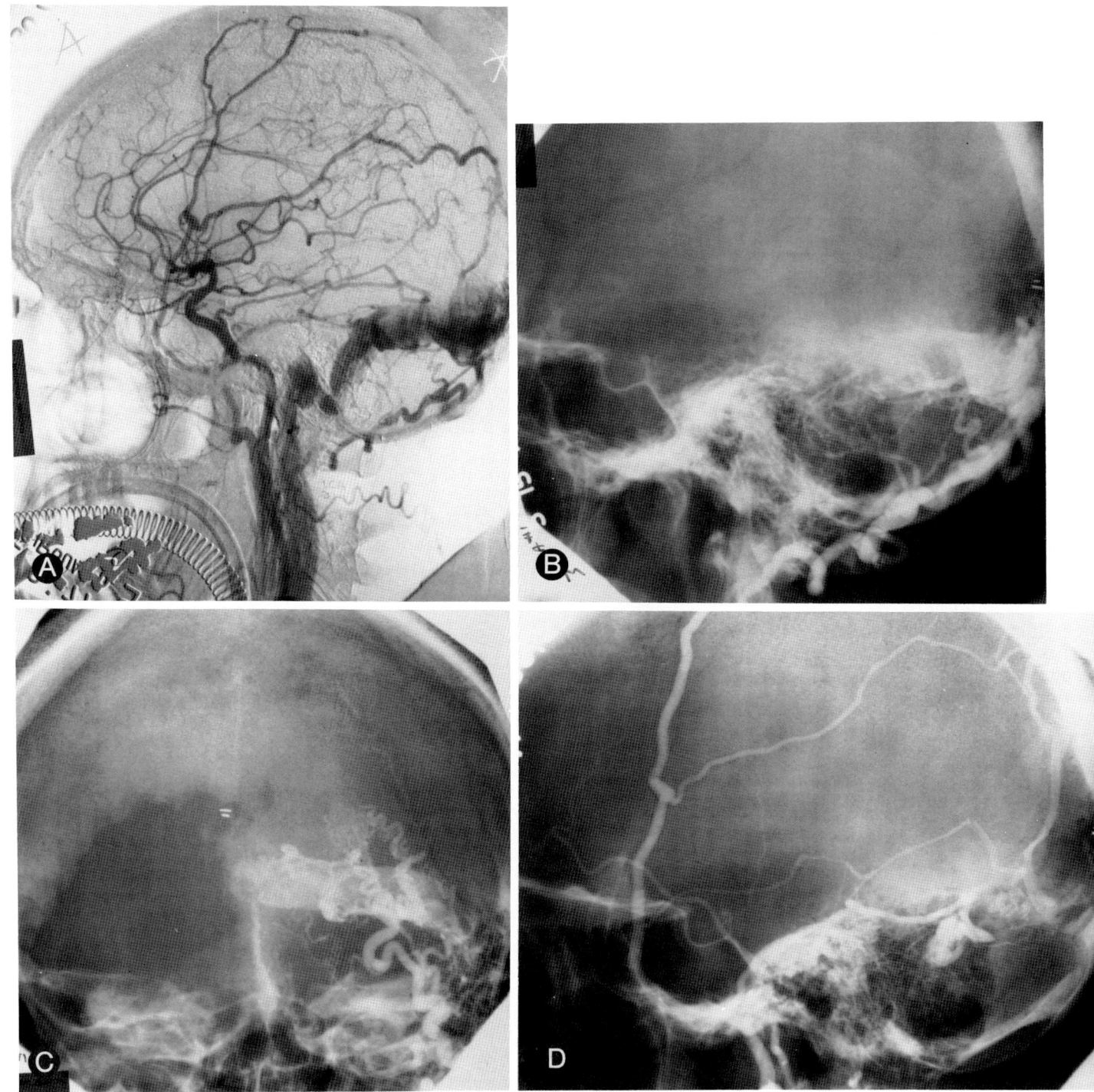

Figure 23.3. Dural arteriovenous malformation. This patient had a previous right dural AVM treated and now presented with a left-sided lesion. **A–D**, The transverse and sigmoid sinus are receiving direct communication from several branches of the hypertrophied occipital artery, the meningeal arteries, the tentorial artery, and the superficial temporal artery.

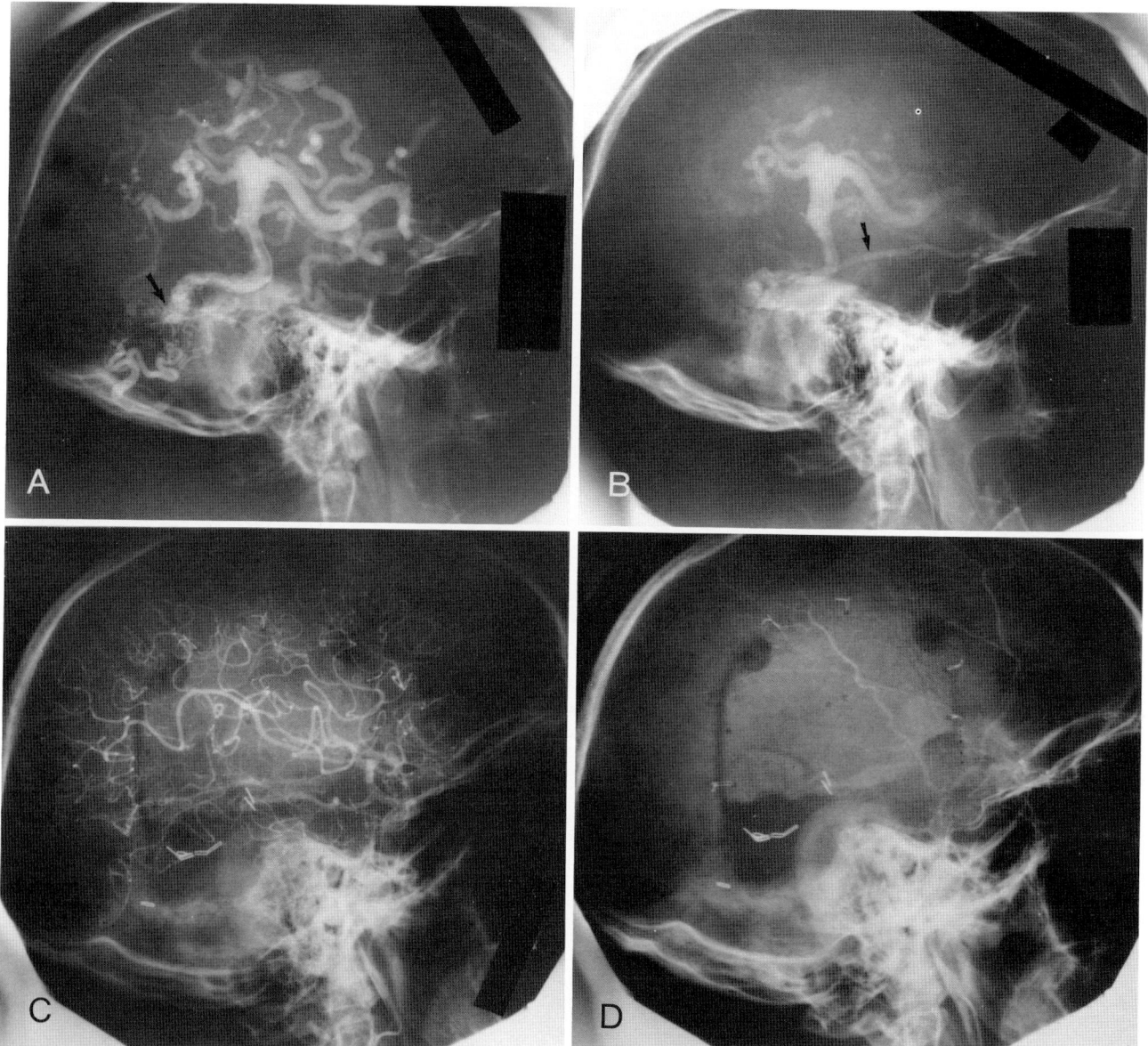

Figure 23.4. Typical AVM of transverse sigmoid sinus in a patient who presented with disabling tinnitus and progressive mild hemispheric symptoms and seizures probably secondary to venous hypertension. **A**, Selective injection of the occipital artery shows the fistula fed by transcranial branches of the occipital artery. The fistula, which is in the transverse sinus (*arrow*), drains through a large cortical vein. Note the greatly distended and abnormal cortical venous drainage system. **B**, Selective middle meningeal injection shows filling of the fistula by an enlarged posterior branch of the middle meningeal artery (*arrow*). **C**, Postoperative internal carotid angiogram shows no residual fistula. **D**, Postoperative external carotid angiogram shows no residual fistula.

rare cases involving the transverse and sigmoid sinuses bilaterally, the prone position with a mastoid-to-mastoid horseshoe-shaped incision is used. The prone position with a long linear incision is used for lesions around the torcula. A bilateral occipital and suboccipital craniotomy is performed, completely isolating ("skeletonizing") the medial aspect of both transverse sinuses and the lower aspect of the sagittal sinus and the torcula (Fig. 23.1).

Results

The authors have treated 8 patients. In 5 with unilateral fistula of the sigmoid-transverse sinus, the sinus

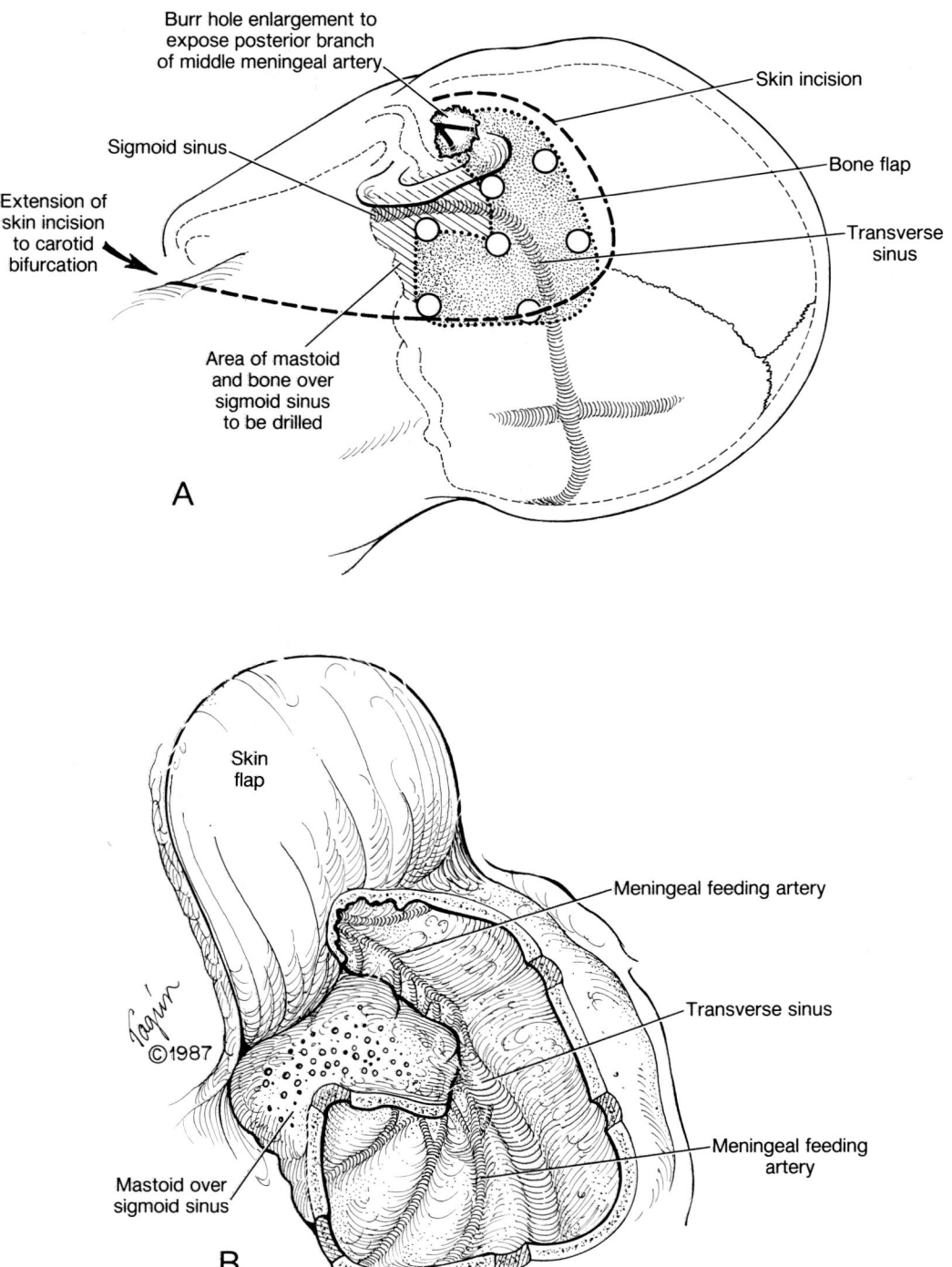

Figure 23.5. Surgical treatment of a dural AVM in the region of the sigmoid and tranverse sinuses. **A**, The patient is positioned supine with a roll under the ipsilateral shoulder and the head turned about 75° or 80° to the opposite side. The incision starts in front of the ear and then curves backward at a height of approximately 3–4 cm above the transverse sinus to a point estimated to be posterior to the medialmost extent of the fistula (usually about the midportion of the transverse sinus). The incision then is brought down in an oblique line toward a point approximately 2–3 fingerbreadths posterior to the mastoid. The incision can stop at that point, or it can continue into the neck to expose the carotid bifurcation, if the latter maneuver is thought to be helpful, which it almost always is in cases of large fistulas. The skin and the muscle are then turned forward to expose the bone. Large occipital branches will be interrupted at this stage. The bone often has a sievelike appearance where arterial vessels have gone through from the back of the scalp flap. One must be very careful to stop bleeding from the bone with bone wax, which can be a very tedious process. **B**, There are two choices to remove the bone flap: One could remove a small craniotomy flap above the sinus and then perform a craniectomy below the sinus. The second option (and the author's preference) is to remove the bone above and below the sinus as a single bone flap after making multiple burr holes and very carefully separating the dura from the bone. Some of the burr holes may be placed strategically over the known location of large meningeal branches, which can then be cauterized through the burr hole. This is particularly true of the relatively constant posterior branch of the middle meningeal artery that can be dealt with by enlarging a temporal burr hole placed just above

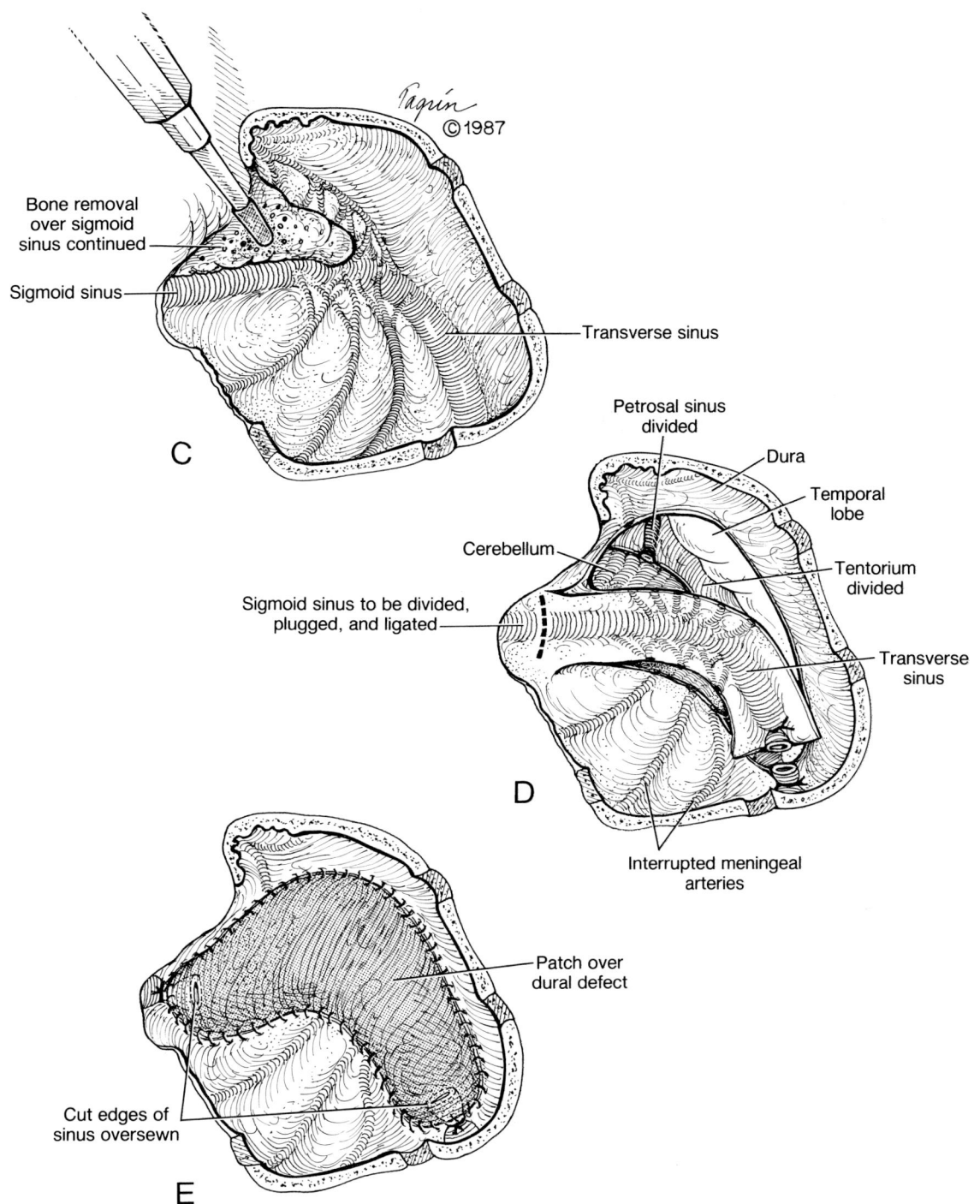

the ear. **C**, The mastoid and the posterolateral portion of the petrous bone are drilled so as to expose the dura lateral and anterior to the sigmoid sinus. Many small arterial feeders come to the fistula through the petrous bone and have to be dealt with, usually with bone wax, at this stage. **D**, The dura is opened above the transverse sinus and lateral and anterior to the sigmoid sinus as far down as possible. One then has two choices: If the sinus is going to be left intact and there are any tentorial feeders, the tentorium must be cut, starting from medially on the transverse sinus and coming laterally across the superior petrosal sinus to the petrous bone. Extreme care must be taken not to injure any of the draining veins from the temporal lobe, particularly if one is dealing with the dominant temporal lobe. For this reason, it may be best to incise the tentorium from the posterior fossa with the surgeon working from below rather than from under the temporal lobe. The second choice is to excise the sinus completely. The authors prefer to do this only when the sinus is either partially or completely occluded or when the venous drainage is retrograde into the brain from the fistula. In either of these circumstances, there is little danger of venous infarction to the temporal lobe by excision of the sinus. When this is done, the sinus can be doubly ligated and divided medially, and as one gradually retracts on the pedicle of dura and sinus, the tentorium can be divided from medial to lateral to the sigmoid sinus. The sigmoid sinus can then be plugged with muscle and ligated. **E**, The dural defect can be closed with a patch of fascia lata or pericranium.

was excised in 2 and "skeletonized" in 3. One patient had a bilateral sigmoid-transverse sinus fistula; 1 patient with a fistula in the area of the torcula was treated by skeletonization; and 1 patient with a fistula in the area of the tentorial incisura and petrosal sinus was treated by thorough coagulation of the tentorium and division of the arterialized vein draining the fistula into the normal posterior fossa pial venous system. All patients had their symptoms relieved. There were no significant complications. One patient that had only skeletonization of the sinus without excision has developed a very mild recurrent fistula that is being treated expectantly because of the mildness of the symptoms. The rest have had no recurrences, but the follow-up period has been relatively short (1–8 years).

EMBOLIZATION

In some patients, selective embolization of the feeding arteries has resulted in at least a partial obliteration of the fistula. Gelfoam, liquid silicone, Silastic spheres, estrogen, Gianturco coils and Silastic adhesive have been used (10, 12, 15, 21, 26, 27, 35–37, 39). The disadvantages of these methods are the possible further development of feeding arteries from other sources and the risk of emboli entering the venous or vertebral arterial circulation and causing neurologic deficit and scalp necrosis (32).

Results of transvenous endovascular occlusion of transverse-sigmoid sinus lesions have been encouraging, but further experience will be needed to establish this method (E. Russell, personal communication, 1986).

REFERENCES

1. Albright AL, Latchaw RE, Price RA: Posterior dural arteriovenous malformations in infancy. Neurosurgery 13:129–135, 1983.
2. Aminoff MJ, Kendall BE: Asymptomatic dural vascular anomalies. Br J Radiol 46:662–667, 1973.
3. Bitoh S, Sakaki S: Spontaneous cure of dural arteriovenous malformation in the posterior fossa. Surg Neurol 12:111–114, 1979.
4. Bitoh S, Arita N, Fujiwara M, Ozaki K, Nakao Y: Dural arteriovenous malformation near the left sphenoparietal sinus. Surg Neurol 13:345–349, 1980.
5. Brainin M, Samec P: Venous hemodynamics of arteriovenous meningeal fistulas in the posterior cranial fossa. Neuroradiology 25:161–169, 1983.
6. Buchanan TA, Harper DG, Hoyt WF: Bilateral proptosis, dilatation of conjunctival veins and papilloedema: a neuroophthalmological syndrome caused by arteriovenous malformation of the torcular region. Br J Ophthalmol 66:186–189, 1982.
7. Chaudhary MY, Sachdev VP, Cho SH, Weitzner I Jr, Puljic S, Huang YP: Dural arteriovenous malformation of the major venous sinuses: An acquired lesion. AJNR 3:13–19, 1982.
8. Chesna EJ, Naheedy MH, Azar-Kia B: CT demonstration of a dural arteriovenous malformation. Comput Radiol 8:49–52, 1984.
9. Chiras J, Bories J, Leger JM, Gaston A, Launay M: CT scan of dural arteriovenous fistulas. Neuroradiology 23:185–194, 1982.
10. Djindjian R, Cophignon I, Rey A, Theron J, Merland JJ, Houdart R: Superselective arteriographic embolization by the femoral route in neuroradiology. Study of 50 cases. III., Embolization in craniocerebral pathology. Neuroradiology 6:143–152, 1973.
11. Endo S. Koshu K, Suzuki J: Spontaneous regression of posterior fossa dural arteriovenous malformation. J Neurosurg 51:715–717, 1979.
12. Han SS, Parry CE, Simeone FA: Embolization of a dural arteriovenous malformation using Gianturco coils. AJNR 3:341–343, 1982.
13. Handa J, Yoneda S, Handa H: Venous sinus occlusion with a dural arteriovenous malformation of the posterior fossa. Surg Neurol 4:433–437, 1975.
14. Harders A, Gilsbach J, Hassler W: Dural AV malformation of the lateral and sigmoid sinuses as possible cause of trigeminal neuralgia. Case report. Acta Neurochir (Wien) 66:95–102, 1982.
15. Hilal SK, Michelsen JW: Therapeutic percutaneous embolization for extra-axial vascular lesions of the head, neck and spine. J Neurosurg 43:275–287, 1975.
16. Houser OW, Baker HL Jr, Rhoton AL Jr, Okazaki H: Intracranial dural arteriovenous malformations. Radiology 105:55–64, 1972.
17. Houser OW, Campbell JK, Campbell RJ, Sundt TM Jr: Arteriovenous malformation affecting the transverse dural venous sinus—an acquired lesion. Mayo Clin Proc 54:651–661, 1979.
18. Hugosson R, Bergstrom K: Surgical treatment of dural arteriovenous malformation in the region of the sigmoid sinus. J Neurol Neurosurg Psychiatry 37:97–101, 1974.
19. Kataoka K, Taneda M: Angiographic disappearance of multiple dural arteriovenous malformations. Case Report. J Neurosurg 60:1275–1278, 1984.
20. Kosnik EJ, Hunt WE, Miller CA: Dural arteriovenous malformations. J Neurosurg 40:322–329, 1974.
21. Kühner A, Krastel A, Stoll W: Arteriovenous malformations of the transverse dural sinus. J Neurosurg 45:12–19, 1976.
22. Lamas E, Lobato RD, Esparza J, Escudero L: Dural posterior fossa AVM producing raised sagittal sinus pressure: Case report. J Neurosurg 46:804–810, 1977.
23. Lasjaunias P, Lopez-Ibor L, Abanou A, Halimi P: Radiological anatomy of the vascularization of cranial dural arteriovenous malformations. Anat Clin 6:87–99, 1984.
24. Luessenhop AJ: Dural arteriovenous malformations. In Wilkins RH, Rengachary JS (eds): Neurosurgery. New York, McGraw-Hill, 1986, pp 1473–1477.
25. Magidson MA, Weinberg PE: Spontaneous closure of a dural arteriovenous malformation. Surg Neurol 6:107–110, 1976.
26. Malik GM, Pearce JE, Ausman JI, Mehta B: Dural arteriovenous malformations and intracranial hemorrhage. Neurosurgery 15:332–339, 1984.
27. Manaka S, Izawa M, Nawata H: Dural arteriovenous malformation treated by artificial embolization with liquid silicone. Surg Neurol 7:63–65, 1977.
28. Miyasaka K, Takei H, Nomura M, Sugimoto S, Aida T, Abe H, Tsuru M: Computerized tomography findings in dural arteriovenous malformations. J Neurosurg 53:698–702, 1980.
29. Nakada T, Kwee IL, Ellis WG, St. John JN: Subacute diencephalic necrosis and dural arteriovenous malformation. Neurosurgery 17:653–656, 1985.
30. Obrador S, Soto M, Silvela J: Clinical syndromes of arteriovenous malformations of the transverse-sigmoid sinus. J Neurol Neurosurg Psychiatry 38:436–451, 1975.
31. Olutola PS, Eliam M, Molot M, Talalla A: Spontaneous regression of a dural arteriovenous malformation. Neurosurgery 12:687–690, 1983.
32. Spetzler RF, Modic M, Bonstelle C: Spontaneous opening of large occipital–vertebral artery anastomosis during embolization. Case report. J Neurosurg 53:849–850, 1980.
33. Storrs DG, King RB: Management of extracranial congenital arteriovenous malformations of the head and neck. Report of five cases. J Neurosurg 38:584–590, 1973.
34. Sundt TM Jr, Piepgras DG: The surgical approach to arterio-

venous malformations of the lateral and sigmoid dural sinuses. *J Neurosurg* 59:32–39, 1983.
35. Suzuki J, Komatsu S: New embolization method using estrogen for dural arteriovenous malformation and meningioma. *Surg Neurol* 16:438–442, 1981.
36. Vinuela FV, Debrun GM, Fox AJ, Kan S: Detachable calibrated-leak balloon for superselective angiography and embolization of dural arteriovenous malformations. *J Neurosurg* 58:817–823, 1983.
37. Vinuela F, Fox AJ, Pelz DM, Drake CG: Unusual manifestations of dural arteriovenous malformations. *J Neurosurg* 64:554–558, 1986.
38. Waga S, Fujimoto K, Morikawa A, Morooka Y, Okada M: Dural arteriovenous malformation in the anterior fossa. *Surg Neurol* 8:356–358, 1977.
39. Watanabe A, Takahara Y, Ibuchi Y, Mizukami K: Two cases of dural arteriovenous malformation occurring after intracranial surgery. *Neuroradiology* 26:375–380, 1984.

24
Carotid-Cavernous Fistula

Most fistulas between the carotid artery and cavernous sinus are due to trauma but spontaneous communication can occur from a dural arterial malformation or, rarely, from rupture of an intracavernous aneurysm. The lesions caused by trauma are frequently associated with a basal skull fracture. A fistula can also occur from attempting to pass a Fogarty catheter in an effort to remove a thrombus from the internal carotid artery and from surgical procedures near this area (11, 16).

POSTTRAUMATIC FISTULA

Clinical Presentation

Patients with traumatic carotid-cavernous fistula may develop symptoms immediately after trauma or several days or weeks later The usual symptoms are exophthalmos, chemosis, extraocular palsies, visual failure, headache, ocular discomfort, or the hearing of a noise synchronous with the pulse. The bruit is the most common and often the most disturbing symptom, but the changes in the eye may be severe. The exophthalmos is due to engorgement of the arterialized ophthalmic veins. Chemosis results from dilatation and arterialization of the small veins of the conjunctiva and sclera. Diplopia is usually secondary to cranial nerve palsy from direct compression of the nerves as they cross the cavernous sinus but can also be due to direct nerve injury at the time of trauma and mechanical restriction from the increased orbital mass (11). The major threat to vision is probably hypoxia (39). The lowered arterial pressure and elevated venous pressure reduce the ocular perfusion pressure. The hypoxic damage may be irreversible despite control of the fistula. Occasionally, particularly in patients with the more chronic indirect fistula, secondary glaucoma develops and results in increased intraocular pressure and visual loss by this mechanism (3). On rare occasions, neurologic symptoms are associated with the steal of arterial blood from the brain or increased venous pressure in cortical veins (1, 3). Even rarer is the occurrence of intracerebral and/or subarachnoid hemorrhage from a carotid-cavernous fistula (47).

Bilateral fistulas are rare but may occur after trauma (9, 25). A patient with a unilateral carotid-cavernous fistula may present with ipsilateral, contralateral, or bilateral signs (11, 44). Occasionally, there may be no ocular signs. The extent of the involvement is determined by the pattern of venous drainage, which is frequently bilateral.

Angiography

The diagnosis is established by angiography. Characteristic angiographic findings include early dense opacification of the enlarged cavernous sinus, early filling of the ophthalmic or other veins draining the area, and reduced opacification of the intracranial arterial system. Although most posttraumatic fistulas appear to originate directly from one internal carotid artery, bilateral selective internal carotid injections should be done, as well as a vertebral study, to assess collateral circulation and to plan the operative procedure. Because the flow into the fistula with ipsilateral carotid injection is so rapid and voluminous, the precise site and size of the fistula frequently cannot be determined even with rapid early filming after ipsilateral carotid injection. With special techniques, Debrun and colleagues were able to locate the fistula precisely on angiograms in all 54 cases on which they reported (13). In 51 of the patients, vertebral angiography with compression of the carotid artery in the neck on the side of the fistula showed retrograde filling of the internal carotid artery through the posterior communicating artery. Since the carotid artery below the fistula did not fill, it was possible to locate and measure the size of the opening in the internal carotid artery. In patients in whom the posterior communicating artery was too small, a double-lumen balloon catheter was used. The balloon was inflated in the internal carotid artery just above the bifurcation, and contrast was injected through the other lumen. Most of the fistulas occurred in the horizontal or posterior ascending segment of the intracavernous internal carotid artery. The fistulas varied in size from 1–5 mm with an average of 3 mm. Rarely was more than one opening present in the internal carotid artery.

The venous drainage may be anterior through the superior ophthalmic vein, posterior through the inferior or superior petrosal sinus, superior through the sylvian vein, inferior into pterygoid plexus, and contralateral into the opposite cavernous sinus and its tributaries through the intercavernous plexus. There may be only one draining vein or any combination. Debrun et al also noted that in posttraumatic fistulas there was no contribution from external carotid branches, which is in striking contrast to the findings in spontaneous fistulas (13).

Treatment

Indications for surgical treatment are preservation of vision, relief of cranial nerve palsies, elimination of the bruit, and restoration of the orbit and its contents to normal while cerebral ischemia is avoided. Hemorrhage, either intracranial or into the sphenoid sinus, is very rare. Spontaneous remission is reported to occur in 5–10% of patients (11).

Prior to the development of catheter techniques, the preferred operative treatment for carotid-cavernous fistula was trapping of the fistula combined with muscle embolization (11, 19, 20, 30). This involved a frontotemporal craniotomy for occlusion of the internal carotid artery proximal to the ophthalmic artery or, if this was not possible, occlusion of both the ophthalmic and intracranial carotid artery and then muscle embolization in the internal carotid artery, followed by ligation of that artery (Hamby procedure) (19).

During the past few years, several techniques have been developed to obliterate the traumatic carotid-cavernous fistula, first by occluding the internal carotid artery by a balloon catheter (36) and more recently by occluding the fistulas with preservation of internal carotid flow (2, 5, 13, 17, 23, 26, 27, 32, 38, 40, 42).

There are three types of treatment to consider in a patient with a carotid cavernous fistula: (a) intraarterial detachable balloon catheter, (b) intravenous detachable balloon catheter, and (c) surgical approach with various adjuncts. For treatment with the intraarterial detachable balloon, the catheter is introduced into the internal carotid artery by direct puncture or transfemoral catheterization and enters the cavernous sinus through the hole in the wall of the artery. The balloon is inflated and detached to occlude the fistula, leaving the artery patent. The use of a latex detachable balloon has been described by Serbienko and Debrun et al (12, 40) and of a calibrated-leak balloon and bucrylate by Kerber (26). Taki et al have used a balloon that can be detached by a polyvinyl alcohol tube that dissolves when heated by a special radiofrequency system (42).

The intravenous detachable balloon technique has been used to treat carotid-cavernous fistulas that drain anteriorly through the superior ophthalmic vein or posteriorly through the inferior petrosal sinus (29, 32). This technique is particularly helful in patients in whom the ipsilateral carotid artery has been occluded in an unsuccessful attempt to treat the fistula. The injection of fibrin glue through the superior ophthalmic vein to occlude a carotid-cavernous fistula has also been reported (22).

The direct surgical approach to the cavernous sinus has been described by Parkinson (35). He and others have surgically occluded the fistula with the patient under cardiac arrest and deep hypothermia (25). Dolenc has described a similar approach and has used it successfully without cardiac arrest or hypothermia (14). Hosobuchi reported the use of electrothrombosis (23). Mullan described the use of thrombogenic needles or bronze wire to induce thrombosis (32). Debrun et al plugged the cavernous sinus with pieces of muscle (13). Samson et al injected isobutyl-2-cyanoacrylate into the cavernous sinus at craniotomy with closure of the fistula (38).

Debrun et al described the use of detachable balloon catheters in treating 54 patients with traumatic carotid-cavernous fistula (13). All three approaches listed above were used. The results of this treatment are summarized in Table 24.1. In 45 patients, treatment consisted of intraarterial balloon catheterization; in 7 patients this was combined with either a venous or surgical approach. One patient was successfully treated by venous approach alone, and one patient was treated by surgery after the venous approach failed. In 50 of 54 patients, total occlusion of the fistulas was accomplished with this balloon technique (Fig. 24.1). In some patients, more than one procedure was required to complete the occlusion. In 2 patients, the fistula recurred and was treated with a second balloon. In 2 patients with previous surgery, the cavernous sinus was punctured under direct vision and a balloon detached. There was often a minor stenosis from the balloon or a small false aneurysm; these were asymptomatic findings. The

Table 24.1.
Results of Treatment in 54 Patients with Carotid-Cavernous Fistula with Use of Detachable Balloon Catheters[a]

Total occlusion of the fistula	50 (93%)
Preservation of internal carotid flow	32 (59%)
Mortality (sepsis)[b]	1 (2%)
Complications	
Venous pouch or false aneurysm	
Small	19 (35%)
Large—requiring treatment	5 (10%)
Oculomotor palsy	
Transient	10 (19%)
Permanent	1 (2%)
Hemiparesis	
Transient[c]	2 (4%)
Permanent[d]	1 (2%)

[a] From Debrun G, Lacour P, Vinuela F, Fox A, Drake CG, Caron JP: Treatment of 54 traumatic carotid-cavernous fistulas. *J Neurosurg* 55:678–692, 1981.
[b] Patient had increased eye symptoms after venous catheterization and then had surgical procedure.
[c] In one patient this was associated with intraoperative injection of bucrylate.
[d] Occurred after surgical intracranial ligation of incompletely occluded fistula.

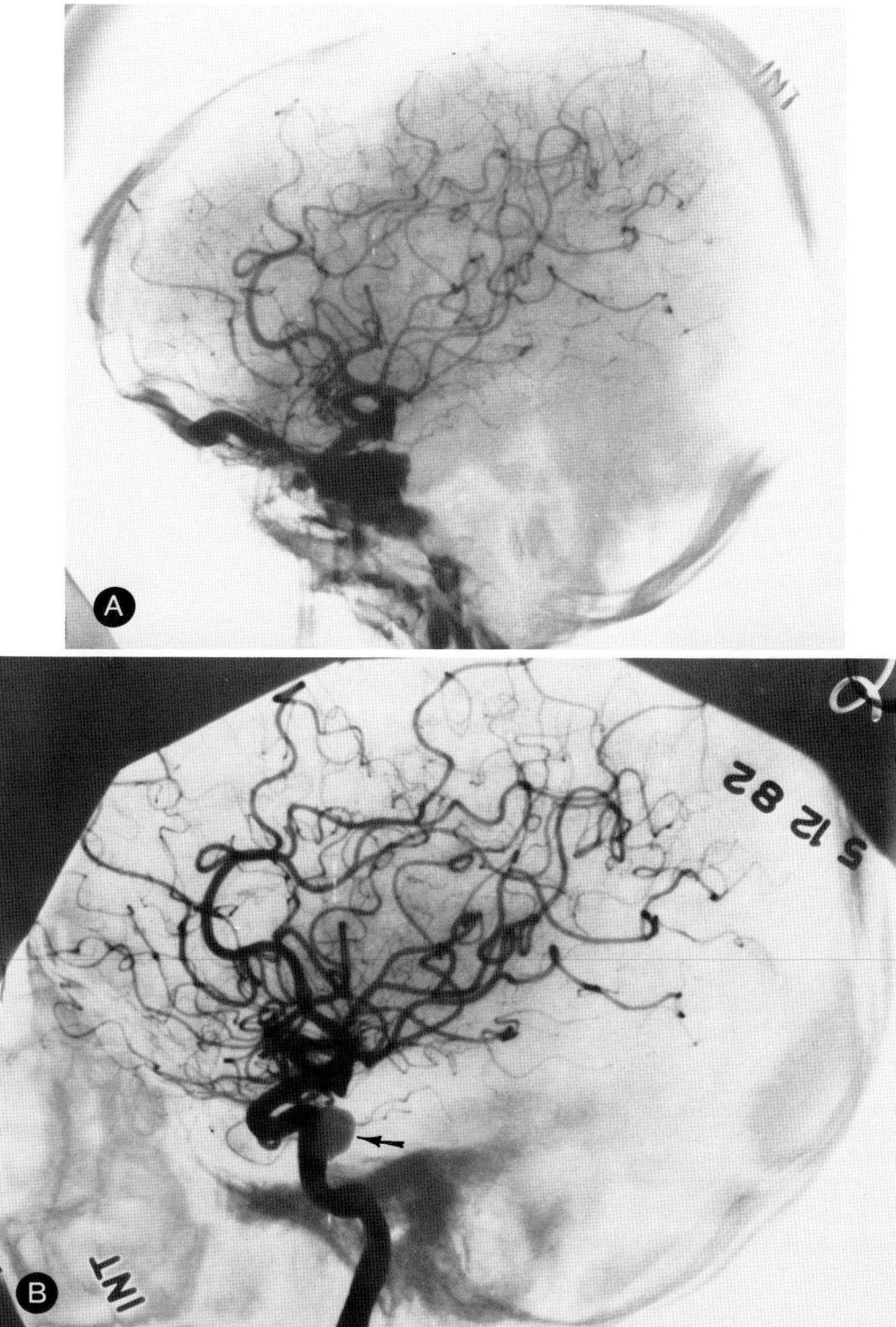

Figure 24.1. Posttraumatic carotid-cavernous fistula. **A**, Lateral angiogram demonstrates a carotid-cavernous fistula with anterior drainage into the superior ophthalmic vein. **B**, Complete occlusion of the fistula after treatment with an intraarterial detachable balloon (*arrow*). The internal carotid circulation is preserved. (These pictures are reproduced through the courtesy of Dr. Gerard Debrun, who treated the patient).

stenosis tended to diminish on follow-up angiography. In 3 patients in whom both the fistula and the internal carotid artery were originally occluded by the balloon, the superior portion of the fistula was later found to be open. This is a potentially serious complication because the patient can develop ischemic symptoms due to steal of blood through the fistula; therefore, these patients had intracranial ligation of the supraclinoid portion of the internal carotid artery. In all patients, the goal was to preserve circulation in the internal carotid artery, but this was not possible in 22 cases. The reasons for this are listed in Table 24.2.

The complications from Debrun et al are listed in Table 24.1 (13). There was one death due to sepsis in a patient who had both a venous catheterization and a surgical procedure. Venous pouch or false aneurysm occurs when the balloon has deflated too quickly but the fistula usually remains occluded. Small pouches cause no symptoms, but large pouches may cause intractable retro-orbital pain or oculomotor palsy. If these symptoms develop, it is necessary to occlude the internal carotid artery and neck of the false aneurysm with a second detachable balloon. This had to be done in 5 of 24 patients who developed a venous pouch or false aneurysm. With the use of nondeflatable balloons filled with silicone, this complication should decrease. The incidence of hemiparesis is small, but an occasional patient may not tolerate the temporary balloon occlusion performed prior to the permanent occlusion. In such patients, a bypass graft may be indicated (18, 41).

In the rare patient with bilateral carotid-cavernous fistulas the detachable balloon technique may also be used (13). Laws et al (27) treated one such patient by combining balloon techniques with direct exposure of the fistula through a trans-sphenoidal approach.

At the present time, the initial treatment of choice for the patient with a posttraumatic carotid-cavernous fistula is to try to occlude the fistula with preservation of internal carotid artery flow by a detachable balloon placed in the fistula through the internal carotid artery. In special cases, such that of the patient with occlusion of the ipsilateral carotid artery, a transvenous placement of the balloon or direct surgical approach may be necessary (46). As new techniques develop, they must be carefully evaluated. For example, there is not yet enough experience to determine whether the injection of a rapidly polymerizing plastic via a catheter or directly into the cavernous sinus at operation will give better results (13, 26, 38).

SPONTANEOUS FISTULA

The symptoms due to spontaneous carotid-cavernous fistula are often mild and may not develop abruptly. Mild unilateral headache, discomfort in the eye, or diplopia due to sixth nerve paresis may antedate the typical orbital signs by many months. Gradually, dilated conjunctival vessels and proptosis may develop. A bruit is noted by the patient in no more than one-half of the reported cases (3, 7, 11, 31).

Careful angiographic studies have shown that most of these spontaneous fistulas are secondary to a dural arteriovenous malformation (see Chapter 23) (11, 15, 34, 43, 45). As such, they are low-flow and low-pressure fistulas. The fistulas in these cases can be from cavernous branches of the internal carotid artery, from dural branches of the external carotid artery, or from a combination of both (3). Spontaneous direct fistulas between the internal carotid artery and the cavernous sinus are exceptionally rare (8). On rare occasion, rupture of an intracavernous aneurysm is the cause, but in this case the fistula is usually of the high-flow, high-pressure type, and the symptomatology is abrupt and dramatic as in cases of traumatic fistulas (3, 48).

Most patients with spontaneous fistula are middle-aged, postmenopausal women (11, 43). However, onset may also occur during pregnancy (45). In the review of the literature by Pang et al, all patients were over 20 years of age except for one infant (34).

Complete selective internal and external carotid and vertebral angiography is essential. In 16 cases of spontaneous carotid-cavernous fistulas, Debrun et al found a contribution from the external carotid artery in all except one case of a ruptured cavernous aneurysm (13). External carotid branches that may supply the fistula include terminal meningeal branches of the internal maxillary, ascending pharyngeal, and pterygopalatine arteries (3, 33, 34, 48). The inferolateral trunk is the usual feeding branch when the internal carotid artery also supplies the fistula.

Spontaneous resolution of the fistula may occur in patients with dural arteriovenous shunts (24). Newton and Hoyt reported that 5 of 11 such fistulas resolved completely (33). Spontaneous improvement

Table 24.2.
Reasons for Internal Carotid Occlusion when Attempting to Preserve Carotid Circulation in 22 Patients with Carotid-Cavernous Fistulas[a]

Failure to enter cavernous sinus	7
False aneurysm with symptoms	5
Cavernous sinus entered but fistula could not be occluded	4
Previous surgery	2
Balloon occluded artery below fistula	1
ICA[b] thrombosis from procedure	1
ICA stenosis from balloon and traumatic dissection	1

[a] Modified from Debrun G, Lacour P, Vinuela F, Fox A, Drake CG, Caron JP: Treatment of 54 traumatic carotid-cavernous fistulas. J Neurosurg 55:678-692, 1981.
[b] ICA, internal carotid artery.

was also noted in 2 patients with onset during pregnancy (45). In many patients, symptoms are mild and nonprogressive, and the patient may be followed conservatively (15, 24, 43). Strong indications for treatment are visual loss, a documented progressive increase in intraocular pressure, or the development of progressive ophthalmoplegia (24). Occasionally, the patient is bothered enough by the bruit or by the cosmetic effects of the fistula (proptosis, scleral injection, etc.) that treatment is justified on this basis. The treatment of choice is external carotid embolization (3, 10, 21, 28, 34, 37, 48) (Fig. 24.2).

Various substances, such as Silastic beads, isobutyl-2-cyanoacrylate, and polyvinyl alcohol, can be used (3, 48). Because of the risk of recanalization, it is preferable not to use Gelfoam (3). When the fistula is fed entirely or partially by the internal carotid artery, the treatment may be quite challenging because in these cases it is very difficult to get a balloon selectively in the small branches feeding these dural fistulas. In these cases, if there is no disappearance of internal carotid artery supply following occlusion of external carotid artery feeders, it may be necessary to sacrifice the internal carotid artery by occluding it with a balloon throughout the cavernous segment (3, 48). There is a report of two spontaneous fistulas involving the internal carotid artery that were treated successfully with low-dose irradiation (6). In the rare

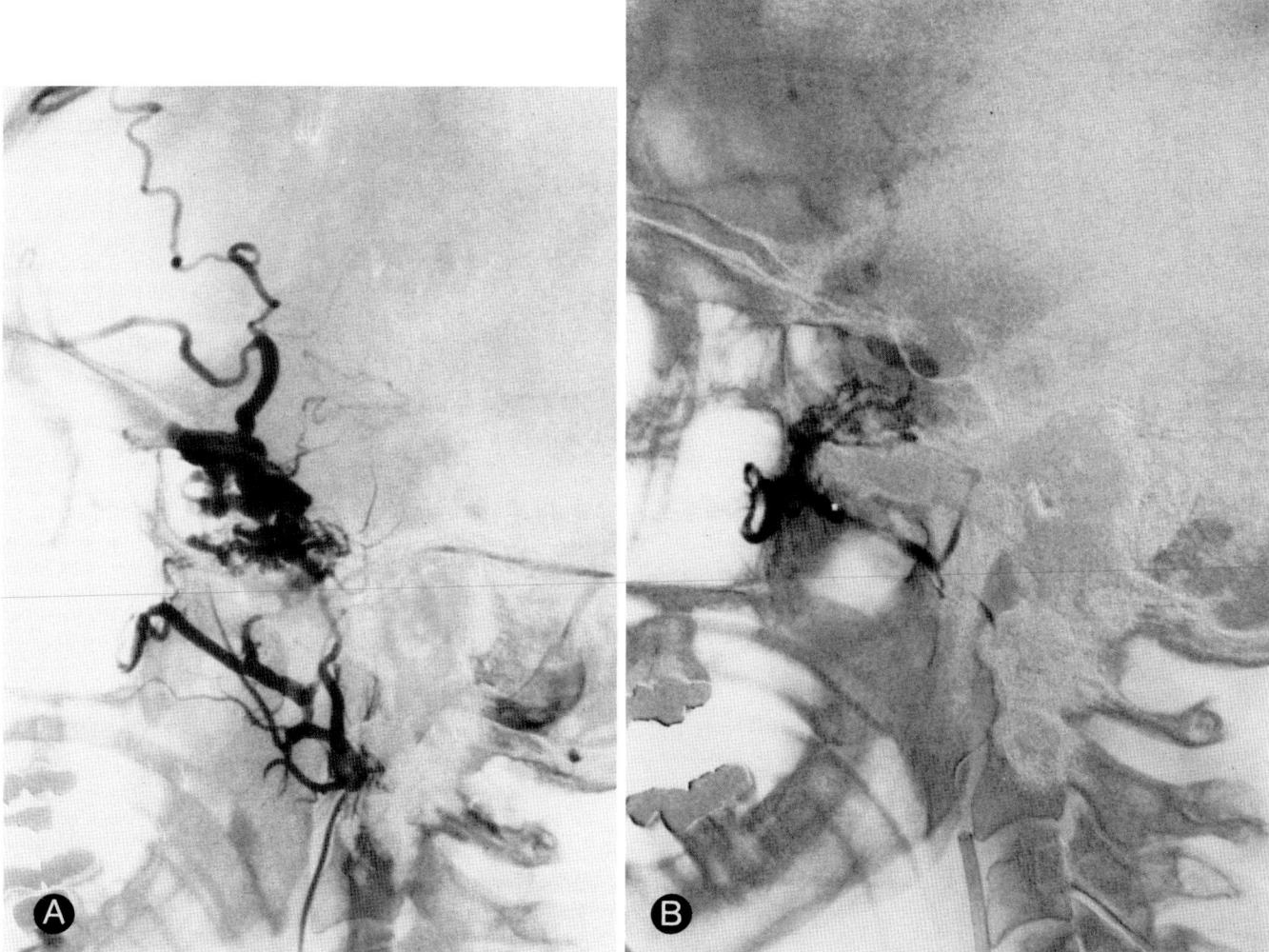

Figure 24.2. Spontaneous carotid-cavernous fistula. **A**, Selective external carotid angiogram reveals a dural arteriovenous malformation with communication into the cavernous sinus. **B**, Selective injection of internal maxillary artery outlines the multiple feeding arteries. **C**, Selective internal carotid angiogram also fills the fistula from small internal carotid artery branches. **D**, Common carotid angiogram after selective embolization of the internal maxillary artery. The external carotid supply is occluded and opacification from the internal carotid artery is much less. (These pictures are reproduced through the courtesy of Dr. Gerard Debrun, who treated the patient.)

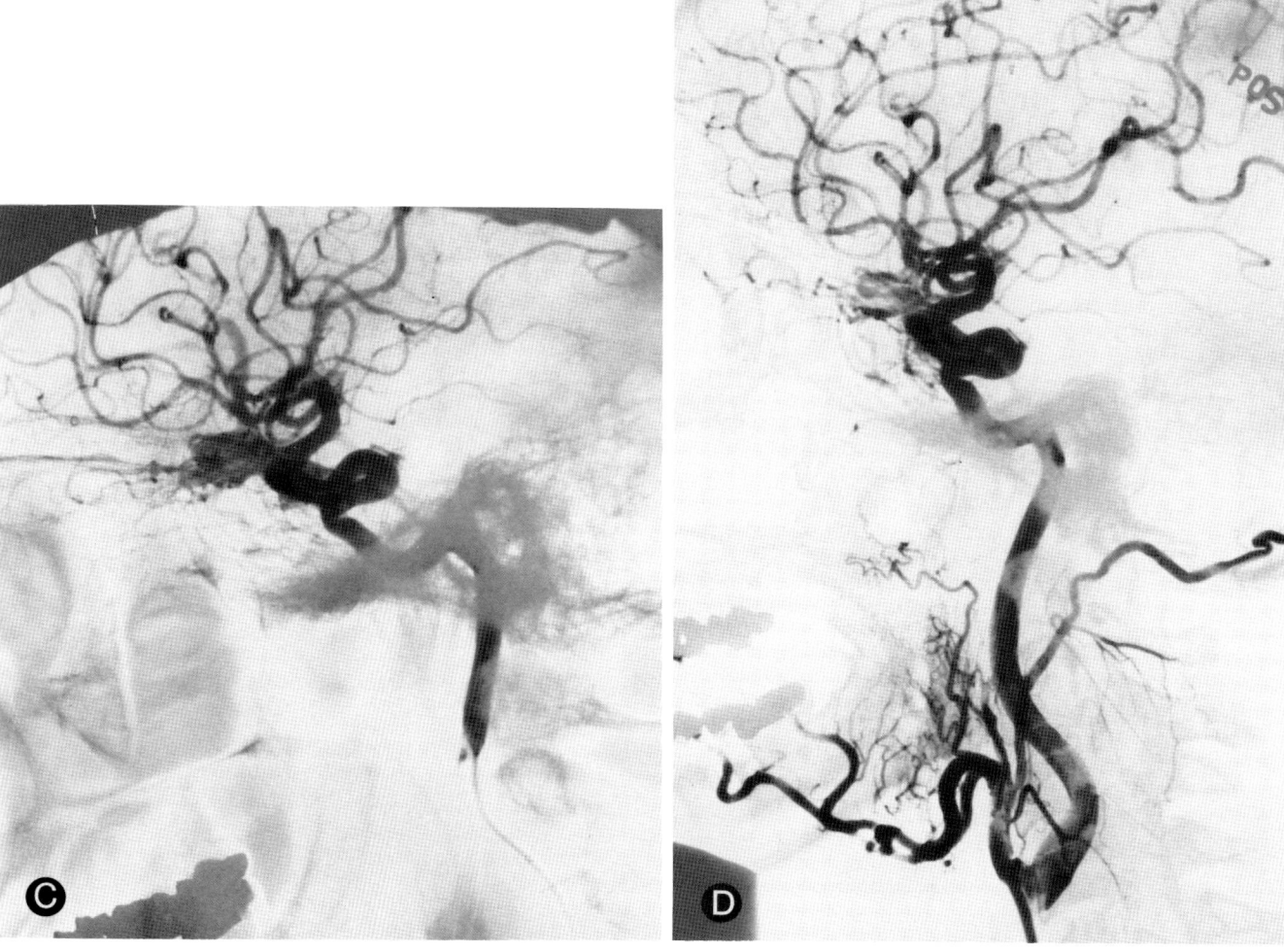

Figure 24.2C and D.

case of a spontaneous high-flow fistula due to a ruptured aneurysm, treatment consists of using a detachable balloon catheter as outlined for traumatic fistula (48).

In one series, 20 patients with spontaneous carotid-cavernous fistulas were treated (48). In this series, 2 of the spontaneous fistulas were due to rupture of a giant intracavernous aneurysm, and 2 patients had bilateral fistulas. Eight patients were treated conservatively, and in two, spontaneous closure of the fistulas occurred. Of the 9 patients with dural fistulas treated with particles and/or isobutyl-2-cyanoacrylate, successful occlusion of the fistula was achieved in 7 and partial occlusion was achieved in 2. Of the 2 fistulas due to rupture of a giant intracavernous aneurysm that were treated with a detachable balloon, preservation of the internal carotid artery was achieved in one. In one patient, a serious neurologic deficit occurred because of embolization of isobutyl-2-cyanoacrylate through the artery of the foramen rotundum into the left middle cerebral artery.

REFERENCES

1. Ambler MW, Moon AC, Sturner WQ: Bilateral carotid-cavernous fistulae of mixed types with unusual radiological and neuropathological findings. Case report. J Neurosurg 48:117-124, 1978.
2. Bank WO, Kerber CW, Drayer BP, Troost BT Maroon JC: Carotid-cavernous fistula: Endarterial cyanoacrylate occlusion with preservation of carotid flow. J Neuroradiol 5:279-285, 1978
3. Barrow DL, Spector RH, Braum IF, Landman JA, Tindall SC, Tindall GT: Classification and treatment of spontaneous carotid-cavernous sinus fistulas. J Neurosurg 62:248-256, 1985.
4. Bartlow B, Penn RD: Carotid-cavernous sinus fistula presenting as a posterior fossa mass. Case report. J Neurosurg 42:585-588, 1975.
5. Benati A, Maschio A, Perini S, Beltramello A: Treatment of post-traumatic carotid-cavernous fistula using a detachable balloon catheter. J Neurosurg 53:784-786, 1980
6. Bitoh S. Hasegawa H, Fujiwara M, Nakao K: Irradiation of

spontaneous carotid-cavernous fistulas. *Surg Neurol* 17:282-286, 1982.
7. Bitoh S, Hasegawa H, Fujiwara M, Nakata M, Sakaki S: Spontaneous carotid-cavernous fistulas. *Neurol Med Chir (Tokyo)* 21:757-764, 1981.
8. Bradac GB, Bender A, Curo G, Debrun G: Report of two cases of spontaneous direct carotid-cavernous fistula. *Neuroradiology* 27:436-439, 1985.
9. Conley FK, Hamilton RD, Hosobuchi Y: Successful surgical treatment of bilateral carotid-cavernous fistulas. Case report. *J Neurosurg* 43:357-361, 1975
10. Costin JA, Weinstein MA, Berlin AJ, Hardy RW, Gutman FA: Dural arterio-venous malformations involving the cavernous sinus, a case report. *Br J Ophthalmol* 62:478-482, 1978
11. Day AL, Rhoton Al Jr: Aneurysms and arteriovenous fistula of the intracavernous carotid artery and its branches. In Youmans JR (ed): *Neurological Surgery*, ed 2. Philadelphia, WB Saunders,1982, pp 1764-1785.
12. Debrun G, Lacour P, Caron JP, Hurth M, Comoy J, Keravel Y: Detachable balloon and calibrated-leak balloon techniques in the treatment of cerebral vascular lesions. *J Neurosurg* 49:635-649, 1978.
13. Debrun G, Lacour P, Vinuela F, Fox A, Drake CG, Caron JP: treatment of 54 traumatic carotid-cavernous fistulas. *J Neurosurg* 55:678-692, 1981.
14. Dolenc V: Direct microsurgical repair of intracavernous vascular lesions. *J Neurosurg* 58:824-831, 1983.
15. Edwards MS, Connolly ES: Cavernous sinus syndrome produced by communication between the external carotid artery and cavernous sinus. *J Neurosurg* 46:92-96, 1977.
16. Eggers F, Lukin R, Chambers AA, Tomsick TA, Sawaya K: Iatrogenic carotid-cavernous fistula following Fogarty catheter thromboendarterectomy. *J Neurosurg* 51:543-545, 1979.
17. Fierstien SB, DeFeo D. Nutkiewicz, A: Complete obliteration of a carotid cavernous fistula with sparing of the carotid blood flow using a detachable balloon chatheter. *Surg Neurol* 9:277-280, 1978.
18. Guegan Y, Javalet A, Eon JY, Vallee B, Pecker J: Extra-intracranial anastomosis preliminary to treatment of carotid artery-cavernous sinus fistula. *Surg Neurol* 10:85-88, 1978.
19. Hamby WB: *Carotid-Cavernous Fistulae*. Springfield, IL, Charles C Thomas, 1966.
20. Hamby WB, Dohn DF: Carotid-cavernous fistulas: Report of thirty-six cases and discussion of their management. *Clin Neurosurg* 11:150-170, 1964.
21. Hardy RW, Costin JA, Weinstein M, Berlin AJ Jr, Gutman FA: External carotid-cavernous fistula treated by transfemoral embolization. *Surg Neurol* 9:255-256, 1978.
22. Hasegawa H, Bitoh S, Pbaski J, Marino M: Closure of carotid-cavernous fistula by use of a fibrin adhesive system. *Surg Neurol* 24:23-26, 1985.
23. Hosobuchi Y: Electrothrombosis of carotid-cavernous fistula *J Neurosurg* 42:76-85, 1975.
24. Ishikawa M, Handa H, Taki W, Yoneda S: Management of spontaneous carotid-cavernous fistulae. *Surg Neurol* 18:131-139, 1982.
25. Johnston I: Direct surgical treatment of bilateral intracavernous internal carotid artery aneurysms. Case report. *J Neurosurg* 51:98-102, 1979,
26. Kerber C: Use of balloon catheters in the treatment of cranial arterial abnormalities. *Stroke* 11:210-216, 1980.
27. Laws ER Jr, Onofrio BM, Pearson BW, McDonald TJ, Dirrenberger RA: Successful management of bilateral carotid-cavernous fistulae with a trans-sphenoidal approach. *Neurosurgery* 4:162-167, 1979.
28. Mahaley MS, Boone SC: External carotid-cavernous fistula treated by arterial embolization: Case report. *J Neurosurg* 40:110-114, 1974.
29. Manelfe C, Bernstein A: Treatment of carotid-cavernous fistulas by venous approach. *J Neuroradiol* 7:13-19, 1980
30. Morley TP: Appraisal of various forms of management in 41 cases of carotid cavenous fistula. In Morley TP (ed): *Current Controversies in Neurosurgery*. Philadelphia, WB Saunders, 1976.
31. Mufti ST: Intracranial external carotid-venous fistulas: A review. *Surg Neurol* 14:203-206, 1980.
32. Mullan S: Experiences with surgical thrombosis of intracranial berry aneurysm and carotid-cavernous fistulas. *J Neurosurg* 41:657-670, 1974.
33. Newton TH, Hoyt WF: Dural arteriovenous shunts in the region of the cavernous sinus. *Neuroradiology* 1:71-81, 1980.
34. Pang D, Kerber C, Biglan AW, Ahn HS: External carotid-cavernous fistula in infancy: Case report and review of the literature. *Neurosurgery* 8:212-218, 1981.
35. Parkinson D: Carotid cavernous fistula: Direct repair with preservation of the carotid artery. Technical note. *J Neurosurg* 38:99-106, 1973.
36. Prolo DJ, Burres KP, Hanbery JW: Balloon occlusion of carotid cavernous fistula: Introduction of a new catheter. *Surg Neurol* 7:209-214, 1977
37. Pugatch RP, Wolpert SM: Transfemoral embolization of an external carotid-cavernous fistula: Case report *J Neurosurg* 42:94-97, 1975.
38. Samson D, Ditmore QM, Beyer CW Jr: Intravascular use of isobutyl-2-cyanoacrylate: Part 2:Treatment of carotid-cavernous fistulas. *Neurosurgery* 8:52-55, 1981.
39. Sanders MD, Hoyt WF: Hypoxia ocular sequelae of carotid-cavernous fistulae. Study of the causes of visual failure before and after neurosurgical treatment in a series of 25 cases. *Br J Ophthalmol* 53:82-97, 1969.
40. Serbienko FA: Balloon catheterization and occlusion of major cerebral vessels. *J Neurosurg* 41:125-145, 1974.
41. Shen AL: Superficial temporal-middle cerebral artery anastomoses in the treatment of a carotid cavernous fistula. *J Neurosurg* 49:760-763, 1978.
42. Taki W, Handa H, Miyake H, Kobayashi A, Yonekawa Y, Yamamura K, Suzuk M, Ikada Y: New detachable balloon technique for traumatic carotid-cavernous fistulae. *AJNR* 6:961-964, 1985.
43. Tanaguchi RM, Goree JA, Odom GL: Spontaneous carotid-cavernous shunts presenting diagnostic problems. *J Neurosurg* 35:384-391, 1971.
44. Theron J, Olivier A, Melanion D, Ethier R: Left carotid-cavernous fistula with right exophthalmus: Treatment by detachable balloon. *Neuroradiology* 27:349-353, 1985.
45. Toya S, Shiobara R, Izumi J, Shinomiya Y, Shiga H, Kimur C: Spontaneous carotid-cavernous fistula during pregnancy or in the postpartum stage: Report of two cases. *J Neurosurg* 54:252-256, 1981.
46. Tress BM, Thomson KR, Klug GL, Crawford B: Management of carotid-cavernous fistulas by surgery combined with interventional radiology. Report of two cases. *J Neurosurg* 59:1076-1080, 1983.
47. Turner DM, Vangilder JC, Mojtahedi S, Peirson EW: Spontaneous intracerebral hematoma in carotid-cavernous fistula. *J Neurosurg* 59:680-686, 1983.
48. Vinuela F, Fox AJ, Debrun GM, Peerless SJ, Drake CG: Spontaneous carotid-cavernous fistulas: Clinical radiological and therapeutic considerations. *J Neurosurg* 62:248–256, 1985.

25
Brain Hemorrhage

The incidence of brain hemorrhage due to hypertension has declined in the United States over the past several years, but the problem of brain hemorrhage remains an important cause of death and disability (24). In Japan, the death rate from cerebral hemorrhage has also dropped, but the problem is still serious and the death rate from hypertensive cerebral hemorrhage per 100,000 population is higher than that in other countries (34).

The advent of the computed tomography (CT) scan has provided us with the ability to determine with accuracy the site and the size of a brain hemorrhage, the degree of surrounding edema, and the presence of ventricular enlargement. In addition, with use of this noninvasive study, patients with brain hemorrhage can now be easily followed.

The syndromes that result from brain hemorrhage are sufficiently characterized to permit their clinical recognition in many patients. However, the clinical and CT criteria for decisions regarding medical and surgical management continue to undergo change (12, 57, 58).

PATHOPHYSIOLOGY

Hypertensive brain hemorrhage tends to occur in specific sites: putamen, thalamus, cerebellum, and pons. Lobar hemorrhage may also be related to hypertension. Hemorrhage in any area of the brain, but especially lobar, may be due to a specific cause but can occur in association with normal blood pressure and with no radiographic evidence of a specific etiologic factor (73). Spontaneous nonhypertensive brain hemorrhage may be associated with aneurysm or arteriovenous malformation (AVM), primary or metastatic brain tumor (38, 42, 45, 64), infarction (40), anticoagulation (11, 38, 47), disease associated with clotting disorders such as leukemia, thrombocytopenic purpura, sickle cell disease (1, 47), and cerebral arteritis such as occurs with collagen vascular diseases (17), amyloid angiopathy (38, 46, 87), and drug abuse (17, 38).

In hypertensive hemorrhage, the most common sources of bleeding are the small penetrating arteries in the base of the brain (the lenticulostriate and thalamoperforating arteries and the paramedian branches of the basilar artery) (20). Although these vessels normally can withstand extremely high pressure without rupture, pathological changes result in weakness. It has been suggested that microaneurysms could be the cause of the hemorrhage, but careful histologic studies indicate that fibrinoid necrosis is usually the etiology of the weakness in the arterial wall (19, 74, 101). The final triggering mechanism for the rupture is not known, although it has been speculated that a sudden increase in blood pressure coincident with factors such as exertion or emotional stress may exceed the tolerance of the vessel wall (103). This notion is supported by the finding that the setting for hemorrhage is usually during activity and infrequently during sleep (59).

The hemorrhage produces both destruction and displacement of tissue. Pathologic studies demonstrate tracking of blood along tissue planes with displacement of tissue (20, 31). This latter effect is often more evident than is the destruction and provides the basis for hope that the ultimate outcome may be considerably better than indicated by the acute deficit. In most cases, the hemorrhage is inferred to be of short duration, irrespective of size when the bleeding ceases. No correlation has been found between hematoma size and blood pressure.

The mechanism of later clinical deterioration is less certain. Rebleeding is rare. In a study with chromium-labeled red cells injected at the time of admission for hypertensive hemorrhage, it was found that patients who died had virtually no evidence of labeling in the original hemorrhage, although the Duret hemorrhages that reflected the postadmission fatal cerebral herniation were easily labeled (28). Occasionally, CT scan will document enlargement of the hematoma, and in a few angiograms performed immediately after admission, extravasation of dye has been seen (52). Edema or ischemic necrosis around the lesion may extend and probably is the chief mechanism for subsequent worsening (15, 59).

Reduction in the hematoma size is accomplished by reparative mechanisms over several months. The process is slow because macrophage activity must go along the rim of the mass to reabsorb the hematoma. Within a year the hematoma site is converted to a slitlike cavity with orange-stained walls representing hemosiderin-laden macrophages surrounded by tissue that appears more or less normal (20).

DIAGNOSTIC STUDIES

CT Scan

Any patient suspected of having a brain hemorrhage should have an immediate CT scan. The scan gives a precise localization of the hemorrhage, outlines its size and configuration, shows the degree of hydrocephalus, indicates ventricular shift or compression, gives an indication of the degree of edema in adjacent brain tissue, and can be repeated as needed for evaluation of the subsequent clinical course (15, 26, 31, 55, 59, 78, 95).

Over several weeks, the high density seen on the CT scan gradually becomes isodense and then changes to a low-density appearance. The change in the scan appearance is due to an alteration of photon absorption rather than actual resorption of the hematoma as shown by CT-autopsy correlation (51). From a few days to some months after hemorrhage, the CT scan with contrast administration will often show a ring-like enhancement around the hemorrhage, which presumably represents the area of edema or local ischemic infarction (96, 102).

There is almost no indication for lumbar puncture in a patient suspected of having brain hemorrhage. It should not be used as a diagnostic study because large hemorrhages can result in transtentorial herniation, and in small hemorrhages, the spinal fluid may be clear. CT scan provides the information needed.

Angiography

When the clinical syndrome and CT scan indicate a typical hypertensive brain hemorrhage, particularly in the putamen, thalamus, cerebellum, or pons, angiography is now rarely indicated. In cases in which hypertension is not the likely cause and in lobar hemorrhages, angiography is needed to help decide whether there is a vascular malformation or tumor (26, 73). However, the procedure may fail to show either of these lesions, particularly in the acute phase. The authors recommend that if initial angiography is negative and no other cause for the hematoma is apparent, the study be repeated in 2–3 months when pressure from the hematoma has subsided. If no abnormality is seen at that time, they would continue to follow the patient with a CT scan at 4–6-month intervals to be certain that an underlying tumor is not being overlooked as a cause for the hemorrhage.

Coagulation Studies

Every patient with brain hemorrhage should have coagulation parameters checked. These should include prothrombin time, partial prothromboplastin time, and platelet count. In patients known to be receiving aspirin, bleeding time should be measured.

MEDICAL TREATMENT

When a diagnosis of brain hemorrhage has been established by CT scan, measures are taken to normalize blood pressure, prevent hemorrhage, reduce mass affect, control edema, and prevent seizures. Since most hemorrhages appear to have stopped before the patient arrives in the hospital, it has been difficult to assess efforts to stop hemorrhage in the occasional case of continued bleeding. Recurrence of hemorrhage is rare, except when the etiology is an aneurysm or amyloid angiopathy (87). Aminocaproic acid has not been recommended.

Hypertension is controlled with drug therapy. The authors do not recommend lowering the blood pressure below normotensive levels, since autoregulation is probably impaired in the brain tissue around the hemorrhage and a significant decrease in cerebral perfusion pressure may produce secondary ischemic damage.

When increased intracranial pressure is suspected, it should be treated vigorously. Steriods may be of help. The authors have noted temporary worsening after discontinuation of high-dose steriod treatment. However, the benefit of this therapy in a large series of cases has not been established. One controlled study showed no benefit, but the majority of patients were in coma or deep stupor (85). Intravenous mannitol is an effective and safe therapy for increased intracranial pressure. Furosemide can be used alone or with mannitol to potentiate its effect. The stuporous or comatose patient must be intubated to ensure adequate ventilation and maintenance of a normal or preferably moderately reduced pCO_2.

Careful management of fluid and electrolytes is required for all patients. One must watch for inappropriate antidiuretic hormone secretion which is not uncommon in these patients. All patients are given anticonvulsant medication.

The best guide to prognosis has been the state of consciousness (7, 48, 68). Patients with small hematomas will generally respond to medical therapy, as will most patients with moderately sized hematomas (10, 11, 59, 71). These patients are awake and can be followed by clinical examination; monitoring of intracranial pressure is usually not necessary. The use of continuous monitoring of intracranial pressure in the management of patients with large hematomas has been reported (16, 66). A subarachnoid bolt or ventricular catheter may be used. The effects of hyperventilation, mannitol, and furosemide can then be closely followed. When these measures are insufficient to control increased intracranial pressure, consideration is given to surgical removal of the hematoma or to treatment with large doses of barbiturates. The latter treatment undoubtedly lowers intracranial pressure in some patients in whom all other measures have failed, but whether it actually alters ultimate outcome is unknown (72).

SURGICAL TREATMENT

Indications

The indications for surgical therapy for brain hemorrhage continue to be modified (12, 56–58). Although clear-cut indications are not yet available for all patients, clinical and CT guidelines for therapy have been proposed (11, 12, 31, 36, 58, 68, 71, 79). The smaller hematomas will generally respond to medical therapy, as will most of the moderately sized hematomas (11, 59, 71). When the hematoma is larger than 3.0 cm in diameter, sugical therapy is considered. There is little to be gained by direct surgery in cases of thalamic hemorrhage, but occasionally a shunt is indicated. In patients with cerebellar hemorrhage, there are distinct indications for surgery which are discussed in the next section. If the patient with a lobar or putaminal hemorrhage is showing signs of increasing neurologic deficit or decreasing state of consciousness in spite of medical therapy, then surgical removal of the hematoma is usually indicated.

Several reports have attempted to determine whether immediate (2, 35, 43, 81) or delayed (7, 65, 70, 84) operation in patients with hypertensive hemorrhage alters long term morbidity. Surgery can be lifesaving in the deteriorating patient (2, 11, 44, 69, 84). It has not been established whether morbidity can be lessened by removal of a hematoma immediately or several days or weeks after onset in a patient with a stable, moderate, or severe neurologic deficit. Reports of single cases and small series suggest that surgery may diminish late morbidity (11, 65, 67, 69, 70, 84, 98).

When a hematoma in any location is associated with a history and finding of severely increased intracranial pressure and brain stem compression, emergency surgery is considered, depending on the findings on CT scan and physical examination. Mannitol (100 gm in 500 ml) is given intravenously over 15–20 minutes while the CT scan is being obtained. Surgery is generally not undertaken if there is massive hemorrhage with loss of pupillary reaction and brain stem function and no response to the medical therapy.

Preoperative Preparation

If the patient has been treated medically for several days, care is taken to be sure that there is adequate hydration and the electrolytes are normal. Prior to induction of anesthesia, a radial artery catheter is placed for continuous monitoring of intraarterial blood pressure and intermittent blood gas determinations. Care is taken to avoid hypertension during induction of anesthesia. A Foley catheter is placed. After induction of anesthesia, a dose 10–20 mg of furosemide is given, and while the craniotomy is being performed, a dose of 50–100 gm of mannitol is infused.

Operative Technique

In putaminal and lobar hemorrhages, the patient is placed in a semilateral position with the head turned to the appropriate side and held with a three-point skeletal fixation headrest. A wide exposure is made and a free bone flap elevated.

The authors operate on cerebellar hemorrhages with the patient in the prone position with his or her head moderately flexed and held with the skeletal fixation headrest. This avoids the risk of hypotension. An occipital burr hole permits ventricular puncture. A midline incision allows a wide suboccipital craniectomy and removal of the posterior rim of the foramen magnum.

With the precise localization from the CT scan, a direct approach to the hemorrhage is usually posible. It is not possible to adequately evacuate an acute hematoma through a ventricular needle or catheter. Direct exposure of the hematoma is required for satisfactory removal. A cortical incision is performed in the appropriate area (Fig. 25.1). For temporal or putaminal lesions, an anterior superior temporal gyrus approach is used. A trans-sylvian approach has been described (82). For parietal-occipital lesions, a superior posterior parietal lobule incision is chosen. For a frontal lesion, the authors prefer a superior frontal gyrus incision anterior to the motor strip. For cerebellar lesions, a paramedian approach is used, depending on the lesion's location. The corticectomy is made 2–3 cm long with the aid of bipolar cautery and microscissors (Fig. 25.2A). Loupes and headlights permit satisfactory visualization. On occasion, the operating microscope is useful if an unexpected AVM is found or there is need to control hemorrhage from a deep vessel.

Evacuation of the hemorrhage is achieved with gentle suction and irrigation (Fig. 25.2B). Sometimes, tumor forceps can deliver a large clot. Most of the hematoma is removed to achieve decompression, but the last adherent bits of colt may be left behind (Fig. 25.3D). This is done to prevent injury and bleeding from the walls of the cavity. Great care is taken to keep instruments, particularly the sucker, away from the adjacent edematous brain tissue. This is aided by the use of self-retaining retractors. Any abnormal-appearing brain tissue should be biopsied.

Hemostasis is achieved by using a bipolar cautery (Fig 25.2C). Occasionally, a clip is needed. Surgicel is used to line the hematoma cavity. Hemostasis must be meticulous to prevent recurrence. The authors raise the blood pressure for 5–10 minutes to 140–150 mm Hg in order to check hemostasis. Great care must be taken to prevent hypertension during the time of clo-

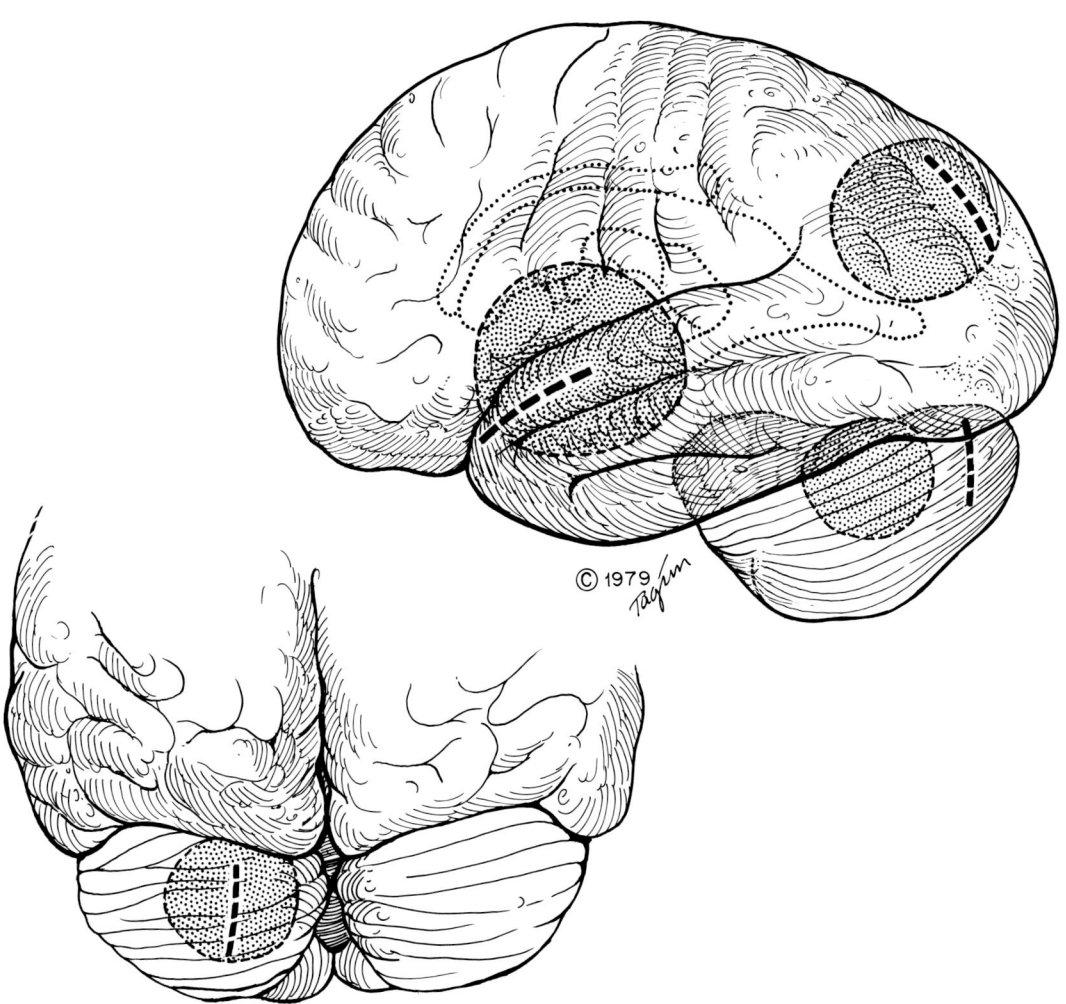

Figure 25.1. Common sites for brain hemorrhage requiring surgical treatment: putamen, lobar (parietal-occipital), and cerebellum. The location of the cortical incisions are outlined for the easiest access with the least trauma to normal brain tissue. (From Crowell RM, Ojemann RG: Surgery for brain hemorrhage. In Mossy J, Reinmuth OM (eds): *Cerebrovascular Disease*. New York, Raven Press, 1981.)

sure, extubation, and immediate postoperative period. Closure is performed in the usual fashion without a drain. In some cases of cerebellar hemorrhage, a ventricular catheter may be left in for a few days.

The removal of a hematoma in both the acute and the chronic stage by CT-guided stereotactic technique has been reported (4, 32, 50). The development of this specialized instrumentation has made possible the subtotal removal of deep hematomas in a few patients in whom the lesion could not be approached by conventional operation without disrupting normal brain tissue. In one report, placement of a catheter was followed by intermittent drainage with the aid of Urokinase (50).

Postoperative Care

Postoperative care must be meticulous in order to prevent recurrence. Blood pressure must be controlled as the anesthesia wears off and must be continuously monitored, particularly during the transfer of the patient from the operating table to the bed and to the recovery room area. Rapidly acting intravenous antihypertensive agents are administered as necessary to keep the blood pressure in the normal range. Steriod medication is continued to control brain swelling. In supratentorial lesions, diphenylhydantoin is started. Electrolytes are checked regularly. If the patient's state of consciousness is reduced, intubation may be continued. The role of continuous intracranial pressure monitoring in postoperative management has not been established, although it probably is of help in comatose patients (72).

If there is any evidence of worsening, a CT scan is indicated. Postoperative complications include recurrence of bleeding, hydrocephalus, infection, and seizures.

SPECIAL CLINICAL PROBLEMS AND GUIDELINES FOR TREATMENT
Putaminal Hemorrhage

The most common site for hypertensive hemorrhages is the putamen. The hemorrhage may remain localized but can track into the white matter, into the frontal or temporal lobe, involve the internal capsule, or rupture into the ventricle. The larger the lesion, the greater the deficit and the worse the prognosis.

The clinical syndrome is well described (21,22, 31, 59). Patients are characteristically up and active when they become aware that something is wrong. Then, a hemiparesis that may progress to a hemiplegia emerges smoothly and steadily, in some cases accompanied by a hemisensory loss, hemianopia, dysphasia if the dominant hemisphere is affected, lack of awareness of the deficit if the nondominant hemisphere is involved, and conjugate deviation of the eyes to the side of the hemorrhage. The syndrome may stabilize at any point or continue to coma and death within a few hours. Of 27 consecutive cases, 62% were characterized by a smooth onset, while 30% were characterized by symptoms that developed so rapidly that observers believed the deficit was nearly maximal at onset (59). None of the patients experienced fluctuation of the deficit. Headache affected only 14% of patients at onset and only 28% at any time, with nearly 72% left free of headache even in the presence of substantial focal neurologic deficit. Only 12% of patients had a stiff neck. On examination, none showed papilledema or subhyaloid preretinal hemorrhages. All patients were affected by some form of motor deficit varying from mild to complete paralysis. Some patients were not fully evaluated for sensory disorder, but approximately 65% of those patients tested showed some alteration in response to pinprick. Fifty-two percent of patients experienced a disorder in conjugate horizontal gaze deviation, 37% had no impairment in eye movement, and 11% showed other disorders in eye funtion, usually associated with midbrain compression.

Most patients with small and many moderately sized hematomas in the putamen make a good re-

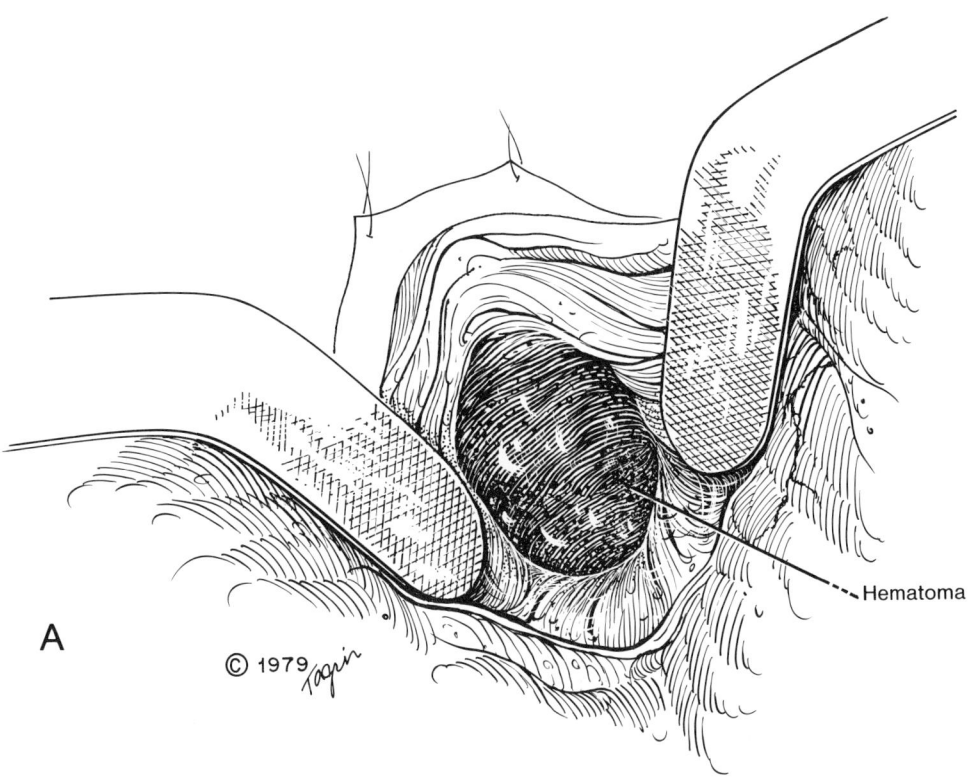

Figure 25.2. Surgical technique for removal of brain hemorrhage. **A,** Exposure of the hematoma after the cortical incision has been made. Self-retaining brain retractors provide gentle steady exposure with minimum trauma. **B,** Removal of hematoma. Careful suction along with irrigation removes the clot with minimal injury to the cavity walls. It is not necessary to remove every last fragment of hematoma from the wall. **C,** Hemostasis is achieved with bipolar coagulation and Surgicel. Abnormal tissue is biopsied (*arrow*). (From Crowell RM, Ojemann RG: Surgery for brain hemorrhage. In Mossy J, Reinmuth OM (eds): *Cerebrovascular Disease*. New York, Raven Press, 1981.)

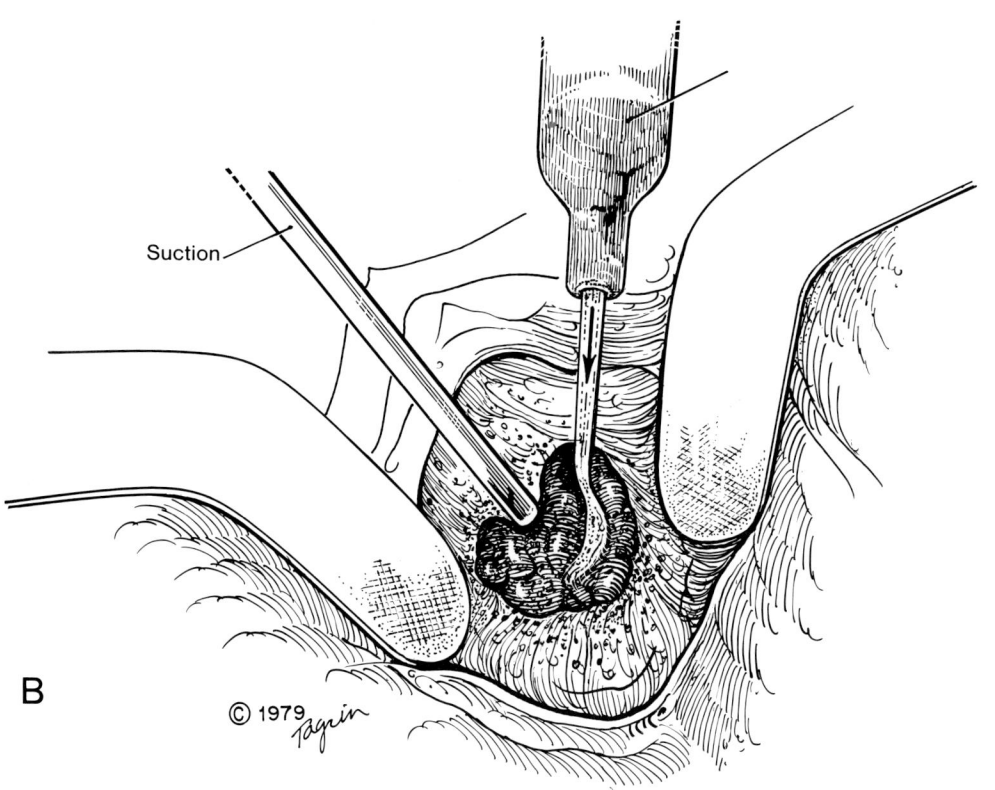

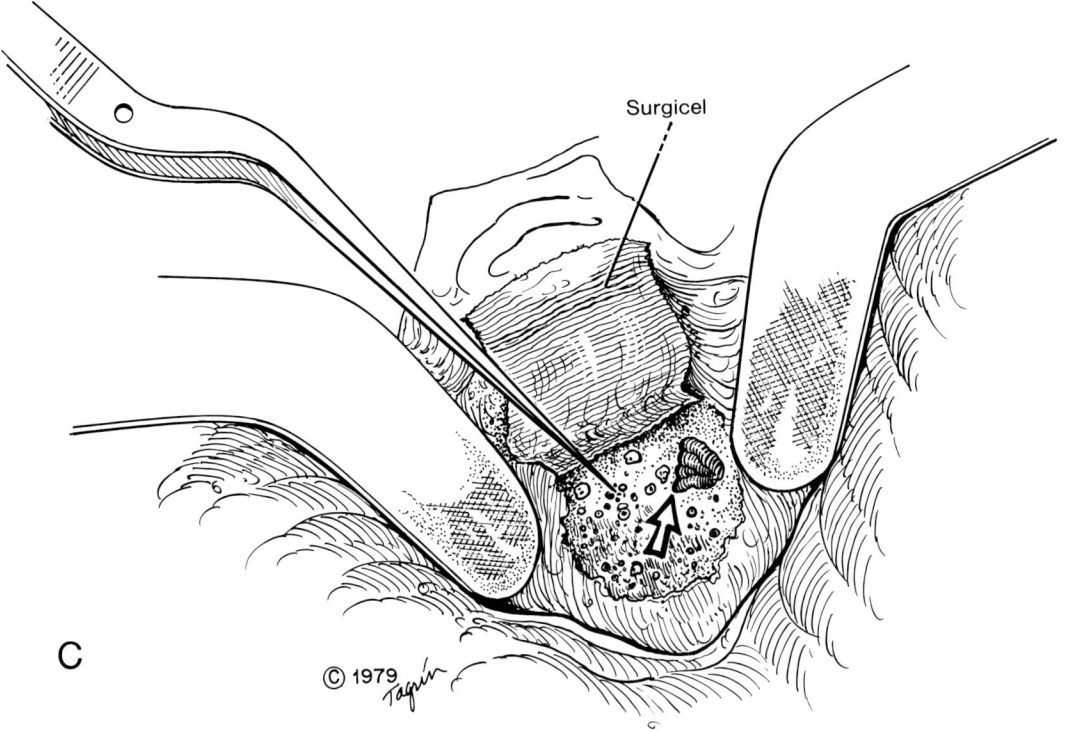

Figure 25.2C.

covery either spontaneously or with medical treatment (57, 90) (Fig. 25.3A and B). With hematomas larger than 3 cm in diameter, the initial treatment is usually medical, but if the patient is showing signs of increasing neurologic deficit or a decreasing state of consciousness in spite of medical therapy, surgical removal of the hematoma is considered (Fig. 25.3C and D).

In an evaluation of the CT scans in 24 patients with putaminal hemorrhage, three groups were defined (31). The first group consisted of patients comatose on admission who were found to have massive hemorrhages and a poor prognosis. The second group consisted of patients who were alert with substantial neurologic deficit and moderately sized hematomas. A few made acceptable recovery, but the majority were left with a significant deficit. The third group consisted of patients who had only mild deficits, were found to have small hemorrhages on the CT scan, and generally made a good recovery. Whether surgery would have improved the outcome in the first two groups is not known, but in other reports, there was no evidence of definite benefit from surgery (36, 57, 90).

Thalamic Hemorrhage

The classic features include, as initial deficit, a hemisensory loss and, if the internal capsule becomes involved, motor weakness (5, 18, 19, 22, 94). Extension into the upper brain stem is common and can cause vertical gaze palsy, retraction nystagmus, skew deviation, loss of convergence, ptosis and miosis, anisocoria, and unreactive pupils. Dysphasia may occur with left-sided hemorrhage. If the hematoma is large, deep coma may be present from the onset. Headache is rare. Compression of the cerebrospinal fluid pathways may cause hydrocephalus.

In 18 patients with hypertensive thalamic hemorrhage, the diagnostic clinical features were limitations of vertical gaze, downward eye deviation, and small but reactive or sluggish pupils (94). All had a contralateral sensory-motor deficit. These findings were confirmed in another report of 23 patients (5). Headache was present in only 20–30% of these patients. The motor deficit was similar to that of patients who suffered putaminal hemorrhage. The sensory deficit was often of striking severity and widely distributed over the limbs, head, face, and trunk on the affected side.

There is a strong correlation between the diameter of the hematoma as seen on CT scan and the recovery (5, 39, 94). Patients with hematomas less than 3 cm in diameter usually survive, and functional recovery is better in patients with these hematomas than in those with larger hematomas, although even with small hematomas there may be significant residual disability (Fig. 25.4).

Direct surgery on the hematoma has generally not been used in patients with thalamic hemorrhage. Hydrocephalus may develop, often acutely, and require placement of ventricular drainage. A permanent shunt will be needed in some patients (5, 39, 89, 94).

Caudate Hemorrhage

Localized hemorrhage may occur in the caudate nucleus due to hypertension or AVM (80, 91). The region is supplied by deep small penetrating arteries. The initial symptoms are similar to those of subarachnoid hemorrhage, since the hemorrhage usually ruptures into the ventricular system. If the hemorrhage extends into the internal capsule focal neurologic deficit may be found. The diagnosis is established by CT scan. With medical therapy, the prognosis for recovery for patients with caudate hemorrhage is good.

Lobar Hemorrhage

Lobar hemorrhage occurs in the subcortical white matter of the cerebral hemispheres (37, 73, 83). About one-third of the hematomas (Fig. 25.5B) result from hypertension; others are associated with metastatic or primary brain tumor, AVMs, anticoagulant therapy (Fig. 25.5A) and blood dyscrasia. The history and findings on admission depend on the location of the hematoma.

Patients whose condition is stable and who are alert or demonstrate mild altered level of consciousness will usually respond to medical therapy. Patients with meduim or large lobar hemorrhages who are obtunded are carefully evaluated and observed, and surgical treatment is undertaken if they fail to improve or show any evidence of progression (11, 13, 37). In as many as 25–30% of patients, no etiology is found on the initial evaluation. These patients will need periodic CT scan and, possibly, angiography to be sure a tumor or AVM is not being overlooked. Magnetic resonance imaging may also be of value in these patients (25, 54).

In young normotensive patients with lobar hemorrhage, surgical exploration to search for a small angiomatous malformation may be indicated, since it has been estimated that this may be the cause of the hemorrhage in 27–53% of such patients (49, 83, 93). Even when an AVM is not seen on the initial angiogram, there is a significant incidence of rebleeding (54, 93) (see Chapter 22).

Cerebellar Hemorrhage

Hemorrhage in the cerebellum causes a life-threatening syndrome which can be reversed by prompt surgical treatment. Classically, the onset of this hemorrhage is sudden, with nausea, vomiting, and inability to stand or walk (23). In a series of 56 patients

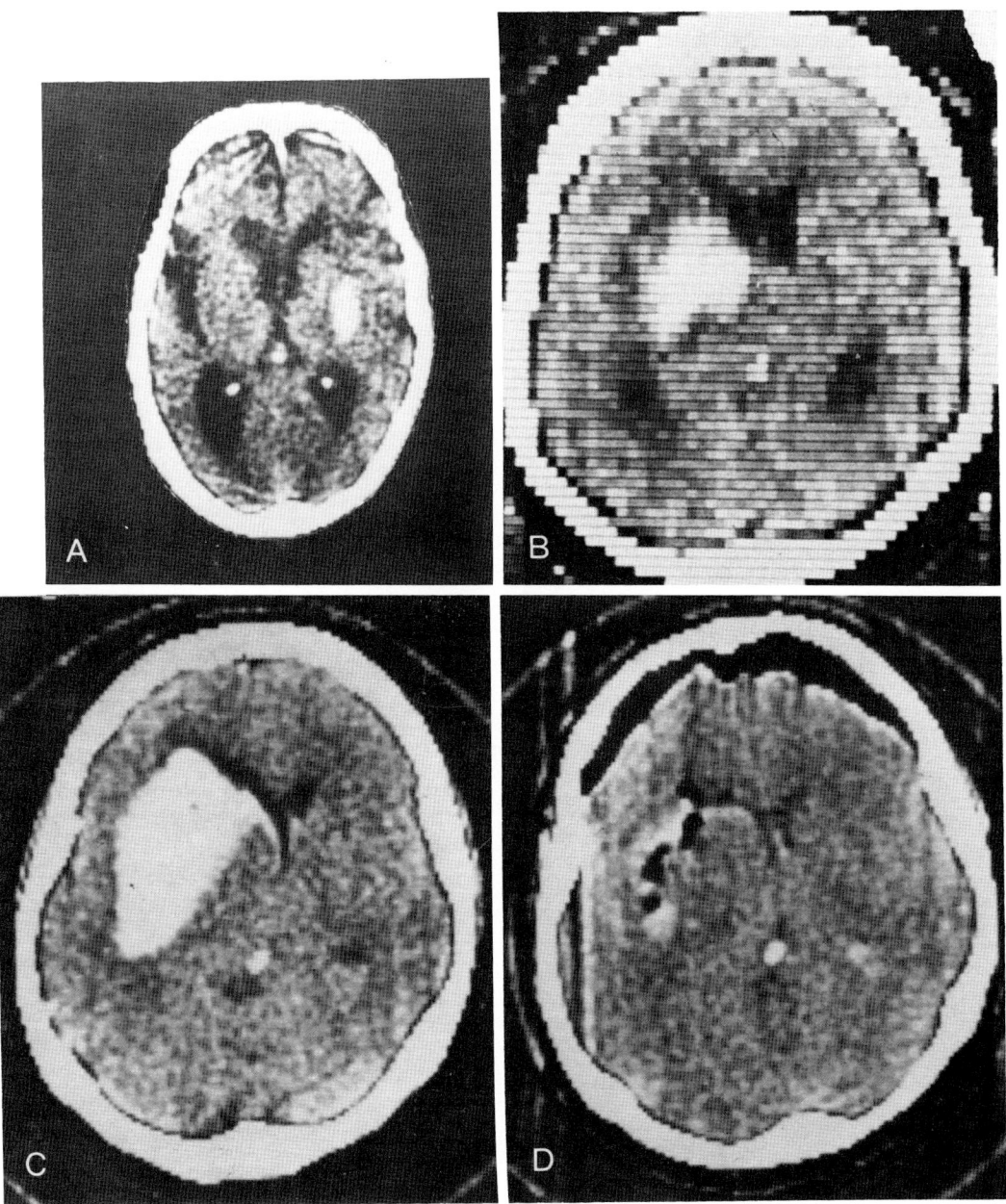

Figure 25.3. Hypertensive putaminal hemorrhage. **A**, Small hematoma. Onset of mild deficit. Treated with steroids. Full recovery. **B**, Moderate hematoma. Onset of severe neurologic deficit that worsened for 1 day, then gradually improved. Speech cleared but residual hemiparesis persisted. **C**, Large hematoma. Sudden onset of neurologic deficit. Stable for 3 days on steroids. Then coma and evidence of increased intracranial pressure. Hematoma removed surgically. **D**, Scan obtained 3 hours postoperatively. There is air in the subdural space anteriorly. The hematoma has been removed, but some hematoma remains on the walls of the cavity. This was left to minimize dusturbance of the surrounding brain tissue. The patient recovered with residual hemiparesis. (From Ojemann RG, Mohr JP: Hypertensive brain hemorrhage. In: *Clinical Neurosurgery*. Baltimore, Williams & Wilkins, 1976, vol 23, chap 17, pp 220–244.)

with cerebellar hemorrhage, headache was present in 74%; dizziness, in 55%; and loss of consciousness at onset, in 14% (63). Examination showed appendicular ataxia in 78%, facial palsy in 60%, and ipsilateral gaze palsy in 54%. No distinctive clinical feature could be delineated in the acute state in noncomatose patients so as to predict those who would survive with minimal or mild disability and those who might progress to brain stem compression and coma.

The cerebellar hematoma represents a special situation regarding treatment. Deterioration due to brain

Brain Hemorrhage

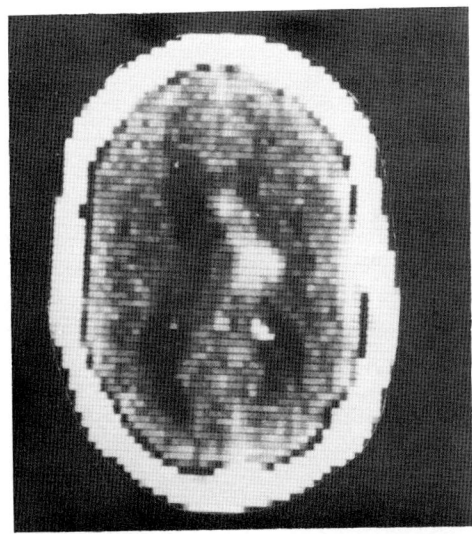

Figure 25.4. Hypertensive thalamic hemorrhage. Patient treated medically. Recovered to moderate neurologic deficit.

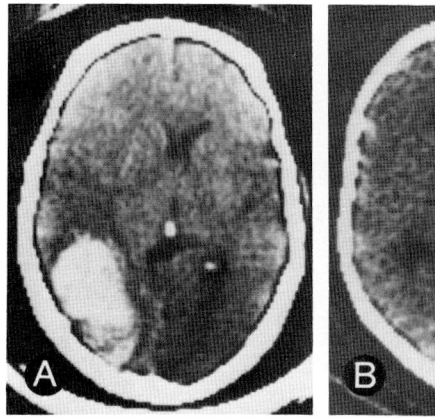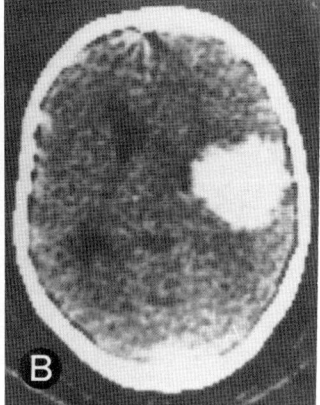

Figure 25.5. Lobar hemorrhage. **A**, Occipital lobe hemorrhage. Patient on coumadin. Patient in coma at the time of hospital admission. Hematoma was removed and patient had good recovery. **B**, Temporal lobe hemorrhage. Patient had mild neurologic signs. Recovery occurred with medical therapy.

stem compression is common, unpredictable and, once set in motion, often irreversible. It is critically important to treat the patient before compression causes (a) alteration in the state of consciousness and (b) an unstable clinical situation. In our experience, 10 of 12 patients who were alert or drowsy preoperatively survived operation, while only 4 of 16 patients who were stuporous or comatose before surgery lived (63). The relationship of the level of consciousness to prognosis and the importance of not delaying surgery in patients with acute cerebellar hematomas has been stressed in other reviews (3, 8, 13, 29). It should be pointed out, however, that even for a patient in deep coma, emergency evacuation of the hematoma can result in good recovery, especially if the time interval between the development of the comatose state and surgery is short. Therefore, operation should not be denied to a patient who is in coma as a result of cerebellar hemorrhage unless there is clinical or CT evidence that the brain stem has been destroyed (29).

In several reports it has been noted that most patients with cerebellar hematoma less than 3 cm in diameter on CT scan usually recover with medical therapy (13, 27, 33, 36, 43, 76, 100) (Fig. 25.6A). These patients generally do not have signs of brain stem compression but are monitored carefully in the intensive care unit. However, once the patient shows signs of brain stem compression, deterioration can proceed at an unpredictable rate, and therefore, operation is indicated even if the hematoma appears smaller than 3 cm (29).

In most patients who develop signs of early brain stem compression, the cerebellar hematoma is 3 cm or greater on the CT scan (33, 43). The authors of this text, as well as others, generally recommend removal of the hematoma if it is larger than 3 cm in diameter on CT scan and if the patient is seen within the first week of the onset of symptoms (10, 11, 33, 63, 76, 100) (Fig. 25.6). Others have questioned the benefit of surgery and prefer to wait, before recommending operation, until signs of progression occur (3, 13, 36). Patients seen a week or more after onset who have a stable neurologic course may be treated with medical therapy but are closely observed.

Pontine Hemorrhage

Pontine hemorrhage is one of the most dramatic and least treatable of all brain hemorrhages. A small hematoma often results in immediate coma, rapid quadriplegia, decerebrate rigidity, pinpoint pupils that may be barely reactive to light, and a variety of ocular motility disturbances. The uncommon smaller hemorrhage may cause the patient to be paralyzed but able to communicate by ocular movements ("locked-in" state). Most patients do not survive the acute phase.

On rare occasions, successful removal of a pontine hematoma has been reported (6, 53, 62). In a review of 24 patients with pontine hematoma due to hypertension, 6 patients with hematoma less than 1.0 cm in diameter as shown on CT scan were reported to have survived, although presently only one is working (75). All patients with hematoma larger than 1.0 cm died, except for one. Four patients had suboccipital craniectomy for removal of the hematoma, and several had ventricular drainage. It was concluded that direct operation was of doubtful value.

Intraventricular Hemorrhage

The degree of intraventricular hemorrhage can be readily recognized on CT scan. Most intraventricular

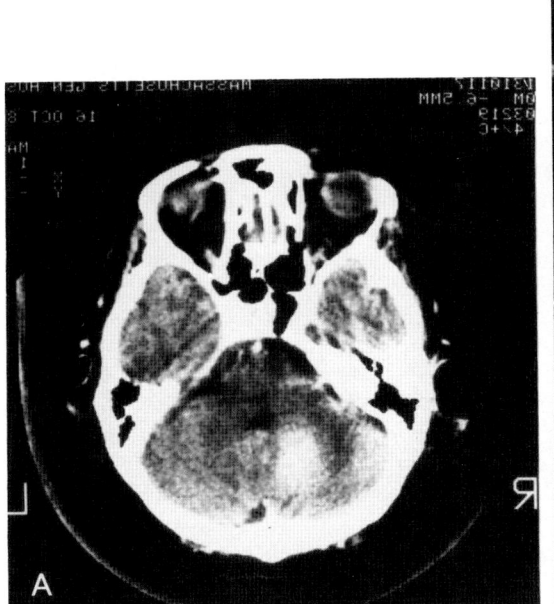
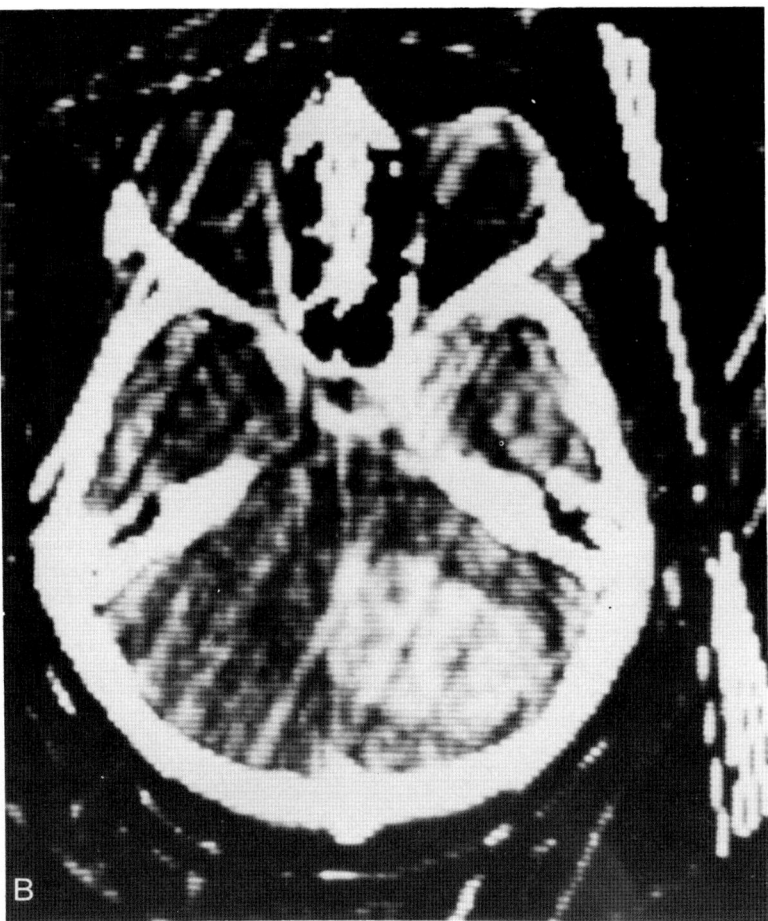

Figure 25.6. Cerebellar hemorrhage. **A**, Hemorrhage less than 3 cm in diameter, located in the medial aspect of the cerebellar hemisphere. Patient recovered on medical therapy. **B**, Large hematoma causing brain stem compression. Emergency surgery was performed to remove the hematoma. Patient recovered over several weeks. (From Mossy J, Reinmuth OM (eds): *Cerebrovascular Disease*. New York, Raven Press, 1981.)

hematomas result from rupture of a parenchymal hematoma into the ventricles, but occasionally, primary intraventricular hemorrhage can occur. The latter, particularly in young normotensive individuals, is most commonly due to cryptic AVM (9,14). Although intraventricular hemorrhage is traditionally thought to be associated with poor prognosis, it can be associated with a relatively benign clinical course.

The spontaneous resolution of intraventricular hemorrhage was originally documented on pneumoencephalogram (60) and has been well demonstrated on CT scan. In a review of 54 patients with intraventricular hemorrhage demonstrated on CT scan, association with a large number of disorders, including hypertension, saccular and mycotic aneurysm, AVM, tumor, and coagulation disorders, was noted (41). In this series, 78% of the cases were associated with intraparenchymal hematoma.

Hypertensive hemorrhage in any of the common sites can rupture into the ventricle. In a report on 32 patients with hypertensive intracerebral hemorrhage, 62% had intraventricular rupture (96). Intraventricular hemorrhage also occurs from rupture of an aneurysm, and these hemorrhages are generally more extensive than those due to other causes.

The guidelines for surgical treatment of this hemorrhage are generally the same as those outlined for treatment of parenchymal hemorrhage. Ventricular drainage has usually not been of help, since the catheter frequently becomes obstructed (41). However, in the rare patient, emergency ventriculostomy can be lifesaving and is indicated when neurologic deterioration appears to be secondary to acute hydrocephalus from intraventricular hemorrhage. In less severe cases, patients who survive the acute phase commonly require placement of a shunt.

Hemorrhage Due to Aneurysm and AVMs

About one-fifth of patients with aneurysmal hemorrhage and one-half of those with hemorrhage from an AVM will have an associated intracerebral hematoma (30). When either aneurysm or AVM is suspected with an intracerebral hematoma, angiography is indicated. The indications for surgical removal are essentially the same as those for other forms of spontaneous intracerebral hemorrhage.

In the aneurysm patient the timing of operation to repair the aneurysm should not be influenced by the intracerebral hemorrhage unless the patient is deteriorating as a result of the mass effect. In patients who require early operation to remove the hematoma, every effort should be made to repair the aneurysm at the same operation so as to prevent postoperative rebleeding.

In patients with a ruptured AVM, the incidence of early rebleeding is low. If the hematoma has to be removed urgently and the AVM is not readily accessible or would require extensive surgery, excision can be delayed for several weeks until brain swelling has subsided. Occasionally, a "cryptic" AVM will be discovered at surgery in a patient with an intracerebral hemorrhage and negative angiogram.

Hemorrhage Due to Tumors

Brain tumor is responsible for about 10% of all spontaneous intracerebral hemorrhages (77). Metastatic tumors, particularly melanoma and glioma, are responsible in the majority of these cases (42, 45, 64, 77, 92) (Fig. 25.7A–D). Pituitary adenomas bleed frequently, but the hemorrhage is usually within the tumor and rarely results in intracerebral hemorrhage (92). Whenever a tumor is suspected as the cause of intracerebral hemorrhage because of clinical, CT, or angiographic findings, the hematoma should be removed, with thorough exploration and biopsy of the wall of the hematoma cavity carried out. If a diag

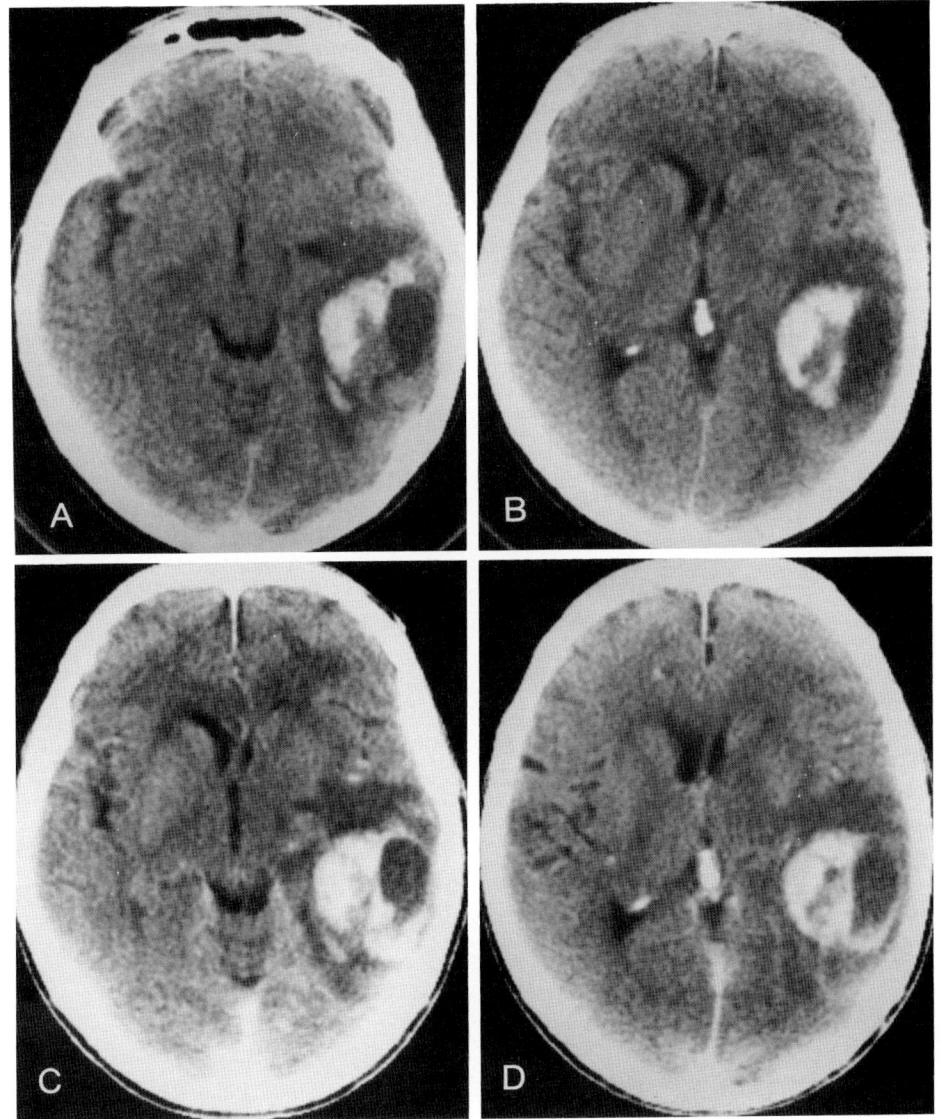

Figure 25.7. Hemorrhage into astrocytoma. Sudden onset of symptoms. **A** and **B**, Plain CT scans of patient with lobar hemorrhage. The irregular margins of the high-density hematoma and, possibly, a cystic area are shown. **C** and **D**, Contrast enhancement around the presumed cystic area. All of these findings are highly suggestive of tumor as the cause of the hemorrhage.

nosis is not established and the suspicion is high, follow-up CT scan and angiography are indicated.

Hemorrhage Due to Amyloid Angiopathy

Amyloid angiopathy is an infrequent cause of spontaneous lobar brain hemorrhage except in a normotensive elderly patient in whom it may be the most frequent cause. Characteristically, the hemorrhages are subcortical, although they can be massive and involve the entire lobe (46, 87, 88). They usually occur in patients over 60 years of age and may be associated with multiple hemorrhages (61, 86, 87). If such a patient has had two or more hemorrhages in different sites, this diagnosis becomes the primary consideration. Whenever amyloid angiopathy is a prominent diagnostic possibility, every effort should be made to treat the patient medically, since surgical evacuation is frequently attended by uncontrollable hemorrhage and postoperative recurrent bleeding. If surgery becomes necessary because of continuing neurologic deterioration despite vigorous medical therapy, care should be taken to disturb the walls of the hematoma cavity as little as possible to avoid further bleeding from the fragile amyloid-laden parenchymal vessels (87).

Hemorrhage Due to Coagulation Disorders

Anticoagulant Therapy

With the widespread use of anticoagulants for treatment of a variety of disorders, the number of patients with brain hemorrhage due to this cause has increased. The majority of patients who develop this complication are found to have either a prothrombin time longer than the therapeutic range or a local lesion such as infarction to account for bleeding (22). In contrast to most other bleeding disorders, an isolated intracerebral hemorrhage in a patient on anticoagulants may occur in the absence of bleeding in other areas of the body.

The initial evaluation and the treatment of coagulation disorders are the same as those described for spontaneous brain hemorrhage. Immediate transfusion of fresh frozen plasma reverses anticoagulation. To maintain hemostasis, parenteral administration of vitamin K_1 (phytonadione) preparation usually restores normal coagulation within 6 hours, except in patients with significant liver disease. With these measures, operation can usually be safely performed (Fig. 25.5A). Prothrombin time should be rechecked postoperatively to guard against rebound effects.

Thrombocytopenia

The normal blood platelet count is 100,000–400,000/mm^3. Thrombocytopenia is diagnosed when the platelet count is less the 80,000/m^3 (1, 95). This condition is a common cause of clotting deficiency. Intracerebral hemorrhage due to thrombocytopenia has been reported in idiopathic thrombocytopenic purpura and in a variety of disease states in which there is secondary thrombocytopenia. Included among the latter are conditions either in which there is failure of production of platelets due to suppression of bone marrow (drugs, speticemia, and metastatic tumor) and myeloinfiltrative conditions (leukemia and multiple myeloma) or in which there is excessive destruction of platelets, as in certain immune reactions or with splenomegaly secondary to hepatic or cardiac failure. The initial symptoms of spontaneous intracranial bleeding in these patients is usually headache followed by deterioration in the level of consciousness. The onset is often insidious, coming on over several days. Usually, the hemorrhage is intracerebral, but subdural hematoma can occur (1).

Surgery is hazardous when the platelet count is below 50,000 and is of concern when the count is 50,000–100,000. It is usually possible to achieve a hemostatic level by a combination of platelet transfusion and administration of corticosteroid drugs that have a number of effects not only on the hemostatic mechanisms but also, in many instances, on the underlying disease process. Guidelines for surgery on the hematoma are the same as those previously stated. In a report on intracranial hemorrhage in children with idiopathic thrombocytopenia purpura, it was recommended that emergency splenectomy be performed prior to neurosurgical intervention (97).

Hemophilia

Hemophilia is due to a deficiency in factor VIII, factor IX, or factor XI, causing a prolonged partial thromboplastin time. The vast majority of patients are deficient in factor VIII; a small number, in factor IX; and a rare patient, in factor XI. The problem has been summarized in several reports (79, 99).

Brain hemorrhage usually is associated with mild trauma, but it can occur spontaneously. Any patient with hemophilia who complians of a persistent headache should have a CT scan. When hemorrhage is confirmed, appropriate replacement treatment should be started immediately. To prevent further spontaneous, intraoperative or postoperative hemorrhage, it is necessary to maintain a minimum level of at least 20% of the deficient factor with transfusions of the appropriate concentrate. If an operation is performed replacement needs to be continued until the incision is healed (61). The indications for operation are the same as those previously outlined.

REFERENCES

1. Almaani WS, Awid AS: Spontaneous intracranial bleeding in hemorrhagic diathesis. Surg Neurol 17:137–140, 1982.
2. Arana-Iniquez R, Wilson E, Bastarrica E, Medici M: Cerebral hematomas. Surg Neurol 6:45–52, 1976.
3. Auer LM, Auer TH, Sayama I: Indications for surgical treat-

ment of cerebellar hemorrhage and infarction. *Acta Neurochir (Wien)* 79:74–79, 1986.
4. Backlund EO, vonHolst H: Controlled subtotal evacuation of intracerebral hematomas by stereotactic technique. *Sug Neurol* 9:99–101, 1987.
5. Barraquer-Bordas L, Illa A, Escartin J, Ruscalleda J, Marti-Vilalta JL: Thalamic hemorrhage. A study of 23 patients with diagnosis by computed tomography. *Stroke* 12:524–527, 1981.
6. Becker DH, Silverberg GD: Successful evacuation of an acute pontine hematoma. *Surg Neurol* 10:263–265, 1978.
7. Benes V, Koukolik F, Obrovska D: Two types of spontaneous intracerebral hemorrhage due to hypertension. *J Neurosurg* 37:509–513, 1972.
8. Brennan RW, Bergland RM. Acute cerebellar hemorrhage. Analysis of clinical findings and outcome in 12 cases. *Neurology* 27:527–532, 1977.
9. Butler AB, Partain RA, Netsky MG: Primary intraventricular hemorrhage. A mild and remediable form. *Neurology* 22:475–487, 1972.
10. Crowell RM, Ojemann RG: Cerebellar hemorrhage. In Buchheit WA, Truex RC Jr (eds): *Surgery of the Posterior Fossa*. New York, Raven Press, 1979, pp 135–142.
11. Crowell RM, Ojemann RG: Surgery for brain hemorrhage. In Mossy J, Reinmuth OM (eds): *Cerebrovascular Disease*. New York, Raven Press, 1981, pp 233–254.
12. Crowell RM, Ojemann RG: Spontaneous brain hemorrhage: Surgical consideration. In Barnett HJM, Mohr JP, Stein BM, Yatsu FM (eds): *Stroke*. New York, Churchill Livingstone, 1986, vol 2, pp 1191–1206.
13. DaPian R, Razzan A, Pasqualin A: Surgical versus medical treatment of spontaneous posterior fossa hematomas: A cooperative study of 205 cases. *Neurol Res* 6:145–151, 1984.
14. Doe FD, Shuangshoti S, Netsky MG: Cryptic hemangioma of the choroid plexus. *Neurology* 22:1232–1293, 1972.
15. Dolinskas CA, Bilaniuk LT, Zimmerman RA, Kuhl DE, Alavi A: Computed tomography of intracerebral hematomas. II. Radionuclide and transmission CT studies of the perihematoma region. *Am J Roentgenol* 129:686–692. 1977.
16. Duff TA, Ayeni S, Levin AB, Javid M: Nonsurgical management of spontaneous intracerebral hematoma. *Neurosurgery* 9:387–393, 1981.
17. Edwards KR: Hemorrhagic complications of cerebral arteritis. *Arch Neurol* 34:549–552, 1977.
18. Fazio C, Sacco G, Bugiani O: The thalamic hemorrhage. An anatomo-clinical study. *Eur Neurol* 9:30–43, 1974.
19. Fisher CM: The pathologic and clinical aspects of thalamic hemorrhage. *Trans Am Neurol Assoc* 84:56–59, 1959.
20. Fisher CM: The pathology and pathogenesis of intracerebral hemorrhage. In Field WS (ed): *Pathogenesis and Treatment of Cerebrovascular Disease*. Springfield, IL, Charles C Thomas, 1961, pp 259–317.
21. Fisher CM: Clinical syndromes in cerebral hemorrhage. In Fields WS (ed): *Pathogenesis and Treatment of Cerebrovascular Disease*. Springfield, IL, Charles C Thomas, 1961, pp 318–338.
22. Fisher CM, Mohr JP, Adams RD: Cerebrovascular diseases. In Wintrobe MM, Thorn GW, Adams RD, Braunwald E, Isselbacher KJ, Petersdorf RG (ed): *Harrison's Principles of Internal Medicine*. New York, McGraw-Hill, 1974, pp 1743–1780.
23. Fisher CM, Picard EH, Polak A, Dalal P, Ojemann RG: Acute hypertensive cerebellar hemorrhage: Diagnosis and surgical treatment. *J Nerv Ment Dis* 140:38–57, 1965.
24. Furlan AJ, Whisnant JP, Elveback LR: The decreasing incidence of primary intracerebral hemorrhage: A population study. *Ann Neurol* 5:367–373, 1979.
25. Gomori JM, Grossman RI, Goldbert HI, Hackney DB, Zimmerman RA, Bilaniuk LT: Occult cerebral vascular malformations: High field MR imaging. *Radiology* 158: 707–713, 1986.
26. Hayward RD, O'Reilly GVA: Computerized tomography and intracerebral hemorrhage. *Am Heart J* 93:126–127, 1977.
27. Heiman TD, Satya-Murti S: Benign cerebellar hemorrhages. *Ann Neurol* 3:366–368, 1987.
28. Herbstein DS, Schaumburg HH: Hypertensive intracerebral hematoma. An investigation of the inital hemorrhage and rebleeding using chromium Cr51-labeled erythrocytes. *Arch Neurol* 30:412–414, 1974.
29. Heros RC: Cerebellar hemorrhage and infarction. *Stroke* 16:17–22, 1981.
30. Heros RC, Zervas NT: Subarachnoid hemorrhage. *Ann Rev Med* 34:367–375, 1983.
31. Hier DB, Davis KR, Richardson EP Jr, Mohr JP: Hypertensive putaminal hemorrhage. *Ann Neurol* 1:152–159, 1977.
32. Higgins AC, Nashold BS: Stereotactic evacuation of large intracerebral hematoma. *Appl Neurophysiol* 43:3–5, 1980.
33. Ito Z, Nakajima K: Surgical treatment of acute cerebellar hemorrhage. In Mizukami et al (eds): *Hypertensive Intracerebral Hemorrhage*. New York, Raven Press, 1983, pp 215–223.
34. Kanaya H: Epidemiology of hypertensive ICH in Japan. In Pia HW, Langmaid C, Zierski J (eds): *Spontaneous Intracerebral Hematomas*. New York, Springer-Verlag, 1980, pp 96–99.
35. Kaneko M, Tanaka K. Shimada T, Sato K, Uemura K: Long term evaluation of ultra-early operation for hypertensive intracerebral hemorrhage in 100 cases. *J Neurosurg* 58:838–842, 1983.
36. Kanno T, Sano H, Shinomya Y, Katuda K, Nasata J, Hoshino M, Mitsuyama F: Role of surgery in hypertensive intracerebral hematoma. A comparative study of 305 nonsurgical and 154 surgical cases. *J Neurosurg* 61:1091–1099, 1984.
37. Kase CS, Williams JP, Wyatt DA, Mohr JP: Lobar intracerebral hematomas. Clinical and CT analysis of 22 cases. *Neurology* 32:1146–1150, 1982.
38. Kase CS: Intracerebral hemorrhage: Nonhypertensive causes. *Stroke* 17:590–595, 1986.
39. Kwak R, Kadoya S, Suzuki T: Factors affecting the prognosis in thalamic hemorrhage. *Stroke* 14:493–500, 1983.
40. Lieberman A, Hass WK, Pinto R, Isom WO, Kupersmith M, Bear G, Chase R: Intracranial Hemorrhage and infarction in antiocoagulated patients with prosthetic heart valves. *Stroke* 9:18–24, 1978.
41. Little JR, Blomquist GA Jr, Ethier R: Intraventricular hemorrhage in adults. *Surg Neurol* 8:143–149, 1977.
42. Little JR, Dail B, Belanger G, Carpenter S: Brain hemorrhage from intracranial tumor. *Stroke* 10:283–288, 1979.
43. Little JR, Tubman DE, Ethier R: Cerebellar hemorrhage in adults. Diagnosis by computerized tomography. *J Neurosurg* 48:575–579, 1978.
44. Luessenhop AJ, Shevlin WA, Ferrero AA, McCullough DC, Barone AM: Surgical management of primary intracerbral hemorrhage. *J Neurosurg* 27:419–427, 1967.
45. Mandybur TI: Intracranial hemorrhage caused by metastatic tumors. *Neurology* 27:650–655, 1977.
46. Mandybur TI, Bates SRD: Fatal massive intracerebral hemorrage complicating cerebral amyloid angiopathy. *Arch Neurol* 35:246–248, 1978.
47. McCormick WF, Rosenfield DB: Massive brain hemorrhage: A review of 144 cases and an examination of their causes. *Stroke* 4:946–954, 1973.
48. McKissock W, Richardson A, Taylor J: Primary intracerebral hemorrhage: A controlled trial of surgical and conservative treatment in 180 unselected cases. *Lancet* 2:221–226, 1961.
49. Margolis G, Odom GL, Woodhall B, Bloor BM: The role of small angiomatous malformations in the production of intracerebral hematomas. *J Neurosurg* 8:564–575, 1951.
50. Matsumoto K, Hondo H: CT-guided stereotaxic evacuation of hypertensive intracerebral hematomas. *J Neurosurg* 61:440–448, 1984.

51. Messina AV, Chernik NL: Computed tomography: The "resolving" intracerebral hemorrhage. Radiology 118:609–613, 1976.
52. Misukami M, Araki G, Mikara H: Arteriographically visualized extravasation in hypertensive intracerebral hemorrhage. Report of seven cases. Stroke 3:527–537, 1972.
53. Murphy MG: Successful evacuation of acute pontine hematoma. J Neurosurg 37:224–225, 1972.
54. New PFJ, Ojemann RG, David KR, Rosen BR, Heros R, Kjellberg RN, Adams RD, Richardson ED: MR and CT of occult vascular malformations of the brain. AJNR 7:771–779, 1986.
55. New PFJ, Scott WR, Schnur JA, Davis KR, Taveras JM: Computerized axial tomography with the EMI scanner. Radiology 110:109–123, 1974.
56. Ojemann RG: Intracerebral and intracerebellar hemorrhage in Youmans JR (ed): Neurological Surgery. Philadelphia, WB Saunders, 1973, vol 2, pp 844–851.
57. Ojemann RG: Spontaneous brain hemorrhage: What treatment should we recommend? Stroke 14:467, 1983.
58. Ojemann RG, Heros RC: Spontaneous brain hemorrhage. Stroke 14:468–475, 1983.
59. Ojemann RG, Mohr JP: Hypertensive brain hemorrhage. Clin Neurosurg 23:220–244, 1975.
60. Ojemann RG, New PFJ: Spontaneous resolution of an intraventricular hemotoma. J Neurosurg 20:899–902, 1963.
61. Okazak H, Reagan TJ, Campbell RJ, Cliniopathologic studies of primary cerebral amyloid angiopathy. Mayo Clin Proc 54:22–31, 1979.
62. O'Lavoire SA, Crockard HA, Thomas DGT, Gordon DS: Brain stem hematoma. A report of six surgical treated cases. J Neurosurg 56:222–227, 1982.
63. Ott KH, Kase CS, Ojemann RG, Mohr JP: Cerebellar hemorrhage: Diagnosis and treatment. A review of 56 cases. Arch Neurol 31:160–167, 1974.
64. Padt JP, DeReuck J, vander Eecken H: Intracerebral hemorrhage as initial symptom of a brain tumor. Acta Neurol Belg 73:241–251, 1973.
65. Paillas JE, Alliez B: Surgical treatment of spontaneous intracerebral hemorrhage. Immediate and long-term results in 250 cases. J Neurosurg 39:145–151, 1973.
66. Papo I, Janny P, Caruselli G, Colnet G, Luongo A: Intracranial pressure time course in primary intracerebral hemorrhage. Neurosurgery 4:504–511, 1979.
67. Pia HW: The surgical treatment of intracerebral and intraventricular hematomas. Acta Neurochir 27:149–164, 1972.
68. Pia HW, Langmaid C, Zierski J (eds): Spontaneous Intracerebral Hematomas. New York, Springer-Verlag, 1980.
69. Ransohoff J, Derby B, Kricheff I: Spontaneous intracerebral hemorrhage. Clin Neurosurg 18:247–266, 1971
70. Richardson A: Surgical therapy of spontaneous intracerebral hemorrhage. In Krayenbull H, Maspes PE, Sweet WH (eds): Progress in Neurological Surgery. Basel, Karger, 1969, vol 3, pp 397–418.
71. Richardson A: Spontaneous intracerebral and cerebellar hemorrhage. In Russell RW (ed): Cerebral Arterial Disease. New York, Churchill Livingstone, 1976, pp 210–230.
72. Rockoff MA, Ropper AH: Treatment of intracranial hypertension in neurological and neurosurgical intensive care. In Ropper AH, Kennedy FK, Zervas NT (eds): Neurological and Neurosurgical Intensive Care. Baltimore, University Park Press, 1983, pp 21–38.
73. Ropper AH, Davis KR: Lobar cerebral hemorrhages: Acute clincial syndromes in 26 cases. Ann Neurol 8:141–147, 1980.
74. Russell DS, Falconer MA, Beck DJK, McMenemey WH: The pathology of spontaneous intracranial hemorrhage. Proc R Soc Med 47:689–704, 1954.
75. Sano K, Ochiai C: Brain stem hematomas: Clinical aspects with reference to indications for treatment. In Pia HW, Langmaid C, Zierski J (eds): Spontaneous Intracerebral Hematomas. New York, Springer-Verlag, 1980, pp 366–371.
76. Sano K, Yoshida S: Cerebellar hematomas. In Pia HW, Langmaid C, Zierski J (eds): Spontaneous Intracerebral Hematomas. New York, Springer-Verlag, 1980, pp 348–356.
77. Scott M: Spontaneous intracerebral hematoma caused by cerebral neoplasms. Report of eight cases. J Neurosurg 42:338–342, 1975.
78. Scott WR, New PFJ, Davis KR, Schnur JA: Computerized axial tomography of intracerebral and intraventricular hemorrhage. Radiology 112:73–80, 1974.
79. Seeler RA, Imana RB: Intracranial hemorrhage in patients with hemophilia. J Neurosurg 39:181–185, 1973.
80. Stein RW, Kase CS, Hier DB, Caplan LR, Mohr JP, Hemmati M, Henderson K: Caudate Hemorrhage. Neurology 34:1549–1554, 1984.
81. Suzuki J, Sato T: Grading and timing of operation in putaminal ICH. In Pia HW, Langmain C, Zierski J (eds): Spontaneous Intracerebral Hematomas. New York, Springer-Verlag, 1980, pp 274–279.
82. Suzuki J, Takaku A: Trans-sylvian approach to putaminal hematomas. In Pia HW, Langmaid C, Zierski J (eds): Spontaneous Intracerebral Hematomas. New York, Springer-Verlag, 1980, pp 384–386.
83. Tanaka Y, Furusa M, Iwasa H, Masuzawa T, Saito K, Sato F, Mizuno Y: Lobar intracerebral hemorrhage: Etiology and long-term follow-up study of 32 patients. Stroke 17:51–57, 1986.
84. Tedeschi G, Bernini FP, Cerillo A: Indications for surgical treatment of intracerebral hemorrhage. J Neurosurg 43:590–595, 1975.
85. Tellez H, Bauer RB: Dexamethasone as treatment in cerebrovascular disease. 1. A controlled study in intracerebral hemorrhage. Stroke 4:541–546, 1973.
86. Tucker WS, Bilbao JM, Klodawsky H: Cerebral amyloid angiopathy and multiple intracerebral hematomas. Neurosurgery 7:611–614, 1980.
87. Tyler KL, Poletti CE, Heros RC: Cerebral amyloid angiopathy with multiple intracerebral hemorrhages. J Neurosurg 57:286–289, 1982.
88. Vinters HV, Gilbert JJ: Amyloid angiopathy: Its incidence and complications in the aging brain. Stroke 12:118, 1981.
89. Waga S, Okada M, Yamamoto Y: Reversibility of Parinaud syndrome in thalamic hemorrhage. Neurology 29:407–409, 1979.
90. Waga S, Yamamoto Y: Hypertensive putaminal hemorrhage: Treatment and results. Is surgical treatment superior to conservative one? Stroke 14:480–485, 1985.
91. Wager S, Fujimoto K, Okada M, Miyazaki M, Tanaka Y: Caudate hemorrhage. Neurosurgery 18:445–450, 1986.
92. Wakai S, Yamakowa K, Manaka S, Takakura K: Spontaneous intracerebral hemorrhage caused by brain tumor. Its incidence and clinical significance. Neurosurgery 10:437–444, 1982.
93. Wakai S, Ueda Y, Inoh S, Nagai M: Angiographically occult angiomas: A report of thirteen cases with analysis of the cases documented in the literature. Neurosurgery 17:549–556, 1985.
94. Walshe TM, Davis KD, Fisher CM: Thalamic hemorrhage: A computed tomographic-clinical correlation. Neurology 27:217–222, 1977.
95. Weisberg LA: Computerized tomography in intracranial hemorrhage. Arch Neurol 36:422–426, 1979.
96. Wiggins WS, Moody DM, Toole JF, Laster DW, Ball MR: Clinical and computerized tomographic study of hypertensive intracerebral hemorrhage. Arch Neurol 35:832–833, 1978.
97. Woerner FJ, Abildgaard CF, French BN: Intracranial hemorrhage in children with idiophathic thrombocytopenic purpura. Pediatrics 67:453–460, 1981.
98. Yashon D, Kosnik EJ: Chronic intracerebral hematoma. Neurosurgery 2:103–106, 1978.
99. Yoshida M, Hayashi T, Kuramoto S, Hiyoshi Y, Yokoyama T: Traumatic intracranial hematomas in hemophiliac children. Surg Neurol 12:115–118, 1979.
100. Zieger A, VonoFakos D, Steudel WT, Dusterbehn G: Non-

traumatic intracerebellar hematomas: Prognostic value of volumetric evaluation by computed tomography. *Surg Neurol* 22:491–494, 1984.
101. Zimmerman HM: Cerebral apoplexy: Mechanism and differential diagnosis. *NY State J Med* 49:2153–2157, 1949.
102. Zimmerman RD, Leeds NE, Naidich TP: Ring blush associated with intracerebral hematoma. *Radiology* 122:707–711, 1977.
103. Zülch KJ: Pathological aspects of cerebral accidents in arterial hypertension. *Acta Neurol Belg* 71:196-221, 1971.

Section 3 SPINAL ARTERIOVENOUS MALFORMATIONS

26

Arteriovenous Malformations of the Spinal Cord

Spinal cord arteriovenous malformations (AVMs) are rare but important lesions because they can cause serious neurologic deficit and can mimic a variety of neurologic conditions. They account for approximately 4% of all intraspinal tumors (30, 63). A review of the literature in 1979 recorded 504 cases (57). The incidence in males is three to four times that found in females (3, 30, 41, 57, 63). Symptoms may occur at any age but are more common during the fourth and fifth decades (2, 41, 61, 63). The majority of these lesions occur in the lower thoracic and lumbosacral segments of the spinal cord; however, they can occur at any level. Most of these lesions are treatable but, if unrecognized and left untreated, they usually result in major disability within a few years.

The first cases of AVMs of the spinal cord were reported at the turn of the century (63). The first operations for "enlarged varicose veins of the spinal cord" were reported by Ellsberg in 1916 (26). In 1926, Foix and Alajouanine described the syndrome of "subacute necrotic myelopathy" with paraplegia evolving subacutely but progressively and leading to death. At autopsy, enlarged veins, sometimes with thrombosis, were found on the spinal cord (27). The landmark monograph on the subject came in 1943 when Wyburn-Mason published his book on vascular abnormalities of the spinal cord (61). He collected 96 cases from the literature, added 16 of his own, and made an attempt to classify these lesions. Radiologically, most cases were diagnosed by Pantopague myelography until 1958, when the first report appeared describing cervical medullary AVMs visualized by vertebral angiography (31). In 1962, Djindjian introduced spinal aortography. A few years later DiChiro introduced selective spinal angiography, which continues to be the definitive diagnostic modality for these lesions. The modern era of treatment of spinal AVMs began with the introduction of microneurosurgical methodology by Yasargil (62) and with the development of angiographic and embolization techniques by DiChiro (13) and Djindjian (19).

PATHOPHYSIOLOGY

Spinal cord AVMs can cause symptoms by hemorrhage (intramedullary, subarachnoid, or subdural), by mechanical compression from distended venous loops (varicosities), by extensive thrombosis of the spinal venous drainage system, by arachnoiditis from previous hemorrhages, by an arterial "steal" phenomenon, or by venous hypertension (2, 17, 35, 38, 40, 41, 45–47). Hemorrhage is the presenting symptom in 15–20% of all patients discovered to have a spinal AVM. The majority of these patients have the intramedullary type of AVM. Symptoms can develop from direct destruction of the spinal cord by the hemorrhage, by compression in those rare cases in which the hemorrhage ruptures into the subdural space and becomes a focal mass, or from subarachnoid hemorrhage. Later arachnoiditis and progressive symptoms can develop from a single or repeated hemorrhages. Thrombosis within the venous coils of the AVM is sometimes found at surgery or autopsy. Whether this mechanism ever results in symptoms by interfering with normal venous drainage from the spinal cord is unknown.

Until a few years ago, it was thought that an arterial "steal" phenomenon accounted for the progressive symptomatology most frequently associated with spinal AVMs (15, 17, 21, 51). This mechanism may account for symptomatology in some patients with the high-flow intramedullary type of AVM in which the arterial supply to the malformation comes directly from the intrinsic arterial supply to the spinal cord, usually by branches of the anterior spinal artery (10, 11, 14, 17, 53, 54). This may also be a mechanism in the rare direct arteriovenous fistulas which the present authors have described (30). However, in the majority of the dorsally located lesions that do not have a significant intramedullary component, the arterial supply to the malformation is separate from the intrinsic arterial supply to the spinal cord (2, 13, 35, 41, 43, 45), and a "steal" phenomenon does not occur. It has been shown that these patients improve by simple ligation of the feeder or feeders to the AVM (35, 45, 46, 60). If the blood supply to the malformation and to the cord were in common, feeder ligation should exacerbate the "steal" rather than improve it.

From the observations of Aminoff et al (1, 2) and Kendall and Logue (35), it has been concluded that the pathophysiology of the majority of spinal AVMs consists of venous hypertension. In many, if not most, of the cases of extramedullary AVMs, the actual arteriovenous shunt is located in the dural sleeve of a spinal root. The true nidus of most of these malformations is small and is fed by separate dural branches of a radicular artery. The fistula then drains intradurally by usually one but occasionally several arterialized veins that, in turn, drain into the normal pial coronal venous plexus in the dorsal aspect of the spinal cord. This plexus of veins then becomes gradually enlarged and tortuous as a result of arterialization and high pressure. What then is observed myelographically and at surgery in the majority of these patients is actually the arterialized draining venous system of a small dural AVM rather than, as was previously thought, the AVM itself (35, 38, 43, 45, 46, 59, 65) (Fig. 26.1).

RADIOLOGIC DIAGNOSIS

Myelography remains the most important screening test (46). Complete spinal myelography with Pantopaque, performed with the patient in the supine position, remains the most sensitive screening test for a suspected spinal AVM. However, the disadvantages of having to inject a high volume of Pantopaque, having to remove the needle to turn the patient into the supine position, the need to perform a second puncture to remove the dye, and the effects of residual Pantopaque on subsequent CT scans and spinal angiography preclude its routine use. Water-soluble dye has the advantage of allowing subsequent CT scanning and does not impair the accuracy of subsequent spinal angiography. The disadvantage is that it may be difficult to obtain a high enough density of dye in the thoracic region to visualize small vessels. The sensitivity of computed tomography (CT) scanning to detect spinal AVMs has been increased by using intravenous contrast enhancement, but there is as yet insufficient experience to know whether this technique will replace myelography as a screening test (14). Another refinement consists of using intrathecal metrizamide and an arterial bolus injection of contrast media during CT scanning (28).

Magnetic resonance imaging (MRI) may prove to be of value as a screening test for spinal AVMs. However, with present methodology caution is in order, since in the only two cases in which the authors have had an opportunity to use MRI, the test was negative even though subsequently a typical dorsal spinal AMV

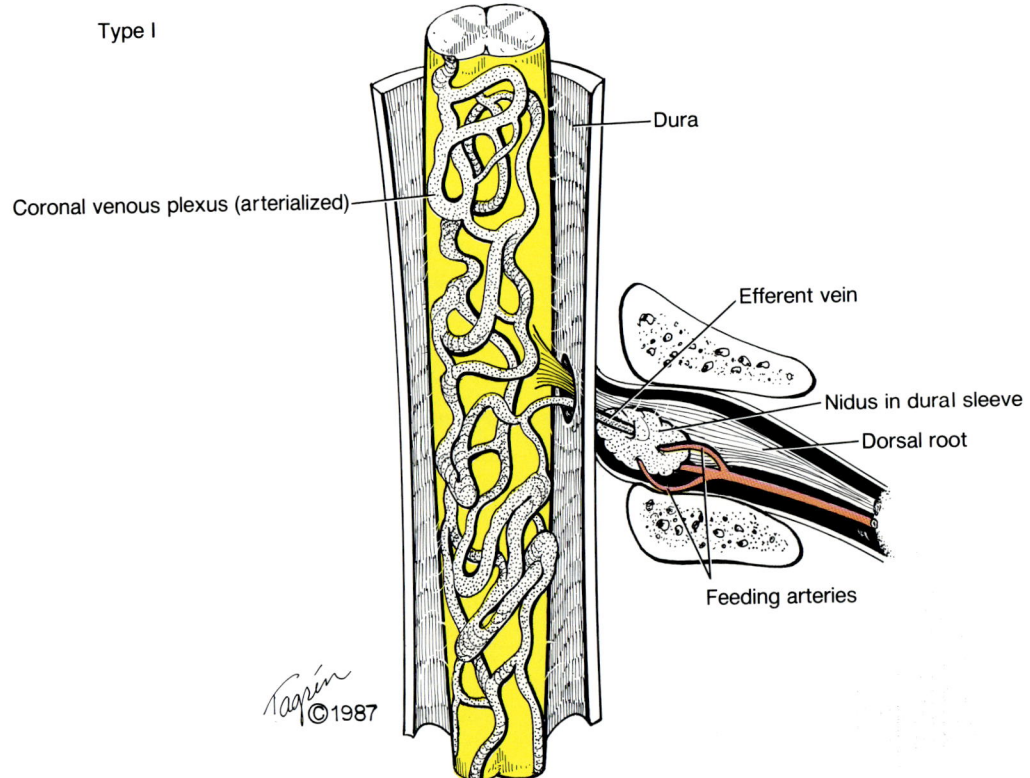

Figure 26.1. Type I spinal AVM. The nidus (or fistula) is located extradurally in relation to the dural sleeve of a nerve root. The nidus (or fistula) drains intradurally through one or more arterialized draining veins that connect with the coronal venous plexus in the dorsal surface of the spinal cord. These arterialized draining veins have traditionally been thought of as the "feeders." The coronal plexus of veins then becomes enlarged and tortuous secondary to arterialization.

was diagnosed by angiography and surgery. The larger intramedullary AVMs and the large varices sometimes associated with these lesions should be readily seen on MRI.

Select spinal angiography remains the definitive test (13, 18, 20, 22, 34, 55). This is a very specialized technique that requires considerable experience to maintain an acceptably low morbidity. It is difficult to estimate the risk of selective spinal angiography, since it depends to a great extent on the vascular anatomy of each patient. However, the procedure is serious enough not to be used routinely as a screening test. It is necessary not only to inject each intercostal vessel but also to inject the hypogastric and internal iliac arteries, since sometimes these malformations are fed by those vessels exclusively (13, 18, 19, 29, 58). Intraarterial digital subtraction angiography may be a useful preliminary test to localize the AVM (24, 37). Usually, the nidus of the AVM cannot be well visualized on this study. Therefore, after the lesion is generally localized, selective injection of the likely feeding arteries is necessary. By combining digital subtraction techniques with superselective angiography, the total amount of dye injected can be minimized, and it is hoped the rate of complications can be reduced (24).

CLASSIFICATION, CLINICAL FEATURES, AND PROGNOSIS

Type I Spinal AVM

The most common type of spinal AVM was initially referred to as "angioma racemosum venosum" by Wyburn-Mason (61). This is the typical long, single-coiled vessel type of malformation that is almost invariably located on the dorsal pial surface of the spinal cord. The actual nidus or true AVM in the great majority of these patients is located in the dural sleeve of a spinal root (Fig. 26.1). The long, coiled vessel observed myelographically and at surgery has all of the histologic characteristics of a typical vein (35).

These lesions have been classified as "type I" (13, 22). They occur most frequently in males in the age range of 40–70 years and are almost always located in the lower thoracic and lumbosacral segments of the spinal cord. There is usually one, occasionally two, and rarely three or more feeders that enter the dura dorsolaterally and drain into the long, coiled vessel that frequently extends for many segments above and, less frequently, below the region of the feeders. This type of AVM is usually of the low-flow variety and angiographically fills relatively slowly.

The clinical features of the type I spinal AVM have been presented and are summarized in Table 26.1 (1, 3, 21, 30, 35, 36, 38, 41, 46, 55, 57, 59–61, 63, 65). The most common syndrome is one of progressive neurologic deterioration with occasional abrupt exacerbations. In about 40% of the patients, there is pain at the time of presentation; this pain can be radicular and simulate typical sciatic pain, be centered at a place remote from the area of the malformation, or occur only in the back. Commonly, there is a history suggestive of neurogenic claudication with exacerbation of the pain and of the neurologic symptoms with exercise. It is likely that under these circumstances the venous hypertension that normally accounts for the progressive symptomatology is exacerbated. This also explains why the symptoms as well as the pain can be exacerbated during pregnancy. Only rarely does the symptomatology develop abruptly, and then the symptoms are usually due to hemorrhage. In approximately 40% of the patients, there is a progressive motor sensory paralysis with or without pain. In about 30%, the course is fluctuating, and in about 15%, the course is one of intermittent exacerbations and remissions resembling demyelinating disease. Cutaneous angiomas, bruits, and true arterial aneurysms are almost never seen with this type of malformation (25, 44). The cerebrospinal fluid shows a slight to moderate increase

Table 26.1.
Type I Spinal AVM

Synonyms:	Long dorsal AVM Single-coiled vessel malformation Angioma racemosum venosum Spinal dural AVM
Pathology:	Dural AVM or fistula in dural sheath of spinal nerve
Pathophysiology:	Arterialization of coronal venous plexus of the spinal cord with subsequent venous hypertension
Sex prevalence:	Males:females 4:1
Age incidence:	40–70 years
Location:	Lower thoracic and lumbosacral cord segments
Hemodynamics:	Slow flow, low pressure
Clinical presentation:	Pain in 40%; frequently exacerbated by exercise Progressive motor/sensory paralysis Hemorrhage infrequent
Prognosis:	90% unable to walk within 5 years of onset of weakness
Treatment:	Surgical occlusion of feeders Surgical excision of dural "nidus" of AVM Embolization of nidus of AVM Removal of long coiled vessel probably not necessary

in protein in about 70% of the patients, with a slight pleocytosis seen in about 10–20%.

The differential diagnosis is extremely important because the symptoms can be confused with a variety of neurologic disorders. Neurogenic claudication, presumed to be caused by lumbar spondylosis, resulted in lumbar laminectomy in two the authors' patients who were subsequently treated for AVM (Fig. 26.2). AVMs are so infrequently a cause of these symptoms that it is not surprising that the first diagnosis considered is usually lumbar spondylosis and the problem is compounded because, with the widespread use of water-soluble dyes, the conus medullaris and the lower thoracic region are often not adequately visualized when myelography is performed for lumbar symptoms. If there are no long tract signs and pain is a prominent feature, the differential diagnosis of spinal AVM from lumbar spondylosis is particularly difficult. However, if there is significant weakness or bladder involvement, neither of which is frequent in early cases of lumbar spondylosis, one should visualize myelographically at least

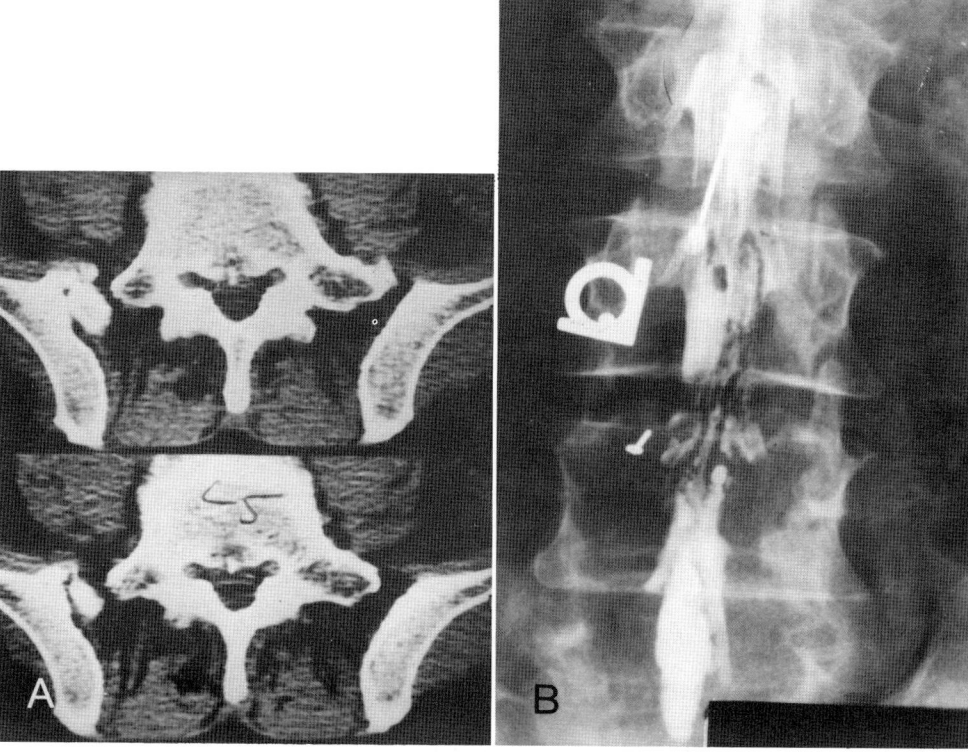

Figure 26.2. Type I thoracolumbar AVM. This 52-year-old man had a clinical history typical of neurogenic claudication (back and leg pain with mild leg numbness and weakness exacerbated by exercise). **A**, Preoperative CT scan confirmed the diagnosis of severe lumbar spondylosis, which was also demonstrated at myelography. After an uneventful L4 and L5 decompressive laminectomy, he developed severe bilateral leg weakness. **B–D**, The myelogram showed persistent waistlike narrowing of the contrast column typical of lumbar spondylosis at L3–L4 and L4–L5. The patient was reoperated immediately, and the laminectomy was extended laterally and superiorly through L3–L4. The dura was opened and the question of arachnoiditis was raised, but no abnormal blood vessels were described. The patient awoke from the second operation almost paraplegic. He was then transferred to the authors. MRI and spinal angiography were "negative" even in retrospect; however, one lumbar intercostal vessel (L1 on the right) and the upper thoracic intercostal vessels were not injected (the study was performed as an emergency at night). Upon review of the myelogram done before the last operation, the question of abnormal vessels in the area of the conus was raised (*arrow* on **D**). However, the authors have seen this appearance from redundant nerve roots or venous compression in patients with severe lumbar spondylosis. Still, because of the desperate neurologic condition (essentially complete paraplegia with a T12 sensory level), a T10–L1 laminectomy was performed in hope of finding a spinal AVM. Indeed, a type I spinal AVM, fed by a feeder piercing the dura adjacent to the right L1 root, was found. The feeder was clipped and the malformation gradually collapsed and turned blue. Nothing else was done. The patient made a dramatic recovery to an ambulatory state and returned to his previous occupation within a 4-month period. Even retrospectively, the authors do not understand the reason for his deterioration at the time of his low lumbar operations. It is possible that exacerbation of venous hypertension in the prone position played a role.

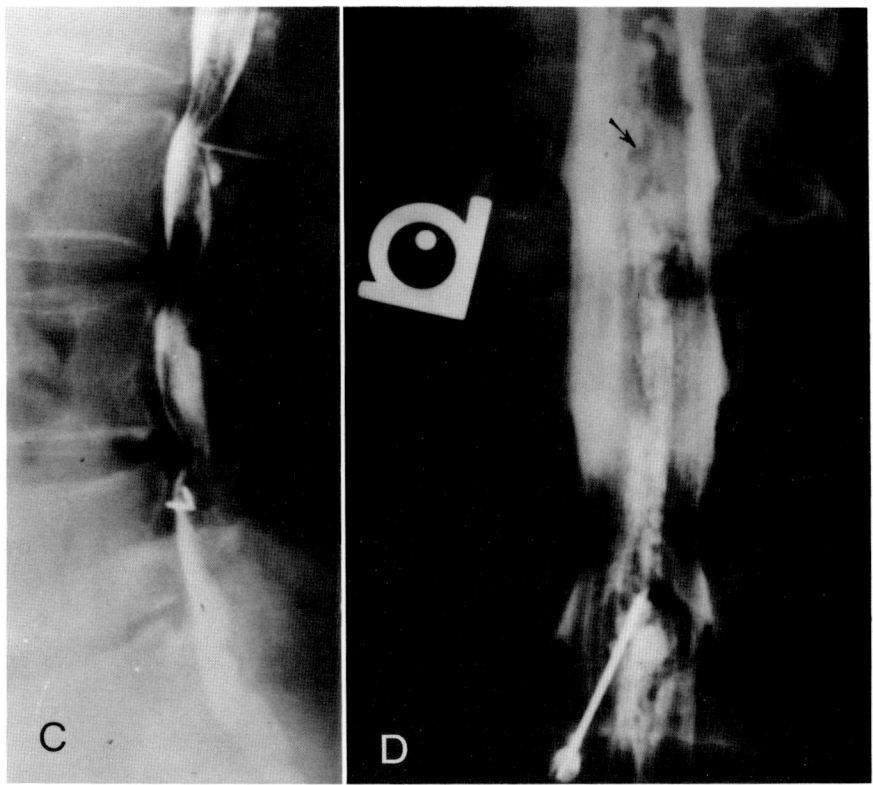

Figure 26.2C and D.

the conus and the lower thoracic area in search for an AVM, even though the patient may have lumbar spondylosis.

The second most common differential diagnostic error is to misdiagnose a spinal AVM as demyelinating disease (Fig. 26.3). This is particularly likely to happen in patients whose course is characterized by remissions and exacerbations. However, demyelinating disease is not common in the age group in which spinal AVMs usually become symptomatic, and spinal AVMs are much more frequent in men than in women, which is the opposite of the sex prevalence for demyelinating disease. If pain is present, the diagnosis of demyelinating disease should not be the primary consideration. In cases of pure spinal symptoms, without ocular or cerebral symptoms, the diagnosis of demyelinating disease should not be made unless a satisfactory myelogram has ruled out the presence of a thoracic or a cervical lesion.

The third most common diagnostic problem is a spinal tumor. Myelography should be diagnostic, but if the diagnosis is still in doubt, spinal angiography should be performed. Other less common initial diagnoses in patients with AVMs are ruptured discs, motor system disease, meningitis, and ruptured cerebral aneurysm in patients who present with subarachnoid hemorrhage.

The prognosis for this type of AVM has been well studied and appears to be very serious. At the time of diagnosis, most patients have had symptoms for a number of years. From the time of onset of leg weakness, about 20% of the patients are unable to walk in 6 months, 50% are unable to walk by 3 years, and 90% are unable to walk by 5 years (4). Of the patients presenting with an abrupt neurologic deficit, half seem to deteriorate progressively over the next several years, whereas the other half remain stable over a period of many years. In the latter cases, the deficit is almost always due to hemorrhage. The risk of rebleeding in patients presenting with hemorrhage is not as well known, but it does not appear to be high. Only 1 of 6 patients in Aminoff's series rebled over a period of 10 years (4).

Type II Spinal AVM

The second type of spinal AVM involves the substance of the spinal cord (Fig. 26.4). The nidus of the malformation is usually intramedullary, although it can be partially intramedullary and partially extramedullary. These lesions have been called "angioma racemosum arteriovenosum" or "angioma arteriovenosum" (61) and "glomus malformation" (41). They account for about 15–20% of all spinal AVMs and occur more frequently in the cervical region but can

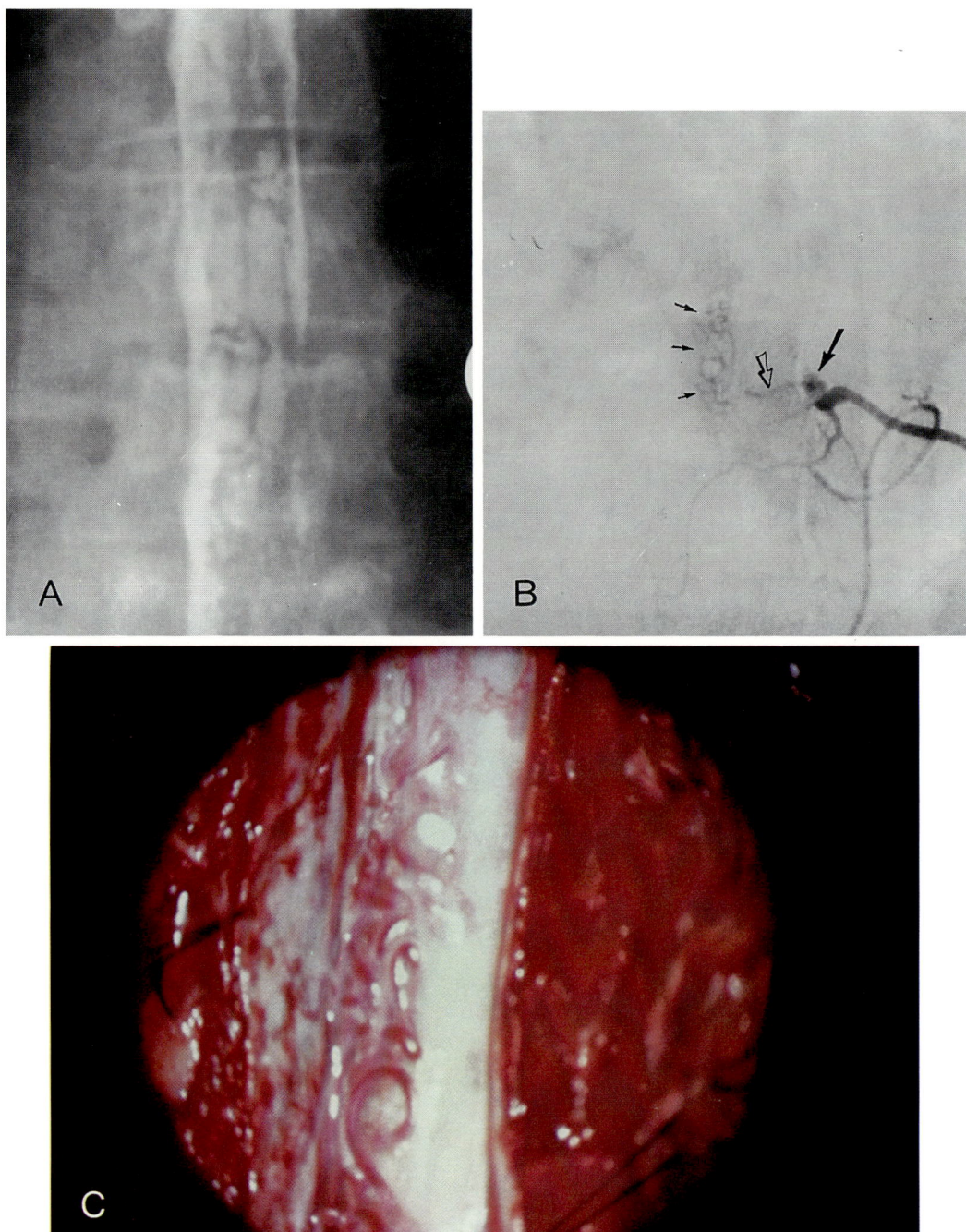

Figure 26.3. Type I thoracic AVM. This 42-year-old man was diagnosed as having multiple sclerosis 7 years prior to admission. At that time he had had a history of fluctuating paraparesis with remissions and exacerbations but with a gradually worsening deficit. A myelogram, done with the patient in the prone position, was reportedly negative. He had been almost paraplegic and wheelchair bound for 5 years when he presented for reevaluation because of gradual loss of his remaining bladder and sexual function. **A**, Repeat myelography with the patient turned to the supine position suggested a spinal AVM. **B**, This was confirmed by spinal angiography which showed a probable small extradural fistula or AVM (*large black arrow*), the "feeder" or arterialized draining vein (*open arrow*), and the arterialized coronal venous plexus (*small arrows*). **C**, At surgery, the expected dorsal arterialized tangle of vessels was found. At that time, being unaware of the more recent pathophysiologic concepts, the authors treated these lesions by "stripping." **D**, The lesion has been partially stripped but is still arterialized, probably because the "feeder" had not yet been clipped. **E**, After further stripping (and probable cauterization of the feeder), the lesion has become blue. The patient improved remarkably in view of the duration and severity of his neurologic deficit. One year after surgery he walks with two canes and has useful bladder and sexual function.

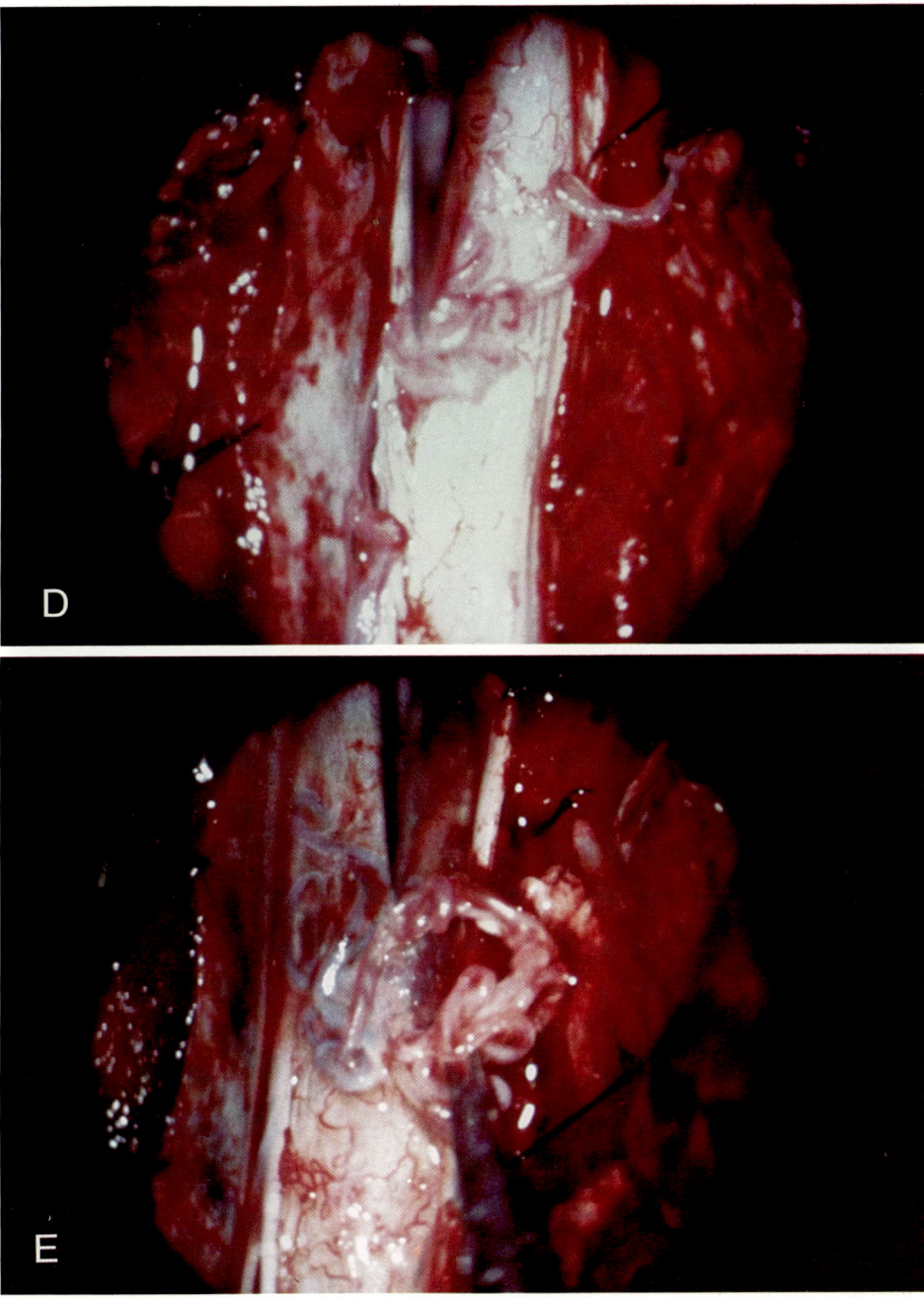

Figure 26.3D and E.

occur throughout the thoracic and lumbrosacral regions. These lesions are as common in males as in females and present with equal frequency throughout adulthood. These are high-flow, high-pressure lesions that opacify rapidly and drain early on angiography (Fig. 26.5). They are mostly fed by branches from the anterior spinal artery and by segmental radicular arteries, but those located in the cervicomedullary junction are usually located dorsally and are fed by branches of the vertebral and posterior inferior cerebellar arteries that reach the lesion from posteriorly, thus making this particular location relatively favorable for surgical excision (41, 62).

The clinical features have been reported and are summarized in Table 26.2 (3, 7, 11, 21, 33, 55, 57, 61, 65). Subarachnoid hemorrhage or intramedullary hemorrhage is more frequent with type II lesions than with type I lesions. True arterial aneurysms, as well as aneurysmally dilated venous varicosities, are frequent (6, 9). The former can result in catastrophic hemorrhage and the latter in symptoms from spinal cord compressions. Drainage is into the coronal ven-

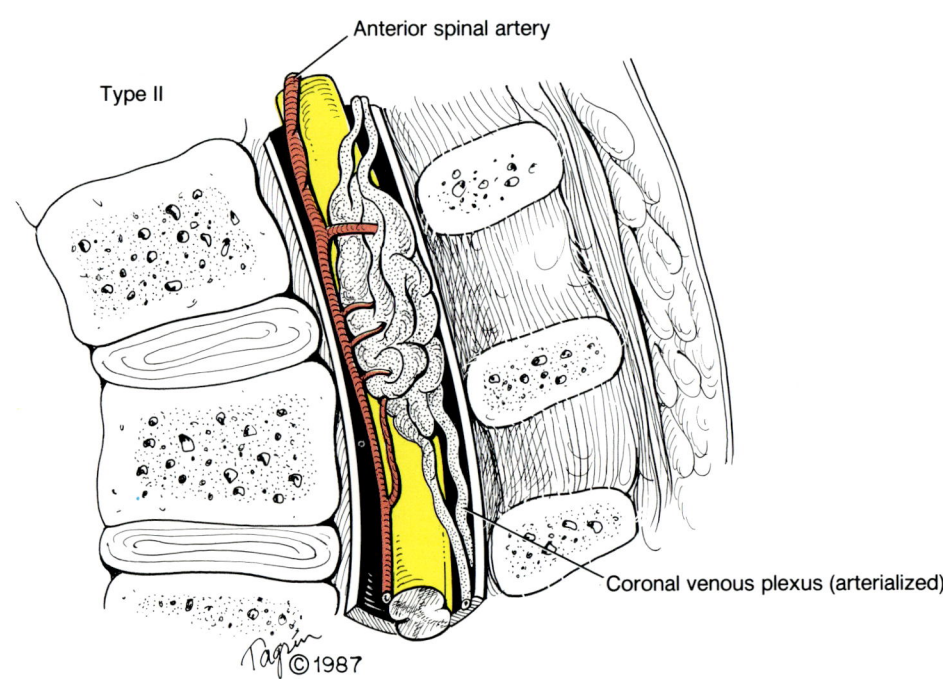

Figure 26.4. Type II spinal AVM. The lesion is usually fed primarily by branches of the anterior spinal artery. The drainage is usually posterior into the coronal venous plexus, which becomes enlarged and tortuous as a result of arterialization.

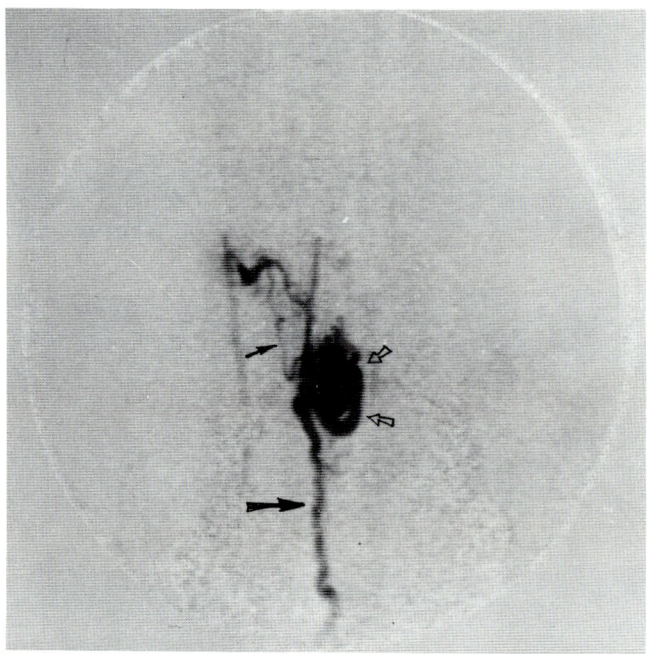

Figure 26.5. Type II intramedullary AVM. This young lady presented with neck pain and minimal numbness and clumsiness of the left arm. The diagnosis of a cervical spinal AVM was made elsewhere by myelography (not available). The illustration is a digital subtraction angiogram that clearly shows a small feeder (*small arrow*) to a high-flow compact intramedullary AVM (*open arrows*) that drains inferiorly by a single large vein (*large arrow*). She was treated conservatively in view of her excellent neurologic status and the risk of quadriplegia from surgery or embolization.

ous plexus; therefore, at a distance from the nidus they may be indistinguishable from type I lesions. However, the dilatation and complexity of the arterialized venous drainage system are much more impressive with the type II lesions than with the type I lesions. Venous hypertension undoubtedly plays a major role in the pathophysiology of the majority of these lesions, just as it does in the type I lesions.

Cutaneous angiomas and angiomatous phakomatoses, such as the Klippel-Trenaunay-Weber syndrome and the Weber-Rendu-Osler syndrome, can rarely be associated with this type of spinal AVM (16, 25). With these lesions, one can occasionally hear an overlying bruit.

Type II AVMs have a less predictable natural history than do type I lesions. Patients who present with a progressive myelopathy usually do poorly and become paraplegic or quadriplegic within a period of several years. Those who present with an abrupt event, usually from hemorrhage, have an uncertain natural history. It is important to keep this in mind because the treatment of these lesions is very difficult.

Type III Spinal AVM

The third type of spinal AVM is the "juvenile spinal malformation" (13, 40, 41, 46, 50, 51). Fortunately, these awesome lesions are uncommon. They occur most frequently in adolescents and young adults, are mostly intramedullary, and have multiple feeders, sometimes involving several vertebral segments. They involve all of the spinal cord, frequently for a long

Table 26.2.
Type II Spinal AVM

Synonyms:	Glomus type of spinal AVM Angioma racemosum arteriosum Intramedullary spinal AVM
Pathology:	Intramedullary or intramedullary and extramedullary true AVM
Pathophysiology:	Venous hypertension Arterial steal—same arterial supply as the spinal cord Hemorrhage—sometimes from associated aneurysms Compression by distended coils and varices
Sex prevalence:	As frequent in males as in females
Age incidence:	About equal frequency throughout adulthood
Location:	Throughout spinal cord
Hemodynamics:	Rapid flow, high pressure
Clinical presentation:	Abrupt deficit due to hemorrhage Progressive motor/sensory paralysis
Prognosis:	Less well known than for type I but probably at least as bad
Treatment:	Very difficult Microsurgical resection ideal but risky Embolization—usually only palliative Partial resection or feeder ligation palliative Cervicomedullary lesions may be favorable for resection because of dorsal feeders from vertebral and posterior inferior cerebellar arteries

segment, and have extraspinal and paraspinal extensions. Their natural history is not well known, but most patients with this type do very poorly. They can present with hemorrhage or progressive paralysis (Figs. 26.6 and 26.7).

Type IV—Direct Spinal Arteriovenous Fistula

The last type of spinal AVM was first described in detail by the present authors (30), although there has been an occasional example found within reported series of spinal AVMs (15, 33). A few more examples of this type of lesion have subsequently been presented (56). These are direct fistulas between the intrinsic blood supply to the spinal cord, usually the anterior spinal artery, and a vein. The result is usually massive aneurysmal dilatation of the venous drainage system. This can result in hemorrhage, cord compression from the dilated varicosities, a "steal" phenomenon, and venous hypertension. Not much is known about the clinical features or prognosis of these lesions, but the one patient who was described by the authors presented with progressive paraparesis and had become unable to walk over a period of about 6 months (Figs. 26.8 and 26.9).

TREATMENT

Type I Spinal AVM

It is fortunate that the type I spinal AVM, which is the most common, is also the easiest to treat. The traditional treatment has been "excision" or stripping of the long, arterialized venous complex (39–41, 50, 62, 64) (Fig. 26.3). There are several problems with this approach. A very long laminectomy may be required because the abnormal venous plexus can extend for many segments. In fact, the abnormal veins may ascend to the base of the skull. Usually, the laminectomy is started where the density of enlarged coils seems to be the highest. The dura is then opened, bringing the coils into view. The arachnoid is opened carefully by using microsurgical techniques because the AVM is always in a subarachnoid location and the arachnoid is often opaque and at times quite adherent to the coils of the AVM. The entire mass of abnormal veins is removed, with care taken to coagulate the tiny vascular connections from the substance of the spinal cord to the venous coils. In the past, it was thought that these small connections were small arterial feeders, but it is most likely that these are the normal small venules draining the substance of the spinal cord into the coronal venous plexus. As the coronal venous plexus becomes arterialized, these small veins become indistinguishable from small arteries. The removal of the venous coils usually stops at the point where the surgeon notices the rest of the vein becoming blue (Fig. 26.3).

The present surgical treatment in most cases consists of excision of the dural fistula, if this is easy to accomplish (35, 38, 45, 46, 59), or interruption of the arterialized veins (feeders) that drain the dural AVM into the subarachnoid coronal venous plexus (35, 38, 45, 59, 65) (Fig. 26.10). There usually is only one but occasionally are two or three (rarely more) of these feeders. The precise location of the dural AVM and its intradural draining veins must be defined by preoperative angiography. When all of the draining veins have been interrupted, the arterialized venous coil becomes soft and, in time, blue. The surgeon must allow sufficient time for venous stasis and bluish discoloration of the veins. The authors have noticed that in some patients it takes about 5–10 minutes for the veins to become blue after the feeders are interrupted. A useful maneuver is to use a temporary clip on the feeder (or feeders) and then observe the arterialized venous coils. If all of the arterialized supply has been occluded, the coils should noticeably change in color within, at the most, 10 minutes (Fig.

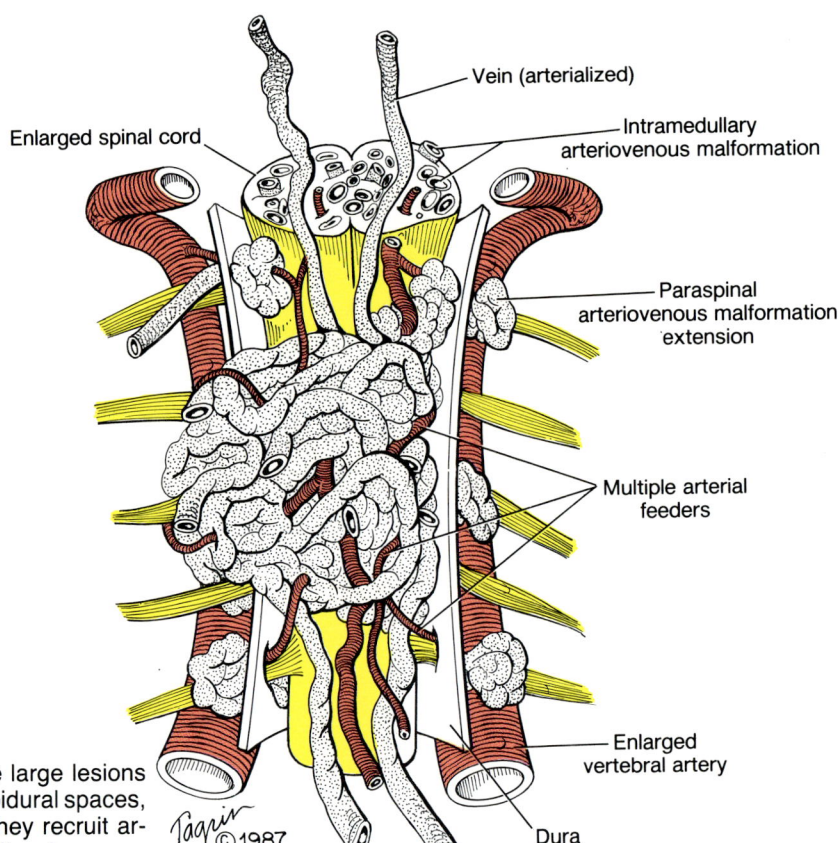

Figure 26.6. Type III spinal AVM. These are large lesions that involve the spinal cord, the subdural and epidural spaces, and the surrounding bone and soft tissues. They recruit arterial feeders from many sources and drain diffusely.

26.10). If this does not occur, one must look for other feeders.

The majority of these patients improve immediately as a result of this procedure, and symptoms do not seem to recur over a period of a few years. However, a longer follow-up will be necessary to determine the incidence of late recurrence. The surest way to avoid a recurrence would be to excise the dural AVM completely. However, sometimes this requires extensive foraminotomy because the dural AVM can be quite peripherally located in the spinal foramen or even beyond it. It seems most reasonable to recommend excision of the dural AVM whenever it is easily accessible through a standard laminectomy and foraminotomy. In cases in which the dural AVM is more peripheral and not readily accessible, one can interrupt the intradural draining veins and follow the clinical response of the patient.

Occasionally, the surgeon is called upon to explore a patient because of the strong clinical and myelographic suspicion of a spinal AVM, even though the lesion cannot be confirmed angiographically—either because spinal angiography is not available at the institution or because, for technical reasons, the angiogram was incomplete or inconclusive. One must then perform the laminectomy over the area in which the venous coils demonstrated by myelography seem to be most prominent. This will usually correspond with the clinical level of dysfunction if such a level can be precisely ascertained from either the motor or, more frequently, the sensory examination. The authors have been in this situation twice, and in both instances the combination of the myelographic findings plus the clinical sensory level allowed them to perform the laminectomy precisely at the area in which the arterialized draining veins were located (Fig. 26.2).

Embolization of spinal AVMs was pioneered by groups in Bethesda and Paris (13, 19, 23, 32). This procedure has evolved into a very specialized field, and because of the relative rarity of these lesions and the technical difficulties and risks involved, only a few centers have accumulated substantial experience. The ideal lesion for embolization is a small dural fistula whose arterial supply is through one or more distinct branches of a radicular artery that are separate from the branches that go on to feed the spinal cord, particularly the artery of Adamkiewicz. Most of these AVMs can be occluded satisfactorily (8, 19, 32, 43, 45). There is considerably more danger involved in the embolization of those lesions fed by a radicular artery that then goes on to supply normal spinal cord, particularly if that radicular artery is the

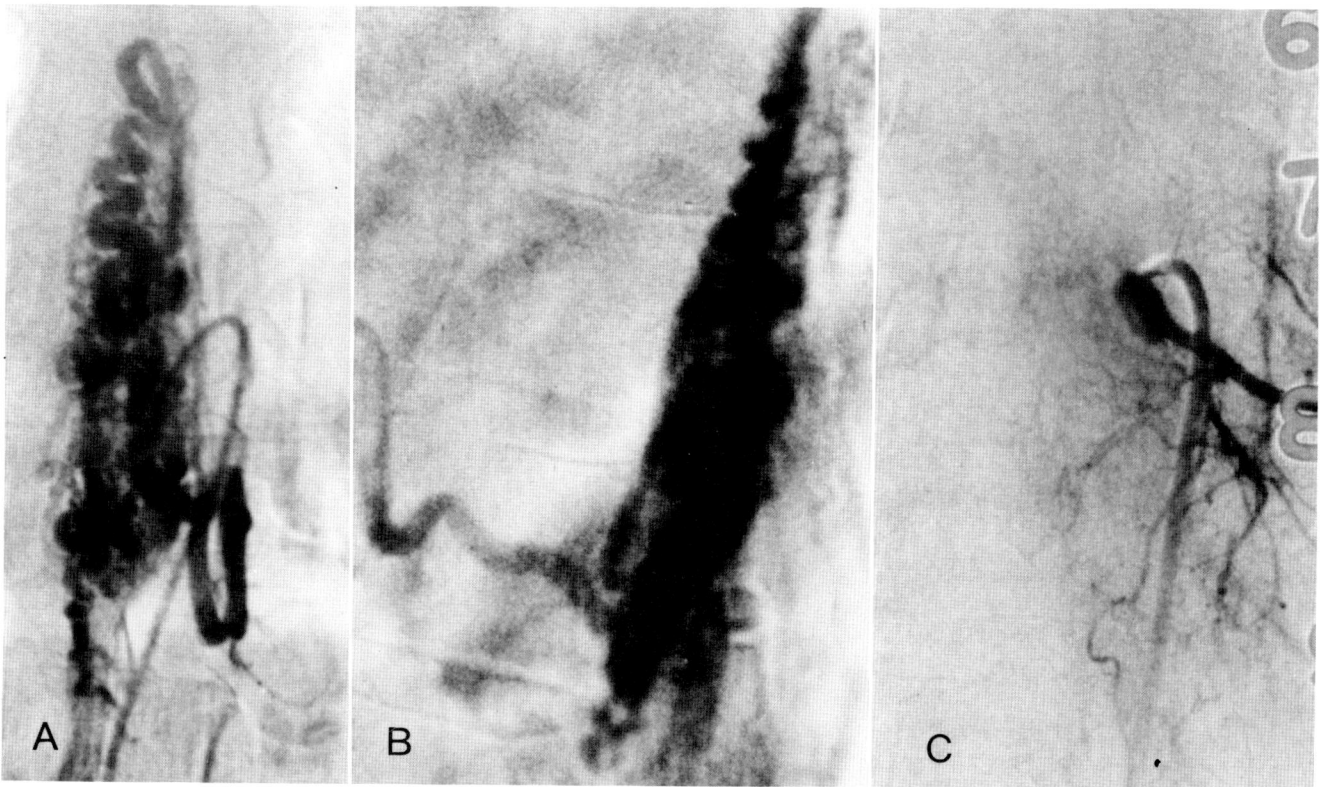

Figure 26.7. Type III spinal AVM. Thoracic AVM of the juvenile type in a patient with a history of subarachnoid hemorrhage and progressive paraparesis. **A** and **B**, Anteroposterior and lateral subtraction films, respectively, during spinal angiography show the large lesion, which was believed to extend beyond the confines of the spinal canal. **C**, The lesion was partially embolized with substantial reduction in flow.

main supply to the anterior spinal artery. The risk of paraplegia is significant, and in the authors' opinion, these cases are best treated surgically. The use of evoked potentials during embolization has been suggested in order to increase its safety (8). However, since the commonly used sensory evoked potentials monitor mainly posterior column sensation, the relevance of this kind of monitoring for the risks of anterior spinal occlusion is questionable. Some prefer to perform the embolization procedures with the patient awake in order to be able to monitor neurologic function directly. However, these are very long tedious procedures, and it is extemely uncomfortable for the patient to be awake throughout.

In summary, the authors recommend surgical excision of the dural AVM or ligation of the arterialized intradural draining veins or so-called "feeders," as the primary form of treatment for most type I spinal AVMs. Simple dural lesions with arterial supply that is completely separate from the intrinsic supply to the cord may be treated by embolization in centers that have attained substantial experience with these techniques. Embolization can also be used for the elderly, debilitated patient who cannot undergo a surgical procedure.

Type II Spinal AVM

The treatment of the intramedullary spinal AVMs is most difficult. The difficulty begins with the decision of whether or not to treat them. Certainly, those AVMs that are found incidentally or because of minor symptoms in patients who are relatively intact neurologically should be left alone (Fig. 26.5). If the patient has a subarachnoid hemorrhage that can be attributed to an intramedullary spinal AVM and has recovered without residual neurologic deficit, the decision of whether to treat becomes much more difficult. The natural history of patients who present with hemorrhage from a spinal AVM is not well known, although it appears that these patients do much better than those who present with progressive neurologic symptoms. For this reason, unless from the surgical point of view the lesion appears to be relatively straightforward, the authors do not recommend surgery. An exception may be in patients with dorsally placed high cervical or cervicomedullary AVMs. It has been suggested that these lesions can be removed quite successfully because their blood supply comes posteriorly from the vertebral and posterior inferior cerebellar arteries and is readily con-

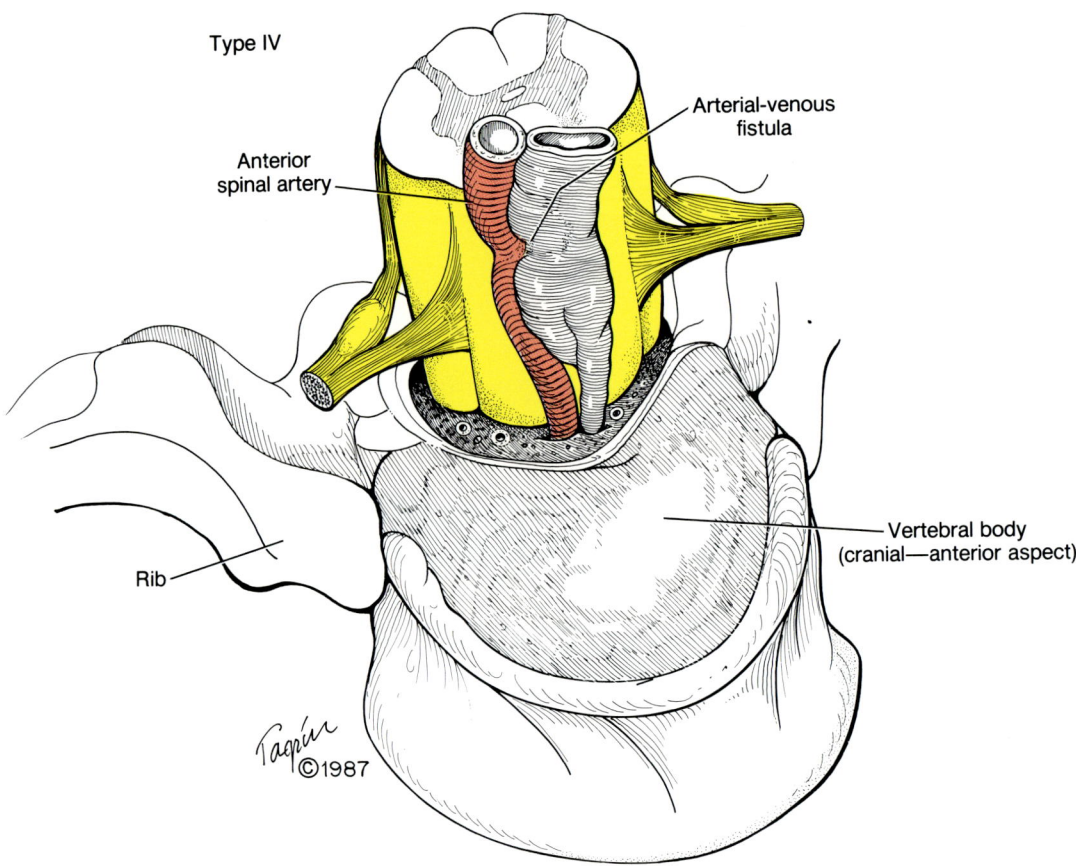

Figure 26.8. Type IV spinal AVM. The lesion is a true intradural fistula involving the intrinsic blood supply to the spinal cord. There is secondary massive venous dilatation. This drawing was made from the operative findings in the patient illustrated in Figure 26.9.

trollable (40). The authors have had no experience with the latter type of lesion.

In patients who are left with a very substantial neurologic deficit from a hemorrhage, it is probably best to wait and see what degree of recovery occurs. If the patient is left with a significant deficit that does not recover and it is thought that the malformation can be removed without producing additional deficit, surgery could be undertaken. The same could be said about embolization in this group of patients.

Patients presenting with progressive paraparesis or quadriparesis should usually be treated at least palliatively. The prognosis in these patients is very poor (4). Treatment may consist of complete surgical excision, if such appears to be feasible without significantly increasing the neurologic deficit, or complete embolization, if that seems to be achievable. If neither of the above can be done safely, a reduction in flow to the AMV can be attempted by either surgical ligation of feeders or by partial embolization. In spinal AVMs, in contradistinction to cerebral AVMs, palliative treatment with decrease in the total volume of the AVM by either surgery or embolization seems to be helpful although not curative treatment. Inasmuch as venous hypertension or spinal cord compression by distended varicosities seems to be the pathogenetic mechanism in most of these patients, a reduction in flow to the lesion should improve both of these situations, and this is probably why it frequently results in improved symptomatology.

Microsurgery has made it possible to excise some intramedullary spinal AVMs without a major worsening in the patient's neurologic condition (11, 40, 41, 46, 48–51, 62–65). This is certainly not surgery to be undertaken lightly, and the patient must be prepared to accept the risk of paraplegia or quadriplegia. As in the case of embolization, it has been suggested that monitoring of evoked potentials may make this surgery safer, but this has not been established (48). Preoperative angiographic delineation of the feeders, which usually come from the anterior aspect of the spinal cord, should be obtained. The techniques involved are identical to those involved in removing intramedullary spinal tumors. The problem is that since the arterial supply comes from the

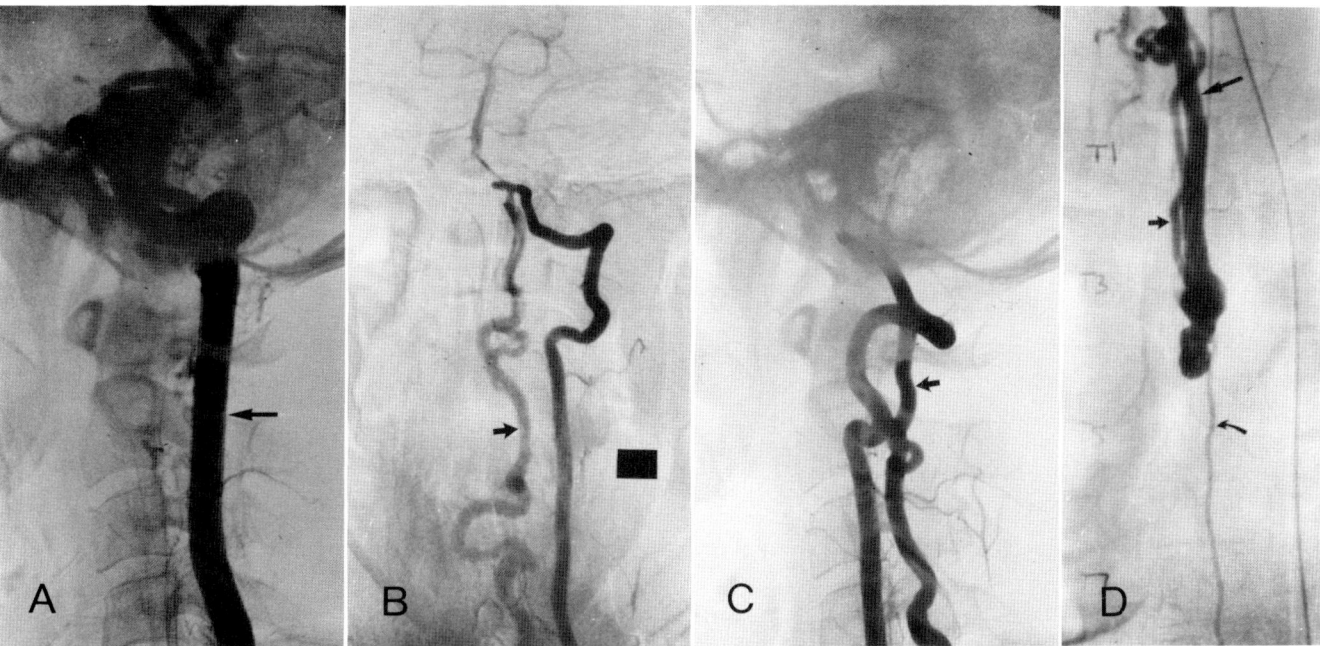

Figure 26.9. Type IV spinal AVM. This patient has been reported in detail (30). He presented with progressive hemiparesis. **A,** On the original angiogram a posterior fossa AVM was suspected because of the large tangle of vessels seen in the posterior fossa. Retrospectively, it became apparent that what he had was a spinal lesion that drained superiorly into the posterior fossa by an enormously enlarged vein (*arrow*). **B** and **C,** Vertebral angiography shows that the lesion was fed by a very enlarged anterior spinal artery (*arrow*). The actual fistula was at the level of T4. **D,** The descending spinal artery (*short arrow*), a small ascending feeder (*curved arrow*), and the large superiorly draining vein (*long arrow*) are identified. The fistula was ligated by a transthoracic approach. The patient deteriorated postoperatively, probably because of thrombosis in the anterior spinal artery or on the draining vein, but over the next several months he recovered most of the lost neurologic function.

front it cannot be controlled until late in the dissection, which creates a major technical hazard. Careful microsurgical techniques and bipolar coagulation are essential for successful excision of intramedullary AVMs.

Embolization rarely results in complete obliteration of intramedullary AVMs, but it can frequently result in significant reduction in the total volume of the lesion (5, 8, 19, 23, 42, 43). The blood flow into the type II lesions is fast and of high volume, and the feeders are sometimes large. Therefore, the malformation exerts a "sump" effect that makes it more amenable to embolization even through the anterior spinal artery (8, 12, 19). Exquisite judgment is required in deciding how far to go in the attempt to reduce the flow to these malformations with embolization.

Type III Spinal AVM

These massive juvenile spinal AVMs have multiple feeders not only from vessels that normally supply the spinal cord but also from arteries supplying the paraspinal tissues and the vertebrae. The prognosis for these patients is very poor. The only treatment available is palliative and consists of staged reduction of the supply to the malformation either by surgical ligation of feeders and partial resection or by embolization or a combination of these methods (Fig. 26.7). The authors have had no surgical experience with these lesions.

Type IV—Direct Spinal Arteriovenous Fistula

Direct arteriovenous fistulas involving the intrinsic supply of the spinal cord can be treated by interruption of the fistula with embolization, by balloon detachment, or by direct surgical interruption of the fistula (30). The case reported by the authors was treated by a transthoracic approach with partial resection of the vertebral body and direct intradural obliteration of the fistula, which involved the anterior spinal artery (Fig. 26.9). A similar approach had been used before in order to ligate the anterior spinal artery in an intramedullary (type II) spinal AVM (52). The treatment for direct fistulas in other locations must be individualized depending on where the fistula is located. There is insufficient experience to make a generalization about the treatment of this type of spinal AVM.

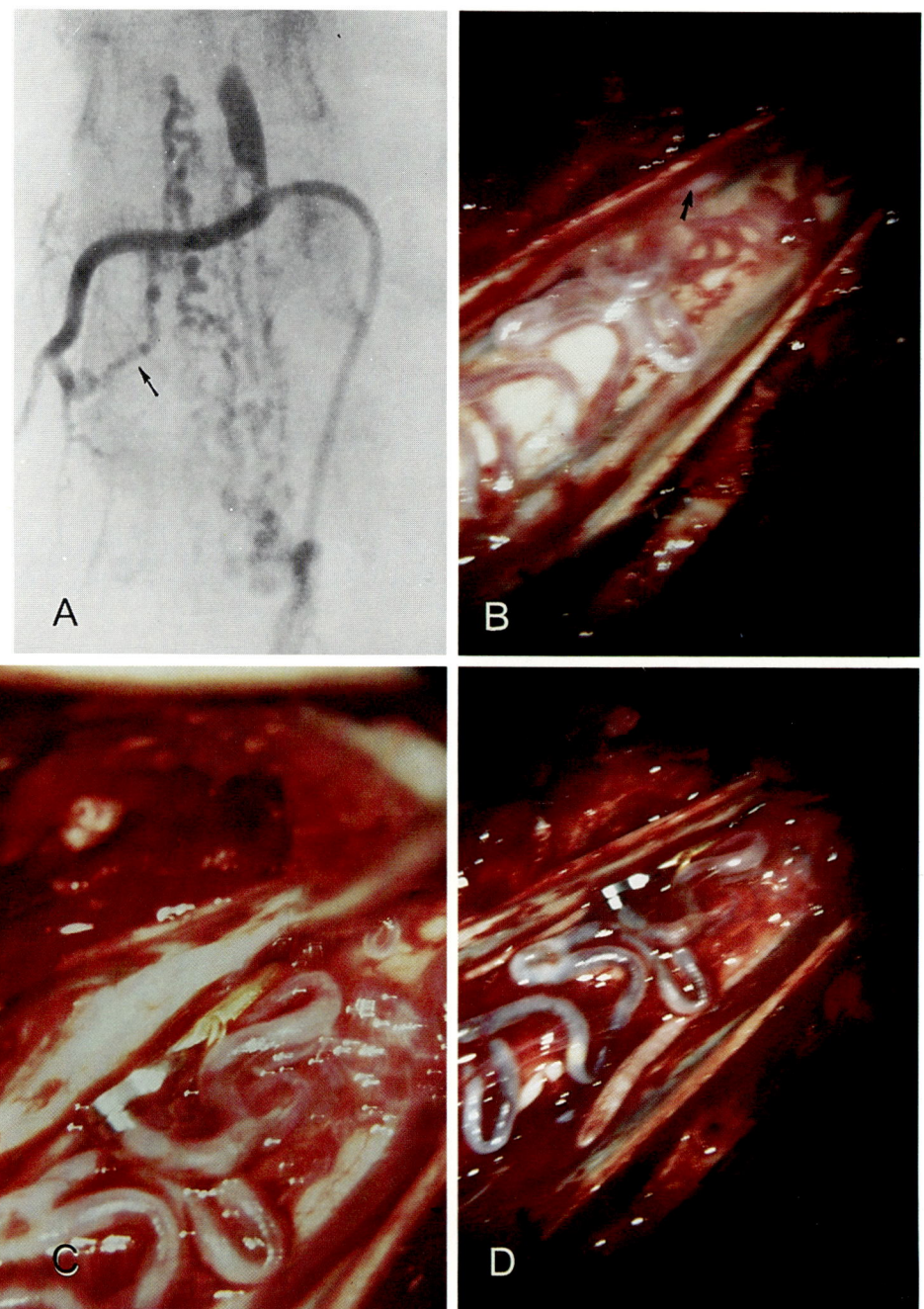

Figure 26.10. Type I spinal AVM treated by feeder ligation. This patient presented with progressive paraparesis, and a spinal AVM was suspected clinically. **A**, The spinal angiogram showed a typical type I AVM with one feeder (*arrow*). **B**, At surgery, the typical coiled dorsal arterialized vessels were found. A single feeder at the level demonstrated angiographically was found (*arrow*). A temporary clip was placed on the feeder and immediately there was a softening of the coils but no change in color. **D**, About 7 or 8 minutes later, the veins became blue. The feeder was then permanently clipped and divided. The patient improved significantly.

RESULTS

The authors' surgical experience with spinal AVMs is summarized in Table 26.3. Patients treated by embolization are not included. During the past 5 years, 10 patients have undergone operations. Six had a type I lesion. Three were treated with removal of the entire arterialized dorsal coil of veins; one was unchanged, and the two others improved. All had presented with a neurologic deficit that was progressive in two and had been relatively stable for a period of about 4 years in the other patient. The other three

Table 26.3.
Spinal AVMs—Surgical Results

	No.	Treatment	Long-Term Result
Type I	3	Excision	1 unchanged, 2 better
	3	"Feeder" ligation	1 unchanged, 2 better
Type II	2	Excision	1 unchanged, 1 better[a]
	1	Decompression	1 unchanged
Type IV	1	Ligation of fistula	1 better[a]
Total	10		3 unchanged, 6 better

[a] Worse immediately after surgery but improved over several months with intensive physical therapy.

patients with type I spinal AVM were treated by laminectomy and intradural interruption of the arterialized draining veins or feeders. One of these patients with advanced paraparesis has remained unchanged for 1 year, and the other two patients improved rather dramatically.

The authors have operated on three patients with type II intramedullary spinal AVMs. In two, the lesion was completely excised; one improved and the other has remained unchanged. The third patient had a very large lesion that was mostly thrombosed. The large thombosed varices were exerting mass effect, and he had extensive arachnoiditis from previous hemorrhages. He was treated by decompression and lysis of adhesions and has remained unchanged.

The ninth patient in the authors' series was the patient with the direct spinal arteriovenous fistula (type IV) that was described above (30) (Fig. 26.9).

REFERENCES

1. Aminoff MJ: Diagnosis and treatment of spinal arteriovenous malformations. Weekly update. Neurol Neurosurg 2:14–20, 1979.
2. Aminoff MJ, Barnard RO, Logue V: The pathophysiology of spinal vascular malformations. J Neurol Sci 23:255–263, 1974.
3. Aminoff MJ, Logue V: Clinical features of spinal vascular malformation. Brain 97:197–210, 1974.
4. Aminoff MJ, Logue V: The prognosis of patients with spinal vascular malformations. Brain 97:211–218, 1974.
5. Ausman JI, Gold LH, Tadavarthy SM, Amplatz K, Chou SN: Intraparenchymal embolization for obliteration of an intramedullary AVM of the spinal cord. J Neurosurg 47:119–125, 1977.
6. Avman N, Ozkal E, Gokben B: Aneurysm and arteriovenous malformation of the spinal cord. Surg Neurol 11:5–6, 1979.
7. Bailey WL, Sperl MP: Angiomas of the cervical spinal cord. J Neurosurg 30:560–568, 1969.
8. Bernstein A, Young W, Ransohoff J, Benjamin V, Merkin H: Somatosensory evoked potentials during spinal angiography and therapeutic transvascular embolization. J Neurosurg 60:777–785, 1984.
9. Caroscio JT, Brannan T, Budabin M, Huang YP, Yahr J: Subarachnoid hemorrhage secondary to spinal arteriovenous malformation and aneurysm. Arch Neurol 37:101–103, 1980.
10. Clavier E, Tadie M, Thiebot J, Presles O, Benazio M: Common origin of the arterial blood flow for an arteriovenous medullary fistula and the anterior spinal artery: A case report. Neurosurgery 18:660–663, 1986.
11. Cogen P, Stein BM: Spinal cord arteriovenous malformations with significant intramedullary components. J Neurosurg 59:471–478, 1983.
12. Decker RE, Stein HL, Epstein JA: Complete embolization of artery of Adamkiewicz to obliterate an intramedullary arteriovenous aneurysm. J Neurosurg 43:486–489, 1975.
13. DiChiro G, Doppman JL, Ommaya AK: Radiology of spinal cord arteriovenous malformations. Prog Neurol Surg 4:329–354, 1971.
14. DiChiro G, Doppman JL, Wener L: Computed tomography of spinal cord arteriovenous malformations. Radiology 123:351–354, 1977.
15. Djindjian M: Les malformations arterio-veineuses de la moelle epiniere et leur traitement. Thesis, University of Paris, 1976.
16. Djindjian M, Djindjian R, Hurth M, Rey A, Houdart R: Spinal cord arteriovenous malformations and the Klippel-Trenaunay-Weber syndrome. Surg Neurol 8:229–237, 1977.
17. Djindjian M, Djindjian R, Hurth M, Rey A, Houdart R: Steal phenomenon in spinal arteriovenous malformations. J Neuroradiol 5:187–201, 1978.
18. Djindjian R: L'Angiographie de la Moelle Epiniere. Paris, Masson et Cie, 1970, pp 161–188.
19. Djindjian R: Embolization of angiomas of the spinal cord. Surg Neurol 4:411–420, 1975.
20. Djindjian R, Faure C: Investigations neuro-radiologique dans les malformations vasculaires medullaires. Neuro-radiol Roentgenol Eur 4:432–434, 1963.
21. Djindjian R, Houdart R, Hurth M: Les Angiomes de la Moelle Epiniere. Paris, Sandoz, 1969.
22. Doppman JL, DiChiro G, Ommaya AK: Selective Arteriography of the Spinal Cord. St Louis, Warren H Green, 1969.
23. Doppman JL, DiChiro G, Ommaya AK: Percutaneous embolization of spinal cord arteriovenous malformations. J Neurosurg 34:48–55, 1971.
24. Doppman JL, Krudy AG, Miler DL, Oldfield E, DiChiro G: Intraarterial digital subtraction angiography of spinal arteriovenous malformations. AJNR 4:1081–1085, 1983.
25. Doppman JL, Wirth FP Jr, DiChiro G, Ommaya AK: Value of cutaneous angiomas in the arteriographic localization of spinal-cord arteriovenous malformations. N Engl J Med 281:1440–1444, 1969.
26. Ellsberg CA: Surgical significance and operative treatment of enlarged and varicose veins of the spinal cord. Am J Med Sci 151:642–652, 1916.
27. Foix C, Alajouanine T: La myelite necroitque subaigue. Rev Neurol 33:1–42, 1926.
28. Guinto FC Jr, Haring JW, Nauta HJW, Hashim H, Pisharodi APM: Dynamic computed tomography scanning with combined metrizamide and arterial bolus injection in arteriovenous malformation of the spinal cord. Surg Neurol 22:181–185, 1984.
29. Heindel CC, Dugger GS, Guinto FC: Spinal arteriovenous malformation with hypogastric blood supply. J Neurosurg 42:462–464, 1975.
30. Heros RC, Debrun GM, Ojemann RG, Lasjaunias PL, Naessens PJ: Direct spinal arteriovenous fistula: A new type of spinal AVM. J Neurosurg 64:134–139, 1986.
31. Hook D, Lidvall H: Arteriovenous aneurysms of the spinal cord; a report of 2 cases investigated by vertebral angiography. J Neurosurg 15:84–91, 1958.
32. Houdart R, Djindjian R, Hurth M, Rey A: Treatment of angiomas of the spinal cord. Surg Neurol 2:186–194, 1974.
33. Hurth M, Djindjian R, Houdart R: Angiome medullaire cervical inextirpable a symptomatologie pseudo-tumorale chez un malade porteur d'une maladie de Rendu-Osler. Etude arteriographique et valeur therapeutique des ligatures multiples. Neurochirurgie 16:287–294, 1970.
34. Kasdon DL, Wolpert SM, Stein BM: Surgical and angiographic localization of spinal arteriovenous malformations. Surg Neurol 5:279–283, 1976.
35. Kendall BE, Logue V: Spinal epidural angiomatous malfor-

mations draining into intrathecal veins. *Neuroradiology* 13:181–189, 1977.
36. Krayenbuhl H, Yasargil MG, McClintock HG: Treatment of spinal cord vascular malformations by surgical excision. *J Neurosurg* 30:427–435, 1969.
37. Levy JM, Hessel SJ, Christensen FK, Crowe JK: Digital subtraction arteriography for spinal arteriovenous malformation. *AJNR* 4:1217–1218, 1983.
38. Logue V: Angiomas of the spinal cord: Review of the pathogenesis, clinical features and results of surgery. *J Neurol Neurosurg Psychiatry* 42:1–11, 1979.
39. Luessenhop AJ, Dela Cruz T: The surgical excision of spinal intradural vascular malformations. *J Neurosurg* 30:552–559, 1969.
40. Malis LI: Microsurgery for spinal cord arteriovenous malformations. *Clin Neurosurg* 26:543–569, 1979.
41. Malis LI: Arteriovenous malformations of the spinal cord. In Youmans JR (ed): *Neurological Surgery*, ed 2. Philadelphia, WB Saunders, 1982, vol 3, pp 1850–1874.
42. Margolis MT, Frenny PC, Kendrick MM: Cyanoacrylate occlusion of a spinal cord arteriovenous malformation. *J Neurosurg* 51:107–110, 1979.
43. Merland JJ, Riche MC, Chiras J: Intraspinal extramedullary arteriovenus fistulae draining into the medullary veins. *J Neuroradiol* 7:271–320, 1980.
44. Miyamoto S, Kikuchi H, Karasawa J, Ikota T, Nagata I: Spinal cord arteriovenous malformations associated with spinal aneurysms. *Neurosurgery* 13:577–580, 1983.
45. Oldfield EH, DiChiro G, Quindlen EA, Rieth KG, Doppman JL: Successful treatment of a group of spinal cord arteriovenous malformations by interruption of dural fistula. *J Neurosurg* 59:1019–1030, 1983.
46. Ommaya AK: Spinal arteriovenous malformations. In Wilkins RH, Rengachary SS (eds): *Neurosurgery*. New York, McGraw-Hill, 1985, vol 2, pp 1495–1499.
47. Ommaya AK, DiChiro G, Doppman J: Ligation of arterial supply in the treatment of spinal cord arteriovenous malformations. *J Neurosurg* 30:679–692, 1969.
48. Owen MP, Brown RH, Spetzler RF, Nash CL Jr, Brodkey JS, Nulsen FE: Excision of intramedullary arteriovenous malformation using intraoperative spinal cord monitoring. *Surg Neurol* 12:271–276, 1979.
49. Patterson RH Jr, Voorhies RM: Surgical approaches to intracranial and intraspinal arteriovenous malformations. *Clin Neurosurg* 25:412–424, 1978.
50. Pia HW: Operative treatment of arteriovenous malformations of the spinal cord. In Carrea R, LeVey D (eds): *Neurological Surgery, with Special Emphasis on Non-Invasive Methods of Diagnosis and Treatment*. Amsterdam, Excerpta Medica, 1978, pp 203–209.
51. Pia HW, Djindjian R (eds): *Spinal Angiomas: Advances in Diagnosis and Therapy*. New York, Springer-Verlag, 1978.
52. Raynor RB, Weiner R: Transthoracic approach to an intramedullary vascular malformation of the thoracic spinal cord. *Neurosurgery* 10:631–634, 1982.
53. Riche MC, Melki JP, Merland JJ: Embolization of spinal cord vascular malformations via the anterior spinal artery. *AJNR* 4:378–381, 1983.
54. Riche MC, Scialfa G, Gueguen B, Merland JJ: Giant extramedullary arteriovenous fistula supplied by the anterior spinal artery; treatment by detachable balloons. *AJNR* 4:391–394, 1983.
55. Richmond IL, Wilson CB: Evaluation and management of spinal cord arteriovenous malformations. *Bull LA Neurol Soc* 43:70–78, 1978.
56. Rosenblum B, Oldfield EH, Doppman J: An anatomic and physiologic basis for the classification of spinal arteriovenous malformations. Presented at the 36th Annual Meeting of the Congress of Neurological Surgeons, New Orleans, 1986.
57. Slade WR Jr: Spinal cord arteriovenous malformations. *Vasc Surg* 13:87–94, 1979.
58. Sugiyama Y, Konda H, Tanabe Y, Sakai N, Yamaja H, Ikeda K: Arteriovenous malformation of the spinal cord and cauda equina fed by branches of the internal iliac artery and associated with vertebral hemangiomas. *Surg Neurol* 18:97–101, 1982.
59. Symon L, Kuyama H, Kendall B: Dural arteriovenous malformations of the spine. Clinical features and surgical results in 55 cases. *J Neurosurg* 60:238–247, 1984.
60. Tobin WD, Layton DD Jr: The diagnosis and natural history of spinal cord arteriovenous malformations. *Mayo Clin Proc* 51:637–646, 1976.
61. Wyburn-Mason R: *The Vascular Abnormalities and Tumours of the Spinal Cord and Its Membranes*. London, Henry Kimpton, 1943.
62. Yasargil MG: Surgery of vascular lesions of the spinal cord with the microsurgical technique. *Clin Neurosurg* 17:257–265, 1970.
63. Yasargil MG: Diagnosis and treatment of spinal cord arteriovenous malformations. *Prog Neurol Surg* 4:355–428, 1971.
64. Yasargil MG, DeLong WB, Guarnaschelli JJ: Complete microsurgical excision of cervical extramedullary and intramedullary vascular malformations. *Surg Neurol* 4:211–224, 1975.
65. Yasargil MG, Symon L, Teddy PJ: Arteriovenous malformations of the spinal cord. In Symon L (ed): *Advances and Technical Standards in Neurosurgery 1984*. New York, Springer-Verlag, 1984, vol 11, pp 62–102.

INDEX

Page numbers in *italics* denote figures; those followed by "t" denote tables.

Abscess, bacterial aneurysm and, 342
ACA. *See* Anterior communicating artery
Accessory nerve, injury to, 67
Acute stroke
  angiography and, 3
  emergency carotid endarterectomy and, 25–31
  fibromuscular dysplasia and, 121
  medical therapy for, 26
  See also Stroke
Adventitia, incision of, 87–89, 96
Age
  aneurysm surgery and, 163
  carotid endarterectomy and, 10
  MCA dissection and, 133
Allcock test, 253
Amaurosis fugax, 15
  dissection and, 125
  EC-IC bypass and, 83
  See also Transient monocular blindness
Amyloid angiopathy, hemorrhage from, 446
Anastomosis
  carotid-subclavian artery bypass, 14
  EC-IC artery bypass graft, 84–94
  occipital artery bypass graft, 113
  vertebral artery and, 110
Anesthesia
  aneurysm surgery and, 164–165
  cardiac arrest and, 35
  carotid endarterectomy and, 36
  endotracheal, 36
Aneurysms
  acquired factors, 148t
  angiography and, 217
  anterior circulation, 147–148, *152*, 190–191, 217–233. *See also* specific artery
  asymptomatic, 163, 289
  AVMs and, 348
  balloon occlusion, 183
  basilar trunk, 116, 217–275
  berry type, 147–148
  brain hemorrhage and, 435
  carotid artery, 19–21, 24, 84–85, 125
    carotid-cavernous fistula and, 427
    ICA, 182, *188*, 191–197, *293*, *312*, 316–317
  cauterization of neck of, 171
  classification of, 148, 165, 175, 252
  clipping of, 170–172, 187–189
  collapse of, 172
  common wall for, *231*
  compressive symptoms, 163, 288
  congenital factors, 147–148
  contralateral, 211
  controlled hypertension and, 165
  deep exposure of, 168
  detection of, 148, 151–153
  dissection and, 135
  distal anterior cerebral artery, 235–239
  dome of, 186–188
  EC-IC bypass and, 83
  edema and, 298
  false, 67
  fungal, 345
  fusiform, *297–298*
  giant, 113, 116, 250, 297, 330–333
  infectious, 147, 337–344
  intracerebral hematoma and, 444–445
  intraoperative rupture of, 172
  large, 249
  metallic injection of, 173, 183
  middle cerebral artery, 241–251
  multiple, 148, 151, 239, 287–288, *290–292*
  natural history of, 153
  neck of, 171–172, *212*, 217, 249
  obliteration of, 171–172
  operative approach, 168–169, *290–292*
  ophthalmic, *200–202*
  paraclinoid, 199–216
  parent artery and, 171
  partially thrombosed, 199
  posterior circulation, 253
  posterior medially projecting, *194*
  pupillary sparing, 184
  puncturing of, 173, 187
  rebleeding peak, 153
  results of surgery, 265t, 330–333
  retraction of, 222
  rupture of, 183, 186, 205, 288, 427
  serpentine, 297, 320, *322*
  significant size of, 163
  site of, 151
  surgical approaches, 163–174
  TIAs and, 2, 104
  timing of surgery, 163–164
  unruptured symptomatic, 288
  vertebral artery, 167, 271–279, *302*, 324, 326, 330
  See also specific artery, location
Aneurysmorrhaphy technique, 148, 170, 307
Angina, unstable, 2
Angiography
  acute stroke and, 26
  broken guide wire, 117
  carotid circulation, 2–4, 95
    asymptomatic bruit and, 80
    neurologic deficits from, 26, 28
    occlusion during, 29
    posterior circulation TIAs, 16–18
    stenosis and, 77, 79
  fibromuscular dysplasia and, 121
  four-vessel, 148, 151–153, 287
  intraoperative, 47
  MCA occlusion and, 138
  occult AVMs and, 403–407
  optimal time for, 15
  postoperative, 62, 95, 173–174
  risk of, 4, 26, 28
  spinal, 451, 455
  string sign, 126, *129*
  three-vessel, 84, 151
  timing of films, 3, 9
  Towne view, 256–257
  vasospasm and, 164
  vertebral artery, 107
  vertebrobasilar ischemia and, 103–104
  See also Digital subtraction angiography; specific artery, disorder, technique
Angiomas
  cavernous, 401–403, *404–405*
  microangiomas, 405
Angioplasty
  patch graft, 55
  percutaneous, 55, 72, 106, 108, 109, 124
Angiotomography, 153
Anterior cerebral artery, *17*
  aneurysms adherent to, 193
  embolic occlusion, 3
Anterior choroidal artery, aneurysm and, 186, 190–191
Anterior circulation, aneurysms of, 147–148, 164, 168, 186. *See also* Aneurysms; specific artery
Anterior clinoid process, paraclinoid aneurysms, *188*, 199–216
Anterior communicating artery
  aneurysms, 164, 168, 217–239
  anterior cerebral complex variants, 222
  bifrontal interhemispheric approach, 233
  bilobed, *229*
  clipping techniques, 227–231
  giant, 320, *322*
  microsurgical dissection of, 217, 221–226
  obliteration of, 226–231
  perforating branches, 222, 225
  postoperative psychoorganic syndrome, 233
  surgical results, 231–233
  symptoms of, 217
Anterior fossa
  access to, 168
  dural AVMs, 415
Anterior hypothalamic region, AVMs in, 378
Anterior inferior cerebellar artery
  basilar trunk aneurysm, 271–275
  subtemporal-suboccipital approach, 253
Anterior scalene muscle, 108–110
Antibiotics
  postoperative, 84
  prophylactic, 47, 164
  See also specific drug, surgery

Anticoagulant therapy
  asymptomatic carotid stenosis and, 79
  brain hemorrhage from, 446
  head injury and, 135
  recurrent embolism and, 137
  thrombosis and, 103
  See also specific drug, surgery
Anticonvulsants, 84. See also Seizures;
    specific drugs
Antidiuretic hormone, 156, 436
Antifibrinolytic agents, 159
Antihypertensive therapy, 104. See also
    Hypertension
Antiplatelet therapy, 8, 12, 95, 122
  asymptomatic carotid stenosis and, 79
  EC-IC bypass and, 84
  postoperative, 62
Aorta
  angiography and, 3, 22, 104
  emboli and, 137
  hypoplasia of, 147
Aphasia, sudden, 140
Arachnoid knives, 166
Arachnoiditis, 451
Argyle carotid shunt catheters, 50
Arm
  TIAs involving, 26
  weakness of, 1, 9
Arteriotomy, 115 123
  closure of, 49
  cortical, 84
  dissected intima and, 131
  for embolus, 139–140
  oval, 90, 111
  patch graft, 46, 52
  posterior cerebral artery, 116
  sutures of, 46
  thrombosis and, 140
Arteriovenous malformations (AVMs),
    148, 347–409
  angiography and, 151
  anterior callosal, 374, 378, *382–383*
  anterior frontal parasagittal, 370
  associated aneurysm, 348
  asymptomatic, 350–351
  basal ganglia, 380
  brain stem, 380–383, *388, 390*
  carotid-cavernous fistula, 427–433
  cerebellar, 383–386, *389, 391*
  classification of, 347
  conservative therapy, 399
  convexity lesions, *349, 352, 357–358, 359–360, 395*
  cryptic, 405
  deep frontal, 374, 378
  deep medial midtemporal, *368–369*
  deep temporal-occipital, 366
  dural, 415–421, 427, 430
  electrothrombosis for, 397
  embolization of, 394–397
  enhanced infarct and, 6
  feeder occlusion, 354
  grading system for, 392
  hemorrhage and, 435
  hypothalamic-basal frontal, 378, 380
  incidence of, 347
  intracerebral hematoma and, 444–445
  intramedullary type of, 451
  intraventricular, 380, *388*
  lateral ventricle atrium, 373

  left parietal, *379–380*
  medial occipital, 370
  natural history of, 350
  occult, 403–408
  parasagittal, 370, *376*
  perfusion breakthrough, 353
  positioning for surgery, 351–359
  postoperative care, 359
  prognosis for, 351
  proton therapy for, 397–398
  radiation for, 397
  radiographic evaluation of, 415–416
  retroatrial, *372*
  right parietal, *354–356, 377*
  of spinal cord, 451–465
  splenial, *367–370, 374–375*
  spontaneous fistulas and, 430
  steal phenomena, 451
  subfrontal, *385*
  subsplenial, 387
  surgical management of, 351–386, 390t,
    417–421
  sylvian, 360–362
  of temporal lobe, 362–367
  thalamic, 380
  trigone, 366
  thrombosed, *408*
  type I spinal, 453–453
  type II intramedullary, *458*
  type III spinal, 459
  type IV spinal, 459
  vein of Galen, 399–401
Arteritis, dissection and, 133
Artery(ies). See specific artery, disorder,
    surgical procedure
Artery of Adamkiewicz, 460
Artery of Huebner, 193
Aspirin therapy
  intraluminal thrombus and, 30
  postoperative, 62, 109
  preoperative, 36
Ataxia, 106t, 143, 383
Atheroma
  dissection, 43–44
  occlusive disease, 2, 57
  See also Carotid endarterectomy
Atherosclerosis, 1, 137
  antegrade thrombosis from, 22
  giant aneurysms and, 297
  medical risk factors, 35
  progression of, 62
  risk factors, 35
  turbulent blood flow and, 77
  ulcerating lesions with, 8
  of vertebrobasilar circulation, 103–109
Atlanto-occipital membrane, 107
Atrial fibrillation, embolism and, 137
Atrial myxomas, aneurysm and, 147
Atropine, 36
Auditory canal, external, 90
Auricular nerve, greater, 38–39

Bacterial endocarditis, 337
  anticoagulation and, 138
  diagnostic studies, 338
Bacterial intracranial aneurysm, 337
  angiogram findings, 344t
  bacteriology in, 338t
  clinical signs, 337–338
  decisions of management, 338

  meningitis and, 344
  multiple, 341
Balloon catheter methods
  basilar occlusion, 386
  detachment of balloon, 140
  dissection and, 131
  internal carotid occlusion, *312–313,* 316
  transluminal angioplasty, 106, 108, 109, 124
Basal ganglia
  AVMs, 362, 380, 399
  hemorrhage, 191
Basal perforating arteries, 217
Basal skull fracture, 427
Basal subarachnoid space, blood in, 151
Basal tumor, EC-IC bypass and, 84
Basal vein of Rosenthal, 197
Basilar artery, 103
  aneurysms, 170
    bifurcation, 116, 168, 253–262, 326
    delayed surgery for, 164
    evaluation of, 253–257
    fusiform, 303
    giant, 116, 326, *328, 332*
    hemorrhage and, 163
    large, 279
    obliteration of, 257–258
    problems of, 258
    results, 265t
    spinal drainage and, 165
  dissection of, 133
  occlusion, 386
  side-to-side anastomosis, 117
  stenosis, 103, *106*
  surgical approaches, 117, 167, 179, 254–259, 261–262, 271–275, 279t
  temporary balloon occlusion, 386
Basilar trunk-superior cerebellar artery
    aneurysm, 263–269
  surgical management, 271–275
  surgical results, 279t
  See also Basilar artery, aneurysms
Berry aneurysms, 147–148
Bifurcation. See specific artery
Bipolar cautery, *212*
Blalock-Taussig anastomosis, 104
Blindness
  giant aneurysm and, 302
  pathological finding, 68t
  postoperative, 183, 216
Blood gases, 165. See also specific
    disease
Blood pressure
  anesthesia and, 36
  monitoring of, 164
  subarachnoid hemorrhage and, 154
  See also Hypertension; Hypotension
B mode scans, 6
Bone
  flap
    closure, 181–182
    internal carotid aneurysm and, 180
    replacement, 90
  removal, 417
  transverse sinus and, 417
  wax, *208,* 210
  See also specific procedure
Booster clips, 171

Botterell classifications, subarachnoid hemorrhage, 150–151
Brachial ischemia, 104
Brachial plexus, 108
Bradycardia, postoperative, 58
Brain
 abscess, 342
 aneurysm surgery. See Aneurysms, surgical approaches
 arterial supply to, 36, 105. See also specific artery
 AVMs and, 347–409, 444–445
 diagnosis techniques. See specific method
 closure, 181–182
 coagulation studies, 436
 hemorrhage, 435–446
  aneurysm-caused, 444–445
  AVM-caused, 444–445
  caudate, 441
  cerebellar, 441–443
  coagulation disorders and, 446
  common sites for, 438
  EC-IC bypass graft and, 95
  hematoma removal, 439
  intraventricular, 443–444
  lobar, 441
  medical treatment of, 436
  pathophysiology, 435
  pontine, 443
  postoperative care, 31, 438
  putaminal, 439–441
  surgery for, 437–438
  thalamic, 441
 hyperemic, 246
 interhemispheric fissure, 236
 intraoperative irrigation, 172
 perioperative injury to, 93, 165
 relaxation of, 165, 180, 218–222, 235
 retraction, 168, 244, 417
 steroids and, 359
 swelling, 140, 143–145, 181, 246, 359
 vascular malformations. See by site, type
 See also specific arteries, disorders, sites
Brain stem
 aneurysm pointing back into, 260
 auditory evoked responses, 103, 255
 AVMs, 380–383, 388, 390, 399
 compression, 143–145, 264, 275
 infarction, 256
 ischemia, 103
 monitoring of, 255
 posterior cerebral artery, 116
 vertebral artery reconstruction, 108
Bridging veins, sacrificing of, 256
Bruit, 427, 431
 B mode scanning and, 6
 carotid, 1–2, 4
  asymptomatic, 2, 77–80
  bilateral, 11
  fibromuscular dysplasia and, 122t
  high-pitched, 77
  phonoangiography of, 6–8
 over subclavian artery, 104
Bulldog clamp, 43
Bypass graft procedures
 carotid ligation and, 182
 extracranial to intracranial, 55

 extrathoracic, 106
 hemorrhage and, 95
 STA-MCA, 131–133
 See also specific artery, procedure

Calcium channel blocker, 158–159
Caloric stimulation, 143
Cardiac arrhythmias, 156
Cardiac surgery
 cardiopulmonary bypass, 307–308
 carotid endarterectomy and, 35
 embolism and, 137
 stroke risk, 80
Carotid artery
 aneurysms of, 308–320
 anterior, 17
 atherosclerosis, 1–31, 35
 auscultation, 1
 bifurcation, 1, 3, 55, 116
  aneurysms, 149, 320, 321
  angiograms of, 7–8
  thrombus, 22, 57
  ulceration at, 4
  unusual anatomy in, 59
 bruit, 1–4
  asymptomatic, 77–80
  bilateral, 11
  fibromuscular dysplasia and, 122
  high-pitched, 77
  perioperative stroke and, 80
  phonoangiography of, 6–8
  severe stenosis and, 3
 cavernous fistula. See Carotid-cavernous fistula
 collateral circulation, 10, 13, 15
 common. See Common carotid artery
 complete occlusion, 53–55
 delayed films and, 9
 diagnostic studies, 2–3
 dissection of, 125–135
 EEG and, 37–38
 emboli and, 137–138
 endarterectomy of. See Carotid endarterectomy
 external. See External carotid artery
 fibromuscular dysplasia of, 121–124
 fistula, 427–433
 internal. See Internal carotid artery
 ipsilateral, 12
 ligation, 216, 308
 loop in, 58-59
 lumen of, 3, 47–48, 51, 54
 noninvasive ultrasound studies of, 6–8
 occlusion of, 8, 9–10, 12, 14, 23, 29t, 53–55, 60, 201, 308–316
 oculoplethysmography, 8
 patch graft, 51–52
 plaque removal, 48
 preoperative deficit, 29t
 proximal external, 44, 47
 reopening and, 14
 risk factors, 35
 siphon, 1, 84
 stenosis, 3, 21–23, 35, 52–53, 55, 80
  acute stroke and, 2
  asymptomatic, 19, 77–80
  bilateral, 17
  B mode scanning and, 6
  at C2 level, 52–53
  degree of, 3

  endarterectomy for, 79–80
  extracranial, 21
  hemodynamic cause, 1
  intraluminal filling defect and, 29t
  posterior TIAs and, 16
  pseudo-occlusions, 3, 10
  residual lumen diameter, 8
  severe, 8
  tandem lesions, 12, 19
  ulceration and, 3
  vertebrobasilar TIAs and, 23
 supraclinoid aneurysms, 318–320
 thrombus, 54, 60–61
 TIAs and, 1, 8, 10–12, 16
 traumatic dissection of, 133–135
 vein grafts and, 97–98
 wall, 125
 See also Carotid endarterectomy
Carotid-cavernous fistula, 54
 aneurysm rupture and, 432
 angiography and, 427–428
 clinical presentation, 427
 detachable balloon catheter treatment, 428–430
 dural AVM and, 431
 internal carotid occlusion and, 430t
 spontaneous, 430–432
 trauma and, 427
 visual loss and, 427
Carotid endarterectomy, 31
 anesthesia and, 36
 asymptomatic aneurysm and, 21
 asymptomatic stenosis and, 79
 bilateral stenosis and, 11
 C2 level stenosis, 52–53
 EEG recording during, 37
  abnormal arterial anatomy, 53
  common carotid stenosis, 55–58
  complete occlusion, 53–54
  complications, 35
 elective, 8
 emergency, 25–31
 external carotid stenosis and, 55
 indications for, 8, 29
 insertion of patch graft, 56
 ipsilateral stroke and, 10
 neck stenosis and, 12
 occlusion, 55–58
 operating room set-up, 39
 postoperative management, 58–67
 preoperative evaluation, 35–36
 prophylactic, 80
 recurrent stenosis and, 70–72
 results of, 10, 29t, 31
 skin incision, 39
 specimen pathology, 67–70
 technical points, 71–72
 technique, 38–50
 tourniquets, 43
 vertebrobasilar symptoms and, 19
Carotid sinus, 42, 58
Carotid-subclavian artery graft, 111–114
Carotodynia, 65
Caudate nucleus
 AVMs, 380
 hemorrhage, 441
Cautery, bipolar, 87, 90, 238
Cavernous angiomas, 347, 401–403
Cavernous sinus
 carotid artery fistula, 427–433

Cavernous sinus—*continued*
    ICA, *215*
    intracavernous aneurysms, 317
    packing of, 183
    spontaneous resolution of lesion, 415
Cerebellar artery
    aneurysm of, 271–275
        basilar trunk-anterior inferior,
            271–275
        distal anterior-inferior, 275
        giant, *331*
        peripheral posterior inferior, 283–285
        subtemporal-suboccipital approach,
            253
        surgical position for, 167
        vertebral-posterior inferior, 279–283
    occipital-posterior inferior bypass, 113,
        115
    posterior inferior, *331*
    superior, 117
Cerebellar hemorrhage, 441–443. See also
    Brain, hemorrhage
Cerebellar infarction, 6, 116, 143
Cerebellar tonsils, 113
Cerebellopontine angle
    aneurysms, 275
    lesions, 383
Cerebellum
    AVMs, *389, 391, 393–394*
    hemorrhage, 435, 437, 441–443
    infarction, 6, 116, 143
    See also Cerebellar artery; specific
        disorders
Cerebral angiography. See Angiography
Cerebral arteries. See specific artery,
    disorder
Cerebral blood flow (CBF)
    acute stroke and, 25
    aneurysm site and, 147
    collateral circulation, 4
    EEG changes and, 37
    embolic occlusion. See Embolism,
        cerebral
    perioperative, 36–38
    reduced, 25
    studies, 83–84
    See also specific arteries, diseases,
        disorders
Cerebral convexity, large AVMs of,
    359–360
Cerebral hemorrhage. See Brain,
    hemorrhage
Cerebral infarction. See Infarction,
    cerebral; Ischemia, cerebral; Stroke
Cerebral ischemia. See Ischemia, cerebral
Cerebrospinal fluid (CSF)
    distal anterior cerebral aneurysms and,
        235
    drainage of, 156–157, 165, 168, 211,
        221
Cervical bruit, differential diagnosis of,
    77t. See also Bruit
Cervical medullary AVMs, 451
Cervical plexus, 38
Cervical spondylosis, 103
Childhood, aneurysms in, 147
Chiropractic manipulation, VA dissection
    and, 135
Choroid plexus, intraventricular AVMs,
    380

Circle of Willis, 103
    aneurysms, 164
    pterional flap and, 168
Circulation
    collateral, 4, 103
    ipsilateral, with intracranial aneurysm,
        19–21
    See also specific artery
Clamps, arterial, 50
Clinoid process, dura overlying, 203. See
    also Paraclinoid aneurysm
Clipping procedures, 50, 227, 306
    aneurysms and, 181, 199–211, *213*
    arterial occlusion and, 173
    middle cerebral artery, 244
    rupture and, 172
    stereotactic, 172
    superficial veins and, 197
    third nerve injury and, 187
    See also specific aneurysm, artery
Clivus, 261
Clotting
    brain hemorrhage and, 435
    deficiency, 446
    EC-MCA bypass grafts and, 95
    intraluminal, 29
Cluster headaches, 65
Coagulation disorders, hemorrhage due
    to, 446
Colloid infusions, 84, 95, 138–139
Coma, 144, 150–151
    intracranial hypertension and, 156
Common carotid artery, 2, 48
    aneurysms, 182–183, 217–233
    arteriotomy, 45, 111, 123
    atheroma, 43–44, 109
    bifurcation of, *41–42*, 138
    bypass graft to subclavian artery,
        106
    end-to-side anastomosis, *114*
    exposure of, 38, 41
    ligation of, 199–200
    nonobstructive irregularity of, 4
    occlusion of, 22, 55–58
    proximal, 57
    stenosis of, 21–23, 55–58
    TIAs with, 21
    transposition of VA, 109
    ulceration in, 15
    vascular clamp and, 43
Common duct dilator, 123
Completed stroke
    EC-IC bypass and, 83
    evaluation of, 22
    See also Stroke
Computed tomography (CT) scans, 4–6
    acute stroke and, 26
    asymptomatic aneurysms and, 148
    neurologic deficits and, 23
    See also specific artery, disease
Confusion state, 137
Congestive heart failure, 35
Consciousness
    altered level of, 2
    cerebral hemorrhage and, 435–436
    dissection and, 133
    infarction and, 31, 144
    See also Coma
Contralateral internal carotid artery
    occlusion, 11–12

Cooperative Study of Subarachnoid
    Hemorrhage and Intracranial
    Aneurysms, 173
Coronary angiography, 35
Coronary artery bypass, 307–308
    angina after, 35
    carotid endarterectomy and, 35, 80
Coronary artery disease, 35
    anesthesia and, 36
    embolism and, 137
    stroke risk, 80
    subarachnoid hemorrhage and, 156
Corpus callosum, AVMs, 374–378, *381*
Cortex
    injury to, 419
    irreversible infarction, 139
Cortical artery, exposure of, *92*
Corticectomy, 168
    around AVM, 352
    frontal, *195*
    in gyrus rectus, 222
    MCA aneurysm, *249*
Coughing, spontaneous dissection and,
    125
Coumadin therapy, 79, 96, 107, 137
    carotid dissection and, 131
    vertebral circulation and, 104
    See also Anticoagulant therapy
Cranial nerve palsy
    carotid-cavernous fistula and, 427
    carotid endarterectomy, 65, 67
    hemorrhage risk and, 149
Cranial nerves, 184
    C3 injury, 187, 255
    compression and, 163
    dysfunction of, 80
    paresis of, 164, 182
    respiration and, 113
Craniectomy, 90, *115*
    decompression of, 145
    suboccipital, 113, 145, 278
Craniotomy, 85
    ACA aneurysms and, 217–221
    cutdown technique, *91*
    flap, 83, 85, 90, 179–180
    frontotemporal, 139
    ipsilateral, 211
    MCA aneurysm and, 242
    parietooccipital, 399
    posterior temporal, *274*
    pterional, 179, 184, 190, *204*, 220, *262*,
        265–266, 362
    scalp incisions, *86–87*
    subtemporal approach, 254
    temporal bone removal and, 362
    unilateral frontal, 217–221
    vein grafts, *98–99*
    See also specific surgical procedure
Cross-compression studies, 299
Crutchfield clamp, placement of, *314–315*
Crystalloid, 36
Cyanoacrylate, embolization, 397
Cystic medial necrosis, 125, 133

Dacron graft, 52, *114*
Decompression, infarction and, 143
Deep temporal AVMs, 362–366
Dehydration, intracranial pressure and,
    154
Dementia, EC-IC bypass and, 83

Demyelinating disease, 455
Descendens hypoglossi nerve, 38, 42, 67
Diabetes mellitus, 35, 62
Diazepam, 36, 164
Diet, 154
Digastric muscle, hypertrophied, 58
Digital subtraction angiography, 4, 104, 148, 153, 299
  after endarterectomy, 62
  giant aneurysms and, 299
  oblique views, 13
  by selective arterial injection, 153
  See also Angiography
Dilation, 72
  fibromuscular dysplasia and, 123
  of proximal common carotid stenosis, 57
  See also Transluminal angioplasty
Diphenylhydantoin, EC-IC bypass and, 84
Diplopia, 106t
Dissection, 180
  cerebral ischemia and, 125
  of internal carotid artery
    clinical manifestations, 125–126
    radiographic findings, 126–131
    spontaneous, 125–133
    traumatic, 133–135
    treatment of, 131–133
  fibromuscular hyperplasia and, 125
  intracranial arteries, spontaneous, 133
  string sign, 129
  of vertebral artery, 135
Distal anterior inferior cerebellar artery, aneurysms of, 275
Distal anterior cerebral artery
  aneurysms, 235–239
  frontal lobe hemorrhage in, 235
  microsurgical dissection, 236–238
  obliteration of, 238
  operative technique, 235–236
  surgical results, 239
Distal common carotid artery. See Common carotid artery
Distal internal carotid artery. See Internal carotid artery
Diuretic medication, potassium deficiency and, 35
Dizziness, TIA and, 1–2
Doll's head maneuver, 143
Doppler imaging
  duplex scanner, 6
  of graft patency, 91
  interpretation of, 6–8
  intraoperative studies, 47
  vertebral stenosis and, 103
Drake clips, 170
Drilling, irrigation and, 203. See also specific procedure
Droperidol, 164
Drowsiness, 150–151
Dura mater
  AVMs of, 415, 420, 424
  closure of, 94
  electrocautery of, 203–205
  embolization and, 424
  grafts, 143
  initial exposure, 180
  opening of, 85, 90, 92, 143, 203, 209, 248, 255, 384, 419

tenting sutures and, 180
  See also specific surgical approach
Dye allergy, 2
Dysarthria, 143
Dysphasia, 80, 150, 441
Dysphonia, 80

Earache, ICA aneurysm and, 182
EC-IC artery bypass graft. See Extracranial-intracranial bypass graft
Edema, 173
  giant aneurysms, 251
  massive cerebral, 297–298
  See also specific disease
EEG. See Electroencephalogram
Ehlers-Danlos syndrome, 147
Elastic, defect in, 147, 148t
Electrocardiogram, stroke and, 26
Electroencephalogram (EEG)
  endarterectomy and, 37, 111
  shunt and, 50
Electrolyte imbalance, subarachnoid hemorrhage and, 156
Electromagnetic flow probe, 91
Electrothrombosis
  AVMs and, 397
  cavernous sinus and, 428
Embolectomy, MCA, 138–140
Embolism, cerebral, 137
  aneurysm and, 19–21, 163
  cardiac source, 2
  cerebellar infarction and, 143
  dilation and, 124
  EC-IC bypass and, 83
  MCA, 29
  proximal internal carotid artery stump, 21
  seizure and, 65
  sitting position and, 367
Embolization
  of AVMs, 394–397
    cyanoacrylate, 397
    dural AVMs, 424
    spinal, 460
  from carotid bifurcation, 1
  See also Balloon catheter methods
Endarterectomy, 8
  dilation and, 124
  heparinized saline and, 46
  intradural, 108
  prophylactic contralateral, 80
  shunt and, 50–55
  stripper, 57
  See also Carotid endarterectomy; by site
Endocarditis, 337
Endocardium
  bacterial aneurysms and, 337
  cerebral emboli and, 137
Epilepsy
  AVMs and, 348
  cortical resection and, 246
  See also Seizures
Epistaxis, 182
External carotid artery, 48, 55
  bypass, 113–117
  delayed films and, 9
  emboli and, 83
  endarterectomy, 55, 62

occlusion of, 15–16, 209
  proximal, 44, 47
  stenosis, 15–16
  TIAs and, 15–16
External carotid-saphenous vein-posterior cerebral artery bypass, 113–117
Extracranial carotid occlusive disease, 9, 15–16. See also Carotid artery
Extracranial-Intracranial Bypass Study, 83
Extracranial to intracranial (EC-IC) artery bypass graft, 83–100
  alternative procedures, 97–99
  anesthesia and, 84
  closure of, 94
  cutdown technique, 87–88
  embolism and, 182–183
  flap technique, 85
  giant aneurysm and, 308
  postoperative management, 94–96
  preoperative evaluation, 84
  pterional approach and, 86
  study, 83
  technique, 85–94
Eyes
  blindness
    giant aneurysm and, 302
    postoperative, 183, 216
    transient monocular, 1
  gaze palsy, 143
  giant aneurysms and, 199
  ocular pulse, 8
  secondary glaucoma, 427

Facial nerves, 116
  damage to, 65, 419
  numbness, 182
  peripheral palsy, 143
  TIAs and, 26
  vein, 38
Fascial band, extrinsic compression, 58
Females, aneurysm incidence, 297
Fentanyl, 165
Fetal vessels, involution of, 147, 148t
Fibromuscular dysplasia
  of internal carotid arteries, 121
    age and sex distribution, 122t
    symptoms of, 121–122
    treatment of, 122
  dissection and, 125, 133
  intracranial aneurysms and, 147
Fingers, numbness of, 1
Fistula, spinal arteriovenous, 459, 463
Flaps. See Scalp flap
Focal cerebral ischemia. See Ischemia, cerebral
Focal hemorrhage. See Hemorrhage
Focal neurologic deficit, 288
Fogarty catheter, 57
Foramen magnum, bone removal and, 278
Forceps
  bipolar coagulating, 166
  See also specific procedure
Frontalis palsy, 254
Frontal lobe
  AVMs, 382–383
  bleeding into, 150
  butterfly hemorrhage, 235
  hematoma in, 235

Frontal lobe—continued
  injury to, 243, 374
  retraction, 180–181, 186, 218–222, 242
Fungal intracranial aneurysms, 345
Furosemide, IV, 165
Fusion, 107

Gaze palsy, 143
Gelfoam, 91. See also specific procedure
Giant aneurysms, 150, 297
  bipolar coagulation and, 209
  booster clips and, 170
  carotid ligation, 216
  carotid occlusion and, 308–316
  cerebellar aneurysm and, 279
  clinical presentation, 297–298
  clipping of, 306. See also Clipping procedures
  delayed surgery for, 164
  hemorrhage and, 163
  indirect surgery for, 172
  intracranial procedure, 303–308
  paraclinoid, 202
  radiologic diagnosis of, 298–300
  spinal drainage and, 165
  surgical results in, 333t
  treatment indications for, 301–303
  unclippable, 140
  visual symptoms of, 199
  See also Aneurysms; by location
Glaucoma, secondary, 427
Glioma
  enhanced infarct and, 5
  hemorrhage, 445
Global aneurysms, 199
Glomus malformation, 455–459
Glycopyrolate, 36
GORE-TEX, patch graft, 47, 52, 113, 114
Graft. See specific procedure, site
Greater auricular nerve, injury to, 65
Greenberg retractor, 166, 168
Guide wire, 117
Gyrus rectus, corticectomy, 168, 222, 225

Hamartomas, 401
Headache
  AVM and, 348
  diagnostic problem and, 149
  dissection and, 125
  hemicranias, 65
  history of severe, 150
  MCA dissection and, 133
  postoperative, 65
  See also specific disorder
Head injury
  intracranial dissection and, 125, 134
  manipulation therapy and, 106–107
Headrest, three-point skeletal fixation, 84
Hearing, damage to, 113, 419
Heart disease. See Cardiovascular disease
Heifetz aneurysm clips, 43
  delayed fracture with, 170
  occlusion with, 84, 87
Hematoma, 5, 173, 246, 435–436
  in basal cisterns, 218
    CT scan and, 151, 287
  caudate, 441
  cerebellar, 441–443
  lobar, 218, 441

  medical treatment of, 436
  occipital lobe, 406
  postoperative care, 438
  subarachnoid, 248
  surgical removal of, 436, 439
  temporal, 246
  thalamic, 441
  wound, 67
  See also Hemorrhage
Hemicranias, 65
Hemicraniectomy, 143–145
Hemilaminectomy, 115
Hemiparesis, 106t, 150
Hemiplegia, sudden, 138, 140
Hemispheric TIAs, 22
Hemodilution, isovolemic, 138
Hemophilia, 446
Hemorrhage, 30, 435–449
  aneurysmal, 148
  antifibrinolytic agents, 155
  arteriotomy and, 46
  AVM and, 350, 353
    occult, 405
    resection and, 353
    spinal, 451, 455
  bacterial endocarditis and, 337
  brain, 435–446
    diagnostic studies, 436
    pathophysiology, 435
    treatment, medical, 436
    treatment, surgical, 437–446
  caudate, 441
  classifications, 150–151
  infarction vs., 26
  intramural, 5
  intraplaque, 70
  intraventricular, 157, 443–444
  lobar, 437, 441
  medical therapy for, 154t
  microaneurysms and, 435
  parenchymal, 347
  pontine, 443
  postoperative, 23, 62, 65
  prevention of, 148
  putaminal, 437
  recurrent, 155
  subhyaloid, 150
  thalamic, 66, 441
  See also Subarachnoid hemorrhage
Hemostasis
  near bypass vessels, 84
  suture line, 91
Hemostat, mosquito, 85
Heparin therapy, 43, 107, 116, 123
  carotid dissection and, 131
  EC-IC bypass and, 84, 89–90
  preoperative use, 8
  reversal of, 47, 100
  short vein graft and, 96–98
  thrombus and, 30
  TIAs and, 26, 28–29
  vertebral circulation and, 104
Herniation, tonsillar, 145
Hippocampus, AVMs of, 364
Homocystinuria, dissection and, 133
Homonymous hemianopia, 113
Horner's syndrome, 106t, 111
Hunt-Hess subarachnoid hemorrhage classifications, 150–151
Hydralazine, 62

Hydrocephalus, 173
  cerebellar AVMs and, 383
  CT scan and, 151
  infarction and, 144
  after subarachnoid hemorrhage, 157
Hypercholesterolemia, 62
Hyperlipidemia, 35
Hypernatremia, with hyperosmolarity, 156
Hypertension, 143
  AVMs and, 452
  brain hemorrhage and, 154, 435–436
  carotid endarterectomy and, 43
  induced, 159
  lacunar, 2
  postoperative, 58–59, 80
  preoperative treatment, 35
Hypertriglyceridemia, 62
Hypoglossal artery, 19
Hypoglossal nerve, 38, 42, 67
Hyponatremia, 156, 158
Hypotension
  drug induced, 255
  fluid and, 58
  induced, 165
  postoperative, 28
Hypothalamic arteries, 222
Hypothalamus, perforating branches and, 228
Hypoxia, carotid-cavernous fistula and, 427

Iliofemoral occlusion, angiograms and, 4
Infancy, aneurysms in, 147, 148t
Infarction, cerebral, 80, 143
  angiograms and, 4
  CT scan and, 1–6, 14, 23
  defined, 143
  EC-IC bypass and, 83
  embolic cause, 137
  healing process, 5
  MRI and, 6–8
  myocardial, 12
  silent, 2
  siphon stenosis and, 12
  stroke and, 5, 12, 23
  thalamic, 187
  vertebral artery, 103
Infectious intracranial aneurysms, 337
Innominate artery
  endarterectomy and, 104, 109
  stenosis, 109
  transthoracic approach, 108
Intercourse, sudden headache and, 153
Internal carotid artery, 2–3, 10, 12, 48, 58
  aneurysm of, 168, 179–197, 293
    anterior choroidal artery, 190–191, 195
    bacterial, 344
    bifurcation, 191–197
    cavernous, 183–184t, 317
    giant, 311
    lateral wall, 211–216
    nongiant, 189t
    paraclinoid, 199–216, 317–318
    petrous, 182, 312, 316–317
    posterior communicating artery, 183–189, 191, 193
    posterior wall, 211–216
    proximal internal, 188

Index

angiographic criteria and, 31, *126*
dissection of, *126, 131–133*
   spontaneous, 125–133
   traumatic, 133–135
distal, 1, 4, *130–131*
fibromuscular dysplasia of, 124
lumen of, 3
MRI and, 6
occlusion of, 3, 5–6, 11, *20*, 31, 53–55, 205
paraclinoid region of, 179, 199–216, 317–318
patency of, 22
petrous portion of, 182, 316–317, 344
proximal, 4, 14–15, *188*
pseudo-occlusion of, *12*
reopening, 14, *20*
stenosis of, *3–4, 7–8*, 11, *19, 27*, 29–30
subclavian artery graft, 113–114
stump embolus into, 16
visualization of, 13–14, 262
Internal carotid-posterior communicating artery aneurysm, 183–189, *191, 193*
Intima, arterial, 57
   common carotid artery, 44
   defect, 125
   flap of, *51*
   increase in fibrous elements, 121
   shunt and, 38
   splitting of, 124, 135
   See also Endarterectomy
Intraaneurysmal detachable balloon technique, 173
Intracranial aneurysms
   instrumentation, 166
   multiple lesions, 287
   obliteration of, 171–172
   positioning, 166–168
   surgical treatment, 163–174
   See also Aneurysms; specific artery
Intraluminal filling defect, 28–30
Intraluminal thrombus, emergency operation for, *64*
Intraventricular hemorrhage, 443
Ischemia, cerebral
   bypass graft and, 83–84
   carotid occlusion and, 2
   CBF regulation and, 36
   collateral circulation and, 25
   dissection and, 28, 125
   fibromuscular dysplasia and, 122t
   focal, 36, 121, 125
   postoperative, 63–65
   risk for, 30
   subarachnoid hemorrhage and, 150t
   See also Transient ischemic attacks; by site
Ischemic necrosis. See Infarction
Ischemic oculopathy, 2, 83
Ischemic stroke. See Stroke
Isoflurane, 36

Jugular vein
   internal, 108–110
   ligation of, 38–40
Juvenile spinal AVMs, 458–459, 463

Kleinert-Kees clips, 84, 90, *93*, 115

Labyrinthine disorder, 143
Lacunar disease, 2
Laryngeal nerve, injury to, 42
Laser, in AVM surgery, 353
Lasix, 235, 248, 417. See also specific surgery
Lateral trans-sylvian approach, MCA aneurysm, 249–250
Latex balloon, embolized, 140. See also Balloon techniques
Leg, 107
   TIAs involving, 26
   weakness of, 1
Lenticulostriate arteries, 243
Ligature, bipolar, 238
Lobar brain hemorrhage, 441, 446
Long vein graft, 97
   CCA to MCA, *98–99*
   external carotid artery to MCA, 100
   vertebral occlusive disease, 104
Low perfusion syndromes, 83
Lumbar puncture
   rebleeding and, 156
   subarachnoid hemorrhage and, 153
Lumbar spondylosis, spinal AVM vs., 454
Lumen, arterial, 50
   bruit and, 77
   carotid, 3, 79
   intraluminal filling defect, 28–30
   irrigation of, 140
   mural thrombus and, 70
   restoration of, *58*
   thrombus, 8
   transluminal angioplasty, 72, 104, 109, 124
Lymph nodes, carotid bifurcation and, 38

MacFadden clip, 170
Magnetic resonance imaging (MRI), 6–8
   clip rotation and, 170
   giant aneurysms and, 300
   infarction and, 143–144
   lacunar disease and, 2
   spinal AVMs and, 452
   TIAs and, 103
Mammary artery, 108
Manipulation, vertebral artery and, 106–10
Mannitol, 116, 165, 235, 248
   prior to clipping, 170
   rebleeding and, 156
Marfan's syndrome, 147
Mayfield headrest, 165–166
MCA. See Middle cerebral artery
Media
   intima stripped from, 125
   saccular dilatations, 121
   splitting of, 124
Medial trans-sylvian approach, MCA aneurysm, 241–246
Melanoma, hemorrhage, 445
Memory, confusion syndrome, 137
Meningeal signs, 150
Meningismus, 150
Meningitis, 344, 455
Mental status, 150
Metzenbaum scissors, 87–88, 113
Microangiomas, 405
Microscope. See Microsurgery

Microsurgery, 90–93, 248
   aneurysm, 165–173
   AVM, 352
   EC-IC bypass, 84–85
   end-to-end anastomosis, 116
   end-to-side anastomosis, 111
   See also specific instruments, surgical procedures
Middle cerebral artery
   anastomosis, 85, 90–93
   aneurysms, 241–*251*
      bacterial, 338
      bifurcation, 139, 244–246
      evaluation of, 242
      giant, *300*, 320–324
      serpentine, 297
      superior temporal gyrus approach, 246
      surgical positioning, *167*, 179
      surgical results, 250–251
      symptoms, 241
   dissection of, 133
   EC-IC bypass grafts, 83–100
      CCA long vein graft, *98–99*
      surgical preparation of, *93*
   occlusion of, 3, 29
      deliberate, 171
      embolectomy for, 137–140
      postoperative, 251
   recipient branch position, 84
   revascularization of, 100
   stenosis, 84
   sylvian fissure AVMs, 360–362
Migraine, dissection and, 133
Mitral stenosis, severe, 137
Motor system disease, 455
   AVMs and, 370, 453
   cortex injury, 168
Moya moya disease, 100
Mural thrombus, *68*, 288
   berry aneurysms and, 147
   dislodgement of, 288
   giant aneurysms, 297
Muslin wrapping, 171–172
Mycotic aneurysms, 337, 345
Myelography, spinal cord AVMs, 452
Myocardial infarction, 35, 108
   cerebral emboli and, 137
   postoperative, 35, 62, 233
   stroke and, 28–29
   vertebrobasilar ischemia and, 103
Myocardial ischemia, 95

Neck, 1, 77 See also Carotid artery
   chiropractic manipulation of, 106–107
   cleavage plane, 225
   dissection and, 125
   hyperextended, 134–135
   internal carotid stenosis in, 12
   operative approach, 22
   See also Carotid artery
Nerve injury, postoperative, 65. See also Cranial nerves
Neurologic deficits
   acute, 26–28
   aneurysm and, 150, 217
   angiograms and, 4
   AVM and, 348
   bypass graft and, 96
   carotid occlusion and, 2, 22–23

Neurological deficits—*continued*
  cerebral infarction and, 1
  compression and, 163
  embolism and, 137
  focal, 288
  pathologic findings, 70t
  perforating artery injury and, 256
  postoperative, 62–63, 173
  recurrent, 23
  spinal AVM and, 455
  spontaneous dissection and, 126
  steal mechanism, 397
  sudden onset, 28
  TIA history and, 26
  unstable syndromes, 26
  See also specific disorder, deficit
Nimodipine, 158–159
Nitroglycerin, 36, 62
Nitroprusside, 84, 95, 255
Nuchal rigidity, 150, 151t
Numbness, of limbs
  carotid artery stenosis and, 9, 95
  TIAs and, 1
Nutrition, 154
Nystagmus, 106t, 143

Occipital artery
  division of, 42
  extradural vertebral artery anastomosis, 113
  microdissection, 113
  posterior inferior cerebellar artery bypass, 104, 113, *115*
  vein graft and, 100
Occipital bone, vein graft and, 100
Occipital lobe, hemorrhage, *443*
Occlusion. *See* specific artery
Occult vascular malformations, 403–407
Ocular abnormalities, cerebellar infarction, 143. *See also* Eyes
Oculoplethysmography 8
Oculosympathetic palsy, dissection and, 125–126
Olfactory tract, *187, 220*
  elevation of, 222
  nerve injury, 211
Omohyoid muscle, 108
Operating room, layout
  aneurysm surgery, 166
  carotid endarterectomy, 39
Ophthalmic artery, 10, 14–15
  aneurysm, 183, 199, *200, 202,* 302
    direct approach for, 216
    giant paraclinoid, 317–318
    injury to, 205, 209
    occluding, 183
  See also Eyes
Ophthalmoplegia, aneurysms and, 183, 302
Optic canal, *205*
  dura overlying, 203
  unroofing of, 209
Optic chiasm, aneurysm and, *229*
Optic nerve, *187, 220*
  clipping injury to, 197
  displacement, 211
  encroachment on, 209
  ipsilateral, 199
  unroofing of, *202*
Orbital circulation, test of, 8

Otitis media, chronic, 316
Otorrhagia, 182
Oxygen extraction fraction studies, 83

Pancuronium, 36, 165
Papaverine, 172
Paraclinoid aneurysm
  carotid ligation, 216
  clinical features, 201t
  contralateral, 211
  giant, *301, 309*
  preoperative evaluation, 199
  surgical management, 199–211
Parahippocampal region, AVMs, 364
Parasagittal AVMs, 370–374, *376*
Park bench position, 167
Patch graft, 46, 51–52, *56,* 113–114
Pentothal, 36
Percutaneous transluminal angioplasty, 55, 72, 104, 106, 109, 124
Perforating arteries
  dissection of, *228*
  importance of, *264*
  injury to, 256
  ischemia, 263
  preservation of, 222, 225
Perfusion breakthrough, 353–354
Periadventitial fibroplasia, 121
Pericallosal arteries
  aneurysm, *236–239*
  dissection of, 236–238
  positioning for surgery, *167,* 179
Periosteum, 90
Peripheral vascular disease, 2, 35. *See also* specific artery
Persantine, 95
Personality changes, postoperative, 233
Petroclinoid ligament, opening of, 185
Petrosal sinus, dural AVMs, 415
Petrous aneurysms, giant, *312,* 316–317
Pharyngeal artery, 42
Phenylephrine, 43, 84
Phenylhydantoin, 95
Phonangiography, of bruit, 6–8, *78*
Photophobia, 150
Phrenic nerve, 108–110
Pituitary adenomas, 445
Plaque, 55
  ulcerated, *69*
  See also Atherosclerosis; Endarterectomy
Platelets
  destruction of, 446
  tranfusion of, 84
Platysma
  closure, 47
  drain, 47
  incised, 38
Polycystic kidneys, 147
Polymers, embolization with, 394
Pons, hematoma, 435, *443*
Positioning, operative, 166–168, 179
Posterior cerebral artery, 253
  aneurysm, 253, 262, 324, *327*
  lateral to brain stem, 116
  thrombus in, 116
  See also specific posterior artery
Posterior circulation, 16, 84, 148. *See also* specific artery

Posterior communicating artery, 184
  ICA wall aneurysms, 214
  location of, 186
  preoperative study of, 187
  aneurysms, 184–189
Posterior fossa
  AVMs, 386
  hemorrhage, 441–443
  ischemia, 103
  mass lesion, 144
Posterior inferior cerebellar artery
  anatomy of, 284
  bypass, 113
  peripheral aneurysms, 283–285
Posterior temporal transtentorial approach, 275
Potts scissors, 43, *46,* 50
Pressors, 95
Propranolol, 58, 164
Protamine sulfate, 47, 100, 116
Proton beam therapy, 397
Proximal internal carotid artery, 1
  aneurysm, *188*
  bruits and, *77*
  severe stenosis, 4
Proximal stump, CA, 55
Pseudoaneurysm, 107
Pseudoxanthoma elasticum, 147
Pterional craniotomy approach, *179,* 262
  anterior-choroidal aneurysm, 190–191
  anterior communicating artery aneurysm and, *220*
  basilar-superior cerebellar artery aneurysms, 265–266
  internal carotid-posterior communicating artery aneurysm, 184
  paraclinoid aneurysm, *204*
  temporal AVMs, 362
  to upper basilar artery, 261–262, 266
Pulmonary artery catheter, monitoring with, 35
Pulmonary disease
  embolism, 159
  obstructive, 35
Pulmonary function tests, preoperative, 35
Putamen, hemorrhage in, 435, 439–441

Radial artery catheter, 84, 94
Radiation therapy, for AVMs, 397
Reconstructive procedures. *See* specific disorder
Recurrent laryngeal nerve, injury to, 67
Reflex bradycardia, carotid sinus, 42
Renal insufficiency, 35
Renograffin, 54
Restenosis, after carotid endarterectomy, *70–72*
Retinal artery
  embolus, 2
  ischemic retinopathy, 15–16
Retraction nystagmus, 441
Retractors, 168
Retrograde femoral catheterization, carotid injection, 3
Revascularization, 103
  emergency, 25
  myocardial, 35
  See also specific artery, procedure

Rheumatic heart disease, 35, 137
Rupture, of aneurysms, 289
  intraoperative, 164, 172
  threat of, 289
  warning symptoms, 148, 150t
Rupture, disc, 455

Saccular aneurysm, 171
Sagittal sinus, occlusion of, 168
Sano multipurpose all angle clip applier, 171
Saphenous vein graft, 47, 51–52, 67, 98, 113
Scalene muscle, anterior, 110
Scalp flap
  aneurysm surgery, 168, 179–180
  necrosis and, 83, 85, 95, 113
  temporalis muscle incision and, 86
Scopolamine, 36, 164
Seizures, 155t, 402
  AVMs and, 347
  intracranial aneurysm, 288
  multiple aneurysms and, 287
  postoperative, 65, 246
  subarachnoid hemorrhage and, 154
  TIA and, 1–2
Septal regions
  AVMs, 378
Serpentine aneurysm, 297, 320, 322
Short vein graft, MCA, 83, 96, 98
Shunt
  endarterectomy 38, 50–51
  external carotid collateral and, 55
  temporary, 111
Sigmoid sinus
  occlusion, 416
  resection of, 417–419
  skeletonized, 419
Silastic stent, 116
Siphon disease, 12, 83
Skew deviation, 441
Sodium nitroprusside, 84, 95, 165, 255
Sodium pentobarbital, 164–165
Somatosensory evoked potentials, craniotomy and, 165, 175
Sphenoparietal sinus, dural AVMs, 415
Spinal aortography, 451
Spinal cord AVMs, 451–469
  direct fistulas, 459
  embolization of, 460–463
  intradural fistula, 462
  intramedullary, 461–462
  misdiagnosis of, 454–455
  pathophysiology of, 451–452
  surgical results, 463–465
  treatment of, 459–469
  Type I, 453–454
  Type II, 453–459
  Type III, 458–459
  Type IV, 459
Spinal myelography, 452
Splenium
  AVMs, 367–370, 374–375
  parasagittal approach to, 373
Steal phenomena, 383, 451
Sternocleidomastoid muscle, 110, 116
Stenosis, 1–11, 21–23
  acute stroke and, 2
  asymptomatic, 19, 77–80
  bilateral, 17

B mode scanning and, 6
endarterectomy for, 79–80
extracranial, 21
intraluminal filling defect and, 29t
measuring degree of, 3
pseudo-occlusion and, 3
pseudostenosis, 10
residual lumen diameter, 8
severe, 8
tandem internal, 19
TIAs and, 16, 23
two planes of view, 6
ulceration and, 3
See also specific artery
Stent, middle cerebral artery, 84
Sternocleidomastoid artery, 42
Sternocleidomastoid muscle, 38–40, 108, 113
Sternotomy, 109
Steroids, preoperative use, 164
Stethoscope, electronic, 148
String sign, 129
Stroke
  acute. See Acute stroke
  anticoagulant therapy and, 79
  bruits and, 2, 77
  carotid artery occlusion and, 62
  completed, 2
  CT scan and, 1–5
  EC-IC bypass and, 83
  embolism and, 1
  in evolution, 26
  hemispheric, 22, 95
  intima injury and, 107
  ischemic, 83
  MRI and, 6
  perioperative, 80
  recurrent, 30
  reversible, 70
  thrombus and, 107
  TIAs and, 10, 23, 80
  vein graft and, 95, 182
  vertebral artery occlusion and, 104t
Stump syndrome, 14–15
  embolus, 61
  endarterectomy for, 61
  thrombus in, 21
Subacute necrotic myelopathy, 451
Subarachnoid catheter, 211
Subarachnoid hemorrhage, 21
  anterior communicating artery aneurysm and, 217
  asymptomatic carotid stenosis and, 19
  basilar trunk aneurysm and, 264, 271
  cardiac arrhythmias and, 156
  cerebellar artery aneurysm and, 279, 283–284
  classifications, 150–151
  clots, 164
  complications of, 155t
  cooperative study, 173–174
  delayed surgery and, 217,233
  diagnosis of, 149–153
  dissection and, 133
  distal anterior cerebral aneurysm and, 235
  electrolyte imbalance and, 156
  etiology of, 147
  fibromuscular dysplasia and, 122t
  headache and, 149

hydrocephalus and, 157
giant aneurysms and, 297
internal carotid artery aneurysms, 191
medical evaluation, 151
multiple aneurysms and, 287
paraclinoid aneurysms and, 199
plain CT scan, 151
postoperative vasospasm, 174
preoperative complications, 159
prevalence of, 147
radiologic diagnosis, 151–153
surgical mortality, 175
surgical treatment, 163
vasoactive substances and, 158–159
vasospasm after, 157–159
warning signs of, 148, 150t
Subarachnoid space. See Subarachnoid hemorrhage
Subclavian arteries
  angiography and, 104
  carotid graft, 111–113
  cervical exposure of, 108
  endarterectomy, 104, 106, 109
  stenosis, 105
Subclavian steal syndrome
  arch angiogram, 107
  clinical syndrome, 104
  management, 104–106
  transluminal angioplasty and, 109
Subclavian vein, 111
Suboccipital exposure, approach to, 275
Subtemporal approach, 254–259, 265
Subtraction studies. See Digital subtraction angiography
Sugita clips, 116, 170, 188, 209. See also specific procedure
Sundt clip, 188, 194
Superficial temporal artery
  exposure of, 84
  irrigation of, 89
  MCA bypass graft, 83, 85, 97–98, 131, 324
  occipital artery and, 100
  surgical preparation of, 85–90
  suture techniques, 92, 94
Superior cerebellar artery
  anastomosis to, 117
  giant aneurysm, 267
  pterional approach to, 268
Superior laryngeal nerve, injury to, 67
Superior sagittal sinus, bridging veins, 235–236
Superior temporal gyrus
  MCA aneurysm, 246–249
  MCA clipping via, 245
  resection of, 250
Superior thyroid artery, 42, 44
Supraclavicular incision, 108
Surgical clips, aneurysm, 170–171. See also Clipping procedures
Sutures
  dural-pericranial tenting, 92
  technique, 91
  See also specific operation
Sylvian fissure
  arachnoid opening and, 184
  AVMs, 360–363
  embolectomy and, 139
  opening, 195

Sylvian fissure—*continued*
  plane of, 250
Sylvian veins, damage to, 250
Syncope, 1–2, 106, 108

Tachycardia, control of, 36
Tandem lesions, 12
Telangiectases, 347
Temporal lobe
  aneurysm adherent to, 186
  AVMs, 362–370
  bleeding into, 150
  deep anterior AVMs, 364–365
  deep temporal-occipital AVMs, 367–368, 369–370
  elevation of, 116
  hematoma, 251
  infarction, 255
  medial aspect resection, 190
  retraction of, 242
Temporalis muscle, 85, 90, 150
Tenting sutures, 180–181
Tetralogy of Fallot, 104
Thalamus
  AVMs, 380
  hemorrhage, 435, 441
Third nerve palsy, 288
Thoracic duct, 108, 111
Thoracotomy, 108
Thrombocytopenia, 446
Thrombophlebitis, 154
Thromboplastin time, 446
Thrombosis
  of aneurysm 173, 183, 297
  AVMs and, 405, 407
  basilar, 103
  carotid artery and, 22
  electrically induced, 173, 183
  formation of, 3
  heart disease and, 137
  intraluminal, 8, 30
  intraoperative graft, 95
  sinus occlusion, 415
  mural. *See* Mural thrombus
  ultrasonic aspirator and, 307
Thyrocervical trunk, 108
Thyroid artery
  superior, 42, 44
TIAs. *See* Transient ischemic attacks
Tonsils
  cerebellar, 145
  intracranial dissection, 134
Torcular region, dural AVM of, 415, 416
Tourniquet, shunt and, 50
Tracheotomy, 67
Transient ischemic attacks (TIAs)
  aneurysm and, 19–21
  angiography for, 3–4
  antiplatelet therapy in, 8, 79
  bruit and, 2
  bypass grafts and, 83, 95–96
  carotid occlusion and, 10–12, 15–16
  clinical presentation, 1–2
  common carotid artery and, 21–23
  crescendo, 26, 29
  CT scans, 4–6

diagnostic studies, 2–6
duration of, 1
embolism and, 4
emergency surgery and, 29
etiology, 2
extrinsic compression and, 58
fibromuscular dysplasia and, 121–122
history of, 2, 26
management, 8–22
multiple aneurysms and, 287
pathologic finding, 68t
pathophysiology, 1
of posterior circulation, 16–19
postoperative, 65
stroke and, 79, 288
subarachnoid hemorrhage and, 150t
surgery for, 8–22
unilateral headache and, 125
unruptured aneurysm, 288
vertebrobasilar, 103
Transient monocular blindness, carotid stenosis and, 1–4, 10
Transluminal angioplasty, 55, 72, 104, 109, 124
Transoral transclival approach, 275
Transpetrosal approach, 275
Transverse foramen, 107
Transverse sinus, 420. *See also* Dura mater
Trauma
  cervical carotid tears, 134
  dissection of intracranial vessels, 133
Trigeminal artery, 19
Trigone
  AVMs, 366
  inferior wall, 366
Trochlear nerve, 253
Tumors
  brain hemorrhage and, 445
  EC-IC bypass and, 83
  intracranial, 85
  spinal, 451, 455

Ulceration, 3
  endarterectomy, 8
  ICA, 8
  two planes of view, 6
Ulnar nerve, 165
Ultrasound studies
  asymptomatic bruit, 77
  carotid circulation, 2, 6–8
  intraoperative, 47

Vagus nerve, 38, 41
  carotid artery and, 42
  injury to, 67
  rootlets of, 284
Variangle clip, 170
Vasospasm
  ACA aneurysym and, 217
  antifibrinolytic agents and, 155
  clinical syndrome of, 158
  early surgery and, 164
  grading of, 153
  postoperative, 173–174
  severity of, 151

subarachnoid hemorrhage and, 157–159
treatment of, 159
unruptured aneurysms and, 293
Vein grafts, 96–98
  dissection and, 131
  saphenous, 47, 51–52, 113
Vein of Galen, aneurysms, 399–401
Vein of Labbé, 255, 271
Venous angiomas, 347, 403–405
Venous stasis retinopathy, 2
Ventricular drainage, 156–157
Ventriculoperitoneal shunting, 156
Ventriculostomy, 157
Vertebral artery
  cerebellar artery aneurysms and, 279–283
  collateral circulation, 103
  deliberate occlusion of, 171
  dissection, 135
  embolus in, 137
  endarterectomy, 104, 108–109
  exposure of, 108
  extracranial, 103
  giant aneurysms, 302, 326
  removal of foreign body from, 117
  revascularization indications, 104t
  stenosis of, 19, 105–106, 330
  subclavian steal and, 104
  surgical positioning in, 167
  surgical results in, 279t
  transposition of, 104, 106, 108–112
  vertebrobasilar aneurysms
    giant, 324–330
    park bench position, 167
Vertebrobasilar circulation, 13
  atherosclerosis of, 103–109
  ischemia, 113
    clinical syndromes, 103
    dissection and, 135
    evolution of, 103–104
    management of, 104
  patterns, 106t
  TIAs, 22–23
  See also Vertebral artery
Vertebrobasilar junction aneurysms, 275–279, 326
Vertebral-posterior inferior cerebellar artery, aneurysms of, 279–283
Vertical gaze palsy, 441
Visual loss
  carotid-cavernous fistula, 427
  paraclinoid aneurysm and, 199
  TIAs and, 1–4, 10
Vocal cord function, loss of, 67

Wallenberg's syndrome, 135, 144
Wound, hematoma, 67

Xylocaine IV, 36

Yasargil clips, 170, 209

Zygoma, 116
  bone flap, 180
  removal of, 255